The Comprehensive
RESPIRATORY THERAPIST
EXAM REVIEW

Entry and Advanced Levels

Fifth Edition

The Comprehensive
RESPIRATORY THERAPIST
EXAM REVIEW

Entry and Advanced Levels

JAMES R. SILLS, MEd, CPFT, RRT
Professor Emeritus
Former Director, Respiratory Care Program
Rock Valley College
Rockford, Illinois

MOSBY
ELSEVIER

MOSBY
ELSEVIER

3251 Riverport Lane
Maryland Heights, Missouri 63043

THE COMPREHENSIVE RESPIRATORY THERAPIST EXAM REVIEW: ISBN-13: 978-0-323-06701-0
ENTRY AND ADVANCED LEVELS

Notice

Knowledge and best practice in this field are constantly changing. As new research and experience broaden our knowledge, changes in practice, treatment and drug therapy may become necessary or appropriate. Readers are advised to check the most current information provided (i) on procedures featured or (ii) by the manufacturer of each product to be administered, to verify the recommended dose or formula, the method and duration of administration, and contraindications. It is the responsibility of the practitioner, relying on their own experience and knowledge of the patient, to make diagnoses, to determine dosages and the best treatment for each individual patient, and to take all appropriate safety precautions. To the fullest extent of the law, neither the Publisher nor the Author assumes any liability for any injury and/or damage to persons or property arising out of or related to any use of the material contained in this book.

ISBN-13: 978-0-323-06701-0

Managing Editor: Billie Sharp
Developmental Editor: Kathleen Sartori
Publishing Services Manager: Julie Eddy
Project Manager: Rich Barber
Design Manager: Kim Denando
Selected Illustrations: Sandra Hogan and Jeanne Robertson

Working together to grow
libraries in developing countries

www.elsevier.com | www.bookaid.org | www.sabre.org

ELSEVIER   BOOK AID International   Sabre Foundation

Printed in the United States

Last digit is the print number: 9 8 7 6 5 4 3 2 1

This book is dedicated to my wife,
Deb,
and our children, **Rachael** *and* **David,**
who make my life full and complete;
the memory of my Mom, who always showed her love and support for me,
and Dad, who taught me through his actions;
our dog, **Abby,** *who takes me for long walks on the Lake Michigan beach;*
and
Carl Hammond,
who taught me respiratory care.

Words to live by:
The journey of 1000 miles begins with a single step.
Confucius

Hope for the best but plan against the worst.

Reviewers

JEFFERY ANDERSON, MA, RRT
Associate Professor/Director, Clinical Education
Respiratory Care
Boise State University
Boise, Idaho

ERIN E. DAVIS MS, MED, RRT-NPS, CPFT
Director of Clinical Education
Our Lady of Holy Cross College
Ochsner Program in Respiratory Care
New Orleans, Louisiana

TONYA EDWARDS, BSRC, RRT
Program Director
Weatherford College
Weatherford, Texas

DOUGLAS S. GARDENHIRE, RRT-NPS
Director of Clinical Education
Georgia State University
Atlanta, Georgia

JOANNE JACOBS, MA, RRT, AE-C
Program Director, Respiratory Therapy Program
Community College of Rhode Island
Lincoln, Rhode Island

ROBERT L. JOYNER, JR., PHD, RRT, FAARC
Associate Professor and Chair Department of Health
  Sciences Director—Respiratory Therapy Program
Salisbury University
Salisbury, Maryland

MARY N. LABICHE, RRT, NPS, MED
Program Director
Our Lady of Holy Cross College
Ochsner Program in Respiratory Care
New Orleans, Louisiana

JOSHUA NEUMILLER, PHARMD, CDE, GCP, FASCP
Assistant Professor
College of Pharmacy
Washington State Unversity
Spokane, Washington

RANDOLPH REGAL, BS, PHARMD
Clinical Assistant Professor
Adult Internal Medicine
University of Michigan Hospital and College of
  Pharmacy
Ann Arbor, Michigan

ROBERT J TRALONGO, MBA, RT, RRT-NPS, CPFT, AE-C
Director, Respiratory Care Program
Molloy College
Rockville Centre, New York

Foreword

The fifth edition of Jims Sills,' **The Comprehensive Respiratory Therapist Exam Review—Entry and Advanced Levels,** has set a new—and high standard—for the "must-have resource" for students preparing for the National Board of Respiratory Care (NBRC) Certified Respiratory Therapist (CRT) and Registered Respiratory Therapist (RRT) examinations. Now only this one book is needed to fully review accurate and current material for the entry-level exam, the advanced-level Written Registry Exam (WRE), and the Clinical Simulation Exam (CSE). In short, this new review book is a wonderful and painless NBRC preparation tool!

Many new features have been added to this edition to enhance the reader's ability to focus in on all the key items considered testable by the NBRC. For example, unique "Exam Hint Boxes" designed to highlight and emphasize important items commonly tested by the NBRC are frequently placed throughout each chapter. These can be downloaded from the book's website for exam preparation or classroom use. Furthermore, at the end of each chapter, the test questions have been updated to reflect the current Entry Level and Written Registry exam items.

Each question includes a reference page that discusses the rationale for each question.

Another special feature is the use of the Internet to take practice examinations that mirror the NBRC total experience. For the student preparing for the CRT exam, the Entry Level pre-and-post-tests have been increased to 160 questions to match the current NBRC exam—20 previewed questions and 140 actual questions. Both the pre-and-post-tests provide the rationale for the right and wrong options for each question. In addition, every time the exams are taken, the software scrambles both the questions and the option sequence—the student never has to take the same practice test twice.

For the student preparing for the RRT exams, the Written Registry pre-and-post-tests have been increased to 115 questions to reflect the actual NBRC exam—15 previewed questions and 100 actual questions. Similar to the Entry Level Exam, each question has the rationale provided for both the right and wrong options, and each time the exams are taken, the test questions and option sequences will be scrambled. The NBRC's Clinical Simulation Exam experience has been matched by the addition of another scenario. Now there are 11 total clinical scenarios—1 previewed and 10 actual ones. Still another important feature are the clinical pathways for the eleven scenarios showing information gathering and decision-making branches. Finally, a great feature for the faculty member is the ability to set up a controlled practice test for the entire class of students. The student's overall performance data is provided for both the instructor and the student.

Again, Jim Sills has provided the field of respiratory care an outstanding contribution! Undeniably, for the reader preparing for any one of the NBRC respiratory examinations, this one textbook provides a complete and current review, a handy format to practice test taking, the opportunity to develop good testing skills and confidence, and, ultimately, the ability to successfully pass any of the NBRC examinations. Jim Sills' clear and precise writing talent in this area is second to none. As we work to meet the future increased respiratory demands placed upon on us by both the patient and the rapidly changing hospital industry, it is a welcomed relief to have this new and timely resource.

Finally, I would like to welcome you to the field of respiratory care, and I wish you the very best on your travels throughout this wonderful and exciting health care profession.

Terry Des Jardins, MEd, RRT
Professor Emeritus
Respiratory Care Program
Parkland College
Champaign, Illinois

Preface

The Comprehensive Respiratory Therapist Exam Review: Entry and Advanced Levels is presented in a restructured Fifth Edition. Where once there were two, now there is one. I've combined the *Entry Level Respiratory Therapist Exam Guide* and the *Advanced Respiratory Therapist Exam Guide* into one convenient review manual. The information in this edition has been updated to cover all items listed as testable by the National Board for Respiratory Care (NBRC) on its *Summary Content Outline for CRT and Written RRT Examinations* released in July 2008. This document lists all testable items for the Entry Level Examination to earn the Certified Respiratory Therapist (CRT) credential and the Written Registry Examination and Clinical Simulation Examination to earn the Registered Respiratory Therapist (RRT) credential. This document is located on our Evolve website: http://evolve.elsevier.com/Sills/resptherapy so that the exam taker may compare what the NBRC has provided and my attempt to cover those items in this book. Whether a student is preparing for the CRT or RRT credential, this book should cover all items.

To prepare students and graduates for the NBRC exams, this book has been updated in the following ways:

(1) new testable items have been added and discussed, (2) items that will no longer be tested have been deleted, (3) chapter "Exam Hints" have been updated to reflect the most commonly tested content of the current exams, (4) the end-of-chapter Self-Study Questions have been updated and revised as necessary, (5) the study mode pre-test and exam mode post-test for the Entry Level Exam and the Written Registry Exam have been updated to reflect current exam content. These four exams and the Clinical Simulation Exam can be accessed online at http://evolve.elsevier.com/Sills/resptherapy. Because the NBRC exams now include extra questions being previewed for possible future use, the exams with this book have been expanded to match the NBRC experience. So, there are now 160 questions on the practice Entry Level Exams, 115 questions on the practice Written Registry Exams, and 11 patient scenarios on the practice Clinical Simulation Exam.

It is my sincere hope that these revisions will help the exam taker to better focus on the key factors that will lead to successfully passing the NBRC's exams.

James R. Sills, MEd, CPFT, RRT

Introduction

INTRODUCTION AND RECOMMENDATIONS FOR EXAM SUCCESS

The National Board for Respiratory Care (NBRC) released the following four documents in July 2008 to help guide test takers:

1. **Entry Level CRT Examination Detailed Content Outline**. This provides details on the testable items and difficulty level of questions found on the Entry Level Examination. This exam must be passed to earn the Certified Respiratory Therapist (CRT) credential.

2. **Therapist Written RRT Examination Detailed Content Outline**. This provides details on the testable items and difficulty level of questions found on the Written Registry Examination. This is one of the two exams that must be passed to earn the Registered Respiratory Therapist (RRT) credential.

3. **Clinical Simulation Examination Detailed Content Outline**. This provides details on the testable items found on the Clinical Simulation Examination. No difficulty levels are provided. This is one of the two exams that must be passed to earn the Registered Respiratory Therapist (RRT) credential.

4. **Summary Content Outline for CRT and Written RRT Examinations**. This combines documents 1 and 2 into a single content outline for both the Entry Level Examination and Written Registry Examination.

All four of these documents can be accessed online at www.NBRC.org. The Summary Content Outline for the CRT and Written RRT Examinations and the Clinical Simulation Examination Detailed Content Outline are included on the Evolve site.

A careful review of documents 1 and 2 shows that the great majority of listed items are testable on both the Entry Level Examination and Written Registry Examination. A relatively small number of items are tested only on the Entry Level Examination or only on the Written Registry Examination.

A careful review of document 3 shows that everything listed as testable on the Entry Level Examination and Written Registry Examination can be tested on the Clinical Simulation Examination.

The purpose of this book is to help you prepare to take and pass the Entry Level Examination (ELE), Written Registry Examination (WRE), and Clinical Simulation Examination (CSE).

There are several assets that will assist you as you prepare:

- Exam hints within the chapters are coded for the ELE, the WRE, or both. These will point out commonly tested items.
- Self-assessment questions appear at the end of each chapter. Answering these questions will allow you to see what you've retained while reading the content of the chapter. (Rationales will be found in Appendices A and B.)
- The online practice tests, both in study mode pretest and exam mode post-test for the Entry Level Exam and the Written Registry Exam will help you analyze your strengths and weaknesses. (These four exams, the Clinical Simulation Exam, and all rationales can be found on the Evolve website.)

It is recommended that the ELE and the WRE Exam pretests be taken and analyzed before beginning the text and studying. After studying, take the exam mode post-test for the ELE, the WRE, and the CSE. All the sample tests are designed to follow the format, question styles, difficulty levels, and relative weight of tested areas as the real exams. The 11 Clinical Simulation Examination problems are the same mix of patient scenarios typically seen on the actual exam.

The text includes **boldface topic headings** followed by two codes. The **first code** (in parentheses) is the NBRC code for that subject taken from the *Summary Content Outline for CRT and Written RRT Examinations*. If the item is testable on both the ELE and WRE, it will simply be shown as: (Code: . . .). If an item is only testable on the ELE, it will be shown as: (ELE code: . . .). If an item is only tested on the WRE, it will be shown as: (WRE code: . . .). Remember that the Clinical Simulation Exam is comprehensive and includes everything testable on the ELE and WRE. My choice of words for topic headings is either the NBRC's or a paraphrasing of it. Occasionally a heading appears without an NBRC code after it. These headings were added to help you understand what the NBRC is testing for. Some discussion of pathologic processes is included in the general discussion of each chapter as they relate to the treatment or procedure that the respiratory therapist performs. It is recommended that you study the major types of adult and infant disease states and abnormal conditions.

The **second code** [in brackets] is the NBRC code for the difficulty level of the questions that will be used to test your understanding of the material. *R* stands for Recall, *Ap* stands for Application, and *An* stands for Analysis. You will find that the NBRC asks questions at these three different levels of difficulty. See below for more discussion on the difficulty levels. The NBRC does not provide a difficulty code for items tested on the Clinical Simulation Exam. Be prepared for any difficulty level in the 11 patient scenarios.

ENTRY LEVEL EXAMINATION

Critical points to remember:

- The Entry Level Examination consists of 160 total questions. 140 are actual questions. The NBRC also includes 20 extra questions being pre-tested for future versions of the examination. These questions are not scored as part of your examination. Since it is not possible to tell the actual from the pretested questions, take each question seriously. The examination is offered in a computer-based testing format through the Internet. Make sure to follow all commands listed on the computer screens so that you do not make any mistakes. You cannot bring a calculator or any other type of test aid device with you. A pencil and blank piece of paper is provided for making notes and calculations.
- You have 3 hours to complete the examination. Do not leave any questions unanswered. There is no penalty for guessing.
- A passing score is listed as 75% or greater (at least 105 correct tested questions; no more than 35 incorrect). However, you could get fewer than 105 correct and still pass because the Application and Analysis questions are weighted more heavily than the Recall ones (see discussion below). Those passing the examination are awarded the Certified Respiratory Therapist (CRT) credential by the NBRC.

WRITTEN REGISTRY EXAMINATION

Critical points to remember:

- The Written Registry Examination is made up of 115 total questions. 100 are actual questions. The NBRC also includes 15 extra questions being pretested for future versions of the examination. These pretested questions are not scored as part of your exam, but, because you will not know which questions are real and which are being pretested, answer all questions to the best of your ability. The examination is offered in a computer-based testing format through the Internet. You cannot bring a calculator or any other type of test aid device with you. A pencil and blank piece of paper is provided for making notes and calculations.
- You will have 2 hours to complete the examination. Do not leave any questions unanswered. There is no penalty for guessing.

- A passing score is listed as 70% or higher (at least 70 correct tested questions; no more than 30 incorrect). However, you can get less than 70 correct and still pass because the Application and Analysis questions are weighted more heavily than the Recall questions (see the following). Those who pass the exam (and the Clinical Simulation Examination) are awarded the Registered Respiratory Therapist (RRT) credential by the National Board for Respiratory Care.

The Entry Level Exam and Written Registry Exam have three difficulty levels to their questions:

Recall [R]

Recall refers to remembering factual information that was previously learned. "Identify" is a commonly used action verb in this type of question. You may be asked to identify specific facts, terms, methods, procedures, principles, or concepts. Prepare for this type of question by studying the full range of factual information, equations, and so on that are seen in respiratory care practice. These types of questions are on the lowest order of difficulty. You either know the answer or you do not; there is little to ponder more deeply. It is very important to have a solid understanding of the factual basis of respiratory care to do well in this and the next two categories of questions.

Application [Ap]

Application refers to being able to use factual information in real clinical situations that may be new to you. "Apply," "classify," and "calculate" are commonly used action verbs in this type of question. You may be asked to apply laws, theories, concepts, and/or principles to new, practical clinical situations. Calculations may have to be performed. Charts and graphs, such as seen in pulmonary function testing or ventilator graphics, may need to be used. This type of question is on a higher order of difficulty than the Recall [R] type. Critical thinking must be applied to the factual information to answer these questions.

Analysis [An]

Analysis refers to being able to separate a patient care problem into its component parts or elements to evaluate the relationship of the parts or elements to the whole problem. "*Evaluate*," "*compare*," "*contrast*," "*revise*," and "*select*" are commonly used action verbs in this type of question. You may be questioned about revising a patient care plan or evaluating therapy. This type of question requires the highest level of critical thinking. You may have to recall previously learned information, apply it to a patient care situation, and make a judgment as to the best way to care for the patient. Frequently you must analyze cross-connections between subject areas to make a patient care decision—for example, interpreting arterial blood gas results and bedside spirometry data to determine a patient's readiness to wean from the mechanical ventilator.

You will find that the NBRC uses two different types of questions on the exam in the following three ways:

One Best Answer (The NBRC calls this "One Best Response" Multiple-Choice.)

This type of question has a stem (the question) followed by four possible answers coded A, B, C, and D. You must select the best answer from among those presented. Only one is clearly best, even though other possible answers may be good. Carefully read the stem to make sure that you do not misunderstand the clear intent of the question. Controversial issues may be questioned. The use of "should" in the stem will clue you in to the need to select the answer that would be selected by the majority of practitioners.

Multiple True-False (The NBRC calls this "Complex" Multiple Choice.)

This type of question has a stem (the question) followed by four or five possible answers coded with Roman numerals I, II, III, IV, and V; four combinations of the answers, coded by letters A, B, C, and D, follow. The stem may ask you to include all true statements or all false statements in the final answer. You must select the letter that represents the correct combination of answers.

No controversial answers should be offered. They are all either clearly correct or incorrect. That is the key to selecting the best answer. Read each possible answer as separate from the others. It is suggested that you mark each possible answer as true or false. Even if you are not sure of every option, you should be able to determine the best answer.

Qualifying words

Qualifying words give direction to the focus of any type of question. They really direct how you should answer the question. Examples of qualifying words, include, but are not limited to: *initially*, *should*, *first*, *most*, *least*. Phrases using qualifying words include: "What would be the *initial* thing to do . . .", "What is the *first* thing . . .," "What is the *most* important thing . . .," and "What is the *least* important thing . . ."

In the past, the NBRC has included some questions with three correct answers and one incorrect answer. The incorrect answer is the one that needs to be selected. The use of "except" will clue you in to this type of question. For example: "The colors of the American flag include all of the following colors EXCEPT: red, white, blue, green. Obviously, the correct answer is the incorrect color, green. Recently, it would appear that the NBRC is phasing out this type of question. However, some are included within the chapter questions and NBRC style exams because of past practice and so that the test taker is familiar with this style of question.

Situational Sets

These are seen on the Entry Level Examination only. Typically, one or two are included at the end of the exam. They will not be seen on the Written Registry Examination. Instead, they have been replaced with the Clinical Simulation Examination for advanced practitioners. The situation sets involve the use of a patient care scenario that may include such information as the patient's history, vital signs, blood gas values, or pulmonary function results. Three to five questions follow that ask you about patient or equipment management. These questions are the "one best answer" or "multiple true-false" types, as discussed above. However, because of the amount of information offered and the critical thinking required, these questions are categorized as being at the Application or Analysis level of difficulty. Carefully read the scenario to fully understand the information. After reading the related question, refer back to the scenario for information that can help you pick the best answer. Do this for each question and also refer to the prior questions for information that may help you with the current one.

Suggestions for Preparing for the Entry Level Examination and Written Registry Examination

1. **Pace yourself** so that you have enough time to get through all of the questions. A good pace is about 50-55 questions per hour. Make a note on your blank paper on any difficult questions that you skip or want to go back to. You can also computer "bookmark" any questions you want to come back to later. The computer-based test will prompt you if any questions have been skipped. Come back to them at the end of the test time. Do not leave any blank questions. You will not be penalized for guessing on the last few questions if you are running out of time.

2. **Completely read each question.** Determine what it is that you are really being asked. Look for qualifying words as discussed above.

3. **Separate the important information** from that which is not important. Many questions contain patient information and data on blood gases, pulmonary function, hemodynamics, ventilator settings, and so on. Disregard what does not pertain to the question being asked. Interpret the important data.

4. **Do not read beyond the question.** Resist the temptation to "psych out" what you think the question writer wants. Use only what is given to you.

5. **Carefully read every answer** that is offered.

6. **Pick the best answer that is offered.** The answer that you might like best may not be offered. Regardless, you must pick from among those that are offered.

7. In **multiple true-false** questions, use the following **strategy**: (1) Find an option that you know to be incorrect and cross off any of the answers that contain it; (2) find an option that you know to be correct and

cross off any answers that do not contain it; (3) find the remaining answer, which must be correct.

8. Again, **answer every question**. There is no penalty for guessing incorrectly.

9. **Take practice exams.** They are available on the NBRC website (NBRC.org) and accompany this text on the online Evolve Learning System (http://evolve.elsevier.com/Sills/resptherapy). Evaluate your strengths and weaknesses and spend more time studying your weak areas. The online tests with this book contain an interactive pretest (study mode) and posttest (exam mode) formatted like the actual examination.

Relative Weights of the Various Tested Areas on the Entry Level Examination and Written Registry Examination

I have attempted to analyze the content of each of the questions on the available Entry Level Examinations and Written Registry Examinations covering the current exam content. Each question has been matched to one of the chapters in this book, listed in the table below. The numbers of questions and percentages are averages and may not be followed exactly on all versions of the examination. However, the relative weights can offer solid guidance as to what content is relatively more important or less important. Study time can be spent accordingly.

TABLE 1   Average Examination Content Found in Each Chapter*

Chapter	Number of Questions ELE	Percentage of Exam Content ELE	Number of Questions WRE	Percentage of Exam Content WRE
1. Patient Assessment and Care Management	10	7%	14	14%
2. Infection Control	4	3%	1	1%
3. Blood Gas Sampling, Analysis, Monitoring, and Interpretation	10	7%	6	6%
4. Pulmonary Function Testing	7	5%	4	4%
5. Advanced Cardiopulmonary Monitoring	2	1%	4	4%
6. Oxygen and Medical Gas Therapy	13	9%	7	7%
7. Hyperinflation Therapy	2	1%	2	2%
8. Humidity and Aerosol Therapy	8	6%	2	2%
9. Pharmacology	11	8%	5	5%
10. Bronchopulmonary Hygiene Therapy	3	2%	3	3%
11. Cardiac Monitoring and Cardiopulmonary Resuscitation	5	4%	5	5%
12. Airway Management	10	7%	6	6%
13. Suctioning the Airway	4	3%	2	2%
14. Intermittent Positive-Pressure Breathing (IPPB)	3	2%	2	2%
15. Mechanical Ventilation of the Adult	40	30%	24	24%
16. Mechanical Ventilation of the Neonate	0	0%	2	2%
17. Home Care and Pulmonary Rehabilitation	3	2%	4	4%
18. Special Procedures	3	2%	6	6%
19. Pathology	2	1%	1	1%
TOTAL	**140**	**100%**	**100**	**100%**

*The number of questions shown reflects the *average* found on past and current NBRC exams. While individual NBRC exams may vary somewhat, the relative importance of broad content areas can be expected to correlate with this table.

Suggestions for maximizing exam preparation time.

1. Spend the majority of your time studying the most heavily tested areas: Chapter 15: Mechanical Ventilation of the Adult; Chapter 1: Patient Assessment and Care Management; Chapter 3: Blood Gas Sampling, Analysis, Monitoring, and Interpretation; Chapter 6: Oxygen and Medical Gas Therapy; Chapter 9: Pharmacology; and Chapter 12: Airway Management. As time permits, study all remaining chapters.

2. Review the Exam Hint topics in all chapters.

3. Thoroughly understand bedside and advanced patient assessment by studying Chapters 1, 3, 4, and

5. This content is important by itself but is also incorporated into questions covering all therapeutic procedures.

4. Arterial blood gas interpretation must be understood to answer questions related to oxygen administration and mechanical ventilation.

5. Pulmonary function testing must be understood to understand how to interpret the results of bronchodilator therapy and assess a patient's need for mechanical ventilation.

6. Bedside patient assessment, blood gas interpretation, and pulmonary function testing must be

understood to assess a patient to make the correct mechanical ventilator adjustments.

7. Chapter 15: Mechanical Ventilation of the Adult, has the most heavily questioned content of all the chapters. You *must* understand mechanical ventilation to do well on the Entry Level Exam, Written Registry Exam, and Clinical Simulation Exam.

CLINICAL SIMULATION EXAMINATION

Critical points to remember:

- The Clinical Simulation Examination (CSE) is composed of 11 broad-based patient scenarios. 10 are actual tested scenarios. The NBRC also includes 1 extra scenario being pretested for future versions of the examination. Because you cannot tell which scenario is being pretested, approach each one seriously.
- These patient cases are designed to evaluate how well the exam taker is able to gather information, evaluate it, and make clinical decisions that relate to simulated real patient situations. The CSE tests well beyond the recollection of simple facts. Box 1 lists the typical types of patient care problems that will be seen. The computer-based examination process is unique. Each clinical simulation problem is designed to flow in the same manner in which actual patient data are delivered and care decisions are made. Therefore, the problems are designed in a branching logic format. This means that there may be more than one way to solve them. To some extent, you choose your own path; however, only one path is best. There may be another path or two that are acceptable. There may be another path or or two that are unacceptable.
- The exam taker is allowed 4 hours to complete the exam, which works out to about 20 minutes per problem.

BOX 1   The Typical Mix of 10 Tested Problems Found on the Clinical Simulation Examination

1. Two adult patients with chronic obstructive pulmonary disease (COPD). These patients could have chronic bronchitis, emphysema, and/or asthma. Areas of focus on the simulation include, but are not limited to, pre- and postoperative evaluation, critical care management, mechanical ventilation, pulmonary function testing, home care, rehabilitation, and infection control.
2. One or two adult patients with trauma. These patients could have chest, head, or skeletal injuries; surface burns; smoke inhalation; carbon monoxide poisoning; or hypothermia.
3. One or two adult patients with cardiovascular disease. These patients could have congestive heart failure, coronary artery disease, myocardial infarction, valvular heart disease, or cardiac surgery.
4. One or two adult patients with neurologic or neuromuscular diseases. These patients could have myasthenia gravis,

Guillain-Barré syndrome, tetanus, muscular dystrophy, cerebrovascular accident (stroke), or drug overdosage.
5. One pediatric patient. This patient could have epiglottitis, laryngotracheobronchitis (croup), bronchiolitis, asthma, cystic fibrosis, foreign body aspiration, toxic substance ingestion, or bronchopulmonary dysplasia.
6. One neonatal patient. This patient could require care in the delivery room; need resuscitation; or have infant apnea, meconium aspiration, respiratory distress syndrome, or a congenital heart defect.
7. The *possible* miscellaneous category could involve one adult patient with a medical or surgical problem. This could include head, neck, or thoracic surgery; obesity-hypoventilation syndrome; or acquired immunodeficiency syndrome (AIDS).

There are three components to the clinical simulation problem: (1) the scenario, (2) the information-gathering sections, and (3) the decision-making sections. Each is discussed in turn.

Scenario

The scenario establishes the setting for the patient, and for you, as the respiratory therapist. Typically, it includes the type of hospital, where the patient is within the hospital, and the time of day. General information about the patient, such as name, age, and sex; some general presenting conditions; and a brief history of the illness or event, is given. Your role as a respiratory therapist is described.

You may have to gather more information or may need to make a clinical decision. Determine if the situation is an emergency. If it is, you will have to take immediate steps to help the patient. (The exam taker should assume that any and all services needed to give optimal care are available in any of the patient scenarios.)

Information Gathering Sections

Usually, the respiratory therapist is first directed to an information gathering (IG) section to find out more about the patient. A list of about 15 to 20 parameters from which to choose—for example, vital signs, blood gases, pulmonary function tests, various laboratory studies, and so forth—will be available. You will be instructed to select as many as you believe are important based on what you know at that point in time. Obviously, you should not select information that is unnecessarily risky or irrelevant or that delays important care. Select the desired information. The computer screen will then reveal the data. Interpret the data to make the proper decisions in the next section. When you have finished gathering and interpreting the data, you will be directed to go to a decision-making section. Typically there are two to four information-gathering steps in each clinical simulation problem.

Decision Making Sections

After the selected patient data are analyzed, the test taker is directed to a decision making (DM) section. It is now required that you make a decision on the best care for the patient based on the information that you have at this point in time. Usually you are instructed to "choose only one" from about four to eight options. One of the choices is best, one or two others may be acceptable, and the others are not acceptable. Select the option and the computer will reveal the answer. Usually it will say "Physician agrees. Done" or something to that effect. One or more of the available answers will reveal "Physician disagrees. Make another selection in this section" when it is exposed. This may or may not mean that a bad choice was made. It is possible that the author of the scenario simply does not want to follow that particular course of action.

Occasionally, you will be directed to "select as many as indicated" for the situation with which you are dealing. This involves a scenario in which proper care includes several procedures being done simultaneously with a patient. Again, select the options, and the computer will reveal the answer.

Whether you are directed to make one or several decisions, when finished, you will be instructed to go to a new area. This usually takes you to another information-gathering section. You will now need to evaluate how the patient responded to your earlier decision(s). You will then need to make one or more patient care decisions. Typically, there are 8 to 10 decision-making steps in each clinical simulation pattern. This pattern of information gathering and decision making repeats itself until the problem is ended. You will then go on to the next problem until all 11 have been completed. See the table below for how this unique examination is scored.

Scoring of the Clinical Simulation Problem and Examination

All the options selected on each problem are scored on the following scale. The score is based on how appropriate it is to the condition of the patient at the time it was selected.

Score	Score Rationale
+3	Critically important for good patient care. It is necessary for prompt, proper care. Omitting it would result in the patient being seriously harmed from delays in care, pain, cost, and increased chance of morbidity and/or mortality
+2	Very important for good patient care.
+1	Helpful for good patient care.
0	Neither helpful nor harmful to patient care.
−1	Somewhat counterproductive to good patient care.
−2	Quite counterproductive to good patient care.
−3	Extremely counterproductive to good patient care. Detrimental to prompt, proper care. Its inclusion will result in the patient being seriously harmed from delays in care, pain, cost, and increased chance of morbidity and/or mortality.

Exam Scoring

Each of the 10 actual problems and the pretested problems are individually scored for information-gathering (IG) and decision-making (DM) based on the judgment of the problem author and the examination committee. The scores in these two areas on all 10 actual problems are totaled to give a grand total IG score and a grand total DM score. The examination committee determines the two required scores to pass the Clinical Simulation Examination. These scores may vary from exam to exam, but a score of at least 65% on both exam areas is typically needed to pass the Clinical Simulation Examination.

Suggestions for Preparing for the Clinical Simulation Examination

Things you should do:

1. **Carefully follow all directions.** If instructed to make only one choice, make only one.
2. **Read the scenario carefully** to understand the patient's situation and what you are required to do. Is this an emergency? If it is, you will want to gather only the most vital information needed to make a patient care decision. Quick action will be required to decide on the best care to give. If it is not an emergency, more complete information gathering is called for. Then a more well-considered decision for patient care can be made.
3. **Know the rules for the initiation and changing of mechanical ventilation parameters. In general,** use 10 mL/kg of ideal body weight for the initial tidal volume setting. As discussed in Chapter 15, there may be clinical circumstances when a smaller tidal volume is justified. Make adjustments from there based on arterial blood gas results.

4. **Thoroughly read all options.** For information-gathering sections, it may be helpful to make a list of each desirable option on your paper before making your choices. Choose all the options that will give you important information. You will be penalized for skipping over important data and also for making dangerous or wasteful choices. When you are sure of your selections, reveal them all and then review and interpret them. Avoid the temptation to reveal and interpret one piece of data at a time. You may mistakenly decide not to gather some important information later.

5. Try to **visualize yourself in the real situation** as described. Do what you would do on the job. Make the best choice(s) that you can based on what you know at this point. This is true for both information-gathering and decision-making sections. It may be necessary to go back over past information or choices.

6. It may be helpful to **make a map on your paper** of where you have been for each of the 11 problems. This will help you keep track of past choices. However, the software allows you to go back in the scenario history to review previous selections.

7. **Pace yourself** to get through all 11 problems in the 4-hour time limit. That gives you about 20 minutes per problem. For example, you should be finishing your third problem after 1 hour. Unlike on the ELE or the WRE, you should *not* rush ahead at the end and pick just anything. You will be penalized for incorrect choices.

8. **Take a practice Clinical Simulation Examination.** Eleven practice patient simulations are offered on the Evolve webite (http://evolve.elsevier.com/Sills/resptherapy). Others are available from the NBRC at NRBC.org.

Things you should avoid:

1. **Do not try to jump ahead** in the problem or try to guess what the author is leading to. With the branching logic format, there are several possible pathways. Work only with what you know now and from the past.

2. **Try not to become flustered if you are faced with a scenario you have never experienced** at work. Imagine what you would do if faced with this problem and go from there. Also, do not become frustrated if the choice that you prefer is not available. There may be more than one way to take care of a patient's problems. Make your next best choice and move on.

3. **Do not make changes in patient care unless they are needed.** If a patient is stable with acceptable arterial blood gas values and vital signs, be content to leave the patient as he or she is.

4. **Do not get flustered by patient complications or equipment problems.** They do not necessarily mean that you did anything wrong! They are meant to test your ability to solve problems.

5. **Do not select everything in the information-gathering sections.** You will lose points by choosing unimportant, time-consuming, unnecessarily expensive, or dangerous procedures.

6. **Avoid selecting new or unusual procedures** that you are not familiar with—jet ventilation, for example. You will lower your score if you do not know how to operate the equipment properly.

7. **Do not misinterpret the data you are given.** Avoid assumptions about things that are not spelled out for you.

SUMMARY—GENERAL SUGGESTIONS

1. Take the NBRC's free Entry Level Exam, Written Registry Exam, and Clinical Simulation Exam and the practice tests available online with this text. Evaluate your results to find your strengths and weaknesses.

2. Begin studying about 2 months before the exam. Pace yourself so that everything can be covered in the time that you have. Avoid "cramming" a few days before the examination; these tests demand more than the simple recall of facts.

3. Study the most important and heavily tested areas first. See Table 1 on p. xvi and Box on p. xvii. Spend any remaining time studying less heavily tested topics or disease conditions.

4. Focus on the areas where you are weakest, especially if they are heavily tested.

5. If it is necessary to travel out of your hometown to take the exam, arrive at the city where the test will be given the evening before the exam. Make a practice drive from your motel to the test site and determine where you will park. Check the time required to get there and add more for traffic congestion.

6. Have a good dinner. Avoid alcohol, even if you are nervous, to keep a clear head in the morning.

7. Do not "cram" for the exam back at the motel. Unfortunately, if you are not prepared by now, a few more hours will not really help. If necessary, brush up on only a few test areas.

8. Set the alarm to get you up in plenty of time to be ready. Get a good night's sleep. Avoid sleeping pills.

9. Eat a good meal before the exam. Minimize caffeine. You will have plenty of adrenaline running through your system to keep you awake while taking the test!

10. Attempt to relax with the self-confidence that comes from knowing that you are well prepared.

IMPORTANT ADDRESSES AND PHONE NUMBERS

For information on the examination processes, taking free practice exams, purchasing other practice exams, scheduling an exam date and location (linking to Applied Measurement Professionals), and getting a copy of the exam detailed content outlines, contact:

National Board for Respiratory Care
18000 W. 105th Street
Olanthe, Kansas 66061-7543
Toll free: 888-341-4811
Telephone: (913) 895-4900
Fax: (913) 895-4650
Internet address: http://www.nbrc.org

For information on examination sites and to schedule an exam, purchasing practice exams, getting a copy of exam content outlines, and state credentialing requirements contact:

Applied Measurement Professionals
18000 W. 105th Street
Olanthe, Kansas 66061-7543
Telephone: (913) 895-4600
Fax: (913) 895-4650
Candidate support telephone: 888-341-4811
Internet address: http://www.goamp.com

For information on accredited respiratory care educational programs, contact:

Committee on Accreditation for Respiratory Care
1248 Harwood Road
Bedford, Texas 76021-4244
Toll free: 800-874-5615
Telephone: (817) 283-2835
Fax: (817) 354-8519
Internet address: http://www.coarc.com

For information on professional activities and resources, including Clinical Practice Guidelines, contact:

American Association for Respiratory Care
9425 N. MacArthur Boulevard
Suite 100
Irving, Texas 75063-4706
Telephone: (972) 243-AARC (2272)
Fax: (972) 484-2720
E-mail: info@aarc.org
Internet address: http://www.aarc.org

Contents

1 | Patient Assessment and Care Management

Note 1: This book is written to cover every item listed as testable on the *Entry Level Examination (ELE)*, *Written Registry Examination (WRE)*, and *Clinical Simulation Examination (CSE)*.

The listed code for each item is taken from the National Board for Respiratory Care's (NBRC) **Summary Content Outline for CRT (Certified Respiratory Therapist) and Written RRT (Registered Respiratory Therapist) Examinations** (http://evolve.elsevier.com/ Sills/resptherapist/). For example, if an item is testable on both the ELE and WRE, it is shown simply as (Code:...). If an item is testable only on the ELE, it is shown as (ELE code:...). If an item is testable only on the WRE, it is shown as (WRE code:...).

Following each item's code, the difficulty level is indicated for the questions on that item on the ELE and WRE. (See the Introduction for a full explanation of the three question difficulty levels.) **Recall [R]** level questions typically expect the exam taker to recall factual information. **Application [Ap]** level questions are harder, because the exam taker may have to apply factual information to a clinical situation. **Analysis [An]** level questions are the most challenging because the exam taker may have to use critical thinking to evaluate patient data to make a clinical decision.

Note 2: *A review of the most recent Entry Level Examinations (ELE) has shown that an average of 9 questions out of 140 (7% of the exam) cover patient assessment and care management. A review of the most recent Written Registry Examinations (WRE) has shown that an average of 15 questions out of 100 (15% of the exam) cover patient assessment and care management. Of these 15 questions, an average of 11 cover patient assessment and an average of 4 cover care management. Typically, 9 of the patient assessment questions deal with adult patients. The remaining two patient assessment questions deal with neonatal or pediatric patients. The Clinical Simulation Examination is comprehensive.*

Note 3: *The Entry Level Examination has shown an average of 2 questions that directly cover a cardiopulmonary pathology issue; the Written Registry Examination has shown an average of 1 question. It is beyond the scope of this book to cover all the cardiopulmonary diseases and conditions that befall patients for whom respiratory therapists may provide care. It is recommended*

that asthma, chronic obstructive pulmonary disease (COPD; emphysema or chronic bronchitis or both), pneumonia, pneumothorax, flail chest, congestive heart failure with pulmonary edema, myasthenia gravis, Guillain-Barré syndrome, head (brain) injury with increased intracranial pressure, pediatric croup and epiglottitis, infant respiratory distress syndrome, acute respiratory distress syndrome (ARDS), and smoke inhalation with carbon monoxide poisoning be studied. Some limited discussion of these topics is covered in this book. The Written Registry Examination frequently ask questions about the respiratory therapy procedures that patients with these types of problems are receiving. In addition, the 11 Clinical Simulation Examination scenarios are built around the care of patients with these types of diseases and conditions. See Box 1 in the Introduction.

PART 1. PATIENT ASSESSMENT

MODULE A

Review the patient's chart for the following data and recommend the following diagnostic procedures based on current information

Note: The following discussion involves noninvasive, bedside activities that apply to adults in most respiratory care settings. Some assessment items have been placed in later chapters, because they are procedure specific. Topics that relate to neonates and children are included in Module H.

1. Review the patient's history: present illness, admission notes, progress notes, diagnoses, respiratory care orders, medication history, do not resuscitate (DNR) status, and previous patient education (Code: IA1) [Difficulty: ELE is R; WRE: Ap]

a. Patient history

Review the complete initial patient history and note the following:

1. Date of history taking
2. Patient data: name, age, gender, race, and occupation
3. Primary complaints

4. Secondary complaints
5. Present illness history and symptoms
6. Family history
7. Medical history of cardiopulmonary disease(s), including smoking history, cough, sputum production, and activities of daily living
8. Review of body systems

It is important that the respiratory therapist obtain a *brief* history before beginning therapeutic procedures. Determine how the patient has been doing since the last treatment. Has there been a change in dyspnea, cough and secretions, chest pain, and so on? This will help guide therapy as effectively as possible.

b. Admission notes

The attending physician writes up his or her key findings and how they are related to the reason the patient was admitted to the hospital.

c. Progress notes

Review the physician's, nurse's, and respiratory therapist's patient progress notes before seeing the patient and beginning the therapeutic procedure. Look for any cardiopulmonary or other organ-system changes that will have an impact on the patient's ability to take the treatment. You may need to revise the therapy, get different equipment, or seek help. Check for new patient care orders if the physician notes a change in the patient's care plan.

d. Diagnoses

After the medical history, physical exam, and laboratory tests are completed, the patient will be placed into one of the following four diagnostic categories. Refer to Table 1-1 for examples of each category:
- Crisis/acute onset of illness
- Intermittent but repeated illness
- Progressive worsening
- Mixed patterns/multiple problems

e. Current respiratory care orders

Physician orders must have the patient's name, date, time, complete and proper orders for each therapeutic procedure, and the physician's signature. Verbal orders from the physician to the nurse or respiratory therapist must follow hospital guidelines and include the preceding information. Incomplete, improper, or questionable orders must be confirmed by calling the physician for clarification or correction.

f. Medication history

Note the respiratory medications that the patient is currently taking. In addition, note any medications used to help manage cardiovascular, renal, or neurological problems that may also affect the patient's respiratory status.

TABLE 1-1	Patient Illness Categories	
Category	**Examples**
Crisis/acute onset of illness	Trauma, heart attack, allergic reaction, aspiration of a foreign body, pneumothorax, pulmonary embolism, and some pneumonias
Intermittent but repeated Illness	Asthma, chronic bronchitis, congestive heart failure, angina pectoris, myasthenia gravis, and some pneumonias
Progressive worsening	Congestive heart failure, chronic bronchitis, emphysema, and upper respiratory tract infection leading to bronchitis or pneumonia
Mixed patterns/ multiple problems	Chronic obstructive pulmonary disease and cystic fibrosis complicated by multiple problems, mucous plugging or infection; mixes of congestive heart failure and chronic lung disease; mixes of neuromuscular and lung disease; mixes of renal failure and congestive heart failure with chronic lung disease

g. Do not resuscitate (DNR) status

The physician, patient, and family should determine the patient's cardiopulmonary resuscitation status. A patient with a terminal condition, such as end-stage chronic obstructive pulmonary disease (COPD), often will choose not to be resuscitated. If it has been determined that the patient does not want to be resuscitated, his or her DNR status should be clearly posted in the chart and in the patient's room. All members of the health care team should be aware of the patient's decision.

h. Previous patient education

If the patient has asthma or COPD and has been admitted before, check for any record of a respiratory therapist teaching the patient about the disease and how it can be better managed.

2. Review the results of the patient's physical examination and vital signs (Code: IA2) [Difficulty: ELE: R; WRE: Ap]

Review the results of the physical examinations performed by physicians, nurses, and respiratory therapists. Review the following organ systems:
- Pulmonary
- Cardiovascular
- Neuromuscular
- Renal

a. Current vital signs

Review the current vital signs in the patient's chart. Compare them with the admission vital signs and what you observe in the patient now. Look for a change in pattern that suggests either worsening or improvement in the patient.

b. Temperature

The textbook "normal" oral body temperature is 98.6° F (37° C). However, some range from 96.5° F to 99.5° F (35.8° C to 37.4° C) is normal. Make sure the patient has not eaten any hot or cold foods recently and has not been smoking before taking an oral temperature.

A rectal or core temperature is commonly taken in very sick patients, because it is more accurate and reliable. The normal rectal temperature is 97.5° F to 100.4° F (36.4° C to 38° C). Some variance is normal, but less so than with oral temperatures. Axillary temperatures are used as a last resort in stable patients. These run 1° F lower than oral temperatures and are less accurate and reliable.

The variations in temperature noted depend on the time of day, activity level and, in women, stage of the menstrual cycle. For example, a lower body temperature is normal when a person is in a deep sleep. An oral temperature higher than 99.4° F (37.4° C) in a patient with a history of respiratory disease indicates a fever. Typically, it can be caused by atelectasis or a pulmonary or systemic infection. Patients commonly are treated to keep their temperature below 103° F, if possible. In general, a rectal temperature below 97° F (36° C) is considered hypothermic. In some procedures, such as open-heart surgery, a patient's temperature is lowered to reduce metabolism and oxygen needs. The rectal temperature must be kept above 90° F (32° C) to prevent cardiac dysrhythmias caused by the cold.

c. Respiratory rate

The respiratory rate (f for frequency) is the number of breaths the patient takes in 1 minute. The number is counted by looking at or feeling the chest or abdominal movements, or both. The normal rate varies with age (Table 1-2). It is assumed that the patient is resting but awake and has a normal temperature and metabolic rate. A respiratory rate above or below normal is cause for alarm.

Hyperthermia (fever), acidemia, hypoxemia, fear, anxiety, and pain cause a patient to breathe more rapidly. Hypothermia, alkalemia, and hyperoxia in a patient breathing on hypoxic drive, sedation, and coma cause a patient to breathe more slowly.

Remember that even in healthy people, considerable variation is found in the respiratory rate. It is best to consider the respiratory rate and the patient's tidal volume and minute volume to get a more complete impression of

TABLE 1-2	Normal Resting Respiratory Rates	
Age (Years)	Male	Female
0	31 ± 8	30 ± 6
1-2	26 ± 4	27 ± 4
2-4	25 ± 4	25 ± 3
5-7	22 ± 2	21 ± 2
8-11	19 ± 2	19 ± 2
12-14	19 ± 2	18 ± 2
15-16	17 ± 3	18 ± 3
17-18	16 ± 3	17 ± 3
Older	16 ± 3	17 ± 3

Modified from Eubanks DH, Bone RC: *Comprehensive respiratory care,* ed 2, St Louis, 1990, Mosby.

how the patient is breathing. Carefully measure the respiratory rate of any patient with cardiopulmonary disease or with a respiratory rate outside the normal range. The rate should be checked as often as needed to monitor the patient's condition.

d. Blood pressure

The blood pressure (BP) is the result of the pumping ability of the left ventricle (made up of the heart rate and stroke volume), arterial resistance, and blood volume. Normal BP results when all three factors are in balance with each other. If one factor is abnormal, the other two have some ability to compensate. For example, if the patient has lost a lot of blood, the body attempts to maintain BP by increasing both arterial resistance and the heart rate.

Normal Blood Pressures

- Adults: lower than 120/80 mm Hg
- Infants and children younger than 10 years old: 60 to 100/20 to 70 mm Hg

As with the other vital signs, some variation in BP is noted among individuals. It is important to know the patient's normal BP to compare it with the current value. Carefully measure the BP in any patient who has cardiopulmonary disease or a history of hypotension or hypertension.

Hypotension in the adult is a systolic BP of less than 80 mm Hg. Recommend a BP measurement for any patient who has a history of hypotension, appears to be in shock, has lost a lot of blood, has a weak pulse, shows mental confusion, is unconscious, or has low urine output.

Hypertension in the adult is a systolic BP of 140 mm Hg or greater or a diastolic BP of 90 mm Hg or greater, or both. Carefully measure the BP of any patient with a history of hypertension, bounding pulse, or symptoms of a stroke (mental confusion, headache, and sudden weakness or partial paralysis). Fear, anxiety, and pain also cause the patient's BP to increase temporarily.

e. Heart/pulse rate

The heart/pulse rate (HR) is the number of heartbeats per minute. It can be counted by listening to the heart tones with a stethoscope or by feeling any of the common sites where an artery is easy to locate. Table 1-3 shows the normal pulse rates based on age. It is assumed that the patient is alert but resting when the pulse is counted. Carefully measure the heart/pulse rate in any patient with cardiopulmonary disease or any of the aforementioned conditions for hypotension or hypertension.

3. Serum electrolytes and other blood chemistries

a. Review the results of the patient's serum electrolyte levels and other blood chemistries (Code: IA3) [Difficulty: ELE: R; WRE: Ap]

b. Recommend blood tests, such as the potassium level, to obtain additional data (WRE code: IC1) [Difficulty: WRE: R, Ap, An]

The serum (blood) electrolytes are measured in most patients when they are admitted to the hospital and as needed thereafter. This is to determine whether the values are within the normal ranges listed in Table 1-4. Any abnormality should be promptly corrected so that the patient's nervous system, muscle function, and cellular processes can be optimized. Diet and a number of medications can affect the various electrolytes. Most abnormalities can be corrected by dietary adjustments or, if necessary, by oral or intravenous supplementation.

1. Potassium (K⁺)

Potassium is the most important electrolyte to monitor because of its effect on general nerve function and cardiac function. Hyperkalemia is a high blood level of potassium. It causes the following electrocardiographic (ECG)

changes: high, peaked T waves and depressed S-T segments; widening QRS complex; and bradycardia. Hypokalemia is a low blood level of potassium. It causes the following ECG changes: flat or inverted T waves, depression of the S-T segments, premature ventricular contractions (PVCs), and ventricular fibrillation (if severe enough). Chapter 11 offers a more complete discussion of ECG interpretation.

Exam Hint 1-1 (WRE)

Hypokalemia can be caused by the use of diuretic medications such as furosemide (Lasix). Signs of hypokalemia include the cardiac rhythm disturbances noted previously and muscle weakness. In addition, a metabolic alkalosis is found when the results of an arterial blood gas analysis are interpreted. Be prepared to recommend the administration of potassium if the serum level is low.

2. Chloride (Cl⁻)

Hyperchloremia is a high blood level of chloride, which causes significant prolongation of the ST segment and the QT interval on the ECG. Hypochloremia is a low blood level of chloride, which shortens the QT interval and perhaps widens and rounds off the T waves on the ECG.

3. Sodium (Na⁺)

Hypernatremia is a high blood level of sodium. It might be seen in a patient who is dehydrated or who has lost many gastrointestinal secretions because of vomiting, nasogastric tube drainage, or diarrhea. Hyponatremia is a low blood sodium level, which might be seen in a patient who is fluid overloaded.

4. Bicarbonate (HCO₃⁻)

Altered bicarbonate levels are commonly seen in patients with pulmonary conditions. The kidneys of patients with a chronically elevated arterial partial pressure of carbon dioxide (PaCO₂) typically retain bicarbonate to moderate

TABLE 1-3	Normal Pulse Rates According to Age
Age	**Beats/min**
Birth	70-170
Neonate	120-140
1 year	80-140
2 years	80-130
3 years	80-120
4 years	70-115
Adult	60-100

From Eubanks DH, Bone RC: *Comprehensive respiratory care,* ed 2, St Louis, 1990, Mosby.

TABLE 1-4	Normal Serum Electrolyte and Glucose Levels
NORMAL ELECTROLYTE VALUES*	
Chloride (Cl⁻)	95-106 mEq/L
Potassium (K⁺)	3.5-5.5 mEq/L
Sodium (Na⁺)	135-145 mEq/L
Calcium (Ca⁺⁺)	4.5-5.5 mEq/L
Bicarbonate (HCO₃⁻)	22-25 mEq/L
NORMAL GLUCOSE VALUES*	
Serum or plasma	70-110 mg/100 mL (dL)
Whole blood	60-100 mg/100 mL (dL)

*These values may vary somewhat among references.

the respiratory acidosis caused by the elevated carbon dioxide level. Conversely, the kidneys of patients with a chronically decreased $PaCO_2$ level excrete bicarbonate to moderate the respiratory alkalosis caused by the decreased $PaCO_2$ level.

5. Calcium (Ca^{++})

Hypercalcemia is an elevated calcium level, which may be associated with patients taking diuretics. ECG changes associated with an increased calcium level include a shortened QT interval and widened, rounded T waves. Hypocalcemia is a decreased calcium level. It causes ECG changes such as lengthening of the S-T segment and the QT interval.

6. Glucose

The blood glucose level is important to monitor, because it directly relates to how much glucose is available to the patient for energy for daily activities. The normal values are listed in Table 1-4. Hypoglycemia is a low blood level of glucose; it can mean that the patient is malnourished. Hyperglycemia is a high blood level of glucose; this may indicate that the patient has diabetes mellitus or Cushing's disease or is being treated with corticosteroids. More specific testing must be done to prove the diagnosis.

4. Complete blood count

a. Review the results of the patient's complete blood count (Code: IA3) [Difficulty: ELE: R; WRE: Ap]

b. Recommend a complete blood count for additional data. (Code: IC1) [Difficulty: WRE: R, Ap, An]

A complete blood count (CBC) is routinely done for all hospitalized patients, as well as for patients seen for a variety of illnesses and for routine physical examinations. The red blood cell (RBC, or erythrocyte) count, white blood cell (WBC, or leukocyte) count, and differential (Diff) provide a great deal of information about the hematologic system and many other organ systems.

The key normal values for the RBC count are listed in Table 1-5. The hemoglobin and hematocrit values also are important, because they directly relate to the patient's oxygen-carrying capacity. Decreased hemoglobin and hematocrit values indicate that the patient is anemic. An anemic patient has less oxygen-carrying capacity, and as a result, more stress is placed on the heart during exercise. Hypoxemia resulting from a cardiopulmonary abnormality places this patient at great risk. A transfusion is indicated if the hematocrit is below the level the physician considers clinically safe.

An increased number of circulating erythrocytes indicates that the patient has polycythemia. When this is seen as a response to chronic hypoxemia from COPD, cyanotic congenital heart disease, or another disorder, it is labeled *secondary* polycythemia. This patient is at added risk

| TABLE 1-5 | Normal Hemoglobin, Hematocrit, and Red Blood Cell Counts for Adults and Children* |

Gender	Adult	Infant	Child
HEMOGLOBIN (g/100 mL [g/dL])			
Female	12.0-16.0	12.2-20.0	11.2-13.4
Male	13.5-18.0	Same	Same
HEMATOCRIT (mL/100 mL [mL/dL])			
Female	38%-47%		
Male	40%-54%		
RED BLOOD CELL COUNT (in millions/mL)			
Female	4.2-5.4	5.0-5.1	4.6-4.8
Male	4.6-6.2	Same	Same

*These values may vary somewhat among references.

| TABLE 1-6 | White Blood Cell and Differential Counts* |

WHITE BLOOD CELL COUNT (mm^3)	
Adult	4,500-11,000
Infant and child	9,000-33,000
DIFFERENTIAL COUNT	
Segmented neutrophil	40%
Lymphocytes	20%
Monocytes	2%
Eosinophils	0%
Bands	0%
Basophils	0%

*These values may vary somewhat among references.

because the thickened blood causes an increased afterload against which the heart must pump. These patients also are more prone to blood clots. With supplemental oxygen or other clinical treatment to increase the arterial partial pressure of oxygen (PaO_2) to at least 55 to 60 torr, the erythrocyte and hematocrit levels, over time, return to normal.

The key normal leukocyte count and differential are listed in Table 1-6. A normal leukocyte count and a normal differential reveal two things about the patient. First, no active bacterial infection is present. Second, the patient's body is able to produce the normal number and variety of WBCs to combat an infection.

A mild to moderate increase in the leukocyte count is called *leukocytosis*. It is seen as a WBC count of 11,000 to 17,000 per cubic millimeter (mm^3). Usually, the higher the count, the more severe the infection. A WBC count above $17,000/mm^3$ is seen in patients with severe sepsis, miliary tuberculosis, and other overwhelming infections. When a patient has an acute, severe bacterial infection, the WBC differential count shows an increased number of neutrophils. Exceptions to this are patients who are elderly, those who have acquired immunodeficiency syndrome (AIDS), and those with other immunodeficiencies. These patients may have an infection but show only a mildly elevated WBC count.

Leukopenia is a low absolute WBC count of 3,000 to 5,000/mm³ or less. An acute viral infection can cause a mild to moderate decrease in the neutrophil count. A patient with a low WBC count is at great risk of bacterial or other infections.

5. Review the patient's coagulation study results (Code: IA3) [Difficulty: ELE: R; WRE: Ap]

Coagulation studies are routinely done for many hospitalized patients; for those who are to have surgery; and for those who have or are suspected of having a blood-clotting disorder. Also, many medications speed or slow clotting time (so-called blood thinners). It is important to review a patient's coagulation studies before drawing a blood sample or performing a procedure that may lead to bleeding. Table 1-7 lists normal coagulation study results. If the patient's clotting time is increased, the individual is at risk of bleeding. Be prepared to apply pressure to a blood sampling site (especially and arterial one) longer than expected.

6. Gram stain results, culture results, and antibiotic sensitivity results

a. Review the patient's Gram stain results, culture results, and antibiotic sensitivity results (Code: IA3) [Difficulty: ELE: R; WRE: Ap]

The first step in the microbial analysis of sputum, mucus, or other body fluids or tissues is a Gram stain. Gram staining is a special process for colorizing bacteria that divides them into two groups. Gram-positive (g⁺) bacteria are stained violet. These are the most common types of bacteria that cause bronchitis and pneumonia. In general, penicillin or related drugs and sulfa-type antibiotics kill gram-positive bacteria. Gram-negative (g⁻) bacteria are

stained pink. These organisms, unfortunately, are found in many of the sickest and weakest patients. Often the only way to kill gram-negative bacteria is with a specific antibiotic to which they have been proven sensitive. So-called broad-spectrum antibiotics, such as tetracycline, also may be used.

After Gram staining of the sample of fluid or tissue, a culture and sensitivity (C & S) study is performed. Culturing involves actively growing the organism or organisms to determine what they are. In a sensitivity test, the cultured organism is exposed to a variety of antimicrobial drugs. The goal is to determine which drug or drugs kill the pathogen most effectively. The patient then is treated with that antibiotic. It may take 1 to 3 days to get back the C & S results.

Gram staining cannot be used to identify *Mycobacterium tuberculosis* (TB) bacteria. Instead, the Ziehl-Neelson stain must be used. This is an *acid-fast* stain, and it gives the TB bacteria a red coloration. Other pathogens, such as viruses, protozoa, and fungi, cannot be identified by Gram staining. Protozoa and fungi must be identified with specialized stains. Fungi and *M. tuberculosis* may take 6 to 8 weeks to culture.

b. Recommend a Gram stain and C & S study for additional data (Code: IC4) [Difficulty: ELE: R, Ap; WRE: An]

Whenever an infection is suspected, it is important to obtain a sample of fluid or tissue from the site in question. This patient material is tested for possible bacterial infection by Gram staining and C & S study. Whenever bronchitis or pneumonia is suspected, it is important to obtain a mucus or sputum sample for evaluation. A sample of mucus suctioned from the lungs should show only pulmonary organisms. Sputum is the mix of mucus from the lungs and saliva from the mouth; therefore the organisms found in it may have come from either place. If the patient has pleural fluid, that also must be sampled. Often a blood sample also is taken to look for evidence of septicemia.

Note: The following two items have been listed as testable on the previous NBRC Content Outlines. They are included here in case they are tested again.

7. Review the patient's urinalysis results

A urine sample routinely is taken from every patient admitted to the hospital and from pregnant women and presurgical patients. Much information about the functioning of the kidneys and other metabolic processes can be gathered from the urinalysis results. A urinalysis also is done for diagnostic purposes in patients with abdominal or back pain, hematuria, and chronic renal disease. Table 1-8 lists the normal findings for a urinalysis. Any abnormal findings should be further investigated to discover the cause.

TABLE 1-7 Normal Coagulation Study Results		
Test Name	**Normal Value**	**Critical Value**
Bleeding time	1-9 min	>15 min
Prothrombin time (PT or Pro-time)	11.0-12.5 sec; 85%-100%	>20 sec
Partial thromboplastin time (PTT)	60-70 sec	>100 sec
Activated partial thromboplastin time (APTT)	30-40 sec	>70 sec

TABLE 1-8	Normal Urinalysis Results
Test Item	**Normal Value**
Appearance	Clear
Color	Amber yellow
pH	4.6-8.0 (average 6.0)
Specific gravity	Adult: 1.005-1.030 (usually 1.010-1.025)
	Newborn: 1.001-1.020
White blood cells	0-4
Red blood cells	0-2

8. Review the patient's pleural fluid study results

If a patient has had a thoracentesis procedure to remove pleural fluid, the fluid is sent to the laboratory for further analysis. The fluid may turn out to be watery, bloody, infected, or lymphatic. See Chapter 18 for a complete discussion of the types of pleural fluids.

MODULE B
RADIOGRAPHIC IMAGING

Note: It is beyond the scope of this text to cover all the features of normal radiographic images. Review standard textbooks for this as needed. This discussion is limited to items listed as testable by the NBRC.

1. Review the patient's imaging findings (Code: IA6) [Difficulty: ELE: R; WRE: Ap]

Look for the results of radiographs (x-rays), computed tomography (CT) scans, and magnetic resonance imaging (MRI) studies of the chest or upper airway. If possible, view these results to gain a better understanding of the patient's condition. (Although not specified by the NBRC, the following should be studied, if possible: positron emission tomography [PET] scans, ventilation/perfusion [V/Q] scans of the lungs, angiograms, and barium swallow studies.)

2. Recommend radiographic and other imaging studies to obtain additional data (Code: IC2) [Difficulty: ELE: R, Ap; WRE: An]

a. Chest radiograph

A *chest radiograph* should be recommended in the following situations:

- After an endotracheal or tracheostomy tube has been placed or repositioned
- After the jugular/subclavian route has been used to insert a central venous pressure (CVP) or pulmonary artery (Swan-Ganz) catheter

- After a chest tube has been placed in the pleural space to remove air or fluids
- Hemoptysis (bloody sputum) is noted
- A sudden deleterious change is noted in the patient's cardiopulmonary condition
- The balloon on the pulmonary artery (Swan-Ganz) catheter has been inflated for a prolonged period, and a pulmonary infarct is suspected
- A pneumothorax is suspected

Exam Hint 1-2 (ELE, WRE)

Expect to see at least one question on the *Entry Level Examination* and the *Written Registry Examination* in which the respiratory therapist should recommend a chest radiograph to rule out or confirm a pneumothorax. Signs and symptoms that the patient may have a pneumothorax include the following: sudden chest pain with an increase in dyspnea and shortness of breath (SOB), absent breath sounds over a lung field, tracheal deviation and heart sounds shifted to the side opposite the pneumothorax, asymmetrical chest movement, hyperresonant percussion noted over the pneumothorax, a sudden increase in peak pressure or plateau pressure or both on the patient's ventilator, or air in the soft tissues, or a combination of these.

b. Upper airway radiograph

An *upper airway radiograph* (anterior or lateral or both) should be recommended for a patient who presents with indications of upper airway obstruction. This can include:

- Aspirated foreign body
- Laryngeal edema
- Laryngeal tumor
- Laryngotracheal bronchitis (LTB or croup) versus epiglottitis (see Module H for more information)

c. CT scan

A *CT scan* provides a more detailed image than a conventional radiograph. It is able to depict abnormalities of the lungs and mediastinum. Indications include, but are not limited to, the following:

- Tumor
- Hematoma
- Abscess and cyst
- Pleural effusion
- Aortic or other vascular abnormalities (after an intravenous contrast material has been administered)

d. MRI scan

An *MRI scan* provides images of body organs without the use of radioactive materials. The images are created when the powerful magnet of the MRI machine is turned on and off, affecting the way hydrogen atoms align within the body. A limitation of MRI is that the patient cannot have any metallic implants. In addition, most mechanical ventilators cannot be used during an MRI scan because the magnetic field will interfere with the unit. Indications for an MRI scan include, but are not limited to, the following:

- Imaging of the head, spinal cord, and surrounding structures
- Imaging of the heart and great vessels
- Imaging of the kidneys, liver, and other organs

Although not specified by the NBRC, the following should be studied, if possible: PET scans, V/Q scans of the lungs, angiograms, and barium swallow studies.

e. PET scan

A **PET scan** is performed using a radioactive substance that is either inhaled or given intravenously. As the radioactive substance breaks down in the target organ, it emits a positron (a positive electron). When the positron combines with an electron, they annihilate each other with the release of two gamma rays. Detectors outside the body identify the origin of the gamma rays and can determine the functioning and metabolism of the target organ. Indications for a PET scan include, but are not limited to, the following:

- Determining the regional metabolism of the heart and brain
- Measuring the size of a myocardial infarction
- Measuring the effects of treatment on a cancerous tumor
- Determining pulmonary perfusion or ventilation

f. Ventilation/perfusion ($\dot{V}/\dot{Q}$) scan

A **ventilation/perfusion ($\dot{V}/\dot{Q}$) scan** is used to identify where air moves into the lungs during breathing and blood flows through the lungs. A **ventilation scan ($\dot{V}$ scan)** is performed to verify or refute the clinical suspicion that a patient has an area of the lung or lungs that is underventilated. Abnormal ventilation is seen in the case of a bronchial obstruction from a tumor or foreign body or with an alveolar problem, such as atelectasis, consolidation, or emphysema. Radioactive xenon (^{133}Xe) is mixed with oxygen and inhaled to show the lung fields. A special scanner is used to pick up the radioactivity through the chest wall. Areas of normal ventilation can be compared with underventilated areas.

A **perfusion scan ($\dot{Q}$ scan)** is performed to verify or refute the clinical suspicion that a patient has an area of pulmonary circulation that is underperfused. Abnormal perfusion is seen in the case of a pulmonary embolism, tumor, or vascular problem, such as pulmonary hypertension. Radioactive technetium ($^{99\,m}$Tc) is injected into the patient's venous system, where it is filtered out by the

pulmonary circulation. As previously described, a special scanner is used to pick up the radioactivity through the chest wall. Areas of normal perfusion can be compared with underperfused areas. The ventilation scan and perfusion scan tests can be done singly or as a set.

Comparing the ventilation and perfusion results side by side enables the physician to look for areas of mismatching. Normally, ventilation and perfusion match fairly closely and result in a 1 : 1 mix of air and blood at the alveolar capillary membrane. A pulmonary embolism results in a $\dot{V}/\dot{Q}$ ratio of 2 (or greater):1 (or less), because normal ventilation is present, and perfusion is reduced or absent. An obstructed airway with resulting atelectasis results in a $\dot{V}/\dot{Q}$ ratio of 1 (or less):2 (or greater), because ventilation is reduced or absent, and perfusion is normal.

g. Angiogram

An **angiogram** involves the placement of a catheter into an artery or a vein. Commonly, a radiopaque dye is injected so that the flow of blood through the vessel can be observed. If a blockage is found, a balloon at the tip of the catheter may be inflated (balloon angioplasty) to flatten the blockage. Indications for an angiogram include, but are not limited to, the following:

- Check blood flow through the carotid arteries and into the brain
- Check blood flow through the coronary arteries and the chambers of the heart
- Check blood flow through the pulmonary arteries when perfusion study results are inconclusive
- Perform a procedure to remove a blockage from an artery (this could include balloon angioplasty, laser atherectomy, or embolectomy)

h. Barium swallow (esophagogram)

A **barium swallow (esophagogram)** enables a radiographic image to be taken of the esophagus, stomach, and small intestine. Indications for a barium swallow include, but are not limited to, the following:

- Dysphagia
- Noncardiac chest pain
- Gastroesophageal reflux

3. Review the chest radiograph to determine the quality of the imaging (WRE code: IB7a) [Difficulty: R, Ap, An]

a. Patient identification

It is standard practice for the patient's name and identification number to be incorporated into the chest radiograph (chest radiograph film).

b. Patient positioning

The patient is positioned between the radiograph machine and the film cassette so that the electromagnetic (x-ray) radiation penetrates the patient's body, hits the film, and provides the desired view of the internal organs. Figure 1-1 shows the most common radiographic projections used for patients with cardiopulmonary problems. Examples of some of these positions are shown in this chapter.

If possible, the patient should be moved to the radiography department, and the chest radiograph should be taken from the *posterior to anterior* (*posteroanterior, P-A,* or *PA*) *position.* The patient's chest is placed against the film cassette with the shoulders rolled forward. Because radiographs penetrate from back to front, the size of the heart is close to normal. Normally, the patient is instructed to take in and hold a deep breath. This reveals more clearly the lung fields, heart, and other structures. This may be contrasted with a chest radiograph taken after the patient has exhaled completely. If the patient has been correctly positioned perpendicular to the film cas-

Figure 1-1 Common radiographic projections of the chest to evaluate the heart and lungs. **A,** Anteroposterior (AP) projection; **B,** Posteroanterior (PA) projection; **C,** Lateral projections; **D,** Right anterior oblique (RAO) position; **E,** PA oblique projection, left anterior (LA) projection; **F,** AP oblique position, left posterior oblique (LPO) position; **G,** AP oblique projection, right posterior oblique (RPO) position; **H,** Left lateral decubitus; **I,** Right lateral decubitus; **J,** Dorsal decubitus; **K,** Ventral decubitus. *(From Long BW, Frank ED, Ehrlich RA: Radiography essentials for limited practice, ed 3, St. Louis, 2010, Saunders).*

sette, the radiograph image will show the clavicle bones to be symmetrical.

If a portable chest radiograph must be taken because the patient is too ill to be moved from his or her bed, the *anterior to posterior* (*anteroposterior, A-P,* or *AP*) *position* must be used. The radiographs penetrate the body from front to back. This should be noted in the chart, because this view of the organs shows the heart's size to be larger than that seen in a PA radiograph.

The standard *lateral view* is taken with the patient standing upright with both arms raised above the head and the left side against the film cassette. This is done because the heart is left of center in the chest. A lateral view is used to see behind the heart and hemidiaphragms. It can be combined with an AP or a PA view to localize lesions within the chest. This view also is used to measure the patient's anterior-to-posterior chest diameter. This is often enlarged in patients with air trapping from emphysema.

The *oblique position* provides a third angle for viewing the internal chest structures. This is especially helpful when the physician is checking the heart borders, mediastinal structures, hilar structures, and lung masses.

The *lateral decubitus position* enables fluid within the pleural space to be viewed. As little as 25 to 50 mL of fluid can be detected in an adult as it flows to the horizontal position. An air/fluid level in a lung cavity (cyst) also can be evaluated by the shifting of the fluid line by gravity. The *dorsal decubitus position* is used to help identify a small pneumothorax in an infant.

The *lordotic (apical lordotic) position* is used when the upper lung fields must be viewed without the clavicles and first and second ribs obscuring them. The apices, right middle lobe, and lingula can be clearly seen.

Make sure, when viewing any chest radiograph, that you are looking at the film correctly. That is, the film should be viewed as if you were looking directly at the patient's chest. For example, in a PA or AP film, if you reached out your right hand, you would touch the image of the patient's left shoulder. To help with correct viewing, the film should show the letter L over the patient's left shoulder (on your right as you look at the film). Note that sometimes the film will show the letter R over the patient's right shoulder (on your left as you look at the film).

c. Exposure

The radiology technologist is responsible for exposing the patient to x-rays long enough to acquire the proper exposure of the internal organs. In all chest radiograph positions, the patient must take and hold a deep breath without moving as the picture is taken. If the patient is on a mechanical ventilator when an AP chest radiograph is obtained, a sigh breath should be delivered and held by the respiratory therapist to inflate the lungs fully.

It must be understood that the image seen on a chest radiograph film is the negative, or reverse, image of the densities of the structures within the chest. When viewing an radiograph film, a range of shadings will be seen progressing from white to black. *Radiopaque* items are very dense. They absorb most radiographs, preventing them from striking the film, and therefore appear white on the film. *Radiolucent* items have little density. They absorb few radiographs, allowing them to strike the film, and therefore appear dark on the film. Altogether, four densities are seen on a chest radiograph:

1. Air

Because air is the least dense substance, it blocks very few radiographs; most hit the film in the cassette. This causes the film to turn black. Notice that the film around the patient's body is completely black. Because the normal lungs are air filled with little tissue, they appear almost black. Normally some lung tissue markings can be seen as wispy white shadows. Air in the stomach or intestine also appears dark compared with the surrounding tissues.

2. Tissue

The tissues of the lungs, heart, diaphragm, breasts, and so on partially block the radiographs. This results in white shadows of varying opacity, depending on the density of the tissues. For example, the heart appears as a fairly solid white organ. Fluid also partially blocks radiographs. A pleural effusion is seen as a white shadow around one or both lungs.

3. Bone

The calcium in bone makes it dense enough to block most x-ray penetration; therefore the ribs, clavicles, and vertebrae are seen as fairly solid white lines. Broken ribs can be easily identified by the misalignment of their shadows.

4. Metallic

Bullets, wire sutures, metal plates, artificial heart valves, and coins completely block all radiograph penetration. This results in a sharply outlined white shadow. Medical devices, such as an endotracheal or a tracheostomy tube, nasogastric tube, or heart catheter, contain materials that completely block radiographs. Therefore these radiopaque items can be easily seen within the patient on a chest radiograph.

When the radiograph is obtained with the proper penetration and exposure, the intervertebral spaces of the spinal column are just visible. If the film is underexposed (the overall color of the film and body tissues is too white), the carina or an internal catheter may not be seen. If the film is overexposed (the overall color of the film and body tissues is too black), the air-filled lung fields will be too black, and it may not be possible to detect a pneumothorax.

4. Recommend and review the patient's chest radiograph to evaluate and monitor the patient's response to respiratory care procedures (Code: IIIE1) [Difficulty: ELE: R, Ap; WRE: An]

A chest radiograph should be taken whenever a significant change occurs in the patient's cardiopulmonary condition or whenever an invasive thoracic procedure is performed (chest tube insertion, endotracheal intubation, or placement of a pulmonary artery catheter).

5. Look for the presence of, or any changes in, pneumothorax (ELE code: IB7c) [Difficulty: R, Ap, An]

Free air that leaks into the interstitial spaces of the lung or body cavities is abnormal in any patient. Causes of an air leak include barotrauma/volutrauma (alveolar rupture related to the use of a mechanical ventilator), a ruptured bleb (congenital or acquired blister on the visceral pleura), puncture wound through the chest wall, and needle puncture through the pleural space during the insertion of a CVP or pulmonary artery catheter via the subclavian or jugular vein. Once air under pressure is forced through a bronchial or alveolar tear into the interstitial tissues, it tends to follow the path of least resistance. This may result in air being found in any of the following areas, singly or in combination.

a. Pneumothorax

Pneumothorax is air in the pleural space. The lung tends to collapse toward the hilum. A pneumothorax is identified on the chest radiograph as an area of black, indicating air that surrounds the collapsed lung. No lung markings are visible in the air-filled space, and the edge of the lung can be seen (Figure 1-2). If the air is under sufficient pressure to shift the lung and mediastinal structures to the opposite side, the condition is called a *tension pneumothorax*. This is a serious condition that can lead to the death of the patient if it is not quickly identified and treated. A pleural chest tube is always placed into the affected side to remove the air so that the lung can re-expand.

In addition, the following are other locations where free air can be found:

b. Subcutaneous emphysema

Subcutaneous emphysema is air found in the soft tissues, such as the skin, axilla, shoulder, neck, or breast, of the affected side. In extreme cases, the air forces its way into skin and soft tissues throughout the body. Scattered dark areas (air pockets) appear in the various soft tissues on the chest radiograph (Figure 1-3). *Pneumomediastinum* is air in the mediastinal space (Figure 1-3). *Pneumopericardium* is air in the pericardial space (Figure 1-4). Both of these conditions can be very serious. Cardiac tamponade is

Figure 1-2 Frontal radiograph of an adult male with a left-sided tension pneumothorax. The edge of the collapsed lung is shown *(arrows)*. Note how the mediastinum is shifted to the right, the right lung is compressed, and the left hemidiaphragm is depressed. *(From Des Jardins TR: Clinical manifestations of respiratory disease, ed 5, St Louis, 2006, Mosby.)*

Figure 1-3 Frontal radiograph of a neonate showing subcutaneous emphysema in the shoulders and neck area. Other abnormal air in the patient's chest includes a pneumomediastinum, which outlines the right lobe of the thymus gland *(arrow)*, and a left anterior pneumothorax. *(From Carlo C: Neonatal respiratory care, St Louis, 1988, Mosby.)*

Figure 1-4 Frontal radiograph of a neonate showing a pneumopericardium that resulted from pulmonary interstitial emphysema. Note the dark outline of air around the heart. Chest tubes have been placed to remove air from around the heart and the right pleural space from an earlier pneumothorax. An endotracheal tube also is seen. *(From Koff PB, Eitzman DV, Neu J: Neonatal and pediatric respiratory care, St Louis, 1988, Mosby.)*

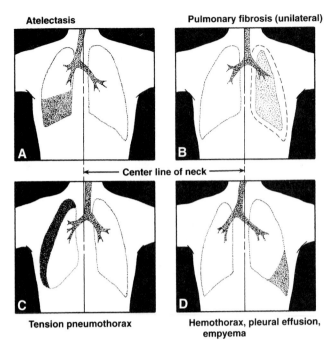

Figure 1-5 Conditions causing tracheal deviation and mediastinal shift (simulated chest radiograph findings). **A,** Unilateral atelectasis with tracheal deviation toward the affected lung. **B,** Unilateral pulmonary fibrosis with tracheal deviation toward the affected lung. **C,** Tension pneumothorax with tracheal deviation away from the affected lung. **D,** Pleural fluid with tracheal deviation away from the affected lung. The normal lung expands more than the abnormal lung during inspiration.

created if the pressure around the heart is great enough to interfere with its function. *Pneumoperitoneum* is air in the peritoneal space. This condition can be dangerous in an infant if a large enough volume of air is below the diaphragm and its movement is limited. *Pulmonary interstitial emphysema (PIE)* is air that has disseminated throughout the interstitial spaces of the injured lung or lungs. The lungs appear "bubbly" on the chest radiograph (Figure 1-4). The air may further leak into any of the previously listed locations. PIE is most commonly seen in infants with infant respiratory distress syndrome (RDS) who require mechanical ventilation (MV).

Exam Hint 1-3 (ELE)

The NBRC often has a question about how to identify the location of an endotracheal tube on a chest radiograph. The distal tip of the tube should be seen in the middle of the trachea. An endotracheal tube that has been inserted too deeply will enter the right mainstem bronchus.

---

6. Look for the presence of, or any changes in, mediastinal shift (Code: IB7f) [Difficulty: ELE: R, Ap; WRE: An]

The mediastinum is the area between the lungs that contains the heart and great vessels, trachea, hilar structures, and esophagus. In the neonate, the heart and other mediastinal structures should be approximately in the center of the chest, with the left ventricle to the left of center. In the adult, the majority of the heart and mediastinal structures should be left of center in the chest. A shift of the mediastinum (and heart) is abnormal, as shown in several conditions in Figures 1-2 and 1-5. Either atelectasis or pulmonary fibrosis, if unilateral and great enough, can result in a shift *toward* the problem area. Tension pneumothorax results in a shift *away* from the problem area. Fluid in the pleural space, if great enough, results in a shift *away* from the problem area.

7. Look for the position of indwelling tubes and catheters (Code: IB7d) [Difficulty: ELE: R, Ap; WRE: An]

All medical devices placed into the body are made of radiopaque material. They can be seen on a chest radiograph as a white object or line.

Chest tubes are placed to remove any abnormal collection of air or fluid from the thoracic cavity so that the function of the heart and lungs returns to normal. A pleural chest tube is placed to remove air or fluid from the pleural space (see Figure 1-4). The insertion site and depth of insertion of the tube depend on the patient's disorder. (See Chapter 18 for more discussion on the placement of pleural chest tubes.)

A mediastinal or pericardial chest tube is placed to remove air or fluid from either of these spaces (see Figures 1-4 and 1-6). Cardiac tamponade can result from the pressure of either air or fluid compressing the heart. Most postoperative open-heart surgery patients have one or more mediastinal chest tubes in place for several days to remove any blood from around the heart. The insertion site is below the sternum, and the tube or tubes are placed posterior to the heart in the pericardial or mediastinal space or both.

On the chest radiograph, a nasogastric tube appears as a white line from the patient's nose or mouth through the esophagus and into the stomach (on the left side below the diaphragm). A feeding tube may be placed as a nasogastric tube or may be surgically placed through the abdominal wall and into the stomach or small intestine. A white line on the radiograph shows its position.

A cardiac pacemaker is placed in two ways. An external pacemaker is identified on the chest radiograph by the

Figure 1-6 Frontal radiograph of an adult postoperative open-heart surgery patient with several medically necessary devices. A properly placed pulmonary artery (Swan-Ganz) catheter is noted to loop through the right side of the heart and out into the right pulmonary artery. The catheter tip is marked *CT*. Other foreign bodies include a properly placed endotracheal tube (marked *TT*), sternal wire sutures, ECG chest leads on each shoulder, and pericardial chest tubes (marked *ChT*). *(From Wilkins RL, Dexter JR, Heuer A: Clinical assessment in respiratory care, ed 6, St Louis, 2010, Mosby.)*

long electrode leads that run through a vein in the right arm, through the superior vena cava, and into the right ventricle. The battery and control unit of an internal pacemaker are placed under the skin below a clavicle. The electrode leads run through the superior vena cava into the right ventricle.

The various venous catheters (pulmonary artery catheter, central venous pressure [CVP] catheter, umbilical artery catheter [UAC], and umbilical vein catheter [UVC]) should be seen on the chest radiograph from their insertion points to their end points. (See Figures 1-6 and 1-7 for the placement of several catheters.)

8. Look for the presence of, or any changes in, consolidation (ELE code: IB7c) [Difficulty: R, Ap, An]

A *consolidation* is a filling of the alveoli with fluid from a pulmonary infiltrate, aspirated vomitus, blood, or water. It is often segmental or lobar. A pulmonary infiltrate occurs when blood plasma (water) passes from the pulmonary vascular bed into the lung tissues. Usually this fluid moves into the lung, because the alveolar capillary membrane is damaged. On a chest radiograph, an infiltrate often appears as a faint white blurring of the lung and other associated structures. Consolidation is noticed on the chest radiograph as a dense white shadow, because fluid has completely replaced the air. The mediastinum and heart are seen in their normal locations. Figure 1-8 shows a PA and lateral chest radiograph, indicating consolidation in each of the segments of both lungs. Air bronchograms also may be noticed on a radiograph that reveals consolidation.

9. Look for the positions of, or any changes in, the hemidiaphragms (Code: IB7f) [Difficulty: ELE: R, Ap; WRE: An]

The normal infant's and adult's AP or PA chest radiograph reveals a domed shape to the hemidiaphragms, with the edges turning down to acute costophrenic angles. A lateral chest radiograph reveals the same domed shape with the edges turning down to acute costophrenic angles. The edges of the hemidiaphragms should be smooth; any dips or peaks indicate an abnormality.

Both hemidiaphragms, and each separately, can be either elevated or depressed, depending on the condition of the lungs (underinflated or overinflated [hyperinflation]) and the abdominal contents. The following are commonly encountered clinical situations:

- *Unilateral elevation:* Atelectasis and pulmonary fibrosis (see Figure 1-5) decrease the lung's volume; an enlarged liver pushes up on the right hemidiaphragm.
- *Unilateral depression:* Excessive pleural fluid, tension pneumothorax (see Figure 1-2), check-valve

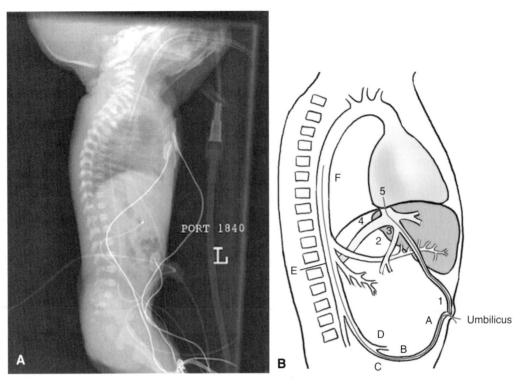

Figure 1-7 Lateral radiograph **(A)** and diagram **(B)** of the course of umbilical venous and arterial catheters. The umbilical venous catheter enters through the umbilicus and passes through the umbilical vein *(1)*, portal vein *(2)*, ductus venosus *(3)*, and inferior vena cava *(4)* and stops in the right atrium *(5)*. The umbilical arterial catheter enters through the umbilicus and passes through the umbilical artery *(A)*, hypogastric artery *(B)*, internal iliac artery *(C)*, common iliac artery *(D)*, and abdominal aorta *(E)*, and stops in the thoracic aorta *(F)*. *(From Wilkins RL, Dexter JR, Heuer A:* Clinical assessment in respiratory care, *ed 6, St Louis, 2010, Mosby.)*

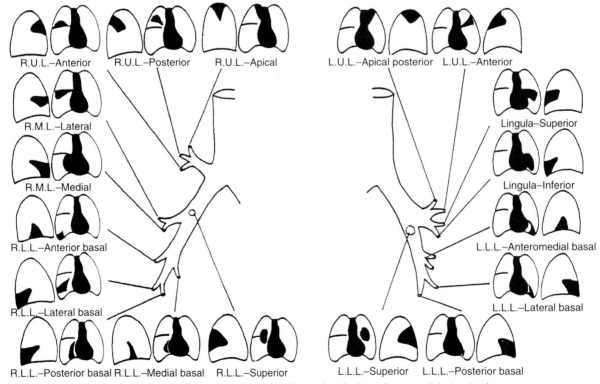

Figure 1-8 Simulated frontal and lateral radiographic findings for consolidation in the various segments of both lungs. *LLL,* Left lower lobe; *LUL,* left upper lobe; *RLL,* right lower lobe; *RML,* right middle lobe; *RUL,* right upper lobe. *(From Cherniack RM, Cherniack L:* Respiration in health and disease, *ed 3, Philadelphia, 1983, WB Saunders.)*

bronchial obstruction from a foreign body, or an airway tumor can cause unilateral depression.

- *Bilateral elevation:* Free abdominal fluid, as seen with peritoneal dialysis, can push up on both hemidiaphragms.
- *Bilateral depression:* Asthma attack and COPD (Figures 1-9 and 1-10) result in overinflation of both lungs and depression of both hemidiaphragms.

In a person with asthma, bronchitis, or emphysema (COPD), and in a newborn with meconium aspiration, both lungs are overinflated and both hemidiaphragms are depressed. Other radiographic findings include widened intercostal spaces; hyperlucent lung fields; a small, vertical heart; a small cardiothoracic diameter; and decreased vascularity of peripheral areas of the lungs, with enlarged hilar vessels. The lateral chest radiographic findings in the patient with COPD are the same, and they include anterior bowing of the sternum, increased retrosternal air space, and kyphosis. In any of the previously mentioned conditions, improvement should result in a return of the hemidiaphragm or hemidiaphragms to a position closer to normal.

10. Look for the presence of, or any changes in, pleural fluid (ELE code: IB7c) [Difficulty: R, AP, An]

Pleural fluid typically is shown on a PA or AP film as obscuring the costophrenic angle. This is because gravity tends to draw the fluid to the lowest level. Often this results in an obscuring or a blunting of the costophrenic angle of the affected side (Figure 1-11). In some cases, an air/fluid level is seen within the intrapleural space. The term *meniscus* is used to describe the upward curve seen in the fluid part of this intrapleural air/fluid level. Small amounts of fluid sometimes can be better visualized by taking a lateral decubitus radiograph. If the fluid is able to move freely in the pleural space, it shifts in a few minutes to the lower side (Figure 1-12). An empyema that is loculated (fixed) by adhesions does not move when the patient lies on his or her side. If large amounts of fluid are removed by a thoracentesis procedure, a chest radiograph should be taken to confirm the removal of fluid, the re-expansion of the lung, and that a pneumothorax did not result.

Figure 1-9 Frontal radiograph of an adult with advanced chronic obstructive pulmonary disease (COPD). Both lungs are overinflated and hyperlucent. The ribs are spread more widely than normal. Often these patients have a cardiothoracic ratio that is smaller than normal because the heart is elongated and the lateral chest diameter is increased. *(From Wilkins RL, Dexter JR, Heuer A: Clinical assessment in respiratory care, ed 6, St Louis, 2010, Mosby.)*

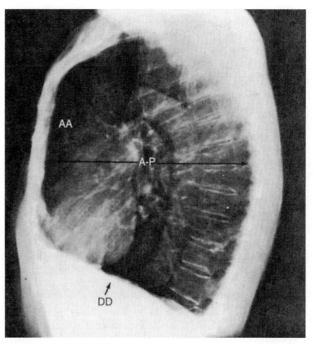

Figure 1-10 Lateral radiograph of an adult with advanced chronic obstructive pulmonary disease. Note the characteristic shape of a "barrel chest" from the overinflated lungs. The anteroposterior (AP) diameter of the chest is increased. *AA* marks an increased anterior air space between the heart and sternum. The angle of the manubrium and body of the sternum is more obtuse than normal. *DD* marks depressed hemidiaphragms that are flattened. *(From Wilkins RL, Dexter JR, Heuer A: Clinical assessment in respiratory care, ed 6, St Louis, 2010, Mosby.)*

Figure 1-11   Frontal radiograph of an adult showing a small pleural effusion in the right chest. Note how the costophrenic angle and hemidiaphragm are obscured by the white shadow of fluid. *(From Wilkins RL, Dexter JR, Heuer A:* Clinical assessment in respiratory care, *ed 6, St Louis, 2010, Mosby.)*

Figure 1-12   Lateral decubitus radiograph of an adult showing the shift of a small pleural effusion to the now-dependent part of the pleural space. The layer of fluid is marked by arrows. *(From Wilkins RL, Dexter JR, Heuer A:* Clinical assessment in respiratory care, *ed 6, St Louis, 2010, Mosby.)*

11. Look for the presence of, or any changes in, pulmonary edema (ELE code: IB7c) [Difficulty: R, Ap, An]

Pulmonary edema is watery fluid (plasma) that has leaked out of the pulmonary capillary bed into the interstitial

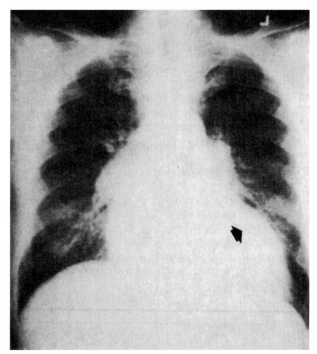

Figure 1-13   Frontal radiograph of an adult showing pulmonary edema, increased pulmonary vascular markings, and an enlarged left ventricle. The cardiothoracic diameter is increased, and the arrow shows where the border of the left ventricle normally would be seen. *(From Des Jardins T, Burton GG:* Clinical manifestations and assessment of respiratory disease, *ed 5, St Louis, 2006, Mosby.)*

spaces and alveoli. It is most commonly caused by left ventricular failure (also known as *congestive heart failure*), but it can be the result of fluid overload, pulmonary capillary damage, or decreased osmotic pressure in the blood from a low level of protein.

Pulmonary edema appears on a PA or AP chest radiograph as fluffy, white infiltrates in either or both lung fields. These tend to be seen more extensively in the lower lobes as a result of gravity pulling the fluid to the basilar vessels, where it leaks out. If the root cause is left ventricular failure, the vessels in the hila also are engorged, and the left ventricle is enlarged (Figure 1-13). A worsening problem results in more fluid leaking into the lungs and the appearance of more white infiltrates on succeeding chest radiographs. Once the problem has been corrected, the lungs return to normal as the fluid is reabsorbed and removed.

12. Look for the presence of any foreign bodies (Code: IB7e) [Difficulty: ELE: R, Ap; WRE: An]

A foreign body is anything that is not naturally found in the chest. Metallic objects (e.g., bullets or swallowed or aspirated coins or metal buttons) are easily noticed, because they completely block any radiograph penetration through the chest and are clearly outlined on the film as solid, white shadows (Figure 1-14). Nonmetallic foreign objects (e.g., plastic pieces from toys and foods, such as peanuts) are much more difficult to identify, because they have about the same densities as normal body tissues. Determining the exact location of a foreign body may require taking PA, lateral, and oblique chest radiographs. Lung volumes can be compared by taking inspiratory and expiratory films. A CT scan may be the most successful method of finding a nonmetallic foreign body.

13. Check the chest radiograph for the position of the patient's endotracheal or tracheostomy tube (Code: IB7b) [Difficulty: ELE: R, Ap; WRE: An]

The distal ends of these tubes should be seen within the lumen of the trachea and about midway between the larynx and the tracheal bifurcation to the right and left mainstem bronchi (see Figures 1-4 and 1-6 for endotracheal tube placement). The proximal end of the tracheostomy tube (or transtracheal oxygen catheter) is seen on the film coming out of the surgical insertion site in the suprasternal notch. The distal end should be centered

within the trachea above the carina (see Figure 1-6). All these tubes are made of a radiopaque material or have a line of radiopaque material embedded in them so that they can be easily seen on the radiograph.

Care must be taken not to push the endotracheal tube deeper into a bronchus (usually the right) or to pull it out. The tracheostomy tube and transtracheal oxygen catheter are less likely to be displaced if they receive proper care. Another radiograph should be taken to check the position of any of these tubes if clinical evidence suggests that a position may have changed.

Note: The following items have been listed as testable on previous exams and should be reviewed, if possible.

14. Check the chest radiograph for a sign that the cuff on the endotracheal or tracheostomy tube is overinflated

A properly inflated cuff fills the space between the tube and the patient's trachea so that an airtight seal is made. If the cuff is overinflated, it places excessive pressure on the trachea. This can cause it to dilate and be seen as a wider dark area than the rest of the tracheal air column.

Figure 1-14 Foreign body obstruction in an 18-month-old girl. **A,** Frontal radiograph with the solid white disk of a coin clearly seen in the hypopharynx. **B,** Lateral view of the chest with the edge of the coin seen as a solid white line. *(From Hunter TB, Bragg DG: Radiologic guide to medical devices and foreign bodies, St Louis, 1994, Mosby.)*

If this is noticed, the cuff pressure should be measured. Excessive pressure should be reduced to a safer level.

15. Check the chest radiograph for the size and patency of the patient's major airways

The trachea and both the right and left mainstem bronchi should be seen on a properly taken chest radiograph. They appear as straight, dark air columns in contrast to the white shadows of the various surrounding tissues. A white shadow within the airway may be a foreign body or a tumor. A lung tumor that presses on an airway causes the airway to narrow or be occluded.

16. Look for the presence of, or any changes in, atelectasis

Atelectasis is the collapse of alveoli; no air is found in them. This problem is commonly seen postoperatively in the lower lobes of patients who have had abdominal or thoracic surgery and who do not breathe deeply because of pain. The radiograph of atelectasis shows an increase in lung markings and a decrease in the lung volumes. If it is one sided, the mediastinum may shift toward the affected side (see Figure 1-5, *A*). If it is bilateral, the mediastinum is properly located. If it is severe enough, the lungs appear a uniform white (Figure 1-15).

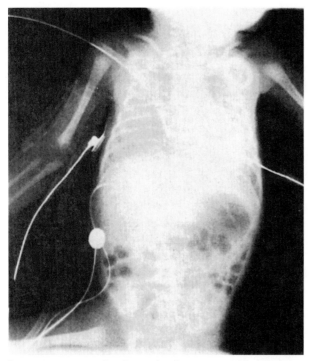

Figure 1-15 Frontal radiograph of a neonate with severe atelectasis from infant respiratory distress syndrome (RDS). Also note the right pleural chest tube and wires to various monitoring systems. *(From Des Jardins T, Burton GG: Clinical manifestations and assessment of respiratory disease, ed 5, St Louis, 2006, Mosby.)*

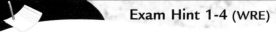

Exam Hint 1-4 (WRE)

Past exams have had at least one question that requires the identification of the cause of an abnormal chest radiograph. Typically the question refers to a patient who has a pneumothorax or pleural effusion. In addition, expect a question that requires the identification of the location of an endotracheal tube or the tip of a CVP catheter or pulmonary artery catheter. Also be prepared for questions related to recommendation of a chest radiograph to check for a foreign body obstructing the upper airway or a bronchus.

MODULE C
Interview the patient

1. What is the patient's level of consciousness or sedation? (Code: IB5a) [Difficulty: ELE: R, Ap; WRE: An]

One common way to evaluate a patient's level of consciousness is to categorize him or her as alert, stuporous, semicomatose, or comatose.

a. Alert

This is the normal mental state. The patient is conscious or can be fully awakened from sleep by calling his or her name. The patient can voluntarily ask logical questions and answer questions logically. The conversation is relevant to the topic under discussion. The patient's movements and actions are willful and purposeful.

b. Stuporous or lethargic

The patient is sleepy or seems to be in a trance. He or she can be aroused to respond with willful, purposeful movements and actions, but the patient may be slow. The patient may not respond to questions in a totally appropriate way.

c. Semicomatose

The patient does not perform requested movements or actions. The patient does not answer questions in an appropriate way. He or she responds defensively to pain. For example, if the right arm is pinched, it is withdrawn. Posturing of semicomatose patients includes the following:

1. Decerebrate

Legs are extended; arms are extended and rotated either inward or outward.

2. Decorticate

Legs are extended; arms are flexed, and the forearms may be rotated either inward or outward.

3. Opisthotonic

Legs, arms, and neck are extended, and the body is arched forward.

d. Comatose or coma

The patient has no spontaneous, oriented responses to the environment. Pain causes no defensive movement, but an increase in the heart and respiratory rates may occur.

Another common way to evaluate a patient's level of consciousness is to use the Glasgow Coma Scale (GCS). With this scale, a range of 3 to 15 points is possible; the larger the total number, the more normal the patient. A score of 15 is achieved in a patient normally awake and alert; a score of 3 is found in an unresponsive patient. Table 1-9 presents the details of the scale.

2. Is the patient oriented to time, place, and person? (Code: IB5a) [Difficulty: ELE: R, Ap; WRE: An]

Time refers to the patient knowing the calendar date, the day of the week, and the time of day. Ask the patient, "Do you know what day of the week it is? Do you know what the date is?" (The patient must be able to see a calendar.) "Do you know what time it is?" (The patient must be able to see a clock.) If the patient can answer these questions, he or she is oriented to time. If not, inform and show him or her. Tell the patient that you will return at a certain time. Ask the same questions when you return.

Place refers to the patient knowing where he or she is located (e.g., hospital, nursing care unit, extended care facility, home). Ask the patient, "Do you know where you are?" If the patient knows, he or she is oriented to place. If not, inform the patient of the location. Tell the patient that you will return at a certain time. Ask the same question when you return.

Person refers to the patient knowing his or her own name, address, and telephone number. The patient also should know the names of obviously important people. Ask the patient, "Do you know who the president (or the physician) is?" If not, inform the patient. Tell the patient who you are and what your job is. When you return for your next treatment, ask the patient if he remembers who you are and what you do. If the patient remembers who the president (or the physician) is and your name or job, he or she is oriented to person.

Orienting a stuporous or lethargic patient to person, place, and time may encourage the individual to cooperate more in his or her care. Pain-relieving and sedative drugs, stroke, injury to or edema of the brain, and other illnesses may cause disorientation to person, place, or time.

3. What is the patient's emotional state? (Code: IB5a) [Difficulty: ELE: R, Ap; WRE: An]

Acute illness or injury with great pain may result in some patients feeling fear, anxiety, or panic. Because of these feelings, the patient may be unable to concentrate closely on what you are telling him or her. This can result in directions not being understood or followed. It is important to tell the patient that you are there to help and that you need the patient to calm down so that you can help.

Chronic illness has been approached by a number of authors from varying points of view. Table 1-10 gives a presentation of a patient's reaction to chronic illness. Substitute "respiratory therapists" for "nurses" as needed.

A patient's statements and actions that indicate the *disbelief* stage of adaptation include the following:

- "I don't have (fill in the disease or condition)."
- "There is nothing really wrong with me."
- "The laboratory results are wrong."
- "The equipment is faulty."
- "The doctor/nurse/therapist is incompetent."
- Refusal to take medications.
- Refusal to take treatments or follow other physician orders.

TABLE 1-9	Glasgow Coma Scale	
Test Parameter	**Response**	**Score***
EYES		
Open	Spontaneously	4
	To verbal command	3
	To pain	2
	No response	1
BEST MOTOR RESPONSE		
To verbal command	Obeys command	6
Moves arms to	Localizes pain	5
painful stimulus	Flexion—withdrawal	4
of knuckles	Flexion—abnormal	3
against sternum	movement (decorticate rigidity)	
	Extension—abnormal movement (decerebrate rigidity)	2
	No response	1
BEST VERBAL RESPONSE (MAY AROUSE BY PAINFUL STIMULUS IF NECESSARY)		
	Oriented and converses	5
	Disoriented and converses	4
	Inappropriate words used	3
	Incomprehensible sounds	2
	No response	1

From Teasdale G, Jennett B: *Management of head injuries,* Philadelphia, 1981, FA Davis.
*The total is obtained by adding the scores in all three areas. The range is 3 to 15.

TABLE 1-10   Teaching-Learning Process in Adaptation to Chronic Illness

Stages of Adaptation	Patient's Behavior	Nurse's Behavior	Nurse's Facilitation of the Teaching-Learning Process
Disbelief	Denies threatening condition to protect self and conserve energy; refuses to accept diagnosis; may claim to have something else; may behave so as to avoid the issue; may seem to accept diagnosis but avoids feelings about it	Allows patient to deny illness as he or she needs to; functions as noncritical listener; accepts patient's statements of how he or she feels; helps clarify patient's statements; does not point out reality	Orients all teaching to the present, not to tomorrow or next week; teaches as he or she does other nursing activities; assesses patient's level of anxiety; assures patient that he or she is safe and being observed carefully; explains all procedures and activities to the patient; gives clear, concise explanations; coordinates activities to include rest periods
Developing awareness	Uses anger as a defense against being dependent and against guilt about being sick	Listens to patient's expressions of anger and recognizes them for what they are; explores own feelings about illness and helplessness; does not argue with patient; gives dependable care with an attitude that it is necessary	Does not give anxious patient long lists of facts; continues development of trust and rapport through good physical care; orients teaching to present; explains symptoms, care, and treatment in terms of the fact that they are necessary now; does not mention long-range care needs
Reorganization	Accepts increased dependence and reorganizes relationships with significant others; members of patient's family may also use denial while they adapt to what patient's illness means to them	Establishes climate in which family and friends can express feelings about patient's illness; does not solve patient's problems but helps build communication so that patient and family can work together to solve problems	Assures family that patient is all right and safe; uses clear, concise explanations; does not argue about need for care
Resolution	Acknowledges changes seen in self; identifies with others with same problem	Encourages expression of feelings, including crying; understands own feelings of loss	Brings groups of patients with same illness together for group discussions; has a recovered person visit patient; teaches patient what he or she wants to learn (or perceives he or she needs to learn) first
Identity change	Defines self as an individual who has undergone change and is now different; "There are limits to my life because I have a disease."	Understands own feelings about patient becoming independent again	Realizes that as patient's own perceived needs are met, more mature (more progressive) needs will surface; is prepared to answer patient's questions as they arise
Successful adaptation	Can live comfortably or resignedly with himself or herself as a person who has a specific condition	Initiates closure of nurse-patient relationship	Has helped develop a relationship with the patient in which the nurse is a guide with whom the patient can consult when he or she wishes

From Kenner CV, Guzzetta CE, Dossey BM: *Critical care nursing: body—mind—spirit,* Boston, 1981, Little, Brown.

A patient's statements and actions that indicate the *developing awareness* state of adaptation include the following:

- "The doctor/nurse/therapist doesn't know what he or she is doing."
- "It's all their fault."
- "Why is this happening to me?"
- The patient is angry about his or her illness.
- The patient may strike out verbally or physically at staff members.
- Some patients who do not get angry withdraw into a depression and wish to be left alone.

A patient's statements and actions that indicate that he or she is progressing from the *reorganization* to the *successful adaptation* stage include the following:

- "I'll never be able to do that again." (Fill in the activity.)
- "I have to get on with my life."
- "At least I'm still alive and can do this for myself."
- The patient may be sad and cry often.
- The patient may invent a nickname for his or her defect or diseased body part.
- The patient accepts the disability and focuses on his or her abilities.
- The patient works with family and others in planning for the future.

4. What is the patient's ability to cooperate? (Code: IB5a) [Difficulty: ELE: R, Ap; WRE: An]

You should be able to judge the patient's ability to cooperate. This should be based on his or her responses to your questions on level of consciousness; orientation to time, place, and person; and emotional state. An alert patient should be able to understand and follow directions. He or she should be able to take an effective treatment or cooperate in a procedure. Conversely, if the patient truly refuses the treatment or procedure, it should not be forced. Contact the patient's nurse or physician about the refusal. The physician must then decide what to do.

An alert but panicked, fearful, or anxious patient may be unable to cooperate fully until he or she is calmed by understanding who you are, what you are there to do, and why the treatment or procedure is important. Try to reassure the patient to improve cooperation.

If the patient appears alert but does not follow what you are saying, check to see whether he or she is deaf or does not speak English. An effective way to communicate must be found. Writing materials, a picture board, or a sign language interpreter is needed to communicate with a patient who is deaf. A native language translator will be needed to communicate with a patient who does not speak English.

A stuporous or very lethargic patient may be roused if you talk louder or shake the person gently. He or she may

or may not be able to cooperate fully. The practitioner may have to modify the treatment plan or how it is administered to compensate for the patient's lack of cooperation.

Pain relievers and sedatives may make a normally alert patient seem stuporous. If the patient has not been medicated, check with the nurse or physician to see what may have recently changed in the patient's condition.

A semicomatose patient may present the greatest problems in providing treatment or performing a procedure. These patients do not cooperate in any way but are unlikely to fight treatment either. In addition, some of their involuntary body posturings make correct positioning impossible. You must modify your equipment or procedure to accommodate the patient's inability to cooperate.

5. Does the patient complain of dyspnea? (Code: IB5c) [Difficulty: ELE: R, Ap; WRE: An]

Dyspnea is the patient's subjective feeling of shortness of breath (SOB) or labored breathing. This is normal after vigorous exercise but abnormal in a resting patient. Orthopnea is the condition in which a patient must sit erect or stand to breathe comfortably. Lying flat causes dyspnea.

Box 1-1 classifies the degrees of dyspnea, and Table 1-11 lists different kinds of dyspnea, including orthopnea. Only class I is normal dyspnea (on severe exertion). Classes II to V are progressively severe and limiting for the patient. Any orthopnea is abnormal, and the more the patient must sit up to breathe, the more limited the patient.

The following are examples of questions to ask in evaluating dyspnea:

1. "How far can you walk before you feel short of breath?"
2. "How many flights of stairs can you climb before you experience SOB?"
3. "How far can you walk when walking as fast as your spouse?"
4. "Is there anything you do that makes the SOB worse?"
5. "Is there anything you do that makes the SOB better?"
6. "How long does the SOB last after you stop to rest?"
7. "Is the SOB worse at any particular time of the day?"
8. "Is the SOB worse at any particular time of the year?"

The following are examples of questions to ask in evaluating orthopnea:

1. "Do you wake up at night with SOB?"
2. "Does your nighttime SOB get better after you sit up on the side of your bed or in a chair?"
3. "Do you get SOB when lying down to take a nap?"

BOX 1-1   Degrees of Dyspnea

Class I   Dyspnea only on rigorous exertion ("appropriate" dyspnea)

Class II   Able to keep pace with person of same age and build on level ground without breathlessness but not on inclines

Class III   Able to walk a mile at own pace without dyspnea but cannot keep pace on level ground with normal person

Class IV   Dyspnea present after walking about 100 yards on level ground or ascending 1 flight of stairs

Class V   Dyspnea on low-level activity or at rest

Modified from Burton GG: Practical physical diagnosis in respiratory care. In Burton GG, Hodgkin JE, editors: *Respiratory care: a guide to clinical practice*, ed 2, Philadelphia, 1984, JB Lippincott.)

TABLE 1-11	Causes of Dyspnea Related to Preferred Body Position	
Type of Dyspnea	**Clinical Correlations**
Orthopnea (must sit up to breathe; often occurs at night as paroxysmal nocturnal dyspnea)	Congestive heart failure
Obstructive sleep apnea (periodically stops breathing, particularly when lying on back)	Obesity; obstructive sleep apnea syndromes
Emphysematous habitus	Chronic obstructive pulmonary disease (COPD)
Platypnea	Pleural effusion; dyspnea associated with various body positions
Orthodeoxia	Pulmonary fibrosis; improvement in dyspnea when patient lies flat

From Burton GG: Patient assessment procedures. In Barnes TA, editor: *Respiratory care practice*, Chicago, 1990, Mosby.

4. "Do you use extra pillows behind your head and back to help you not get SOB at night or during a nap?"

5. "How many pillows do you need to keep you from getting SOB at night or when taking a nap?"

Dyspnea, like pain, is based on the patient's level of discomfort. Some patients may complain of dyspnea, whereas others may not. The therapist can get an impression of the patient's dyspnea by how many words can be spoken continuously. A patient with severe dyspnea cannot complete even a short sentence on a single breath.

6. What is the patient's sputum production like? (Code: IB5c) [Difficulty: ELE: R, Ap; WRE: An]

a. Time of maximal and minimal expectoration

Interview the patient to determine the following:

1. Time of maximal expectoration

Ask the patient, "When do you cough up the most? For example, is it in the morning; after eating spicy foods; after a breathing treatment; after smoking, work, or other exposure to dusts?"

2. Time of minimal expectoration

Ask the patient, "When do you cough up the least? For example, during certain nonallergic seasons of the year, after a breathing treatment, after consuming milk or milk products?"

b. Quantity

Some practitioners prefer to know of a specific amount such as a teaspoon, tablespoon, 10 mL, and so on. Others prefer to use subjective measures, such as "a little" or "a lot." Interview the patient to determine the following:

1. How does the quantity of sputum relate to the times of maximal and minimal expectoration and the patient's lifestyle?

Ask the patient, "Is there anything you do that increases or decreases the amount you cough out?" For example, the patient states that he coughs up 20 mL after breathing treatments but can cough up nothing after eating a bowl of ice cream.

2. Does the amount coughed up change in a cyclical way?

Ask the patient, "Do you cough up the most in the mornings or at night? Is there a work or lifestyle habit that changes how much you cough up? Is there a seasonal allergic condition that influences your asthma and sputum production?"

c. Adhesiveness of the sputum

Interview the patient to determine the following:

1. Are there times of the day or things that you do in the day that seem to result in your secretions becoming thicker or thinner?

2. Do your medications (like acetylcysteine [Mucomyst]) make the secretions easier to cough out?

3. Do some foods make your secretions easier to cough out?

7. What is the patient's exercise tolerance? (Code: IB5c) [Difficulty: ELE: R, Ap; WRE: An]

Exercise tolerance refers to how active a person can be before feeling the need to slow down or stop. A normal person at rest should feel no difficulty breathing. During vigorous exercise, a person should be aware that he or she is working harder than normal to breathe. This is to be expected. However, after recovering from exercise, the work of breathing should again be easy.

In a person with cardiopulmonary disease, *work of breathing* (WOB) refers to the patient's subjective feeling of how difficult it is to breathe during a given activity. Patients with acute or chronic lung disease often feel that they are breathing with some difficulty with little or no activity. Because this is a subjective feeling of the patient, it is helpful to have the patient quantify it. Ask the patient to rate his or her WOB on a 1-to-10 scale with 1 being easy breathing and 10 being extremely difficult.

If bronchospasm or secretions have increased, the patient will tell you that his or her WOB has worsened. If medications such as bronchodilators or mucolytics are effective, the patient should feel that his or her breathing is easier. Because of this, the patient can exercise more vigorously.

MODULE D

Use *observation* (inspection) to determine the patient's overall cardiopulmonary condition

1. Evaluate the patient's general appearance (Code: IB1a) [Difficulty: ELE: R, Ap; WRE: An]

Start by quickly inspecting the patient from head to toe, including how he or she is dressed and found in the room. Ideally, this is done without the patient knowing that he or she is being observed. The patient who does not have cardiopulmonary disease should be able to lie flat in bed or on either side without any breathing difficulty. The patient with one-sided lung disease may prefer to lie with the good side down. This might be the case with lobar pneumonia, pleurisy, or broken ribs. The patient with severe airway obstruction, as seen in asthma, bronchitis, or emphysema, tends to sit up in a chair or on the edge of the bed and use locked arms and shoulders for support. This enables the patient to use accessory muscles (Figure 1-16). The patient with orthopnea will not want to lie down flat because of the resulting SOB. This is commonly seen in patients with congestive heart failure and pulmonary edema.

CLINICAL MANIFESTATIONS

- Use of accessory muscles to breathe
- Pursed-lip breathing
- Minimal or absent cough
- Leaning forward to breathe
- Barrel chest
- Digital clubbing
- Dyspnea on exertion (late sign)

A

B

Figure 1-16 Typical posture seen in patients using accessory muscles of respiration. The shoulders are locked so that the accessory muscles can be used more effectively. *(Adapted from Burton GC, Hodgkin JE, editors: Respiratory care, ed 2, Philadelphia, 1984, Lippincott, Williams and Wilkins.)*

2. Determine whether the patient is cyanotic (Code: IB1a) [Difficulty: ELE: R, Ap: WRE: An]

Cyanosis is an abnormal blue or ashen gray coloration of the skin and mucous membranes. It is most easily seen in white persons by looking at the lips and nail beds. It can be seen in darker pigmented people by looking at the inner portion of the lip, the inner portion of the lower eyelid, and the nail beds. Commonly, cyanosis is said to be caused by hypoxemia, and that the more bluish a patient's color, the more hypoxemic he or she is. This often is the case, but cyanosis is not an accurate measurement of a patient's oxygenation. To be safe, a patient with cyanosis should have an arterial blood gas sample drawn for PaO_2 measurement or a pulse oximetry (SpO_2) measurement performed to evaluate oxygenation.

3. Determine whether the patient is diaphoretic (Code: IB1a) [Difficulty: ELE: R, Ap; WRE: An]

Diaphoresis is profuse sweating. It normally is seen after vigorous exercise. A patient is expected to sweat after a stress test or even an oxygen-assisted walk. Diaphoresis in a patient who is resting in bed should be investigated. When the body is severely stressed, it releases adrenaline into the bloodstream. Diaphoresis is one of many bodily effects caused by the release of the hormone adrenaline. Similar sweating may be seen if a large enough dose of the drug epinephrine is given.

Diaphoresis is a nonspecific sign of serious cardiopulmonary difficulties. It may be seen any time the patient is in shock or hypoxemic. Patients with a myocardial infarct are commonly diaphoretic. The practitioner should promptly evaluate the diaphoretic patient's pulse, respiratory rate, blood pressure, and arterial blood gases.

4. Determine whether the patient has clubbing of the fingers (Code: IB1a) [Difficulty: ELE: R, Ap; WRE: An]

Clubbing of the fingers (also known as *digital clubbing*) is an abnormal thickening of the ends of the fingers. It also

can occur in the toes. The key finding is an angle of more than 160 degrees between the top of the finger and the nail when seen from the side. Clinically, you will notice both a lateral and an AP thickening of the ends of the fingers (Figure 1-17 shows a comparison of normal fingers and clubbed fingers). The fingernail and toenail beds may be cyanotic.

The underlying cause is not completely understood but at least in part seems to be chronic hypoxemia. This results in arteriovenous anastomosis with thickening of the tissues. The list of diseases in which clubbing is seen includes COPD, bronchogenic carcinoma, bronchiectasis, sarcoidosis, and infective endocarditis.

5. Determine whether the patient has edema (Code: IB1a) [Difficulty: ELE: R, Ap; WRE: An]

Edema is an abnormal accumulation of fluid in the interstitial spaces of the tissues and potential spaces of the body. Peripheral edema is seen when fluid leaks from the capillary bed into the tissues beneath the skin in the ankles and feet or along the back when the patient is lying supine in bed. The extent of the edema is measured by pressing a finger into the tissues. Normal skin springs back, whereas edematous skin is pitted or depressed. The pitting edema is graded as 1+ for less than $1/4$-inch (mild), 2+ for $1/4$- to $1/2$-inch (moderate), and 3+ for $1/2$- to 1-inch (severe) indentation. Obviously, the deeper the pitting, the more peripheral edema the patient has.

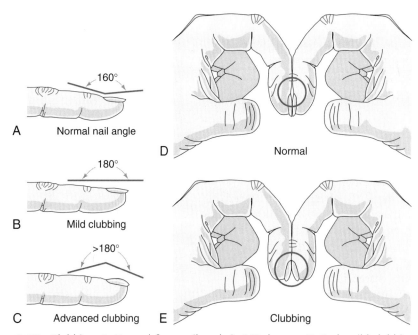

Figure 1-17   Clubbing. **A,** Normal fingernail angle is 160 degrees. **B,** Early mild clubbing appears as a flattened angle between nail and skin (180 degrees). **C,** Advanced clubbing shows a rounded (clubbed) fingertip and nail. To assess clubbing by Schamroth's diagnostic method (**D** and **E**), place the nails of the second digits together. Obliteration of the normal diamond-shaped space between the nails is an abnormal finding, signifying clubbing. *(From Copstead-Kirkhorn LC, Banasik JL:* Pathophysiology, *ed 4, St Louis, 2010, Saunders.)*

Peripheral edema is most commonly seen in patients with congestive heart failure and those who have a fluid overload. Patients with septicemia often have peripheral edema because the blood-borne pathogen (usually *Staphylococcus*) causes abnormal capillary leakage.

Many patients with edema from heart failure also have excessive venous distention of the neck veins. The internal jugular vein and external/anterior jugular vein are observed in the normal patient by having him or her lie supine with the head elevated 30 degrees. The crest of the vein column should be seen just above the border of the mid-clavicle. Make a rough measure of the intravascular volume and CVP by pressing on the veins at the base of the neck. The returning blood should fill the veins and make them distend (Figure 1-18). When the pressure is released, the veins should return to their previous level of distention just above the level of the mid-clavicle. Increased venous distention is noted when the veins stand out at a level above the clavicle. This is seen in patients with right-sided heart failure (cor pulmonale), cardiac tamponade, fluid overload, and COPD and when high airway pressures and positive end-expiratory pressure (PEEP) are needed for mechanical ventilation. The more the veins are distended, the more the patient is compromised.

It is not normal for the veins to collapse below the clavicle when the obstructing finger is removed. If this is seen, the patient should then have his or her head laid flat. Normally, when flat, the external jugular vein should be seen as partially distended. If the vein collapses on inspiration, low venous pressure is confirmed, and the patient probably is hypovolemic. This is commonly seen with dehydration, hemorrhage, or increased urine output after the use of diuretics.

A patient with heart failure also commonly has decreased capillary refill. Capillary refill is the time needed for blood to refill the capillary bed after it has been forced out. The procedure is to pinch the finger or toenail until it blanches and then release the pressure. The pink color of the nailbed should return in less than 3 seconds. Any delay in the return to pink color indicates reduced blood flow to the extremities. Cyanotic nail beds also are seen with reduced blood flow. Examples of conditions that result in decreased capillary refill include decreased cardiac output, low blood pressure from any cause, and the use of vasopressor medications.

6. Determine the patient's chest wall movement (Code: IB1a) [Difficulty: ELE: R, Ap; WRE: An]

Normal infants and adults have symmetrical chest movement when breathing at rest or during exercise. All breathing efforts are best observed when the patient is sitting up straight or standing erect and shirtless. Ideally, look at the patient from the front, back, and both sides to see the symmetry. In female patients, it may be necessary to observe only the uncovered back to judge chest movement. Any kind of asymmetrical chest movement is abnormal. The asymmetrical movement may result from an

Figure 1-18 Evaluating distention of the external jugular vein. These photographs show a patient with right-sided heart failure. Note that the left photograph shows the external jugular vein distended above the level of the clavicle. The right photograph shows how pressing a finger over the external jugular vein results in its further filling with blood and distending. In a normal person, when the pressure is released, the vein collapses to just above the superior border of the midclavicle. See the text for further discussion. *(From Daily EK, Schroder JS: Techniques in bedside hemodynamic monitoring, ed 5, St Louis, 1994, Mosby.)*

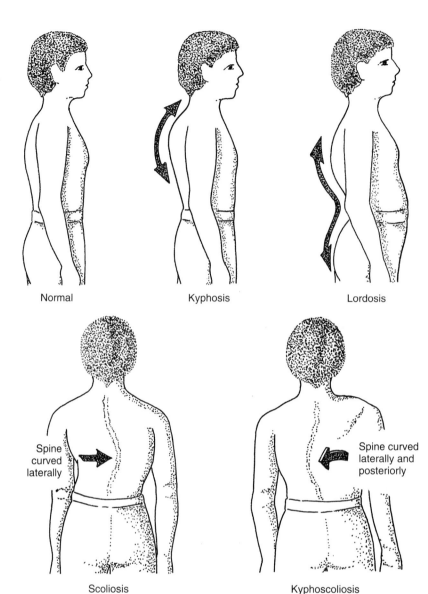

Figure 1-19 Normal and abnormal spinal curves. The patient should sit or stand erect during examination.

Normal   Kyphosis   Lordosis

Spine curved laterally

Spine curved laterally and posteriorly

Scoliosis   Kyphoscoliosis

abnormality of the chest wall or abdomen or from a pulmonary disorder.

a. Thoracic scoliosis or kyphoscoliosis

Several variations on curvature of the spine are found. *Kyphosis* is an exaggerated AP curvature of the upper portion of the spine. *Lordosis* is an exaggerated AP curvature of the lower portion of the spine. Scoliosis is either a right or left lateral curvature of the spine. *Kyphoscoliosis* is either a right or left lateral curvature combined with an AP curvature of the spine.

Figure 1-19 shows the back view of a patient with thoracic scoliosis or kyphoscoliosis. The patient with scoliosis in Figure 1-19 tends to have more chest movement on the right side because of the right spinal curvature. The left side of the chest and left lung would inflate more than the right if the spine curved to the left. These same findings are seen in a patient with kyphoscoliosis.

b. Flail chest

The flail segment moves in the opposite direction from the rest of the chest (this is also known as *paradoxical movement*). That is, with inspiration, the flail segment moves inward while the rest of the chest moves outward, and during expiration, the flail segment moves outward as the rest of the chest moves inward. As the ribs heal, the segment stabilizes and moves with the rest of the chest.

c. Pneumothorax

The side with the collapsed lung does not move as much as the chest wall over the normal lung (see Figure 1-2).

d. Atelectasis/pneumonia

The side with the atelectasis or pneumonia does not move as much as the chest wall over the normal lung (see Figure 1-5).

Normally, an adult's diaphragm moves downward several centimeters toward the abdomen during inspiration as the chest wall moves outward. This is seen when the abdomen protrudes as its contents are forced forward. The chest and abdomen should rise and fall together during quiet and vigorous breathing efforts. In two conditions, this normal chest and abdominal movement does not occur.

First, in patients with emphysema, severe air trapping, and a barrel chest, the diaphragm is depressed and flat rather than domed because of the air that is trapped in the lungs. On inspiration, the diaphragm still contracts, but it is unable to displace the abdominal contents downward to permit air to be drawn into the lungs. These patients do not have the expected abdominal movement during inspiration. They use the accessory muscles of inspiration to assist breathing.

Second, the normal movement does not occur in any condition in which airway resistance is increased or lung compliance is decreased. The greater negative intrathoracic pressure needed to draw the tidal volume into the lungs can cause the chest wall to collapse inward as the abdominal contents are displaced outward. The result is a kind of "seesaw" or paradoxical movement relation between the chest wall and abdomen. On inspiration, the chest wall may move inward as the abdomen moves outward. Patients with RDS typically demonstrate this because the premature neonate's rib cage is relatively compliant compared with the stiff lungs (Figure 1-20).

Exam Hint 1-5 (WRE)

Frequently a question relates to physical signs that a patient has a pneumothorax. This could include asymmetrical chest movement. The chest wall on the side with the pneumothorax will not move as much as the normal side during breathing.

---

7. Determine whether the patient uses accessory muscles when breathing (Code: IB1a) [Difficulty: ELE: R, Ap; WRE: An]

Accessory muscles of respiration should not be needed during passive, resting breathing. They are normally used when a person is breathing vigorously during exercise. A dyspneic patient likely will use them even when resting; this indicates that the WOB is greatly increased. The primary accessory muscles of inspiration are the intercostal, scalene, sternocleidomastoid, trapezius, and rhomboid muscles. The abdominal muscles are used during active expiration. The easiest accessory muscles of inspiration to observe in action are the sternocleidomastoids from the front and side of the patient and the trapezius

from the back of the patient (Figure 1-21). Their use is not specific for any one condition but is commonly seen in an adult patient with emphysema (see Figure 1-16).

Contraction of the dilator nares muscles (so-called nasal flaring) during inspiration further opens the nasal passages. A person breathing comfortably should have little or no nasal flaring. A person who is exercising vigorously may show nasal flaring in an attempt to reduce airway resistance. Nasal flaring is abnormal in a patient resting in bed, and it is a sign of increased work of breathing, especially in a neonate. Examples of conditions in which nasal flaring is seen include RDS (see Figure 1-20), acute respiratory distress syndrome (ARDS), and any condition in which pulmonary compliance is decreased or airway resistance is increased.

When a person with cardiopulmonary disease is using the inspiratory accessory muscles, intercostal or sternal retractions often are seen. A normal person breathing at rest should not have any retractions. That same person may have some minor retractions during vigorous exercise. Retractions of any kind are abnormal in any patient of any age who is resting in bed. Retractions are commonly seen in conditions in which airway resistance is increased or lung compliance is decreased. Both increase a patient's WOB. The patient must generate a more negative intrathoracic pressure to breathe, and as a result, the various soft tissues are drawn inward during inspiration.

Intercostal retractions are noticed when the soft tissues between the ribs are drawn inward during inspiration as the chest wall moves outward. Suprasternal retractions are noticed when the soft tissues *above* the sternum are drawn inward during an inspiration as the chest wall moves outward. Substernal retractions are noticed when the soft tissues *below* the sternum are drawn inward during an inspiration as the chest wall moves outward (see Figure 1-20). Conditions in which retractions are seen include RDS, ARDS, pulmonary edema, pneumonia, asthma, bronchitis, and emphysema.

8. Determine the patient's breathing pattern (Code: IB1a) [Difficulty: ELE: R, Ap; WRE: An]

The various respiratory patterns can be identified by their characteristic respiratory rate, respiratory cycle, and tidal volume. Figure 1-22 shows a normal adult breathing pattern, and Figure 1-23 shows examples of normal and abnormal breathing patterns.

a. Eupnea (normal breathing)

1. Normal respiratory rate for the age of the patient (see Table 1-2)
2. Normal respiratory cycle. When timing the flow of air into and out of the lungs, the inspiratory/

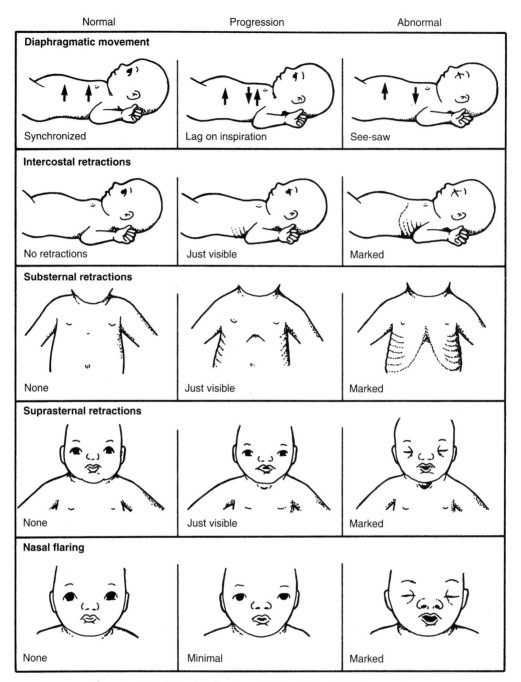

Figure 1-20   Physical indications of labored breathing in a newborn.

expiratory (I:E) ratio is about 1:2. A pause of variable time may follow exhalation of the tidal volume. This could change the true I:E ratio from 1:2 to 1:4

3. Tidal volume is normal for the size of the patient. (See Chapter 4 for calculation of a predicted tidal volume.) Inspiration is achieved without the use of accessory muscles of inspiration; exhalation is passive

4. A person usually sighs every few minutes; especially when inactive. A sigh breath typically is about 1.5 times as large as a tidal volume. It is thought to help prevent atelectasis. Frequent sighing may indicate a problem

b. Hypopnea (shallow breathing)

1. Respiratory rate usually somewhat slower than normal

Figure 1-22 Eupnea. Pause is the time from the end of exhalation to the beginning of inspiration. *I,* Inspiratory time; *E,* expiratory time.

Figure 1-21 Sternocleidomastoid and trapezius accessory muscles of respiration.

Figure 1-23 Representative drawings of normal and abnormal respiratory patterns. *(Modified from Seidel HM, Ball JW, Dains JE, et al: Mosby's guide to physical examination, ed 6, St Louis, 2006, Mosby.)*

2. Normal respiratory cycle
3. Tidal volume decreased for the size of the patient
4. Possible causes: deep sleep, sedation, coma, hypothermia, alkalemia, restrictive lung disease
5. May be combined with bradypnea

c. Hyperpnea (deep breathing)

1. Respiratory rate may be normal or somewhat faster
2. Normal respiratory cycle
3. Tidal volume increased for the size of the patient
4. Possible causes: acidemia, fever, pain, fear, anxiety, increased intracranial pressure
5. May be combined with tachypnea

d. Bradypnea (slow breathing)

1. Slower than normal respiratory rate
2. Expiration may be longer than normal as a result of a longer pause
3. Tidal volume may be decreased for the size of the patient
4. Possible causes: deep sleep, sedation, coma, hypothermia, alkalemia
5. May be combined with hypopnea

e. Tachypnea (rapid breathing)

1. Faster than the normal respiratory rate
2. Inspiration may be faster than normal with the help of inspiratory accessory muscles. Expiration may be shorter than normal, and expiratory accessory muscles may be used to force the air out faster. The pause seen in eupnea is absent. The I:E ratio may be 1:2 or less
3. Tidal volume may be increased for the size of the patient
4. Possible causes: acidemia, fever, pain, anxiety, increased intracranial pressure
5. May be combined with hyperpnea

f. Obstructed inspiration

1. Normal to slower respiratory rate
2. Inspiratory time is equal to or longer than expiratory time. Inspiration is aided by use of the inspiratory accessory muscles. Expiration is passive
3. Tidal volume may be normal or larger or smaller than normal, depending on how the patient adapts to the increased WOB. A slower rate most commonly is seen with a larger tidal volume
4. Possible causes: croup, epiglottitis, foreign body aspiration with partial airway obstruction, postextubation laryngeal edema, airway tumor, or airway trauma

g. Obstructed expiration with or without air trapping

1. Normal to slower respiratory rate
2. Expiratory time is longer than normal. Accessory muscles of inspiration and expiration may be used
3. Tidal volume may be normal or decreased for the size of the patient
4. Possible causes: asthma, emphysema, bronchitis, cystic fibrosis, bronchiectasis, airway tumor, or airway trauma. In severe cases, such as status asthmaticus, incomplete exhalation may cause air trapping

h. Kussmaul's respiration (rapid, large breaths)

1. Faster than normal rate
2. I:E ratio approaches 1:1. Both inspiratory and expiratory accessory muscles may be used
3. Tidal volume is increased for the size of the patient
4. Probable cause: acidemia (pH, 7.2 to 6.95) from diabetic ketoacidosis

i. Cheyne-Stokes respiration (waxing and waning tidal volumes)

1. The respiratory rate varies from normal to faster and may include short periods of apnea
2. The respiratory cycle is normal or approximates it, except if the patient has periods of apnea
3. The tidal volumes increase and decrease over a variable time cycle. A 20-second cycle is fairly common. Periods of apnea may occur between the decreased tidal volumes
4. Possible causes: head injury, stroke, increased intracranial pressure, or congestive heart failure

j. Biot's respiration (unpredictably variable)

1. The respiratory rate may be slow with deep breaths or rapid with shallow breaths; sighing is common. Periods of apnea occur between the periods of breathing
2. The respiratory cycle varies considerably, with periods of apnea
3. Tidal volume may be larger or smaller than normal
4. Possible causes: meningitis, head (brain) injury, brain tumor, increased intracranial pressure

k. Ataxic respiration (unpredictably variable)

1. The respiratory rate varies considerably, with abrupt periods of apnea

2. The respiratory cycle varies considerably, with periods of apnea
3. Tidal volume varies unpredictably between larger and smaller than normal
4. Possible causes: lesion of the medullary respiratory centers, head (brain) injury, brain tumor, increased intracranial pressure

l. Apnea (cessation of breathing at the end of exhalation)

1. Apnea that lasts long enough to result in hypoxemia, bradycardia, and hypotension must be treated aggressively. Artificial respiration, with or without supplemental oxygen, must be started immediately
2. It is important to evaluate the patient's previous breathing pattern to determine the cause of the apnea. Normal breathing followed by apnea could result from a heart attack, stroke, or upper airway obstruction. An abnormal breathing pattern followed by apnea could be the result of worsening of the original problem
3. Evaluate the previous tidal volume variation for the reasons previously listed
4. Possible causes: airway obstruction, heart attack, stroke, or head (brain) injury

9. Determine the kind of cough the patient has (Code: IB1c) [Difficulty: ELE: R, Ap; WRE: An]

a. Normal cough

A normal cough has four parts:
1. The person takes a deep breath.
2. The epiglottis and vocal cords close to keep the air trapped within the lungs.
3. The abdominal and other expiratory muscles contract to increase the air pressure in the lungs.
4. The epiglottis and vocal cords open to allow the compressed air to escape explosively and remove any mucus or foreign matter.

All components must work individually and in a coordinated manner for the patient to have an effective cough. The following are possible variations used by patients who for some reason cannot cough normally.

b. Serial cough

All actions of a normal cough take place, except that the patient performs a series of smaller coughs rather than a single large one. This method of coughing may be used by postoperative patients who have too much abdominal or thoracic pain to cough normally. As the pain lessens, the patient should be able to cough normally.

c. Midinspiratory cough

All actions of a normal cough take place, except that the patient does not take as deep a breath. This midinspiratory cough can also be called a *huff cough*. Patients with emphysema and chronic bronchitis (COPD) sometimes use this to help prevent airway collapse when they cough.

A midinspiratory/huff cough also is used by patients with artificial airways. Because they cannot close the epiglottis and vocal cords, they can only take a large breath and blow out with as much force as possible. This can be an effective way to remove watery secretions.

d. Huff cough

Patients with artificial airways use this method. They cannot close the epiglottis and vocal cords, therefore they can only take a large breath and blow out with as much force as possible. This still is an effective way to remove watery secretions.

e. Assisted cough

This patient needs direct help from the therapist. The patient is given a deep breath by means of intermittent positive pressure breathing (IPPB) machine or manual ventilator. The therapist then helps the patient blow the air out quickly by pushing on the abdominal area to move the diaphragm up. This procedure is limited to conscious patients with neuromuscular defects who cannot cough effectively on their own.

10. Determine the quantity and characteristics of the patient's sputum (Code: IB1c) [Difficulty: ELE: R, Ap; WRE: An]

a. Quantity

Normally, a person is not aware of mucus production. The mucociliary escalator moves mucus toward the throat, where it is unconsciously swallowed. Normally mucus is uninfected and clear or white.

Typically, infections causing bronchitis or pneumonia result in the production of large amounts of mucus. The patient reports coughing and "spitting up." This mixture of mucus from the lungs and saliva from the mouth is called *sputum*. Any increase in mucus or sputum production, to the extent that the patient is aware of it, is abnormal.

As mentioned earlier, some practitioners prefer to use subjective measurements of sputum production, such as "a little," "a medium amount," or "copious." Objective measurements, such as a teaspoon, a tablespoon, or 5, 10, or 15 mL, for example, are preferred to quantify production. A marked measuring cup is needed to do this.

Note any changes in the amount of sputum the patient produces. This is best done in a timed manner, such as production per hour or per shift. It also is wise to correlate sputum production with breathing treatments or other procedures that may increase or decrease its production or clearance.

b. Characteristics

Homogeneity is best determined by letting a sputum sample stand in a test tube for several hours so that it stratifies. This is an important test to perform in a patient with a pulmonary infection or bronchiectasis. Normal sputum separates into a relatively thin surface layer of gel that floats on a lower layer of water (sol). The patient with a pulmonary infection or bronchiectasis has more viscous sputum because it contains dead bacterial cells, dead white blood cells, and cellular debris from the infected lung tissues. These cells settle over time to the bottom of a sputum sample and create a third layer of sediment. Figure 1-24 shows how this layering looks in the sputum from a patient who has a pulmonary infection that eventually clears up. Table 1-12 explains other details of sputum characteristics.

Note: The following item was listed as testable on previous exams and should be studied, if possible.

Exam Hint 1-6 (WRE)

Usually one question requires the therapist to evaluate the patient's sputum. Examples: (1) a change from white or yellow to green indicates pneumonia; (2) a lung abscess is likely when the sputum is green and foul smelling; and (3) pink-tinged, bubbly (frothy) secretions are found with pulmonary edema.

11. Determine whether the patient has muscle wasting

Muscle wasting is an abnormal condition of decreased muscle mass. Muscle wasting can be generalized or localized, depending on the underlying cause. The term *cachectic* refers to an emaciated patient whose arms and legs are thin; the shoulder, elbow, and knee joints are prominent; and the ribs are clearly outlined by deep intercostal spaces. The following are examples of conditions in which muscle wasting is seen.

a. Chronic obstructive pulmonary disease

COPD (emphysema and bronchitis) often results in muscle wasting because the patient is using an unusually large number of calories through the act of breathing. In addition, these patients often do not eat well, because a full stomach restricts the movement of the diaphragm

Figure 1-24 Evaluation of the homogeneity of sputum in the infected patient.

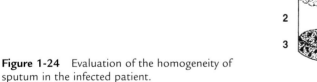

1. Gel layer: thicker than normal

2. Sol layer: thinner in ratio to gel layer than normal

3. Cellular debris: dead bacteria, WBCs, other cells

NOTE: The total volume of sputum is greatly increased

1. Gel layer: reducing toward normal

2. Sol layer: returning to normal ratio with gel layer

3. Cellular debris: thinning out as fewer dead cells are being coughed out

1. Gel layer: normal volume

2. Sol layer: normal volume and ratio with the gel layer

NOTE: The total volume of sputum is reduced to normal; also, there is no third layer of cellular debris

TABLE 1-12	Sputum Characteristics				
Sputum Type	**Color**	**Contents**	**Illnesses**	**Odor**	
Bloody (hemoptysis)	Red	Blood	Bronchogenic carcinoma; pulmonary hemorrhage; lung abscess; tuberculosis; pulmonary infarction	Typically none	
Frothy or bubbly	Clear or pink	Water; plasma proteins; red blood cells	Pulmonary edema	Typically none	
Mucoid	Clear or white	Water; complex sugars; glycoproteins; some cellular debris	Asthma; chronic bronchitis	Typically none	
Mucopurulent	Light to medium yellow	Decreased water and complex sugars; increased cellular debris and causative organisms (if applicable); organisms are usually aerobes	Chronic and acute bronchitis	Typically none but may exist, depending on organism	
Purulent	Dark yellow or green	Decreased water; greatly increased cellular debris and causative organisms (usually aerobes); complex sugars	Bronchiectasis; lung abscess; pneumonia	Depending on organism, along with clearance of mucus; also may be foul tasting to the patient; odor usually not offensive	
Purulent (fetid)	Dark yellow or green	Decreased water; may contain some blood; greatly exaggerated cellular debris and causative organisms (frequently anaerobes); complex sugars	Bronchiectasis; lung abscess; cystic fibrosis	Offensive odor	

From DiPietro JS: *Clinical guide for respiratory care and cardiopulmonary disease,* Acton, Mass, 1998, Copley Custom Publishing.

and worsens the WOB and SOB. Because of this, they frequently are malnourished or undernourished.

b. Lung cancer

Lung cancer or other cancers usually result in a loss of muscle mass. This is because the growing tumor consumes many calories that then are not available to the normal body tissues. These patients usually also have thin arms and legs with prominent joints in advanced disease.

c. Neurologic injuries

Neurologic injuries, such as transsection of the spinal cord, result in atrophy of the affected muscles. Atrophy of the muscles is a decrease in size resulting from lack of use. This is an unavoidable consequence of the permanent loss of nerve input to the affected muscles. For example, transsection of the spinal cord at the first lumbar vertebra (L1)

results in loss of nerve input to the legs. The patient is a paraplegic. In time, the muscles of the legs atrophy; however, if the arms are exercised, they retain normal muscle mass. If the patient has a spinal transection that results in the loss of nerve input to both the arms and legs (quadriplegia), all of the limbs atrophy.

MODULE E

Use *palpation* to determine the patient's complete respiratory condition

1. Determine the patient's pulse rate, rhythm, and force (Code: IB2a) [Difficulty: ELE: R, Ap; WRE: An]

The HR is most commonly counted by palpating the following locations: carotid, femoral, radial, and brachial arteries and apical pulse of the heart (Figure 1-25). The apical pulse normally is located in the area of the left midclavicular line in the fifth intercostal space. The apical pulse is also known as the point of maximal impulse (PMI). The location indicates the apex of the heart (left ventricle). Other arterial sites, such as the temporal, dorsalis pedis, and posterior tibial, can be used but are more difficult to find. The pulse should be counted for a minimum of 30 seconds; counting for 1 minute provides the most accurate measure of HR.

Palpating a pulse at any of the aforementioned sites reveals the timing between the heartbeats. This rhythm is normally regular in people who are at rest or exercising at a steady level. The rhythm is felt and mentally timed as the pulse rate is counted. The period between beats should be about the same.

The respiratory effort may have some influence on the rhythm. Fairly common in children and sometimes in adults, the heart rhythm and rate increase on inspiration and decrease on expiration. This sinus arrhythmia is not really abnormal. It is caused when the negative intrathoracic pressure during inspiration draws blood more quickly into the thorax and heart. The opposite may be true during mechanical ventilation with a high peak pressure or mean airway pressure. Then the heart rhythm and rate may slow during inspiration and speed up during expiration. In any other case, an irregular rhythm indicates some sort of cardiac problem. An electrocardiogram is needed to help determine the specific cause.

The force of the pulse is an indicator of the strength of the heart's contraction and BP. Normally each heartbeat should be felt with the same amount of force. A "thready" or variable force felt with each heartbeat is usually a sign of heart disease. Atrial fibrillation is an example of an irregular heart rhythm that results in an irregular force. The irregular rate and rhythm cause variable volumes of blood to be pumped with each contraction. A large volume of blood is felt as a strong pulse, whereas a small volume of blood is felt as a weak pulse.

A "bounding" or greater than normal force felt with each beat is usually a sign of hypertension. In either case, for safety's sake, the BP should be measured and compared with the patient's previous BP to see if a change has occurred.

2. Determine whether the patient has asymmetrical chest movements when breathing (Code: IB2b) [Difficulty: ELE: R, Ap; WRE: An]

Normally the lungs and chest move together in symmetry throughout the respiratory cycle. Asymmetrical chest wall movement during inspiration indicates a lung or chest wall problem. If the patient does not have an abnormal chest wall configuration, the problem has to be in the lungs. Less air is getting into the affected lung area or areas; therefore the chest wall does not move out as far as the chest wall over the normal lung. This is a nonspecific finding of lung disease but is also seen in pneumonia, bronchial or lung tumor, and pneumothorax.

The therapist's hands should be placed over the patient's chest to assess for asymmetrical chest movement (Figure 1-26). The thumbs should touch at the end of expiration. The patient then is instructed to breathe in deeply as the therapist looks and feels for asymmetrical movement. In Figure 1-26, A and B show the movement of the anterior apical lobes, C and D show the movement of the anterior middle and lower lobes, E and F show the movement in the posterior lower lobes, and G and H show the movement of the costal margins.

3. Determine whether the patient has tactile fremitus (Code: IB2b) [Difficulty: ELE: R, Ap; WRE: An]

Tactile fremitus is a vibration felt through the chest wall when the patient speaks. Normally, when a sound is

Figure 1-25 Determining the position of the apical pulse. **A,** Technique for locating the apical pulse by palpation. **B,** Location of the apical pulse. *(From Eubanks DH, Bone RC: Comprehensive respiratory care, ed 2, St Louis, 1990, Mosby.)*

created in the larynx, its vibration is carried throughout the tracheobronchial tree to the lung parenchyma and to the chest wall. The intensity of the vibration or its absence gives the practitioner important information about the patient's condition.

Figure 1-27 shows different methods of detecting tactile fremitus. Some practitioners may prefer to use their fingertips, as in *A* and *B*, whereas others prefer the ulnar edge of the open or closed hand, as in *C* and *D*. The practitioner should feel all areas of the patient's chest for tactile fremitus to detect any variations and should touch the chest over both lung fields to compare their symmetry as well as anterior and posterior differences (see Figure 1-27, *E* and *F*). Figure 1-28 shows the posterior and anterior locations for the evaluation of tactile fremitus. Start with the supraclavicular fossae and proceed to alternate intercostal spaces. An attempt must be made to preserve the adult female patient's modesty when

evaluating the anterior locations. The patient may be asked to lift the breast so that the examiner can palpate beneath it.

The procedure for evaluating tactile fremitus is to have the patient say "99" in a normal voice as the practitioner's fingers or hands are moved from location to location. This procedure is also called *palpation for bronchophony*. The "99" should be spoken at least once for each location to determine any variations. Having the patient speak more loudly or deeply should increase the intensity of the vibrations felt. The intensity of the vibrations directly relates to the density of the underlying lung and chest cavity. Conditions that increase density result in more intense vibrations. Conversely, conditions that decrease density result in less-intense vibrations. Vibrations also are reduced when they are blocked from penetrating through to the surface. Table 1-13 presents conditions that alter tactile fremitus.

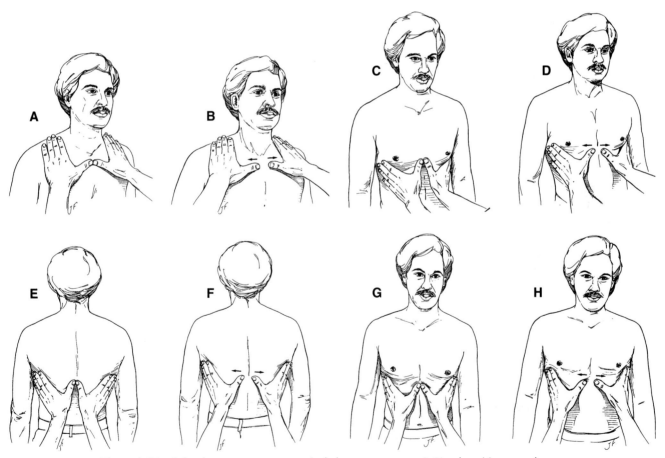

Figure 1-26   Palpation to access symmetrical chest movements. **A,** Hand position over the apical lobes during expiration. **B,** Apical movement during inspiration. **C,** Hand position over the middle and lower lobes during expiration. **D,** Middle and lower lobe movement during inspiration. **E,** Hand position over the posterior middle lobes during expiration. **F,** Movement of the posterior middle lobes during inspiration. **G,** Hand position to check for movement of the costal margins during expiration. **H,** Costal movement during inspiration. *(From Eubanks DH, Bone RC:* Comprehensive respiratory care, *ed 2, St Louis, 1990, Mosby.)*

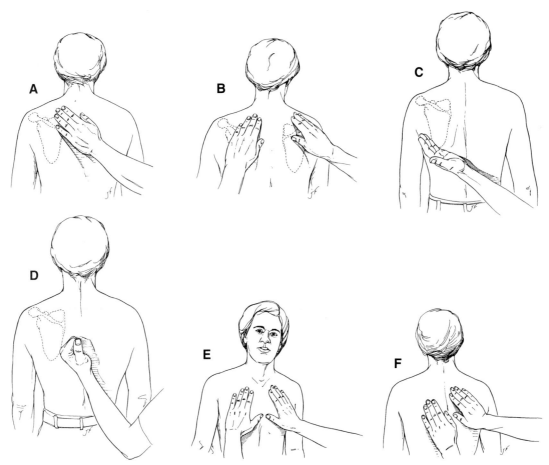

Figure 1-27   A to **D,** Techniques for detecting tactile fremitus. **E** and **F,** Anterior and posterior placement of the hands to detect tactile fremitus. *(From Eubanks DH, Bone RC: Comprehensive respiratory care, ed 2, St Louis, 1990, Mosby.)*

Figure 1-28   A, Locations on the posterior chest for detecting tactile fremitus and performing percussion. **B,** Locations on the anterior chest for detecting tactile fremitus and performing percussion. *(From Swartz MH: Textbook of physical diagnosis, ed 6, Philadelphia, 2010, Saunders.)*

TABLE 1-13	Abnormal Tactile Fremitus	
Increased		**Decreased**
UNILATERAL		**UNILATERAL**
Pneumonia		Pneumothorax
Atelectasis		Pleural effusion
Consolidation		Bronchial obstruction
BILATERAL		**BILATERAL**
Pulmonary edema		Thick chest wall (fat or muscle)
Acute respiratory distress syndrome		Chronic obstructive pulmonary disease

A   **B**

Figure 1-29   **A** and **B,** Detecting the position of the trachea by pressing the index finger into the suprasternal notch. *(From Eubanks DH, Bone RC:* Comprehensive respiratory care, *ed 2, St Louis, 1990, Mosby.)*

4. Determine whether the patient has rhonchial fremitus, indicating secretions in the airway (Code: IB2b) [Difficulty: ELE: R, Ap; WRE: An]

Rhonchial fremitus, also known as *palpable rhonchi,* is a type of tactile fremitus noticed when vibrations from airway secretions can be felt through the chest wall as the patient breathes. They are abnormal because they indicate that the patient has a significant secretion problem. Palpable rhonchi are not detected in a patient with clear airways. Having the patient cough or suctioning the airway to remove secretions results in the reduction or complete elimination of palpable rhonchi. Remember that an airway that is completely occluded by a mucus plug or foreign body will *not* reveal palpable rhonchi, because no airflow is present. Breath sounds also are absent in this area.

Different methods are available for detecting palpable rhonchi. Some therapists may prefer to use their fingertips, whereas others prefer to use the edge of the open or closed hand. It is important to assess all areas of the patient's chest to detect the exact location or locations of the secretions.

5. Determine whether the patient has crepitus (Code: IB2b) [Difficulty: ELE: R, Ap; WRE: An]

Crepitus (or crepitation) is the sound heard when an area with subcutaneous emphysema is gently pressed. The dry crackling-like sound resembles that of the breakfast cereal Rice Krispies in milk. A stethoscope can be used to help focus the sound to the exact location. In extreme instances, the unaided ear can detect the sound. As the fingers of one hand are sequentially pressed into the affected area, the subcutaneous air is felt to move away from the pressure points.

Subcutaneous emphysema is air under the skin that has leaked from a damaged lung. The skin appears puffy or edematous; this is most commonly seen in the tissues on the side of the leaking lung. The pressurized air dissects through the tissues, following the path of least resistance, and is most likely found under the skin in the axilla, neck, chest wall, and breast. In extreme cases, air is found under the skin throughout the body.

Although not dangerous, crepitus is a serious finding because it indicates that the patient has a pulmonary air leak. It may be accompanied by pneumothorax, pneumomediastinum, or pulmonary interstitial emphysema. A chest radiographic examination should be done immediately if the crepitation is a new finding.

6. Determine whether the patient has any tracheal deviation (Code: IB2b) [Difficulty: ELE: R, Ap; WRE: An]

Normally the trachea is in a midline position within the neck and thorax. The location of the trachea is found by having the patient look straight ahead and gently inserting the index finger into the suprasternal notch of an upright or supine patient (Figure 1-29). The trachea should be detected in the midline, with soft tissues on both sides. A trachea that is shifted off to one side is abnormal and can be caused by the following (see Figure 1-5):
- Atelectasis, which causes the trachea to be pulled *toward* the affected side
- Pulmonary fibrosis, which causes the trachea to be pulled *toward* the most affected side
- Tension pneumothorax, which causes the trachea to be pushed *away* from the affected side
- Hemothorax, pleural effusion, and empyema, which push the trachea *away* from the affected side

Correction of the underlying pulmonary problem results in the trachea returning to its normal midline position.

7. Determine whether the patient has any tenderness (Code: IB2b) [Difficulty: ELE: R, Ap; WRE: An]

Tenderness is an increased local sensation of pain when the chest is gently hit with the ulnar area of the fist. This tapping is done in a symmetrical pattern over the posterior and anterior lung areas and normally should not cause any pain. Intercostal tenderness is felt at the site of an inflamed pleura. Local tenderness and a history of trauma to an area of the chest lead to the conclusion of musculoskeletal pain. A chest radiograph might be indicated to determine whether any ribs have been fractured. The absence of chest wall tenderness should lead to a further investigation as to the cause of the chest pain. Consider angina pectoris (hypoxic heart pain).

MODULE F

Use *auscultation* to determine the patient's complete respiratory condition

1. Breath sounds

a. Determine whether the patient has bilaterally normal breath sounds (Code: IB4a) [Difficulty: ELE: R, Ap; WRE: An]

Three types of normal breath sounds are found (Figure 1-30):

1. *Normal* breath sounds are also called *vesicular.* These normal breath sounds are heard over all areas of normally ventilated lungs. Normal breath sounds have been variously described as "leaves rustling" or "like a gentle breeze." These faint sounds are made as air is moved through the small airways of the lungs during the breathing cycle. The inspiratory to expiratory (I:E) ratio is about 3:1. The inspiratory sound is louder than the expiratory sound, and there is no pause between inspiration and expiration

2. *Bronchial* breath sounds are also called tracheal. These normal breath sounds are heard over the trachea and main bronchi. Bronchial breath sounds have been described as being louder, harsher, and higher pitched than normal. They have a fairly uniform pitch on inspiration and expiration, with a distinct pause in the transition of flow. The I:E ratio is about 1:1.5

3. *Bronchovesicular* sounds are a cross between bronchial and vesicular.

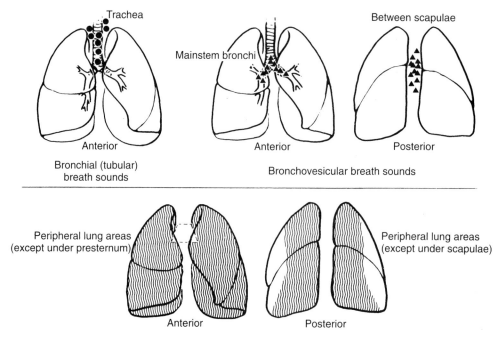

Figure 1-30   Breath sounds heard over the normal chest. *(From Lehrer S: Understanding lung sounds, Philadelphia, 1984, WB Saunders.)*

Bronchovesicular sounds are more muffled than bronchial but louder than vesicular and have the same pitch throughout inspiration and expiration. The I:E ratio is about 1:1

Bronchial and bronchovesicular breath sounds are abnormal if heard in any other areas except those mentioned here. When these sounds are heard over areas that should be normal vesicular, it is a sign of consolidation or atelectasis with a patent airway.

b. Determine whether the patient has abnormal breath sounds (Code: IB4a) [Difficulty: ELE: R, Ap; WRE: An]

The following discussion is limited to variations in normal vesicular breath sounds. The abnormal presentation of bronchial and bronchovesicular breath sounds was discussed earlier.

1. Increased normal vesicular breath sounds

a. Found most often in children and in debilitated adults because their thinner chest walls transmit the sounds better

b. Increased breath sounds are commonly described as harsh

2. Decreased normal vesicular breath sounds

a. Most commonly caused by a pleural effusion, hemothorax, or empyema because of fluid between the lung and the stethoscope (see Figure 1-5, *D*)

b. Pulmonary fibrosis resulting from decreased airflow (see Figure 1-5, *B*)

c. Emphysema resulting from decreased airflow

d. Pleural thickening resulting from dampening from the thicker pleural tissues

Exam Hint 1-7 (ELE)

Remember that when an intubated patient has breath sounds from the right lung but breath sounds are absent from the left lung, the endotracheal tube has been placed into the right mainstem bronchus.

3. Greatly decreased or absent normal vesicular breath sounds

a. Pneumothorax caused by the lung being forced away from the chest wall (see Figure 1-5, *C*)

b. Severe atelectasis (see Figure 1-5, *A*) or severe bronchospasm that results because little or no air is moving into the alveoli

c. Endotracheal tube placement into a bronchus instead of the trachea. In this case, the right bronchus is most commonly intubated; therefore the breath sounds are absent over the left lung

d. Large pleural effusion

e. Obese patient

Exam Hint 1-8 (ELE)

Expect to see at least one question that deals with identifying the presence of abnormal breath sounds. With proper treatment of the underlying problem, breath sounds should return to normal.

4. Unequal normal vesicular breath sounds

a. Pneumonia, consolidation, or atelectasis that decreases airflow into a segment or lobe

b. Foreign body or tumor in a bronchus that decreases airflow to the distal lung

c. Spinal or thoracic deformity that reduces airflow to the underlying lung. The term *adventitious* is used to describe collectively all types of abnormal breath sounds.

5. Wheezing

Wheezing (also known as *wheeze* and *rhonchi*) has the following features or characteristics:

- They are continuous sounds.
- They are more commonly heard on expiration than inspiration.
- Low-pitched, polyphonic expiratory wheezing is commonly associated with secretions in the airways. A common term for these sounds is *rhonchi*. Common pulmonary conditions include bronchitis, pneumonia, or any other secretion-causing problem. Coughing or tracheal suctioning often causes these sounds to be modified or eliminated.
- High-pitched, *monophonic* expiratory sounds are commonly associated with closure of one large airway. This is commonly found with an airway tumor.
- High-pitched, *polyphonic* expiratory sounds are commonly associated with closure of many small airways. The term *wheeze* is commonly used to describe these sounds caused by bronchospasm in an asthmatic patient. Coughing or tracheal suctioning is unlikely to eliminate these high-pitched sounds. Effective treatment with bronchodilating medications should make the wheezing diminish and vesicular sounds return.

6. Crackles (rales)

Crackles have the following features or characteristics:
- They are discontinuous sounds.
- They are more commonly heard on inspiration than expiration.
- They may be caused by the sudden opening of collapsed airways. Early inspiratory crackles are heard in patients with obstructive lung diseases such as chronic bronchitis, bronchiectasis, asthma, and emphysema. Late inspiratory crackles are heard in patients with atelectasis, pneumonia, pulmonary edema, or fibrosis.
- They may be caused by air passing through secretions and are heard as a repeated sound during the same phase of the respiratory cycle.

Exam Hint 1-9 (ELE)

Severe stridor is a respiratory emergency, because the airway may rapidly close completely. The patient usually is intubated to provide a secure airway.

7. Stridor

Stridor is heard as a harsh, monophonic, high-pitched inspiratory sound over the larynx. (It is not the normal tracheal sound.) It has these features or characteristics:
- Stridor can often be heard without a stethoscope.
- Common pediatric conditions include acute epiglottitis, laryngotracheobronchitis (croup), and laryngomalacia (congenital stridor).

Exam Hint 1-10 (WRE)

Usually at least one question concerns the interpretation of breath sounds or identifying a situation that might cause an abnormal breath sound. Examples include (1) absent breath sounds over an area of pneumothorax; (2) absent breath sounds over the left lung when an endotracheal tube has been misplaced into the right mainstem bronchus; (3) stridor over the larynx of a patient with epiglottitis or laryngeal edema. Remember that severe stridor is a respiratory emergency, because the airway may rapidly close completely. Nebulized racemic epinephrine may be given. If there is no improvement, the patient usually is intubated to provide a secure airway; (4) wheezing in a patient with asthma. Effective medication treatment results in less wheezing and an improved patient. However, understand that ineffective medication treatment results in less wheezing because the patient is getting worse.

- Common adult conditions include postextubation laryngeal edema and a laryngeal tumor.
- When stridor is heard on inspiration and expiration, it commonly is caused by an aspirated foreign body, tracheal stenosis, or a laryngeal tumor.

8. Friction rub

A friction rub (also known as a *pleural* friction rub) is the sound caused by the rubbing together of the inflamed and adherent visceral and parietal pleura, as seen in pleurisy. It is heard through a stethoscope and is described as loud and grating, clicking, or the creaking of old leather. The inspiratory sound frequently is reversed from the expiratory sound as the pleural tissues rub against each other in the opposite direction.

A friction rub is heard most commonly over the lower lung areas. Commonly, the sound is found at the site where the patient complains of pleural pain on breathing. Coughing and suctioning do not affect it. The causes include pulmonary infarct or any pneumonia that leads to an abscess or empyema.

2. Heart sounds

a. Determine the patient's heart sounds (Code: IB4b) [Difficulty: ELE: R, Ap; WRE: An]

The patient's heart rate and rhythm can easily be determined by listening at the point of the apical pulse (see Figure 1-25). Heart sounds are caused by the closing of the four heart valves during a cardiac cycle. The first heart sound, S_1, is heard as a "lub" sound when the mitral (bicuspid) and tricuspid valves close after the ventricles contract during systole. The second heart sound, S_2, is heard as a "dup" or "dub" sound when the pulmonary semilunar and aortic valves close after the ventricles relax during diastole. Obviously, if a heart sound cannot be detected, the patient should be assessed for cardiac arrest. Begin cardiopulmonary resuscitation (CPR) if needed.

b. Determine the patient's heart rhythm (Code: IB4b) [Difficulty: ELE: R, Ap; WRE: An]

A steady rhythm has approximately equal amounts of time between ventricular contractions. It is considered normal to have a slight increase in the HR and faster rhythm during an inspiration than during an expiration. This is caused by the increase in blood brought into the chest during the inspiration when the intrathoracic pressure is more negative. The opposite pattern might be seen when a patient is being mechanically ventilated with high peak-airway pressures. This indicates that the venous return to the heart is decreased during a mechanically delivered inspiration.

Any sudden variations in rate and rhythm not related to the respiratory cycle are abnormal. Occasionally, a third (S_3) or fourth (S_4) heart sound is heard. A patient with these extra sounds is described as having a "gallop" rhythm. This pathologic finding is usually noted in patients with congestive heart failure.

It is difficult to determine the origin of most dysrhythmias (arrhythmias) solely on the basis of their sound patterns. A diagnostic 12-lead electrocardiogram (ECG) is indicated (see Chapter 11 for details). A premature ventricular contraction (PVC) can be noted by the following rhythm characteristics: (1) the heartbeat is premature, and (2) a complete compensatory pause is noted between the PVC and the following normal beat. The complete compensatory pause is the time interval of two normal heartbeats. (See the representative rhythm strip [Figure 11-36] in Chapter 11.)

3. Determine the patient's blood pressure (Code: IB4c) [Difficulty: ELE: R, Ap; WRE: An]

Measure a blood pressure on any patient to establish a baseline normal value and whenever you think a significant increase or decrease in the BP might be present. The BP should be the same on any arm or leg. However, an arm typically is used. Place the proper cuff around the arm and inflate the cuff pressure above the patient's normal value. Place the diaphragm of the stethoscope over the brachial artery, and slowly let the air out of the cuff. The first distinct sound heard as the blood flows through the artery is the systolic pressure. The last distinct sound heard is the diastolic pressure. Clinical practice is needed to determine BP accurately.

MODULE G

> **Use percussion to determine the patient's overall cardiopulmonary status (Code IB3) [Difficulty: ELE: R, Ap; WRE: An]**

Percussion of the chest is performed to determine normal and abnormal densities of the lungs and related structures. It must be performed properly to be a reliable diagnostic tool. There are two generally accepted methods of performing percussion. Both must be performed with equal force and speed, or the resulting sound will reflect the technique rather than the condition of the lungs. Do not percuss over a woman's breast tissue.

Immediate percussion involves striking the tip of the middle finger of one hand directly onto the chest wall in a symmetrical pattern. This is useful for finding large general differences in density and for finding landmarks such as the sternum and other bony structures, the liver, and the heart. Mediate percussion involves striking the tip of the middle finger of one hand onto the central section of the middle finger of the other hand (Figure 1-31). The finger to be struck is fitted firmly between the ribs in a

Figure 1-31 Technique for performing mediate chest percussion. *(From Shapiro BA et al: Clinical application of respiratory care, ed 4, St Louis, 1991, Mosby.)*

symmetrical pattern, as shown in Figure 1-28. Mediate percussion is better for precisely locating an abnormal area and is used in the following discussions.

1. Determine the patient's diaphragmatic excursion

It is helpful to determine the patient's diaphragmatic excursion during both normal tidal volume breathing and during maximal inspiration and expiration. Both hemidiaphragms should move the same amount during both the normal and maximal efforts. It should be remembered that, because of the liver, the right hemidiaphragm usually is found to be about 1 cm higher than the left.

The following procedure determines diaphragmatic excursion during tidal volume breathing:

1. The patient should be sitting up straight, exhale passively, and hold.
2. Percuss down the posterior chest to find the level of both hemidiaphragms. The air-filled lungs have a resonant sound, whereas the more solid tissues below the lungs have a dull sound.
3. Have the patient inhale a normal tidal volume and hold.
4. Percuss down the posterior chest to find the level of both hemidiaphragms.
5. Note the range of movement on both sides by the intercostal space when the dull sound was heard at the end of expiration and at the end of inspiration. During a quiet tidal volume breath, the adult's hemidiaphragms move down about 1.5 cm on both sides. For example, the dull sound was heard at the ninth intercostal space at the end of exhalation and the tenth intercostal space at the end of inspiration.

The following procedure determines diaphragmatic excursion during maximal expiratory and inspiratory (vital capacity) breathing:

1. The patient should be sitting up straight, exhale as completely as possible, and hold.
2. Percuss down the posterior chest to find the level of both hemidiaphragms. The air-filled lungs have a resonant sound, whereas the more solid tissues below the lungs have a dull sound.
3. Have the patient inhale as completely as possible and hold.
4. Percuss down the posterior chest to find the level of both hemidiaphragms.
5. Note the range of movement on both sides by the intercostal space when the dull sound was heard at the end of expiration and at the end of inspiration. During the vital capacity effort, the adult's hemidiaphragms move down about 5 cm on both sides. For example, the dull sound was heard at the seventh intercostal space at the end of exhalation and the eleventh intercostal space at the end of inspiration (Figure 1-32).

Box 1-2 shows conditions that can affect the position of one or both hemidiaphragms.

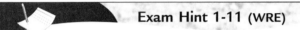

Exam Hint 1-11 (WRE)

There is usually one question that relates to an abnormal percussion note. Know that a hyperresonant percussion note is heard over an area of pneumothorax.

2. Determine whether the patient has areas of altered resonance

Mediate percussion with proper technique should be performed over the posterior and anterior areas of the chest while avoiding breast tissue (see Figure 1-28). The usual pattern is to proceed from the top down and side to side to compare for symmetrical sounds. The shoulders should be rolled forward when percussing the posterior chest to move the scapulae as much out of the way as possible. Table 1-14 shows the different types of percussion notes, their common characteristics, and example locations. Figure 1-33 shows the location of the normal percussion sounds over the anterior chest.

BOX 1-2   Conditions that Affect the Position of the Hemidiaphragms

ELEVATED
Unilateral
Atelectasis (on the affected side)
Paralysis of the hemidiaphragm (on the affected side)
Enlarged liver (right side only)

Bilateral
Third semester of pregnancy
Obesity
Ascites
Atelectasis (if bilateral)

DEPRESSED
Unilateral
Pneumothorax (on the affected side)
Check-valve obstruction to exhalation (on the affected side)
Pleural effusion (on the affected side)

Bilateral
COPD*
Asthma attack

---

*COPD is chronic obstructive pulmonary disease; a combination of chronic bronchitis and emphysema.

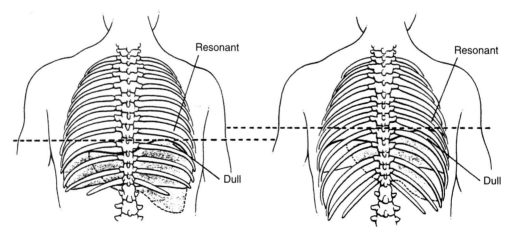

Figure 1-32 Excursion of the hemidiaphragms can be determined by percussing the patient's posterior chest. This should be done at the end of inspiration (as shown on the left) and expiration (as shown on the right). The change from a resonant (lung) sound to a dull (abdominal) sound indicates the border of the hemidiaphragm on each side. *(From Swartz MH: Textbook of physical diagnosis, ed 6, Philadelphia, 2010, Saunders.)*

TABLE 1-14 Percussion Notes and Characteristics

Percussion Notes	Relative Intensity	Relative Pitch	Relative Duration	Example Locations
Resonant/resonance	Loud	Low	Long	Normal lung
Flat/flatness	Soft	High	Short	Sternum, spine, scapula
Dull/dullness	Medium	Medium	Medium	Liver, heart
Tympanic/tympany	Loud	High	Longer	Stomach air
Hyperresonant/hyperresonance	Very loud	Low	Long	Bilateral: emphysema, asthma
				Unilateral: pneumothorax, bleb

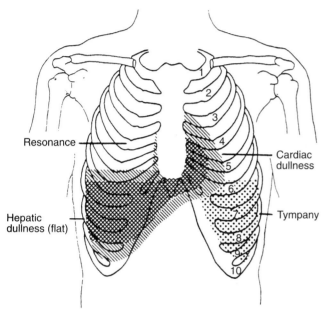

Figure 1-33 Areas over the normal anterior thorax where resonance, dullness, tympany, and flatness can be heard during percussion. *(From Prior JA, Silberstein JS, Stang JM: Physical diagnosis, ed 6, St Louis, 1981, Mosby.)*

A hyperresonant sound is always abnormal when found over lung areas. It indicates that more air than normal is present. Although emphysema can cause hyperresonance, a pneumothorax usually is the cause. Be careful not to confuse hyperresonance with the normal sound of tympany found over an air-filled stomach. An increase in the density of the underlying lung or related structures results in a dull sound at an abnormal location. This sound is associated with pneumonia, consolidation, or atelectasis when the alveoli are fluid filled or airless; with tumor; and with pleural fluid, such as effusion, blood, pus, or chyle. Dullness over the heart and liver is normal.

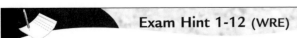

Exam Hint 1-12 (WRE)

Usually at least one question deals with interpretation of a newborn's given Apgar score. Also, be able to determine the Apgar score based on given information and interpret the patient's condition based on the score.

MODULE H
Neonatal and pediatric assessment

1. Review the perinatal/neonatal patient's chart for the following data

a. Review the maternal and perinatal/neonatal history and data (Code: IA1) [Difficulty: ELE: R, Ap; WRE: An]

Perinatal refers to the period toward the end of a pregnancy and for up to 4 weeks after the birth of the infant.

1. Antenatal assessment (assessment during the pregnancy)

The medical and personal history of the mother is obviously important, because it directly relates to the health of the fetus she is carrying. The mother's age is important, because women younger than 16 years and older than 40 years are more likely to have a high-risk pregnancy. This is especially true if a woman older than 40 years is having her first child. *Gravida* is the term that refers to pregnancy; *primigravida* refers to a woman with her first pregnancy. *Para* is the term that refers to the woman delivering a potentially live infant; *primipara/primiparous* refers to a woman's first delivery of an infant. Box 1-3 lists a number of maternal and other factors that can result in the anticipation of a high-risk infant being born. It must be noted that about 25% of high-risk infants are born without any indication of a problem in the history.

2. Intrapartum assessment (assessment during labor)

Some of the labor and delivery/obstetric factors that can adversely affect the delivery process include premature labor (less than 38 weeks' gestation), postmature labor (greater than 42 weeks' gestation), prolapsed umbilical cord, and cesarean section. The fetal heart rate (FHR, or fetal heart tones) usually is monitored to determine how the fetus is tolerating the stress of labor and delivery.

The FHR should range from 120 to 160 beats/min, and it is normally variable with the fetus's waking and sleeping

---

BOX 1-3   Some Factors Associated with a High-Risk Newborn Infant

MATERNAL FACTORS

Maternal age younger than 16 or older than 40 years
Low socioeconomic status
Poor nutrition
Lack of medical care during pregnancy
Smoking, drug or alcohol abuse
Underweight or overweight
Abnormal fetal growth
Hereditary anomalies
Vaginal bleeding early in pregnancy
Low maternal urinary estriol
Polyhydramnios or oligohydramnios
Toxemia of pregnancy/pre-eclampsia
Previous history of infant(s) with jaundice, respiratory distress, or previous premature delivery
Chronic disease
Hypertension unrelated to pregnancy
Diabetes mellitus
Cardiovascular
Pulmonary
Anemia
Renal

LABOR AND DELIVERY/OBSTETRIC FACTORS

Premature rupture of the membranes
Prolonged rupture of the membranes (>24 hr)
Premature labor (<38 weeks' gestation)
Postmature labor (>42 weeks' gestation)
Rapid or prolonged labor
Prolapsed umbilical cord
Previous or primary cesarean section
Breech or other abnormal presentation
Analgesia and anesthesia

FETAL FACTORS

Multiple births
Meconium in amniotic fluid
Abnormal fetal heart rate or rhythm
Fetal acidosis
Prematurity or postmaturity
Small or large for gestational age
Rh factor sensitization
Congenital malformation
Immature lecithin/sphingomyelin (L/S) ratio or negative phosphatidylglycerol (PG) test
Birth trauma

---

periods. The FHR can be measured externally through the mother's abdominal wall. During a contraction of the uterus, the FHR commonly slows to near or less than 120 beats/min. This occurs because of vagus nerve stimulation during compression of the head into the birth canal (Figure 1-34, *A*). The FHR returns to normal when the contraction is over. This normal decrease and increase in the FHR related to uterine contractions is called *early deceleration* or *type I dips.*

Late deceleration, or *type II dips,* are seen when the FHR slows sometime after the contraction begins and does not return to normal until sometime after the contraction is over (Figure 1-34, *B*). This is often caused by uteroplacental insufficiency from compression of the vessels in the placenta. It is frequently associated with low Apgar scores and fetal asphyxia and acidosis.

Variable deceleration is seen when the FHR slows and increases in an unpredictable pattern in comparison with the contractions (see Figure 1-34, *C*). This pattern is more commonly seen than late deceleration and is believed to be caused by compression of the umbilical cord by a body part. During the compression, little or no blood reaches the fetus. It also is often associated with low Apgar scores and fetal asphyxia and acidosis.

With late and variable deceleration, the mother's HR and BP should be monitored. Treatment includes giving the mother supplemental oxygen and placing her in a head-down, left lateral position. If the fetus is thought to be at risk of asphyxia, a cesarean section must be performed.

Other heartbeat irregularities are not related to labor and delivery. Tachycardia of greater than 160 beats/min can be associated with infection, fetal immaturity, congenital heart malformations, and the effects of maternal drugs. Bradycardia of less than 120 beats/min and decreased beat-to-beat variability (fixed heart rate) are seen with fetal asphyxia and distress.

3. Postpartum or neonatal assessment

Some of the fetal factors that can adversely affect the newborn include multiple births, meconium in the amniotic fluid, abnormal FHR or rhythm, prematurity or postmaturity, small or large size for gestational age, congenital malformation, and birth trauma.

4. Resuscitation and vital signs

All newborns require some level of resuscitation. This is usually limited to suctioning amniotic fluid out of the nose and mouth, drying the skin, providing warmth, and the tactile stimulation that comes from these procedures. Newborns with moderate Apgar scores may need to breathe in some supplemental oxygen until they are more vigorous and ventilating better. The newborn with a low Apgar score requires CPR. Table 1-15 lists the vital signs seen in a normal newborn.

5. Weight

The relationship between birth weight and gestational age is important to evaluate. In general, an infant between the 10th and 90th percentiles of normal weight for gestational age is within normal limits. Any infant either large or small for gestational age is at increased risk of compli-

Figure 1-34   Fetal heart rate patterns showing normal early deceleration **(A)**, abnormal late deceleration **(B)**, and variable deceleration **(C)**.

cations during and after delivery. Large post-term infants and small preterm infants are especially at risk.

b. Review the results of the neonate's lecithin/sphingomyelin ratio test (Code: IA9) [Difficulty: ELE: R; WRE: Ap]

To determine the lung maturity of the fetus, a sample of amniotic fluid must be obtained by amniocentesis. The maturity of the fetus's lungs can be determined by evaluating three components of surfactant released by the developing alveolar type II cells. Recall that in a premature neonate without sufficient surfactant in the lungs, infant respiratory distress syndrome probably will develop.

The first test of lung maturity is the lecithin/sphingomyelin (L/S) ratio. This test is a comparison of the relative amounts of these two surfactant components. In general, the more lecithin compared with sphingomyelin, the more mature the lungs. Usually a significant increase in the lecithin level occurs at about 35 weeks of gestation. A

weakness of the L/S ratio test is that borderline values are difficult to interpret, and false-positive values are sometimes found.

The second test involves determining the presence of phosphatidylglycerol (PG) in the amniotic fluid. It appears at about 36 weeks of gestation and increases through the duration of the pregnancy. The laboratory reports PG as either present or absent from the sample of amniotic fluid. Its presence always indicates lung maturity. Table 1-16 provides more information about the interpretation of these two tests.

c. Review the patient's Apgar scores (Code: IA9) [Difficulty: ELE: R; WRE: Ap]

The Apgar scoring system is used in the delivery room to provide a general evaluation of how a newborn infant is responding. The five parameters judged are heart rate, respiratory effort, muscle tone, reflex response, and color. Table 1-17 shows how the five parameters are scored on a scale of 0, 1, and 2. The newborn is evaluated soon after birth to calculate a 1-minute Apgar score. A 5-minute evaluation and Apgar score also are calculated. The infant is rated as good if the score is 7 to 10; fair if the score is 4 to 6; and poor if the score is 0 to 3. If the 5-minute score is less than 7, the newborn is rescored every 5 minutes up to 20 minutes after the delivery.

TABLE 1-15	Normal Newborn Vital Signs	
Characteristic	**Normal Range**	
Heart rate	>120 beats/min <160 beats/min	
Blood pressure	Systolic	**Diastolic**
1,000-2,000 g birth weight	55 mm Hg	30 mm Hg
>3,000 g birth weight	65 mm Hg	40 mm Hg
Respiratory rate	30-60 breaths/min Periodic breathing with apneic spells of <10 sec common; should not be associated with bradycardia or cyanosis	
Temperature	Keep abdominal skin temperature at 36.5° C Keep rectal (core) temperature between 35.5° and 37.5° C	

TABLE 1-16	Lecithin/Sphingomyelin (L/S) Ratio and Phosphatidylglycerol (PG) as Markers of Fetal Lung Maturity
Clinical Finding	**Interpretation**
L/S ratio ≥2:1 (2.0)	Mature lungs; <5% chance of RDS
L/S ratio 1.5:1 (1.5)	Transitional lungs; about a 50% chance of RDS
L/S ratio ≤1:1 (1.0)	Immature lungs; about a 90% chance of RDS
PG present	Mature lungs
PG absent	Immature lungs

RDS, Infant respiratory distress syndrome.

TABLE 1-17	Apgar Scoring Chart			
Sign		**0**	**1**	**2**
Heart rate		Absent	Slow (<100 beats/min)	>100
Respiratory effort		Absent	Weak cry, hypoventilation	Good strong cry
Muscle tone		Limp	Some flexion of extremities	Well flexed
Reflex response		No response	Grimace	Cough, sneeze, or cry
Response to catheter in nostril or to other cutaneous stimulation				
Color		Blue, pale	Body pink, extremities blue	Completely pink

d. Review information on the patient's gestational age (Dubowitz score) (Code: IA9) [Difficulty: ELE: R; WRE: Ap]

The Dubowitz score is made up of 11 physical and 10 neurologic criteria that develop at a set rate during gestation. Ballard and co-workers modified the scoring system by simplifying it to six physical and six neurologic criteria. Figure 1-35 shows the criteria, scoring system, and scale for rating the maturity of the newborn. A score of 35 to 45 indicates that the infant was born between 38 and 42 weeks of gestation; this is a normal score for a term infant. A premature infant has a score of less than 35, and a post-term infant has a score of greater than 45. The maturity rating scale can be used to estimate gestational age accurately within 2 weeks.

2. Use *inspection* (observation) to determine the perinatal or neonatal patient's overall cardiopulmonary status

a. Determine the patient's Apgar scores (Code: IB1d) [Difficulty: ELE: R; WRE: Ap, An]

Review the previous information and Table 1-17 as needed. Shortly after birth, the neonate's HR, respiratory effort,

Neuromuscular maturity

	−1	0	1	2	3	4	5
Posture							
Square window (wrist)	>90°	90°	60°	45°	30°	0°	
Arm recoil		180°	140°-180°	110°-140°	90°-110°	<90°	
Popliteal angle	180°	160°	140°	120°	100°	90°	<90°
Scarf sign							
Heel to ear							

Physical maturity

								Maturity rating	
								score	weeks
Skin	Sticky, friable, transparent	Gelatinous red, translucent	Smooth, pink, visible veins	Superficial peeling and/or rash, few veins	Cracking, pale areas, rare veins	Parchment, deep cracking, no vessels	Leathery, cracked, wrinkled	−10	20
Lanugo	None	Sparse	Abundant	Thinning	Bald areas	Mostly bald		−5	22
Plantar surface	Heel-toe 40-50 mm:−1 <40 mm:−2	>50 mm No crease	Faint red marks	Anterior transverse crease only	Creases ant. 2/3	Creases over entire sole		0	24
								5	26
Breast	Imperceptible	Barely perceptible	Flat areola, no bud	Stippled areola, 1-2 mm bud	Raised areola, 3-4 mm bud	Full areola, 5-10 mm bud		10	28
								15	30
Eye/Ear	Lids fused loosely: −1 tightly: −2	Lids open; pinna flat; stays folded	Slightly curved pinna; soft; slow recoil	Well-curved pinna; soft but ready recoil	Formed and firm instant recoil	Thick cartilage ear stiff		20	32
								25	34
Genitals male	Scrotum flat, smooth	Scrotum empty; faint rugae	Testes in upper canal; rare rugae	Testes descending; few rugae	Testes down; good rugae	Testes pendulous; deep rugae		30	36
								35	38
Genitals female	Clitoris prominent; labia flat	Prominent clitoris; small labia minora	Prominent clitoris; enlarging minora	Majora and minora equally prominent	Majora large; minora small	Majora cover clitoris and minora		40	40
								45	42
								50	44

Figure 1-35   Ballard modification of the Dubowitz Gestational Age Assessment. *(From Ballard JL, Khoury JC, Wedig K: New Ballard Score, expanded to include extremely premature infants, J Pediatr 119:417, 1991.)*

muscle tone, reflex response, and color are evaluated and each is given a score of 0, 1, or 2. The total of all five parameters is the 1-minute Apgar score. This score is a good index of how the newborn tolerated the delivery process. The 5-minute Apgar score is a good index of how the newborn's cardiopulmonary system is adjusting from fetal to adult conditions. A low 5-minute Apgar score is associated with increased mortality in the first month of life. Survivors have a high risk of mental impairment and cerebral palsy.

Exam Hint 1-13 (WRE)

Know the indication (suspected pneumothorax) and interpretation of the transillumination procedure results.

b. Determine the patient's gestational age (Dubowitz score) (Code: IB1d) [Difficulty: ELE: R; WRE: Ap, An]

The descriptions of gestational development for the criteria of physical maturity are listed in Figure 1-35. As can be seen, more points are earned for each step of gestational development. A term infant will score 3 or 4 points for each of the 12 criteria. The illustrations of gestational development for the criteria of neurologic/neuromuscular maturity can be seen in the figure; however, because the infant must be manipulated to perform the rating, the following descriptions can be helpful.

1. Posture

The infant should be supine and quiet. Simply observe how the infant positions the arms and legs. The more mature infant fully flexes the elbows, hips, and knees.

2. Square window

Flex the hand at the wrist. Exert gentle pressure to have the wrist flex as much as possible. The more mature infant has full flexibility of the hand against the forearm.

3. Arm recoil

With the infant supine, fully flex the forearms for 5 seconds. Then fully extend the forearms by pulling on the hands. When released, the more mature infant quickly returns the forearms to full flexion.

4. Popliteal angle

The infant must lie supine with the pelvis flat on the examining surface. The lower leg is flexed onto the thigh, and the thigh is fully flexed to the abdomen. One hand is used to hold the thigh in the flexed position, and the other hand is used to extend the lower leg. The angle between the thigh and lower leg is then measured. The

more mature infant has less joint flexion and a smaller angle.

5. Scarf sign

With the infant supine, take one of the infant's hands and extend it as far as possible across the neck toward the opposite shoulder. The infant is scored as follows:

0 = The elbow reaches the opposite anterior axillary line.
1 = The elbow reaches closer to the opposite anterior axillary line than the midline of the chest.
2 = The elbow reaches midway between the opposite anterior axillary line and the midline of the chest.
3 = The elbow reaches the midline of the chest.
4 = The elbow does not reach the midline of the chest.

6. Heel-to-ear maneuver

The infant should be supine on the examining table with the pelvis flat. Take the infant's foot in one hand and move it as near to the head as possible. Do not force it! The more mature infant has less joint flexibility and is unable to move the foot as near the head as a less mature infant.

c. Assess the patient's cardiopulmonary condition by viewing the results of transillumination of the chest (Code: IB1d) [Difficulty: ELE: R; WRE: Ap, An]

Transillumination of the chest is a test performed on a neonate to identify the presence of a pneumothorax. The room is darkened, and a bright light from a flashlight is placed against the patient's chest. When free air is around the collapsed lung, the light creates a "halo" effect through the neonate's thin chest wall. This confirms the pneumothorax.

Exam Hint 1-14 (CSE)

A past version of the *Clinical Simulation Examination* included a scenario with a pediatric patient in which the respiratory therapist had to make a differential diagnosis between croup and epiglottitis. The care of the patient was then tested. The *Clinical Simulation Examination* includes one neonatal and one pediatric patient scenario.

3. Inspect the patient's face to identify the presence of macroglossia (Code: IB1b) [Difficulty: ELE: R, Ap; WRE: An]

Macroglossia is an excessively large tongue that often is seen to protrude out of the mouth. It can partially obstruct the neonate's upper airway and may be associated with inspiratory stridor. Macroglossia is associated with Down syndrome, Beckwith-Wiedemann syndrome, and several metabolic disorders. Immediate treatment may require the placement of an oropharyngeal airway. See Chapter 12 for more discussion.

4. Inspect a lateral neck radiograph to evaluate the following:

Note: The following discussion usually applies to a child but can also apply to an adult.

a. Look for the presence of epiglottitis (Code: IB8) [Difficulty: ELE: R, Ap; WRE: An]

Epiglottitis is an inflammation of the epiglottis and surrounding supraglottic structures. It is a medical emergency. It usually is diagnosed on the basis of the history and physical examination and results in the child being intubated. A lateral neck radiograph of an epiglottitis shows a white haziness in the supraglottic area. This is the swollen epiglottis, and it is sometimes obvious enough to be called the "thumb sign." This is seen when the usually thin epiglottis is swollen and looks like the end of the thumb. It must be emphasized that under no circumstances should the child be laid supine for the neck radiograph, because this can result in the swollen epiglottis fatally closing over the opening to the trachea. Allow the child to sit upright in the most comfortable position. (Figure 1-36 shows the epiglottis and a lateral neck radiograph of the epiglottis. Table 1-18 lists the general history and physical findings for distinguishing between epiglottitis and laryngotracheobronchitis.)

b. Look for the presence of subglottic edema (Code: IB8) [Difficulty: ELE: R, Ap; WRE: An]

Subglottic edema is an inflammation of the subglottic mucous membranes of the larynx, trachea, and bronchi. This condition is also known as *laryngotracheal bronchitis*

Figure 1-36   Drawing of the normal upper airway is shown in the middle. Contrast it with **(A)** epiglottitis and **(B)** laryngotracheobronchitis (croup). *EP,* Epiglottis; *SEP,* swollen epiglottis; *STT,* swollen tracheal tissue; *TG,* tongue; *TR,* trachea; *VC,* vocal chords. *(From Des Jardins TR: Clinical manifestations of respiratory disease, ed 5, St Louis, 2006, Mosby.)*

(LTB) and *croup*. Subglottic edema usually is treated with inhalation of a cool aerosol in a mist tent and racemic epinephrine for mucosal vasoconstriction. A lateral neck radiograph of subglottic edema shows a white haziness in the subglottic area. This is the swollen laryngeal and tracheal tissue, and it is sometimes obvious enough to be called the "pencil sign" or "steeple sign." This is seen when the usually blunt end of the trachea at the vocal cords is thinned to a narrow point by the swollen mucous membrane (Figure 1-36 shows subglottic edema, and Figure

TABLE 1-18	General History and Physical Findings of Laryngotracheobronchitis (LTB) and Epiglottitis	
Clinical Finding	LTB	Epiglottitis
Age	3-36 mo	2-4 yr
Onset	Slow (24-48 hr)	Abrupt (2-4 hr)
Fever	Absent	Present
Drooling	Absent	Present
Lateral neck radiograph	Haziness in subglottic area	Haziness in supraglottic area
Inspiratory stridor	High pitched and loud	Low pitched and muffled
Hoarseness	Present	Absent
Swallowing difficulty	Absent	Present
White blood cell count	Normal (viral)	Elevated (bacterial)

From Des Jardins TR: *Clinical manifestations and assessment of respiratory disease,* ed 5, St Louis, 2006, Mosby.

1-37 shows a lateral neck radiograph image of this problem).

c. Look for the presence and position of any foreign bodies (Code: IB8) [Difficulty: ELE: R, Ap; WRE: An]

A history of sudden breathing difficulty, cough, and inspiratory stridor combined with a physical examination of the patient usually points to aspiration. A lateral neck radiograph or PA or AP chest and neck radiograph or both often help confirm the presence and position of a foreign body. See Figure 1-14 for an AP chest and neck radiograph image. The clearly seen solid white shape of the foreign body indicates that the object is metallic (a coin).

Plastic toy pieces and foods such as peanuts are much harder to see on a neck radiograph than are metallic objects, because their densities are closer to those found in the body. Obstructing plastic toys and food are more easily identified by looking for a narrowing or distortion of the dark air column of the upper airway and trachea.

Airway narrowing also can be caused by a tumor. This can be either a growth within the lumen of the airway or a growth from outside of the trachea or bronchi that forces it to collapse.

Figure 1-37 Lateral neck radiographs in children showing **(A)** normal upper airway during an inspiration; **(B)** laryngotracheobronchitis (croup) with haziness of the subglottic trachea from mucosal edema; and **(C)** epiglottitis with a swollen, rounded epiglottis. Areas marked *E* show the epiglottis; areas marked *S* show the subglottic trachea. *(From Koff PB, Eitzman DV, Neu J, editors: Neonatal and pediatric respiratory care, St Louis, 1988, Mosby.)*

Exam Hint 1-16 (WRE)

Usually one question deals with patient or family teaching. This could involve assessing a patient's or family member's learning needs, developing a teaching plan, or assessing the patient's or family member's understanding of what was taught.

BOX 1-4   Fluid Intake and Urine Output for Normal Adults

Normal, minimal daily water requirement for an adult patient is ~1,500-2,000 mL

Average urine output is 0.5-1.0 mL/kg/hr

Polyuria is a urine output of >1,500 mL/hr

Oliguria is a urine output of <400 mL in 24 hr

Anuria is a urine output of <100 mL in 24 hr

MODULE I

Evaluate and monitor the patient's objective and subjective responses to respiratory care

1. **Monitor and record the patient's vital signs (Code: IIIE6) [Difficulty: ELE: R, Ap; WRE: An]**

2. **Monitor the patient's heart rhythm (Code: IIIE6) [Difficulty: ELE: R, Ap; WRE: An]**

3. **Auscultate the patient's breath sounds, and interpret any changes (Code: IIIE11) [Difficulty: ELE: R, Ap; WRE: An]**

4. **Recommend and review a chest radiograph (Code: IIIE1) [Difficulty: ELE: R, Ap; WRE: An]**

5. **Look for changes in the patient's sputum characteristics (Code: IIIE5a) [Difficulty: ELE: R, Ap; WRE: An]**

6. **Recommend measurement of the patient's electrolytes (potassium), hemoglobin, complete blood count, other chemistry values, or a combination of these (Code: IIIE8) [Difficulty: ELE: R, Ap; WRE: An]**

All of the preceding topics were discussed earlier in this chapter. Review them as necessary. They must be applied to all respiratory care procedures as presented in the following chapters.

7. **Review data on the patient's fluid balance (intake and output) (Code: IA7a) [Difficulty: ELE: R; WRE: Ap]**

Fluid intake and output (I and O) should be approximately equal in a normal person with a properly functioning heart and kidneys. Fluid intake includes liquids that the patient drinks or is given by nasogastric tube and intravenous fluids. Output includes urine output and fluid loss from vomiting, the nasogastric tube, or diarrhea. Intake and output usually are measured over each 8-hour shift. Insensible water loss through perspiration and breathing usually is ignored in adults, because the amount lost is relatively small and can only be estimated. Insensible water loss can be a risk in the low-birth-weight infant. Prevent this by keeping the infant's environmental tem-

perature within 1° C of the body temperature (neutral thermal environment, or NTE). Supplemental oxygen should be humidified.

8. **Evaluate the patient's fluid balance (Code: IIIE6) [Difficulty: ELE: R, Ap; WRE: An]**

Intake and output should be monitored closely in any patient who has a history of heart or kidney problems or who has a current serious cardiopulmonary disorder. Do this by adding all the patient's intake (e.g., oral, intravenous) and output (e.g., urine, blood work) for each 8-hour shift. Box 1-4 shows the normal adult values for fluid intake and urine output; see Table 1-8 for the normal values for urine specific gravity and other urinalysis information.

The dehydrated patient will likely show some or all of the following signs and symptoms: tachycardia, hypotension, high urine specific gravity, oliguria (low urine output), low CVP and pulmonary capillary wedge pressure (PCWP), tenting of the skin when pinched, and mental confusion. This patient needs more fluid.

Often a patient with heart or kidney failure has a decreased output compared with input. This can lead to fluid overload problems, with peripheral or pulmonary edema and heart failure. The patient will likely show some or all of the following signs and symptoms: tachycardia, hypertension, low urine specific gravity, increased urine output, increased CVP and PCWP, peripheral edema in the dependent parts of the body, and pulmonary edema with breath sounds revealing crackles/rales. This patient needs to be fluid restricted and sodium restricted. If a patient is given a diuretic medication, the urine output can greatly increase to exceed the intake. Remember that the loss of 1 L of fluid results in the patient losing 1 kg (2.2 pounds) of weight.

PART 2. CARE MANAGEMENT

MODULE A

Respiratory Care Plan

1. **Assess the patient's learning needs (Code: IB6) [Difficulty: ELE: R, Ap; WRE: An]**

Based on the previously gathered information, the respiratory therapist should be able to determine what the patient understands of his or her condition and what the patient needs to be taught. This assessment could take place in a hospital, long-term care facility, or the patient's home.

a. Age-appropriate teaching

The patient is taught based on his or her age and ability to understand. This is most important with small children. They commonly have these fears when hospitalized:

- *Fear of abandonment (separation anxiety)*. Small children are afraid of being abandoned in the hospital by their parents.
- *Fear of the unknown*. Equipment and procedures must be explained so that the child will not be left to use his or her imagination.
- *Fear of punishment*. Children may imagine that their illness is a punishment for doing something wrong.
- *Fear of bodily harm*. Explain a procedure so that the child understands what is going to happen.
- *Fear of death*. Children who are sick but expected to recover need to understand that they will get better. It is all right for children to feel afraid. Talking about those feelings or fear of death should be encouraged.

b. Language-appropriate teaching

Use nonmedical terms whenever possible. The patient's native language must be used so that he or she will understand the situation. A translator may be needed.

c. Education level

Patients should be taught in a manner and at a level that is matched to their education and knowledge of their medical condition.

d. Prior disease knowledge

The patient should be taught, as needed, about his or her condition.

e. Medication knowledge

The patient should be taught, as needed, about his or her medication or medications, including how the medication is to be taken (e.g., metered-dose inhaler with spacer).

Exam Hint 1-17 (WRE)

Usually one question deals with checking for an advance directive or implementing the patient's wishes.

2. Interview the patient to determine whether any advance directives exist, such as DNR status (Code: IB5f) [Difficulty: ELE: R; WRE: Ap, An]

An advance directive is an advance declaration by a patient who is so hopelessly and terminally ill that he or she does not wish to be connected to life-support equipment. This statement could preclude the use of a mechanical ventilator, kidney dialysis equipment, cardiac pacemaker, or other means of artificially prolonging life. The advance directive also can declare that the patient does not want to be resuscitated if a cardiac arrest should occur. This is commonly called a *do-not-resuscitate (DNR) order,* and it should be clearly noted in the patient's chart. The advance directive legal document should be part of the patient's medical record. The document may also be known as a *living will* in some states. A related legal document is the Durable Power of Attorney for Health Care. This document assigns another person, such as a relative or close friend, the right to make medical decisions when the patient is unable to do so. This can include stopping or withdrawal of medical treatment and the DNR order. Always be sensitive to a patient's feelings about such a personal and difficult decision. The patient's emotional state may very well determine his or her readiness for an advance directive. A related issue is the patient's ability to cooperate based on his or her emotional and physical condition.

Exam Hint 1-18 (ELE, WRE)

The NBRC is known to ask questions about commonly encountered cardiopulmonary pathologies. Take the time to study at least the following: asthma, emphysema and chronic bronchitis (chronic obstructive pulmonary disease [COPD]), bacterial pneumonia, tension pneumothorax, and heart failure with pulmonary edema.

3. Interview the patient to determine his or her level of pain (Code: IB5b) [Difficulty: ELE: R, Ap; WRE: An]

It has been shown that unmanaged pain can slow a patient's recovery from trauma or surgery. Because pain is a subjective feeling, only the patient can determine how severe the pain is. Some patients have a low pain threshold and report pain sooner and at a higher level than individuals with a high pain threshold. Therefore the acceptable way to determine the pain level is to have the patient rate it. Commonly, the patient is told to self-rate a pain level of 0 when no pain is felt and to assign a number up to a pain level of 10 for the most severe pain possible. Additionally, the patient should be asked to point with one finger to the area with the greatest pain. After the patient has been given a pain medication, and it has had time to take effect, the patient again is asked to rate the pain on the 0-to-10 scale. If the patient can tolerate the new pain level, it may not be necessary to give more medication. However, if the pain is still too great, additional medication may be given, if allowed within the physician's orders for pain management.

4. Interview the patient to determine his or her nutritional status (ELE Code: IB5d) [Difficulty: ELE: R]

Many patients with chronic illnesses are unable to prepare nutritious meals regularly. Because of this, the patient may appear thin and emaciated (cachectic). The chronically sick patient may also be dehydrated. This can make it more difficult for the patient to cough out secretions. Realize that malnutrition may not be the primary reason for the patient's appearance. Therefore consider other causes, such as cancer, COPD, and paralysis. See the earlier discussion on muscle wasting, as well as further discussion in Chapter 17.

5. Interview the patient to determine his or her social history, such as smoking, substance abuse (Code: IB5e) [Difficulty: ELE: R; WRE: Ap]

Because smoking tobacco is a cause of COPD, and asthma is exacerbated by tobacco smoke and other airborne irritants, it is important to interview the patient or the

patient's family about the home environment. In addition, inhaling illegal substances, such as marijuana and crack cocaine, and "huffing" from household aerosol cleaning agents can cause lung injury. If patients are assured that their responses will be kept strictly confidential within the medical record, they may be more willing to discuss these topics. If the patient is taking addictive substances, the care plan must include ways to deal with any addiction-related issues.

6. Analyze the available information to determine the patient's pathophysiologic state (Code: IIIH1) [Difficulty: ELE: R, Ap; WRE: An]

The limitations of this text prevent an in-depth discussion of the various cardiopulmonary conditions and disorders that befall the patients to whom respiratory therapists provide care. However, some discussion of cardiopulmonary conditions is included in the following chapters as the respiratory therapies are presented. Table 1-19 summarizes some of the key physical examination findings associated with commonly encountered clinical conditions.

Exam Hint 1-19 (ELE, WRE)

Be prepared to use the information from the respiratory care plan to help make decisions on patient care. Expect questions that relate to what would be the best recommendations for care.

TABLE 1-19	Common Physical Findings in Selected Pulmonary Conditions			
Condition	**Inspection**	**Palpation**	**Percussion**	**Auscultation**
Asthma and COPD	Hyperinflated chest / Use of accessory muscles	Decreased expansion / Decreased fremitus	Hyperresonance / Low diaphragms	Long expiratory time / Wheezes
Atelectasis (lobar)	Inspiratory lag on affected side	Decreased fremitus / Trachea and heart shifted *toward* affected side	Dullness	Absent breath sounds
Consolidation (pneumonia)	Possible inspiratory lag or splinting on affected side	Rhonchial fremitus	Dullness	Bronchial breath sounds / Bronchophony / Pectoriloquy
Pleural effusion (large)	Inspiratory lag on affected side	Decreased fremitus	Dullness	Absent breath sounds
Tension pneumothorax	Inspiratory lag on affected side	Absent fremitus / Trachea and heart shifted *away* from affected side	Hyperresonance	Absent breath sounds

Modified from Hinshaw HC, Murray JF: *Diseases of the chest*, ed 4, Philadelphia, 1980, Saunders.
*COPD is chronic obstructive pulmonary disease; a combination of emphysema and chronic bronchitis.

The NBRC has released information on the mix of patient problems that will be found on the 11 Clinical Simulation Examination problems. See Box 1 in the Introduction for this list and the categories of diseases included on the test. It is highly recommended that a pathology book be reviewed for guidance on how these disease conditions (e.g., COPD, asthma, heart failure) are managed.

7. Review the interdisciplinary patient and family care plan (Code: IIIH2b) [Difficulty: ELE: R, Ap; WRE: An]

8. Review the planned therapy to establish the therapeutic plan (Code: IIIH2a) [Difficulty: ELE: R, Ap; WRE: An]

9. Determine the appropriateness of the prescribed therapy and goals for the identified pathophysiologic state (Code: IIIH3) [Difficulty: ELE: R, Ap; WRE: An]

10. Recommend changes in the therapeutic plan when indicated (Code: IIIH4) [Difficulty: ELE: R, Ap; WRE: An]

For the patient to receive the best care possible, the respiratory therapist must know the indications, contraindications, complications, and hazards of the respiratory care procedures the patient will receive. The patient must be assessed before, during, and after the treatment or procedure to determine whether it was effective. The key goal of an appropriate care plan is to treat the patient's condition in the best way possible. Modifications to the care plan must be made as needed as the patient's condition changes.

The respiratory therapist should be a member of the patient care team (i.e., the physician, nurse, and others) in deciding how best to care for the patient. The following steps are necessary in developing the respiratory care plan for any patient:

1. Determine an expected outcome or goal or goals.
2. Develop a plan to achieve success.
3. Decide how to measure whether the goal or goals have been achieved.
4. Plan a timeline to measure the patient's progress.
5. Document the patient's response to care and the final outcome.

When the patient has recovered sufficiently from illness or injury, a discharge plan will be needed to help in the transition to home or a long-term recovery facility. Typically, the discharge plan includes the following:

- Patient evaluation that determines the patient is ready for discharge. The patient needs to have recovered sufficiently to leave the hospital.
- Determination of the best place for the patient to go for further recovery and the necessary patient care resources. It must be determined whether the patient can go home or should go to an extended care facility. If the patient is to go home, it must be determined whether the family can provide the necessary care. If not, arrangements must be made for home care respiratory therapists and nurses.
- Determination that the patient's financial resources are adequate. If not, social services must be contacted to work with the patient's insurance company or other financial support agencies.

11. Conduct health management education programs (WRE code: IIIH9) [Difficulty: Ap, An]

The most recent Written Registry Examinations have had questions that relate to the management and education of the patient with asthma. It also is recommended that the management and education of a patient with COPD be studied. The bibliography includes information on standard references on these two subjects.

12. Explain the planned therapy and goals to the patient in understandable (nonmedical) terms to achieve the best results from the treatment or procedure (Code: IIIA6) [Difficulty: ELE: R, Ap; WRE: An]

Avoid using technical and medical terms unless the patient has a medical background or asks you about the specifics of what you are doing. Generally, it is best to describe the procedure in common terms that do not demean the intelligence of the patient.

Describe the procedure in steps rather than as a whole process from beginning to end. Demonstrate each step for the patient. Ask if the patient has any questions, and answer them or redemonstrate. Coach the patient to perform each step and to correct any problems. Describe and demonstrate the next step and the next, until the procedure has been completed.

13. Stop the treatment or procedure if the patient has an adverse reaction to it (Code: IIIF1) [Difficulty: ELE: R, Ap; WRE: An]

Patient safety should always be an important consideration during the treatment or procedure. The respiratory therapist should know the complications and hazards of any patient care activity that is performed. These are discussed in the following chapters. Be prepared to stop the treatment or procedure if the patient has an adverse reaction to it. Additionally, be prepared to recommend to the physician that the treatment or procedure be discontinued if it is likely to result in additional adverse reactions.

14. Discontinue treatment based on the patient's response (Code: IIIG1i) [Difficulty: ELE: R, Ap; WRE: An]

Typically three reasons are found for a patient's treatment to be discontinued. First, the patient has recovered and no longer needs the treatment or procedure. It is expensive and wasteful to perform unnecessary treatments. Second, the patient has had an adverse reaction and is likely to have an adverse reaction every time the treatment or procedure is repeated. For example, the patient's BP goes too high whenever he is placed in a head-down position for postural drainage. Third, the patient's condition is terminal, and the patient or responsible family member wants all treatment to be stopped.

MODULE B
Respiratory Care Protocols

1. Develop respiratory care protocols (Code: IIIH6b) [Difficulty: ELE: R, Ap; WRE: An]

2. Apply respiratory care protocols to patient care situations (Code: IIIH8) [Difficulty: ELE: R, Ap; WRE: Ap]

3. Monitor the outcomes of respiratory care protocols (Code: IIIH7b) [Difficulty: ELE: R, Ap; WRE: An]

Respiratory care protocols are set treatment plans designed to manage certain patient care conditions. They have been developed to improve the quality of patient care by ensuring that the necessary treatments or procedures are delivered as quickly and appropriately as possible. Common respiratory care protocols include oxygen therapy, aerosolized bronchodilator therapy, hyperinflation therapy (incentive spirometry versus intermittent positive-pressure ventilation), and aspects of mechanical ventilation and weaning. A patient-driven protocol is one in which the patient is appropriately able to take charge of this aspect of his or her care. The respiratory therapist instructs the patient and monitors that the patient is able to perform the care correctly. Examples could include incentive spirometry and bronchodilator therapy by a metered-dose inhaler with a reservoir unit. A therapist-driven protocol would be one in which the respiratory therapist is responsible for implementing and changing care within the protocol's guidelines. Examples include making ventilator changes to correct arterial blood gas abnormalities and weaning a patient from the ventilator.

The goal of all protocols is to restore the patient's condition to as close to normal as possible. When it is not possible to restore to normal conditions, acceptable conditions must be listed as the target for care. The patient must be evaluated before, during, and after a protocol is used to determine whether improvement has occurred. Based on the results of the patient assessment, the care can be upregulated (increased) or downregulated (decreased). Protocol information is listed, as indicated, in later chapters of this text.

4. Communicate the outcomes of therapy, and change the therapy based on the protocol (Code: IIIA5) [Difficulty: ELE: R, Ap; WRE: An]

5. Interact with a case manager (Code: IIIK5) [Difficulty: ELE: R, Ap; WRE: An]

Inform the patient's physician, nurse, case manager, and supervising therapist if any serious question or problem occurs with the patient. Routine communication should occur as needed between these people and any other caregiver.

Exam Hint 1-20 (WRE)

Usually one question deals with the implementation or evaluation of a patient care protocol.

MODULE C
Quality Assurance and Quality Control

1. Develop quality improvement programs (Code: IIIH6a) [Difficulty: ELE: R; WRE: Ap, An]

2. Perform respiratory care quality assurance (Code: IIIH5) [Difficulty: ELE: R, Ap; WRE: An]

3. Monitor the outcomes of quality improvement programs (Code: IIIH7a) [Difficulty: ELE: R; WRE: Ap, An]

Quality improvement (QI) refers to the processes used to identify areas of needed improvement in patient care services. Quality assurance (QA) refers to any evaluation of services provided and the results achieved compared with accepted standards. These standards are developed through a process called *benchmarking*, wherein agreement is reached on fair and reasonable patient care criteria and outcomes. The later chapters of this text provide information on quality control procedures in the NBRC-specified areas.

MODULE D
Maintain records and communicate information

Record any therapy given and the results of the therapy in conventional medical terminology. This needs to be done as required in any health care facility or setting and/or as required by regulatory agencies.

1. Accept and verify patient care orders (Code: IIIA3) [Difficulty: ELE: R; WRE: Ap, An]

An authorized physician may write clinically appropriate patient care orders. Depending on institutional policy, a nurse practitioner (NP) or physician assistant (PA) may also write patient care orders. In addition, a credentialed respiratory therapist (or registered nurse) may accept a verbal order for patient care, either in person or over the telephone, from a physician, NP, or PA. To help ensure accuracy, the verbal order should be repeated back to the physician for confirmation. The respiratory therapist writes the verbal order into the patient's chart and signs it. Later, the physician, NP, or PA must co-sign the order to make it official. Typically, an uncredentialed respiratory therapist (student or recent graduate) is not permitted to accept a verbal order.

A respiratory therapist must not perform an order that is factually incorrect (e.g., has an incorrect drug dosage) or that could harm the patient (e.g., reducing the delivered oxygen percentage in a patient who is hypoxic). The respiratory therapist must directly contact the ordering physician to discuss the questionable order for clarification.

2. Specify the therapy administered, date, time, frequency of therapy, medication, and ventilatory data (Code: IIIA1a) [Difficulty: ELE: R; WRE: Ap]

3. Apply computer technology to document patient management (ELE code: IIIA4a) [Difficulty: R, Ap]

4. Apply computer technology to monitor workload assignments (ELE code: IIIA4b) [Difficulty: R, Ap]

5. Apply computer technology to patient safety initiatives, such as drug dispensing, order entry (Code: IIIA4c) [Difficulty: ELE R, Ap; WRE: An]

Many institutions now make use of computers for all aspects of patient care and management of the Respiratory Care Department. Each authorized person (e.g., RT, nurse) has an alphanumeric pass code that must be used to gain access to each of the computer systems. Only authorized individuals are able to review patient information or add to it. These systems also restrict who can get patient medications.

6. Record and evaluate the patient's response to the treatment(s) or procedure(s), including the following:

a. Record and interpret the patient's vital signs: heart rate and rhythm, respiratory rate, blood pressure, body temperature, and pain level (Code: IIIA1b4) [Difficulty: ELE: R, Ap; WRE: An]

b. Record and interpret the patient's breath sounds (Code: IIIA1b3) [Difficulty: ELE: R, Ap; WRE: An]

c. Record and interpret the type of cough the patient has, sputum production, and sputum characteristics (Code: IIIA1b3) [Difficulty: ELE: R, Ap; WRE: An]

d. Note and interpret any effects of therapy or adverse reactions the patient had to treatment(s) or procedure(s) (Code: IIIA1b1) [Difficulty: ELE: R, Ap; WRE: An]

e. Note and interpret the patient's subjective and objective responses to therapy (Code: IIIA1b1) [Difficulty: ELE: R, Ap; WRE: An]

See the earlier discussions on these topics. Later chapters include more specific information based on the treatment performed.

f. Recheck any math work and make note of incorrect data (Code: IIIA1b2) [Difficulty: ELE: R, Ap; WRE: An]

Errors made in charting must be corrected by drawing a single mark through the error and writing in the correct information. Some prefer that the error be further clarified by writing in "error" next to it and adding initials. Never erase or use any covering material over an error.

Exam Hint 1-21 (ELE, WRE)

Often one question concerns the proper way to document patient care or how to document a charting error. Remember that a charting error should never be hidden or covered up. Typically, the error is identified, the correct information is written, and the charting therapist signs his or her name.

---

7. Communicate information regarding the patient's clinical status to appropriate members of the health care team (Code: IIIA2a) [Difficulty: ELE: R, Ap; WRE: An]

Inform the patient's nurse or physician and the supervising therapist if a serious question or problem occurs with the patient. Routine communication should occur, as needed, between these people and any other caregivers.

8. Communicate information relevant to coordinating patient care and discharge planning (e.g., scheduling, avoiding conflicts, and sequencing of therapies) (Code: IIIA2b) [Difficulty: ELE: R, Ap; WRE: An]

Common scheduling problems include eating times and when the patient must go to another department, such as radiology or physical therapy. Some procedures, such as giving aerosolized medications and performing chest physiotherapy, should be performed before eating. Typically, the discharge plan includes the following:

- Patient evaluation that determines the patient is ready for discharge. The patient needs to have recovered sufficiently before leaving the hospital.
- Determination of the best place for the patient to go for further recovery and the necessary patient care resources. It needs to be determined if the patient can go home or should go to an extended care facility. If the patient is to go home, it needs to be determined if the family can provide the necessary care. If not, arrangements for home care respiratory therapists or nurses will be needed.
- Determination that the patient's financial resources are adequate. If not, social services will need to be contacted to work with the patient's insurance company or other financial support agencies.

BIBLIOGRAPHY

Aloan CA, Hill TV, editors: *Respiratory care of the newborn and child,* ed 2, Philadelphia, 1997, Lippincott-Raven.

American Association for Respiratory Care: Clinical practice guideline: discharge planning for the respiratory care patient, *Respir Care* 40:1308, 1995.

Barkauskas VH, Stoltenberg-Allen K, Baumann LC, et al: *Health physical assessment,* St Louis, 1994, Mosby.

Barnes TA, editor: *Core textbook of respiratory care practice,* ed 2, St Louis, 1994, Mosby.

Burton GC, Hodgkin JE, Ward JJ, editors: *Respiratory care: a guide to clinical practice,* ed 4, Philadelphia, 1997, Lippincott-Raven.

Carlo C: *Neonatal respiratory care,* St Louis, 1988, Mosby.

Cherniack RM, Cherniack L: *Respiration in health and disease,* ed 3, Philadelphia, 1983, WB Saunders.

Clochesy JM, Breu C, Cardin S et al, editors: *Critical care nursing,* ed 2, Philadelphia, 1996, WB Saunders.

Czervinske MP, Barnhart SL: *Perinatal and pediatric respiratory care,* ed 3, St Louis, 2010, WB Saunders.

Daily EK, Schroeder JS: *Techniques in bedside hemodynamic monitoring,* ed 4, St Louis, 1989, Mosby.

Des Jardins TR, Burton GG: *Clinical manifestations and assessment of respiratory disease,* ed 5, St Louis, 2006, Mosby.

DiPietro JS, Mustard MN: *Clinical guide for respiratory care practitioners,* Norwalk, Conn, 1987, Appleton & Lange.

Erickson B: *Heart sounds and murmurs: a practical guide,* ed 3, St Louis, 1997, Mosby.

Eubanks DH, Bone RC: *Comprehensive respiratory care,* St Louis, 1985, Mosby.

Fink JB, Hunt GE, editors: *Clinical practice in respiratory care,* Philadelphia, 1999, Lippincott-Raven.

Hess DR, Kacmarek RM: *Essentials of mechanical ventilation,* New York, 1996, McGraw-Hill.

Hess DR, MacIntyre NR, Mishoe SC et al, editors: *Respiratory care principles and practice,* Philadelphia, 2002, WB Saunders.

Kacmarek RM, Mack CW, Dimas S: *The essentials of respiratory therapy,* ed 3, St Louis, 1990, Mosby.

Kenner CV, Guzzetta CE, Dossey BM: *Critical care nursing: body-mind-spirit,* Boston, 1981, Little, Brown.

Koff PB, Eitzman DV, Neu J, editors: *Neonatal and pediatric respiratory care,* ed 2, St Louis, 1993, Mosby.

Lehrer S: *Understanding lung sounds,* Philadelphia, 1984, WB Saunders.

Levitsky MG, Cairo JM, Hall SM: *Introduction to respiratory care,* Philadelphia, 1990, WB Saunders.

National Asthma Education Program: *Expert Panel Report 2: guidelines for the diagnosis and management of asthma.* Bethesda, Md, Publication No. 97-4051, April, 1997, National Heart, Lung, and Blood Institute, National Institutes of Health.

National Heart, Lung, and Blood Institute and World Health Organization Global Initiative for Chronic Obstructive Lung Disease (GOLD): Global strategy for the diagnosis, management and prevention of chronic obstructive pulmonary disease: executive Summary, *Am J Respir Crit Care Med* 163:1256, 2001.

Oblouk DG: *Hemodynamic monitoring: invasive and noninvasive clinical monitoring,* Philadelphia, 1987, WB Saunders.

Pagana KD, Pagana TJ: *Manual of diagnostic and laboratory tests,* ed 3, St Louis, 2006, Mosby.

Peters RM: Chest trauma. In Moser KM, Spragg RG, editors: *Respiratory emergencies,* ed 2, St Louis, 1982, Mosby.

Rau JL, Pearce DJ: *Understanding chest radiographs,* Denver, 1984, Multi-Media Publishing.

Shapiro BA, Kacmarek RM, Cane RD et al, editors: *Clinical application of respiratory care,* ed 4, St Louis, 1991, Mosby.

Stillwell SB, McCarter RE: *Pocket guide to cardiovascular care,* ed 2, St Louis, 1994, Mosby.

Tilkian AG, Boudreau CM: *Understanding heart sounds and murmur,* ed 4, Philadelphia, 2001, Saunders.

Whitaker K: *Comprehensive perinatal and pediatric respiratory care,* ed 2, Albany, NY, 1997, Delmar.

Wilkins RL, Hodgkin JE, Lopez B: *Lung sounds: a practical guide,* ed 3, St Louis, 2004, Mosby.

Wilkins RL, Dexter JR, Heuer A: *Clinical assessment in respiratory care,* ed 6, St Louis, 2010, Mosby.

Wilkins RL, Stoller JK, Kacmarek RM, editors: *Egan's fundamentals of respiratory care,* ed 9, St Louis, 2009, Mosby.

Wyka KA, Mathews PJ, Clark WF, editors: *Foundations of respiratory care,* Albany, NY, 2002, Delmar.

SELF-STUDY QUESTIONS FOR THE ENTRY LEVEL EXAM   *See page 582 for answers*

1. You have finished charting on your patient when you notice that an error was made. You should do which of the following?
   A. Tell the nurse so that she will tell the physician.
   B. Tell the nurse so that she will chart the correct information.
   C. Place a line through the error, initial it, and write in the correct information.
   D. Have your supervisor chart the correct information.

2. In listening to a patient's lungs, you notice bronchial breath sounds in her right lower lobe. These would indicate which of the following?
   A. Normal lungs
   B. Pneumothorax
   C. Consolidation in her right lower lobe
   D. Pleural effusion in her right lower lobe

3. You are called to start a new aerosolized medication treatment. After reading the physician's order, you notice that the drug dosage is outside the normal department guidelines. You should do which of the following?
   A. Give the treatment as ordered.
   B. Contact the physician to confirm that the order is indeed correct.
   C. Give the treatment as ordered, and leave a note in the chart asking for clarification for the next treatment.
   D. Have the nurse rewrite the order.

4. You are called to the Emergency Department to help care for a patient who was in a car accident and has chest injuries, including broken ribs. While palpating her neck, you feel a crepitation. What is the most likely cause of this?
   A. She has a laryngeal tumor.
   B. Blood is in the back of her throat.
   C. She has aspirated a tooth.
   D. She has an air leak from her lung.

5. You are called to help in the evaluation of a 55-year-old male patient. You notice the following signs and symptoms: oral temperature of 40° C (104.5° F), diaphoresis, respiratory rate of 22, the use of accessory muscles of respiration, and palpable rhonchi in the right lower lobe. You would suspect which of the following diagnoses:
   A. Bacterial pneumonia
   B. Heart attack
   C. Pneumothorax
   D. Viral pneumonia

6. Since being told of the diagnosis of cancer, a patient has become argumentative about his care and threatens to hit the nurse and therapist. He should be evaluated for

A. Language barrier problems
B. Hypercarbia
C. Emotional state
D. Hypoxemia

7. To help determine your patient's level of consciousness, you should ask which of the following questions?
   1. "Do you know what day this is?"
   2. "Can I see your identification wristband?"
   3. "Do you know where you are?"
   4. "How are you feeling today?"
   5. "Do you know who the president is?"
   A. 2, 4
   B. 3
   C. 5
   D. 1, 3

8. To help you determine whether your patient has orthopnea, you would ask which of the following?
   A. "How many flights of stairs can you climb before you become short of breath?"
   B. "Do you know who the governor is?"
   C. "Do you need to use extra pillows behind your head and back to keep from getting short of breath when you sleep?"
   D. "Do any particular foods seem to make it harder for you to cough up your secretions?"

9. In observing an infant's chest configuration, you notice that it is the same size in both the AP and lateral dimensions. This would indicate that the patient has
   A. A normal chest
   B. Funnel chest/pectus excavatum
   C. Pulmonary emphysema with air trapping
   D. Lordosis

10. In examining your patient, you notice that she has greatly diminished breath sounds in her right lower lobe, and her trachea has shifted to the right. These signs indicate which condition?
    A. Right-sided pneumothorax
    B. Right-sided atelectasis
    C. Left-sided pneumothorax
    D. Left-sided pneumonia

11. In palpating your patient for symmetrical chest movements, you notice that his left side does not move as much as his right side. This indicates that he has which condition or conditions?
    1. Emphysema
    2. Congestive heart failure
    3. Left-sided pneumonia
    4. Left-sided pneumothorax
    5. Right-sided pneumonia
    A. 1, 2
    B. 3, 4
    C. 4, 5
    D. 2

12. You are called to the Emergency Department to help evaluate a pediatric patient. On entering the room, you observe the patient's breathing effort and can hear a harsh, high-pitched sound on inspiration. Which of the following is true?
    A. Sounds are tracheal and normal.
    B. Sounds are bronchovesicular and not normal.
    C. Sounds are stridorous and indicate a respiratory emergency.
    D. Sounds are bronchial and indicate a respiratory emergency.

13. You are called to evaluate a patient's breathing pattern. You notice that the patient's tidal volumes go from small to large to small and then stop for 10 seconds before starting up again. The pattern repeats itself. This patient's breathing pattern would best be called
    A. Eupnea
    B. Obstructed expiration
    C. Kussmaul's respiration
    D. Cheyne-Stokes respiration

14. A tension pneumothorax is identified by which of the following?
    1. **Chest x-ray film shows a shift of the mediastinum toward the affected lung.**
    2. **Chest x-ray film shows elevation of the hemidiaphragm on the affected side.**
    3. **The patient's vital signs suddenly deteriorate.**
    4. **Chest x-ray film shows a depression of the hemidiaphragm on the affected side.**
    5. **Chest x-ray film shows a shift of the mediastinum away from the affected lung.**
    6. **Vital signs are essentially unchanged.**
    A. 1, 2, 6
    B. 3, 4, 5
    C. 1, 2, 3
    D. 1, 3, 4

15. Your patient is complaining of localized pain over the lower right area of the chest while breathing. When you auscultate her chest, you hear a rasping noise at her point of pain on both inspiration and expiration. This is most likely
    A. Pleural friction rub
    B. Normal breath sounds
    C. Wheeze
    D. Rhonchi

16. Your patient has distended external jugular veins, even though her head and body are raised 45 degrees above her legs. This would indicate that she
    A. Is hypertensive
    B. Is fluid overloaded
    C. Has emphysema
    D. Is dehydrated

17. Tactile fremitus would be reduced in all of the following conditions EXCEPT
    A. Pneumothorax
    B. COPD
    C. Pulmonary edema
    D. Pleural effusion

18. A frail, thin patient known to have lung cancer is admitted to the hospital. His family members are also present. What should be asked of them to make sure the proper level of care is delivered?
    A. The last time he ate
    B. The last time he had a bowel movement
    C. Whether any advance directives have been documented
    D. Whether he has brought his home care medications with him

19. It is most important to ask a patient with a broken ankle from a recent slip on an icy sidewalk about which of the following?
    A. Level of pain
    B. Level of consciousness
    C. Work of breathing
    D. Emotional state

20. All of the following could result in a mediastinal shift on a chest x-ray film EXCEPT
    A. Right-sided hemothorax
    B. Bilateral lower lobe pneumonia
    C. Left-sided tension pneumothorax
    D. Right lower lobe atelectasis

21. A patient who is suffering respiratory distress would exhibit all of the following EXCEPT
    A. Normal respiratory rate
    B. Nasal flaring
    C. Intercostal retractions
    D. Use of accessory muscles of inspiration

SELF-STUDY QUESTIONS FOR THE WRITTEN REGISTRY EXAM   *See page 604 for answers*

1. An adult patient with a history of smoking has shown an increased anteroposterior diameter and depressed hemidiaphragms on a PA chest radiograph. It is most likely that the patient
   A. Has pulmonary fibrosis.
   B. Has emphysema.
   C. Would have normal findings if an AP chest radiograph were taken.
   D. Has left ventricular failure.

2. After 2 days of vomiting and diarrhea caused by the flu, a 50-year-old patient is admitted. Her ECG shows five PVCs in 1 minute and flat T waves. What laboratory test would you recommend?
   A. Urinalysis
   B. Arterial blood gas analysis
   C. Electrolytes
   D. Complete blood count

3. A 48-year-old patient with an extensive smoking history usually coughs out about 20 mL of sputum every day. He developed a "chest cold" 4 days ago and has noticed increased shortness of breath and thicker secretions. What should be done at this time?
   A. Have him increase the flow on his home oxygen concentrator.
   B. Get a sputum sample for a culture-and-sensitivity study.
   C. Have him perform a 6-minute walk test.
   D. Perform percussion to determine the hemidiaphragm positions.

4. A recently home-delivered baby is brought in to the Emergency Department by the paramedics. The physician asks you to help evaluate her condition. Normal vital signs for a term newborn include all of the following EXCEPT:
   A. Heart rate of 130/min
   B. Rectal temperature of 36.5° C
   C. Blood pressure of 64/40 mm Hg
   D. Respiratory rate of 20/min

5. You are assisting with the delivery of a high-risk infant. After evaluating the infant, you give it a 5-minute Apgar score of 8 and recommend that the assisting nurse and physician:
   A. Give the infant supplemental oxygen.
   B. Give the mother supplemental oxygen.
   C. Begin bag-mask rescue breathing on the infant.
   D. Give the infant to the mother as soon as possible for bonding.

6. You are called to the Pediatrics Department to help in the evaluation and care of a 4-year-old girl who has been sick with a bad cold for the past 2 days. The nurse shows you a lateral neck radiograph of the child and asks for your opinion. You notice a clear air column through the upper airway but a pointed narrowing of the tracheal air column below the larynx. You tell the nurse that you suspect the child has
   A. Laryngotracheobronchitis
   B. Aspirated a coin
   C. Epiglottitis
   D. Bilateral upper lobe pneumonia

7. A young adult who had surgery for a deviated nasal septum was accidentally given 2 L of intravenous fluid in 1 hour. Which of the following signs cause you to suspect that the patient is fluid overloaded?
   1. Tachycardia
   2. Bradycardia
   3. High urine specific gravity
   4. Peripheral edema in the dependent parts of the body
   5. Low urine specific gravity
   A. 1, 4, 5
   B. 3, 4
   C. 1, 3
   D. 2, 5

8. Patients with heart or lung disease commonly have shifting of mediastinal structures. In evaluating patients with cardiopulmonary disease, which of the following could result in a mediastinal shift being seen on a chest radiograph?
   1. Right-sided hemothorax
   2. Bilateral lower lobe pneumonia
   3. Left-sided tension pneumothorax
   4. Right lower lobe atelectasis
   5. Fibrosis of the left lung
   A. 3
   B. 4, 5
   C. 1, 2, 3
   D. 1, 3, 4, 5

9. The radiologist remarks to you during the viewing of a 65-year-old patient's posteroanterior (PA) chest radiograph that the patient has an enlarged left side of the heart. This indicates to you that:
   A. The patient has an athletic heart.
   B. The patient has a left pleural effusion.
   C. The patient has an abnormal heart.
   D. The patient has a left middle lobe infiltrate.

10. A patient has acute respiratory distress syndrome (ARDS) and is significantly hypoxemic. It is likely that the patient will exhibit all the following EXCEPT
   A. A normal respiratory rate
   B. Nasal flaring
   C. Intercostal retractions
   D. Use of accessory muscles of inspiration

11. An adult patient with a history of COPD and left ventricular failure has been hospitalized. A series of

diagnostic procedures is being performed. The preferred radiographic position to minimize distortion of the heart is
  A. Anteroposterior
  B. Posteroanterior
  C. Lateral
  D. Oblique

12. A patient who is intubated has been moved from the Operating Room to the Intensive Care Unit. Concern is voiced that the endotracheal tube has been moved. What is the best way to determine its location?
  A. Palpate the larynx.
  B. Listen to stomach sounds.
  C. Percuss the patient's chest.
  D. Get a chest radiograph.

13. A 65-year-old patient with repeated episodes of congestive heart failure has a chest radiograph taken. It shows the left costophrenic angle to be blunted with an air/fluid level with a meniscus in the left lower lung area. How should this be interpreted?
  A. Pleural effusion of the left lung
  B. Pulmonary edema of the left lung
  C. Pneumonia of the left lung
  D. Pulmonary embolism of the left lung

14. A 3-day-old newborn is brought into the Emergency Department with her father after they were involved in an automobile accident. The newborn is showing signs of respiratory distress with cyanosis and tachycardia. What test would you recommend to determine whether she has a pneumothorax?
  A. Arterial blood gases
  B. Apgar score
  C. Transillumination
  D. Thoracentesis

15. You have been assisting with the insertion of a flow-directed, balloon-tipped pulmonary artery catheter. After the procedure, a chest radiograph was taken. It would be acceptable to take a mixed-venous blood sample from the catheter if the tip were found in the
  A. Right pulmonary artery
  B. Superior vena cava
  C. Aortic arch
  D. Right ventricle

16. The respiratory therapist has instructed a 16-year-old asthma patient in the proper use of a metered-dose inhaler with reservoir and the bronchodilator medication. The patient has shown the proper drug administration and breathing pattern. What should be recommended now?
  A. Continue to administer the treatment because the patient is a minor.
  B. Have the parent administer the treatment because the patient is a minor.
  C. With the parent's permission, begin a patient-driven medication protocol.
  D. Delegate the treatments to a nurse.

17. You are assisting in the delivery of a high-risk neonate. At 1 minute after birth, the following are noted:
  • Heart rate is 90 beats/min.
  • There is a weak cry.
  • Arms and legs show some flexion.
  • The baby grimaces when a nasal catheter is inserted into a nostril.
  • Extremities are blue with a pink body (acrocyanosis).
  You would give the neonate an Apgar score of:
  A. 3
  B. 5
  C. 7
  D. 9

18. An elderly patient with congestive heart failure has been treated with the diuretic furosemide (Lasix). Which serum electrolyte is the most important to monitor in this situation?
  A. Potassium
  B. Chloride
  C. Calcium
  D. Sodium

19. After feeling a sudden chest pain and shortness of breath while lifting weights, a 37-year-old man drove himself to the Emergency Department. After starting oxygen therapy on the patient, the respiratory therapist performed a physical exam. Pertinent findings included a hyperresonant percussion note on the right side and tracheal shift to the left. Based on these findings, what is the patient's most likely problem?
  A. Broken ribs on the right side
  B. Right-sided pneumothorax
  C. Broken clavicle on the right side
  D. Acute myocardial infarction

2 Infection Control

Note 1: This book is written to cover every item listed as testable on the *Entry Level Examination (ELE), Written Registry Examination (WRE),* and *Clinical Simulation Examination (CSE).*

The listed code for each item is taken from the National Board for Respiratory Care's (NBRC) **Summary Content Outline for CRT (Certified Respiratory Therapist) and Written RRT (Registered Respiratory Therapist) Examinations** (http://evolve.elsevier.com/Sills/resptherapist/). For example, if an item is testable on both the ELE and the WRE, it will be shown simply as (Code: …). If an item is testable only on the ELE, it will be shown as (ELE code: …). If an item is testable only on the WRE, it will be shown as (WRE code: …).

Following each item's code will be the difficulty level of the questions on that item of the ELE and WRE. (See the Introduction for a full explanation of the three question difficulty levels.) **Recall (R)** level questions typically expect the exam taker to recall factual information. **Application (Ap)** level questions are more difficult because the exam taker may have to apply factual information to a clinical situation. **Analysis (An)** level questions are the most challenging because the exam taker may have to use critical thinking to evaluate patient data to make a clinical decision. For example, [Difficulty: ELE is R, Ap; WRE is An].

Note 2: A review of the most recent Entry Level Examinations (ELE) has shown that an average of four questions (out of 140), or 3% of the exam, will cover infection control issues. A review of the most recent Written Registry Examinations (WRE) has shown that an average of two questions (out of 100), or 2% of the exam, will cover infection control issues. The Clinical Simulation Examination is comprehensive and may include everything that should be known or performed by an advanced level respiratory therapist.

MODULE A

Follow infection control policies and procedures (e.g., Standard Precautions) (Code: IIB5) [Difficulty: ELE: Ap; WRE: An]

1. Hand washing or cleansing

Hand washing or cleansing is probably the single most important procedure for reducing the spread of infection. Washing with plain soap and warm tap water is acceptable in most cases. Antimicrobial soap should be used if called for in the infection control protocol. In many institutions, an isopropyl alcohol and skin softener/cleansing agent is used unless the hands are obviously contaminated. When contaminated with body fluids, the hands should be washed. In any case, respiratory therapists should wash or cleanse their hands before and between each patient contact. The following times are recommended when working in a general patient care area:

- When coming on duty
- When hands are obviously soiled or after contamination by blood or other patient body fluids. Hands should be washed, rather than using a cleansing agent, if a patient has an antibiotic-resistant infection, such as methicillin-resistant *Staphylococcus aureus* (MRSA).
- Before contact with the face and mouth of a patient, especially if the patient has an artificial airway
- Before setting up equipment or pouring medicines
- When leaving an isolation area or handling contaminated articles from an isolation area
- After handling soiled dressings, sputum containers, urinals, bedpans, catheters, etc.
- After removing patient care gloves. When working in a restricted area, such as the operating room, burn unit, or neonatal intensive care unit, policy may require hand washing before putting on gloves and entering the unit, as well as after removing the gloves.
- After personal use of the toilet
- After using hands to cover a cough and after blowing or wiping the nose
- Before eating or serving food
- On completion of duty

The most common bacterial organisms spread by personal contact are *Staphylococcus aureus, Escherichia coli,* and *Streptococcus* species. Suspect personal contact and poor hand cleansing whenever a patient has one of these infections.

Exam Hint 2-1 (ELE, WRE)

Past examinations have asked about the importance of hand washing and the indications for it to prevent the spread of infection.

2. Standard precautions

Standard (formerly called *Universal*) Precautions are designed for the care of all patients, regardless of their diagnosis or presumed infection status. Barriers such as gloves and masks and other procedures are used to prevent contact with body fluids. This approach to patient care has been adopted because of the concern of health care workers and the public that the human immunodeficiency virus (HIV), hepatitis B, or other deadly pathogens may be spread unknowingly by contact. Box 2-1 includes specific standard precaution guidelines established by the Centers for Disease Control and Prevention (CDC) and the Occupational Safety and Health Administration (OSHA).

3. Respiratory hygiene/cough etiquette

To contain respiratory secretions, anyone with signs and symptoms of a respiratory infection should be told to do the following:

- Cover nose and mouth when coughing or sneezing.
- Use tissues to contain secretions.
- Throw away used tissues in the nearest waste container.
- Cleanse the hands after contact with respiratory secretions. An alcohol-based hand rub should be used when hand washing cannot be done.
- Wear a surgical mask and sit at least 3 feet away from others.
- Droplet Precautions should be used by health care workers when working with a patient who is showing signs and symptoms of a respiratory infection.

4. Respiratory care equipment and procedures

The following guidelines are recommended to minimize the spread of infection by equipment and procedures. Follow the manufacturer's specific guidelines when applicable:

a. Each patient should have his or her own equipment.
b. Disposable equipment should be discarded after use.
c. Reusable equipment should undergo high-level disinfection or should be sterilized between patients.
d. Equipment such as O_2 masks, large-volume nebulizers, and aerosol tubing should be changed every 24 hours.
e. Ventilator breathing circuits should be changed only when they are visibly soiled with secretions or blood. If a heat-moisture exchanger is used for humidification, it may be kept with the circuit for at least 48 hours unless visibly soiled.
f. Sterile water should be used for procedures, and the unused portion should be discarded after 24 hours.

BOX 2-1 Standard Precautions to Prevent the Spread of Infection

EXCLUSION FROM PATIENT CONTACT

Any health care worker with exudative skin lesions should not work in the direct care of patients.

BARRIERS

1. Gloves should be worn under these conditions: during direct contact with blood, body fluids, secretions, mucous membranes, and wounds; when handling all items or surfaces contaminated by blood or body fluids; when performing venipuncture; or when handling intravenous catheters or monitoring devices.
2. Gloves must be changed between patients or if the gloves become torn or punctured, as with a needle-stick injury.
3. Hands should be washed immediately after the gloves are removed; the hands and any other body areas must be washed immediately if contaminated by blood or other body fluid.
4. Masks, eye goggles, or face shields, as well as gowns or aprons, should be worn when a procedure is performed that may lead to the splashing or splattering of blood, secretions, or body fluids.
5. Contaminated masks, goggles, face shields, gowns, and aprons should be removed and disposed of properly.
6. Contaminated worker uniforms should be left at the hospital for cleaning.

NEEDLE AND INSTRUMENT PRECAUTIONS

1. Care should be taken when needles and sharp instruments are handled.
2. Used needles and sharp instruments should be placed into puncture-resistant containers for proper disposal; reusable needles should be placed into a puncture-resistant container for transport.
3. No attempt should be made to manually recap arterial blood gas or other needles, remove them from the syringe, or bend or cut them (needle-covering systems or methods of pushing the needle into a rubber cube are used widely; these require the use of only one hand with no touching of the needle).

PATIENT SPECIMENS

1. Blood and body fluids should be placed into leak-proof, sturdy plastic bags for transportation to the laboratory.
2. The laboratory requisition form should be placed on the outside of this bag.

CARDIOPULMONARY RESUSCITATION

1. Mouth-to-mouth breathing should be avoided even though no evidence suggests that saliva transmits human immunodeficiency virus infection.
2. Mouth-to-valve mask resuscitators and manual resuscitators (bag-valve) should be readily available for use in ventilating patients.

g. Add water to reservoir systems immediately before use.
h. Discard any unused water in a reservoir system before refilling.
i. Drain and discard any water collected in tubing; do *not* drain water back into the reservoir.
j. Medications should be stored under the conditions set by the manufacturer, should be discarded if they appear abnormal, and should be discarded on the expiration date.
k. Unused portions of medications should be discarded after 24 hours.
l. Sterile syringes should be used when measuring medications.
m. Sterile suction catheters should be used and sterile gloves worn whenever the patient's airway is suctioned.

Exam Hint 2-2 (ELE, WRE)

Past examinations have questioned the types of routine procedures that should be performed to control the spread of infection through respiratory care equipment.

5. Implement transmission prevention protocols

Transmission prevention protocols are used for patients known or suspected to be infected or colonized with epidemiologically significant pathogens, which are spread through airborne or droplet transmission or by contact with dry skin or contaminated surfaces. These protocols are used in addition to Standard Precautions. The following are general guidelines and specific diseases or conditions established by the CDC for the three types of patient isolation categories. Hospitals may establish extra standards and post them at the door to the patient's room.

a. Airborne precautions

Airborne Precautions are used in addition to Standard Precautions for patients with known or suspected illnesses transmitted by airborne droplet nuclei (these include pulmonary tuberculosis [TB], varicella [chickenpox], rubeola [measles], and avian influenza [flu]), and when severe acute respiratory syndrome (SARS) is known or strongly suspected.

1. Room placement

Patients under Airborne Precautions must be placed in an airborne isolation room (AIR). This room must have a negative airflow versus that of the corridor, with 6 to 12 air changes per hour. Room air can be vented outside of the building, or it can be recirculated through a high-efficiency particulate air (HEPA) filter.

2. Gloves and hand washing

Use Standard Precautions.

3. Respiratory protection

a. If a patient is known to have or is suspected of having TB or SARS, a National Institute for Occupational Safety and Health (NIOSH)-approved respirator mask (N-95, N-99, or N-100) must be worn by all caregivers who enter the room. If the caregiver cannot wear an N-95 mask, a powered air protection respirator (PAPR) must be worn.
b. If a patient is known to have or is suspected of having varicella or rubeola, a NIOSH-approved respirator mask (N-95 or higher) must be worn by all *susceptible* caregivers who enter the room.

4. Eye protection

Health care workers should wear goggles or a face shield when within 3 feet of the patient.

5. Patient transport

a. Transport personnel must wear a NIOSH-approved respirator mask (N-95 or higher).
b. The patient must wear an isolation mask while out of his or her room.

6. Patient equipment

Use Standard Precautions.

b. Droplet precautions

Droplet Precautions are used in addition to Standard Precautions for patients known to have or suspected of having serious illness transmitted by large-particle droplets such as human influenza (flu), invasive *Haemophilus influenzae* (type b), *Neisseria meningitidis* disease including meningococcal bacteremia and meningitis, *Mycoplasma pneumoniae*, and *Bordetella pertussis*. A patient with *possible* SARS also is placed into this group until the condition is ruled out. (If SARS is confirmed, the patient is kept under Droplet, Airborne, Contact, and Standard Precautions.)

1. Room placement

A private room is preferred, but patients with the same infection may be placed in the same room.

2. Gloves and hand washing

Use Standard Precautions.

3. Gown

Use Standard Precautions.

4. Respiratory protection

a. Use Standard Precautions.

b. Caregivers must wear an isolation mask if working within 3 feet of the patient.

5. Patient transport

a. Transport personnel must wear an isolation mask if working within 3 feet of the patient.
b. The patient must wear an isolation mask while out of his or her room.

6. Patient equipment

Use Standard Precautions.

c. Contact precautions

Contact Precautions are used in addition to Standard Precautions for patients known to have or suspected of having epidemiologically important organisms that can be transmitted by direct contact with environmental surfaces, such as patients with SARS, avian flu, diarrhea, inadequately contained wound infection, or localized herpes zoster (shingles).

1. Room placement

A private room is preferred, but patients with the same infection may be placed in the same room.

2. Gloves and hand washing

a. Wear gloves when entering the patient's room.
b. Change gloves after contact with any contaminated item.
c. Remove gloves and wash hands before leaving the patient's room.

3. Gown

a. Wear a gown when entering the patient's room if you anticipate substantial contact with the patient, environmental surfaces, or patient items.
b. Remove the gown and wash hands before leaving the room.

4. Respiratory protection

Use Standard Precautions.

5. Patient transport

a. Limit transportation of the patient from the room. The patient must wear a clean gown.
b. If transportation is required, caregivers must wear a gown and gloves.

6. Patient equipment

a. Each patient should have his or her own dedicated noncritical equipment (thermometer, commode, blood pressure cuff, sphygmomanometer, stethoscope, etc.).
b. Clean and disinfect all patient care equipment after the patient has been discharged.

6. Implement infectious disease protocols (Code: IIB4) [Difficulty: ELE: Ap; WRE: An]

a. Avian flu (avian influenza)

Avian flu (also called "bird flu") is caused by influenza type A viruses that primarily infect poultry. Although human infections are rare, persons in contact with infected poultry or who inhale infected aerosolized droplets from infected poultry can become infected. A person who presents with a severe febrile respiratory illness and has traveled within the past 10 days from an area with an avian flu outbreak (usually China or a Southeast Asian country) should be suspected of having avian flu. Standard Precautions and Droplet Precautions are implemented for the patient. These precautions are continued for 14 days after the symptoms begin, or until (1) it is proven that the patient does not have avian flu, or (2) a different diagnosis is established.

See the previous discussion on Standard Precautions, respiratory hygiene/cough etiquette, and Droplet Precautions for guidance on how to prevent the spread of this infection. In addition, all health care workers should be immunized against influenza.

b. Severe acute respiratory syndrome (SARS)

Severe acute respiratory syndrome (SARS) is caused by a corona virus (CoV). (Thus, the common abbreviation, SARS-CoV.) This rare but serious pulmonary infection is spread by respiratory droplets through close person-to-person contact. If a person has a serious pneumonia or acute respiratory distress syndrome (ARDS) with an unknown cause and has traveled to China or a Southeast Asian country within the past 10 days, SARS infection should be considered until another cause cannot be found.

See the previous discussion on Standard Precautions, respiratory hygiene/cough etiquette, and Droplet Precautions for guidance on how to prevent the spread of this infection.

MODULE B

Recommend vaccinations (Code: IIIG4k) [Difficulty: ELE: R; WRE: Ap]

1. Pneumovax

The Pneumovax 23 (pneumococcal vaccine polyvalent) vaccine provides protection against the 23 most prevalent or invasive types of *Streptococcus pneumoniae* bacteria. Patients with serious chronic illness should be immunized to prevent them from developing this very dangerous type of pneumonia. Guidelines for immunization include the following:

In any *immunocompetent* person 2 years of age or older who fits the following conditions:

- 50 years of age or older
- Chronic cardiovascular disease (congestive heart failure and cardiomyopathies)
- Chronic pulmonary disease (chronic obstructive pulmonary disease, asthma with chronic bronchitis)
- Diabetes mellitus
- Alcoholism or chronic liver disease
- Cerebrospinal fluid leaks
- Sickle cell disease
- Splenectomy
- Persons who live in special environments or social settings (Alaskan Natives and certain American Indian populations)

In any *immunoincompetent* person 2 years of age or older who has one of the following conditions:
- Human immunodeficiency virus (HIV) infection
- Leukemia
- Lymphoma
- Hodgkin's disease
- Multiple myeloma
- Generalized malignancy
- Renal failure or nephrotic syndrome
- Receiving immunosuppressive chemotherapy including corticosteroids
- Organ or bone marrow transplant

Revaccination is recommended in the following circumstances as long as at least 5 years have passed since the first vaccination:
1. An immunocompetent person 65 years of age or older
2. An immunoincompetent person who is at highest risk for a serious pneumococcal infection or who has a rapid drop in pneumococcal antibody levels

A third vaccination is not recommended. In general, vaccination should be performed at least 2 weeks before certain medical procedures such as elective splenectomy or immunosuppressive therapy are started. The Pneumovax 23 intramuscular or subcutaneous injection can be given at the same time as the influenza vaccination, as long as a different arm is used for each injection.

2. Influenza

Seasonal influenza (flu) vaccination begins in September or October of each year but can be given later if necessary. Two ways to be immunized are available, and each method provides protection against three strains of flu virus. The intramuscular injection vaccine contains inactivated or killed virus and is given to healthy people and those with medical conditions. The inhaled vaccine is given only to healthy individuals between 5 and 49 years of age; pregnant women are excluded.

The flu vaccine is recommended for the following groups:
- Children 6 to 59 months of age
- A woman who will be pregnant during the flu season

- Those who will be 50 years or older
- Anyone 6 months of age or older with a chronic heart or lung condition, including asthma
- Anyone with difficulty breathing or swallowing caused by brain injury or disease, spinal cord injury, seizure disorder, or neuromuscular disease
- Anyone who has been hospitalized or needed regular doctor visits in the past year because of chronic medical conditions such as diabetes, kidney disease, hemoglobin abnormalities, or a weakened immune system
- Those between 6 months and 18 years of age in need of regular aspirin therapy who might therefore be at risk for Reye's syndrome if they get the flu
- Residents of nursing homes or similar facilities
- Family members and caregivers of children younger than 6 months of age and anyone at risk for severe complications from influenza
- Any health care worker

The influenza vaccination injection and Pneumovax 23 intramuscular or subcutaneous injection can be given at the same time as long as a different arm is used for each injection.

MODULE C
Decontaminate respiratory care equipment

Decontamination is the process of disassembling, washing (to remove dried secretions or other debris), rinsing, and disinfecting or sterilizing used patient care equipment. The process results in the equipment being free of any pathogens, so that it can be used with another patient. Obviously, once disinfected, the equipment must be reassembled aseptically and stored for future use.

1. Choose the appropriate agent and method for disinfection and sterilization (ELE code: IIB1) [Difficulty: ELE: Ap, An]

a. Disinfection

Disinfection is a procedure that significantly reduces the microbial contamination of the equipment that has been processed. All disinfection processes destroy the vegetative form (the cell) of pathogenic organisms, including the vast majority of respiratory system pathogens. However, a few *Bacillus*-type bacteria are difficult to kill because they have a particularly tough cell wall or have spores for reproduction. Spores are analogous to seeds in that they grow into bacteria under the right conditions and are resistant to drying, heat, and many chemicals that kill the bacterial cell. Therefore a spore-forming organism may be able to reproduce itself after the cells have been killed. Obviously, disinfection can be used only on equipment that is *not* contaminated by spore-forming bacteria. Knowing what pathogen has infected the patient, if possible, can help the clinician determine the appropriate disinfection (or sterilization) method to be used on contaminated equipment.

Some disinfecting agents kill different kinds of organisms, depending on the length of exposure time.

Another consideration in selecting the appropriate disinfection method is how the equipment will be used in patient care. Equipment or instruments that do not directly touch the patient (e.g., an electrocardiograph machine) are classified as *noncritical* (low risk of spreading infection) and can undergo low-level disinfection. Low-level disinfectants are agents capable of killing some vegetative bacteria, fungi, and lipophilic viruses. Equipment or instruments that touch surface mucous membranes and the skin but do not penetrate them are listed as *semicritical* and must undergo *high-level* disinfection (e.g., laryngoscope blades, a bronchoscope). Agents that kill all microorganisms except bacterial spores are classified as high-level disinfectants.

A third consideration in choosing the best disinfection method is the type of equipment that requires decontamination. Certain processes and agents can be used only on certain types of equipment. Table 2-1 lists the various ways of disinfecting reusable patient care equipment decontaminated in the hospital.

The fourth consideration to take into account is the location of the patient. The previous discussion relates to patients in the hospital or a long-term care facility. Home care patients typically will not use these methods because of the high costs. Instead, the plastics used in home care medication nebulizers, etc., usually are cleansed in the following way:

1. Disassemble as needed.
2. Run hot water from the tap to eliminate as many organisms as possible. Clean the sink.
3. Use hot water to wash the equipment in a detergent solution.
4. Place the equipment into an acetic acid (white vinegar) solution for disinfection. It should soak for 60 minutes. (Grocery store–purchased white vinegar contains 5% acetic acid. However, it may be diluted with three parts of water to produce a 1.25% solution.) After use, the acetic acid must be thrown away because it will no longer be effective.
5. After soaking, the equipment should be rinsed in hot water and placed on a clean towel to air dry.

A 1.25% or higher percentage solution is classified as a low-level disinfectant and will kill most vegetative bacteria (including *Pseudomonas aeruginosa*) and some fungi and viruses. However, *Mycobacterium tuberculosis*, nonlipid viruses, and spores will not be killed.

Exam Hint 2-3 (ELE, WRE)

Expect to see one question about using white vinegar or acetic acid to disinfect equipment in the home. The percentage of acetic acid specified in the NBRC question should not matter.

b. Sterilization

Sterilization is a procedure that destroys all living microbial organisms and renders them unable to reproduce. All sterilization procedures destroy the vegetative forms and spores of all microscopic organisms. Examples of spore-forming bacteria include *Bacillus anthracis* (anthrax), *Clostridium botulinum* (botulism), *C tetani* (tetanus), and *C perfringens* (gas gangrene). Any equipment or instruments that penetrate body tissue (e.g., a surgical scalpel) are listed as "critical" (high risk of spreading infection) and must be sterilized before use on another patient. As was discussed previously, the method of sterilization depends on the type of equipment under consideration. Table 2-2 lists various methods of sterilization for reusable supplies and patient care equipment decontaminated in the hospital.

2. Disinfect or sterilize respiratory care equipment (ELE code: IIB1) [Difficulty: ELE: Ap, An]

As was previously discussed, the choice of whether to disinfect or sterilize equipment depends on how it is used clinically, what type of pathogen is involved, and from what material the equipment is made. Most respiratory pathogens are not spore-formers, so low-level or high-level disinfection is acceptable. Either a glutaraldehyde solution or pasteurization is used in most departments for disinfecting plastic masks, hoses, etc.

Any department that processes its own equipment must have adequate facilities for receiving used equipment and for its disassembly, cleansing, packaging, and distribution. First, a "dirty" area must exist where contaminated equipment is brought for disassembly, scrubbing of secretions or blood, and rinsing. Equipment then is placed into the glutaraldehyde solution or a pasteurizing machine. After that, equipment is taken to a "clean" area to be rinsed, dried, reassembled, and placed into plastic bags for storage. Care must be taken not to recontaminate the equipment during this procedure. Items that must be sterilized usually are just processed through the dirty area before being sent to the central supply department, where equipment is sterilized according to the criteria shown in Table 2-2.

3. Monitor the sterilization process to ensure its effectiveness (ELE code: IIB1) [Difficulty: ELE: Ap, An]

The term *surveillance* describes the monitoring of equipment to ensure that the disinfection or sterilization process was successful and that in-use equipment is not a source of patient contamination. Processing (chemical) indicators are used to ensure that disinfection or sterilization was done correctly. Examples include special tapes used to hold the wrapping around packages of equipment

TABLE 2-1	Methods of Disinfection Used in the Hospital Setting for Respiratory Care–Related Equipment

Method	Conditions	Microbes effective against					Comments
		Bacteria	TB	Spores	Viruses	Fungi	
LOW- AND INTERMEDIATE-LEVEL DISINFECTION							
Pasteurization	Complete immersion in water heated to 70° C (170° F) for 30 min	Yes	Yes	No	Yes	Yes	Used with rubber and many plastics used in respiratory care, especially those that are sensitive to a high temperature. **Avoid use** with any item that cannot be immersed or will be damaged at this temperature.
Alcohols (70% ethyl or 90% isopropyl)	Complete immersion for several minutes or pooling of alcohol on the equipment	Yes	Yes	No	Lipophilic only	Yes	Used with metallic or plastic surfaces of large pieces of equipment that cannot be disinfected by any other means. Also may be used with most plastics. **Avoid use** with any item that cannot be immersed or will absorb or be damaged by the alcohol.
Iodines (iodine or iodophor with 70% ethyl alcohol)	Complete immersion for several minutes or pooling of the solution on the equipment	Yes	Yes	No	Yes	Yes	Used with metallic or plastic surfaces of large pieces of equipment that cannot be disinfected by any other means. Also may be used with most plastics. **Avoid use** with any item that cannot be immersed or will absorb or be damaged by the alcohol.
HIGH-LEVEL DISINFECTION: GLUTARALDEHYDE SOLUTIONS							
Alkaline glutaraldehyde (Cidex, Cidex 7, Sporicidin)	Complete immersion for 10 min	Yes	Yes	No	Yes	Yes	Used with rubber and many plastics used in respiratory care, especially those that are heat sensitive. Care must be taken to thoroughly rinse items after disinfection. **Avoid use** with any item that cannot be immersed or will absorb the solution.
Acid glutaraldehyde (Sonacide)	Complete immersion for 20 min	Yes	Yes	No	Yes	Yes	Used with rubber and many plastics used in respiratory care, especially those that are heat sensitive. Care must be taken to thoroughly rinse items after they have been disinfected. **Avoid use** with any item that cannot be immersed or will absorb the solution.

TB, Tuberculosis.

TABLE 2-2   Methods of Sterilization Used in the Hospital Setting for Respiratory Care–Related Equipment

Method	Conditions	Comments
Steam autoclave	Autoclave chamber with an internal steam pressure of 15 lb per sq in, 121° C (250° F), 15 min	Used with glass, cloth, bandages, unsharpened stainless steel instruments, ventilator bacteria filters. **Avoid use** with many plastics used in respiratory care, rubber, dextrose solutions, sharpened stainless steel instruments, electrical devices, or machines.
Dry heat	Autoclave chamber at 160° C-180° C (320° F-356° F), 2-hr use	Used with glass or sharpened stainless steel instruments. **Avoid use** with many plastics used in respiratory care, rubber, dextrose solutions, electric devices, or machines.
Ethylene oxide gas	Specific guidelines vary depending on the manufacturer of the chamber and the supplies or equipment being sterilized. In general, a gas concentration of 800-1000 mg/L must be kept for 3-4 hr at 50%-100% relative humidity and 49° C-57° C (120° F-135° F). Great care must be taken to pre-dry all items before gassing and to properly aerate them after sterilization.	Used with heat-sensitive and moisture-sensitive items, as are many plastics in respiratory care equipment. **Avoid use** with supply pouches or plastic films, such as aluminum foil, nylon, thermoplastic resin (Saran), Mylar, cellophane polyamide, polyester, or other films that are not penetrated by the gas, or with PVC that has been sterilized previously by the manufacturer with gamma radiation.
GLUTARALDEHYDE SOLUTIONS		
Alkaline glutaraldehyde (Cidex, Cidex 7, Sporicidin)	Complete immersion. Cidex products for 10 hr; Sporicidin for 6 hr and 45 min	Used with rubber and many plastics in respiratory care, especially those that are heat sensitive; care must be taken to thoroughly rinse items after they have been cleansed. **Avoid use** with any item that cannot be immersed or that will absorb the solution.
Acid glutaraldehyde (Sonacide)	Complete immersion for 1 hr at 60° C (140° F)	Use with rubber and many plastics used in respiratory care, especially those that are heat sensitive; care must be taken to thoroughly rinse items after they have been cleansed. **Avoid use** with any item that cannot be immersed or that will absorb the solution.

PVC, Polyvinyl chloride.

being autoclaved or placed into ethylene oxide. These tapes turn color when the autoclave has reached the proper temperature, or when the correct concentration of ethylene oxide has been reached. The color change shows the user that the package was processed correctly; therefore the package contents are probably sterile.

Another example is a biologic indicator placed into the wrapped package before sterilization. These biologic indicators are bacterial spores that are killed only if the required conditions are met. For example, the spores of *Bacillus subtilis* are placed onto strips of paper to be killed by ethylene oxide gas. After the equipment and spores have been sent through the sterilization process, the spores are placed into conditions favorable for growth. If no growth occurs, they are dead; therefore no other living organisms survived.

Equipment held in storage or being used in patient care also is randomly sampled for contamination. A sample is taken in three ways for culturing of possible organisms in three ways. The first involves wiping a sterile swab onto an equipment surface, and then rubbing it over a plate of growth medium or placing it into a tube of liquid broth. The second, which is used to check inside lengths of tubing, necessitates pouring a liquid broth through the tube and into a sterile container. The third involves sampling the aerosol that a nebulizer produces. A hose usually is attached to the outlet of the nebulizer. The other end of the hose is connected to a funnel, which is attached to a culture plate, where the droplets impact. In all three examples, the growth of any organism in the growth medium indicates a form of contamination. The laboratory then determines whether the organism is pathogenic. If so, measures must be taken to improve the disinfection or sterilization process.

MODULE D
Biohazardous materials

1. Make sure that biohazardous materials are handled properly (Code: IIB2) [Difficulty: ELE: Ap; WRE: An]

A respiratory therapist is most likely to come into contact with biohazardous materials in the form of infectious waste, body fluids, or needles and syringes. All must be handled and disposed of properly to keep the practitioner and the patient safe. Although hospital policies will vary, infectious waste and body fluids usually are placed into a red bag. The bag is removed from the patient care area and incinerated to ensure that all pathogens are killed.

Needles, syringes, or any sharp objects are placed into a sharps container, which also is red and usually is marked with a biohazard symbol. Every patient room should have a sharps container, so that used needles and syringes can be disposed of easily. If at all possible, the needle should not be recapped after use. Instead, simply drop the used needle and syringe into the slot on the container. Never force anything into the container or put a finger into it. When full, the sharps container should be sealed closed and removed for proper disposal.

BIBLIOGRAPHY

American Association for Respiratory Care (AARC): Guidelines for the prevention of nosocomial infections, *AARTimes*, Dallas, Sept. 1983.

American Respiratory Care Foundation (ARCF): Guidelines for disinfection of respiratory care equipment used in the home, *Respir Care* 33:801, 1988.

Carter C, Stone MK: Respiratory microbiology, infection, and infection control. In Hess DR, MacIntyre NR, et al, editors: *Respiratory care principles and practice*, Philadelphia, 2002, WB Saunders.

Centers for Disease Control (CDC): Interim recommendations for infection control in health-care facilities caring for patients with known or suspected avian influenza, May 21, 2004: http://www.cdc.gov/flu/avian/professional/infect-control.htm

Chatburn RL, Kallstrom TJ, Bajaksouzian S: A comparison of acetic acid with a quaternary ammonium compound for disinfection of hand-held nebulizers, *Respir Care* 33(3):179-187, 1988.

Eubanks DH, Bone RC: *Comprehensive respiratory care*, ed 2, St Louis, 1990, Mosby.

Fink JB: Infection control and safety. In Fink JB, Hunt GE, editors: *Clinical practice in respiratory care*, Philadelphia, 1999, Lippincott Williams & Wilkins.

Gordon SM: Principles of infection control. In Wilkins RL, Stoller JK, Kacmarek RM, editors: *Egan's fundamentals of respiratory care*, ed 9, St Louis, 2009, Mosby.

Johnson & Johnson Medical: *Cidexplus, 28-day solution*, Arlington, TX, 1999.

Merck & Co., Inc: *Pneumovax 23 (pneumococcal vaccine polyvalent)*, Whitehouse Station, NJ, July 2008.

OSF Saint Anthony Medical Center, *Infection control precautions*, Rockford, IL, 1998.

Pagana KD, Pagana TJ: *Mosby's manual of diagnostic and laboratory tests*, St Louis, 1998, Mosby.

U.S. Department of Health and Human Services: Public health guidance for community-level preparedness and response to severe acute respiratory syndrome (SARS), version 2: Supplement I: *Infection control in healthcare, home, and community settings*, January 8, 2004.

U.S. Food and Drug Administration (FDA): Influenza: Vaccination still the best protection, September-October 2006: http://www.fda.gov/fdac/features/2006/506_influenza.html.

Washington JA: Infectious disease aspects of respiratory therapy. In Burton GG, Hodgkin JE, Ward JJ, editors: *Respiratory care*, ed 4, Philadelphia, 1997, Lippincott-Raven.

SELF-STUDY QUESTIONS FOR THE ENTRY LEVEL EXAM   *See page 583 for answers*

1. A hospitalized patient who recovered from a *Clostridium botulinum* infection received several respiratory care services. How should a nondisposable plastic pulmonary function testing mouthpiece be sterilized before being reused?
    A. Steam autoclave for 15 minutes.
    B. Soak in glutaraldehyde solution for 10 hours.
    C. Pasteurize for 20 minutes.
    D. Soak in an alcohol solution for 15 minutes.

2. Select all of the following that can be used in the home to reduce the chance of bacterial growth in a small-volume nebulizer or other respiratory care equipment.

    1. Soak the equipment in white vinegar.
    2. Put the equipment in the oven, and turn on the broiler for 10 minutes.
    3. Rinse a nebulizer in salt water (normal saline) after each use.
    4. Wash the equipment in hot water with a detergent.

    A. 1, 4
    B. 1, 2
    C. 1, 3, 4
    D. 1, 2, 3, 4

3. After use of a mechanical ventilator has been discontinued, what is the best method to sterilize the reusable main-flow bacteria filter?
    A. Wrapping it and soaking it in acetic acid
    B. Pasteurization
    C. Glutaraldehyde soak
    D. Steam autoclaving

4. A batch of respiratory care equipment has gone through the gas sterilization process with ethylene oxide. Routine surveillance of the equipment shows that spores of *Bacillus subtilis* have survived the process. What should be done next?
    A. Use the equipment because this organism does not cause illness.
    B. Aerate the gas as usual, and put into use.
    C. Resterilize the equipment, and check for destruction of the spores.
    D. Wipe off the equipment with 70% alcohol to remove the spores from the equipment.

5. A retired home care patient living on a fixed income needs to be able to disinfect her respiratory therapy equipment. Which of the following would be best for her?
    A. Acetic acid
    B. Acid glutaraldehyde
    C. Ethylene oxide system
    D. Warm, soapy water

6. What is the most cost-effective way for a respiratory care department to disinfect large amounts of reusable plastic tubing and oxygen masks?
    A. 70% ethyl alcohol
    B. Steam autoclave
    C. Pasteurization
    D. Dry heat

7. A contaminated Bird Mark 7 intermittent positive-pressure breathing (IPPB) unit must be sterilized before use with another patient. What is the best method?
    A. Pasteurization
    B. Ethylene oxide
    C. 10-Hour soak in glutaraldehyde
    D. Steam autoclave

8. A 58-year-old patient had an exacerbation of his COPD related to spring allergies. As he is being prepared for discharge from the hospital, what should the respiratory therapist recommend?
    A. Get an influenza vaccination as soon as possible.
    B. Get a tuberculosis skin test as soon as possible.
    C. Have a throat swab performed to check on a possible *Streptococcus* infection.
    D. Get an influenza vaccination in the fall.

SELF-STUDY QUESTIONS FOR THE WRITTEN REGISTRY EXAM

See page 606 for answers

1. A home care company has found that several of its tracheostomy patients have *Escherichia coli* tracheal infections. What is the most likely cause of the infections?
    A. Poor hand-washing technique by visiting respiratory therapists
    B. Contaminated tracheostomy tubes from the manufacturer
    C. Contaminated bottles of sterile water from the manufacturer
    D. Poor hand-washing technique by patients' family members

2. A respiratory therapist notices that two people in the Emergency Department waiting room are coughing regularly. All of the following should be done EXCEPT
    A. Have the two coughing people sit near each other to minimize their contact with other people in the waiting room.
    B. Have each person wear a face mask while waiting.
    C. Give facial tissues to the two people.
    D. Have both people sit at least 3 feet away from anyone else.

3. A patient has been confirmed to have SARS. Which of the following should be implemented to prevent the disease from spreading?
    1. The patient's health care workers must wear an N-95 face mask.
    2. The patient must wear an N-95 face mask in his/her room.
    3. Airborne Precautions are used.
    4. The patient is placed in a positive air pressure room.
    5. Contact Precautions are used.
    A. 2, 5
    B. 1, 4
    C. 1, 3, 5
    D. 1, 2, 3, 4, 5

4. A home care respiratory therapist is setting up a continuous home oxygen system for a 52-year-old patient with congestive heart failure. Besides teaching the patient about her condition and how to properly use the oxygen system, which of the following should the therapist recommend?
    A. Get the severe acute respiratory syndrome (SARS) vaccination.

B. Get the pneumovax vaccination if it has not been given already.
C. Soak the nasal cannula in a glutaraldehyde solution for 1 hour every day.
D. If the patient has already received the pneumovax vaccination, she should get a booster.

5. A 47-year-old man who recently returned from a business trip to Hong Kong has a high fever and other signs and symptoms of pneumonia. SARS-CoV is among the conditions being investigated. While the patient is being evaluated, what preventative measures should be taken?
   1. Standard Precautions
   2. Contact Precautions
   3. Droplet Precautions
   4. Airborne Precautions
   A. 1, 4
   B. 1, 3
   C. 2, 4
   D. 1, 2, 3, 4

6. An annual influenza vaccination should be given, to all of the following groups EXCEPT
   A. Health care workers
   B. People 50 years of age and older
   C. Children and adults with asthma
   D. Infants younger than 6 months of age

3 Blood Gas Sampling, Analysis, Monitoring, and Interpretation

Note 1: This book is written to cover every item listed as testable on the *Entry Level Examination (ELE), Written Registry Examination (WRE),* and *Clinical Simulation Examination (CSE).*

The listed code for each item is taken from the National Board for Respiratory Care's (NBRC) **Summary Content Outline for CRT (Certified Respiratory Therapist) and Written RRT (Registered Respiratory Therapist) Examinations** (http://evolve.elsevier.com/Sills/resptherapist/). For example, if an item is testable on both the ELE and the WRE, it will simply be shown as: (Code:...). If an item is only testable on the ELE, it will be shown as: (ELE code:...). If an item is only testable on the WRE, it will be shown as: (WRE code:...).

Following each item's code will be the difficulty level of the questions on that item on the ELE and WRE. (See the Introduction for a full explanation of the three question difficulty levels.) **Recall [R]** level questions typically expect the exam taker to recall factual information. **Application [Ap]** level questions are harder because the exam taker may have to apply factual information to a clinical situation. **Analysis [An]** level questions are the most challenging because the exam taker may have to use critical thinking to evaluate patient data to make a clinical decision.

Note 2: A review of the most recent Entry Level Examinations (ELE) has shown an average of 10 questions (out of 140), or 7% of the exam, that cover blood gas sampling, analysis, monitoring, and interpretation. A review of the most recent Written Registry Examinations (WRE) has shown an average of 5 questions (out of 100), or 5% of the exam, that cover blood gas sampling, analysis, monitoring, and interpretation. The Clinical Simulation Examination is comprehensive and may include everything that should be known by an advanced level respiratory therapist.

MODULE A

Make a recommendation to obtain a blood sample for blood gas analysis (Code: IC8) [Difficulty: ELE: R, Ap; WRE: An]

Blood can be sampled from a systemic artery, pulmonary artery, or "arterialized" capillary to determine a patient's oxygen and carbon dioxide pressures, acid-base status (pH), and related values. As is discussed later, a pulmonary artery sample is taken to learn a patient's mixed venous

values, and an "arterialized" capillary sample is taken from a neonate when an arterial sample cannot be obtained. Arterial blood gas (ABG) is the term commonly used when discussing drawing a sample of blood from a patient's systemic artery.

There are three broad, general indications for this recommendation:

- To check a patient's oxygenation status (PaO_2)
- To check a patient's acid-base status (pH)
- To check a patient's ventilation status ($PaCO_2$)

Some specific indications follow.

1. Cardiac failure
   a. Congenital defect
   b. Heart attack (myocardial infarction)
   c. Congestive heart failure with or without pulmonary edema

2. Chronic obstructive pulmonary disease (COPD)
   a. Asthma
   b. Emphysema
   c. Bronchitis
   d. Bronchiectasis

3. Any pneumonia that causes hypoxemia

4. Trauma
   a. Broken ribs
   b. Flail chest
   c. Pneumothorax
   d. Hemothorax
   e. Upper airway trauma

5. Ventilatory failure
   a. Overdosage of sedatives or pain relievers
   b. Stroke or head (brain) injury
   c. Spinal cord injury
   d. Neuromuscular diseases such as myasthenia gravis or Guillain-Barré syndrome

6. Airway obstruction
   a. Foreign-body aspiration
   b. Laryngotracheobronchitis (croup)
   c. Epiglottitis

7. Miscellaneous

a. Smoke inhalation

b. Carbon monoxide poisoning

c. Near-drowning

d. Infant respiratory distress syndrome (RDS)/hyaline membrane disease

e. Acute respiratory distress syndrome (ARDS)

f. The patient does not have an indwelling arterial line

g. A shunt percentage calculation or alveolar-arterial O_2 pressure difference [$P(A-a)O_2$)] calculation must be made

h. Cardiopulmonary resuscitation

Exam Hint 3-1 (ELE)

Expect at least one question in which the respiratory therapist is expected to recommend that either an arterial blood gas sample or a pulse oximeter reading be performed.

MODULE B
Obtain a blood sample

1. Blood gas sampling device selection and preparation

A properly prepared sampling device is essential to obtaining a blood sample that accurately reflects the patient's physiologic values.

a. Get the appropriate blood gas sampler

Obtaining an ABG sample generally involves selecting a prepackaged, sterile blood gas kit that contains the following:

- A variety of short-bevel needles: 23 or 24 gauge for radial or dorsalis pedis puncture and a 22 gauge for brachial or femoral puncture
- 3-mL syringe; many kits contain a syringe prepared with heparin as an anticoagulant
- If needed, liquid sodium or lithium heparin with an appropriate concentration
- Alcohol or iodophor (Betadine) wipes to clean the puncture site

If a blood gas kit is not available, an appropriate individual needle, 3-mL syringe, and liquid sodium or lithium heparin must be obtained. These should be available at any nursing station or from the respiratory care department.

A capillary blood gas (CBG) sample requires the following:

- Several heparinized glass capillary tubes with a volume of at least 100 µL
- Metal filing (flea) to place into each capillary tube, if needed

- Plastic caps or clay to seal the tubes
- Magnet to draw the metal filing back and forth in the tube to mix the blood, if needed
- Lancet to make incision
- Moist, warm (42° C) cloth or diaper to wrap around the puncture site; or a chemical warmer
- Sterile cotton balls and bandage to place over the puncture site to aid clotting
- Isopropyl alcohol swabs (70%) to clean the puncture site
- Clean gloves to protect the practitioner's hands from any contact with spilled blood

In addition, if the blood sample cannot be analyzed within 30 minutes, place it into an ice-water mix in a cup to chill the blood.

b. Put the equipment together and make sure that it works properly

To assemble a blood gas syringe, use sterile technique to screw the selected needle onto the syringe. If the syringe does not contain heparin, it must be added. Do this by aspirating liquid heparin through the needle into the syringe. Coat the inside of the syringe with heparin by tipping the needle up, pulling the plunger back, and pushing the plunger forward to squirt the excess heparin out of the needle. This ensures that the needle and dead space of the needle are filled with heparin, and the inside of the syringe is coated.

Make sure that the needle is tightly screwed onto the syringe. The plunger should easily slide within the barrel of the syringe. A blood clot or debris within the needle plugs it and prevents this. Replace and safely dispose of a needle that is obstructed.

c. Make sure no air bubbles are in the syringe

Any bubbles of room air can result in errors in the patient's measured values. For example, if the patient was breathing room air, an air bubble would result in the measured oxygen level being too high. In addition, since there is virtually no carbon dioxide in room air, an air bubble would reduce the patient's measured carbon dioxide level and increase the pH. If an air bubble is found in the syringe, tilt it so that the needle is up. The bubble will rise by itself or may be raised by tapping the syringe. Push the plunger into the syringe to eject the air bubble. Cap off the hub of the syringe or needle to prevent air from entering the syringe.

d. Use the proper amount of heparin

This is a concern only when liquid heparin is added to a needle and syringe. Aspirate about 1 mL of 10 mg/mL or 1000 units/mL sodium heparin through the needle into the syringe. Pull the plunger back to coat the inside of the syringe. Push the plunger forward to squirt the excess heparin out through the needle. The values of a 2- to 4-mL sample of blood should not be affected by this concentration. Remember that inadequate heparin can cause the blood sample to clot. Excessive heparin can alter the blood gas values by reducing the pH and the carbon dioxide level and increasing the oxygen level.

e. Promptly cool the blood gas sample

If the sample cannot be analyzed within 30 minutes of being drawn, it should be placed in an ice-water bath. Failure to do so results in the blood's living cells consuming the available oxygen and producing carbon dioxide, which lowers the pH. Obviously, this results in incorrect measured values.

2. Manipulate arterial catheters by order or protocol (WRE code: IIA20b) [Difficulty: WRE: R, Ap, An]

a. Select the appropriate catheter

An arterial catheter (also called an arterial line) is a flexible catheter that is placed into a peripheral artery for the purposes of sampling blood or continuously monitoring the patient's blood pressure, or both. The blood-sampling procedure is explained in the following discussion. Chapter 5 contains a discussion on blood pressure monitoring and illustrations of how the monitoring system is assembled. The radial artery is the most common site for catheter insertion. Alternate arterial sites may be used if needed.

An adult's radial artery is usually catheterized. To do so, a short needle covered with a flexible plastic catheter (an angiocatheter) is selected. Usually the needle is 23 or 24 gauge. After the angiocatheter is inserted into the artery, the needle is removed, and the catheter is left in the artery.

A newborn with a severe cardiopulmonary problem should have the catheter inserted into either of the umbilical arteries. Usually, a long, flexible umbilical artery catheter (UAC) is placed into the patient and advanced into the aorta (see Figure 1-7). If indicated, this should be done as quickly as possible after birth, before arterial spasm prevents the catheter from being advanced. If the patient weighs more than 1250 g, a 6-French (6 Fr) catheter is used; a 3.5 Fr catheter is used if the neonate weighs less than 1250 g. Besides obtaining blood samples and monitoring the blood pressure, one can give the newborn glucose or a blood transfusion through the catheter. A neonatal patient also may have the umbilical vein catheterized.

b. Put the equipment together and make sure that it works properly

Arterial catheters come as single units in sterile packaging. Additional stopcocks, tubing, flush solution, and an automatic solution drip device are needed. These are discussed in Chapter 5 in some detail.

c. Troubleshoot any problems with the equipment

See the discussion in Chapter 5.

3. Get a blood sample from an arterial catheter (Code: IB9f and IIIE2b) [Difficulty: ELE: R, Ap; WRE: An]

The steps for obtaining an arterial blood sample include the following:

1. Tell a conscious adult patient that you are going to take a blood sample from the arterial catheter.
2. Put gloves on both hands.
3. Remove the dead-ender cap (or syringe) from the sample (side) port on the three-way stopcock between the catheter and the intravenous (IV) tubing.
4. Screw a sterile 5- to 10-mL syringe to the sample port for removing the IV solution from the catheter. (A smaller syringe should be used for a neonate.)
5. Turn the stopcock off to the IV tubing (Figure 3-1).
6. Pull a waste sample of IV solution and blood into the syringe. (The amount withdrawn and discarded depends on the dead space volume from the tip of the catheter to the side port. Studies indicate that between 2.5 and 6 times this volume should be removed. Typically, this is ≤5 mL in an adult and even less in a neonate.)
7. Turn the stopcock off to all ports by turning it halfway between any two ports.
8. Attach a preheparinized sterile syringe to the sample port, turn the stopcock open to the syringe, and withdraw about 2 to 3 mL of arterial blood to be analyzed.
9. Turn the stopcock off to all ports by turning it halfway between any two ports.
10. Remove the blood-sample syringe, and cap off the syringe to seal it.
11. If liquid heparin is used in the syringe, roll the syringe to mix it with the blood.
12. If it will be more than 30 minutes until analysis, place the blood sample into an ice-water bath.
13. Turn the stopcock toward the sample port so that the IV solution runs into the catheter.
14. Fast flush any blood in the catheter back into the patient.
15. Screw the dead-ender cap (or syringe) onto the sample port.
16. Remove gloves, and properly dispose of them and any other waste materials. Wash your hands.

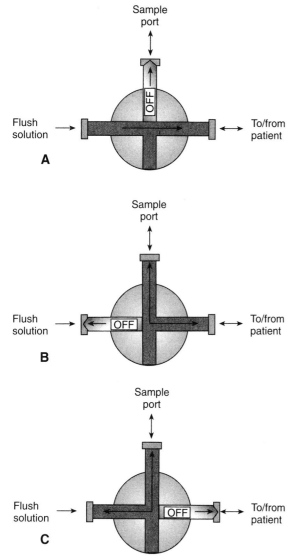

Figure 3-1   A three-way stopcock for use in an arterial line system. **A,** The normal operating position of the stopcock that allows fluid to flow to the patient (and the blood pressure to be monitored if assembled for continuous blood pressure monitoring). **B,** The stopcock position that allows blood to be withdrawn from the patient through the sample port. The flush solution port is closed. **C,** The stopcock position for flush solution to go to the sample port to clear out any blood. When the stopcock is turned to a 45-degree angle between any two ports, all of the ports are closed. *(From Wilkins RL, Stoller JK, Kacmarek RM: Egan's fundamentals of respiratory care, ed 9, St Louis, 2010, Mosby.)*

4. Perform an arterial puncture to obtain a blood sample for analysis (Code: IB9f and IIIE2a) [Difficulty: ELE: R, Ap; WRE: An]

A number of possible variations on the technique exist. The following is a general but thorough listing of the steps and any important related information.

a. Check for a valid physician order.

b. Check the patient's chart for pertinent information on supplemental oxygen being used, bleeding disorders such as hemophilia, and use of anticoagulant medications. It is important to check the patient's clotting time because a hematoma will result in a patient with a slow clotting time if extra time is not spent holding the puncture site.

c. Collect necessary equipment:
  - Ice-water in a cup
  - A 3-mL glass or plastic syringe
  - Appropriate needle(s)
  - Heparin, if needed
  - 70% isopropyl alcohol or iodophor swabs to clean the puncture site and a sterile 4 × 4-inch gauze pad to hold over the puncture site to aid clotting
  - A seal for the needle or syringe to prevent room air contamination
  - Clean gloves to protect the practitioner's hands from any contact with spilled blood
  - Eyeglasses or goggles

d. Introduce yourself and your department to the patient. Identify the patient. Explain what you are there to do. Gain the patient's confidence so that he or she will offer full cooperation.

e. Select the puncture site. The following choices are listed in order from most to least favorable: radial, brachial, dorsalis pedis, and femoral. If the radial site is selected, try to puncture the left wrist if the patient is right-handed or vice versa.

f. If the radial or pedal sites are selected, the Allen's test (also known as the modified Allen's test) must be performed to ensure that adequate collateral flow is present in case the artery becomes clotted because of the procedure.

1. Radial artery site

See Figure 3-2 for the basic procedure. Circulation to the hand is stopped by pressing both the radial and the ulnar arteries closed. Releasing the pressure over the ulnar artery should result in the hand flushing within 5 to 15 seconds. This is a positive test result and proves that the ulnar artery has adequate circulation to the hand. If the hand does not flush within 15 seconds of the release of the ulnar artery, the circulation is inadequate, and the radial artery of that wrist must not be punctured. Another site must be evaluated for puncture.

2. Dorsalis pedis artery site

Press down on the dorsalis pedis artery to occlude it. Press on the nail of the great toe so that it blanches. Release the pressure on the nail, and watch for a rapid return of color. This normal test finding confirms that a good blood flow exists through the posterior tibial and lateral plantar arteries. It is safe to draw a sample from the site. A slow

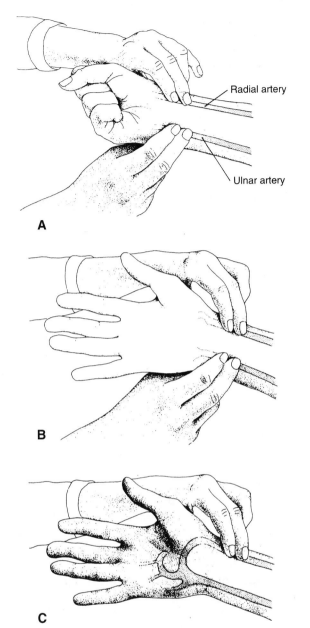

Figure 3-2 The modified Allen's test. **A,** The hand is clenched into a tight fist, and pressure is applied to the radial and ulnar arteries. **B,** The hand is opened (but not fully extended); the palm and fingers are blanched. **C,** Removal of the pressure on the ulnar artery should result in flushing of the entire hand. *(From Shapiro BA, Peruzzi WT, Kozlowski-Templin R: Clinical application of blood gases, ed 5, St Louis, 1994, Mosby.)*

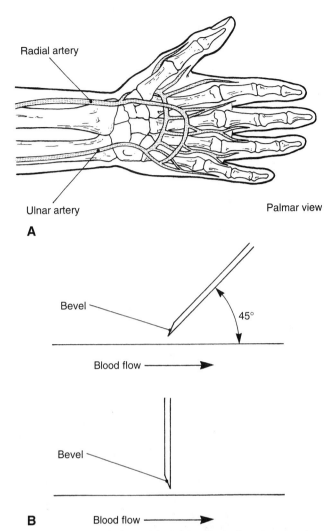

Figure 3-3 **A,** Radial arterial position in the lower arm and wrist. **B,** Bevel and needle positioning for radial arterial puncture and other arterial punctures, respectively. *(From Lane EE, Walker JF: Clinical arterial blood gas analysis, St Louis, 1987, Mosby.)*

return of blood flow indicates poor circulation; another site must be chosen.

g. **Prepare the equipment and the puncture site by using sterile technique.**
   1. If necessary, draw up the heparin solution, flush the syringe with it, and discard the excess.
   2. If a radial or brachial site is selected, the joint should be hyperextended with a folded towel to help stabilize it.

3. **Clean the site by wiping the area with an alcohol or iodophor swab in a widening spiral motion that starts at the desired puncture site.**
4. **Put on gloves and goggles.**
5. **Some prefer to anesthetize the puncture site with a 0.8- to 1.0-mL injection of 0.5% to 2% lidocaine (Xylocaine) into the skin.** Others think that this is unnecessary because the lidocaine injection itself will cause pain. If an anesthetic is used, wait about 2 minutes for it to take effect before puncturing the skin.

h. **Draw the blood sample.**
   1. Hold the syringe like a pencil. The radial and dorsalis pedis arteries should be entered from a 45-degree angle; the brachial and femoral arteries should be entered from a 90-degree angle (Figure 3-3). Use the first two fingers of your free hand to

palpate the pulse and hold the artery still. The bevel of the needle should be up as it enters the skin.

2. Tell the patient that he or she will "feel a stick."

3. The needle should enter the skin quickly to minimize pain. Carefully advance the needle into the artery. A pulsatile flow is seen with each heartbeat. If unsuccessful, withdraw the needle to the skin, change the angle as needed, and reinsert it into the artery.

4. Withdraw about 1 to 2 mL of blood before removing the needle.

5. Press the sterile gauze onto the puncture site for 2 to 5 minutes. Check the site to ensure that clotting has occurred. Hold longer if necessary. An assistant may help with this.

6. While holding the site, seal the syringe or safely cover the needle.

7. If liquid heparin was added to the syringe, roll it to mix the heparin and blood.

8. If the blood sample will not be analyzed within 30 minutes, place the syringe into an ice-water mix. (Failure to cool the blood sample results in a decrease in the PaO_2 value, an increase in the $PaCO_2$ value, and a decrease in the pH value.)

9. Label the syringe with the date, time, patient's name, oxygen percentage, and temperature if abnormal. Some departments may also add the patient's age and the position in which he or she was sitting or lying when the sample was drawn because of the effects they may have on oxygenation.

10. Have the sample promptly analyzed. The patient's blood gas results should be accurate if the blood sample is analyzed within 10 to 15 minutes if not iced and within 60 minutes if iced.

11. Properly dispose of gloves and waste materials, and wash your hands.

12. Return in 20 minutes to recheck the puncture site for a hematoma and good distal circulation.

5. Perform arterialized capillary blood gas sampling (Code: IB9g and IIIE2c) [Difficulty: ELE: R, Ap; WRE: An]

Occasionally, a sample of arterialized capillary blood from a patient must be obtained for blood gas analysis. The usual clinical situation is a neonate who has a pulmonary problem that warrants evaluation. However, because of the neonate's small arteries, a sample cannot be drawn. The steps and key points to keep in mind during the sampling procedure follow.

a. **Select a highly vascularized and well-perfused site. Usually the heel is selected, but the great toe, earlobe, and finger also are acceptable.**

b. **Warm the heel (or other site) with a warm towel or heat lamp for about 5 to 10 minutes; 42° C is ideal. Warming vasodilates the vessels and "arterializes" the capillary blood supply.**

c. **After warming, unwrap the site, and wipe it with an antiseptic pad.**

d. **Use a pediatric lance to deeply puncture the outer edge of the heel (Figure 3-4). Blood should flow freely without squeezing the area. Wipe away the first blood drop with a sterile gauze pad. The blood will be "dearterialized" if it is squeezed out with venous blood, and the sample will be useless for blood gas analysis.**

e. **Insert a preheparinized capillary tube (0.075 to 1.0 mL) deeply into the drop of blood. The blood should easily flow through the tube and, ideally, a second sample tube is filled.**

f. **Seal both ends of the tubes.**

g. **Use a magnet to draw the metal filing (flea) back and forth in the tubes to mix the blood, if needed.**

h. **Unless the blood samples will be analyzed within 30 minutes, place the sealed tubes into an ice-water bath.**

Figure 3-4 Puncture sites on an infant's heel for obtaining an arterialized capillary blood sample. Avoid the posterior tibial artery that runs through the center of the foot. *(From Walsh B, Czervinske MP, Di Blasi RM:* Perinatal and pediatric respiratory care, *ed 3, St Louis, 2010, Mosby.)*

Exam Hint 3-2 (ELE, WRE)

Commonly tested areas involve the ABG technique and possible hazards to it. Patient hazards include blood vessel trauma, hematoma, arterial clot formation, arteriospasm, and infected puncture site. In addition, the therapist may receive an accidental needle puncture injury.

i. Send the samples to the laboratory for analysis along with the proper paperwork unless point-of-care analysis is performed.

j. Apply pressure to stop the bleeding. Complications include infection, bone spurs, and laceration of the posterior tibial artery.

MODULE C

Analyze blood gas values

1. Manipulate a point-of-care blood gas analyzer by order or protocol (Code: IIA10) [Difficulty: ELE: R, Ap; WRE: An]

a. Select the appropriate point-of-care blood gas analyzer

A point-of-care (POC) blood gas analyzer can be used as an alternative to a centrally located analyzer. This is especially helpful when a patient is being transported, or when the data are very quickly needed at the bedside. The blood gas values of PaO_2, $PaCO_2$, and pH are typically obtained from either a POC analyzer or a standard blood gas analyzer. These standard units are acceptable for all patient care situations except when carbon monoxide poisoning is known or suspected. Neither the POC nor the standard blood gas analyzer is able to measure carboxyhemoglobin (COHb). A CO-oximeter is needed to measure the patient's level of carboxyhemoglobin in carbon monoxide cases. Some POC analyzers also can measure levels of serum electrolytes and other commonly needed patient values such as blood glucose, hemoglobin, and hematocrit levels.

b. Put the equipment together and make sure that it works properly (CSE code: IIA10)

POC analyzers can be powered through a self-contained battery or by plugging the unit into a standard alternating current electrical outlet. The units have single-use disposable cartridges that include the electrodes and calibration reagents and will hold waste samples. The following discussion covers the basic principles of operation of the electrodes in POC and standard centrally located analyzers.

1. pH electrode

The modern pH electrode has existed since the mid-1950s and is usually referred to as the *Sanz electrode* after its principal inventor. The basic principle behind the pH analyzer is its ability to measure the voltage (potential for electrical flow) between two different solutions. This is based on the different hydrogen ion (H^+) concentrations between the solutions that reflect their relative pH values. The reference electrode is immersed in a solution with a pH of 6.840 that fills a glass or plastic chamber. The blood sample, of unknown pH, is placed in a separate measuring chamber called a *cuvette*. These two chambers are separated by a special glass membrane that contains metals and sodium ions (Na^+), thus making it pH sensitive. Both chambers are kept at a stable 37° C temperature. See Figure 3-5 for a graphic representation of the pH electrode. When blood or a quality control (QC) material is introduced into the cuvette, the potential exists for hydrogen ions to replace the sodium ions in the pH-sensitive glass if the two pHs are different. The replacement is proportional to the difference in the two pHs.

2. PCO_2 electrode

The partial pressure of carbon dioxide (PCO_2) is measured in a modified pH electrode. This was first designed in the mid-1950s by Stow and further perfected by Severinghaus. Accordingly, these units are now referred to as *Severinghaus electrodes*, or sometimes as *Stow-Severinghaus electrodes*. In Figure 3-6, the electrode is depicted in cross section. It has a reference half-cell and a measuring half-cell that are enclosed within pH-sensitive glass and electrically connected by an electrolyte contact bridge. The blood sample is introduced into a cuvette heated to 37° C.

The principle of operation is based on the amount of CO_2 found in the blood sample that diffuses through the silicone elastic membrane. The CO_2 chemically combines with the bicarbonate solution to change the pH of the solution by the release of H^+. This change in H^+ concentration creates a voltage difference between the measuring and reference half-cells that is proportional to the amount of CO_2 found in the patient's blood sample.

3. PO_2 electrode

This unit is completely different from the others mentioned. It was developed in the late 1950s by Clark and thus is usually called a *Clark electrode*. It is also sometimes known as a *polarographic electrode* because of the basis of its operation. Figure 3-7 is a drawing of key features of the unit. A phosphate-KCl buffer solution surrounds the silver anode. A thin membrane separates the blood-filled cuvette from direct contact with the electrode but allows oxygen molecules to diffuse slowly through to contact the platinum wire cathode. The whole unit is heated to 37° C. The term *polarographic* comes from the addition of about 0.7 volt to the cathode to make it slightly "polarized" or negative compared with the anode. This is needed to ensure that oxygen is rapidly chemically reduced (that it gains electrons) at the cathode. This creates an electrical current directly proportional to the number of reduced oxygen molecules.

It must be understood that the partial pressure of oxygen (PO_2) being measured is derived from oxygen that is dissolved in the plasma. It does not come from the hemoglobin found in the erythrocytes (red blood cells). The reported value for the saturation of oxygen in the hemoglobin (SaO_2) is calculated by using a mathematical

Figure 3-5   Key components of the pH electrode. **A,** A voltage develops across the pH-sensitive glass when a difference exists in the hydrogen ion concentration between the two solutions. **B,** Two separate half-cells are used for the measuring electrode and the reference electrode. **C,** The addition of a KCl contact bridge and voltmeter completes the electrical circuit and enables the pH of the patient's blood sample to be measured. *(From Harrison BA, Shapiro C: Clinical application of blood gases, ed 4, St Louis, 1989, Mosby.)*

Figure 3-6   Schematic illustration of the modern PCO_2 electrode. (Note that the space between the elastic membrane and the nylon spacer is greatly enlarged for clarity.) *(From Harrison BA, Shapiro C: Clinical application of blood gases, ed 4, St Louis, 1989, Mosby.)*

Figure 3-7   Schematic illustration of the Clark electrode for measuring PO_2. *(From Harrison BA, Shapiro C: Clinical application of blood gases, ed 4, St Louis, 1989, Mosby.)*

table. Under normal conditions, the calculated SaO_2 value is the same as or close to the true SaO_2 value. Carbon monoxide (CO) poisoning is the only commonly seen clinical situation during which a calculated saturation can be incorrectly high. If carbon monoxide poisoning is suspected or known, the patient's blood sample should be analyzed on a CO-oximeter unit.

c. Troubleshoot any problems with the point-of-care blood gas analyzer

POC analyzers are designed to self-calibrate and display information on their operation. Replace a testing cartridge that is not properly functioning. Recharge a battery that is running low on reserve power.

d. Perform quality control procedures for a blood gas analyzer (Code: IIC1) [Difficulty: ELE: R, Ap; WRE: An]

1. Quality control

Quality control (QC) refers to creating a measurement and documentation system to confirm the accuracy (precision) and reliability of all blood gas measurements. Accuracy or precision means that the measured physiologic values truly reflect the actual physiologic values. Reliability means that a high degree of confidence exists so that the measured values represent the patient's actual physiologic values. Both are critically important if the blood gas results are to be used to make correct clinical decisions.

2. Quality assurance

Quality assurance (QA) refers to the broader concern that the results of the blood gas measurement are not only accurate and reliable but also clinically useful. To help ensure this, the Clinical Laboratory Improvement Amendments of 1988 (CLIA 88) require that the department have written policies and procedures on items including record keeping, equipment maintenance, staff training, and the correction of errors.

3. Calibration

Calibration is the systematic standardization of the graduations of the blood gas analyzer against known values to ensure consistency. Proper calibration of the electrodes is essential to the accuracy of the blood gas values. Some general calibration steps are discussed later. The manufacturer's guidelines must be followed for the specific steps in calibration.

4. Quality control materials

A variety of QC materials are available to calibrate the electrodes for PO_2, PCO_2, and pH measurements. Their uses vary. Each of the following materials has its advantages, disadvantages, and limitations. The manufacturer of a particular brand or model of blood gas analyzer may require that a specific type of material be used in its units.

Aqueous buffers are water based and are used to check pH and PCO_2 measurements; they cannot be used to check PO_2 measurements. Commercially prepared gases are used to check PO_2 and PCO_2 measurements; they cannot be used to check pH measurements. The following CO_2 mixes may be used: 0, 5%, 10%, and 12%. The following O_2 mixes may be used: 0, 12%, 20%, 20.95% from room air, 21%, and 100%.

Tonometered liquids are exposed in the laboratory to known oxygen and carbon dioxide gas mixes until the liquids are saturated and have the same partial pressures as the gases. Three types of tonometered liquids are used. First, using human or animal serum or whole blood is the most accurate method available and is used mainly to obtain PO_2 and PCO_2 levels. Although whole human blood cannot be used for pH measurements, a bovine blood product can be used to obtain all three values. Second, assayed liquids are non–water-based liquids that are pretonometered by the manufacturer and are available in sealed glass vials. They can be used to obtain PO_2, PCO_2, and pH measurements. These are very popular because of the advantages of speed and simplicity. Third, oxygenated fluorocarbon-based emulsions (perfluorinated compounds) can be used to obtain PO_2, PCO_2, and pH measurements. They are considered as accurate as whole blood without its associated risks.

5. Levey-Jennings charts

The Levey-Jennings charts (also known as *Shewhart/Levey-Jennings* or *quality control [QC] charts*) are used to record the results of each calibration procedure. They are similarly designed with time plotted on the horizontal scale and the analyte (PO_2, PCO_2, or pH) on the vertical scale. The vertical scale for each analyte has a central value for what is normally expected. On both sides of this normal value are standard deviation (SD) points, showing movement away from what is expected. When an analyte electrode is operating within the acceptable limits, it is said to be in control. In general, if an analyte is within 2 SDs of the normal value, it is considered to be in control.

An out-of-control situation exists whenever a single calibration value or a series of calibration values is outside established limits. A random error is an unpredictable aberration in precision that occurs when the QC material is sampled. A systematic error shows an accuracy problem and is much more serious. It must be investigated, corrected, and documented. Figure 3-8 shows an example of both random error and systematic error. Rules have been established for determining whether the error is random or systematic (Table 3-1).

6. pH electrode

NOTE: *These and the following guidelines are based on CLIA standards or widely reported industry standards. The various brands and models of blood gas analyzers may have different frequencies of calibration requirements, depending on their Food and Drug Administration (FDA)-approved manufacturers' studies.*

a. One-point calibration
1. Should be done before every sample is analyzed if one-point calibration is not automatically performed every 30 minutes
2. Performed with the near-normal QC material of 7.384 ± 0.005 pH used to set the balance potentiometer
3. Recommended every 30 minutes
4. Should be rechecked after a suspicious pH result; the blood sample should then be rerun

Figure 3-8 Levey-Jennings quality control chart for PaCO₂. The central horizontal line represents the mean value of 40 torr. The next lower and higher horizontal lines show 1 standard deviation (1 SD) value from the mean. The second most distant lower and higher horizontal lines are 2 SDs from the mean. The most distant horizontal lines are 3 SDs from the mean. The bottom number scale indicates 8-hour work shifts. *Open circles*, Calibration values that are within 2 SDs of the mean value. They are considered to be in control. *Black circles*, Calibration values that are out of control. *A* represents a random error and *B* a systematic error. *(From Shapiro BA, Peruzzi WT, Kozlowski-Templin R: Clinical application of blood gases, ed 5, St Louis, 1994, Mosby.)*

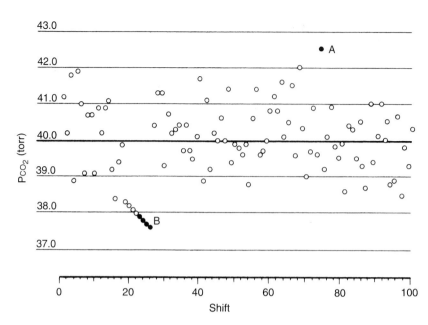

TABLE 3-1	Westgard's Rules for Determining When an Analyzer Is Not Functioning Properly

Rule name	Levey-Jennings chart
RANDOM ERROR	
1-2 SDs	The measurement is more than 2 SDs but not more than 3 SDs from the mean.
1-3 SDs	The measurement is more than 3 SDs from the mean.
R*-4 SDs	Two consecutive measurements are 4 SDs or more apart.
SYSTEMATIC ERROR	
2-2 SDs	Two consecutive measurements are either 2 SDs above or 2 SDs below the mean.
4-1 SDs	Four consecutive measurements are either 1 SD above or 1 SD below the mean.
7-trend	Seven consecutive measurements are on only one side of the mean; each measurement is progressively more out of control.
10-mean	Ten consecutive measurements are on only one side of the mean.

Modified from Lane EE, Walker JF: *Clinical arterial blood gas analysis*, St Louis, 1987, Mosby.
SDs, standard deviations.

b. Two-point calibration
1. Should be done at least once every 8 hours when patient samples are being analyzed
2. Recommended for every 25 patient samples
3. Performed with the slope potentiometer set with a QC material of 6.840 ± 0.005 pH (this is the same pH as the reference electrode solution)

4. Performed with the balance potentiometer set with a QC material of 7.384 ± 0.005 pH

c. Three-point calibration
1. Should be done at least every 6 months on existing equipment
2. Should be done whenever a new electrode is put into use
3. Covers the physiologic range to confirm linearity: QC materials of 6.840 ± 0.005, 7.384 ± 0.005, and 7.874 ± 0.005 pH are used

7. PCO₂ electrode

a. One-point calibration
1. Should be done before every sample is analyzed if one-point calibration is not automatically performed every 30 minutes
2. Performed with 5% ± 0.03% CO_2 used to set the balance potentiometer
3. Recommended every 30 minutes
4. Should be rechecked after a suspicious PCO₂ result; the blood sample should then be rerun

The CO_2 can be directly in contact with the electrode, tonometered with an aqueous material or blood, or premixed in aqueous buffers, assayed liquids, or fluorocarbon-based emulsion.

b. Two-point calibration
1. Should be done at least once every 8 hours when patient samples are being analyzed
2. Recommended for every 25 patient samples
3. Performed with 10% ± 0.03% CO_2 to set the slope potentiometer
4. Performed with 5% ± 0.03% CO_2 to set the balance potentiometer

c. **Three-point calibration.**

1. Should be done at least every 6 months on existing equipment
2. Should be done whenever a new electrode is put into use
3. Covers the physiologic range to confirm linearity; three PCO_2 values between 0 and 80 mm Hg should be determined
4. Room air or a gas cylinder containing up to 0.03% CO_2 can be used to set the 0 point

8. PO_2 electrode

a. **One-point calibration**

1. Should be done before every sample is analyzed if one-point calibration is not automatically performed every 30 minutes
2. Performed with 12% ± 0.03% O_2 used to set the balance potentiometer; some analyzers are designed to use 20% ± 0.03% O_2 from a gas cylinder or draw room air (20.95% oxygen) into the unit
3. Recommended every 30 minutes

4. Should be rechecked after a suspicious PO_2 result; the blood sample should then be rerun

The O_2 can be directly in contact with the electrode, tonometered with an aqueous material or blood, or premixed in aqueous buffers, assayed liquids, or fluorocarbon-based emulsion as discussed.

b. **Two-point calibration**

1. Should be done at least once every 8 hours when patient samples are being analyzed
2. Should be done whenever readjustment of one-point calibration is greater than 3 torr
3. Recommended for every 25 patient samples
4. Performed with 0 ± 0.03% O_2 to set the slope potentiometer
5. Performed with 12% ± 0.03% O_2 to set the balance potentiometer; some analyzers are designed to use 20% ± 0.03% O_2 from a gas cylinder or draw room air (20.95% oxygen) into the unit

c. **Three-point calibration**

1. Should be done at least every 6 months on existing equipment
2. Should be done whenever a new electrode is put into use
3. Should be done to confirm linearity whenever the PO_2 value could be more than 150 torr, assuming that the balance point is set on room oxygen content; the third point should be set on 100% ± 0.03% O_2 from a gas cylinder

Exam Hint 3-5 (WRE)

Often a question relates to QC. It could include reanalyzing a blood gas sample with suspicious results, rechecking out-of-control calibration results (greater than 2 SDs), or using two analyzers for cross referencing.

BOX 3-1   Electrode Precision and Calibration Gases

ELECTRODES

pH ±0.01 unit

P_{CO_2} ±2% (approximately ±1 mm Hg at 40 torr)

P_{O_2} ±3% (approximately ±2.5 mm Hg at 80 torr)

If the P_{O_2} is >150 torr, the precision is approximately ±10% unless three-point calibration is performed.

CALIBRATION GASES

"Low" gas: 0% O_2 (+0.03%), 5% CO_2 (±0.03%), balance N_2

"High" gas: 12% or 21% O_2, 10% CO_2 (both ±0.03%), balance N_2

Suggested three-point gases: 100% O_2 (−0.03%), 0% CO_2 (+0.03%)

N_2, Nitrogen; P_{CO_2}, pressure of carbon dioxide; P_{O_2}, pressure of oxygen.

9. Miscellaneous topics

10. Calibration gas cylinders

For economic reasons, the low-percentage oxygen and carbon dioxide gases are placed together in one cylinder, and the high-percentage oxygen and carbon dioxide gases are placed together in a second cylinder. Box 3-1 summarizes the normal precision of the electrodes discussed and the gases used in their calibration. A cylinder containing 100% oxygen and no carbon dioxide can be used for three-point calibration.

11. Temperature correction

Temperature correction refers to mathematical adjustment of a patient's Pa_{O_2}, Pa_{CO_2}, and pH values if his or her temperature is not 37° C. Remember that blood gas analyzers are calibrated at 37° C because it is normal body temperature. If the patient has a fever, the oxygen and carbon dioxide partial pressures in the blood will be greater than those found during the blood gas analysis. Conversely, the hypothermic patient will have lower oxygen and carbon dioxide partial pressures in the blood than those found during the blood gas analysis. The pH value will shift in the opposite direction from the P_{CO_2} value. Usually this small shift in values is ignored. However, because some physicians may specify that their patient's blood gases be temperature corrected, the patient's temperature should be listed on the blood gas slip. It is a simple mathematical process to temperature correct the

blood gas results. Most modern analyzers perform temperature correction automatically when programmed to do so. However, because the patient's values are not usually affected in a clinically significant way, temperature correction is not currently recommended.

e. Perform quality control procedures for a point-of-care blood gas analyzer (Code: IIC3) [Difficulty: ELE: R, Ap; WRE: An]

The general principles of QC and QA discussed with standard blood gas analyzers apply to point-of-care (POC) analyzers as well. Remember to flush the electrode membrane after each use, if possible, to prevent protein buildup. If protein buildup occurs, the response time is longer than normal. Follow the manufacturer's guidelines to change an electrode membrane as needed. Make sure that no air bubbles are under the membrane or within the tubing through which the blood travels. Rerun the calibration for any of the electrodes and reanalyze the sample if you are suspicious of the result. If the electrode does not calibrate close to the reference buffer solutions or gases, it should not be used.

In a random-error situation, the practitioner likely made a simple error when introducing the material or running the analyzer. Common problems include an air bubble injected into the unit or incomplete flushing of the previous sample. Usually flushing out any residual blood and then carefully injecting more of the current patient blood samples will correct the problem. Run the analyzer again to obtain new patient values or run the same patient sample through another analyzer and compare the two sets of results.

A systematic error usually indicates a problem with the analyzer, QC materials, or processes. Examples of systematic errors include misanalyzed CO_2 or O_2 standards for calibration; contaminated QC materials; or deteriorated oxygen, carbon dioxide, or pH electrode function. Each of these must be investigated until the problem is found and corrected. The unit cannot be used again until after it is proven to work properly and to give accurate results.

f. Perform blood gas analysis (Code: IB9j and IIIE3c) [Difficulty: ELE: R, Ap; WRE: An]

Modern blood gas analyzers are simple to operate. Follow the manufacturer's guidelines for insertion of the blood sample. Perform the specified steps in the analysis. Print out the results. Many current units run a self-diagnosis if any problems appear. Correct any identified problems as discussed above.

1. CO-oximeter/hemoximeter

a. Perform quality control procedures on the CO-oximeter/hemoximeter (Code: IIC1) [Difficulty: ELE: R, Ap; WRE: An]. The unit is preassembled by the manufacturer. Practical experience with a unit is recommended to understand how to add a patient blood sample and perform calibration duties. (See Figure 3-9 for a schematic drawing of a CO-oximeter.) A thallium-neon hollow cathode lamp emits light in the infrared-visible range. A device called a monochromator contains four filters and rotates through the light beam. Each filter allows only one specific wavelength to pass through it. These four monochromatic wavelengths correspond to the three isosbestic points, discussed later (shown in Figure 3-10) and 626.6 nm. This last wavelength is poorly absorbed by all four hemoglobin moieties. It is used to find the maximal difference in absorption so that the relative amounts of the hemoglobin species can be determined.

When a blood sample is placed into the cuvette, the same four wavelengths are passed through it. The amount of absorbance at each wavelength is measured and compared with the absorbance at each wavelength by a reference sample solution (see the following discussion). The computer integrates the data and calculates the total hemoglobin concentration and the amounts of the four hemoglobin moieties.

Total hemoglobin (THb) concentration should be calibrated when the unit is installed, at regular intervals suggested by the manufacturer, after the sample tubing is changed, after the cuvette is disassembled or changed, and whenever a suspicious reading is seen. Calibration is done by filling the cuvette with a special dye produced by the manufacturer and analyzing it by following the prescribed steps.

Routine calibration is done every 30 minutes. The unit obtains and stores absorbance readings at the four different wavelengths from a "blank" solution in the reference detector. When the same blank solution is added to the sample cuvette, the same four wavelengths are measured. Their absorption levels are normally identical. The same procedure is performed after every patient sample is analyzed.

The following are examples of common problems and their solutions:

- Incomplete hemolysis of the blood sample causes the light to scatter off cell fragments and lipids. Sickle cells (as in sickle cell anemia) are difficult to disrupt and may cause false oxyhemoglobin and carboxyhemoglobin readings if extra time is not taken for hemolysis. Follow manufacturer's guidelines on the procedure for hemolyzing the red blood cells.
- More than 10% methemoglobin may cause errors in the measurement of all hemoglobin moieties. Sulfhemoglobin also causes false readings. The practitioner may need to gather additional information from the chart or laboratory regarding the patient's levels of these abnormal hemoglobin moieties. CO-oximetry should probably not be performed on

Figure 3-10   Spectral analysis of the hemoglobin moieties (species). O_2Hb is oxyhemoglobin, COHb is carboxyhemoglobin, RHb is reduced hemoglobin, and MetHb (METHb) is methemoglobin. Point *A* shows the triple isosbestic point at 548 nm for O_2Hb, COHb, and RHb. Point *B* shows the double isosbestic point at 568 nm for O_2Hb and RHb. Point *C* shows the double isosbestic point at 578 nm for RHb and COHb. A fourth wavelength at 626.6 nm is used for comparison purposes. *(From Shapiro BA, Peruzzi WT, Kozlowski-Templin R: Clinical application of blood gases, ed 5, St. Louis, 1994, Mosby.)*

Figure 3-9   CO-oximeter basic components. **A,** Thallium-neon hollow cathode light source. **B,** Lens and mirror. **C,** Monochromator with four specific wavelength filters. **D,** Light-beam splitter that diverts half of the light to the reference detector and half to the cuvette. **E,** Reference wavelength detector. **F,** Patient sample cuvette. **G,** Sample wavelength detector. **H,** Temperature-regulated block set at 37° C. *(From Shapiro BA, Peruzzi WT, Kozlowski-Templin R: Clinical application of blood gases, ed 5, St Louis, 1994, Mosby.)*

blood samples with abnormal levels of methemoglobin or sulfhemoglobin.

- Intravenous dyes such as methylene blue, Evans blue, and indocyanine green used in various cardiac studies can absorb the same wavelengths of light used to identify the various forms of hemoglobin. The presence of these dyes results in a lower measurement of oxyhemoglobin than is actually present. Check the patient's chart for a record of dyes used. CO-oximetry should probably not be used for blood gas analysis on patients who have these dyes in their systems.

- Failure to reprogram the analyzer for fetal hemoglobin instead of adult hemoglobin may produce false results. Remember to check the chart for the patient's age. Reprogram the analyzer for fetal hemoglobin for any sample taken from an infant who is only a few weeks old.

- The presence of lipid particles in the blood causes light scattering and results in a reading that is falsely high in total hemoglobin and percentage of methemoglobin and falsely low in percentage of oxyhemoglobin and percentage of carboxyhemoglobin. Follow the laboratory's guidelines to determine when a patient's blood lipid value is too high for accurate use of the CO-oximeter.

- Air bubbles or incomplete hemolysis of blood in the cuvette causes an absorbance error. Air bubbles must be flushed out and the blood sample inserted again and reanalyzed. Make sure that all blood samples are hemolyzed according to the manufacturer's guidelines.

- Blood clots in the sample tubing prevent blood from flowing through to the cuvette. If a sample cannot be inserted into the unit, suspect and check for a blood clot. Remove any clotted tubing, replace it, and confirm that the CO-oximeter is working properly.

b. Perform CO-oximetry/hemoximetry (Code: IB9j and IIIE3c) [Difficulty: ELE: R, Ap; WRE: An]. Most hospitals have a CO-oximeter in addition to a blood gas analyzer. A CO-oximeter should be used to analyze a blood gas sample whenever carbon monoxide poisoning is known or suspected. In addition, a CO-oximeter gives a complete analysis of the relative amounts of the different types of patient hemoglobin.

CO-oximeters also are called spectrophotometric oximeters and are the most accurate method available to measure the four different hemoglobin moieties (species or variations in the hemoglobin molecule). These hemoglobin species include the following:

- Oxyhemoglobin (HbO_2 or O_2Hb), which carries oxygen to the tissues, and reduced hemoglobin (HbR or RHb), which has given up its oxygen and picked up carbon dioxide

- Carboxyhemoglobin (HbCO or COHb), which is nonfunctional because of the tightness with which carbon monoxide binds to the hemoglobin

- Methemoglobin (HbMet or MetHb), which is nonfunctional because the Hb molecule is unable to combine reversibly with oxygen

- Sulfhemoglobin (HbS or SHb), which is similar to the HbMet and is also nonfunctional

- In addition, a CO-oximeter can measure the fetal hemoglobin (HbF or FHb) found in a newborn infant instead of adult oxyhemoglobin

Each of these hemoglobin moieties has a unique spectroscopic "fingerprint" of absorbed light-wave frequencies. See Figure 3-10 for the spectral analysis of the various forms of hemoglobin.

Follow the manufacturer's guidelines on rewarming the blood sample to body temperature, hemolyzing the sample, and inserting it into the measurement cuvette. Failure to do so may result in incorrect patient values.

The principle of operation of a CO-oximeter is the comparison of the relative absorbances of four wavelengths of light by oxyhemoglobin, reduced hemoglobin, and carboxyhemoglobin. This is done by comparing the absorptions at the three isosbestic points (at which the moieties being compared have equal absorption) and a wavelength point at which the greatest difference in absorption between the two moieties is found. By computer integration of the data, the relative proportions of oxyhemoglobin, reduced hemoglobin, and carboxyhemoglobin are determined. If the total is less than 100% of the hemoglobin present, the difference has to be methemoglobin (or, rarely, sulfhemoglobin). The unit then provides data on total hemoglobin; percentages for oxyhemoglobin, reduced hemoglobin, carboxyhemoglobin, and methemoglobin; and total amounts for them in grams per deciliter of blood. Some units also calculate O_2 content.

Exam Hint 3-6 (ELE, WRE)

If a patient is known to have or suspected of having carbon monoxide poisoning (e.g., removed from inside a burning building), a CO-oximeter should be used for blood gas analysis. A standard or POC blood gas analyzer or pulse oximeter should not be used. These instruments cannot detect or measure carboxyhemoglobin.

MODULE D

Interpret blood gas analysis results to determine how the patient is responding to respiratory care

1. Review the chart for any blood gas results (Code: IA5) [Difficulty: ELE: R; WRE: Ap]

Look in the chart for any blood gas results, including arterial, capillary, or mixed venous. Any patient may have had an arterial sample analyzed. A neonate also may have had an arterialized capillary sample analyzed. A patient with a pulmonary artery catheter may have had a mixed venous sample analyzed.

2. Interpret the results of arterial blood gas analysis (Code: IB10j, IB10f, and IIIE4a) [Difficulty: ELE: R, Ap; WRE: An]

If the blood sampling equipment preparation, the sampling procedure, and blood gas analyzer operation were all done properly, the respiratory therapist and physician can believe that the blood gas results are accurate and reliable. However, if there was a problem with any aspect of obtaining and analyzing the blood gas sample, that sample must be discarded and a new sample obtained and analyzed.

A number of authors have written extensively on how to interpret ABGs. The system proposed by Shapiro and associates (1994) has been found to be both practical and relatively easy to understand. Most of the following discussion and tables are based on this system. This does not mean that if one has learned another system, he or she is at any disadvantage for taking the National Board for Respiratory Care (NBRC) examination.

TABLE 3-2	Age-Based Acceptable Levels of Partial Pressure of Oxygen in Arterial Blood (PaO$_2$) When Breathing Room Air (21% Oxygen) at Sea Level
Age	**PaO$_2$**
NEWBORN	
Acceptable range	40 to 70 torr
CHILD TO ADULT	
Normal	97 torr
Acceptable range	>80 torr
Hypoxemia	<80 torr
OLDER ADULT	
60-year-old	>80 torr
70-year-old	>70 torr
80-year-old	>60 torr
90-year-old	>50 torr

Modified from Shapiro BA, Peruzzi WT, Kozelowski-Templin R: *Clinical application of blood gases,* ed 5, Chicago, 1994, Mosby-Year Book.

Exam Hint 3-7 (WRE)

The *Written Registry Examination* includes specific questions about ABG interpretation. The exam also incorporates blood gas results into other questions that relate to any respiratory care technique or procedure, such as oxygen therapy for a patient with chronic obstructive pulmonary disease (COPD) and adjustment of mechanical ventilation. In addition, often a question requires the interpretation of mixed venous blood gases or arterialized capillary blood gases. The examinee must be proficient in all aspects of blood gas interpretation to do well on the advanced NBRC examinations.

a. Assessment of oxygenation

Hypoxemia or hypoxia can rapidly become life threatening. This will often be first seen when the patient develops cardiac arrhythmias, unstable vital signs, and mental confusion or unconsciousness. Table 3-2 shows the normal PaO$_2$ values for the newborn, child to adult, and the elderly when room air (almost 21% oxygen) is inhaled at sea level. These values decrease progressively as altitude increases. However, under most clinical conditions, this is not a factor unless working in a high-altitude setting.

A general rule is that any patient is seriously hypoxemic if the PaO$_2$ is less than 60 torr on room air. See Table 3-3 for guidelines on judging the seriousness of hypoxemia. Once hypoxemia is recognized, it must be corrected. The

TABLE 3-3	Evaluation of Hypoxemia

CONDITIONS: ROOM AIR IS INSPIRED; THE PATIENT IS YOUNGER THAN 60 YEARS*		
Hypoxemia	PaO$_2$	SaO$_2$
Mild	60-79 torr	90-94%
Moderate	40-59 torr	75-89%
Severe	<40 torr	<75%

CONDITIONS: SUPPLEMENTAL O$_2$ IS INSPIRED; THE PATIENT IS YOUNGER THAN 60 YEARS	
Hypoxemia	PaO$_2$
Uncorrected	Less than room air acceptable limit
Corrected	Within room air acceptable limit (<100 torr)
Excessively corrected	>100 torr

Modified from Shapiro BA, Peruzzi WT, Kozelowski-Templin R: *Clinical application of blood gases,* ed 5, Chicago, 1994, Mosby-Year Book. *Subtract 1 torr of O$_2$ from limits of mild and moderate hypoxemia for each year older than 60. A PaO$_2$ value of <40 torr indicates severe hypoxemia in any patient at any age.

most obvious way to correct hypoxemia is to give supplemental oxygen. The clinician must realize that oxygen alone will not correct the hypoxemia if the patient is hypoventilating (increased PaCO$_2$), has heart failure, or is unable to carry or make use of the oxygen. In general, try to keep the patient's PaO$_2$ level between 60 and 100 torr.

Shapiro and associates (1994) suggested the following formula, in which FiO_2 is the fraction of inspired oxygen, for determining whether the patient will be hypoxemic on room air: "If PaO_2 is less than $FiO_2 \times 5$, the patient can be assumed to be hypoxemic on room air."

Figure 3-11 shows a normal oxyhemoglobin dissociation curve. The saturation value is important to know because it shows how much hemoglobin is saturated with oxygen. Several important points of correlation exist between the SaO_2 and the PaO_2. (Calculated saturation values can be misleadingly high if the patient has inhaled carbon monoxide. In this situation, it is best to measure the saturation directly on a CO-oximeter–type blood gas analyzer.)

Figure 3-12 shows a number of factors that can influence the oxyhemoglobin dissociation curve and how oxygen associates and dissociates from hemoglobin. In a patient with normal oxygenation, these factors are not clinically significant. However, when the PaO_2 level is less than 60 torr and the SaO_2 level is less than 90%, these factors can become an important consideration. As can be seen, a left-shifted oxyhemoglobin dissociation curve results in a lower PaO_2 value at any given saturation. This results in even less oxygen being delivered to the tissues.

Exam Hint 3-8 (WRE)

True shunt or venous admixture leading to ventilation/perfusion mismatching are the two most common clinical findings leading to hypoxemia.

b. Assessment of carbon dioxide and pH

The pH is the next important value to interpret because extreme acidemia/acidosis and alkalemia/alkalosis can be life threatening. The carbon dioxide value is important to interpret because it has a direct effect on the pH and indirectly affects the oxygen level. A high or low $PaCO_2$ level, by itself, is not life threatening.

Table 3-4 shows normal values for pH and $PaCO_2$ and the acceptable ranges around the mean or average. Table 3-5 shows the most widely acceptable therapeutic ranges for pH and $PaCO_2$. Values that fall outside of these ranges present a progressively greater risk to the patient.

Table 3-6 shows the definitions of Shapiro and associates for alkalemia and acidemia from a respiratory cause. An acute change in the patient's ventilation causes the following when starting from a $PaCO_2$ of 40 torr:
- If the $PaCO_2$ level increases by 20 torr, the pH decreases by 0.10 unit.
- If the $PaCO_2$ level decreases by 10 torr, the pH increases by 0.10 unit.

Thus the body can be seen as better able to compensate with metabolic buffers for a respiratory acidosis than a respiratory alkalosis.

Metabolic effects are evaluated by interpreting either the bicarbonate (HCO_3^-) value or the base excess/base

Figure 3-11 The oxygen (oxyhemoglobin) dissociation curve plots the relation between hemoglobin saturation (*y*-axis) and plasma PaO_2 level (*x*-axis). *A*, 75% saturation and a PaO_2 of 40 torr are normally seen in venous blood. *B*, 85% saturation and a PaO_2 of 50 torr are the minimal levels that should be allowed in a chronically hypoxemic patient. *C*, 90% saturation and a PaO_2 of 60 torr are the minimal levels that should be allowed in an acutely hypoxemic patient. *D*, Hemoglobin in the pulmonary capillaries adjacent to normal alveoli will become 100% saturated when the PaO_2 level reaches 150 torr. *(Modified from Lane EE, Walker JF: Clinical arterial blood gas analysis, St Louis, 1987, Mosby.)*

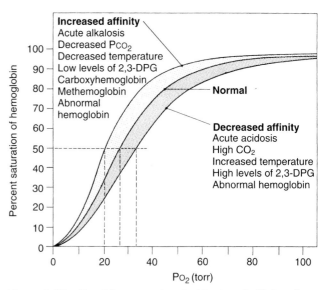

Figure 3-12 Conditions associated with altered affinity of hemoglobin for O_2. P_{50} is the PaO_2 value at which hemoglobin is 50% saturated, normally 26.6 torr. A lower than normal P_{50} value represents increased affinity of hemoglobin for O_2; a high P_{50} value is seen with decreased affinity. Note that variation from the normal is associated with decreased (low P_{50} value) or increased (high P_{50} value) availability of O_2 to tissues *(dashed lines)*. *Shaded area*, The entire oxyhemoglobin dissociation curve under the same circumstances. *(From Lane EE, Walker JF: Clinical arterial blood gas analysis, St Louis, 1987, Mosby.)*

TABLE 3-4	Normal Laboratory Ranges for Partial Pressure of Carbon Dioxide in Arterial Blood ($PaCO_2$) and pH		
	Mean	**1SD***	**2SDs**
$PaCO_2$	40.00	8-42 torr	35-45 torr
pH	7.40	7.38-7.42	7.35-7.45

Modified from Shapiro BA, Peruzzi WT, Kozelowski-Templin R: *Clinical application of blood gases*, ed 5, Chicago, 1994, Mosby-Year Book. *SD*, standard deviation.

TABLE 3-5	Acceptable Clinical Ranges for Partial Pressure of Carbon Dioxide in Arterial Blood ($PaCO_2$) and pH
$PaCO_2$	30-50 torr*
pH	7.30-7.50

Modified from Shapiro BA, Peruzzi WT, Kozelowski-Templin R: *Clinical application of blood gases*, ed 5, Chicago, 1994, Mosby-Year Book. *This is the range for patients with an acute change. It does not apply to patients with long-standing disease, such as chronic obstructive pulmonary disease. These patients may have $PaCO_2$ values greater than 50 torr.

TABLE 3-6	Naming Unacceptable Values for Partial Pressure of CO_2 in Arterial Blood ($PaCO_2$) and pH	
$PaCO_2$ >45 torr	Respiratory acidosis/alveolar hypoventilation/ventilatory failure
pH <7.35	Acidemia
$PaCO_2$ <35 torr	Respiratory alkalosis/alveolar hyperventilation
pH >7.45	Alkalemia

Modified from Shapiro BA, Peruzzi WT, Kozelowski-Templin R: *Clinical application of blood gases*, ed 5, Chicago, 1994, Mosby-Year Book.

deficit (BE/BD) value. Both reveal whether any metabolic effect on the pH exists. Normal values are as follows:
- HCO_3^-: 24 mEq/L
- BE/BD: 0 mEq/L; ±1 mEq/L is often listed as the normal range

Values indicating metabolic alkalosis of a primary or secondary nature are as follows:
- Bicarbonate level greater than 24 mEq/L
- BE greater than 0 or greater than +1 mEq/L

Values indicating metabolic acidosis of a primary or secondary nature are as follows:
- Bicarbonate level less than 24 mEq/L
- BE less than 0 or greater than −1 mEq/L (i.e., −5 mEq/L); some laboratories report this as a BD or negative BE.

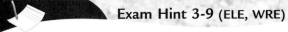

Exam Hint 3-9 (ELE, WRE)

The NBRC uses BE for base excess (regardless of whether it has a positive or negative value) and HCO_3^- for bicarbonate.

Exam Hint 3-10 (ELE)

Expect to see several arterial blood gas questions that require the interpretation of acid-base balance and oxygenation. For example, identify that a patient with COPD has an elevated carbon dioxide level and a pH in the low-normal range with a compensated respiratory acidosis. Also, expect to see ABG values included in questions about the adjustment of oxygen therapy and mechanical ventilation.

TABLE 3-7	Clinical Terminology for Arterial Blood Gas Measurements
Clinical Terminology	**Clinical Findings**
Respiratory acidosis/ alveolar hypoventilation/ ventilatory failure	$PaCO_2$ >45 torr
Acute ventilatory failure	$PaCO_2$ >45 torr; pH <7.35
Chronic ventilatory failure	$PaCO_2$ >45 torr; pH 7.36-7.40
Respiratory alkalosis/ alveolar hyperventilation	$PaCO_2$ <35 torr
Acute alveolar hyperventilation	$PaCO_2$ <35 torr; pH >7.45
Chronic alveolar hyperventilation	$PaCO_2$ <35 torr; pH 7.41-7.45
Acidemia	pH <7.35
Acidosis	Pathophysiologic condition in which the patient has a significant base deficit (plasma bicarbonate level below normal)
Alkalemia	pH >7.45
Alkalosis	Pathophysiologic condition in which the patient has a significant base excess (plasma bicarbonate level above normal)

Modified from Shapiro BA, Peruzzi WT, Kozelowski-Templin R: *Clinical application of blood gases*, ed 5, Chicago, 1994, Mosby-Year Book.

Tables 3-7 to 3-9 show definitions of terms and classifications of the various acid-base states. As stated earlier, there are other systems for interpreting blood gases. All are probably satisfactory for interpretation purposes and preparing for the NBRC examinations.

TABLE 3-8	Evaluation of Ventilatory and Metabolic Effects on Acid-Base Status

EVALUATION OF PaCO$_2$

$PaCO_2$ >45 torr	Respiratory acidosis/alveolar hypoventilation/ventilatory failure
$PaCO_2$ 35-45 torr	Acceptable alveolar ventilation
$PaCO_2$ <35 torr	Respiratory alkalosis/alveolar hyperventilation

EVALUATION OF PaCO$_2$ IN CONJUNCTION WITH pH*

Acceptable Alveolar Ventilation ($PaCO_2$ from 35 to 45 torr)

pH >7.50	Metabolic alkalosis
pH 7.30-7.50	Acceptable pH
pH <7.30	Metabolic acidosis

Alveolar Hypoventilation ($PaCO_2$ >45 torr)

pH >7.50	*Partially compensated* metabolic alkalosis
pH 7.30-7.40	*Chronic* ventilatory failure
pH <7.30	*Acute* ventilatory failure

Alveolar Hyperventilation ($PaCO_2$ <35 torr)

pH >7.50	*Acute* alveolar hyperventilation
pH 7.40-7.50	*Chronic* alveolar hyperventilation
pH 7.30-7.40	*Compensated* metabolic acidosis
pH <7.30	*Partially compensated* metabolic acidosis

Modified from Shapiro BA, Peruzzi WT, Kozelowski-Templin R: *Clinical application of blood gases*, ed 5, Chicago, 1994, Mosby-Year Book.
$PaCO_2$, partial pressure of CO_2 in arterial blood.
*Some authors use a narrower pH range for these classifications.

3. Interpret the results of CO-oximetry/hemoximetry blood gas analysis (Code: IB10j and IIIE4b) [Difficulty: ELE: R, Ap; WRE: An]

If the blood sampling equipment preparation, the sampling procedure, and blood gas analyzer operation were all done properly, the respiratory therapist and physician can believe that the blood gas results are accurate and reliable. However, if there was a problem with any aspect of obtaining and analyzing the blood gas sample, that sample must be discarded and a new sample obtained and analyzed.

The CO-oximeter type blood gas analyzer gives values for oxyhemoglobin (O$_2$Hb), reduced hemoglobin (RHb), carboxyhemoglobin (COHb), and methemoglobin (MetHb)/sulfhemoglobin (SHb). Each of these hemoglobin moieties can be displayed in terms of grams per deciliter, percentage of the whole, and added together for a total hemoglobin (THb) value. Table 3-10 shows normal adult hemoglobin values. The amounts of carboxyhemoglobin and methemoglobin should be subtracted from the total hemoglobin amount to find the amount of functional hemoglobin. Any increase in the COHb or MetHb levels above those listed is abnormal and results in even less normal hemoglobin to carry oxygen. The patient with carbon monoxide poisoning is at greatest risk. A COHb level of 30% saturation or greater can be fatal. By subtraction, the O$_2$Hb (SaO$_2$) level can be no greater than 70% with a resulting PaO$_2$ of less than 40 torr.

TABLE 3-9	Primary Blood Gas Classification			
	O$_2$	pH	Bicarbonate	BE*
VENTILATORY IMBALANCE				
Acute alveolar hypoventilation	I	D	N	N
Chronic alveolar hypoventilation	I	N	I	I
Acute alveolar hyperventilation	D	I	N	N
Chronic alveolar hyperventilation	D	N	D	D
METABOLIC IMBALANCE				
Uncompensated acidosis	N	D	D	D
Partially compensated acidosis	D	D	D	D
Uncompensated alkalosis	N	I	I	I
Partially compensated alkalosis	I	I	I	I
Compensated acidosis or alkalosis	I or D	N	I or D	I or D

Modified from Shapiro BA, Peruzzi WT, Kozelowski-Templin R: *Clinical application of blood gases*, ed 5, Chicago, 1994, Mosby-Year Book.
D, decreased; *I*, increased; *N*, normal range; *BE*, base access.

TABLE 3-10	Normal Hemoglobin Values for Adults
Total hemoglobin (THb)	Men: 13.5-18.0 g/dL
	Women: 12.0-16.0 g/dL
	15.0 g/dL is often listed as an average for both
Oxyhemoglobin	94-100% of THb (reported as SaO_2*) of 94-100%
Carboxyhemoglobin	Nonsmokers: <1.5% (0.225 g/dL) of THb
	Smokers: 1.5-10% of THb
Methemoglobin	0.5-3% (0.075-0.45 g/dL) of THb
Oxygen content (arterial sample)	15-23 g/dL

g/dL, grams per deciliter (sometimes listed as g/100 mL); SaO_2, O_2 saturation in arterial blood.

EXAMPLE 1

The following example shows how to calculate the amount of functional hemoglobin and saturation for a patient with normal COHb and MetHb levels:

$$
\begin{array}{r}
15.0 \text{ g total Hb} \\
-0.225 \text{ g COHb} \\
\hline
14.775 \text{ g} \\
-0.15 \text{ g MetHb} \\
\hline
14.625 \text{ g functional Hb}
\end{array}
$$

$$
\begin{array}{r}
100\% \text{ potential saturation of } O_2\text{Hb in arterial blood} \\
-1.5\% \text{ saturation of COHb} \\
\hline
98.5\% \\
-1.5\% \text{ saturation MetHb} \\
\hline
97\% \text{ saturation of arterial blood (SaO}_2 \text{ of 97\%)}
\end{array}
$$

EXAMPLE 2

The following example is for a patient with an elevated COHb level and a normal MetHb level:

$$
\begin{array}{r}
15.0 \text{ g total Hb} \\
-3.0 \text{ g COHb} \\
\hline
2.0 \text{ g} \\
-0.15 \text{ g MetHb} \\
\hline
11.85 \text{ g functional Hb}
\end{array}
$$

$$
\begin{array}{r}
100\% \text{ potential saturation of } O_2\text{Hb in arterial blood} \\
-20\% \text{ saturation of COHb} \\
\hline
80\% \\
-1.5\% \text{ saturation MetHb} \\
\hline
78.5\% \text{ saturation of arterial blood (SaO}_2 \text{ of 78.5\%)}
\end{array}
$$

Exam Hint 3-11 (ELE, WRE)

If a significant difference is found in hemoglobin saturation values between the pulse oximeter, standard or POC analyzer, and a CO-oximeter, suspect that the patient has an elevated CO level. Only the CO-oximeter value will be accurate if the patient has CO poisoning.

TABLE 3-11	Normal and Abnormal Mixed Venous Blood Gas Values

NORMAL VALUES

Average:	$S\bar{v}O_2$, 75%; $P\bar{v}O_2$, 40 torr; $P\bar{v}CO_2$, 46 torr; pH 7.35
Range:	$S\bar{v}O_2$, 76-70%; $P\bar{v}O_2$, 43-37 torr; $P\bar{v}CO_2$, 46-44 torr; pH 7.36-7.34

CRITICALLY ILL PATIENT

	$P\bar{v}O_2$ (torr)		$S\bar{v}O_2$ (%)	
	Average	Range	Average	Range
Excellent cardiovascular reserves	>37	40-35	>70	75-68
Limited cardiovascular reserves	>32	35-30	>60	68-56
Failure of cardiovascular reserves	<30	<30	<56	<56

Modified from Shapiro BA, Peruzzi WT, Kozelowski-Templin R: *Clinical application of blood gases*, ed 5, St Louis, 1994, Mosby.

4. Mixed venous blood gases

a. Review the patient's chart for mixed venous blood gas results (Code: IA5) [Difficulty: ELE: R; WRE: Ap]

A mixed venous blood sample can be taken from the pulmonary artery of any patient who has a pulmonary artery (Swan-Ganz) catheter. This is a true mixed venous sample and should not be confused with a blood sample taken from an arm vein or other venous site. The symbol $P\bar{v}$ is the prefix for venous blood gas values of oxygen and so forth. In general, a typical patient has the following mixed venous blood gas values: $S\bar{v}O_2$, 75%; $P\bar{v}O_2$, 40 mm Hg; $P\bar{v}CO_2$, 46 mm Hg; and pH 7.35. (Table 3-11 provides details on normal venous blood gas values and their interpretation in patients with cardiovascular disease.)

b. Interpret the results of mixed venous blood gas analysis to evaluate the patient's response to respiratory care (Code: IB10j and IIIE4a) [Difficulty: ELE: R, Ap; WRE: An]

If the blood sampling equipment preparation, the sampling procedure, and blood gas analyzer operation were all done properly, the respiratory therapist and physician can believe that the blood gas results are accurate and reliable. However, if there was a problem with any aspect of obtaining and analyzing the blood gas sample, that sample must be discarded and a new sample obtained and analyzed.

In the critically ill patient, it is just as important to measure the mixed venous blood gases as it is to measure the ABGs. The venous blood gas values reveal what has happened as the arterial blood has passed through the body. Oxygen has been extracted, and carbon dioxide has been added to the blood. The difference between the arterial and venous oxygen levels reflects oxygen consumption by the body as well as cardiac output.

Because of this, the most critical venous blood gas values to measure are the $S\bar{v}O_2$ and $P\bar{v}O_2$. It is generally accepted that a $P\bar{v}O_2$ value of less than 30 torr or an $S\bar{v}O_2$ value of less than 56% indicates that the patient has tissue hypoxia. Both values can be obtained by analyzing a mixed venous blood sample taken through a pulmonary artery catheter. If the patient has a fiberoptic catheter, the $S\bar{v}O_2$ value can be monitored continuously. This is extremely helpful if the patient is unstable or having frequent changes in inspired oxygen or ventilator settings. (Pulmonary artery catheters are discussed in more detail in Chapter 5.)

5. Arterialized capillary blood gases

a. Review the patient's chart for arterialized capillary blood gas results (Code: IA5) [Difficulty: ELE: R; WRE: Ap]

This method of obtaining a blood gas sample is limited to neonatal patients when an arterial sample cannot be obtained.

b. Interpret the results of capillary blood gas analysis to evaluate the patient's response to respiratory care (Code: IB10g and IIIE4a) [Difficulty: ELE: R, Ap; WRE: An]

If the blood sampling equipment preparation, the sampling procedure, and blood gas analyzer operation were all done properly, the respiratory therapist and physician can believe that the blood gas results are accurate and reliable. However, if there was a problem with any aspect of obtaining and analyzing the blood gas sample, that sample must be discarded and a new sample obtained and analyzed.

Because this is not a true ABG sample, the following limitations are placed on interpreting the results.
- The capillary pH (c pH) value has a good correlation with the arterial pH value.
- The capillary CO_2 ($PcCO_2$) value correlates with the $PaCO_2$ value about 50% of the time.
- The capillary O_2 (PCO_2) value does not correlate well with the PaO_2 value.

Based on these limitations, an arterialized capillary blood pH value can be clinically useful. The capillary CO_2 value should be viewed with suspicion. It should not be the only parameter monitored to judge the infant's ability to ventilate; however, the combination of a low pH and elevated CO_2 value indicates hypoventilation. Evaluate the infant's vital signs, breathing efforts, chest radiograph, and so on to determine respiratory status.

Unfortunately, the capillary O_2 value is practically useless for judging the infant's oxygenation. Some infants may have a fairly close correlation with the PaO_2 level, whereas others do not. No way is known to predetermine those that will match and those that will not. Many practitioners view a low capillary oxygen level as a sign of clinical hypoxemia. The American Association for Respiratory Care (AARC) Clinical Practice Guideline Oxygen Therapy in the Acute Care Hospital notes that a PCO_2 level of less than 40 torr documents neonatal hypoxemia. An ABG sample remains the best way to determine the patient's respiratory status.

MODULE E
Pulse oximetry

1. Check the patient's chart for previous pulse oximetry results (Code: IA7e) [Difficulty: ELE: R; WRE: Ap]

Pulse oximetry (SpO_2) spectroscopically analyzes arterial blood to noninvasively determine the percentage of hemoglobin that is saturated with oxygen. It generally is indicated whenever a patient's oxygenation must be monitored. An SpO_2 value of 92% or greater indicates that the patient is adequately oxygenated. Past values should be compared with current readings to monitor the patient's progress or response to treatment.

2. Make a recommendation to perform pulse oximetry (Code: IC8) [Difficulty: ELE: R, Ap; WRE: An]

Pulse oximetry is indicated in the following situations: during anesthesia and intraoperative monitoring of oxygenation, postoperatively when the patient is still sedated, when the patient is receiving sedatives or analgesics that can blunt the airway protective reflexes, during bronchoscopy, during a sleep study, and for evaluating the effectiveness of oxygen therapy. An exception to the use of first-generation pulse oximetry is when there is known or suspected carbon monoxide poisoning.

3. Manipulate a pulse oximeter by order or protocol (ELE code: IIA22) [Difficulty: ELE: R, Ap, An]

a. Get an appropriate pulse oximeter and related equipment

Each pulse oximeter reports a percentage of hemoglobin saturation with oxygen (SpO_2). This information and the patient's heart rate are displayed on a light-emitting diode (LED). More expensive units store the information in memory and/or print out a copy of the SpO₂ percentage and pulse rate to be placed into the patient's chart if it is required. A variety of sensors fit the feet or hands of infants, an adult's fingers, the bridge of the nose, the forehead, and the earlobe. Choose a sensor designed to fit the site that is selected.

In most patient care situations a first-generation pulse oximeter can be used. They are readily available and inexpensive to operate. A second-generation pulse oximeter will be needed if a patient is known to have carbon monoxide poisoning and continuous monitoring is required (for example, a Masimo Rad-57 [Irvine, CA] or Rainbow SET). Second-generation pulse oximeters can identify all types of normal and abnormal hemoglobin. However, because of their relative newness and expense, they may not be widely available.

b. Put the equipment together and make sure that it works properly

Follow the manufacturer's suggestions for setup. The newer pulse oximetry systems visually display the strength of the pulse so that the best place for the probe can be found (Figure 3-13). Keep bright light away from the patient site and transducer. Figure 3-14 shows how to apply the finger probe properly.

c. Troubleshoot any problems with the equipment

The pulse signal will not be strong if the patient has poor circulation at the site of the oximeter probe. This can occur if the patient is hypothermic, hypotensive, or receiving a vasoconstricting medication. If the pulse signal is

weak, the pulse oximetry values may not be accurate. See Table 3-12 for common sources of error and their solutions.

4. Perform pulse oximetry on your patient (Code: IB9c and IIIE3b) [Difficulty: ELE: R; WRE: Ap, An]

First-generation pulse oximetry has gained wide acceptance because it offers a way to monitor continuously and noninvasively a patient's oxygenation by following the percentage of hemoglobin saturated with oxygen. The reported SpO₂% is the percentage of oxyhemoglobin.

Pulse oximetry makes practical use of two physical principles. The first is spectrophotometry, which is used to analyze the transmission of wavelengths of light through the blood and body tissues. First-generation pulse oximeters analyze two wavelengths of light. One wavelength is 660 nm, and the other is between 920 and 940 nm, depending on the manufacturer. The 660-nm wavelength can be seen as red and is preferentially absorbed by oxyhemoglobin (O₂Hb). The 920- to 940-nm wavelength is not visible, because it is in the infrared range. It is preferentially absorbed by reduced hemoglobin (RHb). Second-generation pulse oximeters analyze several more wavelengths of light and can evaluate different forms of hemoglobin.

The second principle is plethysmography. It is used to find and then evaluate the amplitude of the arterial pulse waveform. See Figure 3-13 for the plethysmographic arterial waveform. When the pulse oximeter sensor is placed on a patient site, the fingertip for example, the two wavelengths of light shine through the blood, tissues, and bone within the finger. It is important that the sending LED and receiving (photodiode) sensors be opposite each other (see Figure 3-14). Most units have a signal strength display that indicates when the photodiode is receiving a strong signal, and the patient's pulse has been detected. The microprocessor is designed to detect a baseline level of light absorption by the tissues and venous blood,

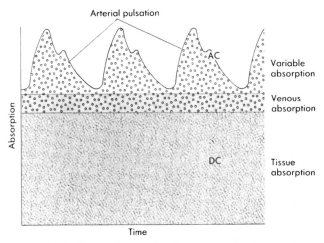

Figure 3-13 Pulse oximetry signal strength. The strong surge of blood through the artery with each heartbeat results in variable absorption of the light emitted by the pulse oximeter. Venous and tissue absorption of light is stable when the heart is at rest. This absorption difference is used to find the patient's artery and measure the heart rate. (*AC,* Variable absorption; *DC,* stable absorption.). *(From Ruppel GL: Manual of pulmonary function testing, ed 9, St Louis, 2009, Mosby.)*

Figure 3-14 Pulse oximetry transducer properly placed on a finger. Fold the OXISENSOR over the end of the digit. Align the other end of the OXISENSOR so that the two alignment marks are directly opposite each other. Press the OXISENSOR onto the skin. Wrap the adhesive flaps around the digit. *(Reprinted with permission of Nellcor Puritan Bennett Inc., Pleasanton, Calif.)*

TABLE 3-12   Sources of Error in Pulse Oximetry

Sources of Error	Remedy
Light interference: xenon lamp, fluorescent light, infrared (bilirubin) light; probe fell off of patient	Cover the probe with an opaque wrap; put the probe back in place on the patient
Low perfusion: low blood pressure, hypothermia, vasoconstricting drugs	Use earlobe, bridge of nose, or forehead instead of finger or toe; discontinue use if still unreliable
Motion artifact	Secure the probe site; ensure that the SpO_2* reading is synchronized with the heart rate
Darkly pigmented patient	Use lightly pigmented site such as tip of finger or toe; SpO_2 value may overestimate PaO_2; discontinue use if still unreliable
Artificial or painted fingernails	Remove acrylic nails; remove black, blue, green, metallic, or frosted nail polish; use a different site
Venous pulsation being read as an arterial pulsation	Loosen a tight sensor; change the finger sensor site every 2-4 hr; loosen the cause of a tourniquet-like effect
The following vascular dyes will cause low SpO_2 readings: methylene blue, indigo carmine, indocyanine green	Do not use SpO_2

PaO_2, partial pressure of O_2 in arterial blood; SpO_2, pulse oximeter.

containing more RHb, as well as the light absorption of arterial blood, containing more O_2Hb. It can then compare the absorptions of the two wavelengths to determine the level of saturated oxyhemoglobin. This is displayed as saturation by pulse oximetry, or SpO_2.

It must be realized that because first-generation pulse oximetry samples only two wavelengths of light, the technology is unable to recognize the presence or quantity of the nonfunctional hemoglobin species of COHb and MetHb. Instead, an ABG sample should be drawn and sent to the laboratory to be passed through a CO-oximeter for a complete fractional hemoglobin analysis. Even healthy persons have small amounts of COHb and MetHB. For this and other technical reasons, manufacturers report the following SpO_2 values for general accuracy at 1 standard deviation (SD) for a general population: ±2% from 100% to 70% saturation, and ±3% from 70% to 50% saturation. Because of these limitations, the following clinical guidelines have been created by a number of authors.

- Do not use pulse oximetry on patients with significant levels of COHb or MetHB.
- If in doubt about abnormal types of hemoglobin, analyze an ABG through a CO-oximeter and compare the true SaO_2 with the SpO_2 from pulse oximetry. Pulse oximetry can be used if the correlation of values is within 4%.
- Question the SpO_2 value when the displayed heart rate is different from the actual heart rate.
- Do not use pulse oximetry when the SpO_2 reading is less than 70%.
- Pulse oximetry can be used on a term neonate or a neonate who weighs 1500 g or more. Smaller neonates should have oxygenation measured by a transcutaneous oxygen monitor. This is because it is too easy to hyperoxygenate a small neonate when small changes in saturation can result in wide swings in PO_2 level. The risk of retinopathy of prematurity (formerly called retrolental fibroplasia) from hyperoxia is too great in the small neonate.

The second-generation pulse oximeters (Masimo Rad-57 or Rainbow SET) analyze 7 to 12 wavelengths of light. Because of this, they can identify and measure the various normal and abnormal types of hemoglobin, such as carboxyhemoglobin (SpCO) from carbon monoxide poisoning and methemoglobin (SpMet) from nitric oxide therapy. These units provide the opportunity to continuously monitor patients with elevated levels of carboxyhemoglobin and methemoglobin as they are being treated. It may not be necessary to draw as many arterial blood gas samples for analysis through a CO-oximeter. If necessary, review the discussion on CO-oximeters and see Figure 3-10 since the principles apply to second-generation pulse oximeters.

Table 3-13 lists common clinical ranges for SpO_2 values. For the aforementioned reasons, with first-generation pulse oximeters the minimum safe values are 2% higher than the corresponding SaO_2 value by CO-oximetry. It is important that the patient have good pulsatile blood flow to the measurement site to obtain an accurate reading.

5. Interpret a patient's pulse oximetry value (Code: IB10c and IIIE4d) [Difficulty: ELE: R, Ap; WRE: An]

The previously healthy patient who has cardiopulmonary failure should have the SpO_2 value kept at 92% or greater to ensure adequate oxygenation. The patient with chronic obstructive pulmonary disease (COPD) can probably tolerate an SpO_2 value as low as 87%. In general, a neonate should have the SpO_2 level kept between 92% and 96%. See Table 3-13 for more specific guidelines. Saturations below these values indicate hypoxemia in most patients.

| TABLE 3-13 | Recommended Clinical Ranges for True Values in Saturation of O_2 in the Hemoglobin (SaO_2), Values in Pulse Oximetry (SpO_2),* and Their Correlation with Values in Partial Pressure of O_2 in Arterial Blood (PaO_2) |

| | Approximate | | |
	SaO_2	SpO_2	PaO_2 (torr)
ADULT			
Acute hypoxemia	90-95%	92-95%[†]	60-95
Chronic hypoxemia	85-90%	87-92%	50-60
NEONATE[‡]			
<1500 g or in the first week of life	About 97%	92-96%	60-70
>1500 g or after the first week of life	90-96%	90-96%	50-70
>1 month of age with chronic lung disease	85-90%	87-92%	50-60

*Based on the patient having normal carboxyhemoglobin and methemoglobin levels. Elevated levels result in an erroneously high SpO_2 reading and unsuspected hypoxemia.

[†]Black patients should have an SpO_2 of 95% maintained to ensure adequate oxygenation.

[‡]Note: The clinical goal with most neonates is to prevent both hypoxemia, defined as a PaO_2 <45 torr, and hyperoxemia, defined as a PaO_2 >90 torr.

Note the site at which the saturation was measured. This is especially important in neonates who may have congenital heart defects. A higher saturation in the right fingers or right earlobe compared with the rest of the body is seen in a neonate who has patent ductus arteriosus (PDA). A higher saturation in the fingers and earlobes as compared with the toes is seen in a neonate who has coarctation of the aorta.

Exam Hint 3-12 (ELE, WRE)

The patient with carbon monoxide poisoning should *not* be evaluated with a first-generation pulse oximeter because the units are unable to distinguish functional oxyhemoglobin from nonfunctional carboxyhemoglobin. These pulse oximeters show the level of only functional O_2Hb. Use only a CO-oximeter blood gas analyzer on a patient with known or suspected CO poisoning. Clinical examples include a patient removed from an enclosed house fire or a patient removed from a car with the engine running.

Second-generation pulse oximeters can measure and display both functional hemoglobin (SpO_2) and nonfunctional hemoglobin (SpCO and SpMet). They can be used to monitor patients with carbon monoxide poisoning.

Exam Hint 3-13 (WRE)

Usually a question is related to an inaccurately low pulse oximeter reading caused by poor local perfusion. See Table 3-12 for this and other examples of causes of inaccurate readings.

MODULE F
Transcutaneous oxygen monitoring

NOTE: Transcutaneous monitoring (TCM) involves the continuous monitoring of oxygen, carbon dioxide, or both as they diffuse through the skin. Each gas has its own individual electrode, and a combined electrode exists for both gases.

1. Review the patient's chart for a transcutaneous oxygen ($PtcO_2$) value (Code: IA7e) [Difficulty: ELE: R; WRE: Ap]

Transcutaneous oxygen monitoring ($PtcO_2$, $tcPO_2$, or TcO_2) enables any patient's oxygenation status to be followed on a continuous basis. In practice, neonates are monitored much more often than adults. Check the chart for a record of the patient's transcutaneous oxygen values. It is particularly important to compare the PaO_2 value with the $PtcO_2$ value. In addition, note what the $PtcO_2$ values are when the inspired oxygen is changed, the patient's airway is suctioned, or changes are made in continuous positive airway pressure (CPAP) or mechanical ventilation. Avoid clinical situations that have previously resulted in hypoxemia.

2. Recommend transcutaneous oxygen monitoring for additional data (Code: IC8) [Difficulty: ELE: R, Ap; WRE: An]

$PtcO_2$ monitoring has been used for the following purposes:
- To monitor oxygenation during transportation of an unstable neonate within the hospital or between two hospitals
- To monitor intraoperative and postoperative oxygenation
- To monitor oxygenation during changes in the inspired oxygen and during changes in mechanical ventilation, and to detect hypoxemia during an equipment failure
- To help detect a right-to-left shunt. When a neonate has a patent ductus arteriosus (PDA), the $PtcO_2$ level is higher in the right upper chest than in the left upper chest, abdomen, or thighs.
- To help detect a coarctation of the aorta. When this defect is present, the $PtcO_2$ value is higher in the right and left upper chest than in the abdomen or thighs.
- To determine the response to an oxygen challenge test by a patient with congenital heart disease

3. Manipulate a transcutaneous oxygen monitor by order or protocol (ELE code: IIA22) [Difficulty: ELE: R, Ap, An]

a. Get the necessary equipment to perform transcutaneous oxygen monitoring

The electrode used for monitoring the patient's transcutaneous oxygen level is a miniaturized and modified Clark-type polarographic electrode similar to that used in the blood gas analyzer (Figure 3-15). Some authors describe it as a Huch or Hellige electrode, named after two researchers who modified the original Clark electrode for their work with pediatric patients.

b. Put the transcutaneous oxygen monitor together and make sure that it works properly

Always follow the manufacturer's recommendations for the assembly and care of the equipment. Select the proper electrode for the monitor based on the physician's order for evaluating transcutaneous oxygen, carbon dioxide, or both together.

c. Troubleshoot any problems with the equipment

Problems usually associated with too much electrode drift include electrode or membrane surfaces contaminated by debris such as blood or sweat, an improperly applied membrane, a worn-out membrane, an air bubble beneath the membrane, improper gas exposed to the membrane during the calibration, exhausted electrolyte solution

Figure 3-15 Schematic drawing of the modified Clark electrode used to monitor transcutaneous oxygen tension. *1*, O-ring to hold the membrane to the electrode; *2*, polypropylene membrane permeable to oxygen; *3*, silver anode that surrounds the platinum cathode; *4*, electrolyte chamber with solution held in place by the polypropylene membrane; *5*, heating element; *6*, platinum cathode; *7*, electrolyte solution of sodium bicarbonate and sodium chloride held between the membrane and electrode; and *8*, negative temperature coefficient (NTC) resistor that serves to regulate the temperature of the sensor. *(From Shapiro BA, Peruzzi WT, Kozlowski-Templin R: Clinical application of blood gases, ed 5, St Louis, 1994, Mosby.)*

in the electrode, or inaccurate calibration values. After correcting a problem, the calibration procedure should be repeated.

4. Perform quality control procedures on a transcutaneous oxygen monitor (Code: IIC7) [Difficulty: ELE: R, Ap; WRE: An]

Always follow the manufacturer's recommendations for the assembly and care of the equipment. Select the proper electrode for the monitor based on the physician's order for evaluating transcutaneous oxygen, carbon dioxide, or both together.

a. Calibration

Two-point calibration must be performed with oxygen percentages that will cause PO_2 values beyond the clinical range that can be expected. Usually the first calibration point is a "zero" point because the electrode is exposed to no oxygen in a nitrogen-filled chamber. This point is usually quite stable. The second calibration point is found when the electrode is exposed to room air (20.95% or 0.2095 oxygen). Always follow the manufacturer's written procedures during the calibration process. Generally, when environmental conditions include a fairly stable room temperature of 25° C and 50% relative humidity, the following equation can be used to predict the room air calibration point:

$$\text{Calibration } Ptc_{O_2} = P_B \times 0.2095$$

in which P_B is the local barometric pressure and 0.2095 is the oxygen fraction found in room air. Expose the electrode to room air to determine whether it matches the calculated calibration value. Adjust the instrument to match the calibration Ptc_{O_2} if necessary. It is recommended that the room air calibration point be rechecked every 24 hours when in continuous use, after changing the membrane, or after changing the electrolyte solution. A variation of up to ±5 torr is acceptable and can be corrected by adjusting the reading on the instrument. If the variation is greater than ±5 torr, the zero point and room air calibration procedures should be repeated.

5. Perform transcutaneous oxygen (PtcO₂) monitoring (Code: IB9b) [Difficulty: ELE: R, Ap; WRE: An]

a. Site selection

Care must be taken to select the best site for the electrode. A bad site will give incorrect information that can lead to mistakes in patient care. See Box 3-2 for a listing of site selection guidelines.

b. Skin and electrode preparation and application of the skin electrode

An airtight seal between the skin and electrode is necessary for accurate readings. An air leak (21% oxygen) will

---

BOX 3-2 Optimal Sites and Sites to Avoid with Transcutaneous Gas Monitoring

OPTIMAL NEONATAL SITES
Upper part of the chest
Right upper chest if a preductal $PtcO_2$ value is desired
Abdomen
Inner aspect of either thigh

OPTIMAL ADULT SITES
Upper part of the chest
Inner aspect of the upper arm

SITES TO AVOID
Large fat deposit
Bony prominence
Pressure point
Thick skin
Skin edema
Hands and feet

CONDITIONS IN WHICH TRANSCUTANEOUS MONITORING SHOULD NOT BE USED
Locally cold skin or general, deep hypothermia
Locally decreased peripheral perfusion or general hypotension
Patient receiving vasoconstricting drugs such as tolazoline or dopamine
Cardiac index less than 1.9 $L/min/m^2$ of body surface area
Halothane anesthesia will give erroneously high transcutaneous O_2 values unless a Teflon membrane is used.

$PtcO_2$, Pressure of transcutaneous oxygen.

falsely increase or decrease the $PtcO_2$ reading from the patient's actual value. A room air leak will always cause a decrease in the $PtcCO_2$ reading. The following steps should be taken to ensure that the skin site and electrode are prepared and an airtight seal is ensured:

1. Clean the skin. Usually, cleaning with an alcohol swab is enough to remove perspiration. Oily skin should be cleaned with soap and water.
2. Adults may need to have hair shaved from the site.
3. Adults may have dead skin cells removed by placing sticky adhesive tape against the site and pulling it off.
4. Prepare the electrode according to the manufacturer's guidelines. This usually includes placing a drop of the electrolyte solution on the electrode surface and placing a gas-permeable membrane with a double adhesive ring over the electrode.
5. The other side of the adhesive ring is pressed against the monitoring site to form an airtight seal.
6. As the electrode warms the skin, the patient values will fluctuate. Stabilization usually requires several

minutes, after which the patient values should be clinically useful.

c. Limitations and patient precautions

Because the electrode is heated, it must be rotated to a different skin site on a routine basis. The general manufacturer's guidelines for site rotation are every 4 to 6 hours for neonates weighing between 1000 and 2500 g; every 3 to 5 hours for neonates weighing between 2500 and 3500 g; and 2 to 4 hours for neonates weighing more than 3500 g, pediatric patients, and adult patients. As a safety precaution, change the electrode on all patients at least every 4 hours, or at least every 3 hours if the patient is hypothermic. The manufacturer's range in times is based on the relative thickness of the patient's skin and the different electrode temperatures. It is important to adjust the site-rotation times on an individual patient basis. Some may tolerate longer times, and others will need more frequent rotations.

Care must be taken when removing the adhesive ring and electrode. It is possible to tear the thin, delicate skin of a premature neonate. Loosen the adhesive by running the edge of an alcohol wipe along the side that is being gently pulled up. After the electrode is removed, it is important to examine the skin; it is normal to see a red circle. This warmed, vasodilated area will stay red for some time and will gradually fade away, with no scarring or permanent injury. Rarely, the skin will have overheated and a blister is seen; this is a second-degree burn. Obviously, future site rotations must be made more frequently. Do not use this site again. Treat it as a burn, and avoid any further injury that might break the skin and lead to an infection.

6. Interpret transcutaneous oxygen monitoring values to evaluate the patient's response to respiratory care (Code: IB10b) [Difficulty: ELE: R, Ap; WRE: An]

It has been found that heating the electrode speeds the diffusion of oxygen through the skin. Heating also provides a closer correlation with the patient's PaO_2 value. However, it must be remembered that the $PtcO_2$ value is not the same as the PaO_2 value. Current recommendations are that any unit should give $PtcO_2$ values that are within $\pm 15\%$ of the PaO_2 values over the operating range of the instrument. The values should then correlate within $\pm 15\%$ as the patient's condition changes. This should always be confirmed.

An arterial blood gas sample should be drawn for PaO_2 every time transcutaneous oxygen monitoring is started. The PaO_2-$PtcO_2$ gradient can then be calculated as the difference between the two. For example, if the patient's PaO_2 value is 100 torr, the $PtcO_2$ value should be no less than

85 torr. If the $Ptco_2$ level decreases to 70 torr, the PaO_2 level should have decreased to no lower than 85 torr. Because of this close correlation, the patient's trend can be monitored with some assurance of accuracy. In addition, ABG samples do not need to be drawn as frequently for the PaO_2 measurement. This trending relation holds true for changes in the patient's pulmonary condition. It does not, however, hold true when the patient has cardiovascular problems such as hypotension, hypothermia, peripheral vascular disease, or cardiogenic shock with decreased tissue perfusion.

Always follow the manufacturer's recommendations for the proper electrode temperature. In general, the temperature ranges from 42.5° C for a 1000-g infant to 44° C for a 3500-g infant. A pediatric patient can tolerate a temperature of 44° C, whereas an adult can have an electrode temperature of 45° C. The higher temperatures are needed in older patients because their skin is thicker. Studies have shown that when the neonate's PaO_2 level is greater than 100 torr, the $PtcO_2$ value underestimates it. This can lead to dangerous hyperoxemia. For this reason, it is recommended that the $PtcO_2$ level be kept at less than 90 torr. In the adult, less correlation is found between the PaO_2 and $PtcO_2$ values because of the thicker skin found in adults. The $PtcO_2$ value can still be used in the adult to follow trends in oxygenation, but the practitioner must realize that a decrease in the $PtcO_2$ value can be a result of hypoxemia, a decreased cardiac output, or cutaneous vasoconstriction. An arterial blood gas sample must be drawn to further evaluate the patient's status.

a. Correlation of $PtcO_2$ and local power consumption

As mentioned previously, the electrode is heated to above body temperature. The amount of electrical current needed to keep the electrode at a constant temperature depends on the temperature of the blood and the speed at which the blood passes beneath the electrode. This is known as local power consumption or simply local power (LP). A change in the LP value and $PtcO_2$ value can be used to indicate what is happening to the patient. For example:

- A normal LP seen with a decreased $PtcO_2$ value indicates that the patient's pulmonary problem has worsened.
- A normal LP seen with an increased $PtcO_2$ value indicates that the patient's pulmonary problem has improved.
- A decreased LP seen with a decreased $PtcO_2$ value indicates that the patient's cardiac output has worsened.
- An increased LP seen with an increased $PtcO_2$ value indicates that the patient's cardiac output has improved.

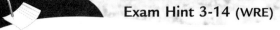

Exam Hint 3-14 (WRE)

If a sick neonate has normal cardiovascular status, the PaO_2 and $PtcO_2$ values should correlate with each other (but not be identical) as the patient's pulmonary condition changes. For example, the neonate has infant respiratory distress syndrome. The PaO_2 and $PtcO_2$ values probably will not correlate when the patient has cardiovascular problems. For example, the neonate is hypotensive with low cardiac output.

MODULE G
Transcutaneous carbon dioxide monitoring

1. Review the patient's chart for a transcutaneous carbon dioxide value (Code: IA7e) [Difficulty: ELE: R; WRE: Ap]

Transcutaneous carbon dioxide monitoring ($PtcCO_2$, $tcPCO_2$, or $TcCO_2$) enables any patient's ventilation status to be monitored on a continuous basis. In practice, neonates are monitored much more often than adults. Check the chart for a record of the patient's transcutaneous carbon dioxide values. It is particularly important to correlate these values with any ABG values, which allows comparison between the $PaCO_2$ and the $PtcCO_2$ measurements. In addition, note the $PtcCO_2$ values when changes are made in CPAP or mechanical ventilation. Avoid clinical situations that have previously resulted in hypoventilation.

2. Recommend transcutaneous carbon dioxide monitoring for additional data (Code: IC8) [Difficulty: ELE: R, Ap; WRE: An]

$PtcCO_2$ monitoring has been used for the following purposes:
- To monitor ventilation during transportation of an unstable infant within the hospital or between two hospitals
- To monitor intraoperative and postoperative ventilation
- To monitor ventilation during changes in mechanical ventilation such as tidal volume, rate, minute ventilation, mechanical dead space, or a combination of these
- To detect hypoventilation during an accidental disconnection from the ventilator

3. Manipulate a transcutaneous carbon dioxide monitor by order or protocol (ELE code: IIA22) [Difficulty: ELE: R, Ap, An]

a. Get the necessary equipment to perform transcutaneous carbon dioxide monitoring

The electrode used for monitoring the patient's transcutaneous carbon dioxide level is a miniaturized and

Figure 3-16 Schematic drawing of the modified Stow-Severinghaus electrode used to monitor transcutaneous carbon dioxide tension. *1*, Epoxy resin; *2*, glass electrode with a chlorinated silver wire, a buffer solution (the inner liquid), and a pH-sensitive glass membrane; *3*, negative temperature coefficient (NTC) resistor that serves to regulate the temperature of the sensor; *4*, O-ring to hold the membrane to the electrode; *5*, electrolyte chamber with solution held in place by the polypropylene membrane; *6*, electrolyte solution of sodium bicarbonate and sodium chloride held between the membrane and electrode; *7*, polypropylene membrane permeable to carbon dioxide; *8*, heating element; and *9*, silver/silver chloride reference electrode. *(From Shapiro BA, Peruzzi WT, Kozlowski-Templin R: Clinical application of blood gases, ed 5, St Louis, 1994, Mosby.)*

modified Stow-Severinghaus–type electrode similar to the ABG electrode (Figure 3-16).

b. Put the transcutaneous carbon dioxide monitor together and make sure that it works properly

Always follow the manufacturer's recommendations for the assembly and care of the equipment. Select the proper electrode for the monitor based on the physician's order for evaluating transcutaneous carbon dioxide.

c. Troubleshoot any problems with the equipment

Problems usually associated with too much electrode drift include electrode or membrane surfaces contaminated by debris such as blood or sweat, an improperly applied membrane, a worn-out membrane, an air bubble beneath the membrane, improper gas sample exposed to the membrane during the calibration, exhausted electrolyte solution in the electrode, or inaccurate calibration values. After correcting a problem, the calibration procedure should be repeated.

4. Perform quality control procedures on a transcutaneous carbon dioxide monitor (Code: IIC7) [Difficulty: ELE: R, Ap; WRE: An]

Two-point calibration must be performed with carbon dioxide percentages that cause PCO_2 values beyond the

expected clinical range. Usually the electrode is exposed to 5% and 10% carbon dioxide from prepared cylinders. Always follow the manufacturer's written procedures during the calibration process. Generally, when environmental conditions include a fairly stable room temperature of 25°C and 50% relative humidity, the following equation can be used to predict the two calibration points:

$$\text{Calibration } PtcCO_2 = (P_B \times CO_2\% \text{ used}) - (XCO_2 \times \text{electrode temperature factor})$$

in which P_B is the local barometric pressure; $CO_2\%$ is the carbon dioxide fraction exposed to the electrode, either 10% (0.10) or 5% (0.05); and XCO_2 is the correction factor used to equilibrate the $PtcCO_2$ to $PaCO_2$. (This is discussed later.)

a. Electrode temperature factor

This is a factor determined by the manufacturer based on the electrode temperature. It is usually heated to 44° C.

Expose the electrode to 10% carbon dioxide in a sealed chamber to determine whether it matches the calculated calibration value. Adjust the instrument to match the calibration $PtcCO_2$ if necessary. Next, expose the electrode to 5% carbon dioxide in the sealed chamber. Again, adjust the instrument to match the calibration $PtcCO_2$ if necessary. It is recommended that the two-point calibration points be rechecked every 24 hours when in continuous use, after changing the membrane, or after changing the electrolyte solution. A variation of up to ±4 torr is acceptable and can be corrected by adjusting the reading on the instrument. If the variation is greater than ±4 torr, the two-point calibration procedures should be repeated.

5. Perform transcutaneous carbon dioxide ($PtcCO_2$) monitoring (Code: IB9b) [Difficulty: ELE: R, Ap; WRE: An]

The information on skin-site selection and so forth presented in the preceding discussion of transcutaneous oxygen monitors applies here, as well. As with the transcutaneous oxygen electrode, it has been found that heating the $PtcCO_2$ electrode speeds the diffusion of carbon dioxide through the skin. Always follow the manufacturer's recommendations for the proper electrode temperature. In general, the temperature is 44° C in both neonates and adults. It must be remembered that the $PtcCO_2$ value is not the same as the $PaCO_2$ value. An arterial blood gas sample should be analyzed for $PaCO_2$ value every time transcutaneous carbon dioxide monitoring is started. Unlike transcutaneous oxygen monitoring, the correlation between $PaCO_2$ and $PtcCO_2$ values is as good in adult patients as in neonatal patients. In addition, it is not as easily influenced by changes in the patient's skin blood flow.

6. Interpret transcutaneous carbon dioxide monitoring values to evaluate the patient's response to respiratory care (Code: IB10b) [Difficulty: ELE: R, Ap; WRE: An]

The net effect of heating the carbon dioxide electrode and skin results in the $PtcCO_2$ readings being 1.2 to 2 times (120% to 200%) greater than the $PaCO_2$ values. Commonly, an average multiplier of 1.6 is found. The actual value varies among patients and can be found by dividing the $PtcCO_2$ value by the $PaCO_2$ value.

For example, a patient has a $PaCO_2$ level of 40 torr and a $PtcCO_2$ level of 64 torr. Calculate the gradient between the arterial and transcutaneous values:

$$\text{Gradient} = \frac{PtcCO_2}{PaCO_2} = \frac{64}{40} = 1.6$$

As long as the patient's cardiovascular status is fairly stable, the $PaCO_2$ value can be calculated by dividing the $PtcCO_2$ value by 1.6. For example, if the patient's $PtcCO_2$ value increases to 80 torr, calculate the $PaCO_2$ value in the following manner:

$$PaCO_2 = \frac{PtcCO_2}{1.6} = \frac{80}{1.6} = 50 \text{ torr}$$

Rather than perform these calculations every time a change occurs in the patient's status, some practitioners divide the CO_2 values found during the calibration procedure by 1.6. This results in "real" $PaCO_2$ values being given continuously on the monitor. This change must be clearly communicated to all staff members to avoid confusion between the original $PtcCO_2$ values and values that have been reduced to "arterialize" them.

MODULE H
Respiratory care plan

1. Analyze available information to determine the patient's pathophysiologic state (Code: IIIH1) [Difficulty: ELE: R, Ap; WRE: An]

Many patients with pneumonia or other pulmonary conditions will have significant hypoxemia despite receiving supplemental oxygen. The alveolar-arterial oxygen pressure difference [$P(A-a)O_2$] can be used to help determine what might be causing the hypoxemia.

2. Difference between the alveolar oxygen level and the arterial oxygen level

a. Calculate the difference between the alveolar oxygen level and the arterial oxygen level (ELE code: IB9i) [Difference: ELE: R, Ap]

This gap between the alveolar oxygen level and the arterial oxygen level is called the alveolar-arterial oxygen pressure difference [$P(A-a)O_2$]. Measurement of this gap or difference gives an important indication of the seriousness of the patient's condition.

Perform the following to determine the alveolar-arterial O_2 pressure difference [$P(A-a)O_2$]:
1. Note the patient's inspired oxygen percentage.
2. Draw and analyze an ABG sample. Note the patient's PaO_2 and $PaCO_2$ values.
3. Note the patient's temperature. This is needed to determine the patient's pulmonary water vapor pressure (PH_2O). The value of 47 torr (mm Hg) is used if the patient's temperature is normal. Check published tables for the pulmonary water vapor pressure if the patient's temperature is higher or lower than normal.
4. Measure the local barometric pressure (P_B) in torr (mm Hg).
5. If possible, calculate the patient's respiratory exchange ratio. If this cannot be done, use the standard value of 0.8.
6. Calculate the patient's PAO_2 value. The formula presented here is the most commonly used of several versions:

$$PAO_2 = [(P_B - PH_2O)F_IO_2] - \frac{PaCO_2}{0.8}$$

In which:
- PAO_2 is the pressure of alveolar oxygen.
- P_B is the barometric pressure of air. This is 760 torr (mm Hg) at sea level; it decreases as the altitude increases.
- PH_2O is the pressure of water vapor in the lungs. This is 47 torr (mm Hg) at the normal temperature of 98.6° F/37° C. Remember that water vapor pressure increases if the patient has a fever and decreases if the patient is hypothermic.
- FIO_2 is the fractional concentration (percentage) of inspired oxygen. Use whatever percentage of oxygen your patient is inhaling:

$$\frac{PaCO_2}{0.8} = \text{effect of carbon dioxide and the patient's metabolism}$$

The factor of 0.8 is based on how much oxygen a normal person uses in 1 minute and how much carbon dioxide is produced in 1 minute. The symbols for this metabolic value are *R* for respiratory exchange ratio and

RQ for respiratory quotient. The following calculation is based on a normal person's metabolism:

$$R \text{ or } RQ = \frac{\dot{V}_{CO_2}}{\dot{V}_{O_2}} = \frac{200\,mL/min}{250\,mL/min} = 0.8$$

Because many sick patients do not react as expected, the factor has a range of 0.6 to 1.1, depending on oxygen consumption and carbon dioxide production. Assume that the factor is 0.8 unless you are told otherwise or measure otherwise.

7. Subtract the patient's PaO_2 value from the PAO_2 value to determine the $P(A\text{-}a)O_2$.

b. Interpret the results of the P(A-a)O₂ calculation (Code: IB10i) [Difficulty: ELE: R, Ap; WRE: An]

When interpreting the patient's value, remember that the $P(A\text{-}a)O_2$ level in a normal young person should be no greater than 15 torr. The difference slowly increases as a normal person ages (see Figure 3-17). Lung disease causes the value to increase significantly. The following are examples of some conditions in which the measurement of the $P(A\text{-}a)O_2$ level aids in diagnosis or treatment:

- Patients who are hypoxemic because they are hypoventilating (increased CO_2 concentration) have a normal $P(A\text{-}a)O_2$ value when breathing room air. The hypoxemia can be corrected by increasing ventilation. Supplemental oxygen results in an expected increase in PaO_2 level.

- Any condition in which a low ventilation-to-perfusion ratio is found show an elevated $P(A\text{-}a)O_2$ measurement when the patient is breathing room air. Supplemental oxygen results in an increase in PaO_2 level; however, the increase is not as dramatic as that seen in the hypoventilating patient. Examples include asthma, bronchitis, emphysema, or any other condition in which unequal distribution of air into and out of the lungs but relatively normal perfusion is found.

- Any shunt-producing disease or condition. Examples include ARDS and right-to-left anatomic shunt, such as could be seen in a ventricular septal defect. The $P(A\text{-}a)O_2$ value becomes greater as the oxygen percentage is increased. It is commonly accepted that a $P(A\text{-}a)O_2$ value of more than 350 torr, when 80% to 100% oxygen is administered, indicates that the patient is experiencing refractory hypoxemia. The patient probably needs to be supported by a mechanical ventilator. Commonly, positive end-expiratory pressure (PEEP) is administered so that the oxygen percentage can be reduced to a safer level.

- Any disease producing a diffusion defect. Pulmonary fibrosis from any cause results in a wider than normal $P(A\text{-}a)O_2$ range. Supplemental oxygen results in an increase in the PaO_2 level, but not as great an increase as desired.

The following examples are offered to aid in the calculation of $P(A\text{-}a)\,O_2$ and the interpretation of the results.

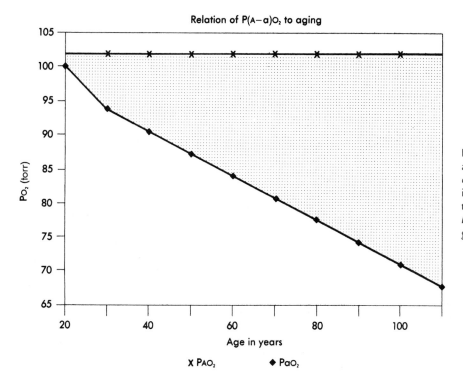

Relation of P(A−a)O₂ to aging

Po₂ (torr) vs *Age in years*

X PAO₂   ◆ PaO₂

Figure 3-17 The relation of $P(A\text{-}a)O_2$ to aging. As the PaO_2 level naturally decreases with age, the $P(A\text{-}a)O_2$ level increases at the rate of approximately 3 torr per decade beyond 20 years. *(From Lane EE, Walker JF: Clinical arterial blood gas analysis, St Louis, 1987, Mosby.)*

EXAMPLE 1

You are working in a major teaching hospital in Miami. The patient's physician asks you to calculate the $P(A-a)O_2$ on a 30-year-old patient. The following conditions exist:

- $P_B = 760$ torr
- $P_{H_2O} = 47$ torr because your patient's temperature is $98.6°\,F/37°\,C$
- $F_IO_2 = 0.21$ because the patient is breathing room air
- $PaCO_2 = 40$ torr from ABGs
- $PaO_2 = 90$ torr from ABGs
- $R = 0.8$

$$PAO_2 = ([P_B - P_{H_2O}]F_IO_2) - PaCO_2/0.8$$

$$PAO_2 = ([760-47]0.21) - 40/0.8$$

$$PAO_2 = ([713]0.21) - 50$$

$$PAO_2 = (150) - 50$$

$$PAO_2 = 100\,torr$$

$$P(A-a)O_2 = 100 - 90 = 10\,torr$$

Interpretation: A $P(A-a)\,O_2$ value of 10 torr is normal for a patient of this age. It is normal to see a difference between the alveolar and arterial oxygen levels that starts in the range of 4 to 12 torr and slowly increases with age (Figure 3-17).

EXAMPLE 2

You are working in a major teaching hospital in Denver. You are asked to calculate the alveolar-arterial difference in oxygen on a 40-year-old patient. The following conditions exist:

- $P_B = 710$ torr
- $P_{H_2O} = 50$ torr because your patient's temperature is $100°\,F/38°\,C$
- $F_IO_2 = 0.35$ because the patient is breathing 35% oxygen by mask
- $PaCO_2 = 55$ torr from ABGs
- $PaO_2 = 65$ torr from ABGs
- $R = 0.85$

$$PAO_2 = ([P_B - P_{H_2O}]F_IO_2) - PaCO_2/0.8$$

$$PAO_2 = ([710-50]0.35) - 55/0.85$$

$$PAO_2 = ([660]0.35) - 65$$

$$PAO_2 = (231) - 65$$

$$PAO_2 = 166\,torr$$

$$P(A-A)O_2 = 166 - 65 = 101\,torr$$

Interpretation: The difference of 101 torr is elevated even though this patient is older than the patient in Example 1.

Exam Hint 3-15 (ELE, WRE)

Performing the above calculation has been tested on previous exams. Know that a widened alveolar-arterial (A-a) gradient indicates pulmonary disease. Diseases that cause true shunt or venous admixture result in a ventilation/perfusion mismatch. Giving supplemental oxygen may have little beneficial effect on the patient's oxygenation.

3. Determine the appropriateness of the prescribed therapy and goals for the identified pathophysiologic state (Code: IIIH3) [Difficulty: ELE: R, Ap; WRE: An]

As part of the patient care team, you may need to evaluate the patient's blood gas values and other parameters to make a recommendation. For example, a patient with carbon monoxide poisoning is best treated by administering 100% oxygen through a nonrebreather mask. Pure oxygen reduces the half-life of COHb to 60 to 90 minutes. A first-generation pulse oximeter should not be used to measure this patient's saturation of oxyhemoglobin. These units are unable to identify COHb and will give misleadingly high saturation values for O_2Hb.

ABG analysis remains the "gold standard" by which all other values are judged. Typically, the arterial sample is analyzed through a standard blood gas analyzer. A CO-oximeter is needed if the patient has carbon monoxide poisoning. Mixed venous and capillary blood-sample analysis is limited in clinical application, but very helpful in the right patient situation. However, these offer only momentary insight into the patient's condition.

Pulse oximetry and transcutaneous oxygen monitoring offer continuous information on the patient's oxygenation status. Transcutaneous carbon dioxide monitoring allows continuous monitoring of the patient's ventilation. As with all technology, these units have advantages, disadvantages, and limitations. It is up to the practitioner to make the correct choices. Some unstable patients can best be monitored through the combination of periodic evaluation of ABGs and these noninvasive continuous monitoring systems.

Exam Hint 3-16 (ELE, WRE)

Be prepared to make a recommendation regarding adjustment of the patient's inspired oxygen based on the PaO_2 (or related) value. Also be prepared to make a recommendation regarding adjustment of the patient's mechanical ventilation settings for tidal volume, rate, minute volume, mechanical dead space, or a combination of these based on the $PaCO_2$ (or related) value.

4. Terminate the procedure if the patient has an adverse reaction to it (Code: IIIF1) [Difficulty: ELE: R, Ap; WRE: An]

The hazards associated with drawing a sample of arterial blood were presented earlier. If a puncture site is not suitable, a different site must be selected. The possible burn hazard of transcutaneous monitoring was presented earlier. If blistering occurs at the probe site, move it to a different site.

5. Recommend discontinuing the procedure based on the patient's response (Code: IIIG1i) [Difficulty: ELE: R, Ap; WRE: An]

If blistering occurs at every transcutaneous monitoring probe site, the patient's skin is likely too sensitive to increased heat. Be prepared to recommend that transcutaneous monitoring be discontinued.

6. Maintain records and communication on the patient's pulse oximetry values (Code: IIIA1b5) [Difficulty: ELE: R, Ap; WRE: An]

Pulse oximetry values and their interpretation were covered earlier.

BIBLIOGRAPHY

Aloan CA, Hill TV, editors: *Respiratory care of the newborn and child*, ed 2, Philadelphia, 1997, Lippincott-Raven.

American Academy of Pediatrics: Task force on transcutaneous oxygen monitors, *Pediatrics* 83(1):122, 1989.

American Association for Respiratory Care: Clinical practice guideline: blood gas analysis and hemoximetry: 2001 revision and update, *Respir Care* 46:498-505, 2001.

American Association for Respiratory Care: Clinical practice guideline: transcutaneous blood gas monitoring for neonatal and pediatric patients: 2004 revision and update, *Respir Care* 49(9):1069-1072, 2004.

American Association for Respiratory Care: Clinical practice guideline: transcutaneous blood gas monitoring for neonatal and pediatric patients, *Respir Care* 39(12):1176, 1994.

American Association for Respiratory Care: Clinical practice guideline: capillary blood gas sampling for neonatal and pediatric patients, *Respir Care* 39(12):1180, 1994.

American Association for Respiratory Care: Clinical practice guideline: oxygen therapy in the acute care hospital, *Respir Care* 36(12):1410, 1991.

American Association for Respiratory Care: Clinical practice guideline: pulse oximetry, *Respir Care* 36(12):1406, 1991.

American Association for Respiratory Care: Clinical practice guideline: sampling for arterial blood gas analysis, *Respir Care* 37(8):913, 1991.

American Association for Respiratory Care: Clinical practice guideline: in-vitro pH and blood gas analysis and hemoximetry, *Respir Care* 38(5):505, 1993.

Barnes TA, editor: *Textbook of respiratory care practice*, ed 2, St Louis, 1994, Mosby.

Blanchette T, Dziodzio J, Harris K: Pulse oximetry and normoximetry in neonatal intensive care, *Respir Care* 36(1):25, 1991.

Bohn DJ: Ask the expert, *Respiratory Tract* 9, Feb 1988.

Branson RD, Hess DR, Chatburn RL, editors: *Respiratory care equipment*, ed 2, Philadelphia, 1999, Lippincott Williams & Wilkins.

Burton GC, Hodgkin JE, Ward JJ, editors: *Respiratory care: a guide to clinical practice*, ed 4, Philadelphia, 1997, Lippincott-Raven.

Cairo JM, Pilbeam SP: *Mosby's respiratory care equipment*, ed 8, St Louis, 2010, Mosby.

Czervinske MP: Arterial blood gas analysis and other cardiopulmonary monitoring. In Koff PB, Daily KE, Schroeder JS, editors: *Techniques in bedside hemodynamic monitoring*, ed 4, St Louis, 1989, Mosby.

Eitzman D, Neu J: *Neonatal and pediatric respiratory care*, ed 2, St Louis, 1993, Mosby.

Elser RC: Quality control of blood gas analysis: a review, *Respir Care* 31(9):807, 1986.

Federal government releases CLIA '88 final regulations, *AARC Times* 16(4):76, 1992.

Fell WL: Sampling and measurement of blood gases. In Lane EE, Walker JF, editors: *Clinical arterial blood gas analysis*, St Louis, 1987, Mosby.

Fink JB, Hunt GE, editors: *Clinical practice in respiratory care*, Philadelphia, 1999, Lippincott-Raven.

Garza D, Becan-McBride K: *Phlebotomy handbook*, ed 4, Stamford, Conn, 1996, Appleton & Lange.

Instrumentation Laboratories: Operator's manual for the IL282 CO-oximeter, Lexington, Mass.

Jubran A, Tobin MJ: Reliability of pulse oximetry in titrating supplemental oxygen therapy in ventilator-dependent patients, *Chest* 97:1420, 1990.

Lane EE, Walker JF: *Clinical arterial blood gas analysis*, St Louis, 1987, Mosby.

Levitzky MG, Cairo JM, Hall SM: *Introduction to respiratory care*, Philadelphia, 1990, WB Saunders.

Madama VC: *Pulmonary function testing and cardiopulmonary stress testing*, ed 2, Albany, NY, 1998, Delmar.

Mahoney JJ, Hodgkin JE, Van Kessel AL: Arterial blood gas analysis. In Burton GG, Hodgkin JE, Ward JJ, editors: *Respiratory care: a guide to clinical practice*, ed 4, Philadelphia, 1997, Lippincott-Raven.

Malley WJ: *Clinical blood gases: assessment and intervention*, ed 2, St. Louis, Elsevier Saunders, 2005.

Martin RJ: Transcutaneous monitoring: instrumentation and clinical applications, *Respir Care* 35(6):577, 1990.

Mathews P, Conway L: Arterial blood gases and noninvasive monitoring of oxygen and carbon dioxide. In Wyka KA, Mathews PJ, Clark WF, editors: *Foundations of respiratory care*, Albany, NY, 2002, Delmar.

Mohler JG, Collier CR, Brandt W: Blood gases. In Clausen JL, editor: *Pulmonary function testing guidelines and controversies*, Orlando, 1984, Grune & Stratton.

Moran RF: Assessment of quality control of blood gas/pH analyzer performance, *Respir Care* 26(6):538, 1981.

Moran RF: CLIA regulations. I. The cure might be worse than the disease, *AARC Times* 14(11):41, 1990.

Moran RF: CLIA regulations. II. An analysis of some technical requirements, *AARC Times* 14(12):25, 1990.

Nelson CM, Murphy EM, Bradley JK, et al: Clinical use of pulse oximetry to determine oxygen prescriptions for patients with hypoxemia, *Respir Care* 31(8):673, 1986.

Novametrics Medical Systems: product literature on transcutaneous monitoring, Wallingford, Conn.

Peters JA, Hodgkin JE, Collier CA: Blood gas analysis and acid-base physiology. In Burton GG, Hodgkin JE, Ward JJ, editors: *Respiratory care: a guide to clinical practice*, ed 3, Philadelphia, 1991, JB Lippincott.

Ruppel G: *Manual of pulmonary function testing*, ed 9, St Louis, 2009, Mosby.

Salyer JW: Pulse oximetry in the neonatal intensive care unit, *Respir Care* 36(1):17, 1991.

Walsh B, Czervinske MP, Diblasi RM: *Perinatal and pediatric respiratory care*, ed 3, St. Louis, 2010, Saunders.

Wilkins RL: Analysis and monitoring of gas exchange. In Wilkins RL, Stoller JK, Kacmarek RM, editors: *Egan's fundamentals of respiratory care*, ed 9, St Louis, 2009, Mosby.

Shapiro BA, Kacmarek RM, Cane RD, et al, editors: *Clinical application of respiratory care*, ed 4, St Louis, 1991, Mosby.

Shapiro BA, Peruzzi WT, Kozlowski-Templin R: Clinical application of blood gases, ed 5, St Louis, 1994, Mosby.

Sonnesso G: Are you ready to use pulse oximetry? *Nursing* 21(8):60, 1991.

Walton JR, Shapiro BA: Value and application of temperature-compensated blood gas data, *Respir Care* 25(2), 1980.

Welch JP, DeCesare R, Hess D: Pulse oximetry: instrumentation and clinical applications, *Respir Care* 35(6):584, 1990.

Whitaker K: *Comprehensive perinatal and pediatric respiratory care*, ed 2, Albany, NY, 1997, Delmar.

White GC: *Equipment theory for respiratory care*, ed 3, Albany, NY, 1999, Delmar.

SELF-STUDY QUESTIONS FOR THE ENTRY LEVEL EXAM   *See page 583 for answers*

1. Before drawing a blood gas sample from the radial artery, you should perform which test of adequate perfusion?
   - A. Allen's test
   - B. Modified Allen's test
   - C. Blood pressure measurement
   - D. $P(A-a)O_2$

2. A patient is brought into the emergency department after being rescued from a house fire. She is unconscious and has facial burns. The physician believes that she is suffering from smoke inhalation. What would you recommend as the best way to evaluate her?
   - A. ABGs analyzed through a CO-oximeter
   - B. Pulse oximetry
   - C. ABGs analyzed through a standard blood gas analyzer
   - D. $PtcO_2$ monitor

3. You are ordered to draw a blood sample from your patient's radial artery. You test for adequate circulation by having the patient make a fist while you put pressure over his ulnar and radial arteries. The patient's hand is then opened, and pressure is released from the ulnar artery. His hand color returns within 15 sec. This would indicate that
   - A. The patient's radial circulation is adequate
   - B. The patient's radial circulation is inadequate
   - C. The patient's ulnar circulation is adequate
   - D. The patient's ulnar circulation is inadequate

4. You are working in the intensive care unit when you notice that an arterial blood sample has been sitting out for 40 min. It was not put in ice-water. You could expect the blood gas analysis to be affected in which ways?
   1. Increased PaO_2
   2. Increased $PaCO_2$
   3. Decreased PaO_2
   4. Decreased $PaCO_2$
   5. Increased pH
   6. Decreased pH
   - A. 1, 2, 6
   - B. 3, 4, 5
   - C. 2, 3, 6
   - D. 3, 4, 6

5. You would recommend an arterial puncture to obtain a sample for blood gas analysis under which of the following conditions?
   1. To measure the patient's PaO_2 level after a change in the patient's inspired O_2 concentration
   2. Suspected CO poisoning
   3. To measure the patient's $PaCO_2$ level after a change in the patient's minute volume
   4. After the patient has been admitted to the emergency department with a tension pneumothorax
   5. During a cardiopulmonary resuscitation attempt
   - A. 1, 2
   - B. 1, 3
   - C. 2, 3, 4
   - D. 1, 2, 3, 4

6. Safety guidelines for the protection of the therapist who is drawing an ABG sample include which of the following?
   1. Put a glove on the hand used to draw the sample.
   2. Put a glove on the hand with which you feel the pulse.
   3. Put gloves on both hands.
   4. Wear goggles.

A. 3, 4
B. 1, 4
C. 2
D. 3

7. A 50-year-old patient has a PaO_2 value of 72 torr when breathing room air. You would interpret this as
   A. Normal for a person of his age
   B. Mild hypoxemia
   C. Moderate hypoxemia
   D. Severe hypoxemia

8. An acute rise in $PaCO_2$ level from 40 to 50 torr would result in the following change in pH:
   A. Rise of 0.10 unit
   B. Fall of 0.05 unit
   C. Fall of 0.10 unit
   D. Rise of 0.05 unit

9. Interpret the following blood gas drawn from a patient who is breathing 40% O_2: PaO_2, 54 torr; SaO_2, 87%; pH, 7.37; $PaCO_2$, 62 torr; bicarbonate, 38 mEq/L; and base excess, +11 mEq/L.
   1. Corrected hypoxemia
   2. Uncorrected hypoxemia
   3. Metabolic alkalosis
   4. Uncompensated metabolic acidosis
   5. Compensated respiratory acidosis
   A. 1, 4
   B. 1, 3
   C. 2, 4
   D. 2, 5

10. Interpret the following blood gas drawn from a patient who is breathing 35% O_2: PaO_2, 86 torr; SaO_2, 90%; pH, 7.29; $PaCO_2$, 37 torr; bicarbonate, 17 mEq/L; and base excess, −8 mEq/L.
    1. Corrected hypoxemia
    2. Uncorrected hypoxemia
    3. Compensated metabolic acidosis
    4. Uncompensated metabolic acidosis
    5. Compensated respiratory acidosis
    A. 2, 4
    B. 1, 4
    C. 2, 5
    D. 1, 3

11. Interpret the following blood gas drawn from a patient who is breathing 21% O_2: PaO_2, 117 torr; SaO_2, 98%; pH, 7.57; $PaCO_2$, 20 torr; bicarbonate, 24 mEq/L; and base excess, +1 mEq/L.
    1. Normal oxygenation
    2. Excessively corrected hypoxemia
    3. Uncompensated respiratory alkalosis
    4. Uncompensated metabolic acidosis
    5. Compensated respiratory and metabolic alkalosis
    A. 2, 3
    B. 2, 4
    C. 1, 3
    D. 1, 4

12. Interpret the following blood gas drawn from a patient who is breathing 60% O_2: PaO_2, 72 torr; SaO_2, 94%; pH, 7.18; $PaCO_2$, 50 torr; bicarbonate, 18 mEq/L; and base excess, −10 mEq/L.
    1. Uncorrected hypoxemia
    2. Corrected hypoxemia
    3. Uncorrected respiratory acidosis
    4. Uncorrected metabolic acidosis
    5. Combined metabolic and respiratory acidosis
    A. 1, 5
    B. 2, 5
    C. 2, 3
    D. 2, 4

13. Interpret the following blood gas drawn from a patient who is breathing 24% O_2: PaO_2, 57 torr; SaO_2, 91%; pH, 7.45; $PaCO_2$, 22 torr; bicarbonate, 16 mEq/L; and base excess, −6 mEq/L.
    1. Corrected hypoxemia
    2. Uncorrected hypoxemia
    3. Compensated respiratory alkalosis
    4. Uncompensated respiratory alkalosis
    5. Combined metabolic and respiratory acidosis
    A. 1, 3
    B. 1, 4
    C. 2, 3
    D. 2, 5

14. Which of the following would indicate that a patient's tissues are adequately oxygenated?
    A. PaO_2, 85 torr
    B. $P\bar{v}O_2$, 30 torr
    C. $S\bar{v}O_2$, 75%
    D. SaO_2, 90%

15. Blood gas analyzer calibration values are considered to be *in control* if they are
    A. Within 1 SD of the norm
    B. Within 2 SDs of the norm
    C. Within 3 SDs of the norm
    D. Within 4 SDs of the norm

16. A 50-year-old patient with emphysema seems to be tiring after 30 min into a weaning attempt on a Briggs adapter (T piece). The best way to evaluate her ventilatory status is by
    A. Checking her PaO_2 value
    B. Measuring a $PtcCO_2$ value
    C. Checking her $PaCO_2$ value
    D. Performing a bedside vital capacity measurement

17. Your patient has Guillain-Barré syndrome and pneumonia. The patient has just been placed on 35% O_2 by mask. The physician asks for your suggestion on the best way to evaluate the patient's overall ability to breathe. You would recommend
    A. Doing a full set of pulmonary function tests
    B. Drawing an arterial blood sample for analysis
    C. Performing pulse oximetry

D. Performing pulse oximetry and a force vital capacity measurement

18. You are called to evaluate a patient who is using a pulse oximeter. Upon entering the room, you notice a black woman with an oximeter probe on her right earlobe. The monitor shows a weak pulse signal and a fluctuating SpO_2 value. Which of the following would you do in an attempt to correct the problem?
    1. Try monitoring from a fingertip.
    2. Switch to a probe over the bridge of the nose.
    3. Cover the probe with an opaque wrap.
    4. Switch the probe to the left earlobe.
    A. 2
    B. 1, 3
    C. 2, 4
    D. 3

19. You are working with a postanesthesia patient who is on a $PtcCO_2$ monitor. The correlation factor between the $PaCO_2$ and $PtcCO_2$ is 1.4. The patient's previous $PtcCO_2$ level was 63 torr. The nurse has called you because it is now 75 torr. The patient's approximate $PaCO_2$ value would be calculated as
    A. 63 torr
    B. 75 torr
    C. 54 torr
    D. 105 torr

20. A 35-year-old patient with pneumonia is receiving mechanical ventilation with positive end-expiratory pressure (PEEP). You are ordered to calculate and interpret the patient's $P(A-a)O_2$ level. The following conditions exist:

    $P_B = 750$ torr. Normal is 760 torr for sea level.

    $P_{H_2O} = 54$ torr because your patient's temperature is 104° F/40° C. Normal is 47 torr for a normal temperature.

    $F_{IO_2} = 0.5$ for 50% inspired oxygen. Normal is 0.21 for room air.

    $PaCO_2 = 36$ torr

    $PaO_2 = 60$ torr

    Respiratory Exchange Ratio $= 0.8$

    $$PAO_2 = [(P_B - P_{H_2O})F_{IO_2}] - \frac{PaCO_2}{0.8}$$

    Based on the listed conditions, what is the patient's PAO_2 value?
    A. 312 torr
    B. 303 torr
    C. 101 torr
    D. 95 torr

21. Based on the listed conditions, what is the patient's $P(A-a)O_2$ value?
    A. 248 torr
    B. 243 torr
    C. 232 torr
    D. 41 torr

22. How should the patient's $P(A-a)O_2$ results be interpreted?
    A. There is an error; check the blood gas analyzer.
    B. Normal oxygenation for 50% oxygen being inspired
    C. Normal for a patient of this age
    D. Larger than normal difference

SELF-STUDY QUESTIONS FOR THE WRITTEN REGISTRY EXAM   *See page 606 for answers*

1. A 50-year-old male patient is being treated for a pulmonary embolism. He is receiving 50% O_2 by mask. The results of a $P(A-a)O_2$ study indicate that his alveolar-arterial difference is 205 torr. What is the best interpretation of this study?
    A. It should be repeated because these results are not physiologically possible.
    B. It is within the normal range.
    C. The alveolar-arterial difference is increased.
    D. The patient's condition is improving.

2. A 56-year-old woman with an acute myocardial infarction is being prepared for ambulance transportation from a rural hospital to a medical center for care. She is receiving oxygen at 8 L/min to a nonrebreathing mask, has intravenous lines for potassium replacement and cardiac medications, has an arterial catheter in place, and is on continuous electrocardiogram monitoring. Which of the following would be most beneficial in assessing her cardiopulmonary status during the transportation?
    A. Second-generation pulse oximeter
    B. CO-oximeter
    C. Point-of-care blood gas analyzer with expanded capabilities
    D. Pressure transducer for continuous blood pressure measurement

3. A premature neonate breathing room air has a $PtcCO_2$ electrode placed on her right thigh and a $PtcO_2$ electrode placed on her left thigh. Both have been showing stable readings over the last hour. After the patient was moved about for nursing care it is noticed that the $PtcO_2$ electrode value has increased. The $PtcCO_2$ electrode value is unchanged. What could explain this?
    A. The $PtcO_2$ electrode has pulled loose from the skin.

B. The inspired oxygen percentage has been decreased.

C. The patient's pulmonary condition has improved.

D. The patient is hyperventilating.

4. After performing a modified Allen's test on a patient's right wrist, it is found to take 25 seconds for the patient's hand to regain its color. What should be done now?

A. Perform an Allen's test on the right wrist.

B. Draw an arterial blood sample on the right wrist.

C. Draw an arterial blood sample on the left wrist.

D. Perform a modified Allen's test on the patient's left wrist.

5. A 45-year-old patient is brought by ambulance into the emergency department from a business where there is a carbon monoxide leak. The patient is obtunded and has an irregular pulse rate. Which of the following is the least important to evaluate at this time?

A. Pulse oximeter value from a first-generation unit

B. 12-lead electrocardiogram

C. ABGs analyzed through a CO-oximeter

D. Glasgow coma analysis

6. For which of the following conditions should an arterial line be inserted?

1. **Septic shock with vasopressor therapy**

2. **Suspected carbon monoxide poisoning**

3. **ARDS requiring mechanical ventilation with PEEP**

4. **Anxiety-induced hyperventilation**

A. 1, 2

B. 1, 3

C. 2, 3, 4

D. All of the above

7. A 45-year-old patient has been admitted to the emergency department after having smoke inhalation from a house fire. He is wearing a nonrebreather mask set at 10 L/min of oxygen. The most appropriate way to evaluate his oxygenation status is by

A. Pulse oximetry with a first-generation unit

B. Transcutaneous oxygen probe

C. Running an ABG sample through the blood gas analyzer

D. Running an ABG sample through the CO-oximeter

8. You are working in the neonatal intensive care unit with a premature neonate who has a transcutaneous carbon dioxide monitor. The correlation factor between the $PaCO_2$ and $PtcCO_2$ is 1.5. The patient's $PtcCO_2$ value is 53 torr. The patient's approximate $PaCO_2$ value would be calculated as

A. 80 torr

B. 51.5 torr

C. 35 torr

D. 33.5 torr

9. Interpret the following blood gas drawn when the patient was breathing 45% oxygen: PaO_2, 64 torr; SaO_2, 91%; pH, 7.38; $PaCO_2$, 59 torr; HCO_3^-, 39 mEq/L; and BE, +12 mEq/L.

1. **Corrected hypoxemia**

2. **Uncorrected hypoxemia**

3. **Metabolic alkalosis**

4. **Compensated respiratory acidosis**

5. **Metabolic acidosis**

A. 1, 4

B. 1, 3

C. 2, 5

D. 2, 4

10. Interpret the following blood gas drawn when the patient was breathing 30% oxygen: PaO_2, 82 torr; SaO_2, 94%; pH, 7.32; $PaCO_2$, 39 torr; HCO_3^-, 16 mEq/L; and BE, −6 mEq/L.

1. **Corrected hypoxemia**

2. **Uncorrected hypoxemia**

3. **Compensated metabolic acidosis**

4. **Uncompensated metabolic acidosis**

5. **Compensated respiratory acidosis**

A. 2, 4

B. 1, 4

C. 2, 5

D. 1, 3

11. Interpret the following blood gas drawn when the patient was breathing 24% oxygen: PaO_2, 125 torr; SaO_2, 99%; pH, 7.52; $PaCO_2$, 25 torr; HCO_3^-, 25 mEq/L; and BE, +1 mEq/L.

1. **Normal oxygenation**

2. **Excessively corrected hypoxemia**

3. **Uncompensated respiratory alkalosis**

4. **Uncompensated metabolic acidosis**

5. **Combined respiratory and metabolic alkalosis**

A. 2, 3

B. 2, 5

C. 1, 3

D. 1, 4

12. Interpret the following blood gas drawn when the patient was breathing 40% oxygen: PaO_2, 75 torr; SaO_2, 93%; pH, 7.15; $PaCO_2$, 55 torr; HCO_3^-, 20 mEq/L; and BE, −8 mEq/L.

1. **Uncorrected hypoxemia**

2. **Corrected hypoxemia**

3. **Uncorrected respiratory acidosis**

4. **Uncorrected metabolic acidosis**

5. **Combined metabolic and respiratory acidosis**

A. 1, 5

B. 2, 5

C. 2, 3

D. 2, 4

13. Interpret the following blood gas drawn when the patient was breathing 30% oxygen: PaO_2, 65 mm Hg;

SaO$_2$, 91%; pH, 7.44; PaCO$_2$, 25 mm Hg; HCO$_3^-$, 17 mEq/L; and BE, −7 mEq/L.

1. Corrected hypoxemia
2. Uncorrected hypoxemia
3. Compensated respiratory alkalosis
4. Uncompensated respiratory alkalosis
5. Combined metabolic and respiratory acidosis

A. 1, 3
B. 1, 4
C. 2, 3
D. 2, 5

14. Which of the following clinical values indicates that a patient's tissues are hypoxemic?
   A. PaO$_2$ of 55 torr
   B. P$\bar{v}$O$_2$ of 25 torr
   C. S$\bar{v}$O$_2$ of 80%
   D. SaO$_2$ of 88%

15. You are working with a neonate in an incubator. She is being monitored with a transcutaneous oxygen electrode on her right upper chest. An hour ago, the patient's oxygen value was 52 torr, and now it is 115 torr. The nurse tells you that no change has occurred in the neonate's condition. What is the most likely explanation of this difference?
   A. The patient has a patent ductus arteriosus.
   B. Air has leaked under the electrode.
   C. The temperature inside the incubator has been increased.
   D. The patient's cardiac output and lung condition have improved.

16. A 17-year-old patient is receiving mechanical ventilation because of apnea resulting from a drug overdose. While the patient is breathing 25% oxygen, the following ABG values are analyzed:

   PaO$_2$ of 155 torr

   SaO$_2$ of 100%

   pH of 7.42

   PaCO$_2$ of 41 torr

   HCO$_3^-$ of 26 mEq/L

   BE of +2 mEq/L

What action should now be taken?
   A. Reduce the patient to 21% oxygen.
   B. Maintain the patient on the present settings.
   C. Recheck the blood gas analyzer.
   D. Increase the tidal volume to hyperventilate the patient.

4 Pulmonary Function Testing

Note 1: This book is written to cover every item listed as testable on the *Entry Level Examination (ELE), Written Registry Examination (WRE),* and *Clinical Simulation Examination (CSE).*

The listed code for each item is taken from the National Board for Respiratory Care's (NBRC) **Summary Content Outline for CRT and Written RRT Examinations** (http://evolve.elsevier.com/Sills/resptherapist/). For example, if an item is testable on both the ELE and WRE, it is shown simply as (Code:...). If an item is testable only on the ELE, it is shown as (ELE code:...). If an item is testable only on the WRE, it is shown as (WRE code:...).

Following each item's code, the difficulty level is indicated for the questions on that item on the ELE and WRE. (See the Introduction for a full explanation of the three question difficulty levels.) **Recall [R]** level questions typically expect the exam taker to recall factual information. **Application [Ap]** level questions are more difficult, because the exam taker may have to apply factual information to a clinical situation. **Analysis [An]** level questions are the most challenging, because the exam taker may have to use critical thinking to evaluate patient data to make a clinical decision.

Note 2: A review of the most recent Entry Level Examinations (ELE) has shown that an average of 7 questions out of 140 (or 5% of the exam) covers pulmonary function testing. A review of the most recent Written Registry Examinations (WRE) has shown that an average of 4 questions out of 100 (or 4% of the exam) covers pulmonary function testing. The Clinical Simulation Examination (CSE) is comprehensive and may include everything that should be known by an advanced-level respiratory therapist.

MODULE A

Review the patient's record for data on the following tests

1. Pulmonary function results (Code: IA4) [Difficulty: ELE: R; WRE: Ap]

Be prepared to review the results of all types of pulmonary function test (PFT) results. This chapter covers the PFTs listed by the NBRC and other PFTs that have been tested by the NBRC.

2. Respiratory monitoring (Code: IA7c) [Difficulty: ELE: R; WRE: Ap]

Patients at risk of respiratory failure, such as those with neurologic disease, should have their breathing monitored regularly. Respiratory monitoring could include checking a patient's respiratory rate, tidal volume, minute volume, inspiratory/expiratory (I:E) ratio, maximum inspiratory pressure, maximum expiratory pressure, and airway graphics.

3. Pulmonary mechanics (e.g., maximum inspiratory pressure, vital capacity) (Code: IA7b) [Difficulty: ELE: R; WRE: Ap]

According to Madama (1998), pulmonary mechanics tests are used to assess the function of the patient's pulmonary/thoracic system under dynamic conditions. In other words, when air is moving. This could include the spirometry tests as well as lung compliance or airway resistance tests.

4. Lung compliance (Code: IA7d) [Difficulty: ELE: R; WRE: Ap]

Lung compliance usually is measured in patients with stiff lungs (as found with pulmonary fibrosis) or overly compliant lungs (as found with emphysema).

5. Airway resistance (Code: IA7d) [Difficulty: ELE: R; WRE: Ap]

Patients with asthma or chronic bronchitis may need to have airway resistance measured as part of their bronchodilator therapy management. Airway resistance decreases if the proper type and amount of medication are taken.

6. Work of breathing (Code: IA7d) [Difficulty: ELE: R; WRE: Ap]

Work of breathing (WOB) is the patient's subjective feeling about his or her difficulty in breathing. A normal person without cardiopulmonary disease would not feel any difficulty in breathing at rest. However, a person with cardiopulmonary disease, such as COPD or congestive heart failure, would feel an increased work of breathing, even at rest. The patient would say that he or she feels "short of breath" (SOB).

MODULE B

Bedside spirometry

1. Perform bedside spirometry tests

a. Recommend lung mechanics (bedside spirometry) tests to obtain additional data (Code: IC7) [Difficulty: ELE: R, Ap; WRE: An]

The bedside lung mechanics tests typically include the following:

- Lung volumes and capacities except for those requiring the residual volume (RV).
- Spirometry for nonforced or slow vital capacity (SVC).
- Forced vital capacity (FVC) and flow values derived from the FVC. These values are needed to determine the degree of impairment in patients with obstructive diseases.
- Maximum inspiratory pressure (MIP) and maximum expiratory pressure (MEP). These values indicate the patient's overall respiratory muscle strength.

Other common bedside tests are also presented in this section. Bedside spirometry tests are indicated in a patient who is showing signs of breathing difficulty and the physician and respiratory therapist are considering the need for mechanical ventilation. For example, a patient with a progressive neuromuscular disease or worsening cardiopulmonary condition would show a smaller vital capacity and MIP and MEP as he or she weakens. Conversely, as a mechanically ventilated patient improves, bedside spirometry is used to evaluate the patient's spontaneous breathing for weaning.

The more advanced spirometry tests, such as flow-volume loop, timed expiratory volumes, and maximum voluntary ventilation, are included later in the chapter with the pulmonary function laboratory tests.

b. Perform any of the bedside spirometry tests (Code: IIIE7) [Difficulty: ELE: R, Ap; WRE: An]

Discussion of the steps to perform and interpretation of the tests follow.

2. Tidal volume

a. Perform the procedure (Code: IB9d) [Difficulty: ELE: R; WRE: Ap, An]

The tidal volume (V_T) is the volume of gas breathed out in each respiratory cycle. Realize that individual tidal volumes are rarely identical. Figure 4-1 shows several different tidal volumes before and after a nonforced (slow) vital capacity (VC). For that reason, it is recommended that the tidal volumes be accumulated for 1 minute (thus providing a minute volume [$\dot{V}_E$]) and the respiratory rate (f) counted. An average V_T is found by dividing the $\dot{V}_E$ by the f. If this cannot be done, find the average volume of at least six breaths. The average predicted tidal volume for a resting, afebrile, alert adult should be about

3 to 4 mL/lb of ideal body weight *or*

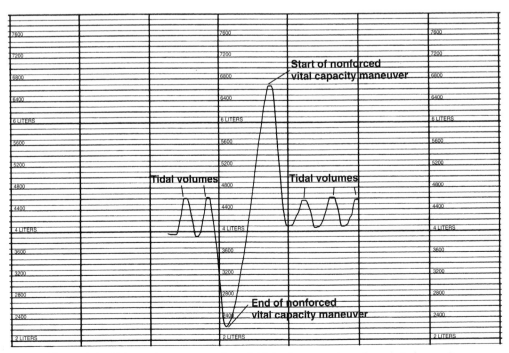

Figure 4-1   Volume-time curve tracing of tidal volumes and nonforced vital capacity.

7 to 9 mL/kg of ideal body weight

For example, the predicted tidal volume range of a 154-lb (70-kg) patient is calculated as follows:

$$3 \text{ to } 4 \text{ mL/lb} \times 154 \text{ lb} = 462 \text{ to } 616 \text{ mL}$$

$$7 \text{ to } 9 \text{ mL/kg} \times 70 \text{ kg} = 490 \text{ to } 630 \text{ mL}$$

The patient should be allowed to relax before the test is performed so that the measured volume is accurate and not enlarged because of any undue stress or excitement. Keeping the instructions and demonstration simple and easy to follow help reduce the patient's anxiety. Some patients will not tolerate a full minute's tidal volume measurement. In that case, measure the accumulated tidal volumes for as long as possible and divide by the number of respirations to obtain the average.

b. Interpret the results (Code: IB10d) [Difficulty: ELE: R, Ap; WRE: An]

A tidal volume that is larger or smaller than expected for the patient's size requires further evaluation. A small tidal volume may be seen in patients who have a low metabolic rate, are asleep or in a coma, have a neuromuscular disease that make them unable to breathe deeply, or are alkalotic. A large tidal volume may be seen in patients with a high metabolic rate, fever, dead space–producing diseases such as a pulmonary embolism, increased intracranial pressure, or acidotic conditions.

c. Monitor the tidal volume and respiratory rate (Code: IA7c) [Difficulty: ELE: R; WRE: Ap]

A patient with a progressive neuromuscular disease or worsening cardiopulmonary disease should have the tidal volume, respiratory rate, and other bedside spirometry values monitored closely. If the patient's condition worsens, mechanical ventilation may have to be started. The frequency of monitoring varies with the patient's condition. For example, every shift initially and hourly if the patient is critical. Conversely, as a mechanically ventilated patient improves, bedside spirometry is used to evaluate the patient's spontaneous breathing for weaning.

d. Monitor inspiratory/expiratory ratio (WRE code: IA7c) [Difficulty: ELE: R; WRE: Ap]

The I:E ratio is the ratio of the patient's inspiratory time to the expiratory time. It can be simply measured at the bedside with a stopwatch. Again, make sure the patient is relaxed and breathing in the normal pattern to get an accurate timing. Measure several of the patient's inspiratory times and expiratory times to figure an average for each. A spirometer that gives a printout is needed if a more complete analysis of the patient's breathing pattern is necessary.

A normal, spontaneously breathing patient has an I:E ratio of 1:2 to 1:4. A prolonged inspiratory time often is seen in patients with an upper airway obstruction. A prolonged expiratory time often is seen in patients with asthma or chronic obstructive pulmonary disease (COPD). Any abnormal I:E ratio should be investigated. For example, patients with Kussmaul's respiration, Cheyne-Stokes respiration, or Biot's respiration will have unusual I:E ratios.

Exam Hint 4-1 (ELE)

The National Board of Respiratory Care (NBRC) is known to test the examinee's ability to calculate (1) the T_I and T_E from a given I:E ratio and f, and (2) the I:E ratio from a given T_I and T_E. These examples should help.

1. Calculate the patient's T_I and T_E when the I:E ratio is 1:2 and f is 12/min.
   a. $\dfrac{60 \text{ sec/min}}{12 \text{ breaths/min}} = 5 \text{ sec/respiratory cycle}$

   b. $\dfrac{5 \text{ sec/respiratory cycle}}{3 \text{ parts of I and E}} = 1.66 \text{ sec for 1 part}$

   c. $T_I = 1 \text{ part} = 1.66 \text{ sec}$
   d. $T_E = 2 \text{ parts} = 3.32 \text{ sec}$
2. Calculate the neonatal patient's I:E ratio when the T_I is 0.3 sec and the T_E is 0.9 sec.
   a. I:E = I/E = 0.3/0.9 sec
   b. I/E = 1/3 (The I:E ratio is 1:3.)

---

3. Minute volume

a. Perform the procedure (Code: IB9d) [Difficulty: ELE: R; WRE: Ap, An]

The minute volume ($\dot{V}E$) is the volume of gas exhaled in 1 minute. It usually is a more stable value than are individual tidal volumes. The minute volume is found by adding the accumulated tidal volumes for 1 minute. A simple handheld spirometer often is used to accumulate the tidal volume breaths. If the patient cannot perform the test for 1 minute, do it for 30 seconds and double the value.

b. Interpret the results (Code: IB10d) [Difficulty: ELE: R, Ap; WRE: An]

The predicted range for a minute volume in a resting, afebrile, alert adult should be 5 to 10 L/min. The wide range is found in part because the minute volume is a product of two factors: tidal volume and respiratory rate. It is possible for either one or both of these factors to be normal, abnormally high, or abnormally low. For these reasons, the minute volume must be evaluated along with the tidal volume and respiratory rate to reach any conclusion about the patient's condition. The same factors that have an impact on the tidal volume affect the patient's minute ventilation.

4. Alveolar ventilation

a. Perform the procedure (Code: IB9d) [Difficulty: ELE: R; WRE: Ap, An]

Alveolar ventilation (V_A) is the amount of tidal volume that reaches the alveoli. It is calculated by subtracting the physiologic dead space (anatomic plus alveolar dead space) from the measured exhaled tidal volume. For a bedside test, it is possible to subtract only the estimated anatomic dead space. It is estimated at 1 mL/lb, or 2.2 mL/kg of ideal body weight. The alveolar dead space measurement requires sophisticated equipment, which usually is available only in the pulmonary function testing laboratory. Clinically normal people have very little alveolar dead space.

EXAMPLE 1

A 154-lb (70-kg) person has a measured tidal volume of 500 mL and an estimated anatomic dead space of about 154 mL.

$$\text{Calculated alveolar ventilation} = 500\ \text{mL} - 154\ \text{mL} = 346\ \text{mL}$$

The minute alveolar ventilation ($\dot{V}_A$) is the volume of gas that reaches the alveoli in 1 minute. It is found by multiplying the alveolar volume by the respiratory rate in 1 minute.

EXAMPLE 2

A 154-lb (70-kg) person has a measured tidal volume of 500 mL and an estimated anatomic dead space of about 154 mL. The respiratory rate is 14/min.

$$\text{Calculated alveolar ventilation} = 346\ \text{mL}\ (500\ \text{mL} - 154\ \text{mL}).$$

$$\text{Calculated minute alveolar ventilation} = 14 \times 346\ \text{mL} = 4{,}844\ \text{mL}$$

b. Interpret the results (Code: IB10d) [Difficulty: ELE: R, Ap; WRE: An]

The following examples show how the patient's alveolar ventilation can vary considerably because of changes in the respiratory rate and tidal volume, even though the minute volume remains unchanged. These examples are included to show the importance of alveolar ventilation on the patient's arterial partial pressure of carbon dioxide ($PaCO_2$) values.

EXAMPLE 1

Normal patient: $f = 12$, tidal volume = 500 mL, anatomic dead space = 154 mL

$$\text{Minute alveolar ventilation}\ (\dot{V}_A) = 12 \times (500\ \text{mL} - 154\ \text{mL})$$
$$= 12 \times 346\ \text{mL}$$
$$= 4{,}152\ \text{mL}$$

This patient should have a normal carbon dioxide level.

EXAMPLE 2

Tachypneic patient: $f = 24$, tidal volume = 250 mL, anatomic dead space = 154 mL

$$\text{Minute volume} = 12 \times 250\ \text{mL} = 6000\ \text{mL}$$

$$\text{Minute alveolar ventilation}\ (\dot{V}_A) = 24 \times (250\ \text{mL} - 154\ \text{mL})$$
$$= 24 \times 96\ \text{mL}$$
$$= 2{,}304\ \text{mL}$$

This patient should have a high carbon dioxide level.

EXAMPLE 3

Bradypneic patient: $f = 6$, tidal volume = 1,000 mL, anatomic dead space = 154 mL

$$\text{Minute volume} = 6 \times 1{,}000\ \text{mL} = 6{,}000\ \text{mL}$$

$$\text{Minute alveolar ventilation}\ (\dot{V}_A) = 6 \times (1000\ \text{mL} - 154\ \text{mL})$$
$$= 6 \times 846\ \text{mL}$$
$$= 5{,}076\ \text{mL}$$

This patient should have a low carbon dioxide level.

5. Maximum inspiratory pressure

a. Perform the procedure (Code: IB79n [Difficulty: ELE: R, Ap; WRE: An]

The maximum inspiratory pressure (MIP) is the greatest amount of negative pressure the patient can create when inspiring against an occluded airway. It also is known as *negative inspiratory force* (NIF). The following factors affect the test results: strength of the diaphragm and accessory muscles of inspiration, lung volume when the airway is occluded, ventilatory drive, and the length of time the airway is occluded. MIP is most commonly used to determine the weanability of mechanically ventilated patients. In addition, it is used to help monitor the strength of patients with a neuromuscular disease.

A study of the literature reveals that a number of measurement devices have been assembled and that different bedside techniques have been used to determine the effort of a patient breathing naturally, an intubated patient, and a patient breathing with assistance from a mechanical ventilator. Branson and colleagues (1989) and Kacmarek and colleagues (1989) make a strong case for the use of a double one-way valve to connect the intubated patient to the manometer (Figure 4-2). Use of the one-way valve lets the patient exhale but prevents an inhalation when the practitioner occludes the opening. This forces the patient to inhale from closer to residual volume with

Figure 4-2 Two systems for measuring maximal inspiratory pressure (MIP) in a patient with an artificial airway. System **A,** Simple occlusion. *A,* Pressure manometer; *B,* connecting tubing; *C,* port to be occluded during MIP; *D,* connection of the adapter to the manometer; *E,* port to connect to the patient's airway. System **B,** One-way valve. *A,* Pressure manometer; *B,* connecting tubing; *C,* inspiratory port to be occluded during the MIP effort; *D,* expiratory port; *E,* port to be connected to the patient's artificial airway. *(From Kacmarek RM, Cycyk-Chapman MC, Young-Palazzo PJ, et al: Determination of maximal inspiratory pressure: a clinical study and literature review, Respir Care 34:868, 1989.)*

each breathing effort. These researchers also recommend that the patient make inspiratory efforts for 15 to 20 seconds.

Steps in the MIP procedure for a normally breathing patient include the following:

1. Obtain a pressure gauge capable of measuring at least −60 cm H_2O pressure.
2. Have the patient sit upright. Place a note in the chart if the patient is lying down.
3. Describe the procedure to the patient.
4. Simulate a demonstration of the procedure.
5. Place nose clips over the patient's nose. Have the patient seal the lips and teeth around the mouthpiece and breathe through the open port.
6. Tell the patient to exhale completely. Seal the port when residual volume has been reached.
7. Tell the patient to breathe in as hard as possible and hold it for 1 to 3 seconds.
8. Reteach if necessary.
9. Repeat until at least three good efforts have been performed. Record the greatest stable value seen

after the first second of effort. This eliminates any artifact created by the cheeks or by chest wall movement.

b. Interpret the results (Code: IB10n) [Difficulty: ELE: R, Ap; WRE: An]

Patients of either gender and of any age should be able to generate at least −60 cm H_2O. This is enough to offer assurance that the patient has enough strength and coordination to protect the airway, take a deep breath, and cough effectively. Patients with neuromuscular diseases, diseases of the respiratory muscles, thoracic injury or abnormality, and chronic obstructive lung diseases tend to have decreased strength. The patient who cannot generate at least −20 cm H_2O is at risk. This patient probably does not have the strength to cough effectively. Depending on the blood gas values and other physical parameters, the patient may need to be intubated and maintained on a mechanical ventilator.

Black and Hyatt (1969) published MIP prediction formulas for spontaneous breathing in nonintubated adults 20 to 86 years old who are breathing from residual volume; these formulas are presented in Table 4-1. The values are in centimeters of water pressure (cm H_2O). As can be seen, the older the patient, the lower the predicted negative inspiratory force.

TABLE 4-1	Age and Gender in Predicting Negative Inspiratory Force	
Age and Gender	**Lower Limits of Normal**
Males: 143 − (0.55 × age)	−75 cm H_2O
Females: 104 − (0.51 × age)	−50 cm H_2O

c. Monitor the patient's MIP (Code: IA7b) [Difficulty: ELE: R; WRE: Ap]

A patient being weaned from mechanical ventilation or with a deteriorating neuromuscular condition should have the MIP measured on a regular, frequent basis. If the patient's pressure is only −20 cm H_2O, the physician should be notified. Mechanical ventilation is probably needed.

It is important to monitor any patient for signs of undue stress and hypoxemia, such as tachycardia, bradycardia, ventricular dysrhythmias, hypertension, hypotension, and decreasing saturation on pulse oximetry. If any of these are seen, the procedure should be stopped and the patient reoxygenated and ventilated. Some patients achieve their best effort on the first or second inspiration and have decreasing effort as they continue trying. This is probably because of fatigue. Stop the procedure and record the best effort.

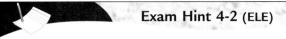

6. Maximum expiratory pressure

a. Perform the procedure (Code: IB9n) [Difficulty: ELE: R, Ap; WRE: An]

The maximum expiratory pressure (MEP) is the greatest amount of positive pressure the patient can create when expiring from total lung capacity (TLC) against an occluded airway. It also is known as a *maximum expiratory force* (MEF). The following factors affect the test results: patient cooperation and effort, strength of the expiratory muscles, lung volume when the airway is occluded, ventilatory drive, and the length of time the airway is occluded. The MEP is used to determine the weanability of mechanically ventilated patients and to monitor the strength of patients with a neuromuscular disease.

As with the MIP test, a study of the literature reveals that a number of measurement devices have been assembled and that different bedside techniques have been used to determine the effort of a patient breathing naturally and the effort of one who is intubated and breathing by way of a mechanical ventilator. A strong case can be made for the use of a double one-way valve to connect the intubated patient to the manometer (see Figure 4-2). Use of the one-way valves lets the patient inhale but prevents an exhalation when the practitioner occludes the expiratory opening. This forces the patient to exhale from closer to TLC with each breathing effort. However, the expiratory efforts should not be held for longer than 3 seconds. This test is similar to the Valsalva maneuver and can cause a reduction in cardiac output because of the high intrathoracic pressure.

Steps in the MEP procedure for a normally breathing patient include the following:

1. Obtain a pressure gauge capable of measuring at least +60 cm H$_2$O pressure.
2. Have the patient sit upright. Place a note in the chart if the patient is lying down.
3. Describe the procedure to the patient.
4. Simulate a demonstration of the procedure.
5. Place nose clips over the patient's nose. Have the patient seal the lips and teeth around the mouthpiece and breathe through the open port.

6. Tell the patient to inhale completely. Seal the port when TLC has been reached.
7. Tell the patient to breathe out as hard as possible. Hold it for 1 to 3 seconds.
8. Reteach if necessary.
9. Repeat until at least three good efforts have been performed. Record the greatest stable value seen after the first second of effort. This eliminates any artifact created by the cheeks or chest wall movement.

It is important to monitor any patient for signs of undue stress and hypoxemia, such as tachycardia, bradycardia, ventricular dysrhythmias, hypotension, and decreasing saturation on pulse oximetry. If any of these is seen, the procedure should be stopped and the patient reoxygenated and ventilated.

b. Interpret the results (Code: IB10d) [Difficulty: ELE: R, Ap; WRE: An]

Clinically normal people of either gender and of any age should be able to generate at least 80 cm H$_2$O. Patients with neuromuscular diseases, thoracic injury or abnormality, and COPD tend to have decreased strength. An MEP of +40 cm H$_2$O is probably enough to offer assurance that the patient has enough strength and coordination to cough effectively to clear secretions. However, depending on the blood gas values and other physical parameters, the patient may need to be intubated and maintained on a mechanical ventilator.

Black and Hyatt published MEP prediction formulas for spontaneously breathing, nonintubated adults 20 to 86 years old who are breathing from TLC; these formulas are presented in Table 4-2. The values are in centimeters of water pressure. As can be seen, the older the patient, the lower the predicted maximum expiratory force.

TABLE 4-2	Age and Gender in Predicting Maximum Expiratory Force	
Age and Gender	**Lower Limits of Normal**
Males: 268 − (1.03 × age)	+140 cm H$_2$O
Females: 170 − (0.53 × age)	+95 cm H$_2$O

7. Vital capacity

a. Perform the test (Code: IB9d) [Difficulty: ELE: R; WRE: Ap, An]

The nonforced (slow) vital capacity (VC or SVC) is the greatest volume of gas the patient can exhale after the lungs have been completely filled. The therapist should demonstrate the procedure to the patient. He or she must understand that there is no need to blow out fast while emptying the lungs. The measurement device can be a simple handheld spirometer if a printout of the result is not needed. A portable, computer-based spirometer can be used, if needed, to generate a printout of the results or a graphic tracing. Normally at least *three* efforts are made, and the largest is recorded.

b. Interpret the results (Code: IB10d) [Difficulty: ELE: R, Ap; WRE: An]

See Figure 4-1 for a graphic tracing of a nonforced VC. Compare it with the tracing on Figure 4-3, which shows a forced vital capacity (FVC). In a patient without obstructive lung disease, the same volume should be found in a nonforced VC and an FVC. A patient with asthma or chronic obstructive lung disease may have a smaller FVC than nonforced VC because of small airway collapse during the maximum effort. The following discussion on the FVC includes predicted values for male and female patients and guidelines on the interpretation.

c. Monitor the vital capacity (Code: IA7b) [Difficulty: ELE: R; WRE: Ap]

The VC and other simple spirometry values are commonly measured at the bedside in patients with neuromuscular disease and those who are being weaned from mechanical ventilation. A VC that is increasing toward the normal, predicted patient value is a good sign, because it indicates that the patient is recovering. If the VC is decreasing, the patient likely is becoming weaker and will not be able to cough out secretions effectively. Mechanical ventilation may be needed. See Module C for more discussion on the vital capacity. See Chapter 15 for more discussion on how the VC is used to evaluate a patient's need for mechanical ventilation.

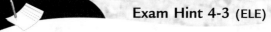

Exam Hint 4-3 (ELE)

A bedside vital capacity test is widely used to help in the assessment of a mechanically ventilated patient's ability to breathe effectively. This issue and weaning guidelines are discussed in Chapter 15. In general, a decreasing VC is a sign that the patient is tired and failing. (Racial adjustment and BTPS correction are not typically done when the VC is used for bedside spirometry.)

8. Forced expiratory volume in one second

a. Perform the test (Code: IB9e) [Difficulty: ELE: R; WRE: Ap, An]

The forced expiratory volume in one second (FEV_1) is the volume exhaled in the first second from a forced vital capacity. It can be measured at the bedside on some portable pulmonary function testing units, but this is most commonly done in the pulmonary function laboratory. The patient is instructed to take in as deep a breath as possible and blow it out as hard as possible. The therapist should demonstrate the procedure. It is not necessary for the patient to push out all air for several seconds until completely empty. The patient should be wearing nose clips and tightly seal the lips around the mouthpiece to prevent leaks. A good patient effort must be repeated three times. The highest recorded value is recorded in liters.

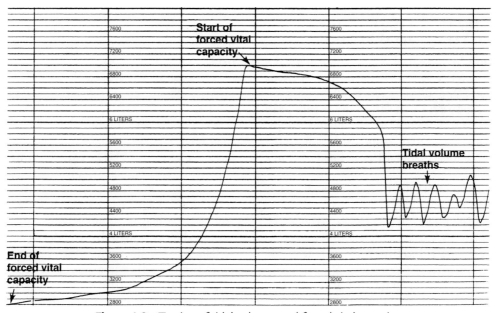

Figure 4-3 Tracing of tidal volumes and forced vital capacity.

b. Interpret the results (Code: IB10e) [Difficulty: ELE: R, Ap; WRE: An]

The FEV_1 and peak flow are the bedside measurements most commonly used to evaluate the response of a patient with asthma or COPD to inhaled bronchodilator medications. If the medication dose is effective, the patient's expiratory flow will increase significantly from the premedication value. See Module C for more discussion on the FEV_1.

9. Peak flow

a. Perform the test (Code: IB9d) [Difficulty: ELE: R; WRE: Ap, An]

The peak flow (PF) or peak expiratory flow rate (PEFR) is the highest flow rate seen in a patient's forced expiratory effort. The PF usually is found at the start of an FVC effort. It can be measured at the bedside on some portable pulmonary function testing units, but it is most commonly done on a portable, disposable peak flowmeter. Select a unit that is appropriate for the patient. An adult peak flowmeter should be able to measure a flow of up to 850 L/min (about 14 L/sec), and a pediatric unit should be able to measure a flow of up to 400 L/min (about 7 L/sec). The patient is instructed to take in as deep a breath as possible and blow it out as hard as possible. The therapist should demonstrate the procedure. It is not necessary for the patient to push out all air for several seconds until completely empty. The patient should tightly seal the lips around the mouthpiece to prevent leaks. Nose clips are recommended but not required. A good patient effort must be repeated three times. Record the highest recorded value in liters per minute (or liters per second, depending on the unit).

b. Interpret the results (Code: IB10e) [Difficulty: ELE: R, Ap; WRE: An]

The peak flow and FEV_1 are the bedside measurements most commonly used to evaluate the response of a patient with asthma or COPD to inhaled bronchodilator medications. If the medication dose is effective, the patient's peak flow will increase significantly from the premedication value. Many peak flowmeters come with adjustable markers for the National Asthma Education Program's "color zone" scheme:

- *Green zone:* Peak flow is 80% to 100% of predicted or personal best.
- *Yellow zone:* Peak flow is 50% to 79% of predicted or personal best.
- *Red zone:* Peak flow is less than 50% of predicted or personal best.

Current asthma guidelines state that if an asthma patient's peak flow is in the green zone, the medications are adequately controlling the asthma. If the peak flow is in the yellow zone, the patient's medications are not adequately controlling the asthma. Increased doses are indicated if ordered by the physician. If the peak flow is in the red zone, the patient's medications are not adequately controlling the asthma. The patient needs more bronchodilator medication. The home care patient should get medical help as soon as possible. Each patient should have his or her individually calculated color zones marked on the peak flowmeter to guide medication usage. The patient should be instructed on the meaning of the zones and the proper use of medications. See Module C for more discussion of the peak flow.

MODULE C
Pulmonary function testing laboratory studies

1. Recommend pulmonary function testing (Code: IC6) [Difficulty: ELE: R, Ap; WRE: An]

Because the pulmonary function testing laboratory has more advanced equipment and specially trained personnel, the more challenging cases requiring a pulmonary diagnosis are sent there for testing. The following tests are either specifically listed as testable by the NBRC or have been tested in recent examinations.

2. Exhaled nitric oxide

a. Perform the test (WRE Code: IB9k) [WRE Difficulty: R, Ap]

Exhaled nitric oxide (eNO) is measured in patients with known or suspected eosinophilic (airway) inflammation. The test has been shown to be most useful for evaluating patients with asthma but may also be of use in patients with COPD. The patient should be told not to eat, drink, or smoke for at least 1 hour before the test. If other pulmonary function tests are scheduled, the exhaled nitric oxide test should be performed first. This is because the other tests, such as spirometry, exercise testing, and methacholine challenge testing, can change the eNo results.

The patient's exhaled breath is analyzed through a chemoluminescent analyzer for the level of nitric oxide in parts per billion (ppb). The patient is instructed to exhale completely (to residual volume), insert the mouthpiece, and inhale as much as possible (to total lung capacity) through the eNO device. The inhaled gas is scrubbed of any NO that may be found in room air. The patient then slowly exhales through the eNO device at a controlled rate of 0.05 L/sec. This results in an exhaled NO plateau of several seconds that is analyzed for the patient's value. The patient must perform at least two acceptable eNO efforts that are within 10% of each other. The two acceptable values are averaged for the final reported value.

b. Interpret the results (WRE code: IB10k) [WRE Difficulty: R, Ap, An]

The following normal ranges have been established for exhalation of a breath at the controlled rate of 0.05 L/sec:

- Adult: 15 to 25 ppb, with an upper limit of normal of 35 ppb.
- Child: 5 to 22 ppb, with an upper limit of normal of 25 ppb.

Actual patient values greater than these indicate increased eosinophilic activity. In other words, a patient with asthma is having more airway inflammation and is not under control. The physician would likely consider increasing the dose of corticosteroids or other controlling medications. In addition, the following conditions have been shown to increase exhaled nitric oxide during an exacerbation: chronic bronchitis (COPD), pneumonia, alveolitis, bronchiolitis obliterans, bronchiectasis, sarcoidosis, or a condition with a chronic cough. Conversely, reduced eNO is found in smokers and patients with cystic fibrosis.

3. Forced vital capacity

a. Perform the test (Code: IB9e and IIIE7a) [Difficulty: ELE: R, Ap; WRE: An]

The FVC is the greatest volume of gas that the patient can exhale as rapidly as possible after the lungs have been completely filled. Normally, the FVC is the same volume as that found in a slow or nonforced VC. Careful instructions, demonstrations, and coaching are needed to ensure that the patient's efforts are the best possible. At least *three* proper efforts must be obtained.

If the measurement instrument does not give a printout, simply record the patient's efforts in the chart. If the measurement instrument does give a printout, include copies of the efforts. See Figure 4-3 for the tracing of a properly performed FVC. The tracing allows comparison of the volumes exhaled in a series of 1-second intervals. Because of this, the tracing often is referred to as a *volume-time curve*. Note that the start of the effort is smooth and without interruption. The initial fast flow of gas from the upper airway is seen as the nearly vertical part of the tracing. The rest of the tracing is smooth without any coughing or other interruptions in the patient's effort. The tracing becomes progressively more horizontal as the end of the effort is reached. Encourage the patient to try to push out as much air as possible as the end approaches. To provide an acceptable FVC, the patient must show maximum effort without coughing or closing the glottis, and the expiratory effort must last at least 6 seconds. The patient's final 2 seconds of expiratory effort should show no appreciable airflow. Each of the three acceptable FVCs must show these traits and close similarity of the patient's efforts.

b. Interpret FVC and spirometry graphics

Figure 4-3 was made on a chain-compensated, water-seal spirometry system. Note how the tracing progresses from the right to the left. The Stead-Wells system shows the same tracing "upside down" compared with the chain-compensated system. The tracing starts on the left and moves to the right (Figures 4-4 and 4-5). Other tracings

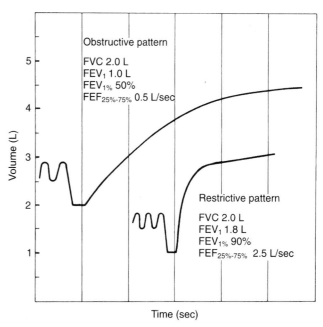

Figure 4-4 Forced vital capacity (FVC) tracings showing an obstructed flow pattern and a restrictive flow pattern. Note that the patient with the obstructed pattern has a slower than normal exhalation, whereas the patient with the restrictive pattern has a faster than normal exhalation. *(From Ruppel G: Manual of pulmonary function testing, ed 6, St Louis, 1994, Mosby.)*

Figure 4-5 Spirometry tracings of normal, obstructed, and restricted patients. Note how the obstructed and restricted patients' volumes and capacities are out of proportion compared with those of the normal patient. *VC,* Vital capacity; *RV,* residual volume; *FRC,* functional residual capacity. *(From Cherniack RM: Pulmonary function testing, Philadelphia, 1977, WB Saunders.)*

may show either the chain-compensated or the Stead-Wells tracings in a mirror image or opposite shape.

Exam Hint 4-4 (ELE, WRE)

The NBRC can show an FVC tracing from any system and expect it to be interpreted. The start of the FVC effort can be determined by the near-vertical portion of the tracing and the relatively small expiratory reserve volume (ERV) compared with the inspiratory reserve volume (IRV). You must be able to determine the various volumes and capacities from a spirometry tracing.

c. Interpret the results (Code: IB10e and IIIE7a) [Difficulty: ELE: R, Ap; WRE: An]

Normal racial differences in the FVC must be taken into consideration. Most modern pulmonary function systems automatically adjust the measured values for racial differences when so programmed by the operator. If not, the predicted values should be mathematically adjusted by the therapist. The predicted normal values, in liters, for the FVC in Caucasian patients were reported by Morris, Koski, and Johnson (1971) as:*

Men: $[(0.148 \times \text{Height in inches}) - (0.025 \times \text{Age})]$
$= 4.24 \,[\text{SD (1 standard deviation)} \, 0.58]$

Women: $[(0.115 \times \text{Height in inches}) - (0.024 \times \text{Age})]$
$= 2.85 \,(\text{SD } 0.52)$

EXAMPLE

Calculate the predicted FVC for a 50-year-old Caucasian man who is 6 feet (72 inches) tall.

$$\begin{aligned} \text{FVC} &= [(0.148 \times \text{Height in inches}) - (0.025 \times \text{Age})] - 4.24 \\ &= [(0.148 \times 72) - (0.025 \times 50)] - 4.24 \\ &= (10.656 - 1.25) - 4.24 \\ &= 9.406 - 4.24 \\ &= 5.166 \, \text{L} \end{aligned}$$

African Americans are known to have a smaller lung capacity than Caucasians of the same height. For this reason, a 10% to 15% adjustment should be made for the predicted FVC and TLC of an African American patient. In other words, the predicted values for this patient are 85% to 90% of those of a comparable Caucasian patient.

Adjustments for Hispanic and Asian populations are not so well documented. It has been reported that the

predicted FVC values should be adjusted downward by 20% to 25% for Asians.

It has been commonly accepted that a measured FVC at least 80% of the predicted FVC is considered to be within normal limits for adults of all races. In addition, the FEV$_1$ and TLC measurements have been included in this 80% of predicted rule. More recent studies by Knudson, Kaltenborn, Knudson, and associates (1987) and Paoletti, Viegi, Pistelli, and associates (1985) suggest that normal values for most tests should be determined by finding the percentage of predicted value above which 95% of the population would be seen (the so-called normal 95th percentile). Even though this method finds 5% (1 in 20) of healthy nonsmokers to be abnormal, it offers more realistic predicted values. It is normal to see a decline in the FVC with age.

Restrictive problems, such as advanced pregnancy, obesity, ascites, neuromuscular disease, sarcoidosis, and chest wall or spinal deformity, can result in a small FVC. Patients with chronic obstructive lung diseases, such as emphysema, bronchitis, asthma, cystic fibrosis, and bronchiectasis, commonly have a small FVC. (Figure 4-5 shows a comparison of the spirometry tracings of a normal, an obstructed, and a restricted patient.)

The limitations of this text prevent a discussion of back-extrapolation to find the start of a less than perfect effort or the calculations for correcting volumes and flows from atmospheric temperature, pressure, saturated (ATPS) to body temperature, pressure, saturated (BTPS). However, most textbooks on pulmonary function testing discuss these topics. Because the BTPS correction reflects the patient's true effort, it is standard practice to report all flows and volumes in BTPS.

Exam Hint 4-5 (WRE)

You may need to calculate how close a patient's FVC or other breathing effort has come to his or her predicted value. This is known as the *patient's percentage of predicted*. It is found by this equation:

$$\frac{\text{Patient's actual test result}}{\text{Patient's predicted test value}} \times 100 = \text{Patient's \% of predicted}$$

For example, in the previous discussion on FVC, it was determined that a patient had a predicted FVC of 5.166 L. Calculate the percentage of predicted if the actual FVC result is 4.65 L.

$$\frac{4.65 \, \text{L}}{5.116} \times 100 = \text{Patient's \% of predicted} = .90 \times 100 = 90\%$$

Therefore, the patient exhaled 90% of predicted FVC and is within the normal range for that test result.

---

*The atmospheric temperature, pressure, saturated (ATPS) to body temperature, pressure, saturated (BTPS) correction has been calculated into these equations.

4. Peak flow

a. Perform the procedure (Code: IB9d) [Difficulty: ELE: R; WRE: Ap, An]

The peak flow is the highest flow rate seen in a patient's forced expiratory effort. Some authors refer to the PF as the peak expiratory flow rate. It usually is seen at the beginning of the FVC effort. The instructions for the test must emphasize that the patient must "blast" the air out as hard and fast as possible. It is not necessary to encourage the patient to empty the lungs completely to residual volume.

For bedside spirometry or home care, the patient's effort is easily measured directly with a handheld peak flowmeter. Usually at least three efforts are required to find two that are acceptably close. PF values that are consistent and low despite variable patient efforts probably indicate a malfunctioning unit that should not be used. It is reasonable to record the patient's effort in liters per second, because the effort takes place in about that much time. However, do not be confused by some measurement instruments and other prediction equations giving the value in liters per minute. Simply multiply or divide by 60 to convert your patient's effort from one time frame to the other. For example, a young man's PF might be recorded as 10 L/sec or 600 L/min. Cherniack and Raber (1972) published the following formulas for predicting PF in liters per second*:

$$\text{Men:} [(0.144 \times \text{Height in inches}) - (0.024 \times \text{Age})] + 2.225$$

$$\text{Women:} [(0.090 \times \text{Height in inches}) - (0.018 \times \text{Age})] + 1.130$$

b. Interpret the results (Code: IB10d) [Difficulty: ELE: R, Ap; WRE: An]

The PF is directly related to height and indirectly related to age. Therefore, the taller the patient, the greater the PF. The PF decreases with age. The PF is a rather nonspecific measurement of airway obstruction. It measures flow through the upper airways and is reduced in patients with an upper airway problem, such as a tumor, vocal cord paralysis, or laryngeal edema.

The PF test is most often given to patients having an asthma attack as a quick and easy measurement of small airway obstruction. Current asthma guidelines state that if the peak flow of a patient with asthma is 80% to 100% of predicted or personal best, he or she is in the green zone. This means that the patient's medications are adequately controlling the asthma. If the peak flow is 50% to 79% of predicted or personal best, he or she is in the yellow zone. This means that the patient's medi-

cations are not adequately controlling the asthma. Increased doses are indicated if ordered by the physician. If the peak flow is less than 50% of predicted or personal best, the patient is in the red zone. This means that the patient's medications are not adequately controlling the asthma. The patient should get medical help as soon as possible.

It is the respiratory therapist's responsibility to calculate the patient's color zones and mark them on the patient's personal peak flowmeter. The therapist must instruct the patient in the meaning of the color zones and the appropriate use of the prescribed inhaled bronchodilator and/or corticosteroid medications.

Timed forced expiratory volume tests

All of the timed forced expiratory volume tests are derived from a properly performed FVC test (see Figure 4-3). When the FVC is done correctly, the following values can be properly calculated and evaluated to determine the patient's condition. As discussed earlier, an FVC within 80% of predicted is interpreted as within normal limits. Therefore, if the results of the following tests show patient values within 80% of predicted, the results are interpreted as being within normal limits.

5. Forced expiratory flow$_{25\%-75\%}$ (FEF$_{25\%-75\%}$)

a. Perform the procedure (Code: IB9u) [Difficulty: ELE: R, Ap; WRE: An]

The FEF$_{25\%-75\%}$ is the mean forced expiratory flow during the middle half of an acceptable FVC (Figure 4-6). The FVC effort to use for this test is the one that has the greatest combination of FVC volume and FEV$_1$. As mentioned earlier, the patient must give his or her best effort. The measurement usually is recorded in liters per second but may be recorded in liters per minute.

b. Interpret the results (Code: IB10u) [Difficulty: ELE: R, Ap; WRE: An]

The results are normally less than in the PF test, because the flow being measured comes from medium-size and small airways (smaller than 2 mm in diameter). The results should decline with age and should be lower in women than in men. A patient with a restrictive lung disease may have a normal or increased value, whereas a low value is seen in a patient with obstructive lung disease. A small FEF$_{25\%-75\%}$ value when the FVC and FEV$_1$ values are normal often is taken to indicate early small airway disease. A normal, 68-kg (150-lb) young man should have values of 4 to 5 L/sec or 240 to 300 L/min. The following formulas were developed by Morris, Koski, and Johnson (1971) and can be used to calculate the predicted values in liters per second:

---

*The ATPS to BTPS correction has been calculated into these equations.

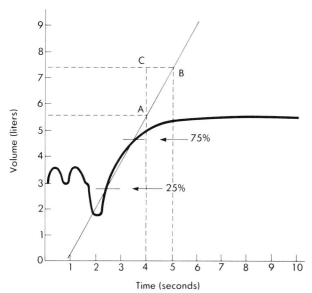

Figure 4-6 One method of determining the 25% to 75% forced expiratory flow (FEF$_{25\%-75\%}$) value from a forced vital capacity (FVC) tracing. First, mark the 25% and 75% points from the start of the effort. These are found by multiplying the FVC value by 0.25 and 0.75, respectively, and measuring from the start of the effort. Second, draw a line through these two points to intersect the dashed time lines at points *A* and *B*. Horizontal dashed lines are added from *A* and *B* to cross the volume scale. The FEF$_{25\%-75\%}$ value is read as the distance between *A* and *C*, or about 2 L/sec. BTPS correct this measurement. *(From Ruppel G: Manual of pulmonary function testing, ed 9, St Louis, 2009, Mosby.)*

$$\text{Men: } [(0.047 \times \text{Height in inches}) - (0.045 \times \text{Age in years})] + 2.513\,(\text{SD } 1.12)$$

$$\text{Women: } [(0.060 \times \text{Height in inches}) - (0.030 \times \text{Age in years})] + 0.551\,(\text{SD } 0.80)$$

6. Forced expiratory volume timed (FEV$_T$)

a. Perform the procedure (Code: IB9u) [Difficulty: ELE: R, Ap; WRE: An]

The FEV$_T$ is the volume of air exhaled from an acceptable FVC in the specified time. The time increments are 0.5, 1, 2, and 3 seconds or more and are listed as FEV$_{0.5}$, FEV$_1$, FEV$_2$, FEV$_3$, and so on. It is important that the FVC have a good start and a maximum effort to the end.

The FEV$_1$ is the measurement most commonly used, along with the FVC, to judge the patient's response to inhaled bronchodilators, for bronchoprovocation testing to screen for asthmatic tendencies, to detect exercise-induced asthma, and for simple screening. BTPS correct all the measured values.

The timed forced expiratory volumes (FEV$_{0.5}$, FEV$_1$, FEV$_2$, FEV$_3$) effectively "cut" the FVC into sections based on how much volume the patient forcibly exhales in 0.5, 1, 2, and 3 seconds. Some patients with severe obstructive

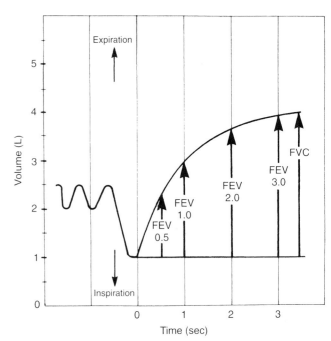

Figure 4-7 Forced vital capacity divided into FEV$_{0.5}$, FEV$_{1.0}$, FEV$_{2.0}$, and FEV$_{3.0}$. *(From Ruppel G: Manual of pulmonary function testing, ed 4, St Louis, 1986, Mosby.)*

lung disease require several more seconds to exhale completely. In these cases, simply keep measuring the volume exhaled in each additional second. Figure 4-7 shows an FVC tracing that is subdivided at 0.5-, 1-, 2-, and 3-second intervals. Some bedside units give a numeric value for some or all of the timed intervals; however, it is best to have a spirometer that produces a printed copy of the patient's FVC effort. The individual volumes can be determined by marking the vertical distance on the volume scale from the baseline (total lung capacity) to the respective arrow tips.

b. Interpret the results (Code: IB10u) [Difficulty: ELE: R, Ap; WRE: An]

The FEV$_T$ values often are reduced in both restrictive and obstructive lung diseases. Patients with a severe restrictive lung disease exhale almost all of their small FVC within the first second. Patients with severe obstructive lung disease show low values at all time intervals, with the volumes at FEV$_2$, FEV$_3$, and so on, becoming progressively smaller. The most commonly evaluated values are the FEV$_1$ and the FEV$_{1\%}$. The following formulas* were developed by Morris, Koski, and Johnson (1971) and can be used to calculate the predicted values for FEV$_1$ in liters:

---

*The ATPS to BTPS correction has been calculated into these equations.

Men: $[(0.092 \times \text{height in inches}) - (0.032 \times \text{age in years})]$
$$- 1.260 \,(\text{SD } 0.55)$$

Women: $[(0.089 \times \text{height in inches}) - (0.024 \times \text{age in years})]$
$$- 1.93 \,(\text{SD } 0.47)$$

7. Forced expiratory volume/forced vital capacity ratio (FEV$_T$/FVC or FEV$_{T\%}$)

a. Perform the procedure (Code: IB9u) [Difficulty: ELE: R, Ap; WRE: An]

The FEV$_T$ to FVC ratio compares, by division, the volume exhaled at 0.5, 1, 2, and 3 (or more) seconds (see Figure 4-7) with the FVC. This results in a series of decimal fractions. These are multiplied by 100 to convert the answers to percentages.

Because each person's FVC is unique, the FEV time interval volumes taken from the FVC also are unique. The division process described previously standardizes the FEV time interval results, regardless of the patient's FVC. Therefore, these percentage values can be standardized for all individuals despite different FVCs. The predicted values for normal patients are as follows:

FEV$_{0.5}$ 50% to 60% of the FVC
FEV$_1$ 75% to 85% of the FVC
FEV$_2$ 94% of the FVC
FEV$_3$ 97% of the FVC

b. Interpret the results (Code: IB10u) [Difficulty: ELE: R, Ap; WRE: An]

These values normally decrease slightly in elderly patients. Most patients with normal lungs and airways are still able to completely exhale the FVC within 4 seconds.

Patients with restrictive lung diseases often exhale the FVC more quickly than expected. This happens because these patients have a smaller than normal FVC and stiff lungs, which recoil more quickly than expected to their resting volume. See Figure 4-4 to compare the FVC curves of a patient with restrictive lung disease with the FVC curves of a patient with obstructive lung disease.

Patients with obstructive lung disease take longer than expected to exhale the FVC. As a result, the percentages of the FVC exhaled in the timed intervals listed are lower than normal. Obviously, the lower the percentage exhaled for any timed interval, the worse the obstruction to exhalation. A patient with restrictive lung disease exhales the FVC too quickly, and all of the derived values are higher than expected.

Exam Hint 4-6 (ELE, WRE)

Of all the timed forced expiratory volume tests, the FEV$_1$ is the most important to monitor. An FEV$_1$ of less than 70% of the FVC confirms obstructive lung disease.

---

8. Spirometry before and after inhalation of an aerosolized bronchodilator

a. Perform the procedure (Code: IB9u) [Difficulty: ELE: R, Ap; WRE: An]

The following are common indications for the procedure:

- The patient is known to have asthma or another type of chronic obstructive lung disease.
- The patient has an FEV$_{1\%}$ of less than 70% (unless elderly).
- The effectiveness of a new bronchodilator is being evaluated.

The most commonly administered tests are the PF and FEV$_{1\%}$ from an FVC. Before starting the test, make sure that the patient has not taken a bronchodilating drug in the previous 4 to 6 hours. If no bronchodilating drugs have been administered, the test can be performed. A PF or FEV$_{1\%}$ test is performed and the value or values are measured, and then a fast-onset, sympathomimetic-type drug is given. The medication can be given by intermittent positive-pressure breathing (IPPB), handheld nebulizer, or metered-dose inhaler (MDI), as long as the method is done properly. Wait about 10 to 15 minutes for the medication to take effect and the patient's blood gas values to return to normal. Then repeat the PF or FEV$_{1\%}$ test. The percentage of improvement is calculated using this formula:

$$\text{Percentage of change} = \frac{\text{After drug airflow} - \text{Before drug airflow}}{\text{Before drug airflow}} \times 100$$

b. Interpret the results (Code: IB10u) [Difficulty: ELE: R, Ap; WRE: An]

To prove that the medication is effective, according to the current standard, the patient must have at least a 12% improvement in PF or FEV$_{1\%}$ or both and a 200-mL increase in exhaled volume. (The old standard required a 15% to 20% improvement in flow.) It is not uncommon to see patients with asthma improve much more than this. Other patients may not have this much improvement but do show increases in airflow and FVC and say that they feel better. In these cases, the physician may decide to continue the medication.

Exam Hint 4-7 (ELE, WRE)

A postbronchodilator increase in PF or FEV$_{1\%}$ of at least 15% shows reversible small airway obstruction. This indicates that a patient with asthma or COPD is responding to the inhaled bronchodilator.

9. Bronchoprovocation studies

a. Perform the procedure (Code: IIIE7f) [Difficulty: ELE: R, Ap; WRE: An]

A bronchoprovocation study (also known as *bronchial provocation*) is indicated when a patient has a history indicating asthma or hyperactive airways yet has normal spirometry testing. This means that the patient's FVC and FEV_1 from the forced vital capacity are within normal limits. Other indications for a bronchoprovocation study include assessing the severity of airway hyperresponsiveness; evaluating the risk of asthma developing, including occupational asthma; assessing the effectiveness of medications to control the patient's asthma; and excluding asthma during a diagnostic workup.

The most common testing regimen involves having the patient inhale increasingly higher doses of nebulized methacholine (a cholinergic [parasympathetic] drug) and measuring spirometry results. Because of this, the procedure may be referred to as a *methacholine challenge test.* Occasionally, other factors, such as cold air exercising; inhaling an histamine; or inhaling a targeted antigen, such as animal dander, are substituted for methacholine. In addition, to evaluate the effectiveness of asthma-controlling medications, the physician may order that they be withheld for a specified period. The following discussion is limited to inhaled methacholine.

Testing should not be performed on an at-risk patient, such as someone who (1) has an FEV_1 of less than 50% of predicted, (2) has had a stroke or heart attack within the past 3 months, (3) has uncontrolled hypertension, or (4) has a known aortic or cerebral aneurysm. Remember, above all, that a positive test result indicates that the patient has some level of bronchospasm.

The basic procedure is as follows:

1. Perform a baseline FVC and measure the FEV_1 from it. These results should be within the normal range to justify continuing the testing procedure.
2. Have the patient inhale nebulized normal saline (0.9% NaCl). Repeat the FVC. A decrease in the FEV_1 of 10% or greater is a positive response. See step 6.
3. If the patient is normal, continue as follows: Have the patient inhale 0.03 mg/mL of nebulized methacholine. Repeat the FVC. A decrease in the FEV_1 of 20% or greater is a positive response. (For example, after the methacholine was inhaled, the patient's FEV_1 dropped from 3,000 mL to 2,500 mL.) See step 7.
4. If the patient is normal, continue as follows: Have the patient inhale 0.06 mg/mL of nebulized methacholine. Repeat the FVC. A decrease in the FEV_1 of 20% or greater is a positive response. See step 6.

If the patient is normal, continue as follows:

5. Repeat step 4 with the methacholine dose doubling each time (e.g., 0.12, 0.24, 0.48 mg/mL, and so on). Stop the testing if the patient reaches the maximum methacholine dose of 16 mg/mL.
6. Stop any further testing. Assess the patient's vital signs, breath sounds, and oxygenation. Administer a nebulized, fast-acting bronchodilator medication, such as albuterol (see Chapter 9) if needed. Report the findings to the physician in charge.
7. Repeat spirometry to demonstrate that the patient has returned to his or her baseline values. Do not discharge the patient until he or she has returned to normal.
8. Chart the findings of the testing procedure, including how much methacholine was inhaled and how much the FEV_1 dropped.

b. Interpret the results (Code: IIIE7f) [Difficulty: ELE: R, Ap; WRE: An]

If the patient has the above-specified drop in FEV_1, the physician would interpret that to mean the patient had a positive test and has a bronchospasm-inducing condition. Inhaling a small amount of methacholine with a large drop in FEV_1 indicates a severe reaction. A negative test result is seen if the patient inhales the maximum dose of methacholine (16 mg/mL) without a significant drop in FEV_1.

10. Flow-volume loops

a. Perform the procedure (Code: IB9u) [Difficulty: ELE: R, Ap; WRE: An]

The flow-volume loop is a graphic display of the flow and volume generated during a forced expiratory vital capacity (FEVC) that is immediately followed by a forced inspiratory vital capacity (FIVC). It is used to identify inspiratory or expiratory flow at any lung volume.

As with the FVC test, the patient should be coached to inhale completely and blast the air out until he or she is completely empty. When you are sure that the patient has exhaled to residual volume, coach him or her to inhale as quickly as possible until the lungs are completely full. No hesitation at the start, leaks, glottis closing, or coughing should occur throughout the entire procedure.

The expiratory half of the curve is called the *maximum expiratory flow-volume (MEFV) curve.* It begins at TLC and ends at residual volume. The inspiratory half of the curve is called the *maximum inspiratory flow-volume (MIFV) curve.* It begins at residual volume and ends at TLC. Ideally, the two halves of the loop meet at the TLC. Flow is recorded in liters per second and graphed on the vertical (ordinate, or *y*) axis. Volume is recorded in liters and graphed on the horizontal (abscissa, or *x*) axis. Both flow and volume should be BTPS adjusted.

b. Interpret the results (Code: IB10u) [Difficulty: ELE: R, Ap; WRE: An]

Flow-volume loops have gained great popularity, because the shape of the curve is diagnostic of the patient's condition. In addition, the peak inspiratory and peak expiratory flows can be determined. If the effort can be timed, all the parameters found on the previously discussed volume-time curves can be found on the flow-volume loop. The following examples show a normal flow-volume loop and representative abnormal loops.

1. Normal

A normal flow-volume loop is shown in Figures 4-8 and 4-9. First look at Figure 4-8, in which the various volumes are measured on the horizontal scale. The tidal volume (V_T) of 500 mL is the small loop within the larger VC loop. The ERV and IRV are shown on both sides of the tidal volume. The FVC is shown as the total of all three volumes. Finally, TLC and residual volume (RV) are marked.

Figure 4-9 shows the same normal flow-volume loop in which the various flows are measured on the vertical scale. Starting from TLC with the FEVC, the peak expiratory flow rate is seen as the greatest flow generated; it is about 9 L/sec. Starting from RV with the FIVC, the peak inspiratory flow rate is seen as the greatest flow that is generated; it is about 7 L/sec. It is normal for the PEFR to be greater than the PIFR.

To find the instantaneous flow at any FVC lung volume, the FVC must be divided by 4 to find the 25th, 50th, and 75th percentile points. In Figure 4-8, the FVC is 4,800 mL. Dividing by 4 gives 1,200 mL per quarter of the FVC. These points are marked on the horizontal volume scale. If a vertical (dashed) line is drawn through these three points to the flow-volume tracing, the instantaneous flows at these volumes can be found. *Expiratory flows* are reported as follows:

- Flow at 75% of the FEVC = $\dot{V}_{max75}$ (maximum flow with 75% of the FVC remaining), or $FEF_{25\%}$ (forced expiratory flow with 25% of the FVC exhaled)
- Flow at 50% of the FEVC = $\dot{V}_{max50}$ (maximum flow with 50% of the FVC remaining), or $FEF_{50\%}$ (forced expiratory flow with 50% of the FVC exhaled)
- Flow at 25% of the FEVC = $\dot{V}_{max25}$ (maximum flow with 25% of the FVC remaining), or $FEF_{75\%}$ (forced expiratory flow with 75% of the FVC exhaled)

Inspiratory flows are reported in this way:

- Flow at 25% of the FIVC = $FIF_{25\%}$ (forced inspiratory flow with 25% of the FVC inhaled)
- Flow at 50% of the FIVC = $FIF_{50\%}$ (forced inspiratory flow with 50% of the FVC inhaled)
- Flow at 75% of the FIVC = $FIF_{75\%}$ (forced inspiratory flow with 75% of the FVC inhaled)

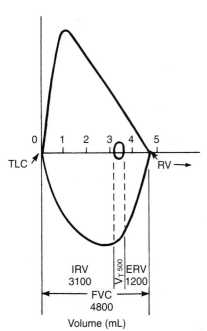

Figure 4-8 Flow-volume loop tracing of a normal adult showing the positions and values of the lung volumes. *ERV,* Expiratory reserve volume; *FVC,* forced vital capacity; *IRV,* inspiratory reserve volume; *RV,* residual volume; *TLC,* total lung capacity.

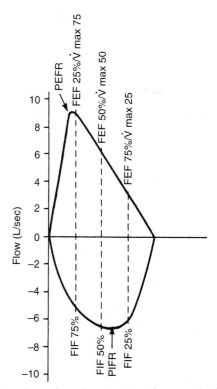

Figure 4-9 Flow-volume loop tracing of a normal adult showing the positions and values of the various inspiratory and expiratory flows. *FEF,* Forced expiratory flow; *FIF,* forced inspiratory flow; *PEFR,* peak expiratory flow rate; *PIFR,* peak inspiratory flow rate.

The PEFR and FEF_{25} or $\dot{V}_{max75\%}$ values should be about the same, because they all measure flow through the large upper airways. Either test is a good gauge of the patient's effort, because it will be low if the patient is not trying hard. The FEF_{50} or $\dot{V}_{max50\%}$ values should approximate the $FEF_{25\%-75\%}$ values, because they both show flow through the medium to small airways in the middle half of the FVC effort. It is normal for the FIF_{50} to be greater than the FEF_{50}. The FEF_{75} or $\dot{V}_{max25\%}$ values are the best indicator of early small airway disease because both show flow through the small airways as the patient approaches the residual volume. Note that the tracing from the FEF_{25} or $\dot{V}_{max75\%}$ point to the residual volume is close to a straight line. In normal patients, the flow decreases in proportion to the decreasing lung volume, resulting in the straight-line tracing. Cherniack and Raber (1972) published formulas for predicting adult MEFV flows in liters per second; see the bibliography.

2. Small airway disease

Examples of conditions that result in disease in the small airways (i.e., those less than 2 mm in diameter) include asthma, chronic bronchitis, bronchiectasis, cystic fibrosis, and emphysema. The obstruction can be from bronchospasm, mucus plugging, or damage to the alveoli and small airways, leading to their collapse on expiration.

Figure 4-10 shows representative flow-volume loops for patients with asthma and emphysema superimposed over a normal flow-volume loop. Note that both loops are shifted to the left, toward the TLC, because the residual volumes are increased. Also note that the flows are decreased more than normal as the patient exhales closer to the residual volume. This "scooped out" appearance is very characteristic of small airway disease. Having the patient inhale a bronchodilator and repeating the flow-volume loop shows the degree of reversibility. Some computer-based systems allow the before and after bronchodilator loops to be superimposed to show further the amount of improvement.

3. Restriction

A restriction can be caused by a pulmonary condition, such as fibrosis; a thoracic condition, such as pleural effusion, pneumothorax, hemothorax, or kyphoscoliosis; or obesity, advanced pregnancy, or ascites pushing up on the diaphragm. Only fibrosis and kyphoscoliosis are permanent. Figure 4-10 shows a representative flow-volume loop for a patient with restrictive lung disease. Note that the volume is small and shifted to the right, toward the small residual volume.

4. Variable intrathoracic obstruction

A variable intrathoracic obstruction can be caused by a tumor or foreign body that partly blocks a bronchus. Figure 4-10 shows a representative flow-volume curve. Note that the FVC volume is almost normal, with a greatly decreased peak expiratory flow rate.

5. Variable extrathoracic obstruction

A variable extrathoracic obstruction can be caused by vocal cord paralysis, laryngeal tumor, or a foreign body that partly obstructs the upper airway. Figure 4-10 shows a representative flow-volume curve. Note that the FVC volume is almost normal, with a greatly reduced inspiratory flow. This same pattern is commonly seen in patients

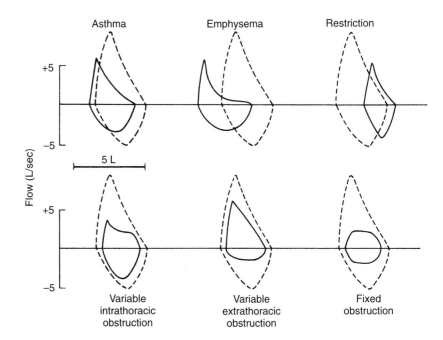

Figure 4-10   A series of abnormal flow-volume loop tracings superimposed over a dashed-line tracing of a normal loop. *(From Ruppel G: Manual of pulmonary function testing, ed 9, St Louis, 2009, Mosby.)*

with obstructive sleep apnea. The $FEF_{50\%}$ will be greater than the $FIF_{50\%}$.

6. Fixed obstruction

A fixed obstruction usually is caused by a tumor in the trachea or a mainstem bronchus. Figure 4-10 shows a representative flow-volume loop. Again, the FVC volume is close to normal. Note the abnormally reduced inspiratory and expiratory flow rates. The tracing looks almost squared off, with the $FEF_{50\%}$ and $FIF_{50\%}$ values being about the same.

Exam Hint 4-8 (WRE)

Expect to see a flow-volume loop that needs to be interpreted for the patient's condition or to find a specific value, such as the vital capacity or peak flow.

11. Maximum voluntary ventilation

a. Perform the procedure (Code: IB9u) [Difficulty: ELE: R, Ap; WRE: An]

The maximum voluntary ventilation (MVV) is the volume of air exhaled in a specified period during a repetitive maximum respiratory effort. It is most commonly done to evaluate a patient's ability to perform a stress test. It also may be used as a preoperative screening test to help determine the patient's chance of pulmonary complications.

The patient should breathe at a volume that is greater than the tidal volume but less than the VC, at a rate of 70 to 120 per minute. The minimum time for the test is 12 seconds. Figure 4-11 shows two different tracings of the MVV effort. The total volume exhaled in the given period is mathematically adjusted for 1 minute so that the derived value is in liters per minute. This is done by multiplying a 5-second effort by 12 or a 12-second effort by 5. The derived value then is BTPS corrected to give the final value.

b. Interpret the results (Code: IB10u) [Difficulty: ELE: R, Ap; WRE: An]

The results of the MVV test are among the most difficult to evaluate. This is because the patient's effort, the condition of the respiratory muscles, lung and thoracic compliance, neurologic control over the drive to breathe, and airway and tissue resistance all have an influence. Abnormalities in any of these can cause the MVV to decrease. Because more than one problem can exist, a decreased MVV does not point out the exact difficulty. A healthy young man can have an MVV of 150 to 200 L/min. Women tend to have smaller values, and the values of both genders decrease with age. Because of the many factors involved in the MVV, normal predicted values may vary by as much as ± 30%. Therefore, unless the MVV is less than 70% of

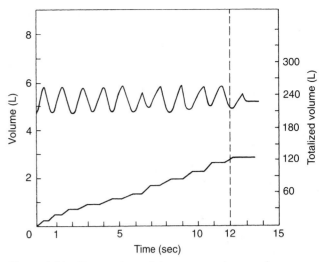

Figure 4-11 Two tracings of the same maximum voluntary ventilation (MVV) effort. The saw-toothed tracing shows each individual volume effort and the respiratory rate. The stair-stepped tracing shows the cumulative volume during the effort. *(From Ruppel G: Manual of pulmonary function testing, ed 6, St Louis, 1994, Mosby.)*

predicted, the patient cannot really be considered abnormal.

Cherniack and Raber (1972) published the following equations* for predicting the MVV in liters per minute:

Males: $[(3.03 \times \text{Height in inches}) - (0.816 \times \text{Age in years})] - 37.9$

Females: $[(2.14 \times \text{Height in inches}) - (0.685 \times \text{Age in years})] - 4.87$

The following considerations are important in the evaluation of an abnormally low MVV value:
1. Did the patient try his or her best? The respiratory therapist must make a professional judgment that the patient made his or her best effort. An objective way of judging this is to multiply the patient's FEV_1 by 35 to estimate the MVV. They should be close to the same volume. For example, if the patient's FEV_1 is 3 L, the estimated MVV is 105 L/min (3 L × 35). An MVV that is much less than this indicates that the patient did not try very hard. Conversely, an MVV value that is much greater than this indicates that the FEV_1 value is too low and should be repeated.
2. What is the condition of the patient's respiratory muscles? Patients with neuromuscular abnormalities probably will not be able to breathe much more deeply than the normal tidal volume or keep up the great effort required for the duration of the test. Because of this, their results will be low.
3. What is the patient's lung/thoracic compliance? Patients with low compliance probably will not be able

---

*The ATPS to BTPS correction has been calculated into these equations.

to sustain the greater than normal workload required by the MVV test. However, some patients are able to compensate for a small tidal volume by increasing their respiratory rate enough to generate an MVV value within normal limits. A printout of the MVV test would show a smaller than expected volume moved at a higher than expected respiratory rate.

4. What is the patient's neurologic control over the drive to breathe? Patients who have had an injury to the brain may have an abnormal drive to breathe. Because of this, they produce a low MVV.

5. What is the patient's airway and tissue resistance? Patients with increased airway resistance usually have a low MVV result. This problem also may cause air trapping and force the patient to stop the effort. Increased tissue resistance, such as is seen in pulmonary edema, obesity, and ascites, also results in a low MVV value.

Despite these difficulties in determining the cause of a decreased MVV value, doing so has proven helpful in preoperative evaluation and cardiopulmonary stress testing. Any patient with a lower than normal MVV value is at an increased risk of postoperative atelectasis and pneumonia. The risks of pulmonary complications related to MVV are low when the patient reaches 75% to 50% of predicted, moderate when the patient reaches 50% to 33% of predicted, and high when the patient reaches less than 33% of predicted. Patients with known moderate to severe COPD usually have to stop exercise testing because of their inability to breathe. An MVV value of less than 50 L/min is a good predictor of this.

12. Single-breath nitrogen washout test and closing volume

Note: This test is not listed in the NBRC's detailed content outlines. However, questions about the test have been included in recent versions of the *Written Registry Examination*.

a. Perform the procedure (Code: IB9u) [Difficulty: ELE: R, Ap; WRE: An]

The single-breath nitrogen washout (SBN$_2$) is used to measure two things: (1) the evenness of the distribution of ventilation into the lungs during inspiration and (2) the emptying rates of the lungs during exhalation. It is a helpful diagnostic test in any adult patient who is known to have or suspected of having obstructive airway disease. The NBRC uses the phrase *nitrogen washout distribution test* for its examinations.

The closing volume is one part of the SBN$_2$ test. It marks the lung volume when small airway closure begins and is used as an early indicator of small airway disease.

The SBN$_2$ test is done by analyzing the nitrogen (N$_2$) percentage exhaled after an inspiratory vital capacity (IVC) of 100% oxygen. It is beyond the scope of this book to go

into detail on all the steps of the procedure; however, the general steps include instructing the patient to perform an IVC test while inhaling oxygen. The patient is told to exhale slowly and evenly until the lungs are empty again, without any breath holding. The exhaled gases are sent through a rapid N$_2$ analyzer to measure the percentage, a spirometer to measure the volume, and a graphing device.

b. Interpret the results (Code: IB10u) [Difficulty: ELE: R, Ap; WRE: An]

Figure 4-12 shows a normal tracing, which shows these phases:

- **Phase I** shows gas exhaled from the anatomic dead space of the upper airway. Because it is made up of 100% oxygen, the nitrogen percentage shows a zero reading.
- **Phase II** shows a mix of dead space gas and alveolar gas. The nitrogen percentage increases rapidly as the pure oxygen is exhaled and nitrogen-rich gas from the alveoli is brought out. The first 750 mL of gas that includes these first two phases is not used in the evaluation of the distribution of ventilation.
- **Phase III** shows a fairly level plateau as alveolar gas from the lower lobes with a stable mix of oxygen and nitrogen is exhaled. Phase III is further evaluated in the following two ways:
  (1) $\Delta N_{2\,750\text{-}1250}$ looks at the increase in the nitrogen percentage found in the 500 mL of gas exhaled between 750 mL and 1,250 mL of the VC. It is normally no more than 1.5% in healthy young adults. It increases to 3% to 4.5% in healthy older adults. Patients with severe airway and lung disease, such

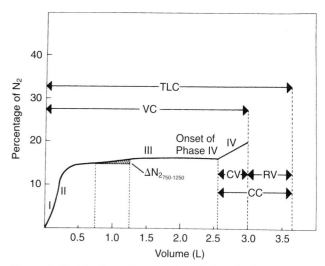

Figure 4-12 Tracing of a normal single-breath nitrogen washout (SBN$_2$) test showing the four phases and other features. *CC,* Closing capacity; *CV,* closing volume; $\Delta N_{2\,750\text{-}1250}$, nitrogen percentage found in the 500 mL of gas exhaled between 750 and 1250 mL of the vital capacity; *RV,* residual volume; *TLC,* total lung capacity; *VC,* vital capacity. (*From Ruppel G: Manual of pulmonary function testing, ed 9, St Louis, 2009, Mosby.*)

as emphysema, may have a finding of 6% to 10% or more.

(2) The slope of phase III is found by drawing a straight line from the point where 30% of the VC is exhaled to the point where phase IV begins. It is normally no more than 0.5% to 1% N_2 per liter of exhaled volume in healthy young adults, but it may vary widely.

- *Phase IV* is seen as a sharp increase in the nitrogen percentage and continues to residual volume. This is seen when the nitrogen-rich gas from the upper airways continues to be exhaled as the basilar airways became compressed and close off near the end of the VC effort.

The start of phase IV is called the *closing volume* (CV). It marks the lung volume when small airway closure begins and is an early indicator of small airway disease. CV does not occur in healthy young adults until after about 80% to 90% of the VC has been exhaled. The closing capacity (CC) is found by adding the closing volume to the residual volume (found by another test). Healthy young adults have a CC that is about 30% of their TLC.

Problems can be indicated as follows: increases in the $\Delta N_{2\ 750-1250}$, the slope of phase III, and especially early onset of phase IV; increased closing volume; and increased closing capacity. The diseases or conditions that can cause these abnormal test results are small airway disease, congestive heart failure with pulmonary edema, and obesity.

13. Functional residual capacity by the helium dilution method

Note: This test is not listed in the NBRC's detailed content outlines. However, questions about interpreta-tion of the results of lung volume tests have been included in recent versions of the *Written Registry Examination*.

a. Perform the procedure (Code: IIIE7c) [Difficulty: ELE: R, Ap; WRE: An]

The functional residual capacity (FRC) is the volume of gas left in the lungs at the end of a normal expiration. It cannot be measured through spirometry. The FRC is needed to calculate a patient's residual volume (RV) and TLC. It is necessary to know a patient's RV, FRC, and TLC to diagnose and determine the severity of obstructive lung disease and restrictive lung disease.

The helium (He) dilution method basically involves diluting the resident gases in the lungs (mainly nitrogen and oxygen) with helium to mathematically determine the FRC. This also is called the *closed-circuit* method, because the patient and circuit are sealed off. Figure 4-13 shows a schematic drawing of the components that make up the circuit. These include a two-way valve to switch the patient from breathing room air to the helium mix, soda lime to absorb the patient's exhaled carbon dioxide from the circuit, a combined carbon dioxide (CO_2) and water vapor absorber to prevent these gases from entering the helium analyzer, the helium analyzer, a variable speed blower to move the gases through the circuit, a spirometer for monitoring tidal volumes, an attached kymograph to trace the patient's breathing pattern, and an oxygen supply to meet the patient's needs. The helium supply is not shown.

It is beyond the scope of this text to cover all the steps in the helium dilution test; however, the following features of the procedure are important to know. Add enough helium to the room air in the circuit to create a 10% to

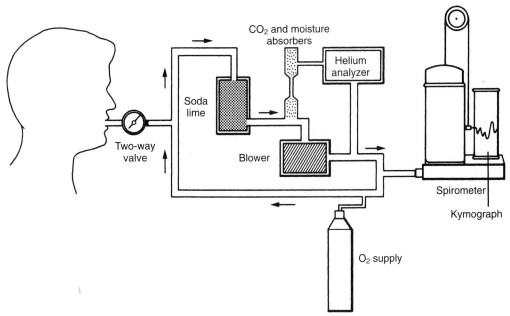

Figure 4-13   Schematic drawing of the key components of a helium dilution system for measuring functional residual capacity. *(From Beauchamp RK: Pulmonary function testing procedures. In Barnes TA, editor: Respiratory care practice, St Louis, 1988, Mosby.)*

15% He mix. At the end of a normal exhalation, the patient is switched to breathing the mix so that the FRC can be determined. The patient breathes the gas mix until the helium is evenly distributed throughout the lungs and the helium percentage is stable. Typically, the test is performed for up to 7 minutes, if needed, to reach an equilibrium point. Extending the test longer may help to reach a stable equilibrium point in abnormal patients. The calculation of RV is rather complex and usually is done through the computer built into the pulmonary function system. Spirometry also must be performed, because the ERV is subtracted from the FRC to find the RV. Commonly the test is repeated. The patient should be allowed to breathe room air for 5 minutes between tests to clear the helium from the lungs. Patients with severe obstructive lung disease may need more time. Bates, Macklem, and Christie (1971) published the following equations* for calculating the normal FRC in liters:

$$\text{Males: } (0.130 \times \text{Height in inches}) - 5.16$$

$$\text{Females: } (0.119 \times \text{Height in inches}) - 4.85$$

Goldman and Becklake (1959) published the following equations* for calculating the normal RV in liters:

$$\text{Males: } [(0.069 \times \text{Height in inches}) + (0.017 \times \text{Age in years})] - 3.45$$

$$\text{Females: } [(0.081 \times \text{Height in inches}) + (0.009 \times \text{Age in years})] - 3.90$$

b. Interpret the results (Code: IIIE7c) [Difficulty: ELE: R, Ap; WRE: An]

A normal young man has an FRC volume of about 2,400 mL. As shown in Figure 4-14, it is composed of the ERV and the RV. The FRC and RV values are invaluable for diagnosing obstructive and restrictive lung diseases. See Figure 4-6 for the relative volumes and capacities for a normal patient, a patient with an obstructive pattern, and a patient with a restrictive pattern. Note that the obstructive patient has a disproportionate increase in the RV, with a resulting decrease in the FVC. The TLC may be normal, as shown, or, more commonly, lung capacity may be increased. The patient with restrictive disease has a proportionate decrease in all the lung volumes and capacities. It is commonly accepted that the normal limits of TLC are about ±20% of the predicted value. This ±20% of the normal limit applies to the FRC and RV values as well. In other words, obstructive lung disease can be diagnosed by an RV, FRC, or TLC that is more than 120% of the predicted value. Common examples of obstructive diseases include asthma, bronchitis, and emphysema. Restrictive lung disease can be diagnosed by an RV, FRC,

---

*The ATPS to BTPS correction has been calculated into these equations.

or TLC that is less than 80% of the predicted value. Examples of restrictive diseases include fibrotic lung disease, air or fluid in the pleural space, obesity, kyphoscoliosis, pectus excavatum, and neuromuscular weakness or paralysis.

The following factors are important to ensure that the measured values are accurate:

- The system must not have any leaks. A leak can result in overestimation of the FRC, because the lost helium results in a lower final helium percentage. A leak also can result in failure of the final helium percentage to stabilize as expected.
- The patient must be breathing on the system long enough for the helium to reach all the lung units and reach equilibrium. Usually this takes about 7 minutes; however, patients with severe obstructive lung disease will need more time and may never reach an equilibrium state. This results in an underestimation of the FRC.

14. Functional residual capacity by the nitrogen washout method

Note: This test is not listed in the NBRC's detailed content outlines. However, questions about interpretation of the results of lung volume tests have been included in recent versions of the *Written Registry Examination*.

a. Perform the procedure (Code: IIIE7c) [Difficulty: ELE: R, Ap; WRE: An]

As discussed in the helium dilution method, the nitrogen (N_2) washout method is used to find the FRC so that the RV can be derived from it and TLC calculated. It is necessary to know a patient's RV, FRC, and TLC to diagnose and determine the severity of obstructive lung disease and restrictive lung disease.

The nitrogen washout method basically involves having the patient breathe in 100% oxygen until all the resident nitrogen is removed from the lungs. It also is called the *open-circuit* method, because the patient inspires as much oxygen as needed to displace the nitrogen to a reservoir for measurement.

Figure 4-15 shows a schematic drawing of the components that make up the automated nitrogen washout system and circuit. These include a solenoid valve to switch the patient from breathing room air to breathing pure oxygen, an oxygen source with demand valve, a nitrogen analyzer with recorder, a pneumotachometer, and a microprocessor that directs all the necessary activities for the test. It is beyond the scope of this text to go into the complete procedure for the test; however, the following features should be known. The circuit is filled with pure oxygen. The patient is switched from room air to oxygen at the end of a normal exhalation so that the nitrogen in the FRC can be determined. Typically, the test is performed for up to 7 minutes or until the nitrogen per-

Volumes: Four primary

A. Tidal volume (V_T). The volume of gas inspired *or* expired during normal respiration.
B. Inspiratory reserve volume (IRV): The maximum volume of gas that can be inspired beyond a normal inspiration.
C. Expiratory reserve volume (ERV): The maximum volume of gas that can be exhaled after a normal expiration.
D. Residual volume (RV): The volume of gas remaining in the lungs after a maximum expiration.

Capacities: Four, which include two or more primary volumes

A. Total lung capacity (TLC): The total amount of gas contained in the lungs after maximum inspiration. Includes all four primary volumes (TLC = V_T + IRV + ERV + RV).
B. Vital capacity (VC): The maximum amount of gas that can be exhaled after a maximum inspiration. Includes three primary volumes (VC = V_T + IRV + ERV).
C. Inspiratory capacity (IC): The maximum amount of gas that can be inspired after a normal expiration. Includes two primary volumes (IC = V_T + IRV).
D. Functional residual capacity (FRC): The total amount of gas remaining in the lungs after normal expiration. Includes two primary volumes (FRC = ERV + RV).

Figure 4-14   Lung volumes and capacities for a clinically normal young man.

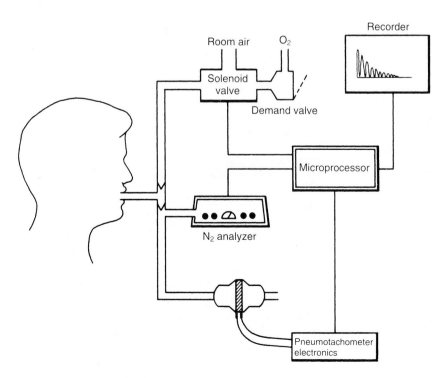

Figure 4-15   Schematic drawing of the key components of the automated nitrogen washout system for measuring functional residual capacity. *(From Beauchamp RK: Pulmonary function testing procedures. In Barnes TA, editor:* Respiratory care practice, *St Louis, 1988, Mosby.)*

centage falls below a target level. This target percentage has been reported by various authors as 1% (best results) up to 3%. Extending the test longer may help to reach a target level in patients with increased airway resistance or an increased lung volume. As before, the calculation of RV is rather complex and is usually done through the computer built into the pulmonary function system. Spirometry also must be performed, because the ERV is subtracted from the FRC to find the RV. Commonly the test is repeated. The patient should be allowed to breathe room air for at least 15 minutes between tests to clear the oxygen from the lungs. Patients with severe obstructive lung disease may need more time.

Predicted patient values for the FRC and RV can be determined with the same equations listed in the previous discussion of the helium dilution method of determining FRC.

b. Interpret the results (Code: IIIE7c) [Difficulty: ELE: R, Ap; WRE: An]

As discussed earlier in the helium dilution test, the FRC and RV values are invaluable for diagnosing obstructive and restrictive lung diseases. When done properly, the helium dilution and nitrogen washout tests reveal similar patient values. If the nitrogen percentage is graphed over time, the shape of the washout curve also can be helpful for evaluating the degree of airway obstruction. Both the normal and abnormal tracings show rapid nitrogen washout from the upper airway dead space. However, as the test continues, a patient with obstructive lung disease shows a progressive slowing of the nitrogen washout rate.

The following considerations are important to ensure that the measured values are accurate:

* The system must not have any leaks. A leak would be noticed as a sudden increase in the nitrogen percentage after a steady decrease. This results in overestimation in the FRC value.
* The patient must be breathing on the system long enough for the nitrogen to be washed out of all the lung units. Usually this takes less than 7 minutes; however, patients with severe obstructive lung disease need more time and may never reach the targeted percentage. This results in underestimation of the FRC.

15. Total lung capacity

Note: This test is not listed in the NBRC's detailed content outlines. However, questions about interpretation of the results of lung volume tests have been included in recent versions of the *Written Registry Examination*.

a. Perform the procedure (Code: IIIE7c) [Difficulty: ELE: R, Ap; WRE: An]

The TLC is the volume of air in the lungs after inhalation of a VC. As discussed earlier, the patient's TLC must be

determined to diagnose obstructive or restrictive lung disease.

See Figure 4-14 for an example of the relationships between lung volumes and capacities. As can be seen, the TLC can be found by adding several combinations of volumes and capacities. Most commonly, it is calculated by adding the FRC to the inspiratory capacity (IC) found through spirometry. However, be prepared to add or subtract various combinations of volumes and capacities to find the TLC.

b. Interpret the results (Code: IIIE7c) [Difficulty: ELE: R, Ap; WRE: An]

The TLC results cannot be interpreted without looking at the volumes and capacities that compose it. Figure 4-5 shows representative TLC patterns for a normal patient and a patient with an obstructive pattern and a restrictive pattern. Note that with the abnormal patterns, the FRC and its components, the ERV and RV, are out of proportion. Patients with emphysema, bronchitis, or asthma often show the obstructive pattern with its large FRC of trapped gas. Patients with fibrotic lung disease, thoracic deformities, or obesity often show the restrictive pattern, with its decreased FRC and other lung volumes.

Some practitioners use the general rule that a TLC more than 120% of predicted indicates an obstructive pattern, and a TLC less than 80% of predicted indicates a restrictive pattern. However, this may be an oversimplification. It is more reliable to calculate the RV to TLC (RV/TLC) ratio. This takes into account the interrelation of the two. Normal healthy adults have an RV/TLC ratio of 0.20 (20%) to 0.35 (35%). An increased RV/TLC ratio is commonly seen in patients with emphysema and an increased RV. However, if the patient's TLC is increased in proportion to the RV, the ratio may be within normal limits. A decreased RV/TLC ratio is commonly seen in patients with fibrotic lung disease. The ratio will be normal, however, if the patient's TLC is decreased in proportion to the RV. Table 4-3 shows the relationship of the lung volumes and capacities, TLC, and the RV/TLC ratio found in a number of conditions.

Exam Hint 4-9 (WRE)

Most examinations have at least one table that must be interpreted to determine whether the patient has obstructive lung disease or restrictive lung disease. The "20% rule" can help with this determination. Obstructive lung disease is identified by lung volumes (TLC, FRC, RV) that are 20% or more *greater* than predicted (more than 120% of predicted). Restrictive lung disease is identified by lung volumes (TLC, FRC, RV) that are 20% or more *smaller* than predicted (less than 80% of predicted).

TABLE 4-3	Lung Volumes and Capacities Seen in Various Disorders						
Disorder	VC	IC	ERV	FRC	RV	TLC	RV:TLC
Asthma or airway disease	D	N	D	N, I	I	N, I*	I
Emphysema	N	N	N	I	I	I	N, I
Diffuse parenchymal disease							
Early	N	N	N	D	N	N	N
Advanced (all volumes and capacities equally reduced)							
Space-occupying lesions	N	N	N	N	D	N	
Obesity	N	N	D	N, I†	N	N	I
Thoracic/skeletal disease	D	D	D	D	N	D	I

Modified from Snow MG: Determination of functional residual capacity, *Respir Care* 34:586, 1989.

D, Decreased; *ERV*, expiratory reserve volume; *FRC*, functional residual capacity; *I*, increased; *IC*, inspiratory capacity; *N*, normal; *RV*, residual volume; *TLC*, total lung capacity; *VC*, vital capacity.

*When airway resistance is greater than about 3.5 cm $H_2O/L/sec$.

†When the weight:height (pounds:inches) ratio is greater than 5:1.

16. Body plethysmography

The body plethysmography unit (sometimes called the *body bubble* or *body box*) is a sealable chamber large enough for an adult to sit inside. Auxiliary equipment includes a differential pressure pneumotachometer, a monitor/storage oscilloscope, a computer, and a recording device (Figure 4-16). The plethysmograph can be used to measure (1) the FRC and, from that, the RV and TLC; (2) lung compliance; and (3) airway resistance. Each of these tests is discussed later.

a. Thoracic gas volume

Note: This test is not listed in the NBRC's detailed content outlines. However, questions about interpretation of the results of lung volume tests have been included in recent versions of the *Written Registry Examination*.

1. Perform the procedure (Code: IIIE7c) [Difficulty: ELE: R, Ap; WRE: An]

The volume of gas measured in the lungs at the end of exhalation by a plethysmograph is called the *thoracic gas volume* (TGV or VTG). When the unit has been accurately calibrated and the test properly performed, the plethysmograph provides a more accurate FRC volume measurement than either the helium dilution or nitrogen washout methods. Once TGV is determined, the RV can be derived from it and the TLC calculated. It is necessary to know a patient's RV, FRC, and TLC to diagnose and determine the severity of obstructive lung disease and restrictive lung disease.

It is not possible to go into a complete discussion of the procedure; however, the following steps are important. The unit must be sealed so that it is airtight during the patient's breathing. The patient is instructed to breathe a normal tidal volume through the pneumotachometer. At the end of exhalation (FRC), a shutter is closed on the pneumotachometer so that no air leaks. The patient is instructed to continue to make tidal volume

Figure 4-16 Schematic drawing of the layout of a body plethysmograph with its components. The patient sits within the sealed plethysmograph chamber for the tests. *(From Ruppel G: Manual of pulmonary function testing, ed 9, St Louis, 2009, Mosby.)*

breathing efforts. The computer integrates the following two pressure changes: (1) a decrease in mouth pressure as the patient attempts to inhale, and (2) an increase in plethysmograph chamber pressure as the patient's chest expands. The patient's TGV is then determined at FRC. Figure 4-17, *A*, shows a normal TGV loop on the oscilloscope. Through spirometry, the patient's ERV, RV, and TLC can be calculated.

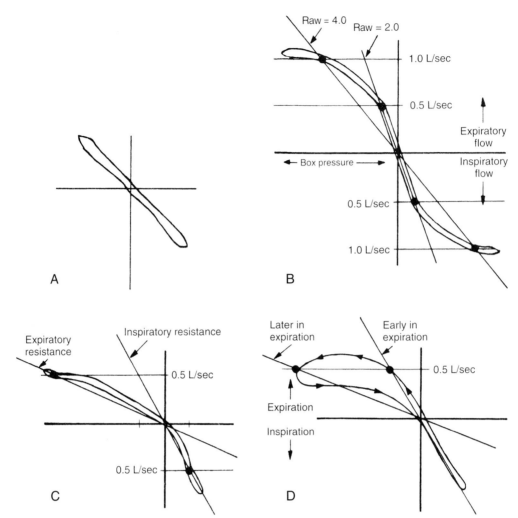

Figure 4-17   Examples of body plethysmography tracings. **A,** A normal thoracic gas volume loop. **B,** A normal inspiratory and expiratory loop for airway resistance (Raw). Note that it is symmetrical. This patient has an Raw of 2 cm H_2O/L/sec at the standard flow of 0.5 L/sec. As the flow increases, the Raw increases as a result of the increased turbulence. The Raw of 4 cm H_2O/L/sec seen at the flow of 1 L/sec should not be recorded as the patient's value. **C,** A patient whose expiratory resistance is greater than the inspiratory resistance. In this case, either both resistances should be recorded in the chart or just the expiratory resistance if only one can be recorded. **D,** A significant difference between early and late expiratory resistance. This is commonly seen in patients with obstructive airway disease, such as emphysema. Record the late resistance, because it better represents the patient's disease condition. *(From Zarins LP, Clausen JL: Body plethysmography. In Clausen JL, editor:* Pulmonary function testing guidelines and controversies, *Orlando, 1984, Grune & Stratton.)*

2. Interpret the results (Code: IIIE7c) [Difficulty: ELE: R, Ap; WRE: An]

The interpretation of the TGV and TLC results from a body plethysmograph are about the same as the interpretation of the FRC and TLC results from the helium dilution or nitrogen washout methods. (Review these earlier discussions if needed.) The only difference would be if the TGV were significantly larger than the FRC. This would

indicate that the patient has trapped gas that was measured only in the plethysmograph. The TGV is commonly larger than the FRC measured by the preceding two methods when the patient has chronic obstructive pulmonary disease (COPD). This is because it includes *all* the gas found in the thorax. That gas may be found in normal alveoli connected by a patent airway to the atmosphere, but the TGV may also include gas trapped in emphysematous blebs and bullae, pneumothorax, pneumomediastinum, and so forth.

b. Lung compliance

1. Recommend the procedure (Code: IC7) [Difficulty: ELE: R, Ap; WRE: An]

Lung compliance (CL) is the volume change per unit of pressure change in the lungs. It is recorded in liters or milliliters per centimeter of water pressure (L[mL]/cm H_2O). A lung compliance test is indicated in a patient with a known or suspected condition that caused the lungs to be either overly compliant (as in emphysema) or noncompliant (as in pulmonary fibrosis).

2. Perform the procedure (Code: IB9n and IIIE7b) [Difficulty: ELE: R, Ap; WRE: An]

The patient must swallow a balloon 10 cm long to the midthoracic level. A catheter connects the proximal end of the balloon to a pressure transducer outside the patient. Air is injected into the balloon, and the transducer is calibrated accurately to measure changes in intrathoracic pressure as the patient breathes. The patient is then placed into a body plethysmograph that is sealed. He or she is told to breathe through the differential pressure pneumotachometer to measure lung volumes. The patient is then instructed to inhale slowly from the resting level (FRC) to TLC. As this is done, the pneumotachometer shutter is periodically closed to measure the intrathoracic pressure decrease at the increasing volumes (Figure 4-18). As the patient slowly exhales from TLC, the shutter is again periodically closed to measure the increasing intrathoracic pressure as the patient returns to FRC volume. Lung compliance is usually calculated from the pressure and volume points of FRC and FRC plus 500 mL (for a tidal volume).

3. Interpret the results (Code: IIIE7b) [Difficulty: ELE: R, Ap; WRE: An]

Normal lung compliance (CL) in an adult is 0.2 L/cm H_2O. Through other methods, the normal adult's thoracic compliance (CT) has been determined also to be 0.2 L/cm H_2O. However, because the lungs tend to collapse smaller and the thorax cage tends to expand out, the two opposing forces offset each other somewhat. Because of this, the lung/thoracic compliance (CLT) is calculated as 0.1 L (or 100 mL)/cm H_2O.

A number of diseases and conditions can affect lung, thoracic, and lung/thoracic compliance. Patients with emphysema are known to have a higher than normal lung compliance. Their lungs are overly distended. Decreased lung compliance is seen in pulmonary fibrosis (from sarcoidosis, silicosis, or asbestosis), lung tumor, pulmonary edema, atelectasis, pneumonia, or decreased surfactant. Decreased thoracic compliance is seen in patients with kyphoscoliosis, pectus excavatum, obesity, enlarged liver, or advanced pregnancy. All these conditions result in small, stiff lungs.

Figure 4-18 Measurement of lung compliance (CL) with the esophageal balloon technique. A balloon is swallowed to the midthoracic level, filled with air, and connected to a pressure transducer to measure intrapleural pressure. The patient sits within a body plethysmograph and breathes through a pneumotachometer to measure mouth pressure and gas flow. The graph shows a tracing for a patient with normal compliance. In contrast, the patient with emphysema has an increased total lung capacity (TLC) and increased compliance; the patient with pulmonary fibrosis has a decreased TLC and decreased compliance. *(From Ruppel G: Manual of pulmonary function testing, ed 9, St Louis, 2009, Mosby.)*

c. Airway resistance

1. Recommend the procedure (Code: IC7) [Difficulty: ELE: R, Ap; WRE: An]

Airway resistance (Raw) is the difference in pressure between the alveoli and the mouth that develops as air flows into and out of the lungs. It is recorded in centimeters of water pressure per liter of gas moved per second (cm H_2O/L/sec). The test is performed on patients with a known or suspected condition of increased airway resistance. These conditions include asthma, emphysema, and chronic bronchitis (COPD). The test confirms the patient's condition. Then it is used to help determine the proper dose of bronchodilator medications to help manage the problem.

2. Perform the procedure (Code: IB9n and IIIE7b) [Difficulty: ELE: R, Ap; WRE: An]

The patient is placed into a plethysmograph that is sealed. He or she is instructed to breathe through a differential pressure pneumotachometer. With the pneumotachometer shutter open, the patient is told to pant several tidal volumes of about 500 mL at a rate of 1 breath per second. Data on flow rate, tidal volume, mouth pressure changes, and chamber pressure changes are recorded and graphed (Figure 4-19). Then the shutter is closed at the patient's resting FRC volume. The patient is told to continue panting at the same volume and rate. Again, flow rate, tidal volume, mouth pressure changes, and chamber pressures are recorded and graphed. The computer integrates the data to calculate the patient's airway resistance during tidal volume breathing.

3. Interpret the results (Code: IIIE7b) [Difficulty: ELE: R, Ap; WRE: An]

Airway resistance is the pressure difference developed per unit of flow. This pressure is required to overcome the friction of moving the tidal volume through the airways to the lungs. It can be thought of as the ratio of alveolar pressure to airflow. It is calculated by this formula:

$$Raw = \frac{\text{Atmospheric pressure} - \text{Alveolar pressure}}{\text{Flow}}$$

Ruppel (2003) reported the normal adult's airway resistance ranges from 0.6 to 2.4 cm H_2O/L/sec. The standard inspiratory and expiratory flow rate during the test is 0.5 L/sec (500 mL/sec). This is to standardize air turbulence during the test. The usual components of airway resistance found in an adult are as follows:

- Upper airway including the nose and mouth (50%)
- Trachea and bronchi larger than 2 mm in diameter (30%)
- Airways less than 2 mm in diameter (20%)

Increased airway resistance is abnormal. It is most readily noticed if the problem is in the upper airway, trachea, or major bronchi, because most resistance is normally found there. Patients with asthma, bronchitis, and emphysema have most of their resistance in the airways that are 2 mm or less in diameter. Because of this, significant disease must be present before a large enough airway resistance is noticed to alert the therapist or physician to

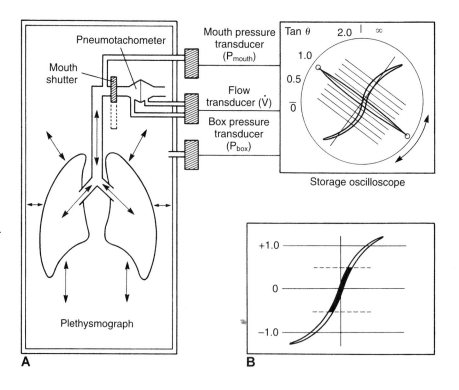

Figure 4-19 Measurement of airway resistance (Raw). **A,** The body plethysmograph in which the patient sits during the test. Tidal volume panting against an open and then closed pneumotachometer shutter is displayed on the storage oscilloscope. **B,** A printout of the pressure changes as the patient pants a tidal volume of 500 mL/sec. *(From Ruppel G: Manual of pulmonary function testing, ed 6, St Louis, 1994, Mosby.)*

the problem. Figure 4-17, *B* through *D*, shows normal and increased expiratory resistance curves. Madama (1998) lists the following airway resistance values and their severity:

Raw (cm H₂O/L/sec)	Severity
2.8 to 4.5	Mild
4.5 to 8	Moderate
Over 8	Severe

17. Diffusing capacity

a. Perform the procedure (Code: IIIE7d) [Difficulty: ELE: R, Ap; WRE: An]

The diffusing capacity (DL or DLCO) tests look at the capacity for carbon monoxide to diffuse through the lungs into the blood. Carbon monoxide is used, because its high affinity for hemoglobin virtually eliminates blood as a barrier to diffusion. The measured value can then be correlated to the ability of oxygen to diffuse through the lungs. This test is indicated when it is important to know the extent of lung disability causing hypoxemia. This is most common with patients having emphysema, but it also is important in patients with fibrotic lung disease.

At the time of this writing, the single-breath carbon monoxide diffusing capacity test (DLCO-SB) is the only version that has a widely adopted standard technique for administration. It is recorded in milliliters of carbon monoxide (CO) per minute per millimeter of mercury at 0° C, 760 mm Hg, and dry standard temperature and pressure (STPD).

The following are key steps in the procedure. A reservoir or spirometer is filled with a mix of 0.3% CO, 10% He, 21% O₂, and the balance of N₂ (Figure 4-20). The patient is connected to the apparatus and breathes room air while being instructed in the test. After the patient is told to exhale completely (to RV), the practitioner switches the patient to the gas mix. The patient is instructed to rapidly inhale an IVC. A shutter automatically closes so that the patient cannot exhale for 10 seconds. This allows time for some of the carbon monoxide to diffuse into the patient's bloodstream.

After the breath hold, the shutter opens, and the patient is told to exhale to resting volume. The equipment is designed to automatically let 750 to 1,000 mL of exhaled gas pass through to the spirometer. The next 500 mL of gas is diverted into the end-tidal gas sampler. This sample is then analyzed for He% and CO%. The remainder of the patient's exhaled volume is passed through into the spirometer. The various measured parameters are integrated into the equations in the computer to give the patient's DLCO-SB value.

This test is done only after the patient has been measured for both RV and TLC. That is because the patient's lung volume directly affects the diffusibility of carbon monoxide.

b. Interpret the results (Code: IIIE7d) [Difficulty: ELE: R, Ap; WRE: An]

Interpretation is limited to the results of the DLCO-SB test. Ruppel (2009) reported that the average resting normal adult DLCO-SB is 25 mL CO/min/mm Hg STPD (standard temperature, pressure, dry, conditions). Gaensler and Wright (1966) reported the following DLCO-SB prediction equations, with values in mL/CO/min/mm Hg STPD:

Males: $[(0.250 \times \text{Height in inches}) - (0.177 \times \text{Age in years})]$
$$+19.93$$

Females: $[(0.284 \times \text{Height in inches}) - (0.177 \times \text{Age in years})]$
$$+7.72$$

It should be noted that a number of other authors have developed their own prediction equations. In general, patients who show DLCO-SB results within ± 20% of the predicted values (80% to 120% of predicted) are considered to be within normal limits. A patient who has actual results that are significantly below the predicted values (<80% of predicted) has a problem with lung diffusion. Figure 4-21 shows a number of common conditions that can lead to poor lung diffusion. The following factors also should be taken into consideration when interpreting the measured values:

- Increased hematocrit and hemoglobin values result in an increased DLCO, whereas decreased values result in a decreased DLCO. An actual value should be used to calculate a patient's DLCO.
- An increased carboxyhemoglobin level results in a decreased DLCO. Patients who smoke should be

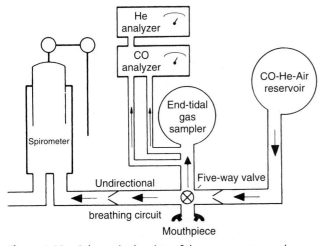

Figure 4-20 Schematic drawing of the components and breathing circuit used to perform a single-breath lung-diffusion test (DLCO-SB). Analysis of the patient's exhaled helium (He) and carbon monoxide (CO) percentages is critical to the test. *(From Ruppel G: Manual of pulmonary function testing, ed 6, St Louis, 1994, Mosby.)*

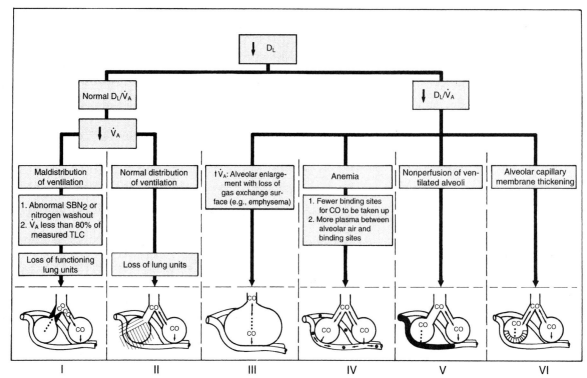

Figure 4-21 Six factors that can cause decreased lung diffusion (DL). Factors I and II result in a decrease in DL that is in proportion to the decrease in alveolar volume. Factors III, IV, V, and VI result in a decrease in DL that is greater than the decrease in alveolar volume. Therefore these later conditions are more harmful to the patient's pulmonary function and well-being. *SBN₂*, Single-breath nitrogen washout; *TLC*, total lung capacity; *Vₐ*, alveolar ventilation. *(From Ayers LN, Whipp BJ, Ziment I: A guide to the interpretation of pulmonary function tests, ed 2, New York, 1978, Roerig.)*

instructed not to smoke the night before the test so that the COHb level will decrease to normal.

- An increased alveolar carbon dioxide level results in a lowered alveolar oxygen level. This, in turn, results in an increased DLCO. A decreased alveolar carbon dioxide level results in a decreased DLCO.
- Increased altitude results in an increased DLCO. This is probably a concern only if the patient is tested in a mountainous area.
- An increased pulmonary capillary blood volume results in an increased DLCO.
- The patient should breathe room air for at least 4 minutes before the test is repeated.
- It is well known that diffusibility is directly related to lung volume. This is the reason that African Americans have lower diffusion rates than Caucasians. To eliminate this as a factor in interpreting the DL value, it is necessary to divide the diffusion value by the TLC. African Americans have the same normal values as Caucasians when this calculation is performed.

MODULE E
Pulmonary function equipment

1. Manipulate water, digital, and aneroid manometers (pressure gauges) by order or protocol (ELE code: IIA16) [Difficulty: ELE: R, Ap, An]

a. Get the necessary equipment for the procedure

Water (or mercury) manometers have a vertical column of the liquid and are commonly used in a blood pressure sphygmomanometer. The pressure units depend on the type of liquid. A water manometer will have units of centimeters of water (cm H₂O) pressure; mercury manometers will have units of millimeters of mercury (mm Hg). The fluid column must be kept vertical for accuracy. An aneroid (spring-loaded) unit should be selected if the pressure gauge cannot be kept in a vertical position. Aneroid manometers can be calibrated in either mm Hg or cm H₂O pressure and look like a Bourdon gauge. Newer, digital manometers will display the measured pressure on a light emitting diode (LED) or other display. (*Note:* The NBRC recently substituted digital for mercury manometers in this section. Mercury manometers are being phased out because of environmental concerns over mercury spills.)

b. Put the equipment together and make sure that it works properly

These pressure gauges come preassembled by the manufacturer. It is necessary to attach the pressure source only to the inlet port on the unit to measure a pressure change. This connection must be airtight, or a leak will occur, and the measured pressure will be less than actually exists. The accuracy of the unit can be checked by opening the inlet port to room air and reading the pressure. A reading of zero should be seen (indicating no pressure change from atmospheric). Next, a known pressure is applied to the gauge. Often this is done by attaching it to a sphygmomanometer and pumping up the pressure to a known level, such as 50 mm Hg. The pressure gauge should show the same.

c. Troubleshoot any problems with the equipment

If, during the calibration procedure, the set pressure does not match the pressure in the gauge, a leak may be present in the system, or the pressure gauge is miscalibrated. Tighten all connections and attempt to calibrate again. Do not use a pressure gauge that cannot be calibrated.

2. Manipulate inspiratory or expiratory force meters (pressure gauges) by order or protocol (ELE code: IIA16) [Difficulty: ELE: R, Ap, An]

a. Get the necessary equipment for the procedure

The maximum inspiratory pressure and maximum expiratory pressure tests are usually recorded in centimeters of water pressure. However, millimeters of mercury can be used. If a centimeters of water pressure gauge is used, it should be able to record a negative and positive pressure of at least 100 cm H_2O. However, a unit that can record $\pm$ 60 cm H_2O is probably adequate.

b. Put the equipment together and make sure that it works properly

No standard setup exists for these devices. See Figure 4-2 for two possible assemblies. The system can be sealed and pressure checked with a known force to make sure that the pressure manometer is accurate and all the connections are airtight.

c. Troubleshoot any problems with the equipment

If, during the calibration procedure, the set pressure does not match the pressure in the gauge, a leak may be present in the system, or the pressure gauge is miscalibrated. Tighten all connections and attempt to calibrate again. Do not use a pressure gauge that cannot be calibrated. The one-way valves must function so that the patient can exhale or inhale only as needed for the test.

3. Manipulate a pressure transducer by order or protocol (ELE code: IIA16) [Difficulty: ELE: R, Ap, An]

a. Get the necessary equipment for the procedure

Pressure transducers are used in the body plethysmograph for measuring mouth pressure and chamber pressure. They come with the unit and are supplied by the manufacturer. Another type of transducer is used with an esophageal balloon when performing a lung compliance measurement. Follow the balloon manufacturer's recommendations for the proper transducer.

b. Put the equipment together and make sure that it works properly

c. Troubleshoot any problems with the equipment

Each type of pressure transducer should be assembled as described by the manufacturer. As seen in Figure 4-22, the

Figure 4-22 Cutaway view of a differential pressure pneumotachometer. Flow is measured as the pressure decreases between *A* and *B,* which are ports leading to a differential pressure transducer. The resistive element may consist of a mesh screen, a network of parallel capillary tubes, or other devices. *(From Beauchamp RK: Pulmonary function testing procedures. In Barnes TA, editor: Respiratory care practice, St Louis, 1988, Mosby.)*

differential pressure transducer has small-bore tubing connecting it before and after a resistive element. These small tubes transmit the pressures before and after the resistance element to the transducer as gas flows through the large, main tube. Make sure that the tubing is properly connected to the main tube and transducer. If a tube were to disconnect, the transducer would give a reading of zero.

4. Manipulate a pneumotachometer respirometer by order or protocol (ELE code: IIA17) [Difficulty: ELE: R, Ap, An]

a. Get the necessary equipment for the procedure

b. Put the equipment together and make sure that it works properly

c. Troubleshoot any problems with the equipment

All pneumotachometers convert one type of physical information or signal to another (e.g., converting an airflow or pressure signal to an electrical signal). Two common types are discussed next. Either type should be acceptable for performing bedside spirometry. Make sure that the unit you select is capable of performing the ordered test. Be sure that you select a unit capable of printing out a hard copy of the patient's test results and spirometry tracings if they are required for the chart.

d. Differential-pressure (flow sensing) pneumotachometer

Some articles refer to a differential pressure pneumotachometer as a *Fleisch-type* device. These units have a resistive element (tubes or mesh screen) in the flow tube. The faster the flow of gas through the flow tube, the greater the pressure difference before and after the resistance. Hoses connect the flow tubes before and after the resistive element to the differential pressure transducer. The transducer converts this pressure difference into an electrical signal. A microprocessor calculates the various patient values from this information (see Figure 4-22).

Assembly requires the addition of the patient's mouthpiece to the inspiratory port so that no air leak occurs. The expiratory port should be kept completely open so that the only obstruction to the patient's airflow is from the resistive element. A volume calibration check is performed by forcing a known amount of air from a super syringe (certified volume standard syringe) through the pneumotachometer. Minimally, several repetitions of a known 3-L volume should reveal identical measured volumes. As long as the measured volumes are within ± 3% or 50 mL (whichever is less), the unit is acceptably accurate.

Common problems with accuracy include an air leak around the mouthpiece; cracked, disconnected, or obstructed pressure-relaying hoses; water condensation or mucus on the resistive element; or obstructed upstream or downstream port. The resistive element is usually heated to minimize any condensation.

e. Heat-transfer pneumotachometer

Some articles refer to a heat-transfer pneumotachometer as a *thermistor-type device* or *hot-wire anemometer*. These units have a heated thermistor that is cooled as the gas flows past it. The temperature transducer automatically increases and measures the flow of electricity to the thermistor to keep it at the required temperature. A microprocessor calculates the various patient values from this information. The earlier discussion on assembly, calibration, and troubleshooting applies to the heat-transfer pneumotachometers, except that no pressure-relaying hoses are present (Figure 4-23).

5. Manipulate bedside screening spirometers by order or protocol (ELE code: IIA25) [Difficulty: ELE: R, Ap, An]

a. Get the necessary equipment for the procedure

Following are typical pulmonary function tests performed at the patient's bedside:
1. Tidal volume (V_T)
2. Vital capacity (either a forced effort [FVC] or a nonforced effort [VC])
3. Peak flow (PF) (the PF requires an initial forced vital capacity effort)
4. Maximum expiratory pressure (MEP)
5. Maximum inspiratory pressure MIP)

The tidal volume and VC volumes can be measured on a handheld, turbine-type flow sensor, such as the Wright respirometer. The patient's peak flow is measured on a dedicated, handheld PF meter. A pressure gauge capable of measuring both positive and negative pressure is used for the MEP and MIP (see Figure 4-2). In addition, there are electrically powered, portable PFT units that contain a micropressor and can measure all of the standard spirometry volumes and flow.

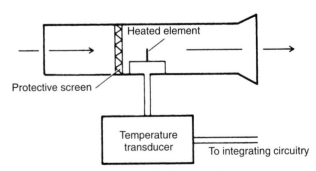

Figure 4-23 Cutaway view of a heat-transfer pneumotachometer. *(From Ruppel G: Manual of pulmonary function testing, ed 6, St Louis, 1994, Mosby.)*

b. Put the equipment together and make sure that it works properly

All of these separate pieces of equipment require additional items, such as patient nose clips and a mouthpiece. A double one-way valve system can also be added to direct gas flow properly through the equipment and to minimize cross-contamination between patients.

c. Troubleshoot any problems with the equipment

All units must work properly and have all ancillary equipment properly connected to be airtight. Any leaks will result in a loss of volume, flow, or pressure respectively. Tighten any loose connections and repeat the procedure if necessary.

6. Manipulate CO, He, O₂, and specialty gas analyzers by order or protocol (Code: IIA26) [Difficulty: ELE: R, Ap; WR: An]

a. Get the necessary equipment for the procedure

These tests are needed for a variety of special purposes, as described earlier, and require the appropriate equipment:
1. Carbon monoxide is analyzed in the single-breath carbon monoxide diffusing capacity test.
2. Helium (He) is analyzed in the single-breath carbon monoxide diffusing capacity test and the helium dilution test to find the FRC.
3. Oxygen (O_2) is analyzed in the single-breath carbon monoxide diffusing capacity test and the helium dilution test to find the FRC.
4. Nitrogen (N_2) is analyzed in the single-breath nitrogen washout test and the nitrogen washout method of finding the FRC.

b. Put the equipment together and make sure that it works properly

Check the label on the tank to be sure it is the correct gas at the correct percentage. Review Table 6-1 for color codings for tanks, if needed. Each specialty gas has its own diameter index safety system (DISS) reduction valve to connect to the tank. A high-pressure hose connects the reduction valve outlet to the pulmonary function testing machine inlet.

c. Troubleshoot any problems with the equipment

The problems that can occur with specialty gas cylinders, pressure-reducing valves, and connecting high-pressure hoses are the same as can occur with oxygen cylinders. Review the discussion in Chapter 6 if needed.

MODULE F
Respiratory care plan

1. Analyze available information to determine the patient's pathophysiologic state (Code: IIIH1) [Difficulty: ELE: R, Ap; WRE: Ap]

Even though a physician must legally determine the patient's diagnosis, a therapist must be able to understand the cause, pathophysiology, diagnosis, treatment, and prognosis for patients with cardiopulmonary disorders. Interpretation of patient data that is tested by the NBRC was discussed earlier. Figure 4-24 shows an algorithm demonstrating several key pulmonary function differences between normal people and those with common pulmonary conditions. The following is a brief summary of the PFT test results that would indicate an obstructive or restrictive lung condition.

a. Obstructive airway disease

The patient with severe obstructive lung disease shows low gas flow at all time intervals. However, a decreased FEV_3 and the $FEF_{25\%-75\%}$ are early markers of small airway disease. Quite commonly, the RV is increased as a result of air trapping. This increases the FRC and often the TLC. Despite the increased lung volume, the patient's diffusing ability is decreased. Examples of conditions that cause obstructive lung disease include asthma, emphysema, bronchitis, and bronchiolitis. Excessive mucus, foreign bodies, and airway tumors also cause bronchospasm and air trapping.

b. Restrictive lung disease

In restrictive lung disease, all lung volumes and capacities are reduced, and lung diffusion is reduced. Expiratory flows such as FEV_1 are increased. Examples of conditions that cause restrictive lung disease include fibrosis, pulmonary edema, hemothorax or pneumothorax, acute or infant respiratory distress syndrome, chest wall deformities, obesity, and various neuromuscular disorders.

Exam Hint 4-10 (WRE)

Most examinations have tested the examinee's understanding and interpretation of data to determine whether a patient has obstructive or restrictive lung disease. This usually involves the assessment of patient data on a table. A key finding in patients with obstructive lung disease is air trapping, which results in an RV, FRC, and TLC greater than 120% of predicted. A key finding in patients with restrictive lung disease is an RV, FRC, and TLC less than 80% of predicted.

2. Determine the appropriateness of the prescribed therapy and goals for the identified pathophysiologic state (Code: IIIH3) [Difficulty: ELE: R, Ap; WRE: Ap]

The care plan depends on the patient's diagnosis and the degree of limitation. If the patient has reversible small airway disease, he or she should be counseled to stop smoking and avoid all airborne irritants. Inhaled or systemic bronchodilators or both should be prescribed to relax the airways as much as possible. If the patient has restrictive lung disease, he or she should also be counseled to avoid any airborne irritants. Whether any medications or other procedures can be performed to offer some relief depends on the specific cause of the patient's disorder.

MODULE G
Quality assurance and quality control

1. Develop outcomes of quality improvement programs (Code: IIIH7a) [Difficulty: ELE: R; WRE: Ap, An]

2. Perform respiratory care quality assurance (Code: IIIH5) [Difficulty: ELE: R, Ap; WRE: Ap]

3. Record and monitor the quality control (QC) data using accepted statistical methods (Code: IIC8) [Difficulty: ELE: R, Ap; WRE: An]

4. Perform quality control procedures for pulmonary function equipment (Code: IIC4) [Difficulty: ELE: R, Ap; WRE: An]

Every pulmonary function testing laboratory must have a quality control (QC)/quality improvement (QI) program. Regular maintenance of equipment and calibration must be performed and documented. The essential components of the program have been established by the American Thoracic Society–European Respiratory Society (ATS-ERS) standards. All of the major equipment manufacturers have adopted these requirements and built them into their equipment and the computer software that monitors calibration and related concerns. If an error is detected by the software or by the respiratory therapist, the problem must be recorded. After the correction has been made, the solution must be documented.

See the earlier discussion on pneumotachometer respirometers for information on calibration and commonly encountered equipment problems with these widely used devices. The following discussion concerns older types of laboratory equipment that does not use a pneumotachometer. All modern laboratories have computers and dedicated software with any PFT equipment.

Volume displacement (also called *positive displacement*) respirometers are mechanical devices. They are called *volume displacement respirometers,* because the patient's exhaled gas fills and moves a sealed bell or accordion-like bellows. These systems are self-contained and sealed rather than open to room air, as are the other devices. They can have residual volume and lung diffusion test hardware added on. The three general categories are discussed here: water-seal spirometers, dry rolling-seal spirometers, and wedge-type spirometers.

a. Water-seal spirometers

Water-seal spirometers are the commonly found chain-compensated and Stead-Wells units made by Collins Medical (see Figure 4-25 for the cutaway appearance of the chain-compensated type). The bell falls and rises as the patient breathes in and out. A pulley system attached to the bell and the marking pens record the patient's efforts on the rotating kymograph paper. Note that the tracing is inverted from the patient's actual breathing effort. The Stead-Wells units have the marking pen attached directly to the bell, and the tracing directly shows the patient's breathing efforts (Figure 4-26). The newer chain-compensated and Stead-Wells units also have microprocessors for calculating patient information.

Gas analyzers for helium, nitrogen, carbon monoxide, and other extra equipment can be added for RV and lung diffusion measurements. The carbon dioxide absorber should be left out of the breathing circuit for FVC tests because it interferes with the fast flow of gas; however, it must be put in line for any testing that will last more than 15 seconds and involves breathing repeatedly into the closed system. Supplemental oxygen must be added to the circuit for any tests that require the patient to breathe repeatedly from the closed system. The following is a checklist for setup and where to look when problem solving:

1. Make sure the water level is correct (not too high or too low).
2. Use a 7-L bell for children and a 14-L bell for adults.
3. Make sure all circuit tubing and one-way valve connections are tight.
4. Check the following kymograph features: paper on correctly; pens contain ink; kymograph speeds are adjustable to 32, 160, and 1920 mm/sec.
5. Make sure the carbon dioxide absorber is out of the circuit for FVC tests and in the circuit for RV and lung diffusion tests.
6. Add oxygen to the system for RV and lung diffusion tests.
7. Make sure the various gas analyzers are calibrated properly.
8. Do not be confused by the various ways the tracing is presented. Always find the start of the FVC by the near-vertical slope of the tracing.

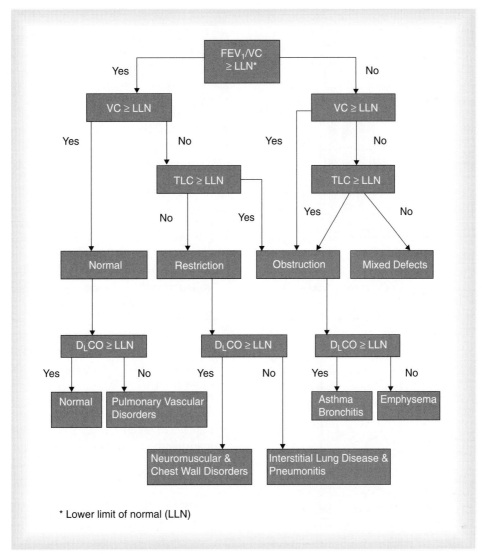

Figure 4-24 An algorithm that can be used to help guide the decision-making process to determine whether a patient is normal (within the lower limit of normal [LLN]) or has one of five different pulmonary conditions. See the text for a discussion of each of the decision making points. *(From Gardner RM, et al:* Computer guidelines for pulmonary laboratories, *Am Rev Respir Dis 134:628, 1986.)*

b. Dry rolling-seal spirometers

Dry rolling-seal spirometers are sometimes called *piston spirometers*. As can be seen in Figure 4-27, these units use a flexible silicone rubber (Silastic) or Teflon-coated rubber seal instead of water. The large volume piston moves in and out as the patient breathes. The patient's efforts can be directly recorded by pen on paper.

Newer units also have microprocessors for calculating the information. They are still rather large and are best suited for the pulmonary function laboratory. These units also can be outfitted with a carbon dioxide absorber and various gas analyzers, so they, too, can be used for the full range of lung function tests. The previous checklists for setup and problem-solving ideas apply in this case except

for items specific to the chain-compensated and Stead-Wells systems.

c. Wedge-type spirometers

Wedge-type spirometers are sometimes called *bellows spirometers* (Figure 4-28). Note that these units have plastic or rubber bellows that are fixed on one side and flexible like an accordion on other sides. The bellows move in and out as the patient breathes. The patient's efforts can be directly recorded by pen on paper. Newer units also have microprocessors for calculating the information.

All the earlier information on the dry rolling-seal spirometers applies here except what is specific to those units. The same setup and problem-solving ideas apply here also.

Figure 4-25 Cutaway view of a chain-compensated water-seal spirometer. *CO,* Carbon monoxide; *CO_2,* carbon dioxide; *He,* helium; *N_2,* nitrogen. *(From Ruppel G: Manual of pulmonary function testing, ed 6, St Louis, 1994, Mosby.)*

Figure 4-26 Cutaway view of a Stead-Wells water-seal spirometer. *CO,* Carbon monoxide; *CO_2,* carbon dioxide; *He,* helium; *N_2,* nitrogen. *(Courtesy Warren E. Collins, Inc, Braintree, Mass.)*

d. Spirometry equipment

Volume-displacement respirometers should have the following quality control procedures performed on a regular basis:

1. Use a super syringe with at least a 3-L capacity to pump air repeatedly into and out of the unit. A reading that is accurate to within ± 3%, or ± 50 mL, must be measured. The flow rates should be varied to ensure that they do not affect the measured volumes. Volumes of 1 and 2 L also should be pumped into the unit to check for linearity.
2. To check for leaks in the circuit, perform the following steps:

A Piston spirometer   **B** Piston spirometer (schematic)

Figure 4-27 Outside **(A)** and cutaway **(B)** views of a dry rolling-seal or piston spirometer. *(From Beauchamp RK: Pulmonary function testing procedures. In Barnes TA, editor: Respiratory care practice, St Louis, 1988, Mosby.)*

    a. Pump a 3-L volume into the bellows.
    b. Close the mouthpiece to the atmosphere to seal the circuit.
    c. Add a weight to the bell to speed up any small leaks.
    d. Turn on the kymograph at a slow speed and put the pen on the paper to record any decrease in volume.
    e. If a leak is noted, locate and seal it.
3. Turn on the kymograph to its various speeds and check its accuracy with a stopwatch. The manufacturer's literature should tell how far the kymograph will travel at its set speeds.
4. Compare the thermometer reading with that of a laboratory-quality unit.
5. Replace or repair any component that fails to meet the manufacturer's standards or those established by the American Thoracic Society–European Respiratory Society (ATS-ERS).

Body plethysmography equipment

(See Figure 4-16 for the basic components of the system.) The plethysmograph chamber must be airtight when the door and all vents are closed. This can be confirmed by attaching a pressure manometer to a chamber port and applying a known volume or pressure into the sealed chamber. The pressures should be identical between the chamber pressure gauges and outside pressure manometer. The differential-pressure pneumotachometer must also read accurately when a known volume is pumped through it. Most manufacturers have a series of calibration check procedures listed in the equipment literature.

Exam Hint 4-11 (WRE)

Commonly, examinations have at least one question that deals with recommending tests for assessing a patient with airway obstruction or evaluating the results of PFTs on a patient with airway obstruction. This can include interpreting a table of data, a volume-time tracing, a flow-volume loop, or calculating the results of a before and an after bronchodilator study.

A Wedge spirometer   **B** Wedge spirometer (schematic)

Figure 4-28 Outside **(A)** and cutaway **(B)** views of a wedge-type spirometer. *(From Beauchamp RK: Pulmonary function testing procedures. In Barnes TA, editor: Respiratory care practice, St Louis, 1988, Mosby.)*

5. Perform quality control procedures for gas analyzers (Code: IIC4) [Difficulty: ELE: R, Ap; WRE: An]

a. Nitrogen washout equipment for measuring functional residual capacity

(See Figure 4-15 for the basic setup and breathing circuit of a nitrogen washout system.) Review the troubleshooting of volume-displacement and pneumotachometer spirometers; they are used with the nitrogen washout procedure to find the FRC. The nitrogen washout–type RV test uses an emission spectroscopy ionization chamber analyzer for nitrogen. It is more commonly called a *Giesler tube ionizer.* It uses a vacuum pump to draw a gas sample into the ionization chamber. The intensity of the light spectrum given off by the ionized nitrogen directly relates to its percentage in the sample. A two-point calibration check should be performed at least every 6 months to check for linearity. It involves the following steps:

1. Draw a room-air sample into the unit and check the nitrogen meter reading. It should read about 78% nitrogen.
2. Adjust the meter reading, if necessary, to the manufacturer's specified value.
3. Turn off the needle valve so that no air can be drawn into the unit.
4. Check to see that the nitrogen meter reading decreases to zero nitrogen as the vacuum pump removes all gas from the ionization chamber.

Linearity (three-point calibration) can be checked by introducing 5% to 10% nitrogen into the unit to see whether the nitrogen meter measures that value. If all three points match, there is even greater confidence in the accuracy of the measurements. Do not use an analyzer that is inaccurate.

b. Helium dilution equipment for measuring functional residual capacity

(See Figure 4-13 for the basic setup of the helium dilution equipment and breathing circuit.) Again, review the troubleshooting of volume-displacement and pneumotachometer spirometers; they are used with the helium dilution procedure to find the FRC. Both the helium dilution FRC test and the lung diffusion tests require the analysis of helium in the gas mixture. A thermal conductivity analyzer typically is used. It operates under the principle of a Wheatstone bridge, in which differences in gas density lead to different cooling rates of heated thermistor beads. The different rates of cooling change electrical resistances and cause different electrical currents to flow. In a helium analyzer, the greater the helium concentration, the faster the thermistor bead cools, and the more electricity flows through the circuit. This is then read off a meter as the helium percentage.

The thermal conductivity helium analyzer should be linear over the clinically used range of helium to an accuracy of $\pm$ 0.2% He. Minimally, a two-point calibration should be performed. A room-air sample can be drawn into the analyzer and should read zero helium. A known helium concentration may then be added and analyzed (for example, heliox, which contains 80% helium and 20% oxygen). A third point can be checked if needed by analyzing another known helium percentage.

BIBLIOGRAPHY

American Association for Respiratory Care: Clinical practice guideline: spirometry—1996 update, *Respir Care* 41:629, 1996.

American Association for Respiratory Care: Clinical practice guideline: single-breath carbon monoxide diffusing capacity, *Respir Care* 44:539, 1999.

American Association for Respiratory Care: Clinical practice guideline: static lung volumes—2001 revision and update, *Respir Care* 46:531, 2001.

American Association for Respiratory Care: Clinical practice guideline: static lung volumes, *Respir Care* 39:830, 1994.

American Association for Respiratory Care: Clinical practice guideline: infant/toddler pulmonary function tests—2008 revision and update, *Respir Care* 53:929, 2008.

American Association for Respiratory Care: Clinical practice guideline: methacholine challenge testing, *Respir Care* 46:523, 2001.

American Association for Respiratory Care: Clinical practice guideline: body plethysmography—2001 revision and update, *Respir Care* 46:506, 2001.

American Association for Respiratory Care: Clinical practice guideline: assessing response to bronchodilator therapy at point of care, *Respir Care* 40:1300, 1995.

American Thoracic Society: Standardization of spirometry—1987 update, *Am Rev Respir Dis* 136:1285, 1987.

Ayers LN, Whipp BJ, Ziment I: *A guide to the interpretation of pulmonary function tests,* ed 2, New York, 1978, Roerig.

Bates DV, Macklem PT, Christie RV: *Respiratory function in disease,* ed 2, Philadelphia, 1971, WB Saunders.

Beauchamp RK: Pulmonary function testing procedures. In Barnes TA, editor: *Respiratory care practice,* Chicago, 1988, Mosby.

Black LF, Hyatt RE: Maximal respiratory pressures: normal values and relationship to age and sex, *Am Rev Respir Dis* 99:696, 1969.

Branson RD, Hurst JM, Davis K Jr, et al: Measurement of maximal inspiratory pressure: a comparison of three methods, *Respir Care* 34:789, 1989.

Buist SA, Ross BB: Predicted values for closing volumes using a modified single-breath nitrogen test, *Am Rev Respir Dis* 111:405, 1975.

Cairo JM: Assessment of pulmonary function. In Cairo JM, Pilbeam SP, editors: *Mosby's respiratory care equipment,* ed 7, St Louis, Mosby, 2004.

Cherniack RM: *Pulmonary function testing,* ed 2, Philadelphia, 1992, WB Saunders.

Cherniack RM, Raber MD: Normal standards for ventilatory function using an automated wedge spirometer, *Am Rev Respir Dis* 106:38, 1972.

Clausen JL, editor: *Pulmonary function testing guidelines and controversies,* Orlando, 1984, Grune & Stratton.

Clausen JL: Clinical interpretation of pulmonary function test, *Respir Care* 34:638, 1989.

Crapo RO: Reference values for lung function tests, *Respir Care* 34:626, 1989.

Douce FH: Pulmonary function testing. In Wilkins RL, Stoller JK, Kacmarek RM, editors: *Egan's fundamentals of respiratory care,* ed 9, St Louis, 2009, Mosby.

Enright PL, Hodgkin JE: Pulmonary function tests. In Burton GG, Hodgkin JE, Ward JJ, editors: *Respiratory care: a guide to clinical practice,* ed 4, Philadelphia, 1997, Lippincott-Raven.

Gaensler EA, Wright GW: Evaluation of respiratory impairment, *Arch Environ Health* 12:146, 1966.

Gardner RM: Pulmonary function laboratory standards, *Respir Care* 34:651, 1989.

Gardner RM, et al: Computer guidelines for pulmonary laboratories, *Am Rev Respir Dis* 134:628, 1986.

Goldman HI, Becklake MR: Respiratory function tests: normal values at median altitudes and the prediction of normal results, *Am Rev Tuberculosis* 79:457, 1959.

Gursel G, Adams AB: Pulmonary function testing. In Hess DR, MacIntyre NR, Mishoe SC, et al, editors: *Respiratory care principles and practice,* Philadelphia, 2002, WB Saunders.

Hess D: Measurement of maximal inspiratory pressure: a call for standardization, *Respir Care* 34:857, 1989.

Holland SA: Pulmonary function testing. In Wyka KA, Mathews PJ, Clark WF, editors, *Foundations of respiratory care,* Albany, NY, 2002, Delmar.

Hunt GE: Diagnostic procedures at the bedside. In Fink JB, Hunt GE: *Clinical practice in respiratory care,* Philadelphia, 1999, Lippincott Williams & Wilkins.

Kacmarek RM, Cycyk-Chapman MC, Young-Palazzo PJ, et al: Determination of maximal inspiratory pressure: a clinical study and literature review, *Respir Care* 34:868, 1989.

Knudson RJ, Kaltenborn WT, Knudson DE, et al: The single-breath carbon monoxide diffusing capacity, *Am Rev Respir Dis* 135:805, 1987.

Knudson RJ, Lebowitz MD, Holberg CJ, et al: Changes in the normal maximal expiratory flow-volume curve with growth and aging, *Am Rev Respir Dis* 127:725, 1983.

Kory RC, Callahan R, Syner JC: The Veterans Administration–Army cooperative study of pulmonary function. I. Clinical spirometry in normal men, *Am J Med* 30:243, 1961.

MacIntyre NR: Diffusing capacity of the lung for carbon monoxide, *Respir Care* 34:489, 1989.

Madama VC: *Pulmonary function testing and cardiopulmonary stress testing,* ed 2, Albany, NY, 1998, Delmar.

Morris JF, Koski A, Johnson LC: Spirometric standards for healthy nonsmoking adults, *Am Rev Respir Dis* 103:57, 1971.

National Institutes of Health: Practical guide for the diagnosis and management of asthma, Pub No 97-4053, Atlanta, 1997, US Department of Health and Human Services.

Paoletti P, Viegi G, Pistelli G, et al: Reference equations for the single-breath diffusing capacity, *Am Rev Respir Dis* 132:806, 1985.

Ruppel G: *Manual of pulmonary function testing,* ed 9, St Louis, 2009, Mosby.

Single breath carbon monoxide diffusing capacity (transfer factor): recommendations for a standard technique, *Am Rev Respir Dis* 136:1299, 1987.

Snow MG: Determination of functional residual capacity, *Respir Care* 34:586, 1989.

Wanger J: *Pulmonary function testing,* ed 2, Baltimore, 1996, Williams & Wilkins.

Zamel N, Altose MD, Speir WA Jr: Statement on spirometry, *Chest* 3:547, 1983.

1. Which of the following statements is/are true of the MEP test?
   1. A pressure of −20 to −25 cm H_2O usually is adequate.
   2. A pressure of +20 to +25 cm H_2O usually is adequate.
   3. A pressure of +40 cm H_2O is usually adequate.
   4. It is a good indicator of the patient's ability to cough.
   5. The patient should hold the effort for 1 to 3 seconds.
   A. 1, 2
   B. 3, 4
   C. 3
   D. 3, 4, 5

2. The predicted FVC value for African Americans is
   A. 10% to 15% higher than that for Caucasians
   B. The same as for Caucasians
   C. 10% to 15% less than that for Caucasians
   D. 20% to 25% less than that for Caucasians

3. Which of the following test results is/are needed to calculate TLC?
   1. FRC
   2. RV
   3. V_T
   4. ERV
   5. IC
   6. VC
   A. 1, 3
   B. 2, 6
   C. 2, 5
   D. 1 and 5, or 2 and 6

4. A normal MEFV loop test would show
   A. $FEF_{50\%}$ less than $FIF_{50\%}$
   B. Predicted lung diffusion ability
   C. $FEF_{50\%}$ greater than $FIF_{50\%}$
   D. A normal FRC

5. A patient with a neuromuscular disease has been having serial bedside spirometry performed. Over the past 4 hours, her VC and MIP values have been decreasing. How should this be interpreted?
   A. Her strength is improving.
   B. She is not performing to the best of her ability.
   C. She has undiagnosed asthma.
   D. Her condition is worsening.

6. An order is received to perform the following bedside spirometry tests on a patient: tidal volume, FVC, and peak flow. Which device would you take with you to perform the tests?
   A. Stead-Wells water-seal spirometer
   B. Maximum inspiratory pressure manometer
   C. Differential pressure pneumotachometer
   D. Body plethysmograph

7. Before a patient does an FVC test, the pneumotachometer should have the following done:
   A. The gas analyzer should be calibrated.
   B. A CO_2-absorbing material should be placed in line with the circuit.
   C. A 3-L volume should be pumped into and out of the circuit to check for leaks.
   D. The kymograph speeds should be checked.

8. To help in the diagnosis of a patient with a questionable history of wheezing and possible asthma, which of the following would be the best test?
   A. Bronchoprovocation study
   B. Flow-volume loop
   C. Before and after bronchodilator study
   D. Raw

9. A patient has just been tested for C_L in a body plethysmograph. Her compliance was determined to be 0.2 L (200 mL)/cm H_2O. Based on this, she most likely has
   A. Asthma
   B. Pulmonary fibrosis
   C. Emphysema
   D. Normal lungs

10. Calculate a patient's inspiratory time and expiratory time when he has an I : E ratio of 2 : 1 and a respiratory rate of 15/min.
    A. 2.7 sec for inspiration and 1.3 sec for expiration
    B. 3.3 sec for inspiration and 1.7 sec for expiration
    C. 1.3 sec for inspiration and 2.7 sec for expiration
    D. 1.7 sec for inspiration and 3.3 sec for expiration

11. When a patient performs an MEP test, it is important that he or she
    A. Blow out all air before starting the effort
    B. Breathe in a V_T and blow out hard
    C. Inhale to TLC and blow out hard
    D. Exhale a V_T breath and inhale as hard as possible

12. A patient weighs 45 kg (100 lb). Her predicted V_T would be
    A. 550 mL
    B. 450 mL
    C. 350 mL
    D. 250 mL

13. You receive an order to calculate your patient's alveolar ventilation. His respiratory rate is 16, and his average V_T is 580 mL. He weighs 170 lb. His alveolar ventilation is
    A. 2720 mL
    B. 410 mL
    C. 750 mL
    D. 510 mL

14. Your patient has an $FEV_{1\%}$ that is calculated to be 80% of his FVC. On the basis of this finding, the patient probably
    A. Is having an asthma attack
    B. Has a laryngeal tumor
    C. Has a fibrotic lung disease
    D. Is clinically normal

    Note: Refer to the figure on p. 147 for questions 15 and 16.

15. Which section of the spirometry tracing represents the FVC?
    A. 2
    B. 3
    C. 4
    D. 5

16. Which section of the spirometry tracing represents the V_T?
    A. 1
    B. 2
    C. 3
    D. 4

17. The VC is made up of
    1. RV
    2. FRC
    3. ERV
    4. V_T
    5. IRV
    A. 2, 4
    B. 3, 4
    C. 1, 2, 3
    D. 3, 4, 5

18. Which of the following are true of the PF measurement?
    1. It is usually seen at the end of the patient's FVC effort.
    2. It increases with height.
    3. It increases with age.
    4. It decreases with age.
    5. It is usually seen at the beginning of the patient's FVC effort.
    A. 1, 2, 3
    B. 2, 4, 5
    C. 1, 2, 4
    D. 4, 5

19. You are having your patient perform the MIP test. His three attempts produce these results: −15 cm H_2O, −45 cm H_2O, and −20 cm H_2O. The best explanation for these values is that
    A. The patient is starting from the FRC.
    B. The equipment has a large leak.
    C. The patient is starting from the RV.
    D. The patient is not trying his best every time.

20. The physician wants to know whether a new bronchodilator would be helpful to his patient with asthma. He orders a before and after bronchodilator study. The patient has the following peak flow values: 7.5 L/min before the medication and 9.4 L/min after the medication. Calculate her percentage change.
    A. 25%
    B. 1.25%
    C. −25%
    D. 80%

SELF-STUDY QUESTIONS FOR THE WRITTEN REGISTRY EXAM   *See page 608 for answers*

1. Complete spirometry is performed on a 50-year-old patient, revealing the following data:

	Predicted	Actual	% Predicted
TLC (L)	5.9	8.1	137
RV (L)	1.1	1.8	164
FVC (L)	5.0	2.6	52
$FEF_{25\%-75\%}$ (L/sec)	4.2	1.5	36
FEV_1/FVC	75%	20%	27

   How should the data be interpreted?
   A. Mild restrictive lung disease
   B. Severe restrictive lung disease
   C. Mild obstructive lung disease
   D. Severe obstructive lung disease

2. A nitrogen washout test for residual volume has been performed on a patient for 7 minutes and has not reached the desired nitrogen percentage. What could explain this situation?

   A. There is an oxygen leak into the system.
   B. The patient has an abnormally high respiratory exchange ratio.
   C. The patient has severe air trapping.
   D. Nitrogen has been absorbed into the patient's tissues.

3. A patient has been scheduled for a battery of pulmonary function tests. He tells you that he is so nervous about the testing that he has smoked four cigarettes in the last 2 hours. Which of the following tests is most likely to be adversely affected by this?
   A. FRC
   B. Lung diffusion
   C. Raw
   D. FVC

4. Which section of the following spirometry tracing represents the inspiratory reserve volume?

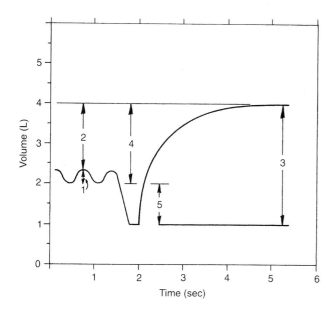

A. 2
B. 3
C. 4
D. 5

5. Which section of the spirometry tracing in question 4 represents the expiratory reserve volume?
   A. 1
   B. 2
   C. 3
   D. 4

6. After spirometry is performed, it is important that patient flow rates be reported at
   A. ATPS
   B. BTPS
   C. STPD
   D. ATPD

7. Your patient is performing a residual volume test on a water-seal spirometer in the pulmonary function laboratory. After breathing on the system for 1 minute, he takes out the mouthpiece and complains of being short of breath. What is the most likely problem in the pulmonary function system?
   A. The carbon dioxide absorber was accidentally left in the circuit.
   B. There is too much water around the spirometer bell.
   C. The carbon dioxide absorber has been left out of the circuit.
   D. Nose clips were left off of the patient.

8. Which of the following studies produces the most accurate determination of the TLC in a patient with severe emphysema?

A. Single-breath nitrogen washout test
B. Seven-minute nitrogen washout test
C. Helium dilution test
D. Body plethysmography test

9. The pulmonary function testing laboratory has recently acquired an exhaled nitric oxide (eNO) analyzer. In which patient population is its use best indicated?
   A. History of COPD
   B. History of asthma attacks
   C. History of ARDS
   D. History of asbestos exposure

10. Before a patient performs a forced vital capacity test, all of the following should be done to the water-sealed spirometer EXCEPT
    A. Make sure the circuit is airtight
    B. Place a carbon dioxide–absorbing material in line with the circuit
    C. Pump a 3-L volume into and out of the circuit to check for leaks
    D. Check the kymograph speeds

11. A properly performed FVC test will not have
    1. Any coughing or leaks
    2. A weak patient effort
    3. An unsatisfactory start to the test
    4. Excessive variability among test results
    A. 1, 2
    B. 2, 3
    C. 1, 2, 4
    D. 1, 2, 3, 4

12. A patient has a suspected diagnosis of asthma. Which of the following tests would be the least helpful in assessing the patient for this condition?
    A. Before and after bronchodilator study
    B. Flow-volume loop
    C. Diffusion study
    D. Bronchoprovocation testing

13. A patient with a history of COPD has been admitted. To help clarify her diagnosis as emphysema or asthma, which of the following should the respiratory therapist recommend?
    A. Flow-volume loop
    B. Maximum voluntary ventilation
    C. Spirometry before and after an inhaled bronchodilator
    D. Peak flow test

14. Based on the flow-volume loops in the following figure, which one represents the most severe small airway obstruction?

A

B

C

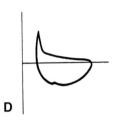

D

    A. Tracing A
    B. Tracing B
    C. Tracing C
    D. Tracing D

15. Based on the flow-volume loops in question 14, which one represents the fixed large airway obstruction?
    A. Tracing A
    B. Tracing B
    C. Tracing C
    D. Tracing D

16. Based on the flow-volume loops in question 14, tracing *A* represents a patient with asthmatic bronchitis, and tracing *C* represents the same patient 1 hour after receiving an inhaled bronchodilator medication. What conclusion can be reached?
    A. The patient's condition is treatable.
    B. The patient is not giving his or her best effort.
    C. The patient's condition has worsened.
    D. The patient needs another bronchodilator treatment.

17. As the PFT lab respiratory therapist, you have received an order to perform exhaled nitric oxide (eNO) analysis, spirometry testing, and residual volume testing on a 10-year-old girl with a history of wheezing and chronic cough. First, you perform the eNO analysis and find the girl's eNO value to be 35 ppb. How should you interpret this information?
    A. The value is within normal limits, and the other testing should continue.
    B. The analyzer must be recalibrated to room air and the test repeated.
    C. The patient's value is increased from normal.
    D. The patient's other tests need to be performed first and the eNO test repeated.

5 Advanced Cardiopulmonary Monitoring

Note 1: This book is written to cover every item listed as testable on the *Entry Level Examination (ELE), Written Registry Examination (WRE),* and *Clinical Simulation Examination (CSE).*

The listed code for each item is taken from the National Board for Respiratory Care's (NBRC) **Summary Content Outline for CRT (Certified Respiratory Therapist) and Written RRT (Registered Respiratory Therapist) Examinations** (see http://evolve.elsevier.com/Sills/resptherapist/). For example, if an item is testable on both the ELE and the WRE, it will simply be shown as: (Code: . . .). If an item is only testable on the ELE, it will be shown as: (ELE code: . . .). If an item is only testable on the WRE, it will be shown as: (WRE code: . . .).

Following each item's code will be the difficulty level of the questions on that item on the ELE and WRE. (See the Introduction for a full explanation of the three question difficulty levels.) **Recall [R]** level questions typically expect the exam taker to recall factual information. **Application [Ap]** level questions are harder because the exam taker may have to apply factual information to a clinical situation. **Analysis [An]** level questions are the most challenging because the exam taker may have to use critical thinking to evaluate patient data to make a clinical decision.

Note 2: A review of the most recent Entry Level Examinations (ELE) has shown an average of 2 questions (out of 140), or 1% of the exam, will cover advanced cardiopulmonary monitoring. A review of the most recent Written Registry Examinations (WRE) has shown an average of 3 questions (out of 100), or 3% of the exam, will cover advanced cardiopulmonary monitoring. The Clinical Simulation Examination is comprehensive and may include everything that should be known by an advanced level respiratory therapist.

MODULE A

Exhaled carbon dioxide analysis

1. Capnography (exhaled CO_2 monitoring)
a. Review capnography data in the patient's chart (Code: IA7e) [Difficulty: ELE: R; WRE: Ap]

Capnography is the analysis of graphic and numeric data from a patient showing the pattern and amount of exhaled carbon dioxide (CO_2). It is wise to look for previous capnography data before measuring the patient's exhaled CO_2 level again. Look for numeric values as well as a printout of the tracing of exhaled CO_2. Be prepared to compare the previous information with the new data to help evaluate the patient's condition. It is also useful to compare the patient's pressure of CO_2 in arterial blood ($PaCO_2$) with the capnography information, even though they should not be expected to be the same.

b. Recommend capnography to obtain additional data (Code: IC10) [Difficulty: ELE: R, Ap; WRE: An]

There are three main reasons to recommend capnography. The first reason is to assess a patient's ventilation. General anesthesia and even conscious sedation can result in a blunting of the patient's normal drive to breathe. Several clinical or pathologic situations (discussed later in this chapter) can result in an abnormal increase or decrease in the carbon dioxide level. Second, capnography helps evaluate the effectiveness of cardiopulmonary resuscitation efforts. See the discussion in Chapter 11. Third, capnography can be used to help identify the proper placement of an endotracheal tube. If the tube is within the patient's trachea or a main stem bronchus, the exhaled tidal volume will contain carbon dioxide. See the discussion in Chapter 12.

c. Perform the bedside procedure (Code: IB9c and IIIE3d) [Difficulty: ELE: R; WRE: Ap, An]

The capnometer is a device that measures the concentration of CO_2 in a gas sample from a patient. The principle of operation of most bedside units is based on carbon dioxide's absorption of infrared light in a narrow wavelength band (4.3 μ). Infrared light at this wavelength is passed through the gas sample to a receiving unit. The difference between what is transmitted and what is received is directly related to how much carbon dioxide is in the gas sample. In other words, the greater the difference between the sent and the received infrared light, the greater the concentration of carbon dioxide in the gas sample.

The capnometer is calibrated by comparing a gas sample without carbon dioxide (possibly room air) with a second gas sample containing a known amount of carbon dioxide. The first gas sample without CO_2 should give a "zero" reading. Adjust the calibration control to zero if needed. The second sample usually contains 5% to 10% carbon dioxide. The capnometer should display a CO_2 level that matches the amount in the known gas sample. Adjust the calibration control as necessary. The carbon dioxide level can be documented as a percent or fraction (F_ACO_2) or as a partial pressure (P_ACO_2).

The capnograph is a strip chart recorder that provides a copy of the patient's exhaled carbon dioxide curve. There are at least two paper speeds that are useful for different purposes. The fast speed is most useful for evaluating sudden changes in the patient's condition. Each individual breath is easily seen (Figure 5-1). The slow speed is most useful for trend monitoring (Figure 5-2).

Two different gas sampling methods exist: mainstream and sidestream. The mainstream method involves having the infrared sensing unit at the airway; usually it is attached directly to the endotracheal/tracheostomy tube. If the patient is on a ventilator, the sampling adapter must be placed between the endotracheal tube and the ventilator circuit (with or without mechanical dead space).

All inspired and expired gas passes through the sensor (Figure 5-3).

The sidestream method employs a capillary tube placed so that a small sampling of the patient's exhaled gas can be drawn into the capnometer for analysis. It is not necessary for the patient's entire breath to pass through the

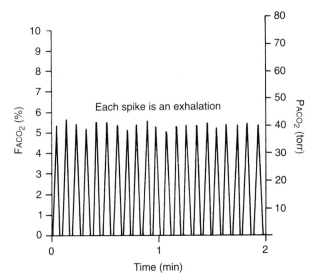

Figure 5-2   Normal capnograph tracing taken at a slow speed. The percentage of exhaled alveolar CO_2 is shown on the left vertical scale as F_ACO_2. The partial pressure of exhaled alveolar CO_2 is shown on the right vertical scale as P_ACO_2. The slow speed results in a blending of parts **A, B,** and **C** of the fast-speed tracing (Figure 5-1). Each spike is part **C** of the curve and marks an exhalation. A slow-speed tracing is more useful in trend monitoring of a patient than a fast-speed tracing.

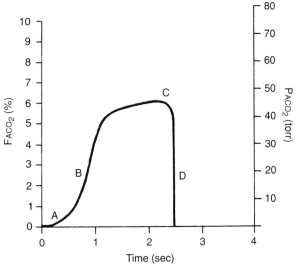

Figure 5-1   Normal capnograph tracing taken at a fast speed. The percentage of exhaled alveolar CO_2 is shown on the left vertical scale as F_ACO_2. The partial pressure of exhaled alveolar CO_2 is shown on the right vertical scale as P_ACO_2. The tracing of exhaled gas can be divided into these four components: *A,* the beginning of exhalation, which shows no carbon dioxide in the upper airway anatomic dead space; *B,* the addition of alveolar gas, rich in carbon dioxide, to the anatomic dead space gas causes a rapid rise in measured CO_2 level; *C,* pure alveolar gas with a stable amount of CO_2 causes a plateau—the end-tidal CO_2 point is shown at **C** just before inspiration; and *D,* inspiration with a rapid drop in carbon dioxide concentration to zero. Compared to a slow-speed tracing, a fast-speed tracing is more useful for determining the cause of a patient's changing condition.

Figure 5-3   Schematic drawing of a mainstream exhaled carbon dioxide analyzer sensor. The infrared sensor is attached to the patient's airway so that all of the exhaled and inhaled gas passes through it. *(From Szaflarski NL, Cohen NH: Heart Lung 20:363-374, 1991.)*

Figure 5-4 Representation of a sidestream capnometry system. A capillary tube is placed into the ventilator circuit to sample the exhaled and inhaled gases.

sampling adapter; therefore it can be used in an unintubated patient by taping the sampling catheter a short distance into a nostril. If the patient is on a ventilator, the sampling adapter must be placed between the endotracheal tube and the ventilator circuit (with or without mechanical dead space). Remember that the patient's exhaled tidal volume (V_T) and minute volume ($\dot{V}_E$) are reduced by the amount that is drawn into the capnometer (Figure 5-4).

d. Interpret the results from the procedure (Code: IB10c, IIIE4e) [Difficulty: ELE: R, Ap; WRE: An]

It is known that carbon dioxide diffuses from the higher concentration in the tissues to the venous blood and to the lungs to be exhaled. Figure 5-5 shows the normal physiology behind capnography. This diffusion or "flow" of CO_2 results in a measurable gradient or difference. In a healthy, upright sitting person, a close relationship exists between carbon dioxide levels in both venous blood and arterial blood and the amount of exhaled carbon dioxide gas. The carbon dioxide level at the end of exhalation is most frequently monitored during patient care. This is called the end-tidal carbon dioxide pressure ($PetCO_2$). When ventilation and perfusion match well, as in a healthy upright person, the gradient between the arterial carbon dioxide level ($PaCO_2$) and the $PetCO_2$ is between 2 and 3 torr, with a range of 1 to 5 torr. The gradient will show the $PetCO_2$ level to be less than the $PaCO_2$ level. This is because the $PetCO_2$ value is an average of exhaled carbon dioxide levels from all lung areas.

Box 5-1 lists normal values of capnography. Three factors influence capnography's use and the interpreta-

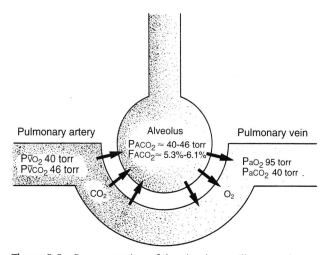

Figure 5-5 Representation of the alveolar-capillary membrane showing the diffusion of oxygen and carbon dioxide and the arterialization of venous blood. Also shown are alveolar CO_2 values measured by capnography.

tion of the results. (1) The first factor is the patient's metabolism. The average resting adult produces about 200 mL of CO_2 per minute, and fever and exercise increase this value. Hypothermia, sleep, and sedation decrease CO_2 production. Exhaled CO_2 is monitored during a cardiopulmonary resuscitation (CPR) attempt to determine the effectiveness of circulation and ventilation attempts and to decide if the efforts should be continued or stopped. If no carbon dioxide is being exhaled despite proper CPR procedures, the physician may conclude that the patient's metabolism has stopped altogether and death has occurred. There would then be nothing to gain by continuing cardiopulmonary resuscitation (CPR) efforts.

BOX 5-1 Normal Blood Gas and Capnography Values (Based on a Sea Level Barometric Pressure of 760 torr)*

$PaCO_2$[†] is 40 torr (range of 35 to 45 torr).

$P\bar{v}CO_2$[‡] is about 46 torr.

The pressure of exhaled alveolar CO_2 (P_ACO_2) ranges from 35 to 43 torr with the breathing cycle.

The pressure of exhaled end-tidal ($PetCO_2$) ranges from 35 to 43 torr. This shows the carbon dioxide level varying between the arterial and mixed venous blood levels. This value normally trends with the $PaCO_2$ level.

The normal trends between the pressure of arterial CO_2 and end-tidal CO_2 is about 2 to 3 torr, with a range of 1 to 5 torr. In other words: $P(a-et)CO_2$ is about 2-3 torr.

The percentage of end-tidal CO_2 (F_ACO_2) is about 4%-6% and trends with the $PaCO_2$ level.

---

*Both P_ACO_2 and F_ACO_2 may be seen listed in the literature as end-tidal CO_2. NOTE: The NBRC uses the abbreviation $P_{ET}CO_2$ for end-tidal CO_2.

[†]$PaCO_2$ is the partial pressure of carbon dioxide in arterial blood.

[‡]$P\bar{v}CO_2$ is the partial pressure of carbon dioxide in mixed venous blood.

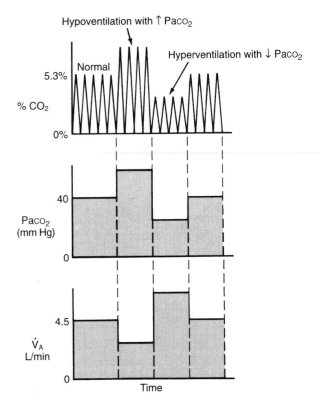

Figure 5-6 Relationship between alveolar ventilation, $PaCO_2$, and exhaled percent CO_2. *(From Pilbeam SP: Mechanical ventilation: physiological and clinical applications, ed 4, St Louis, 2006, Mosby.)*

(2) Although not a major factor, the patient's cardiac output is another factor that influences the use of capnography. Sepsis, which might double a patient's cardiac output, reduces the PCO_2 level only a few torr (millimeters of mercury [mm Hg]). Cardiogenic shock, which reduces the cardiac output, raises the partial pressure of CO_2 (PCO_2) only a few torr.

(3) The third and most important factor is alveolar ventilation. A doubling of alveolar ventilation, under steady-state conditions for carbon dioxide production, results in a halving of the PCO_2 levels in arterial blood and alveolar gas. However, a reduction of alveolar ventilation to half of its previous level will result in the $PaCO_2$ and P_ACO_2 levels being doubled (Figure 5-6).

Tidal volume (V_T) and respiratory rate are directly related to alveolar ventilation. Of the two, tidal volume is more important because it relates to the patient's dead space (V_D) to V_T ratio (V_D/V_T). A decrease in the patient's V_T level results in less alveolar ventilation and a rise in PCO_2 level. Conversely, an increase in the V_T level results in more alveolar ventilation and a drop in the PCO_2 level.

Capnography is most accurate and correlates best with the $PaCO_2$ level if the patient's ventilation and perfusion match. The more ventilation and perfusion mismatching there is, or the more unstable the pulmonary perfusion, the wider or less reliable is the gradient between the patient's arterial carbon dioxide and alveolar carbon dioxide levels. The following procedures should be performed to help understand the patient's condition and interpret the capnography results.

Exam Hint 5-1 (ELE, WRE)

Remember that mm Hg (millimeters of mercury) and torr (Torricelli) are equivalent units of pressure. The National Board of Respiratory Care (NBRC) uses these two units for different items in its questions. It uses mm Hg for blood pressure measurements and torr for blood gas values (such as $PaCO_2$ and $P\bar{v}O_2$). However, in questions referring to capnography, the NBRC has used both mm Hg and torr in its questions that relate to exhaled CO_2 (such as P_ACO_2 and $P_{ET}CO_2$).

Remember that mm Hg (millimeters of mercury) and torr (Torricelli) are equivalent units of pressure. The National Board of Respiratory Care (NBRC) uses these two units for different items in its questions. It uses mm Hg for blood pressure measurements and torr for blood gas values (such as $PaCO_2$ and $P\bar{v}O_2$). However, in questions regarding capnography, the NBRC has used both mm Hg and torr in its questions that relate to exhaled CO_2 (such as P_ACO_2 and $PetCO_2$).

2. Arterial–end-tidal carbon dioxide gradient

a. Perform the bedside procedure (Code: IB9c and IIIE3d) [Difficulty: ELE: R; WRE: Ap, An]

The arterial–end-tidal carbon dioxide gradient [P(a-et) CO_2] is useful, because once it is reliably determined the patient's ventilatory condition can be monitored by capnography alone. Drawing an arterial blood sample to measure the $PaCO_2$ level is less necessary if the patient is stable.

The normal gradient is 2 to 3 torr, with a range of 1 to 5 torr. However, most patients using capnography are not normal. The possible gradient ranges from 6 to 20 torr in unstable patients with cardiopulmonary abnormalities. For example, the patient who is breathing shallowly may have an end-tidal CO_2 level that is greater than the arterial CO_2 level. This is because the patient is not exhaling completely to empty alveolar gas. Therefore determining each patient's own gradient is important.

Follow these steps:

1. Simultaneously draw an arterial blood gas (ABG) sample for $PaCO_2$ measurement and take an end-tidal gas sample for P_ACO_2 measurement.
2. The difference is the P(a-et)CO_2 gradient. The alveolar sample commonly shows a lower CO_2 level than the arterial sample.

EXAMPLE 1

A patient is seen in the recovery room after surgery and has the following PCO_2 levels: $PaCO_2$ = 40 torr, $PetCO_2$ = 36 torr. Calculate the patient's arterial–end-tidal carbon dioxide gradient, as follows:

$$PaCO_2 = 40 \text{ torr}$$
$$PetCO_2 = -36 \text{ torr}$$
$$P(a\text{-}et)CO_2 = 4 \text{ torr}$$

The usefulness of this gradient is demonstrated when monitoring a patient's spontaneous breathing during weaning or making ventilator changes in the tidal volume or minute volume. It may be possible to avoid drawing as many ABG samples.

EXAMPLE 2

The patient in example 1 is seen later and has the following capnography reading: $PetCO_2$ = 54 torr. The patient's $PaCO_2$ level can be easily calculated by addition:

$$PetCO_2 = 54 \text{ torr}$$
$$P(a\text{-}et)CO_2 \text{ gradient} = +4 \text{ torr}$$
$$\text{estimated } PaCO_2 = 58 \text{ torr}$$

It can be concluded that the patient is not breathing as deeply as before. Appropriate action should be taken to awaken the patient, further reverse the anesthesia, or begin artificial ventilation.

b. Interpret the results from the procedure (Code: IB10c, IIIE4e) [Difficulty: ELE: R, Ap; WRE: An]

Review the components of a fast-speed capnography tracing in Figure 5-1 to understand a normal person's expiratory pattern. Figure 5-7 shows eight different abnormal fast-speed capnography tracings. See the figure legend for an explanation of each problem. As the patient returns to normal, the tracing should approach that shown in Figure 5-1.

3. Arterial–residual volume alveolar carbon dioxide gradient

a. Perform the bedside procedure (Code: IB9c and IIIE3d) [Difficulty: ELE: R; WRE: Ap, An]

Have a cooperative patient exhale maximally to residual volume (RV) through the capnography unit. The graphic results will be similar to that shown in Figure 5-8. The usual P(a-RV)CO_2 gradient in a healthy person is about 3 to 5 torr, and should be less than 7 torr. The wider the gradient, the greater is the ventilation to perfusion ($\dot{V}/\dot{Q}$) mismatching. A gradient of more than 13 torr is considered to be markedly abnormal. This may be the case in patients with chronic obstructive pulmonary disease (COPD), pulmonary emboli, left heart failure (LHF), or hypotension.

b. Interpret the results from the procedure (Code: IB10c, IIIE4e) [Difficulty: ELE: R, Ap; WRE: An]

When comparing the normal (solid line) tracing in Figure 5-8 with the $\dot{V}/\dot{Q}$ mismatching (dashed line) tracing, note the increased gradient at end-tidal CO_2. With continued exhalation to residual volume, the left heart failure and COPD patients have a narrowing of the gradient. This can be used clinically to follow these patients' progress and response to treatment. The patient with a large pulmonary embolism will not have such a narrowing of the gradient as he or she exhales to residual volume. This patient's gradient will narrow to normal as the embolism is resolved and the physiologic dead space returns to normal.

Exam Hint 5-2 (ELE, WRE)

Past exams have often had one question that requires the interpretation of capnography results, especially the end-tidal CO_2 value ($PetCO_2$). Examples include a change in alveolar ventilation or shallow breathing.

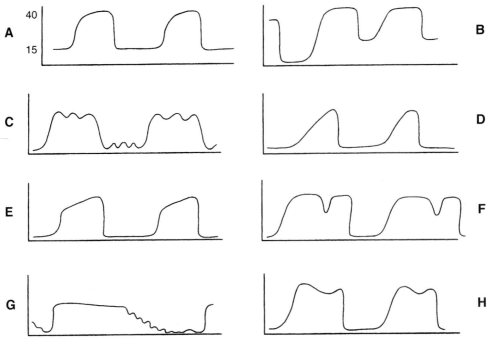

Figure 5-7   A series of abnormal fast-speed capnography tracings. **A,** A mechanically ventilated patient with a malfunctioning exhalation valve. Note that the baseline CO_2 level is elevated because the patient's exhaled breath is measured during an inspiration. Correction of the exhalation valve should result in normal inhalation and exhalation. **B,** This rapidly rising baseline gas pressure and failure to return to baseline is usually seen when moisture or secretions block the capillary tube. Clearing the obstruction enables the patient's gas to again reach the analyzer. **C,** Distortions in the tracing from incomplete exhalation. These may be caused by hiccups, chest compressions during CPR, or inconsistent tidal volume efforts during an asthma attack. **D,** An obstructive lung disease patient with ventilation and perfusion mismatching. There is no alveolar plateau with a stable CO_2 level. Inhaling a bronchodilator should result in the tracing returning closer to normal. **E,** A patient with restrictive lung disease showing no plateau of alveolar gas emptying. This is because the alveoli do not empty evenly. **F,** A sudden drop in carbon dioxide level in the middle of an exhalation indicates that the patient attempted inspiration. This "cleft" is usually seen when a patient who has been pharmacologically paralyzed begins to regain movement. **G,** Uneven carbon dioxide levels seen at the end of exhalation can be caused by the following: (1) the patient's heartbeat pumping fresh blood and CO_2 to the emptying lungs; the cardiogenic oscillations should match the heart rate; (2) the ventilator's exhalation valve is fluttering open and closed. **H,** The alveolar plateau is biphasic. This has been seen in patients with lungs that are different in compliance and ventilation/perfusion matching (e.g., single lung transplantation). *(From Shapiro BA, Peruzzi WT, Templin R: Clinical application of blood gases, ed 5, St Louis, 1994, Mosby.)*

Past exams have often had one question that requires the interpretation of capnography results, especially the end-tidal CO_2 value (PetCO$_2$). Examples include a change in alveolar ventilation, shallow breathing, and CPR attempt.

MODULE B
Dead space to tidal volume ratio

1. Review dead space to tidal volume data in the patient's chart (Code: IA7e) [Difficulty: ELE: R; WRE: Ap]

Dead space is that part of the tidal volume that does not participate in gas exchange (wasted ventilation). A patient's dead space may be anatomic and/or alveolar. The dead space to tidal volume test (V_D/V_T) is performed to document the amount of a patient's dead space. There are several clinical situations, such as a pulmonary embolism, that can justify the procedure. Review previous data before repeating the test to understand if the patient's condition has changed or is abnormal. Be prepared to compare the previous information with the new data to help evaluate the patient's current condition.

2. Perform the bedside procedure (ELE Code: IB9l) [Difficulty: ELE: R, An]

The procedure is the mathematical comparison of a person's dead space volume with tidal volume. Steps in the traditional procedure follow (Figure 5-9):

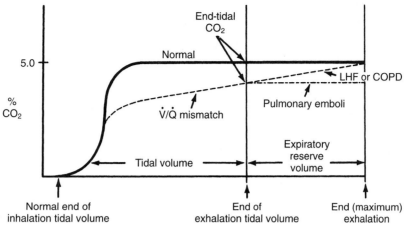

Figure 5-8 Comparison of several fast-speed capnograph tracings showing how the exhaled carbon dioxide level changes as the patient exhales to residual volume. A normal tracing is matched against abnormal tracings of pulmonary emboli, left heart failure (LHF), and chronic obstructive pulmonary disease (COPD). The normal patient has the same end-tidal CO_2 level as residual volume CO_2 level, showing good matching of ventilation and perfusion. LHF and COPD patients have a narrowing of the gradient as residual volume is approached. The patient with a pulmonary embolism keeps the same gradient at the residual volume as that found at the end of the tidal volume. *(From Pilbeam SP:* Mechanical ventilation: physiological and clinical applications, *ed 4, St Louis, 2006, Mosby.)*

Figure 5-9 A schematic presentation of the procedure for gathering patient samples for calculating the dead space to tidal volume ratio (V_D/V_T). An anesthesia or other airtight bag is used to gather all exhaled gas to determine the average exhaled carbon dioxide pressure. An arterial sample is collected for $Paco_2$ determination. *(From Pilbeam SP:* Mechanical ventilation: physiological and clinical applications, *ed 4, St Louis, 2006, Mosby.)*

1. Determine the *average* exhaled CO_2 ($P_{\bar{E}CO_2}$) level by either of these methods:
   a. Collect the patient's entire exhaled gas sample over several minutes in a large airtight bag. Count the number of breaths that occurred. Calculate the average tidal volume breath by dividing the total exhaled volume by the total rate. Put all or part of this gas sample through the blood gas analyzer to determine the PCO_2 value.
   b. Have the patient's exhaled gas pass through a capnometer that can give you an average value (not end-tidal CO_2). The number of breaths should be averaged for greater PCO_2 accuracy. Measure or calculate the patient's average tidal volume over the time of the test.
2. Draw an arterial sample at the same time that you are performing either step 1a or step 1b. Have the blood sample analyzed for $PaCO_2$ level.
3. Calculate the results using either of two methods.

a. Determine the decimal fraction or percentage of dead space

Place both carbon dioxide values into this formula, which is derived from the original Bohr formula:

$$V_D/V_T \; (\text{or } V_D) = \frac{(PaCO_2 - P_{\bar{E}CO_2})}{PaCO_2}$$

In which:

V_D/V_T or V_D = the patient's physiologic dead space

$PaCO_2$ = the patient's arterial carbon dioxide pressure

$P_{\bar{E}CO_2}$ = the patient's average exhaled carbon dioxide pressure

The following example is based on an abnormal adult:

$$PaCO_2 = 45 \text{ torr}$$

$$P_{\bar{E}CO_2} = 18 \text{ torr}$$

$$V_D = \frac{(45-18)}{45}$$

$$= \frac{27}{45} = 0.6$$

The patient's V_D fraction can be recorded as 0.6 or 60%. (Note that this equation must be used when the patient's tidal volume is not known.)

b. Determine the dead space volume

Place both carbon dioxide values into this formula, which is derived from the original Bohr formula:

$$V_D/V_T \; (\text{or } V_D) = \frac{(PaCO_2 - P_{\bar{E}CO_2})}{PaCO_2} \times V_T$$

In which:

V_D/V_T or V_D = the patient's physiologic dead space

V_T = the average exhaled tidal volume

$PaCO_2$ = the patient's arterial carbon dioxide pressure

$P_{\bar{E}CO_2}$ = the patient's average exhaled carbon dioxide pressure

The following example is based on a normal adult:

$$V_T = 500 \text{ mL}$$

$$PaCO_2 = 40 \text{ torr}$$

$$P_{\bar{E}CO_2} = 28 \text{ torr}$$

$$V_D = \frac{(40-28)}{40} = \frac{12}{40} \times 500 = 0.3 \times 500 \text{ mL} = 150 \text{ mL}$$

The patient's physiologic V_D volume = 150 mL. (Note that this equation must be used when the patient's tidal volume is known.)

In addition, the preceding equation allows calculation of the patient's V_D/V_T ratio. In this example, it is 150/500, 0.3, or 30%, depending on how it is written.

The recent advent of *volumetric capnography* technology allows the patient's dead space to be rapidly determined. These units can simultaneously measure the patient's exhaled tidal volume and the variable percentage of carbon dioxide found during the exhalation (Figure 5-10). The computer that is integrated with the volumetric capnography unit then calculates the volume of dead space as a fraction of the exhaled tidal volume. Figure 5-11 shows how volumetric capnography can be set up to measure the dead space of a patient requiring mechanical ventilation. This technology permits the rapid assessment of a patient as treatment is being performed. For example, if a patient had a large pulmonary embolism resulting in significant

Figure 5-10 A graphic representation of the factors involved in the calculation of a patient's dead space volume, or dead space to tidal volume (V_D/V_T) ratio, through volumetric capnography. These units can measure exhaled carbon dioxide (by pressure or percentage) at time intervals as the patient's tidal volume is exhaled. Review Figure 5-1, as needed, for a normal capnograph tracing.

Figure 5-11 Measurement of volumetric capnography on a patient receiving mechanical ventilation. All measurements are taken between the patient's endotracheal tube and mechanical ventilator circuit. The mainstream capnograph sensor sends data on exhaled carbon dioxide concentration to the computer within the capnograph monitor. The pressure and flow sensors send data to the computer to determine the exhaled volume. The computer integrates the information to determine anatomic dead space (white area) and alveolar dead space (black area). With areas *q* and *p* being calculated as equal, the shaded area is alveolar volume where gas exchange occurs.

dead space, a clot-dissolving medication such as streptokinase (Kabikinase or Streptase) or alteplase (Activase) would be given. These "clot buster" medications will rapidly dissolve the patient's pulmonary embolism. With volumetric capnography, the dead space volume can be monitored as it normalizes when blood flow through the lungs is restored.

3. Interpret the results of the V_D/V_T calculation (Code: IB10l) [Difficulty: ELE: R, Ap; WRE: An]

The normal adult's V_D/V_T ratio ranges from 0.2 (20%) to 0.4 (40%). Anatomic dead space is normally greater in men than in women. The normal 3-kg neonate's dead space to tidal volume ratio is 0.3 (30%). Physiologic dead space (also known as respiratory dead space) is gas that is ventilated into the lungs but does not take part in gas exchange. This is because the alveoli are not perfused or are underperfused for the amount of gas that they receive.

Physiologic dead space is composed of the following:
- Anatomic dead space, or the gas in the connecting airways from the nose and mouth to the terminal bronchioles. Generally it is assumed to be about 1 mL/lb of ideal body weight, or 2.2 mL/kg of ideal body weight.
- Alveolar dead space that is composed of nonfunctioning alveoli that are ventilated but not perfused is minimal in a normal person. The previous "normal" adult example has the expected amount of dead space for his or her weight.

The following conditions or pulmonary disorders can cause the ratio to vary from the normal range:

a. Decreased V_D/V_T ratio

1. Lung resection or pneumonectomy, because the airways are removed; the patient will maintain his or her tidal volume in the other lung segments.
2. Asthma attack, because the airways are narrowed.
3. Insertion of an endotracheal or tracheostomy tube, because the upper airway is bypassed.
4. Exercise in the normal, healthy person, because the increased blood pressure increases perfusion of the apices (Zone 1).

b. Increased V_D/V_T ratio

1. Vascular tumor, because of decreased perfusion to ventilated alveoli.
2. Pulmonary embolism, because of lack of blood flow to ventilated alveoli. Consider this if the patient is a

candidate for a pulmonary embolism and suddenly deteriorates.

c. Increased dead space effect with ventilation greater than perfusion ($\dot{V} > \dot{Q}$)

1. Rapid, shallow ventilations, because the upper airway dead space is overventilated compared with the alveoli.
2. Mechanical dead space added to the ventilator circuit. This is an intentional effort to have the patient retain some of his or her exhaled carbon dioxide to correct for a respiratory alkalosis.
3. COPD (bronchitis, bronchiectasis, cystic fibrosis, emphysema), because varying degrees of bronchospasm, mucous plugging, and tissue destruction lead to increased ventilation and perfusion mismatching.

Many clinicians believe that a dead space/tidal volume ratio of 0.6 (60%) or more is an indication for mechanically ventilating the patient. A person who is wasting 60% or more of his or her ventilation will soon tire from the work of breathing and go into ventilatory failure.

Exam Hint 5-4 (ELE, WRE)

Remember that a pulmonary embolism is the most likely cause of a sudden increase in dead space. This concept is usually tested. In addition, there is usually a question that relates to identifying that a COPD patient will have a chronically increased V_D/V_T value.

MODULE C
Hemodynamic monitoring

1. Blood pressure

a. Review blood pressure data in the patient's chart (Code: IA8b) [Difficulty: ELE: R; WRE: Ap]

Systemic arterial blood pressure (BP) is the force exerted against the walls of the arteries when blood is pumped through them. As one of the vital signs, the patient's BP should be found in the chart. Review it to know the patient's normal blood pressure reading, and if it has been stable or variable with the patient's changing condition.

b. Recommend blood pressure measurement to obtain additional data (Code: IC11) [Difficulty: ELE: R, Ap; WRE: An]

The patient's blood pressure, and other vital signs, should be monitored as often as clinically prudent. If the patient's cardiovascular or pulmonary condition is changing frequently, the blood pressure should be measured frequently, even continuously.

c. Perform blood pressure measurement (Code: IB9m, IIIE3e) [Difficulty: ELE: R, Ap; WRE: An]

The general steps in measuring blood pressure were described in Chapter 1. The BP is usually measured on either of the patient's arms. Necessary equipment includes the proper size of blood pressure cuff, a sphygmomanometer to measure the pressure, and a stethoscope to hear the sounds of bloodflow returning through the brachial artery. Figure 5-12 shows the basic elements of the procedure. The cuff is inflated to a pressure that is greater than the patient's systolic pressure. As the pressure in the cuff is gradually decreased, the first sound heard (Korotkoff sounds) is the systolic pressure. The pressure reading at which this sound ceases is the diastolic pressure. Blood pressure measurement can usually be performed manually by a respiratory therapist or other trained health care professional. If BP measurement is needed on a frequent basis, an automated blood pressure measurement system can be set up on the patient's arm. This unit can be programmed to measure the BP on a schedule and can also have high and low blood pressure alarm limits established as a safety feature.

d. Recommend the insertion of an arterial line (WRE code: IC12) [Difficulty: WRE: R, Ap, An]

Recommend that an arterial line (catheter) be inserted in the following situations: (1) the patient needs continuous monitoring of blood pressure, (2) frequent arterial blood samples are needed for blood gas analysis. The arterial line is usually placed into the radial artery of an adult; a newborn will have the line placed into the umbilical artery.

e. Interpret the results of the blood pressure measurement (Code: IB10m, IIIE4c) [Difficulty: ELE: R, Ap; WRE: An]

Review the general discussion on blood pressure in Chapter 1. The following are normal blood pressure values:

Adult: less than 120/80 mm Hg

Infants and children younger than 10 years:
60 to 100/20 to 70 mm Hg

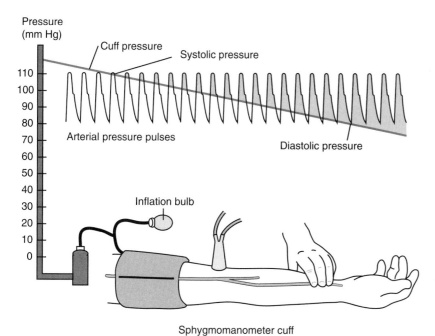

Figure 5-12 Arterial blood pressure is most commonly measured with a sphygmomanometer cuff that is inflated to a pressure greater than the patient's BP. When that happens, no palpable pulse can be felt. As the cuff pressure is gradually decreased, a respiratory therapist can listen, with a stethoscope placed over the brachial artery, for the return of blood flow. The first sound heard is systolic pressure (in this case 110 mm Hg) and the last sound heard is diastolic pressure (in this case 80 mm Hg). *(Modified from Rushmer RF: Cardiovascular dynamics, ed 3, Philadelphia, 1970, Saunders. In Wilkins RL, Dexter JR, Heuer AJ: Clinical assessment in respiratory care, ed 6, St Louis, 2010, Mosby.)*

Patients who have values that are higher or lower than these should be further evaluated. Know the following values since they represent a serious patient problem:

Hypotension in an adult is a systolic BP of less than 90 mm Hg

Hypertension in an adult is a systolic BP of 140 mm Hg or greater, a diastolic blood pressure of 90 mm Hg or greater, or both

2. Central venous pressure (CVP) monitoring

a. Review central venous pressure measurement data in the patient's chart (Code: IA8b) [Difficulty: ELE: R; WRE: Ap]

The central venous pressure (CVP) is the pressure measured in a patient's superior vena cava, just above the right atrium. See Figure 5-13. Review previous patient data to understand whether there is an abnormality. Compare the current data with the earlier information to determine if there has been a change in the patient's condition. See Box 5-2 for normal values.

b. Recommend the insertion of a central venous pressure catheter to obtain additional data (WRE code: IC12) [WRE Difficulty: R, Ap, An]

A single-lumen central venous pressure catheter (also called a CVP line) is inserted into many patients for one

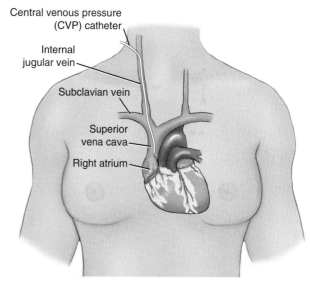

Figure 5-13 Proper position of a central venous pressure (CVP) catheter with its distal tip located in the superior vena cava, just above the right atrium. The catheter can be inserted through the internal jugular vein (as shown) or the subclavian vein. This traditional, single-lumen CVP catheter can be used to measure the pressure on the right side of the heart and to administer fluids or medications.

or more reasons: (1) to monitor the patient's right-sided (right atrium) heart pressure, (2) to rapidly administer a large volume of intravenous fluids, and (3) to administer cardiac medications during a CPR attempt (preferred route). Recently, the development of a triple-lumen

BOX 5-2   Normal Cardiopulmonary Values

ARTERIAL BLOOD PRESSURE (BP)

Adults: less than 120/80 mm Hg

Infants and children younger than 10 years: 60-100/20-70 mm Hg

CENTRAL VENOUS PRESSURE (CVP)

Range for a normal adult is 2-8 cm of water or 1-6 mm Hg

Range for a normal infant is 1-5 mm Hg

Range for a normal neonate is 3 mm Hg or less

PULMONARY ARTERY PRESSURE (PAP)

Range for a normal adult is 15-28/5-16 mm Hg (about 25/10 mm Hg)

Range for a normal adult mean PAP is 10-22 mm Hg

Range for a normal child is 15-30/5-10 mm Hg

Range for a normal neonate is 30-60/2-10 mm Hg

PULMONARY CAPILLARY WEDGE PRESSURE (PCWP)

Range for a normal PCWP (mean) is 6-15 mm Hg (about 8 mm Hg)

CARDIAC OUTPUT

Range for a normal adult is 4-8 L/min

Range for a normal neonate is 0.6-0.8 L/min

STROKE VOLUME

Adults: 50-120 mL/beat

School-age children: 35 mL/beat

Preschoolers: 15 mL/beat

Neonates: 5 mL/beat

CARDIAC INDEX

2.5-4.0 L/min/m^2 of body surface area

ARTERIAL-VENOUS OXYGEN CONTENT DIFFERENCE [C(a-v)O$_2$]

Range of normal is 3.0-5.5 vol % of O$_2$

SHUNT

5% or less of cardiac output

PULMONARY VASCULAR RESISTANCE

80-240 dynes/sec/cm^{-5} or

1-3 mm Hg/L/min

SYSTEMIC VASCULAR RESISTANCE

900-1400 dynes/sec/cm^{-5}

Figure 5-14 New triple-lumen CVP catheter that can be used to continuously monitor the patient's oxygen saturation of central venous blood (S$\overline{c}$vO$_2$) in addition to measuring the right heart pressure and administering fluids and medications. *(From Edwards Lifesciences LLC, Irvine, Calif.)*

CVP catheter with integrated fiberoptic channel (Edwards Lifesciences, LLC) has enabled the continuous monitoring of central venous oxygen saturation (ScvO$_2$), in addition to the previously mentioned uses. See Figure 5-14.

c. Recommend central venous pressure measurement to obtain additional data (Code: IC11) [Difficulty: ELE: R, Ap; WRE: An]

The CVP is measured in order to know the pressure in the right atrium of the patient's heart. This information is used to help evaluate a patient's fluid status and to guide the administration or restriction of more fluids.

d. Perform central venous pressure measurement (Code: IB9e) [Difficulty: R, Ap, An]

The catheter is usually inserted into the right jugular vein or right subclavian vein and advanced to just above the superior vena cava. When set up for monitoring pressure, it measures the right atrial pressure (see Figure 5-15 for how to perform the procedure). Note that the stopcock must be kept at the midchest (midheart) level. Usually a mark is placed at this location (on the patient's chest) for consistency. Raising the stopcock above the mark results in an incorrectly low reading. Lowering the stopcock below the mark results in an incorrectly high reading. See

Figure 5-15 Procedure for determining the central venous pressure (CVP) with a manometer. **A,** Water-column manometer marked in centimeters, IV tubing, and patient in place. The patient must be placed in a horizontal position with the stopcock located at the midchest (midheart) point, as shown by the dashed line. **B,** Turn the stopcock so that the manometer fills with fluid above the expected pressure. **C,** Turn the stopcock off to the IV so that the fluid flows from the manometer into the patient. Look at the stable fluid level for the CVP reading. **D,** Turn the stopcock so that the fluid flows from the IV into the patient. *(From Daily EK, Schroeder JS:* Techniques in bedside hemodynamic monitoring, *ed 5, St Louis, 1994, Mosby.)*

Figure 5-16. Clinical practice is very important in learning how to perform this procedure. It is important that the patient breathes spontaneously if at all possible. Peak pressures during inspiration on a mechanical ventilator may artificially raise the CVP reading. Positive end-expiratory pressure (PEEP) may also raise the CVP reading. If the patient cannot be removed from the ventilator, take the reading during exhalation. Make a note of the settings and that the reading was taken with the patient on the ventilator. Record the data in the patient's chart or flow sheet.

Exam Hint 5-5 (ELE, WRE)

Past exams have asked about the proper placement of the CVP stopcock or arterial pressure transducer at the midchest (midheart) location to ensure accurate pressure measurements. Usually a mark is placed on the patient's chest for a consistent measurement point. Review Figure 5-16 for the effects of misplacement.

Past exams have asked about the proper placement of the CVP stopcock or arterial pressure transducer at the midchest (midheart) location to ensure accurate pressure measurements. Usually a mark is placed on the patient's

chest for a consistent measurement point. Review Figure 5-16 for the effects of misplacement.

e. Interpret the results of the central venous pressure measurement (Code: IB10m, IIIE4c) [Difficulty: ELE: R, Ap; WRE: An]

As noted earlier, the CVP is a measure of the pressure in the right atrium. The two main factors that influence the right atrial pressure are the blood volume returning to it and the functioning of the right ventricle (see Box 5-2 for normal CVP readings).

A decreased CVP reading usually indicates that the patient is hypovolemic. Hypotension confirms this. An increased CVP reading may suggest one of the following possibilities:

- **Fluid overload.** Check for an elevated blood pressure measurement and crackles in the bases of the lungs. Unfortunately, an elevated CVP reading is a late finding with this problem.
- **Tricuspid valve or pulmonic valve insufficiency or stenosis.** Abnormal electrocardiogram or echocardiogram findings or abnormal heart sounds (heart murmur) help to specify the problem.
- **Right ventricular failure.** A right ventricular heart attack can be identified on an electrocardiogram. If

Figure 5-16 The effects of patient position compared to position of the pressure transducer. **A,** When the patient's midchest (midheart) is *above* the pressure transducer, the measured pressure will be *higher* than actual. **B,** When the patient's midchest (midheart) is *below* the pressure transducer, the measured pressure will be *lower* than actual. **C,** True pressures will be measured when the patient's midchest is the same height as the pressure manometer. All hemodynamic pressures (CVP, arterial pressure, pulmonary artery pressure, and pulmonary capillary wedge pressure) will be adversely affected if the patient and manometer heights do not match, as shown in **A** and **B**. *(From Oblouk Darovic G: Hemodynamic monitoring—invasive and noninvasive clinical application, ed 3, Philadelphia, 2002, Saunders.)*

a COPD patient with pulmonary hypertension has right ventricular failure, the condition is called *cor pulmonale*.

- **Cardiac tamponade** (blood filling the pericardium). Watch for a drop in the blood pressure reading, tachycardia, and distended jugular veins. This problem can be rapidly fatal if not quickly corrected.

- **Atrial septal defect or ventricular septal defect with a left to right intracardiac shunt.** These congenital conditions are usually detected in a young child by an abnormal electrocardiogram or echocardiogram finding or an abnormal heart sound (heart murmur).

- **Pulmonary embolism.** This condition should be suspected when a patient who is prone to the problem experiences sudden onset of hypoxemia and clinical deterioration. A pulmonary angiogram showing blocked blood flow through the lung(s) confirms the problem.

Exam Hint 5-6 (ELE, WRE)

Memorize the values listed in Box 5-2. Expect to see several questions in which these values are used as patient data or as options to answer a question. The normal values must be understood to identify abnormal values and know why they are abnormal.

Memorize the values listed in Box 5-2. Expect to see several questions in which these values are used as patient data or as options to answer a question. The normal values must be understood to identify abnormal values and know why they are abnormal.

3. Pulmonary artery pressure monitoring

a. Review pulmonary artery pressure data in the patient's chart (Code: IA8b) [Difficulty: ELE: R; WRE: Ap]

The pulmonary artery pressure (PAP) is the systolic and diastolic pressure found in either pulmonary artery. It can be measured only through a pulmonary artery catheter. (The NBRC often refers to this as a flow-directed pulmonary artery catheter.) Review the patient's previous values before taking another pressure reading to make a comparison. Box 5-2 shows normal cardiopulmonary values.

b. Recommend the insertion of a pulmonary artery catheter for additional data (WRE code: IC12) [WRE Difficulty: R, Ap, An]

To read the PAP, a pulmonary artery catheter (PAC) must be inserted through a vein and passed through the right atrium and right ventricle into the pulmonary artery. The common insertion sites, in descending order of preference, are the basilic vein in either the right or the left arm, the right internal jugular or subclavian vein, or the right or left femoral vein. The pulmonary artery catheter is also commonly called a Swan-Ganz catheter after the inventors who gave their names to a particular brand. The catheters are available in different lengths and diameters for pediatric and adult patients. See Figure 5-17 for a typical adult catheter.

c. Recommend pulmonary artery pressure measurement to obtain additional data (Code: IC11) [Difficulty: ELE: R, Ap; WRE: An]

The PAP is important to measure in patients with severe pulmonary or cardiovascular problems, pulmonary hyper-

tension, myocardial infarction, congestive heart failure, hypertension, and hypotension.

d. Perform pulmonary artery pressure measurement (Code: IB9m, IIIE3e) [Difficulty: ELE: R, Ap; WRE: An]

Figure 5-17 is an illustration of a 7-French quadruple-lumen thermodilution pulmonary artery catheter. Besides measurement of PAP, it is capable of being used to measure cardiac output. Figure 5-18 illustrates how a pulmonary artery catheter could be arranged with a pressure transducer and pressure monitor. Figure 5-19 shows a representation of the series of pressure waveforms seen as the catheter is advanced through the heart and into the wedged position in a branch of the pulmonary artery. Figure 5-20 shows a larger cutaway view of the heart with a PAC and normal heart chambers and related pressures.

To obtain an accurate pulmonary artery pressure measurement, the equipment must be set up and calibrated properly, the distal lumen of the catheter must be patent with a continuous fluid-filled channel from the patient's bloodstream back to the transducer, and the catheter's balloon must be deflated. Clinical practice is important in understanding how to perform this procedure. Record the PAP data in the patient's chart or flow sheet.

e. Interpret the results of pulmonary artery pressure measurement (Code: IB10m, IIIE4c) [Difficulty: ELE: R, Ap; WRE: An]

Again, the PAP is the systolic and diastolic pressure found in the pulmonary artery (see Box 5-2 for normal values). Elevated PAP values are usually seen with the following conditions:

1. Left ventricular failure/congestive heart failure, acute myocardial infarction, or fluid overload. To better determine the pathophysiologic problem, it is necessary to evaluate the following kinds of clinical information:
   a. The patient has a known history of heart disease or of sudden illness suggesting a heart attack.
   b. Crackles are heard in the bases of the lungs.
   c. Decreased static lung compliance is present.
   d. The patient has elevated pulmonary capillary wedge pressure.
   e. Decreased cardiac output and/or low blood pressure is present.
   f. The normal gradient (difference) between pulmonary artery diastolic pressure (PAd) and pulmonary capillary wedge pressure (PCWP) is 5 mm Hg.

EXAMPLE

An adult patient has the following pulmonary artery catheter values: PAP, 35/24 mm Hg; PCWP, 22 mm Hg. Calculate the patient's pulmonary artery diastolic pressure minus pulmonary capillary wedge pressure (PAd-PCWP) gradient as follows:

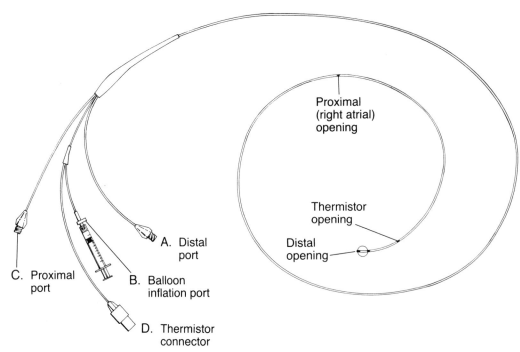

Figure 5-17 A 7-French quadruple-lumen thermodilution pulmonary artery catheter. *A*, Distal port goes to the tip of the catheter. It is used for measuring PAP and PCWP and for sampling blood for $P\bar{v}O_2$ determination. *B*, Balloon inflation port is used to inflate the balloon for inserting the catheter and for obtaining a PCWP reading. *C*, Proximal port is used for measuring central venous pressure and for injecting iced saline for a thermodilution cardiac output study. The iced saline exits from the right atrial opening. *D*, Thermistor connector attaches to the cardiac output computer. A bimetallic wire runs through the catheter to the thermistor opening, where it is exposed to temperature changes of the blood and cold injectate. (NOTE: Not all catheters are capable of measuring cardiac output. Some catheters have other special features such as continuously measuring venous saturation or cardiac pacemaker leads.) *(From Oblouk Darovic G:* Hemodynamic monitoring—invasive and noninvasive clinical applications, *ed 3, Philadelphia, 2002, Saunders.)*

Pulmonary artery diastolic is: 25 mm Hg
Pulmonary capillary wedge pressure is: −22 mm Hg
The PAd-PCWP gradient is: 3 mm Hg

It can be concluded that this person's PAd-PCWP gradient is normal.

2. Pulmonary hypertension from COPD (usually emphysema). To better determine the pathophysiologic problem, it is necessary to evaluate the following kinds of clinical information:
   a. The patient usually has a known history of COPD.
   b. Systolic PAP may exceed 40 mm Hg if the problem is long-standing.
   c. The gradient (difference) between the pulmonary artery diastolic pressure and the pulmonary capillary wedge pressure (PAd-PCWP) is greater than 5 mm Hg.

EXAMPLE

An adult patient has the following pulmonary artery catheter values: PAP, 35/25 mm Hg; PCWP, 8 mm Hg. Calculate the patient's pulmonary artery diastolic pressure

minus pulmonary capillary wedge pressure (PAd-PCWP) gradient as follows:

Pulmonary artery diastolic is: 25 mm Hg
Pulmonary capillary wedge pressure is: −8 mm Hg
The PAd-PCWP gradient is: 17 mm Hg

It can be concluded that this person's PAd-PCWP gradient is elevated.

3. Pulmonary hypertension from a pulmonary embolism. To better determine the pathophysiologic problem, it is necessary to evaluate the following kinds of clinical information:
   a. The patient's history matches that of a sudden onset of shortness of breath and other pulmonary problems.
   b. The systolic PAP is less than 40 mm Hg. This is because the relatively thin-walled right ventricle cannot rapidly increase its muscle mass to increase the driving pressure.
   c. The gradient (difference) between the pulmonary artery diastolic pressure and the pulmonary

Figure 5-18   The various components of the pulmonary artery monitoring system. It includes a fluid source such as normal saline that is pressurized to 300 mm Hg to maintain a flow of fluid through the tubing system. The continuous flush device (made by Sorenson) is designed to allow three drips of fluid per minute through the tubing system; pulling on the fast-flush valve gives a continuous flow of fluid to clear air or blood from the system. The transducer converts a pressure signal to an electrical signal that is sent to the monitor for display as numeric data and a pressure waveform. The high-pressure tubing transfers the patient's pressure accurately to the transducer. The double stopcocks are used to close off the tubing system or sample blood from the patient. This then connects to the distal port of the pulmonary artery catheter. This same monitoring system can be used with an arterial catheter for continuous pressure monitoring and blood sampling.   *(Adapted from Smith RN: Invasive pressure monitoring,* Am J Nurse 9:1514, 1978. Copyright 1978 The American Journal of Nursing. Used with permission in Oblouk Darovic G: Hemodynamic monitoring, *Philadelphia, 1987, WB Saunders.)*

capillary wedge pressure (PAd-PCWP) is greater than 5 mm Hg if the embolism is large.

4. Pulmonary hypertension in the neonate with persistent pulmonary hypertension of the newborn (PPHN) is present. This condition is often seen in the premature neonate with respiratory distress syndrome (RDS). When these neonates become hypoxic, the pulmonary vascular bed constricts. This causes the infant to revert back to fetal circulation. Administering 100% oxygen and hyperventilating the infant usually reverse the processes. The PAP then returns to normal.

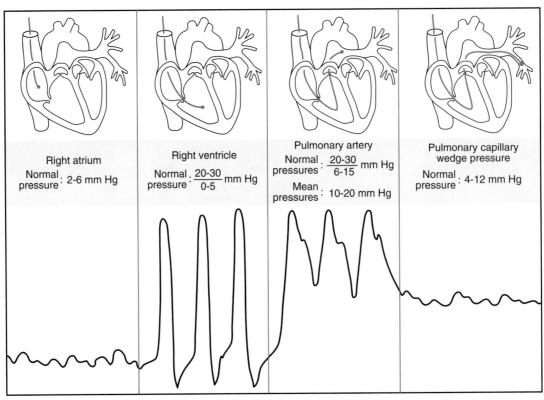

Figure 5-19   Sequence of pressures and pressure waveforms seen as the pulmonary artery catheter advances through the *right atrium, right ventricle,* and *pulmonary artery* until it wedges. Be observant of premature ventricular contractions (PVCs) as the catheter is advanced through the right ventricle. *(From Wilkins RL, Dexter JR, Heuer AJ:* Clinical assessment in respiratory care, *ed 6, St Louis, 2010, Mosby.)*

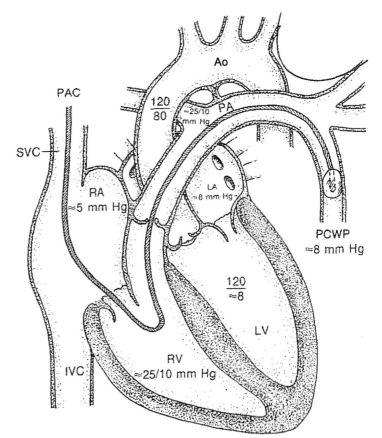

Figure 5-20   Pulmonary artery catheter (PAC) through a heart with normal chamber pressures. *SVC,* Superior vena cava; *IVC,* inferior vena cava; *RA,* right atrium; *RV,* right ventricle; *PA,* pulmonary artery; *PCWP,* pulmonary capillary wedge pressure; *LA,* left atrium; *LV,* left ventricle; and *Ao,* aorta.

Decreased pulmonary artery pressure values are not frequently seen. Patients with hypovolemic shock, anaphylaxis (allergic shock), or excessive use of vasodilating drugs may have a decreased pulmonary artery pressure. The most obvious clinical sign in these patients is a low systemic blood pressure.

Exam Hint 5-7 (ELE, WRE)

Expect to see at least one question requiring the calculation of the PAd-PCWP gradient and at least one question requiring the result to be interpreted.

Expect to see at least one question requiring the calculation of the PAd-PCWP gradient and at least one question requiring the result to be interpreted.

4. Pulmonary capillary wedge pressure monitoring

a. Review pulmonary capillary wedge pressure data in the patient's chart (Code: IA8b) [Difficulty: ELE: R; WRE: Ap]

The pulmonary capillary wedge pressure (PCWP) refers to the pressure measured in the pulmonary capillary bed under no-flow conditions. It is important to review previous patient data before measuring another pressure. Normal values are listed in Box 5-2.

b. Recommend pulmonary capillary wedge pressure measurement to obtain additional data (Code: IC11) [Difficulty: ELE: R, Ap; WRE: An]

Measuring the PCWP is important in patients with severe pulmonary or cardiovascular problems, including pulmonary hypertension, myocardial infarction, congestive heart failure, fluid overload, dehydration, hypertension, and hypotension.

c. Perform pulmonary capillary wedge pressure measurement (Code: IB9m, IIIE3e) [Difficulty: ELE: R, Ap; WRE: An]

A pulmonary artery catheter must be placed into a patient's pulmonary artery for the PCWP to be measured. The PCWP is obtained by inflating the balloon at the tip of the catheter. This obstructs that branch of the pulmonary artery so that the downstream pressure from the left ventricle is seen on the monitor (see Figures 5-19 and 5-20). The balloon volume varies with the diameter of the catheter. The necessary volume is printed on the catheter near where the air is injected into the balloon. For example, the 5-French catheter balloon holds 0.8 mL of air and the 7-French catheter balloon holds 1.5 mL of air. It is important to inject only the required amount of air. Overinflating may burst the balloon or rupture the pulmonary artery. If the balloon wedges at less than the required volume, the catheter is probably too far down in the artery and may need to be withdrawn a short distance. The balloon is only inflated long enough to obtain the PCWP and then the balloon is deflated. Pulmonary infarction will occur if the balloon is left inflated and the blood in the pulmonary artery is stagnant and allowed to clot. Record the PCWP value in the patient's chart or flow sheet.

d. Interpret the results of pulmonary capillary wedge pressure measurement (Code: IB10m, IIIE4c) [Difficulty: ELE: R, Ap; WRE: An]

As noted earlier, the PCWP refers to the pressure measured in the pulmonary capillary bed under no-flow conditions. This pressure reflects downstream pressure from the left side of the heart. At diastole, in the patient without pulmonary hypertension or mitral valve disease, the PCWP parallels left atrial pressure (LAP) and left ventricular end-diastolic pressure (LVEDP). The literature reveals that a variety of terms and initials are used to describe the same physiologic value. Do not be confused by reading about the pulmonary capillary pressure (PCP), pulmonary wedge pressure (PWP), pulmonary artery wedge pressure (PAWP), or wedge pressure.

Elevated PCWP is generally considered to be greater than 10 mm Hg and can indicate the following conditions:

1. **Intravascular fluid overload:** Review the patient's history to see if the patient is in renal failure or has recently received a large amount of oral or intravenous fluids. Perform a physical exam to determine if the patient has edema in the ankles, or in the back if the patient has been lying down. Look for jugular vein distension if the patient has been recumbent. Listen for crackles in the bases of the lungs.
2. **Left ventricular dysfunction with congestive heart failure:** Perform the same steps listed in point 1. In addition, look for a history of chronic heart failure or acute myocardial infarction.
3. **Mitral valve insufficiency:** Blood regurgitating back into the left atrium is shown as an elevated PCWP reading.

These conditions result in serious problems for the patient's lung function. When the PCWP reaches 20 to 25 mm Hg, fluid begins to leak into the pulmonary interstitium. This makes the lungs less compliant and increases the patient's work of breathing. A PCWP of 25 to 30 mm Hg results in frank pulmonary edema and dramatically decreases the patient's PaO_2 level.

Decreased PCWP is generally considered to be less than 4 mm Hg and can indicate the following conditions:

1. **Low intravascular volume (hypovolemia):** Review the patient's history for an illness resulting in dehydration (e.g., vomiting and diarrhea). A physical examination will show tachycardia, low blood pressure, low urine output with a high specific gravity, tenting of the skin when pinched (showing poor turgor), and flat jugular veins when the patient is lying down.

2. **Sepsis:** The patient's history will show infection, usually a septicemia. The physical examination will disclose tachycardia, hypotension, and oliguria, as noted in point 1. A major difference is that the patient will appear to be fluid overloaded because of the peripheral edema. This finding is present when an infectious organism (often *Staphylococcus aureus*) causes a dilation of the peripheral vascular bed and leakage of fluids out of the vascular bed into the tissues. The patient will have weak peripheral pulses and feel warm.

5. Cardiac output

a. Review cardiac output data in the patient's chart (Code: IA8b) [Difficulty: ELE: R; WRE: Ap]

Cardiac output (CO) is the volume of blood pumped in 1 minute. It is calculated as the product of heart rate (HR) for 1 minute and stroke volume (SV): $(CO = HR \times SV)$. CO is a measurement of the heart's pumping ability to meet the body's needs. As always, review previous data before repeating the test. Box 5-2 lists normal values.

b. Recommend a cardiac output measurement to obtain additional data (Code: IC11) [Difficulty: ELE: R, Ap; WRE: An]

A cardiac output measurement is performed on patients with serious cardiovascular disease to assess the condition of the heart. A major change in vital signs or new cardiovascular treatment justifies a measurement. See Figure 5-21 for the interplay of factors that can impact a patient's cardiac output. To measure CO, the patient must have a pulmonary artery catheter in place that is capable of measuring cardiac output.

c. Perform a cardiac output measurement (Code: IB9m, IIIE3e) [Difficulty: ELE: R, Ap; WRE: An]

At the time of this book's publication, there are several cardiac output methods that are commonly utilized in the cardiac catheterization laboratory. They will not be presented here. This discussion is limited to intensive care unit bedside procedures where a respiratory therapist is likely to be involved. A thermodilution cardiac output study involves using one of two special four-lumen pulmonary artery catheters. Both catheter types require additional hardware and supplies, including a computer designed to calculate the CO.

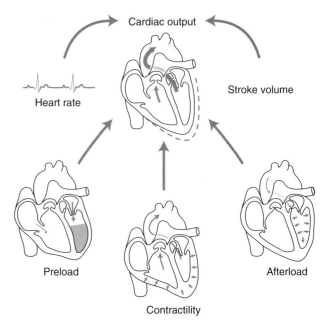

Figure 5-21 Factors that influence cardiac output (CO). CO is the product of heart rate and stroke volume. Stroke volume is determined by preload (blood volume), contractility of each ventricle, and afterload (arterial resistance). *(From Wilkins RL, Dexter JR, Heuer AJ: Clinical assessment in respiratory care, ed 6, St Louis, 2010, Mosby.)*

The first type of thermodilution catheter is used to inject a cool solution into the heart. This cool solution is diluted with the patient's blood. As the blood and cool solution mix passes a thermistor at the catheter tip, the computer calculates the patient's cardiac output based on the time required to pump the cooler blood past the thermistor (see Figure 5-17).

This procedure requires an injectable saline solution or a 5% dextrose, ice-water bath to cool the injectate, necessary tubing and connections, thermometer, 10-mL syringes, and injector system (Figure 5-22). It is beyond the scope of this text to describe all of the steps in the different types of adult and neonatal thermodilution cardiac output procedures. Hands-on experience is necessary. Only the most important and common features are presented here:

- The usual injectate volume is 10 mL. The neonatal injectate volume may be reduced to 3 mL in an attempt to prevent fluid-overloading the patient. The right atrial lumen is used for the injection.
- The usual injectate temperature is 0°C to 4°C. Some clinicians use room air temperature injectate because it is easier to work with. The cold injectate cardiac output result may be more accurate because of the greater difference between its temperature and the patient's body temperature. If the patient is

Figure 5-22 Complete system for performing thermodilution cardiac output studies. *(From Edwards Lifesciences LLC, Irvine, Calif, 1985.)*

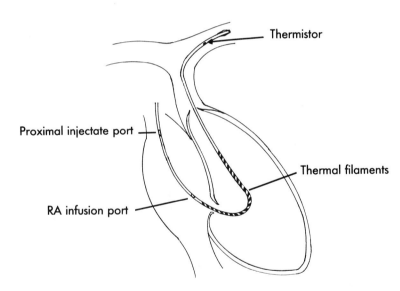

Figure 5-23 View of the right side of the heart showing a continuous cardiac output thermodilution pulmonary artery catheter in proper position. Note the thermal filaments that heat the passing blood. The resulting temperature change is detected by the thermistor in the pulmonary artery. *(From Daily EK, Schroeder JS: Techniques in bedside hemodynamic monitoring, ed 5, St Louis, 1994, Mosby.)*

hypothermic, the cold injectate must be used for greater accuracy.

• Three injections are usually performed. The results are then averaged for the final CO value. Individual CO measurements that vary by more than 10% from each other probably indicate an error in the procedure. A compressed CO_2 "gun" is preferred to hand injection because the injector gun provides a smoother and more reliable injection. The injection must be completed within 4 seconds.

The "cool solution" thermodilution cardiac output procedure has been available for more than 20 years and is widely used clinically. Its main disadvantages are that the CO value is available only intermittently, it is a time-consuming procedure, and patients with heart failure are given significant amounts of additional fluid for each cardiac output calculation.

The second type of thermodilution cardiac output catheter uses a thermal filament (a heated wire) that wraps around the catheter (Figure 5-23). With this catheter, the computer periodically directs electricity to the filament. This results in periodic warming of the blood from the heated wire. The computer calculates the patient's cardiac output by determining the time needed to pump the heated blood past the thermistor at the tip of the catheter. The advantages of the "heated wire" cardiac output catheter are that it gives an updated cardiac output value every 30 seconds, requires no additional time from the nurse or respiratory therapist after the initial setup, and does not add any additional fluid to the patient's intake.

d. Calculate the patient's cardiac output value (ELE code: IB9I) [Difficulty: ELE: R, Ap]

The following formula can be used to calculate a predicted cardiac output for the adult patient. This value can then be compared with the actual patient cardiac output.

$$CO = \frac{BSA \times 125}{0.045}$$

BSA is the body surface area and can be calculated mathematically or determined from a data table (Figure 5-24). See the following discussion on cardiac index for information on calculating BSA.

The following two methods can be used to calculate the patient's cardiac output:

1. A computer calculates the cardiac output (CO) when either thermodilution method is used. As long as the procedural steps are done properly and the patient and catheter variables are programmed into the computer, the results should be reliable. This method is widely used at the bedside.
2. The Fick method of measuring cardiac output is the "gold standard" by which all others are compared. Unfortunately, it is difficult to perform at the bedside and is primarily utilized in the cardiac catheterization laboratory. The patient's inhaled and exhaled gases must be analyzed for P_{O_2} level to calculate his or her

DUBOIS BODY SURFACE CHART

Figure 5-24 DuBois Body Surface Chart (as prepared by Boothby and Sandiford of the Mayo Clinic). *Directions:* To find the body surface of a patient, locate the height in inches (or centimeters) on scale I and the weight in pounds (or kilograms) on scale II. Place a straightedge (ruler) between these two points, which will intersect scale III at the patient's surface area value. *(From Boothby WM, Sandiford RB:* Boston Med Surg J *185:337, 1921.)*

oxygen consumption. In addition, arterial and mixed venous blood samples must be taken and analyzed for oxygen level to calculate the arterial-venous oxygen content difference [C(a-v)O₂]. The following example shows fairly standard values for an adult:

$$CO\ (mL/min) = \frac{oxygen\ consumption\ (mL/min)}{arterial\ O_2\ content\ (vol\%) - venous\ O_2\ content\ (vol\%)}$$

In which:

vol % = volume percent or mL of oxygen/100 mL of blood

Oxygen consumption = 250 mL/min

Arterial oxygen content = 20 vol %

Mixed venous oxygen content = 15 vol %

C(a-v)O₂ = 5 vol %

Therefore:

$$CO = \frac{250\ mL/min}{20\ vol\% - 15\ vol\%} = \frac{250\ mL/min}{5\ vol\%} = \frac{250}{.05}$$
$$= 5000\ mL/min = 5\ L/min$$

e. Interpret the results of the patient's cardiac output measurement (Code: IB10l) [Difficulty: ELE: R, Ap; WRE: An]

As listed in Box 5-2, the healthy, resting adult has a cardiac output in the range of 4 to 8 L/min and a healthy, resting neonate has a cardiac output in the range of 0.6 to 0.8 L/min.

Cardiac output can increase markedly in a person with a healthy heart who is stressed or exercising, has a fever, or has any other reason for an increased metabolism. All these conditions increase the person's demand for oxygen, which is primarily met by increasing cardiac output. (To a lesser extent, the tissues extract more oxygen from the blood.) Sepsis is the one serious condition that results in a high cardiac output.

There are many possible causes of a decreased cardiac output. The most common are hypovolemia, increased peripheral resistance, and heart failure. A patient with low cardiac output often has a low blood pressure. If the cardiac output and blood pressure are too low, the patient will develop metabolic acidosis from peripheral hypoxemia. Death can result if this is not corrected.

6. Stroke volume

a. Review stroke volume data in the patient's chart (Code: IA8b) [Difficulty: ELE: R; WRE: Ap]

Stroke volume (SV) is the volume of blood ejected with each heartbeat. It is the difference between the volume of blood in each ventricle at the end of diastole (preload) and the volume left in the ventricles at the end of systole (after ejection [afterload]). It is helpful to review the patient's previous cardiac output and stroke volume data before performing another SV measurement.

b. Recommend a stroke volume measurement to obtain additional data (Code: IC11) [Difficulty: ELE: R, Ap; WRE: An]

A stroke volume (and cardiac output) measurement is performed on patients with serious cardiovascular disease to assess the condition of the heart. A major change in vital signs or new cardiovascular treatment justifies a measurement. As shown in Figure 5-21, preload, contractility of each ventricle, and afterload can impact a patient's stroke volume.

c. Calculate the patient's stroke volume (ELE code: IB9l) [Difficulty: ELE: R, Ap]

The normal stroke volume is based on a person's age. See Box 5-2 for normal values. Stroke volume can be determined through a cardiac ultrasound procedure or can be calculated from the patient's heart rate and cardiac output measurements.

For example, calculate an adult patient's stroke volume when the heart rate is 100 beats/min and cardiac output is 8 L (8000 mL):

$$SV = \frac{CO}{HR} = \frac{800\ mL}{100\ beats/min} = 80\ mL$$

The stoke volume is not the entire preload volume. The stroke volume portion of the preload that is pumped out of the ventricle is referred to as the *ejection fraction*. Under normal conditions, an adult will have an ejection fraction of 0.6 to 0.75. This means the ventricle ejects a stroke volume that is usually 60% to 75% of the preload volume.

d. Interpret the results of the patient's stroke volume calculation (Code: IB10l) [Difficulty: ELE: R, Ap; WRE: An]

The stroke volume is the same for both ventricles except under pathologic conditions. Usually, however, only the left ventricle is of concern. The Frank-Starling curve shows us that as the heart muscle is stretched with greater volume, it contracts and pumps more completely, resulting in a larger stroke volume. A left ventricle that has been damaged by a myocardial infarction does not pump as effectively and the stroke volume decreases. A drop in stroke volume results in a decrease in cardiac output unless the heart rate can increase to compensate for the difference. This is seen in many patients with heart disease. In addition, when a healthy right ventricle continues to pump more blood than the damaged left ventricle, the unpumped blood backs up into the pulmonary circulation and results in pulmonary edema (congestive heart failure).

7. Cardiac index

a. Review cardiac index data in the patient's chart (Code: IA8b) [Difficulty: ELE: R; WRE: Ap]

The cardiac index (CI) is the cardiac output per square meter of body surface area. Review any previous information on CI before performing another calculation.

b. Recommend a cardiac index measurement to obtain additional data (Code: IC11) [Difficulty: ELE: R, Ap; WRE: An]

If cardiac output is being determined, the CI should also be calculated for additional information on heart function.

c. Calculate the patient's cardiac index value (ELE code: IB9l) [Difficulty: ELE: R, Ap]

Since CI is the cardiac output per square meter of body surface area, both cardiac output and body surface area must be known. Cardiac output is usually measured by the thermodilution cardiac output method via a special pulmonary artery catheter. The body surface area (BSA) can be determined from the DuBois Body Surface Chart as shown in Figure 5-24. The body surface area can also be determined with the following equation:

$$BSA = \frac{1 + \text{weight in kilograms} + (\text{height in centimeters} - 160)}{100}$$

EXAMPLE

A 166-lb/75-kg, 5 feet 10 inches/152-cm man has a cardiac output of 6 L/min. According to the DuBois Body Surface Chart, he has a BSA of 1.92 m^2. His cardiac index is calculated as:

$$CI = \frac{CO}{BSA} = \frac{6 \text{ L/min}}{1.92 \text{ m}^2} = 3.125 \text{ L/min/m}^2$$

d. Interpret the results of the patient's cardiac index calculation (Code: IB10l) [Difficulty: ELE: R, Ap; WRE: An]

A normal, resting cardiac index is 2.5 to 4 L/min/m^2 of BSA. The cardiac index is a much more accurate way of determining if the patient's oxygen demands are being met than by simply looking at the cardiac output. For example, a resting cardiac output of 4 L/min is considered normal. This cardiac output might be fine for a small adult but not for a large one. The CI takes into account the difference in body sizes. A normal cardiac index indicates that the patient is receiving enough oxygen to meet the body's needs. A low cardiac index should be a cause

for concern; it usually indicates that the patient is not getting enough blood and oxygen to his or her tissues. Check to see if the patient's cardiac output and blood pressure are also low and if the patient has hypoxemia or acidemia. If these conditions exist, they must be corrected as quickly as possible to prevent dire consequences. A high cardiac index indicates that the patient is pumping more blood than appears necessary. Investigate why this is occurring. See the earlier discussion on cardiac output and the factors that affect it to understand the factors that affect cardiac index as well.

8. Mixed venous blood sampling

a. Review mixed venous oxygen data in the patient's chart (Code: IA8b) [Difficulty: ELE: R; WRE: Ap]

Mixed venous blood sampling involves taking blood from either the pulmonary artery or the superior vena cava. The gold standard for this procedure involves the analysis of true mixed venous blood taken from the pulmonary artery through a pulmonary artery catheter. The pressure of mixed venous oxygen ($P\bar{v}O_2$) and the saturation of mixed venous oxygen ($S\bar{v}O_2$) represent tissue oxygenation. This is because the blood has returned from the body after having some of its oxygen extracted. (Remember that PaO_2 and SaO_2 represent the supply of oxygen to the tissues.) Another option involves the use of a CVP catheter equipped with fiberoptic technology for the measurement of the saturation of central venous oxygen ($ScvO_2$). As always, the $P\bar{v}O_2$ or $ScvO_2$ value(s) should be reviewed before performing another measurement.

b. Recommend a mixed venous oxygen measurement to obtain additional data (Code: IC11) [Difficulty: ELE: R, Ap; WRE: An]

Recommend a mixed venous oxygen measurement if it is clinically important to know the patient's level of tissue oxygenation. Low $P\bar{v}O_2$, $S\bar{v}O_2$, and $ScvO_2$ values are often seen in patients with heart failure because the slow flow of blood through the tissues results in more oxygen being extracted. In addition, $P\bar{v}O_2$ and $S\bar{v}O_2$ values are needed to calculate a patient's arterial-venous oxygen content difference or shunt percentage.

Because of technical difficulties and increased risks associated with the placement of a pulmonary artery catheter, the placement of a triple-lumen CVP catheter with fiberoptic channel for $ScvO_2$ monitoring may be recommended. This CVP catheter has been found useful in monitoring patients with increased intracranial pressure, heart failure, heart surgery, and severe sepsis. Information from either catheter is very helpful in managing these critically ill patients.

c. Perform mixed venous oxygen measurement (Code: IB10m, IIIE4c) [Difficulty: ELE: R, Ap; WRE: An]

A patient with a functioning pulmonary artery catheter (PAC) can have a sample of blood withdrawn through it and analyzed for the mixed venous oxygen ($P\bar{v}O_2$) value (and the other blood gas values as well). There are currently three methods of performing the bedside procedure.

1. Perform the procedure through the distal lumen of a PAC as it is being inserted

This method is employed when trying to determine whether there is a ventricular septal defect. The procedure is commonly done on neonates with suspected congenital heart defects, but may be used in adults as well. Using sterile technique, blood samples are withdrawn serially from the right atrium, right ventricle, and sometimes from the pulmonary artery.

Normally, the $P\bar{v}O_2$ and $S\bar{v}O_2$ values are the same in all blood samples. The patient with a ventricular septal defect shows a significant increase in $P\bar{v}O_2$ and $S\bar{v}O_2$ values when measurements are taken from the right atrium to the right ventricle and pulmonary artery. This is because the oxygenated blood from the left ventricle is forced though the ventricular septal defect to raise the oxygen value of the right ventricular blood.

2. Use a pulmonary artery catheter with reflectance oximetry capability

These catheters have fiberoptic bundles built into them and use technology similar to that used in pulse oximeters. See Figure 5-25. The processing unit sends two narrow wavebands of light down the transmitting fiberoptic bundle to be illuminated on the passing blood in the pulmonary artery. Oxyhemoglobin in the red blood cells absorbs some of the light. The rest is reflected. The receiving fiberoptic bundle picks up some of this light and transmits it back to the monitoring unit.

$S\bar{v}O_2$ is determined by the monitoring unit based on the light waves that were transmitted and received. Care must be taken when using this catheter in patients with elevated carboxyhemoglobin or methemoglobin levels. As with pulse oximetry, COHb and MetHb will be interpreted as oxyhemoglobin. Thus inaccurately high readings will be seen.

An actual mixed venous blood sample can be taken with this catheter through the distal lumen as described next. The advantage of the reflectance oximetry system is that it provides continuous monitoring of the patient's venous oxygen level. In addition, high and low saturation alarms can be set. If the tip should become lodged in the wall of the artery or if a clot should form at the tip, the $S\bar{v}O_2$ value will drop or fluctuate dramatically. The alarms should warn the clinician of a problem with the equipment.

3. Use the distal lumen of a "standard" pulmonary artery catheter

A true mixed venous blood sample is obtained by withdrawing blood from the distal lumen of the catheter. This is the same lumen that is used for the PAP and PCWP readings. Using sterile technique, a 5- to 10-mL syringe is used to withdraw the heparinized solution in the lumen until about 1 to 2 mL of blood are removed. A second preheparinized syringe is then used to withdraw about 2 mL of mixed venous blood. It is important to withdraw the intravenous (IV) solution and blood at a rate no faster than 0.5 mL per second. Withdrawing at a faster rate can pull preoxygenated blood back through the capillary bed and give falsely elevated oxygen values. After sampling the blood, the lumen must be fast-flushed with the heparinized solution to prevent the blood from clotting (see Figure 5-18). Flush for several seconds until the solution flows freely. This blood sample may be reliably analyzed for $S\bar{v}O_2$, $P\bar{v}O_2$, and $P\bar{v}CO_2$ values.

4. Use a central venous catheter with reflectance oximetry capability

As discussed earlier, this CVP catheter has gained acceptance in monitoring the status of patients with a variety of conditions. Clinical studies have shown that the $ScvO_2$ values will track patient changes in the same direction as $S\bar{v}O_2$ and $P\bar{v}O_2$ values from a PAC. In other words, if the patient's $S\bar{v}O_2$ and/or $P\bar{v}O_2$ values increase (or decrease) so will the $ScvO_2$ values. However, because the $ScvO_2$ values are less consistent than true mixed venous oxygen values, the patient's clinical goal for $ScvO_2$ monitoring is >70% saturation.

d. Interpret the results of the mixed venous blood measurement (Code: IB10m, IIIE4c) [Difficulty: ELE: R, Ap; WRE: An]

This topic is discussed in some detail in Chapter 3. The normal values follow:

$P\bar{v}O_2$ of 40 torr (range of 37 to 43 torr)

$S\bar{v}O_2$ of 75% (range of 70% to 76%)

True mixed venous blood oxygen values are useful for monitoring the patient's oxygen consumption. The most accurate methods of calculating percent shunt and cardiac output (Fick method) use mixed venous blood oxygen values with arterial blood oxygen values. A $P\bar{v}O_2$ value of less than 30 torr or an $S\bar{v}O_2$ value of less than 56% is considered to show tissue hypoxemia. Quick steps must be taken to reverse this. Increase the inspired oxygen percentage as needed. Low stroke volume and cardiac output measurements can be increased by giving digoxin

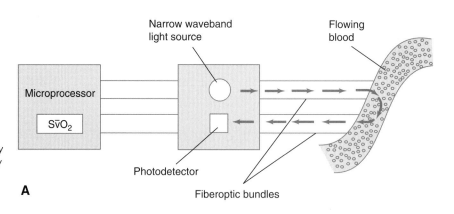

Figure 5-25   Mixed venous oxygen saturation ($S\overline{v}O_2$) can be monitored continuously by reflection spectrophotometry (spectroscopy) in the appropriate pulmonary artery catheter. (Note that the same technology is used in a CVP catheter that measures continuous central venous oxygen saturation [$ScvO_2$].) **A,** Detail of the fiberoptic bundles in the catheter. Specific wavelengths of light are directed at passing blood. Some of the light is absorbed by the passing red blood cells and some is reflected back to the photodetector. The microprocessor calculates the percentage $S\overline{v}O_2$. **B,** Components of the system include (1) microprocessor that connects to the catheter, displays the $S\overline{v}O_2$ % values, and has high and low saturation alarms; (2) strip-chart recorder to copy the saturation values over time; and (3) fiberoptic reflective spectroscopy-type pulmonary artery catheter. The catheter can also be used for measuring pulmonary artery pressure, pulmonary capillary wedge pressure, and cardiac output; and for obtaining a mixed venous blood gas sample. (**A,** *from Rupple GL: Manual of pulmonary function testing, ed 9, St Louis, 2009, Mosby.* **B,** *Courtesy of Abbott Critical Care Systems, Mountain View, Calif.*)

B

(Lanoxin) or other inotropic agents. Low blood pressure can be increased by administering vasopressors such as dopamine hydrochloride (Intropin).

9. Arterial-venous oxygen content difference

a. Review arterial-venous oxygen content difference data in the patient's chart (Code: IA8b) [Difficulty: ELE: R; WRE: Ap]

The arterial-venous oxygen content difference [$C(a-v)O_2$] is a calculation of oxygen consumption by the body. It is the difference between the oxygen content of arterial blood and the oxygen content of mixed venous blood. Box 5-2 lists normal values. As always, check previous values to compare with present values to determine if the patient's condition has changed.

b. Recommend an arterial-venous oxygen content measurement to obtain additional data (Code: IC11) [Difficulty: ELE: R, Ap; WRE: An]

The $C(a-v)O_2$ measurement should be recommended when it is necessary to know a patient's oxygen consumption, such as with heart failure or sepsis management.

c. Perform the arterial-venous oxygen content difference measurement (Code: IB9m, IIIE3e) [Difficulty: ELE: R, Ap; WRE: An]

The following steps must be performed to make the arterial-venous oxygen content calculation:

1. Draw and analyze an arterial blood gas sample.
2. Simultaneously draw and analyze a mixed venous blood gas sample.

3. Determine the patient's hemoglobin value.
4. Place the data into the calculations shown in the next discussion.

d. Calculate the patient's arterial-venous oxygen content difference (ELE code: IB9l) [Difficulty: ELE: R, Ap]

As mentioned in the previous discussion, the arterial-venous oxygen content difference is found by subtracting venous blood oxygen content from arterial blood oxygen content. These two values must first be calculated separately and then subtracted as shown in these three steps:

1. CaO_2 = the content of oxygen in arterial blood = vol % of oxygen in arterial blood (vol % is mL of oxygen/100 mL of blood):

$$CaO_2 = (Hb \times 1.34 \times SaO_2) + (PaO_2 \times 0.003)$$

2. $C\bar{v}O_2$ = the content of oxygen in mixed venous blood = vol % of oxygen in mixed venous blood:

$$C\bar{v}O_2 = (Hb \times 1.34 \times S\bar{v}O_2) + (P\bar{v}O_2 \times 0.003)$$

3. Therefore:

$$C(a\text{-}\bar{v})O_2 = CaO_2 - C\bar{v}O_2$$

EXAMPLE

Your patient has the following clinical data:

$PaO_2 = 95$ torr

$SaO_2 = 97\%$ or 0.97

$P\bar{v}O_2 = 40$ torr

$S\bar{v}O_2 = 75\%$ or 0.75

15 g/dL = the patient's hemoglobin concentration

1.34 = mL of oxygen/g of Hb in the patient (The value of 1.39 mL of oxygen/g of Hb is occasionally used.)

0.003 = the oxygen-carrying capacity of blood plasma per torr PO_2

Therefore:

1. $CaO_2 = (Hb \times 1.34 \times SaO_2) + (PaO_2 \times 0.003)$
   $= (15 \times 1.34 \times 0.97) + (95 \times 0.003)$
   $= (19.5) + (0.3)$
   $= 19.8$ vol %

2. $C\bar{v}O_2 = (Hb \times 1.34 \times S\bar{v}O_2) + (P\bar{v}O_2 \times 0.003)$
   $= (15 \times 1.34 \times 0.75) + (40 \times 0.003)$
   $= (15.1) + (0.1)$
   $= 15.2$ vol %

3. $C(a\text{-}\bar{v})O_2$ difference = $(CaO_2$ of 19.8 vol %) $-$
   $(C\bar{v}O_2$ of 15.2 vol %)
   $= 4.6$ vol %

e. Interpret the results of the patient's arterial-venous oxygen content difference (Code: IB10l) [Difficulty: ELE: R, Ap; WRE: An]

The normal range for the $C(a\text{-}v^-)O_2$ difference is 3 to 5.5 vol %. Measurements in this range show normal levels of oxygen consumption by the tissues, cardiac output, and cardiopulmonary function. (See Figure 5-26 for a

Figure 5-26 Oxyhemoglobin dissociation curve showing normal oxygen saturations and pressures in arterial and venous blood. From these, the normal $C(a\text{-}\bar{v})O_2$ difference of 4.6 vol % can be calculated.

graphic presentation of $C(a-\bar{v})O_2$ on the oxyhemoglobin dissociation curve.) A $C(a-\bar{v})O_2$ difference of greater than 5.5 to 6 vol % is seen in patients with a low cardiac output. As the blood flows more slowly than normal through the tissues, more oxygen is consumed per mL of blood. The $S\bar{v}O_2$ and $P\bar{v}O_2$ values drop and the $C(a-\bar{v})O_2$ difference widens.

A $C(a-\bar{v})O_2$ difference of less than 4 vol % in the healthy patient commonly indicates good cardiovascular reserve with an increased cardiac output. As the blood flows more quickly than normal through the tissues, less oxygen is consumed per mL of blood. The $S\bar{v}O_2$ and $P\bar{v}O_2$ values increase and the $C(a-\bar{v})O_2$ difference narrows. The septic patient may have a narrowed $C(a-\bar{v})O_2$ difference because of peripheral shunting and decreased oxygen consumption by the tissues caused by the infection. The $C(a-\bar{v})O_2$ difference is necessary to accurately calculate the percent of pulmonary shunting as discussed next.

10. Shunt study

a. Review shunt study data in the patient's chart (Code: IA8b) [Difficulty: ELE: R; WRE: Ap]

Shunt $(\dot{Q}s/\dot{Q}t)$ is the amount of blood pumped by the heart that passes through the lungs but does not participate in gas exchange. A pulmonary artery catheter must be inserted into the patient for a shunt study to be performed. Review previous $(\dot{Q}s/\dot{Q}t)$ study results and compare with current information to see if there has been a change in the patient's status. See Box 5-2 for normal values.

b. Recommend a shunt study measurement to obtain additional data (Code: IC11) [Difficulty: ELE: R, Ap; WRE: An]

A shunt study is very useful to find out how much ventilation to perfusion mismatch a patient has. Most patients with refractory hypoxemia and requiring mechanical ventilation have an increased amount of pulmonary shunting. When an optimal positive end-expiratory pressure (PEEP) study is performed, a shunt study should be done with each change in the PEEP level.

c. Perform a shunt study measurement (Code: IB9m, IIIE3e) [Difficulty: ELE: R, Ap; WRE: An]

Steps in the bedside shunt procedure include:
1. Measure the patient's fractional concentration of inspired oxygen (FiO$_2$).
2. Simultaneously draw arterial and mixed venous blood samples.
3. Have both blood samples analyzed for SO$_2$ and PO$_2$ levels.
4. Calculate the percent of shunt as shown next.

d. Calculate the patient's shunt percentage (ELE code: IB9l) [Difficulty: ELE: R, Ap]

Exam Hint 5-8 (ELE)

To date, the NBRC has not included an examination question that requires all of the calculations needed to determine a patient's shunt percentage. However, examinations have included questions that relate to calculating components of the shunt equations. These have included calculating CaO_2, $C\bar{v}O_2$, and $C(a-\bar{v})O_2$.

To date, the NBRC has not had an examination question that requires all of the calculations needed to determine a patient's shunt percentage. However, examinations have had questions that relate to calculating components of the shunt equations. These have included calculating CaO_2, $C\bar{v}O_2$, and $C(a-\bar{v})O_2$.

There are a number of possible variations on the methods and equations for calculating shunt percentage. Only the two most commonly used equations are presented here.

1. Modified clinical shunt equation

$$\dot{Q}_s/\dot{Q}_t = \frac{P(A\text{-}a)O_2 \times 0.003}{C(a-\bar{v})O_2 + [P(A\text{-}a)O_2 \times 0.003]}$$

In which:

PAO_2 = The partial pressure of oxygen in the alveoli calculated from the alveolar oxygen equation

PaO_2 = The partial pressure of oxygen in the arterial blood

0.003 = The oxygen-carrying capacity of blood plasma per mm Hg PO_2

$C(a-\bar{v})O_2$ = The oxygen content of arterial blood minus the oxygen content of mixed venous blood

This formula requires that the patient's hemoglobin be 100% saturated. This does not happen until the PaO$_2$ level reaches 150 torr at any given FiO$_2$. An obvious clinical limitation is that very ill patients never reach 100% saturation even when breathing 100% oxygen. Also, putting patients on more than 80% oxygen, even for just the duration of the test, may lead to some denitrogenation absorption atelectasis. This results in an incorrectly high shunt percentage calculation.

EXAMPLE

Modified clinical shunt equation

The subsequent example shows the modified clinical shunt calculation with the following environmental and patient information:

P_B = Local barometric pressure; 760 torr for sea level in this example

P_{H_2O} = 47 torr; water vapor pressure in the lungs at normal body temperature

FIO_2 = inhaled oxygen percent of 100% or 1.0

PaO_2 = 155 torr

$PaCO_2$ = 40 torr

SaO_2 = 100% or 1.0

$P\overline{v}O_2$ = 40 torr

$S\overline{v}O_2$ = 75% or 0.75

0.8 = The normal respiratory quotient (An exact value can be determined by a metabolic study.)

15 g/dL = The patient's hemoglobin concentration

0.003 = The oxygen-carrying capacity of blood plasma per torr PO_2

1.34 = mL of oxygen/g of Hb in the patient (The value of 1.39 mL of oxygen/g of Hb is occasionally used.)

Preliminary calculations:
1. Oxygen content of arterial blood

$$CaO_2 = (Hb \times 1.34 \times SaO_2) + (PaO_2 \times 0.003)$$
$$= (15 \times 1.34 \times 1.0) + (155 \times 0.003)$$
$$= (20.1) + (0.5)$$
$$= 20.6 \text{ vol \%}$$

2. Oxygen content of mixed venous blood

$$C\overline{v}O_2 = (Hb \times 1.34 \times S\overline{v}O_2) + (P\overline{v}O_2 \times 0.003)$$
$$= (15 \times 1.34 \times 0.75) + (40 \times 0.003)$$
$$= (15.1) + (0.1)$$
$$= 15.2 \text{ vol \%}$$

3. Partial pressure of oxygen in the alveoli: the alveolar oxygen equation is used for this. (Review Chapter 3 if necessary.)

$$PAO_2 = [(P_B - PH_2O) \times FIO_2] - \frac{PaCO_2}{0.8}$$
$$= [(760 - 47) \times 1.0] - \frac{40}{.8}$$
$$= [713] - 50$$
$$= 663 \text{ torr}$$

Final calculation:

$$\dot{Q}_s/\dot{Q}_t = \frac{P(A\text{-}a)O_2 \times 0.003}{C(a\text{-}\overline{v})O_2 + [P(A\text{-}a)O_2 \times 0.003]}$$
$$= \frac{(663 - 155) \times 0.003}{(20.6 - 15.2) + [(663 - 155) \times 0.003]}$$
$$= \frac{(508) \times 0.003}{5.4 + [(508) \times 0.003]}$$
$$= \frac{1.5}{5.4 + 1.5}$$
$$= \frac{1.5}{6.9}$$
$$= 0.217 \text{ or } 21.7\% \text{ shunt}$$

2. Classic shunt equation

This equation is widely used because of the clinical limitations of the clinical shunt equation:

$$\dot{Q}_s/\dot{Q}_t = \frac{CcO_2 - CaO_2}{CcO_2 - C\overline{v}O_2}$$

In which:

CcO_2 = The content of oxygen in the end pulmonary capillary blood

CaO_2 = The content of oxygen in the arterial blood

$C\overline{v}O_2$ = The content of oxygen in the mixed venous blood

The patient should be inspiring 30% oxygen or more to calculate the oxygen content of end pulmonary capillary blood. This much oxygen should cause the PAO_2 value of the ventilated alveoli to reach 150 torr or more, which results in 100% saturation of the hemoglobin of the end pulmonary capillary blood (ScO_2). Most patients who are sick enough to warrant a shunt determination will be on at least 30% oxygen. If not, the ScO_2 value must be determined by using the oxyhemoglobin dissociation curve.

A pulmonary artery catheter is needed to sample mixed venous blood for $P\overline{v}O_2$ and $S\overline{v}O_2$ levels in both of these equations. An arterial blood gas sample is also needed. There are clinical situations in which either of these equations will work and will result in the same answer.

EXAMPLE

Classic shunt equation

The subsequent example shows the classic shunt calculation with the following environmental and patient information:

P_B = Local barometric pressure; 760 torr for sea level in this example

PH_2O = 47 torr; water vapor pressure in the lungs at normal body temperature

F_IO_2 = Inhaled oxygen percent of 30% or 0.3

PaO_2 = 95 torr

$PaCO_2$ = 40 torr

SaO_2 = 97% or 0.97

$P\overline{v}O_2$ = 40 torr

$S\overline{v}O_2$ = 75% or 0.75

0.8 = The normal respiratory quotient (An exact value can be determined by a metabolic study.)

15 g/dL = The patient's hemoglobin concentration

0.003 = The oxygen-carrying capacity of blood plasma per torr PO_2

1.34 = mL of oxygen/g of Hb in the patient (The value of 1.39 mL of oxygen/g of Hb is occasionally used.)

Preliminary calculations:
1. Oxygen content of arterial blood

$$CaO_2 = (Hb \times 1.34 \times SaO_2) + (PaO_2 \times 0.003)$$
$$= (15 \times 1.34 \times 0.97) + (95 \times 0.003)$$
$$= (19.5) + (0.3)$$
$$= 19.8 \text{ vol \%}$$

2. Oxygen content of mixed venous blood

$$C\bar{v}O_2 = (Hb \times 1.34 \times S\bar{v}O_2) + (P\bar{v}O_2 \times 0.003)$$
$$= (15 \times 1.34 \times 0.75) + (40 \times 0.003)$$
$$= (15.1) + (0.1)$$
$$= 15.2 \text{ vol \%}$$

3. Partial pressure of oxygen in the alveoli: the alveolar oxygen equation is used for this:

$$PAO_2 = [(P_B - PH_2O) \times F_IO_2] - \frac{PaCO_2}{0.8}$$
$$= [(760 - 47) \times 0.3] - \frac{40}{0.8}$$
$$= [214] - 50$$
$$= 164 \text{ torr}$$

4. Oxygen content of pulmonary capillary blood

$$CcO_2 = (Hb \times 1.34 \times ScO_2) + (PAO_2 \times 0.003)$$
$$= (15 \times 1.34 \times 1.0) + (164 \times 0.003)$$
$$= 20.1 + 0.492$$
$$= 20.1 + 0.5 \text{ (Rounded off to one decimal place)}$$
$$= 20.6 \text{ vol \%}$$

Final calculation:

$$\dot{Q}_s/\dot{Q}_t = \frac{CcO_2 - CaO_2}{CaO_2 - CvO_2}$$
$$= \frac{20.6 - 19.8}{20.6 - 15.2}$$
$$= \frac{0.8}{5.4}$$
$$= 0.15 \text{ or } 15\% \text{ shunt}$$

d. Interpret the results of the patient's shunt study calculation (Code: IB10l) [Difficulty: ELE: R, Ap; WRE: An]

As noted earlier, shunt is the amount of blood pumped by the heart that does not participate in gas exchange through the lungs. It is wasted cardiac output and wasted effort by the heart. The healthy person has a shunt of 5% or less of cardiac output. This shunted blood has a low oxygen content and dilutes the oxygen content of all the blood. The larger the percentage of shunted blood, the more the heart and body are stressed. Many clinicians believe that an indication for mechanical ventilation is a shunt of 15% to 20%. Most agree that a 30% or more shunt can be life-threatening. The ventilator is used to reduce the patient's work of breathing and oxygen consumption. Also, supplemental oxygen can be more carefully controlled, and PEEP may be added to increase the patient's functional residual capacity (FRC) as needed.

11. Pulmonary vascular resistance

a. Review pulmonary vascular resistance data in the patient's chart (Code: IA8b) [Difficulty: ELE: R; WRE: Ap]

Pulmonary vascular resistance (PVR) is the total resistance of the pulmonary vascular bed to the blood being pumped through it by the right ventricle (afterload). This value may be calculated when other cardiopulmonary studies are performed.

b. Recommend a pulmonary vascular resistance measurement to obtain additional data (Code: IC11) [Difficulty: ELE: R, Ap; WRE: An]

It is valuable to know the PVR in any case where restricted blood flow through the lungs is known or suspected. This could include a patient with COPD, a pulmonary embolism, or persistent pulmonary hypertension of the newborn (PPHN). If therapeutic procedures are effective, the patient's PVR should be decreased toward normal. For example, inhaled nitric oxide (iNO) therapy has been shown effective in reducing the PVR of a newborn with PPHN.

c. Perform the pulmonary vascular resistance measurement (Code: IB9m, IIIE3e) [Difficulty: ELE: R, Ap; WRE: An]

Cardiac output, mean pulmonary blood pressure, and pulmonary capillary wedge pressure must be known to determine the PVR. To gather the necessary hemodynamic information, the patient must have a thermodilution-type cardiac output pulmonary artery catheter. Measure the CO, PAP, and PCWP as described earlier.

d. Calculate the patient's pulmonary vascular resistance (ELE code: IB9l) [Difficulty: ELE: R, Ap]

The patient must have the mean pulmonary artery pressure (PAm), pulmonary capillary wedge pressure (PCWP), and cardiac output (CO) measured and placed into this formula:

$$PVR = \frac{\begin{array}{c}\text{mean pulmonary artery pressure (PAm)} - \\ \text{pulmonary capillary wedge pressure (PCWP)}\end{array}}{\text{cardiac output (CO)}} \times 80$$

The answer will be in units of dynes/sec/cm^{-5}.

e. Interpret the results of the patient's pulmonary vascular resistance calculation (Code: IB10l) [Difficulty: ELE: R, Ap; WRE: An]

The normal range for PVR in an adult is 1 to 3 mm Hg/L/min. Multiplying this value by 80 changes the result to units of dynes/sec/cm^{-5}. PVR is listed this way in some cardiology studies. The normal range of PVR in an adult is between 80 and 240 dynes/sec/cm^{-5}.

With a normal PVR, the difference between the pulmonary artery diastolic pressure and the pulmonary capillary wedge pressure is 5 mm Hg or less. Any of the following can cause an elevated pulmonary vascular resistance:

- Decreased oxygen in the lungs
- Chronic obstructive pulmonary disease (COPD)
- Acute respiratory distress syndrome (ARDS)
- Persistent pulmonary hypertension of the newborn (PPHN)/persistent fetal circulation
- Primary pulmonary hypertension
- Pulmonary embolism
- Excessive positive end-expiratory pressure (PEEP)
- Increased pulmonary blood flow from a left to right intracardiac shunt such as an atrial septal defect or ventricular septal defect

Additional clinical data must be gathered to confirm the diagnosis. An increased PVR is a serious problem because it can lead to right ventricular hypertrophy. The COPD patient is at risk for developing cor pulmonale—right ventricular failure secondary to lung disease and increased pulmonary vascular resistance.

12. Systemic vascular resistance

a. Review systemic vascular resistance data in the patient's chart (Code: IA8b) [Difficulty: ELE: R; WRE: Ap]

Systemic vascular resistance (SVR) is the total resistance of the systemic vascular bed to the blood being pumped through it by the left ventricle (afterload). This value may be calculated when other cardiopulmonary studies are performed.

b. Recommend a systemic vascular resistance measurement to obtain additional data (Code: IC11) [Difficulty: ELE: R, Ap; WRE: An]

Recommend an SVR measurement in a clinical situation where there may be abnormally increased or decreased resistance to blood flow through the body. This may include a patient with hypertension or vasodilation from an anaphylactic reaction.

c. Perform a systemic vascular resistance measurement (Code: IB9m, IIIE3e) [Difficulty: ELE: R, Ap; WRE: An]

Cardiac output, systemic blood pressure, and central venous pressure must be known to determine the SVR. To gather the necessary hemodynamic information, the patient must have a thermodilution-type cardiac output pulmonary artery catheter, arterial line, and central venous pressure line (if this cannot be measured from the pulmonary artery catheter).

d. Calculate the patient's systemic vascular resistance (ELE code: IB9l) [Difficulty: ELE: R, Ap]

The patient must have mean arterial pressure (MAP), central venous pressure (CVP), and cardiac output (CO) measured and placed into the following formula:

$$SVR = \frac{\text{mean arterial pressure (MAP)} - \text{central venous pressure (CVP)}}{\text{cardiac output (CO)}} \times 80$$

The answer will be in units of dynes/sec/cm^{-5}.

e. Interpret the results of the systemic vascular resistance calculation (Code: IB10l) [Difficulty: ELE: R, Ap; WRE: An]

The normal range of SVR in the adult is 15 to 20 mm Hg/L/min. Multiplying this value by 80 changes the result to units of dynes/sec/cm^{-5}. SVR is listed this way in some cardiology studies. When multiplied by 80, an adult's SVR ranges between 770 to 900 and 1400 to 1500 dynes/sec/cm^{-5}.

A patient with hypertension will have an elevated SVR. It will also increase if the patient is given a vasoconstricting drug and decrease if the patient is given a vasodilating drug. Some allergic reactions result in anaphylaxis with a dramatic drop in the SVR and blood pressure despite an increase in the cardiac output.

Exam Hint 5-9 (ELE, WRE)

Know the normal values for pulmonary and systemic vascular resistance. To date, the NBRC has not expected the examinee to perform all of the calculations to determine a patient's PVR or SVR. Know that a patient with COPD or PPHN will have a chronically increased PVR and a patient with a large pulmonary embolism will have a sudden increase in the PVR. With proper treatment, the PVR will decrease toward normal.

There are several ways that the cardiology version of the PVR or SVR values can be found. The preferred versions have units listed in "dynes/sec/cm^{-5}" or "dyne sec/cm^{-5}." However, the NBRC has also listed these values in units of "dynes seconds cm^{-5}," "dynes·seconds·cm^{-5}," and "mm Hg/L/min."

Know the normal values for pulmonary and systemic vascular resistance. To date, the NBRC has not expected the examinee to perform all of the calculations to determine a patient's PVR or SVR. Know that a patient with COPD or PPHN will have a chronically increased PVR and a patient with a large pulmonary embolism will have a sudden increase in the PVR. With proper treatment, the PVR will decrease toward normal.

There are several ways that the cardiology version of the PVR or SVR values can be found. The preferred versions have units listed in "dynes/sec/cm^{-5}" or "dyne sec/cm^{-5}." However, the NBRC has also listed these values in units of "dynes seconds cm^{-5}," "dynes·seconds·cm^{-5}," and "mm Hg/L/min."

MODULE D

Cardiopulmonary monitoring equipment

1. Manipulate capnography equipment by order or protocol (Code: IIA26) [Difficulty: ELE: R; WRE: Ap, An]

a. Get the necessary equipment for the procedure

As discussed earlier, a capnograph is used to measure a patient's exhaled carbon dioxide level and expiratory pattern. There are two different types of capnography systems. Their main difference is in how the gas is sampled from the patient. Figure 5-3 shows the patient connection for a mainstream capnograph. Figure 5-4 shows a sidestream capnograph. Both work equally well if the patient is intubated. The capnography connector is attached between the endotracheal tube and the ventilator circuit or T-piece (Brigg's adapter). The sidestream unit may also be used with a spontaneously breathing patient because the capillary tube may be taped into a patient's nostril for gas sampling.

b. Put the equipment together and make sure that it works properly

The following are components of a capnography system:

- **Airway attachment:** The mainstream and sidestream units must have both inhaled and exhaled gas pass through the sensor or connector, respectively. Connections must be airtight and free of obstructions.
- The **gas sampling capillary tube** of the sidestream unit must be kept clear of water or secretions.
- **Capnometer:** Periodically calibrate the unit with two gases of different CO_2 content. Room air is used for the "zero" value, and either 5% or 10% CO_2 in a preanalyzed cylinder is used for the "high" value. Both values should calibrate within the manufacturer's specifications.
- **Capnograph:** Check that the paper speeds and marker work properly.

c. Troubleshoot any problems with the equipment

Capnography systems cause relatively few problems. The sidestream capnometer units must be kept dry. An external water trap is located between the capillary tube and the capnometer itself. Make sure that the water is drained periodically. Either capnography system can be disconnected from the patient. This is seen as a drop in the exhaled carbon dioxide level to zero. The alarm should activate if it has been set.

d. Perform quality control procedures on capnography equipment (Code: IIC7) [Difficulty: ELE: R, Ap; WRE: An]

As discussed earlier, both capnography units are calibrated using two points. Room air is used to set the zero point, and either 5% or 10% carbon dioxide from a cylinder is used to set the high point. Follow the manufacturer's guidelines regarding how much adjustment for low or high point can be tolerated. Do not use a machine that cannot be properly calibrated.

2. Manipulate pressure transducers by order or protocol (WRE: code: IIA20a) [Difficulty: WRE: R, Ap, An]

a. Get the necessary equipment for the procedure

Hemodynamic monitoring requires a transducer that converts a blood pressure signal into an electrical signal. Select a strain gauge type transducer to do this. The strain gauge transducer uses a fine wire screen that bends proportionately to the pressure put against it.

b. Put the equipment together and make sure that it works properly

Check to see that the wire screen of the transducer is not bent, damaged, or contaminated with old blood or other debris. The transducer's wire cable and monitor-connecting prongs should not be bent or damaged. Carefully insert the prongs into the receiving jack on the monitor.

A disposable, sterile, clear plastic dome should be firmly attached to the transducer. Noncompliant pressure tubing should connect the transducer with the patient's arterial or pulmonary artery catheter. The automatic fluid drip system (Sorenson) should be pressurized to 300 mm Hg. Heparin must be added to the fluid (usually normal saline) to prevent clotting in the patient's catheter. Because this is a continuous fluid "plumbing" system, all connections must be tightly joined to be watertight. There must be a continuous flow of fluid through the tubing system and into the patient's blood vessel. Any air bubbles must be removed or the measured pressure reading will be lower than the actual reading (see Figures 5-18 and 5-27).

The transducer must be kept at the patient's midchest (midheart) level during calibration and measurement. Calibrate the electronics in the monitor by placing known pressures against the fluid system. The electronics should first be adjusted to "zero" pressure by opening the transducer to room air (atmospheric pressure). Adjust the electronic controls as needed. A sphygmomanometer is then used to pressurize the fluid system. A pulmonary artery catheter system is pressurized to relatively low pressures such as 30 and 50 mm Hg. An arterial system is adjusted

Figure 5-27 Schematic diagram of a strain-gauge pressure transducer. The wire mesh resistance wires are arranged like a Wheatstone bridge so that a pressure change results in a proportional change in the electrical resistance. *(From Armstrong PW, Baigrie RS: Hemodynamic monitoring in the critically ill, Philadelphia, 1980, Harper & Row.)*

to higher pressures such as 100 and 150 mm Hg. The monitored pressure should match the sphygmomanometer pressure. If not, adjust the electronic controls on the monitor to match.

c. Troubleshoot any problems with the equipment

As mentioned previously, all connections must be watertight. If not, the IV solution will drip out when it is pressurized. This can also result in the patient's measured pressure readings being less than the true readings. Stopcocks must be opened or closed properly to allow the

patient's pressure to be measured by the transducer. Electronics that will not calibrate to match the known pressures should not be used.

3. Manipulate central venous catheters by order or protocol (WRE code: IIA20b) [Difficulty: WRE: R, Ap, An]

a. Get the necessary equipment for the procedure

Obtain the catheter type and gauge that are requested by the physician. Additional equipment includes a water-column manometer, stopcock, intravenous tubing, and IV solution system. A triple-lumen fiberoptic channel CVP catheter will be needed to measure the patient's $ScvO_2$ values.

b. Put the equipment together and make sure that it works properly

See Figure 5-15 for the traditional assembly of the equipment and the procedure for measuring the central venous pressure (CVP). The equipment must be properly calibrated to ensure that the data are accurate. Calibrating a central venous pressure water-column manometer usually involves only making sure that it reads zero at atmospheric pressure.

c. Troubleshoot any problems with the equipment

Make sure that all connections are watertight. Check the position of the stopcock if the CVP cannot be measured.

4. Indwelling arterial catheters (WRE code: IIA20b) [Difficulty: WRE: R, Ap, An]

a. Get the necessary equipment for the procedure

As discussed earlier, a neonate can have its umbilical artery catheterized. An adult usually has the radial artery catheterized. Following are the general supplies necessary for catheterizing either of these arteries for drawing blood gases and continuously monitoring blood pressure:

- Sterile 20-gauge or 21-gauge needle with a flexible plastic sheath. After placement into the artery, the needle is withdrawn and the sheath is left in place. A neonate needs a long catheter of the correct gauge based on his or her body weight.
- Sterile surgical drape for covering the area surrounding the insertion site.
- Disinfectant such as 70% isopropyl alcohol or Betadine solution.
- Local anesthetic such as 4% lidocaine in a syringe and needle for injection into the insertion site.

- One or two sterile 3- or 5-mL syringes for blood sampling.
- Equipment for setting up a pressurized intravenous drip system so that the catheter does not clot.

b. Put the equipment together and make sure that it works properly

See Figures 5-18 and 5-28 for illustrations of how the pressure transducer, connecting tubing, stopcocks, infusion system, and monitoring electronics are assembled. See Figure 5-29 for a completed radial artery system. Clinical experience is needed with these types of systems.

The process of calibrating the monitor for systemic artery pressures was briefly discussed earlier. Regardless of whether the catheter is placed into a systemic artery, pulmonary artery, umbilical artery, or superior vena cava, the equipment must be properly calibrated to ensure accurate data. When performing two-point calibration, all pressures should read "zero" when exposed to atmospheric pressure. This is the low point. The high point pressure for arterial pressure monitoring is commonly 100 mm Hg.

c. Troubleshoot any problems with the equipment

Table 5-1 lists problems, causes, prevention, and treatment for inaccurate pressure measurements with arterial or pulmonary artery catheters. Table 5-2 specifically lists problems with arterial lines. Figure 5-30 shows common problem areas with arterial lines. Pulmonary artery catheters can have problems in the same areas.

d. Perform arterial line insertion (Code: IB9s) [Difficulty: ELE: R, Ap; WRE: An]

The most widely used arterial line insertion site is the radial artery in the patient's nondominant hand. The procedure for inserting a radial arterial line is very similar to the procedure for drawing a blood sample from the radial artery. See Chapter 3 to review the procedure. As presented previously, the necessary fluid infusion system and pressure monitoring system must be assembled and working properly. A significant difference is the use of a needle with covering catheter, rather than a needle and syringe, to puncture the artery (Figure 5-31). As the needle and catheter enter the artery, bright red blood will pulse out. In rapid succession, withdraw the needle and advance the catheter into the artery (Figure 5-32). Place a gloved fingertip over the proximal hub of the catheter to stop the bleeding. Next, screw the prepared three-way stopcock and high-pressure tubing to the hub of the catheter. Flush some heparinized saline solution through the arterial catheter to prevent any blood from clotting. Make sure the automatic drip system and arterial pressure monitoring system are working properly. The patient's blood pres-

sure should be displayed on the monitor (see Figures 5-28 and 5-29).

e. Interpret the results of the insertion of arterial monitoring lines (Code: IB10s) [Difficulty: ELE: R, Ap; WRE An]

As discussed previously, if the equipment is properly assembled, the pressure readings will be accurate. If the pressure readings are transmitted to a display monitor, the blood pressure waveform can be seen.

5. Manipulate a pulmonary artery catheter by order or protocol (WRE code: IIA20b) [Difficulty: WRE: R, Ap, An]

a. Get the necessary equipment for the procedure

Pulmonary artery catheters are available in several diameter sizes. The smallest can be advanced into a pediatric patient's vein. Most adults will have either a 5-French or a 7-French catheter inserted. Once the appropriate size is determined, select a catheter that provides the information that is needed. A standard 5-French catheter can be used to measure pulmonary artery pressure and pulmonary capillary wedge pressure, and a mixed venous blood sample can be withdrawn from it for analysis. A 7-French thermodilution cardiac output catheter can perform all the functions just mentioned and in addition provide a central venous pressure measurement and measure cardiac output through the computer (see Figures 5-17 and 5-22). A 7-French fiberoptic catheter can measure continuous $S\overline{v}O_2$ as well as PAP, PCWP, CVP, and cardiac output by the thermodilution method. Mixed venous blood can also be sampled for analysis.

b. Put the equipment together and make sure that it works properly

The 5-French and 7-French catheters are packaged self-contained as a single unit. The general assembly of the related tubing circuit and pressure transducer was discussed earlier and illustrated in Figures 5-18 and 5-28. Clinical experience is needed. Make sure that all connections are watertight, the transducer calibrates accurately, and the balloon inflates and deflates properly.

The process of calibrating the monitor for pulmonary artery pressures or systemic artery pressures was briefly discussed earlier. Regardless of whether the catheter is placed into a systemic artery, pulmonary artery, umbilical artery, or superior vena cava, the equipment must be properly calibrated to ensure accurate data. When performing two-point calibration, all pressures should read "zero" when exposed to atmospheric pressure. This is the low point. The high point pressure for pulmonary artery pressure monitoring is commonly 30 mm Hg.

Figure 5-28   Common steps in the assembly of the tubing circuit and pressure transducer to attach to an arterial or pulmonary artery catheter. Sterile technique must be maintained at all times. (NOTE: Individual institutions will vary these steps. Clinical practice is very important in this assembly.) **A,** Obtain a 250 to 500 mL bag of sterile, normal saline. Add 1 to 2 units of heparin per mL of solution. Attach an IV line with a macrodrip chamber. **B,** Insert the solution bag into a pressure bag. Inflate the pressure to about 100 mm Hg to force the fluid through the IV tubing. The pressure bag will be inflated up to 300 mm Hg at the end of this procedure to ensure that 3 drops of fluid flow through the tubing per minute to keep it patent. **C,** Attach the strain gauge pressure transducer to an IV pole. Let it and the monitor warm up. **D,** Attach the IV tubing to the continuous flush device (Sorenson Intraflow). **E,** Screw the continuous flush device into the transducer stopcock. **F,** Backflush the continuous flush device and transducer, with open stopcocks, so that all air is removed and replaced with the saline solution. **G,** Zero and calibrate the pressure transducer and monitor. **H,** Attach high-pressure tubing to the continuous flush device. Flush the air out of it. **I,** Attach the high-pressure tubing to the patient's arterial line or pulmonary artery catheter. Ensure that no air bubbles are present and that there is a continuous saline to blood connection. Accurate patient pressures should now be seen on the monitor. *(From Oblouk Darovic G: Hemodynamic monitoring, Philadelphia, 1987, WB Saunders.)*

Figure 5-29 Example of a complete setup for monitoring the arterial pressure. *(From Daily EK, Schroeder JS:* Techniques in bedside hemodynamic monitoring, *ed 5, St Louis, 1994, Mosby.)*

c. Troubleshoot any problems with the equipment

See Table 5-3 for a listing of the problems seen with pulmonary artery catheters and their causes, prevention, and treatment. Figure 5-30 shows common problem areas with the related pressure tubing and equipment.

6. Manipulate a cardiac output computer by order or protocol (WRE code: IIA20b) [Difficulty: WRE: R, Ap, An]

a. Get the correct cardiac output computer for the procedure

The manufacturers of cardiac output pulmonary artery catheters (e.g., Edwards Laboratories LLC) also make thermodilution cardiac output computers. However, the computer is usually designed only for use with their brand of catheter. Make sure that you have a compatible catheter and computer.

b. Put the equipment together and make sure that it works properly

Figure 5-17 shows a thermodilution cardiac output pulmonary artery catheter. Note the thermistor connection

to the cardiac output computer and the proximal port where the cooled solution is injected. See Figure 5-22 for the assembly of the cardiac output computer to the catheter. In addition, the computer must be programmed with the size of catheter, injectate volume, and injectate temperature.

c. Troubleshoot any problems with the pulmonary artery catheter equipment and cardiac output computer

An error in the cardiac output value can be caused by an error in programming the computer or by not injecting the cooled solution through the proximal port in the required 4 seconds.

7. Manipulate a continuous mixed venous oxygen saturation monitor by order or protocol (WRE code: IIA20b) [Difficulty: WRE: R, Ap, An]

a. Get the correct monitor for the procedure

The manufacturers of continuous mixed venous oxygen saturation pulmonary artery catheters (e.g., Edwards

TABLE 5-1	Inaccurate Pressure Measurements		
Problem	**Cause**	**Prevention**	**Treatment**
Damped waveforms and inaccurate pressures	Partial clotting at catheter tip	Use continuous drip with 1 unit of heparin/1 mL of IV fluid. Hand flush occasionally. Flush with large volume after blood sampling. Use heparin-coated catheters.	Aspirate, then flush catheter with heparinized fluid (*not* in PAW position).
	Tip moving against wall	Obtain more stable catheter position.	Reposition catheter.
	Kinking of catheter	Restrict catheter movement at insertion site.	Reposition to straighten catheter. Replace catheter.
Abnormally low or negative pressures	Incorrect air reference level (above midchest level)	Maintain transducer air reference port at midchest level; rezero after patient position changes.	Remeasure level of transducer air reference and reposition at midchest level; rezero.
	Incorrect zeroing and calibration of monitor	Zero and calibrate monitor properly.	Recheck zero and calibration of monitor.
	Loose connection	Use Luer-Lok stopcocks.	Check all connections.
Abnormally high pressure reading	Pressure trapped by improper sequence of stopcock operation	Turn stopcocks in proper sequence when two pressures are measured on one transducer.	Thoroughly flush transducers with IV solution; rezero and turn stopcocks in proper sequence.
	Incorrect air reference level (below midchest level)	Maintain transducer air reference port at midchest level; recheck and rezero after patient position changes.	Check air reference level; reset at midchest and rezero.
Inappropriate pressure waveform	Migration of catheter tip (e.g., in RV or PAW instead of in PA)	Establish optimal position carefully when introducing catheter initially. Suture catheter at insertion site and tape catheter to patient's skin.	Review waveform; if RV, inflate balloon; if PAW, deflate balloon and withdraw catheter slightly. Check position under fluoroscope and/or radiograph after reposition.
No pressure available	Transducer not open to catheter Amplifiers still on *cal,* zero, or *off*	Follow routine, systematic steps for pressure measurement.	Check system, stopcocks.
Noise or fling in pressure waveform	Excessive catheter movement, particularly in PA	Avoid excessive catheter length in ventricle.	Try different catheter tip position.
	Excessive tubing length	Use shortest tubing possible (<3 to 4 feet).	Eliminate excess tubing.
	Excessive stopcocks	Minimize number of stopcocks.	Eliminate excess stopcocks.

From Daily EK, Schroeder JS: *Techniques in bedside hemodynamic monitoring,* ed 5, St Louis, 1995, Mosby.
PA, pulmonary artery; *PAW,* pulmonary artery wedge; *RV,* right ventricle.

Laboratories LLC) also make the required monitor. However, the monitor is usually designed only for use with their brand of catheter. Make sure that you have a compatible catheter and monitor.

b. Put the equipment together and make sure that it works properly

See Figure 5-25 for a photograph of a continuous mixed venous oxygen saturation pulmonary artery catheter and its connection to the required monitor and analyzer. Make sure the monitor is properly connected to the catheter. Calibrate the equipment as directed by the manufacturer so that accurate patient values will be measured.

c. Troubleshoot any problems with the monitor

Errors can result from the catheter and monitor not being properly connected or the analyzer not being properly calibrated.

TABLE 5-2	Problems Encountered with Arterial Catheters		
Problem	Cause	Prevention	Treatment
Hematoma after withdrawal of needle	Bleeding or oozing at puncture site	Maintain firm pressure on site during withdrawal of catheter and for 5-15 min (as necessary) after withdrawal. Apply elastic tape (Elastoplast) firmly over puncture site. For femoral arterial puncture sites, leave a sandbag on site for 1-2 hr to prevent oozing. If patient is receiving heparin, discontinue 2 hr before catheter removal.	Continue to hold pressure to puncture site until oozing stops. Apply sandbag to femoral puncture site for 1-2 hr after removal of catheter.
Decreased or absent pulse distal to puncture site	Spasm of artery	Introduce arterial needle cleanly, nontraumatically.	Inject lidocaine locally at insertion site and 10 mg into arterial catheter.
	Thrombosis of artery	Use 1 unit of heparin/1 mL of IV fluid	Arteriotomy and Fogarty catheterization both distally and proximally from the puncture site result in return of pulse in more than 90% of cases if brachial or femoral artery is used.
Bleedback into tubing, dome, or transducer	Insufficient pressure on IV bag	Maintain 300 mm Hg pressure on IV bag.	Replace transducer.
	Loose connections	Use Luer-Lok stopcocks; tighten periodically.	"Fast flush" through system. Tighten all connections.
Hemorrhage	Loose connections	Keep all connecting sites visible. Observe connecting sites frequently. Use built-in alarm system. Use Luer-Lok stopcocks.	Tighten all connections.
Emboli	Clot from catheter tip into bloodstream	Always aspirate and discard before flushing. Use continuous flush device. Use 1 unit of heparin/1 mL of IV fluid. Gently flush <2-4 mL.	Remove catheter.
Local infection	Forward movement of contaminated catheter	Carefully suture catheter at insertion site. Always use aseptic technique.	Remove catheter. Prescribe antibiotic.
	Break in sterile technique Prolonged catheter use	Remove catheter after 72-96 hr. Inspect and care for insertion site daily, including dressing change and antibiotic or iodophor ointment.	
Sepsis	Break in sterile technique Prolonged catheter use	Use percutaneous insertion. Always use aseptic technique. Remove catheter after 72-96 hr.	Remove catheter. Prescribe antibiotic.
	Bacterial growth in IV fluid	Change IV fluid bag, stopcocks, dome, and tubing every 24-48 hr. Do not use IV fluid containing glucose. Use sterile dead-ender caps on all ports of stopcocks. Carefully flush remaining blood from stopcocks after blood sampling.	

From Daily EK, Schroeder JS: *Techniques in bedside hemodynamic monitoring*, ed 5, St Louis, 1995, Mosby.

Figure 5-30   Common problem areas with arterial and pulmonary artery catheters. *(From Oblouk Darovic G:* Hemodynamic monitoring—invasive and noninvasive clinical application, *ed 3, Philadelphia, 2002, Saunders.)*

Figure 5-31   Proper positioning of the patient's hand enables the respiratory therapist to insert a needle and covering catheter into the radial artery for the continuous measurement of blood pressure. The therapist is about to insert the needle with catheter (cannula) into the patient. Steps in the cannulation procedure are very much the same as those for an arterial puncture as described in Chapter 3.

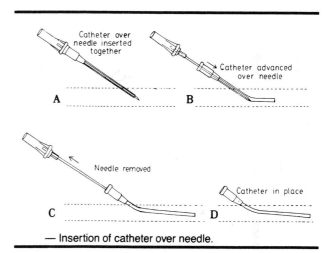

— Insertion of catheter over needle.

Figure 5-32   Steps in the procedure for the percutaneous insertion of an arterial catheter (cannula) for the continuous measurement of arterial pressure. Once the needle and catheter are inserted into the artery, the needle is withdrawn and the flexible catheter is advanced into the artery. The proximal end of the catheter is connected to a tubing circuit and pressure transducer as shown in Figures 5-28 and 5-29. *(From Oblouk Darovic G:* Hemodynamic monitoring, *Philadelphia, 1987, WB Saunders.)*

MODULE E

Respiratory care plan

1. Analyze the available information to determine the patient's pathophysiologic state (Code: IIIH1) [Difficulty: ELE: R, Ap; WRE: An]

Each clinical problem presented in this section requires its own individualized treatment. Be prepared to make recommendations to change the inspired oxygen percentage, give fluids if the patient is dehydrated, give diuretic medications to increase urine output if the patient is fluid overloaded, give vasodilator medications if the patient is hypertensive, or give vasoconstrictor medications if the patient is hypotensive.

See Figure 5-33 for examples of diagnostic pathways. These can be used to help the clinician evaluate all the patient data. The diagnosis or pathophysiologic state can be determined by following the data on a given pathway. Normal values and common conditions associated with abnormal values were discussed earlier in this chapter.

TABLE 5-3 Problems Encountered with Pulmonary Artery Catheters

Problem	Cause	Prevention	Treatment
Phlebitis or local infection at insertion site	Mechanical irritation or contamination	Prepare skin properly before insertion. Use sterile technique during insertion and dressing change. Insert smoothly and rapidly. Use Teflon-coated introducer. Attach silver-impregnated cuff to introducer. Change dressings, stopcocks, and connecting tubing every 24-48 hr. Remove catheter or change insertion site every 4 days.	Remove catheter. Apply warm compresses. Give pain medication as necessary.
Ventricular irritability	Looping of excess catheter in right ventricle	Suture catheter at insertion site; check chest film.	Reposition catheter; remove loop.
	Migration of catheter from PA to RV	Position catheter tip in main right or left PA.	Inflate balloon to encourage catheter flotation out to PA.
	Irritation of the endocardium during catheter passage	Keep balloon inflated during advancement; advance gently.	Advance rapidly out to PA.
Apparent wedging of catheter with balloon *deflated*	Forward migration of catheter tip caused by blood flow, excessive loop in RV, or inadequate suturing of catheter at insertion site	Check catheter tip by fluoroscopy; position in main right or left PA. Check catheter position on radiography film if fluoroscopy is not used. Suture catheter in place at insertion site.	Aspirate blood from catheter; if catheter is wedged, sample will be arterialized and obtained with difficulty. If wedged, slowly pull back catheter until PA waveform appears. If not wedged, gently aspirate and flush catheter with saline; catheter tip can partially clot, causing damping that resembles damped PAW waveform.
Pulmonary hemorrhage or infarction, or both	Distal migration of catheter tip Continuous or prolonged wedging of catheter Overinflation of balloon while catheter is wedged Failure of balloon to deflate	Check chest film immediately after insertion and 12-24 hr later; remove any catheter loop in RA or RV. Leave balloon deflated. Suture catheter at skin to prevent inadvertent advancement. Position catheter in main right or left PA. Pull catheter back to pulmonary artery if it spontaneously wedges. Do not flush catheter when in wedge position. Inflate balloon slowly with only enough air to obtain a PAW waveform. Do not inflate 7Fr catheter with more than 1-1.5 mL of air. Do not inflate if resistance is met.	Deflate balloon. Place patient on side (catheter tip down). Stop anticoagulation. Consider "wedge" angiogram. Intubate with double-lumen ET. Surgery, if severe hemorrhage
"Overwedging" or damped PAW	Overinflation of balloon Eccentric inflation of balloon	Watch waveform during inflation; inject only enough air to obtain PAW pressure. Do not inflate 7Fr catheter with more than 1-1.5 mL of air. Check inflated balloon shape before insertion.	Deflate balloon; reinflate slowly with only enough air to obtain PAW pressure. Deflate balloon; reposition and slowly reinflate.
PA balloon rupture	Overinflation of balloon Frequent inflations of balloon Syringe deflation damaging wall of balloon	Inflate slowly with only enough air to obtain a PAW pressure. Monitor PAd pressure as reflection of PAW and LVEDP. Allow passive deflation of balloon. Remove syringe after inflation.	Remove syringe to prevent further air injection. Monitor PAd pressure.

TABLE 5-3	Problems Encountered with Pulmonary Artery Catheters—cont'd		
Problem	**Cause**	**Prevention**	**Treatment**
Infection	Nonsterile insertion techniques	Use sterile techniques. Use sterile catheter sleeve.	Remove catheter. Use antibiotics.
	Contamination via skin	Prepare skin with effective antiseptic (chlorhexidine). Apply iodophor ointment and sterile gauze dressing daily. Do not use clear semipermeable dressing. Inspect site daily. Reassess need for catheter after 3 days. Avoid internal jugular approach.	
	Contamination through stopcock ports or catheter hub	Use sterile dead-ender caps on all stopcock ports. Change IV solution, stopcock, and tubing every 24-48 hr. Do not use IV solution that contains glucose.	
	Fluid contamination from transducer through cracked membrane of disposable dome	Check transducer domes for cracks. Change transducers every 48 hr. Change disposable dome after countershock. Do not use IV solution that contains glucose.	
	Prolonged catheter placement	Change catheter insertion site every 4 days.	
Heart block during insertion of catheter	Mechanical irritation of His bundle in patients with preexisting left bundle branch block	Insert catheter expeditiously with balloon inflated. Insert transvenous pacing catheter before PA catheter insertion.	Use temporary pacemaker or flotation catheter with pacing wire.

From Daily EK, Schroeder JS: *Techniques in bedside hemodynamic monitoring*, ed 5, St Louis, 1995, Mosby.
ET, Endotracheal tube; *LVEDP*, left ventricular end-diastolic pressure; *PA*, pulmonary artery; *PAd*, pulmonary artery diastolic; *PAW*, pulmonary artery wedge; *RV*, right ventricle.

2. Recommend adjustment of the patient's fluid balance (Code: IIIG1d) [Difficulty: ELE: R, Ap; WRE: An]

The PCWP is often used to guide the administration or limitation of fluids to the patient. It is generally believed that a PCWP of greater than 10 mm Hg indicates fluid overload. If the PCWP is greater than 20 mm Hg, the patient will often progress to pulmonary edema. Fluids should be restricted and diuretic medications (furosemide [Lasix]) given to increase urine output. It is generally believed that a PCWP of less than 4 mm Hg indicates hypovolemia/dehydration. Increase the patient's fluid intake.

3. Determine the appropriateness of the prescribed respiratory care plan and recommend modifications when indicated

a. Determine the appropriateness of the prescribed therapy and goals for the patient's pathophysiologic state (Code: IIIH3) [Difficulty: ELE: R, Ap; WRE: An]

b. Review the planned therapy to establish the therapeutic plan (Code: IIIH2a) [Difficulty: ELE: R, Ap; WRE: An]

c. Recommend changes in the therapeutic plan when indicated (Code: IIIH4) [Difficulty: ELE: R, Ap; WRE: An]

d. Terminate the procedure based on the patient's response to therapy (Code: IIIF1) [Difficulty: ELE: R, Ap; WRE: An]

e. Recommend discontinuing the procedure based on the patient's response to therapy (Code: IIIG1i) [Difficulty: ELE: R, Ap; WRE: An]

A catheter should be withdrawn if the patient develops signs or symptoms of infection at the insertion site.

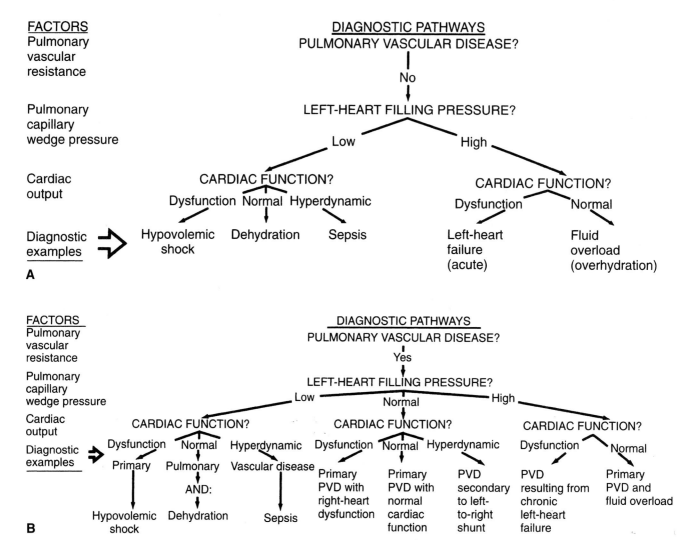

Figure 5-33 Possible diagnostic pathways for patients with **(A)** and without **(B)** pulmonary vascular disease (PVD). In both cases, the pulmonary vascular resistance, pulmonary capillary wedge pressure, and cardiac output are measured. High, normal, or low values lead down different pathways. Previous discussions and clinical experience are needed to determine the final diagnosis. Sepsis may be associated with normal left-heart filling pressures. Primary PVD may be caused by pulmonary emboli, pulmonary artery disease (vasculitis, "primary" pulmonary hypertension), respiratory distress syndromes, hypoxic vasoconstriction, or drugs. *(From Osgood CF, Watson MH, Slaughter MS et al: Respir Care 29[1]:25-34, 1984.)*

4. Record and evaluate the patient's response to the treatment(s) or procedure(s), including the following

a. Record and interpret the following: heart rate and rhythm, respiratory rate, blood pressure, body temperature, and pain level (Code: IIIA1b4) [Difficulty: ELE: R, Ap; WRE: An]

b. Record and interpret the patient's breath sounds (Code: IIIAb3) [Difficulty: ELE: R, Ap; WRE: An]

There is a risk of puncturing the right lung during the insertion of a central venous catheter by way of the subclavian vein (see Figure 5-13). Assess the patient for equal, bilateral breath sounds after this procedure has been attempted. Know the signs and symptoms of a pneumothorax. Review them in Chapter 1, if needed.

c. Recheck any math work and make note of incorrect data (Code: IIIA1b2) [Difficulty: ELE: R, Ap; WRE: An]

Exam Hint 5-10 (ELE, WRE)

Closely review the following concepts because they have been tested on previous examinations.

1. Interpretation of pulmonary artery pressure (PAP): An increased PAP is usually associated with one of the following: fluid overload, heart failure or pulmonary hypertension (increased pulmonary vascular resistance) from COPD (emphysema), pulmonary embolism, or persistent pulmonary hypertension of the newborn (PPHN).

2. Interpretation of pulmonary capillary wedge pressure (PCWP): An increased PCWP is usually associated with one of the following: fluid overload, heart failure, mitral valve insufficiency, cardiac tamponade, or constrictive pericarditis. Treatment for fluid overload and/or heart failure usually includes restriction of fluids and administration of diuretics (Lasix) and digitalis-type drugs (Lanoxin). A decreased PCWP is usually associated with dehydration, treated with increased fluids, or vasodilation, treated with vasoconstricting drugs. When interpreting the PAP and PCWP together, it is very important to calculate the difference between the PAP diastolic pressure and the PCWP. Normally, the difference (or gradient) is 5 mm Hg or less. In other words, if the PAP diastolic pressure minus the PCWP is 5 mm Hg or less, the patient does not have pulmonary hypertension. A gradient of more than 5 mm Hg indicates pulmonary hypertension.

3. Interpretation of cardiac output: A decreased cardiac output is usually caused by hypovolemia, treated with increased fluids, or heart failure, treated with digitalis-type drugs (Lanoxin). Cardiac output may also be decreased on a ventilator-dependent patient with high peak pressures or PEEP level because of the increased intrathoracic pressure. When this is presented in an NBRC question and a request for care is made, the best response is to decrease the PEEP level.

BIBLIOGRAPHY

AARC Clinical Practice Guideline: Capnography/capnometry during mechanical ventilation, 2003 revision & update. *Respir Care* 48(5):534, 2003.

Aggarwal NK, Kiran U, Kapoor PM, Chowdhury UK: Intraoperative central venous oxygen saturation as a surrogate for mixed venous oxygen saturation in patients undergoing cardiac surgery, *J Anesth Clin Pharmacology* 23(1):29-33, 2007.

Anton WR, Raghu G: Measuring end-tidal carbon dioxide tension at maximal exhalation to improve its utility during T-piece weaning trials, *Respir Care* 35(11):1082-1083, 1990.

Bakow ED: A limitation of capnography, *Respir Care* 27(2):167-168, 1982.

Branson RD, Campbell RS: Cardiovascular monitoring. In Branson RD, Hess DR, Chatburn RL, editors: *Respiratory care equipment*, ed 2, Philadelphia, 1999, Lippincott Williams & Wilkins.

Cairo JM: Assessment of cardiovascular function. In Cairo JM, Pilbeam SP: *Mosby's respiratory care equipment*, ed 8, St Louis, 2010, Mosby.

Cairo JM: Hemodynamic monitoring. In Pilbeam SP, Cairo JM: *Mechanical ventilation—physiologic and clinical applications*, ed 4, St Louis, 2006, Mosby.

Carlon GC, Ray C, Miodownik S et al: Capography in mechanically ventilated patients, *Crit Care Med* 16(5):550-556, 1988.

Clark DB, Marshall SG: Mixed venous oxygen saturation measurement. II. General and specific clinical applications, *Respir Ther* 81-86, Nov/Dec 1986.

Daily EK, Schroeder JS: *Techniques in bedside hemodynamic monitoring*, ed 5, St Louis, 1994, Mosby.

Deshpande VM, Pilbeam SP, Dixon RJ: *A comprehensive review in respiratory care*, Norwalk, Conn, 1988, Appleton & Lange.

Divertie MB, McMichan JC: Continuous monitoring of mixed venous oxygen saturation, *Chest* 85(3):423-428, 1984.

Fahey PJ, Harris K, Vanderwarf C: Clinical experience with continuous monitoring of mixed venous oxygen saturation in respiratory failure, *Chest* 86(5):748-752, 1984.

Fink JB, Hunt GE, editors: *Clinical practice in respiratory care*, Philadelphia, 1999, Lippincott-Raven.

Gravenstein JS, Jaffe MB, Paulus DA, editors: *Capnography—clinical aspects*, Cambridge UK, 2004, Cambridge University Press.

Harris K: Noninvasive monitoring of gas exchange, *Respir Care* 32(7):544-557, 1987.

Hess D: Capnometry and capnography: technical aspects, physiologic aspects, and clinical applications, *Respir Care* 35(6):557-576, 1990.

Hess DR, Branson RD: Noninvasive respiratory monitoring equipment. In Branson RD, Hess DR, Chatburn RL, editors: *Respiratory care equipment*, ed 2, Philadelphia, 1999, Lippincott Williams & Wilkins.

Hess D: Respiratory care monitoring. In Burton GC, Hodgkin JE, Ward JJ, editors: *Respiratory care: a guide to clinical practice*, ed 4, Philadelphia, 1997, Lippincott-Raven.

Hunt GE: Diagnostic procedures at the bedside. In Fink JB, Hunt GE, editors: *Clinical practice in respiratory care*. Philadelphia, 1999, Lippincott-Raven.

Jaquith SM: The oximetric opticath: what is it and how can it facilitate nursing management of the critically ill patient? *Crit Care Nurse*, 55-58, May/June 1984.

Kandel G, Aberman A: Mixed venous oxygen saturation: its role in the assessment of the critically ill patient, *Arch Intern Med* 143:1400-1402, 1983.

Kinasewitz GT: Use of end-tidal capnography during mechanical ventilation, *Respir Care* 25(2):169-171, 1982.

Krider SJ: Cardiac output assessment. In Wilkins RL, Sheldon RL, Krider SJ, editors: *Clinical assessment in respiratory care*, ed 4, St Louis, 2000, Mosby.

Krider SJ: Invasively monitored hemodynamic pressures. In Wilkins RL, Sheldon RL, Krider SJ, editors: *Clinical assessment in respiratory care*, ed 4, St Louis, 2000, Mosby.

Malinowski T: Respiratory monitoring in the intensive care unit. In Wilkins RL, Krider SJ, Sheldon RL, editors: *Clinical assessment in respiratory care*, ed 3, St Louis, 1990, Mosby.

Malley WJ: *Clinical blood gases*, ed 2, St Louis, 2005, Saunders.

Marini JJ: Obtaining meaningful data from the Swan-Ganz catheter, *Respir Care* 30(7):572-585, 1985.

Mathews PJ, Gregg BL: Monitoring and management of the patient in the ICU. In Scanlan CL, Wilkins RL, Stoller JK, Kacmarek RM, editors: *Egan's fundamentals of respiratory care*, ed 9, St Louis, 2009, Mosby.

McMichan JC: Continuous monitoring of mixed venous oxygen saturation in clinical practice, *Mount Sinai* J Med 51(5):569-572, 1984.

Nuzzo PF, Anton WR: Practical applications of capnography, *Respir Ther*, 12-17, Nov/Dec 1986.

Oblouk Darovic G: *Hemodynamic monitoring*, Philadelphia, 1987, WB Saunders.

Oblouk Darovic G: *Hemodynamic monitoring—invasive and noninvasive clinical application*, ed 3, Philadelphia, 2002, WB Saunders.

Osgood CF, Watson MH, Slaughter MS et al: Hemodynamic monitoring in respiratory care, *Respir Care* 29(1):25-34, 1984.

Paulus DA: Invasive monitoring of respiratory gas exchange: continuous measurement of mixed venous oxygen saturation, *Respir Care* 32(7):535-543, 1987.

Pilbeam SP: *Mechanical ventilation: physiological and clinical applications*, ed 3, St Louis, 1998, Mosby.

Ragosta M: Textbook of clinical hemodynamics. Philadelphia, 2008, Saunders, Inc.

Reinhart K, Kuhn H, Hartog C, Bredle DL: Continuous central venous and pulmonary artery oxygen saturation in the critically ill, *Intensive Care Med* 30:1572-1578, 2004.

Restrepo RD: Assessment of cardiac output. In Wilkins RL, Dexter JR, Heuer AJ: *Clinical assessment in respiratory care*, ed 6, St Louis, 2010, Mosby.

Ruppel G: *Manual of pulmonary function testing*, ed 9, St Louis, 2009, Mosby.

Shapiro BA, Harrison RA, Cane RD et al: *Clinical application of blood gases*, ed 5, St Louis, 1994, Mosby.

Shapiro BA, Kacmarek RM, Cane RD, et al., editors: *Clinical application of respiratory care*, ed 4. St Louis, 1991, Mosby.

Whitaker K: *Comprehensive perinatal & pediatric respiratory care*, ed 2, Albany, NY, Delmar, 1997.

White GC: *Equipment theory for respiratory care*, ed 4, Albany, NY, Delmar, 2005.

Wiedemann HP: Invasive monitoring techniques in the ventilated patient. In Kacmarek RM, Stoller JK, editors: *Current respiratory care*, Toronto, 1988, BC Decker.

Wilkins RL: Bedside assessment of the patient. In Wilkins, Stoller JK, Kacmarek RM, editors: *Egan's fundamentals of respiratory care*, ed 9, St Louis, 2009, Mosby.

Wilkins RL: Analysis and monitoring in gas exchange. In Wilkins, Stoller JK, Kacmarek RM, editors: *Egan's fundamentals of respiratory care*, ed 9, St Louis, 2009, Mosby.

Wilkins RL, Dexter JR: Assessment of hemodynamic pressures. In Wilkins RL, Dexter JR, Heuer AJ: *Clinical assessment in respiratory care*, ed 6, St Louis, 2010, Mosby.

Wilkins RL, Heuer AJ: Vital signs. In Wilkins RL, Dexter JR, Heuer AJ: *Clinical assessment in respiratory care*, ed 6, St Louis, 2010, Mosby.

1. The waveform sequence seen during the insertion of a pulmonary artery catheter is
   A. RA, RV, PAP, PCWP
   B. RV, RA, PAP, PCWP
   C. RA, RV, PCWP, PAP
   D. Ao, RA, RV, PAP

2. When evaluating a patient's stroke volume, which of the following is true?
   A. It is an indicator of the adequacy of perfusion of the body tissues.
   B. It is the output of blood for 1 minute.
   C. It has a range of 50 to 120 mL in the adult.
   D. It is the resistance to flow.

3. A patient with chronic bronchitis is being monitored with regular measurements of arterial blood gas values and capnometry. The following data are available:

$PaCO_2$	53 torr
PaO_2	67 torr
$P_{ET}CO_2$	33 torr
$P_{\bar{E}}CO_2$	20 torr

   Calculate the patient's V_D/V_T.
   A. 0.30
   B. 0.38
   C. 0.62
   D. 0.71

4. A 40-year-old patient recovering from ARDS is receiving mechanical ventilation with a tidal volume of 650 mL. The patient has an arterial line, a pulmonary artery catheter, and capnometry for monitoring. The following information is gathered after a change in PEEP level:

$PaCO_2$	43 torr
PaO_2	79 torr
$P\bar{v}O_2$	32 torr
$P_{ET}CO_2$	38 torr
$P_{\bar{E}}CO_2$	22 torr

   Calculate the patient's V_D.
   A. 273 mL
   B. 319 mL
   C. 338 mL
   D. 384 mL

5. A 35-year-old patient in the intensive care unit has the following hemodynamic data. Which of these data indicates a problem with the patient?
   A. SVR of 600 dynes/sec/cm^{-5}
   B. CI of 3 L/min/m^2 of body surface area
   C. $P\bar{v}O_2$ of 38 torr
   D. Shunt of 4%

6. A patient with a history of congestive heart failure is inadvertently given intravenous fluids of 2000 mL instead of the ordered amount of 200 mL. Which of the following is most likely to be seen?
   A. Decreased lung markings on chest radiograph
   B. Increased pulmonary capillary wedge pressure
   C. Increased PaO_2
   D. Decreased pulmonary artery pressure

7. A patient hospitalized with leg vein thrombosis experiences sudden shortness of breath. Which of the following should be recommended to evaluate the patient's situation?
   A. Lung compliance
   B. Electrocardiogram
   C. Chest radiograph
   D. V_D/V_T

8. Capnography will be used to monitor a patient's recovery from anesthesia. What gas should be used for the "zero" calibration?
   A. Room air for 0% carbon dioxide
   B. Room air for 21% oxygen
   C. 5% carbon dioxide
   D. The same concentration of anesthetic gas as used with the patient

9. Hypovolemia in an adult patient would be indicated by a PCWP of
   A. 2 mm Hg
   B. 8 mm Hg
   C. 12 mm Hg
   D. 24 mm Hg

10. An adult patient has had a pulmonary artery catheter inserted. A normal PAP pressure in this patient would be
    A. 8 mm Hg
    B. 25/10 mm Hg
    C. 35/15 mm Hg
    D. 120/80 mm Hg

11. The principle of operation of the capnography monitor is
    A. The same as that of the Clark electrode
    B. The same as that of the Severinghaus electrode
    C. Infrared absorption
    D. The same as that of the CO-oximeter

12. Calculate a patient's pulmonary artery diastolic-pulmonary capillary wedge pressure (PAd-PCWP) gradient if the PAP is 30/12 mm Hg and the PCWP is 8 mm Hg.
    A. 38 mm Hg
    B. 12 mm Hg
    C. 8 mm Hg
    D. 4 mm Hg

13. A patient has an end-tidal CO_2 pressure of 30 torr and a $P(a\text{-}et)CO_2$ gradient of 4 torr. The alveolar to end-tidal gradient is in the usual direction. Based on this, his $PaCO_2$ would be estimated as

A. 4 torr
B. 26 torr
C. 30 torr
D. 34 torr

14. Your patient is known to have advanced COPD. When checking his V_D/V_T ratio, you would expect it to be
    A. Unaffected by his condition
    B. Increased
    C. Normal
    D. Decreased

15. A patient is being mechanically ventilated and has a reflectance oximetry pulmonary artery catheter in place. What $S\bar{v}O_2$ value would indicate the patient is oxygenating adequately?
    A. 40%
    B. 50%
    C. 75%
    D. 90%

16. The normal range for the $P(a-et)CO_2$ gradient is
    A. <1 torr
    B. 1-5 torr
    C. More than 15 torr
    D. About 40 torr

17. An adult patient has been admitted for observation after suffering a concussion in a fall. Her arterial blood pressure is found to be 115/78 mm Hg. How should these results be interpreted?
    A. Within normal limits
    B. Hypertension
    C. Hypotension
    D. She has an intracranial bleed.

SELF-STUDY QUESTIONS FOR WRITTEN REGISTRY EXAM
See page 610 for answers

1. A patient with advanced emphysema is admitted to the respiratory intensive care unit. He is placed on a 24% Venturi-type mask and has a pulmonary artery catheter inserted. His initial pulmonary vascular resistance (PVR) is 9 mm Hg/L/min and his PaO_2 is 57 torr. The physician orders him increased to 28% oxygen. The resulting PVR is 5 mm Hg/L/min and PaO_2 is 63 torr. Based on this information, what would you recommend?
    A. Decrease the oxygen to 24%.
    B. Place the patient on a ventilator.
    C. Administer a bronchodilating agent such as albuterol.
    D. Keep the patient on 28% oxygen.

2. Your patient is in the intensive care unit and is being monitored with a pulmonary artery catheter. She has the following parameters: PAP of 35/20 mm Hg, PCWP of 9 mm Hg, central venous pressure of 9 cm of water. You would interpret the data to indicate that she
    A. Has right ventricular failure/cor pulmonale
    B. Has left ventricular failure
    C. Has increased pulmonary vascular resistance
    D. Is hypovolemic

3. A 40-year-old patient receiving mechanical ventilation has an arterial line in place. It is noticed that there is a significant difference between the blood pressure taken by cuff on the left arm and the blood pressure taken by arterial line on the right arm. What could explain this difference?

1. A clot is at the tip of the catheter.
2. There is an air bubble in the arterial line.
3. The ventilator's peak pressure is too high.
4. The patient has a ventricular septal defect.
    A. 1 and 2 only
    B. 2 and 3 only
    C. 1, 3, and 4 only
    D. All of the above

4. An adult patient is receiving mechanical ventilation when the following data are gathered:

	9:00 AM	11:00 AM
PaO_2	75 torr	53 torr
pulmonary vascular resistance	120 dynes/sec/cm^{-5}	340 dynes/sec/cm^{-5}
pulmonary capillary wedge pressure	8 mm Hg	10 mm Hg
pulmonary artery pressure	25/10 mm Hg	42/21 mm Hg

How should the results be interpreted?
    A. Pulmonary edema
    B. Pulmonary embolism
    C. Pneumonia
    D. Cardiac tamponade

5. A patient is receiving mechanical ventilation with the SIMV mode and a mandatory rate of 10/minute. End-tidal carbon dioxide monitoring is being done and the following data are recorded:

	4:00 PM	6:00 PM
Set tidal volume	700 mL	700 mL
Set rate	10	10
$P_{ET}CO_2$	33 torr	41 torr
$PaCO_2$	42 torr	43 torr

How can these data be explained?
   A. Alveolar ventilation has decreased.
   B. Pulmonary edema has developed.
   C. The patient is hyperventilating.
   D. The patient's cardiac output has increased.

6. A patient has had an arterial line inserted. What should be done to ensure that accurate blood pressure readings are obtained?
   1. **Open the stopcock to room air to "zero" the transducer.**
   2. **Make sure that air fills the transducer dome.**
   3. **Have the patient lie flat to measure the blood pressure.**
   4. **Fill the pressure tubing with saline solution.**
   A. 1 and 2 only
   B. 2 and 4 only
   C. 1, 2, and 3 only
   D. 1, 3, and 4 only

7. An unconscious 25-year-old patient is admitted with viral pneumonia, vomiting, and diarrhea. Mechanical ventilation is initiated and a flow-directed pulmonary artery (Swan-Ganz) catheter is inserted. The following data are gathered:

Pulmonary artery pressure	22/8 mm Hg
Pulmonary capillary wedge pressure	3 mm Hg
Central venous pressure	0 mm Hg
Blood pressure	90/60 mm Hg
Pulse	142 beats/min

What is the most likely cause of these findings?
   A. Hypovolemia
   B. High ventilating pressures
   C. Bronchospasm
   D. Rupture of the balloon on the catheter

8. A 3-day postoperative open-heart surgery patient has an arterial catheter in the right radial artery for continuous blood pressure measurements. Because of retained secretions, the respiratory therapist places him into a head-down position for postural drainage therapy. The nurse notices that the patient's blood pressure is less than before being placed into this new position. After the patient is returned to the original position, the blood pressure is the same as it was originally. How can the therapist explain the blood pressure changes?
   A. There was an air bubble in the arterial catheter.
   B. There was a clot in the arterial catheter.
   C. The patient's body was below the level of the pressure transducer.
   D. Postural drainage positions always cause the blood pressure to decrease.

9. A 65-year-old patient has been sick with vomiting and diarrhea for several days. Arterial and pulmonary artery catheters are placed for monitoring blood gases and hemodynamic parameters. ABG values on 30% O_2 show the following: PaO_2, 80 torr; $PaCO_2$, 41 torr; pH, 7.44; bicarbonate, 27 mEq/L. PAC parameters show the following: PAP, 22/8 torr; PCWP, 3 torr. In addition, serum electrolytes show the following: sodium, 156 mEq/L; potassium, 4.5 mEq/L; chlorine, 120 mEq/L. Based on these data, what would you recommend?
   A. Administer a diuretic.
   B. Increase the O_2 percentage.
   C. Administer fluids intravenously.
   D. Give a chronotropic agent such as atropine.

10. A patient with heart failure and pulmonary edema has an initial $P\bar{v}O_2$ value of 35 torr. After being mechanically ventilated and given digitalis, the $P\bar{v}O_2$ value is found to be 41 torr. How should this be interpreted?
   A. Improved tissue oxygenation
   B. No clinical change
   C. Decreased tissue oxygenation
   D. Worsening heart failure

11. A neonatal patient is suspected of having a ventricular septal defect. What could be done to confirm or rule out this condition?
   A. Perform capnography to monitor the $PetCO_2$ level.
   B. Perform a V_D/V_T calculation.
   C. Check the $P\bar{v}O_2$ value from the pulmonary artery.
   D. Check the $P\bar{v}O_2$ value from the right atrium and right ventricle.

12. An adult patient with congestive heart failure needs to have his fluid management and oxygen consumption monitored. What type of catheter should be used for these measurements?
   A. Radial arterial catheter
   B. Umbilical artery catheter
   C. Single-lumen CVP catheter
   D. Triple-lumen $ScvO_2$ CVP catheter

13. As the respiratory therapist assigned to the intensive care unit, you are helping in the care of the following four patients: Mr. Boone is a 28-year-old male being observed after an appendectomy. Mrs. Decker is a 74-year-old female with sepsis. Mrs. Dylan is a 48-year-old female with gastritis who is receiving intravenous fluids for dehydration. Mr. Zawinal is a 42-year-old male with diabetes. The following series of blood pressure measurements (in mm Hg) were taken on these patients:

	10 AM	12 PM	2 AM
Mr. Boone	125/80	122/82	120/78
Mrs. Decker	90/60	105/40	85/45
Mrs. Dylan	88/70	94/75	105/78
Mr. Zawinal	135/98	129/94	125/89

Which of these patient's should have an arterial line placed?

A. Mr. Boone
B. Mrs. Decker
C. Mrs. Dylan
D. Mr. Zawinal

14. A patient with heart failure had an $ScvO_2$ value of 65% an hour ago. He is now showing an $ScvO_2$ value of 60%. How should these results be interpreted?

A. Tissue hypoxia
B. Normal oxygenation
C. Increased cardiac output
D. Decreased pulmonary vascular resistance

6 Oxygen and Medical Gas Therapy

Note 1: This book is written to cover every item listed as testable on the *Entry Level Examination (ELE), Written Registry Examination (WRE),* and *Clinical Simulation Examination (CSE).*

The listed code for each item is taken from the National Board for Respiratory Care (NBRC) **Summary Content Outline for CRT (Certified Respiratory Therapist) and Written RRT (Registered Respiratory Therapist) Examinations** (http://evolve.elsevier.com/Sills/resptherapist/). For example, if an item is testable on both the ELE and the WRE, it will simply be shown as: (Code: . . .). If an item is testable only on the ELE, it will be shown as: (ELE code: . . .). If an item is testable only on the WRE, it will be shown as: (WRE code: . . .).

Following each item's code will be the difficulty level of the questions on that item on the ELE and the WRE. (See the Introduction for a full explanation of the three question difficulty levels.) **Recall (R)** level questions typically expect the exam taker to recall factual information. **Application (Ap)** level questions are harder because the exam taker may have to apply factual information to a clinical situation. **Analysis (An)** level questions are the most challenging because the exam taker may have to use critical thinking to evaluate patient data to make a clinical decision.

Note 2: A review of the most recent Entry Level Examinations (ELE) has revealed that an average of 12 questions (out of 140), or 9% of the exam, will cover oxygen and medical gas therapy. A review of the most recent Written Registry Examinations (WRE) has shown that an average of 7 questions (out of 100), or 7% of the exam, will cover oxygen and medical gas therapy. The Clinical Simulation Examination is comprehensive and may include everything that should be known by an advanced level respiratory therapist.

MODULE A

Ensure that the patient is adequately oxygenated

1. Oxygen administration

a. Recommend changes in the patient's position to minimize hypoxemia (Code: IIIG2a) [Difficulty: ELE: R, Ap; WRE: An]

b. Position the patient to minimize hypoxemia (Code: IIID8) [Difficulty: ELE: R, Ap; WRE: An]

Usually a patient who is short of breath when lying supine should be repositioned to sit more upright in a Fowler's or semi-Fowler's position. This seems to work best in patients with bilateral pulmonary problems such as congestive heart failure or pneumonia. If the patient cannot sit up and the lung problem is one-sided, roll the patient so that the more functional lung is down. The good lung should be positioned up in the following exceptions:

- Undrained pulmonary abscess that should not be drained into the good lung
- Neonatal congenital diaphragmatic hernia in which the good lung should not be compressed by the bowel in the chest cavity
- Pulmonary interstitial emphysema in which, by lying on the bad lung, the air leak and functional residual capacity can be reduced

In either case, always ask the patient whether the new position helps to make breathing easier. If not, reposition the patient until breathing is more comfortable with less shortness of breath. In general, Trendelenburg is not well tolerated. A patient with a closed head injury and brain edema should not be put into the Trendelenburg position.

c. Administer oxygen to achieve adequate respiratory support (ELE code: IIID6) [Difficulty: ELE: R, Ap, An]

Oxygen (O_2) must be administered in doses (up to 100%) that are adequate to treat hypoxemia, decrease the patient's work of breathing, or decrease the work of the heart. Because the U.S. Food and Drug Administration has declared supplemental oxygen to be a drug, a physician's order is required to give it to a patient or to make a change in the percentage. The only exceptions are when recognized protocols exist in your institution to give oxygen under certain limited conditions. For example, all patients with a diagnosed heart attack are given a nasal cannula at

2 L/min, or all patients undergoing cardiopulmonary resuscitation (CPR) receive 100% oxygen.

See Chapter 3 (Module A) for a listing of indications for drawing blood for an arterial blood gas (ABG) measurement. This list should be fairly complete for conditions that justify the need for supplemental oxygen. In general, the goal of giving supplemental oxygen is to keep the patient's PaO_2 level between 60 and 100 torr. Exceptions include carbon monoxide poisoning, severe anemia, and CPR, when the hope is to fully saturate the hemoglobin and increase the plasma oxygen content as much as possible. Oxygen should not be given without proof of hypoxemia or another clinical justification. When those conditions have been corrected, the oxygen percentage should be adjusted accordingly.

Giving supplemental oxygen is not done without risk. Following are oxygen-related problems that may be seen clinically.

1. O₂-induced hypoventilation

This is something to watch for in patients who have an elevated carbon dioxide level and compensated respiratory acidosis caused by severe emphysema, chronic bronchitis, or both (known as chronic obstructive pulmonary disease [COPD]). A common clinical goal is to keep the PaO_2 level between 50 and 60 torr. Check the blood gases frequently for the oxygen and carbon dioxide levels.

2. Retinopathy of prematurity (formerly called retrolental fibroplasia)

This type of blindness is found in some premature neonates who were given high levels of supplemental oxygen. The exact cause is not completely understood but is related primarily to the degree of prematurity. Keeping the PaO_2 in the range of 50 to 60 torr for the first week and at 50 to 70 torr after that should help to prevent the problem.

3. Denitrogenation absorption atelectasis

Giving more than 80% oxygen can result in atelectasis of underventilated alveoli after the oxygen has been taken up by the blood.

4. Central nervous system abnormalities

A patient who is breathing 100% oxygen in a hyperbaric chamber can have muscle tremors and seizures.

5. Pulmonary O₂ toxicity

In general, it appears that patients can breathe up to 50% oxygen for prolonged periods without significant damage. If clinically possible, many practitioners try to limit their patients to no more than 48 to 72 hours of breathing more than 50% oxygen.

Exam Hint 6-1 (ELE)

The NBRC is known to ask questions that relate to the proper use of oxygen and the hazards associated with its use. Expect to see at least one question that deals with the need to decrease the oxygen percentage for a patient with chronic obstructive pulmonary disease (COPD) who has shown an increased $PaCO_2$ when given too much supplemental oxygen.

d. Measure the patient's oxygen percentage, oxygen liter flow, or both (ELE code: IIIE10) [Difficulty: ELE: R, Ap, An]

Always measure the patient's inspired O_2 percentage (FIO_2) if possible. The gas sample should be taken as close as possible to the patient to minimize the chance of dilution from room air. Record the oxygen percentage on the ABG order slip, in the department records, and in the patient's chart if needed. As discussed in Chapter 3, the oxygen percentage must be known before the patient's PaO_2 level can be interpreted.

The oxygen liter flow is all that can be recorded with the following devices: nasal cannula, nasal catheter, simple mask, partial-rebreather mask, nonrebreather mask, and transtracheal oxygen catheter. A direct relation is found between the liter flow and the oxygen percentage, but it is not predictably accurate.

e. Prevent the patient from becoming hypoxemic by using proper technique (ELE code: IIID9) [Difficulty: ELE: R, Ap, An]

Use caution and plan ahead to minimize any time that the oxygen supply to the patient is cut off or reduced. When changing equipment of any kind, have the replacement set up and tested for proper function before replacing the current setup.

It is well known that suctioning the airway reduces the patient's oxygen level. This can result in dangerous dysrhythmias. Remember to increase the patient's inspired oxygen percentage about 1 minute before, during, and for at least 1 minute after suctioning. It is acceptable and safe to give 100% oxygen to an adult for short periods like this. Remember to reduce the oxygen percentage or liter flow to the previous level once the patient is stable after the procedure. Reanalyze the percentage if possible.

2. Manipulate oxygen and specialty gas analyzers by order or protocol (Code: IIA26) [Difficulty: ELE: R, Ap; WRE: An]

a. Get the necessary equipment for the procedure

b. Put the equipment together and make sure that it works properly

c. Troubleshoot any problems with the equipment

Because so many different models are available, consult an equipment book or the manufacturer's literature for details of the various analyzers. All portable, hand-held analyzers fall into one of the following categories: electric, physical/paramagnetic, and electrochemical.

1. Electric analyzers

These analyzers basically operate by comparing the cooling effects of an oxygen-enriched gas sample on a heated wire versus the cooling effects of a room air gas sample on a heated wire. The oxygen-enriched gas cools faster than the room air gas. This is known as the principle of thermal conductivity. Each sample must be drawn into the analyzer through a capillary line. These analyzers are designed to work only in oxygen and nitrogen gas mixes. Do not use them around flammable gases such as those found in anesthesia. Failure to calibrate can be caused by a weak battery, a plugged capillary line, or a defect in an electrical component.

2. Physical/paramagnetic analyzers

These analyzers make use of the fact that oxygen is attracted toward a magnetic field (paramagnetic property). The more oxygen is in a sample gas, the more the magnetic field is altered. These units can be used with all types of gases and are safe in the operating room with flammable and explosive anesthetics. A silica gel–filled container is in line with the capillary tube to dry out the sample gas before it gets to the analyzing chamber. Failure to calibrate can be caused by water or by a defect in the analyzing chamber, a weak battery, or a plugged capillary line.

3. Electrochemical analyzers: polarographic and galvanic fuel cell

Both polarographic and galvanic fuel cells make use of the fact that each oxygen molecule accepts up to two electrons and becomes chemically reduced. The more oxygen is in the gas sample, the more electrons are released from an oxidizing electrolyte solution. This is measured as an electrical current that is proportional to the oxygen percentage. These analyzers can monitor continuously and display the oxygen percentage. Both types are safe by themselves in the presence of flammable gases, but the added alarm systems are powered electrically and may make the units unsafe. Polarographic analyzers use a battery to polarize the gas sampling probe. Because of this, they have a faster response time than do the galvanic fuel cell types. Galvanic fuel cell analyzers do not need a battery for power. However, they usually include alarms that are battery powered.

Failure to calibrate either type can be caused by a weak battery, an exhausted supply of chemical reactant in the gas sampling probe, an electronic failure, or a damaged membrane over the probe. A damaged or torn probe will allow water, mucus, or blood onto the probe. The galvanic units must have their probes kept dry to be read accurately. Both types are pressure sensitive. High altitude causes them to display a lower-than-true oxygen percentage, and high pressure as seen in a ventilator circuit with positive end-expiratory pressure (PEEP) causes the units to display a higher-than-true oxygen percentage.

4. Specialty gas analyzers

Specialty gas analyzers (helium, nitrogen, and carbon monoxide) are used mainly with pulmonary function testing procedures and are discussed in Chapter 4. It may be necessary to use a helium analyzer if a helium and oxygen mix is given to a patient.

Nitric oxide (NO) is delivered through the INOvent delivery system (Datex-Ohmeda, Inc., Madison, WI). It is able to deliver set amounts of therapeutic NO and to continuously monitor the amount of NO given to the patient along with nitrogen dioxide (NO_2) and oxygen.

3. Perform quality control procedures for oxygen analyzers (Code: IIC2) [Difficulty: ELE: R, Ap; WRE: An]

A two-point calibration procedure is done on all oxygen analyzers by sampling room air, adjusting a calibration control if necessary to have the unit show 21% oxygen (first point or low oxygen check), sampling 100% oxygen, and adjusting a calibration control if necessary to have the unit show 100% oxygen (second point or high oxygen check). When room air is sampled again, the analyzer should read 21% oxygen. In general, always follow the manufacturer's guidelines for setup and calibration. If an analyzer does not pass the two-point calibration check, it should not be used.

MODULE B
Storage, hardware, and distribution of medical gases

1. Manipulate oxygen and other gas cylinders, bulk storage systems, and manifolds, by order or protocol (ELE code: IIA9a) [Difficulty: ELE: R, Ap, An]

a. Get the necessary equipment for the procedure

b. Put the equipment together and make sure that it works properly

c. Troubleshoot any problems with the equipment

1. Oxygen and other gas cylinders

The different types of gases in cylinders are identified by the color code of the cylinder and the cylinder label. Note that only E cylinders have mandatory color coding. Color codings on the other cylinders are voluntary but usually are followed by the manufacturers. However, always read the label to be sure of the contents of the cylinder. The most important cylinder colors to remember are those of oxygen and air, but all are included in Table 6-1 for the sake of completeness.

Exam Hint 6-2 (ELE)

The NBRC is known to ask the examinee to calculate how long a certain cylinder lasts at a given gas flow. To date, only the durations of E-, H-, and K-sized oxygen cylinders have had to be calculated.

To review how to calculate the duration of flow for a particular type of cylinder, see Table 6-2 for the cylinder duration factors, the following equation, and the following examples.

$$\text{Minutes of flow (divide by 60 to calculate hours)} = \frac{\text{Gauge pressure in psig} \times \text{Cylinder factor}}{\text{Liter flow}}$$

1. Calculate the duration of flow of an E cylinder with 1500 pounds per square inch gauge (psig) that is running at 6 L/min.

$$\begin{aligned}\text{Minutes of flow}\\ \text{(divide by 60 to}\\ \text{calculate hours)}\end{aligned} = \frac{1500 \text{ psig} \times 0.28}{6 \text{ L}}$$

$$= \frac{420}{6}$$

Minutes of flow = 70 (1.16 hr, or 1 hr and 10 min)

2. Calculate the duration of flow of an H cylinder with 1950 psig that is running at 9 L/min.

$$\begin{aligned}\text{Minutes of flow}\\ \text{(divide by 60 to}\\ \text{calculate hours)}\end{aligned} = \frac{1950 \text{ psig} \times 3.14}{9 \text{ L}}$$

$$= \frac{6123}{9}$$

Minutes of flow = 680.33 (11.34 hr, or 11 hr and 20 min)

2. Bulk storage systems

The bulk liquid oxygen (LOX) storage system is the main source of a hospital's oxygen. A reducing valve is used to decrease the gas pressure to 50 pounds per square inch gauge (psig) before it is piped throughout the hospital for easy access. Alarms will sound if the pressure is low or too high. Pressure relief valves will open if the pressure is greater than 75 psig. Zone valves are located throughout the hospital so the gas can be turned off if a leak develops or if a fire occurs.

TABLE 6-1	Color Codes for Gas Cylinders
Gas	**Color**
Oxygen	Green (white for international)
Air	Yellow
Helium	Brown
Helium and oxygen	Brown and green (check the label for the percentage of each gas)
Carbon dioxide	Gray
Carbon dioxide	Gray and green (check the label for oxygen and the percentage of each gas)
Nitrous oxide	Light blue
Cyclopropane	Orange
Ethylene	Red

TABLE 6-2	Oxygen Cylinder Duration of Flow Factors
Cylinder Size	**Factor, L/psig**
E	0.28
H	3.14
K	3.14
D	0.16
M	1.36
G	2.41

psig, Pounds per square inch gauge.

3. Manifolds

A manifold is a piping system that connects the bulk storage system and the hospital gas piping system with a bank of H- or K-sized cylinders. These free-standing cylinders are a backup source of oxygen in case the bulk system fails. A 24-hour supply of gas must be available.

The manifold system includes a reducing valve to decrease the gas pressure to 50 psig. Check valves are built into the manifold so that a leak in one cylinder connection cannot result in all of the gas cylinders leaking out.

2. Manipulate adjunct hardware, such as reducing valves, flowmeters, regulators, and high-pressure hose connectors, by order or protocol (ELE code: IIA9a) [Difficulty: R, Ap, An]

a. Get the necessary equipment for the procedure

b. Put the equipment together and make sure that it works properly

c. Troubleshoot any problems with the equipment

1. Reducing valves

Reducing valves are used to reduce the high pressure seen in a bulk oxygen storage system, manifold, or gas cylinder.

One or more stages (pressure-reducing steps) can be used to reach the working pressure of 50 psig. Single-stage reducing valves reach the pressure in a single step. Multiple-stage reducing valves give finer control over pressure and flow by decreasing pressure in the first stage to about 200 psig and to 50 psig in the second stage. Occasionally, three stages are seen. All reducing valves (and regulators [combined reducing valve and flowmeter]) have the following built-in safety features:

- A frangible disk that breaks to release gas pressure in the event of mechanical failure or breakage
- A fusible plug that melts to release gas pressure in the event of a fire
- American Standard Compressed Gas Cylinder Valve Outlet and Index Connections (usually called the American Standard Safety System [ASSS]), which prevent the accidental connection of the wrong reducing valve (or regulator) to a large gas cylinder
- The Pin Index Safety System (PISS) is a special section of the American Standard System that applies to gas cylinders that are E-sized and smaller. It is designed to prevent an accidental connection of the wrong gas to a reducing valve or regulator. These reducing valves and regulators are designed with a specifically pinned yoke to wrap around the valve stem of a gas cylinder. A soft plastic O-ring washer is included to help ensure a tight seal. Figure 6-1 shows the location of the pinholes in the cylinder

valve face. Table 6-3 shows the gases and pinhole positions. It is important to know the positions for oxygen and air; the others are included for the sake of completeness.

It is necessary to "crack" or blow some gas out of a cylinder before putting any reducing valve or regulator onto the cylinder. Do this by attaching the tank wrench to the valve stem and slowly turning the valve stem in a counterclockwise (so-called "lefty-loosy") direction to release some gas. This cracking is done to prevent any dust or debris from being forced into the reducing valve or regulator, which might cause a fire. See Figure 6-2 for a schematic drawing of an "E" tank of oxygen and how its yoke is connected. If the O-ring is missing or the yoke is misaligned on the post, a high-pressure gas leak will occur when the tank is opened with the tank wrench. Close off the tank to stop the leak by turning the tank wrench on the valve stem in a clockwise direction (so-called "righty-tighty"). Investigate the yoke-to-post connection to identify causes of the leak.

2. Flowmeters

Flowmeters are designed to regulate and indicate flow. They come with the following safety features so that they cannot be attached to the wrong reducing valve, regulator, high-pressure hose, or appliance:

- Diameter Index Safety System (DISS) inlets and outlets that are specific to the various gases, so a mixup with the wrong appliance or connector cannot occur. The DISS system applies to flowmeters that attach to all American Standard and DISS reduction valves.
- Flowmeters with quick-connect inlet adapters instead of DISS inlets. These quick-connects are designed specifically for the hospital's piped-in oxygen and air outlets. They are not interchangeable between gases or between manufacturers. Occasionally a piped oxygen outlet will jam open and will let gas rapidly escape. Insert the proper flowmeter into

Figure 6-1   Locations of the Pin Index Safety System holes in the cylinder valve face. *(Modified from Branson RD, Hess DR, Chatburn RL: Respiratory care equipment, ed 2, Philadelphia, 1999, Lippincott Williams & Wilkins.)*

TABLE 6-3	Pin Index Safety System Gases and Pinhole Locations

Gas	Pinhole Locations
Oxygen	2-5
Air	1-5
Oxygen/carbon dioxide (≤7%)	2-6
Oxygen/carbon dioxide (>7%)	1-6
Oxygen/helium (not >80% helium)	2-4
Oxygen/helium (helium >80%)	4-6
Nitrous oxide	3-5
Ethylene	1-3
Cyclopropane	3-6

Figure 6-2 Details of an "E" size tank of oxygen and its yoke connector. **A,** A cross section through the stem (also called the control valve) of the tank shows its key features. **B,** A three-dimensional view shows how the yoke with its two pins aligns with the corresponding pin holes (locations 2 and 5) on the yoke. The plastic washer ensures a seal between the gas outlet on the stem and the yoke. (Not shown is the regulator that attaches to the yoke. See Figure 6-9.) **C,** A tank wrench that is attached to the valve stem (also called a control valve). Turn the wrench in a counterclockwise direction to open the tank and allow gas flow; close the tank to stop gas flow by turning the wrench in a clockwise direction. *(Redrawn from Sills JR: Respiratory care for the health care provider, Albany, 1998, Delmar Publishers.)*

the outlet, and turn the flowmeter off. This stops the leak until the defective wall outlet can be repaired.

Flowmeters usually are categorized by how they react to backpressure. To complicate matters further, we must remember that the three different manufactured types of flowmeters may or may not be backpressure compensated:

1. Non–backpressure-compensated (pressure-uncompensated) flowmeters will inaccurately indicate the flow through them in the face of backpressure. Figures 6-3 and 6-4 show non–backpressure-compensated kinetic and Thorpe types of flowmeters, respectively. Note that the Thorpe and kinetic flowmeters have the flow-control valve upstream from the meter. They read accurately if they are kept upright and do not have to "push" against any backpressure. If laid on their sides, the plunger and ball bearing do not indicate the set flow. They both read a lower flow than that actually delivered when faced with a backpressure.

2. The Bourdon flowmeter is designed similarly to the Bourdon gauge in the reducing valve (Figure 6-5). The face piece is marked in liters of flow rather than pressure. It is the flowmeter of choice in a transport situation because it may be laid flat with no effect

Figure 6-3 Kinetic-type non–backpressure-compensated (pressure-uncompensated) flowmeter. *(Modified from McPherson SP: Respiratory care equipment, ed 4, St Louis, 1990, Mosby.)*

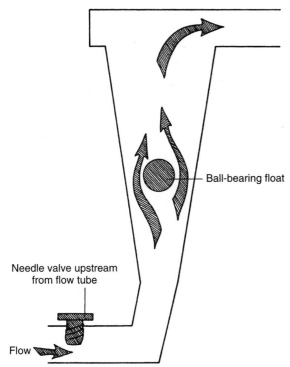

Figure 6-4 Thorpe-type non–backpressure-compensated (pressure-uncompensated) flowmeter. *(Modified from McPherson SP:* Respiratory care equipment, *ed 4, St Louis, 1990, Mosby.)*

Figure 6-5 Bourdon-type non–backpressure-compensated (pressure-uncompensated) flowmeter. *(From McPherson SP:* Respiratory care equipment, *ed 4, St Louis, 1990, Mosby.)*

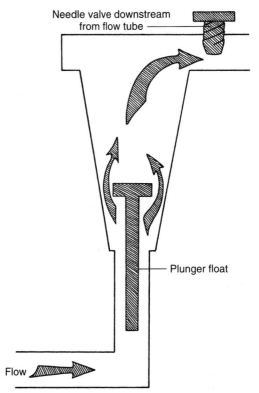

Figure 6-6 Kinetic-type backpressure-compensated (pressure-compensated) flowmeter. *(Modified from McPherson SP:* Respiratory care equipment, *ed 4, St Louis, 1990, Mosby.)*

to its flow if no backpressure is present. These flow-meters will display a higher flow than that actually delivered when faced with a backpressure.

3. Backpressure-compensated (pressure-compensated) flowmeters accurately indicate the flow through them in the face of backpressure. For this reason, they should be used whenever possible. Figures 6-6 and 6-7 show backpressure-compensated kinetic

and Thorpe types of flowmeters, respectively. Note that both of these flowmeters have the flow-control valve downstream from the meter. Because of this, they read accurately in the face of backpressure as long as they are kept upright. Besides reading the label, this simple test enables the practitioner to tell whether a flowmeter is backpressure compensated:

1. Make sure the flowmeter is turned off.
2. Plug the flowmeter into a gas outlet.
3. If the float or ball bearing bounces, the flowmeter is backpressure compensated.

d. Perform quality control procedures for flowmeters (Code: IIC6) [Difficulty: ELE: R, Ap; WRE: An]

When a quality control procedure for a flowmeter is performed, it is critical that a known flow be sent through it so that the flowmeter can be checked for accuracy. This should be done without any backpressure against the flowmeter. Review the previous discussion on troubleshooting flowmeters for the effects of backpressure on non–backpressure-compensated flowmeters and Bourdon flowmeters. Do not use any flowmeter that does not give an accurate reading.

Figure 6-7   Thorpe-type backpressure-compensated (pressure-compensated) flowmeter. *(Modified from McPherson SP: Respiratory care equipment, ed 4, St Louis, 1990, Mosby.)*

Figure 6-8   Drawing of the key components and features of a single-stage regulator. A regulator is composed of a reducing valve for the high tank pressure and a flowmeter. Gas pressure is shown on the cylinder gauge. Also shown is a Thorpe-type backpressure-compensated flowmeter. *(From Cario J, Pilbeam S: Mosby's Respiratory Therapy Equipment, ed 8, St Louis, 2010, Mosby.)*

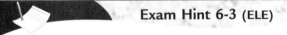

Exam Hint 6-3 (ELE)

Choose a backpressure-compensated flowmeter in all situations except during patient transport, when the oxygen tank and flowmeter might be laid flat. Then a Bourdon flowmeter should be used.

---

1. Regulators

Regulators combine a reducing valve and a flowmeter (Figure 6-8). Everything that has been discussed so far relates to regulators. Bourdon gauge reducing valves usually are seen and can have a second Bourdon gauge added as a flowmeter (Figure 6-9) or a Thorpe or kinetic flowmeter. As mentioned earlier, use a backpressure-compensated flowmeter in all situations except for patient transport.

2. High-pressure hose connectors

These connectors and other adapters connect high-pressure hoses, flowmeters, and oxygen appliances. They have DISS inlets and outlets so that the gases cannot be cross-fitted to the wrong equipment.

3. Manipulate pulse-dose oxygen-conserving devices by order or protocol (ELE code: IIA9b) [Difficulty: R, Ap, An]

a. Get the necessary equipment for the procedure

Three types of intermittent-flow oxygen-conserving devices are available: pulse-dose oxygen delivery devices (PDODs), demand oxygen delivery systems (DODSs), and hybrid units. All are used in the home care setting and save money by delivering oxygen to the patient only during inspiration. These units take the place of a regulator and flowmeter that deliver a steady flow of oxygen to the patient.

The characteristics of each unit will vary depending on the manufacturer. However, the following main operational features are found:

- A pulse-dose system delivers a bolus of oxygen at the start of the inspiratory cycle and shuts off before the end of inspiration.
- A demand system provides a continuous flow of oxygen throughout inspiration.
- A hybrid system combines features of the pulse-dose and demand systems. Cycling mechanisms vary but

Figure 6-9 Drawing of an "E" tank of oxygen showing how the yoke and regulator are connected and their features. A Bourdon-type pressure gauge is shown. Turn the crank to let gas flow through the Bourdon-type non–backpressure-compensated (pressure-uncompensated) flowmeter. A nipple adapter is attached for the connection of small-bore oxygen tubing. If the nipple adapter is unscrewed, a bubble-type humidifier or other oxygen delivery system can be attached. **Note:** This type of regulator is recommended for patient transportation if the "E" tank must be placed horizontally. *(Redrawn from Sills JR:* Respiratory care for the health care provider, *Albany, 1998, Delmar Publishers.)*

Figure 6-10 A pulse-dose oxygen delivery system with its key features shown. A specific type of nasal cannula is needed with this system. One channel transmits the negative pressure from the patient's inspiration back to the demand valve. This negative pressure opens the demand valve to allow a bolus of oxygen to travel down the second channel to the patient to inhale. *(From Cario J, Pilbeam S: Mosby's* Respiratory Therapy Equipment, *ed 8, St Louis, 2010, Mosby.)*

fall into two main categories. First, the unit may be set to time-cycle the oxygen flow on and turn it off. Second, the patient's negative inspiratory pressure will trigger the delivery of oxygen. See Figure 6-10. Depending on the manufacturer, the unit can be used with oxygen tanks, a low-pressure liquid oxygen (LOX)

system, or an oxygen concentrator. Be careful not to place a low-pressure unit on a high-pressure gas source because it will be damaged.

b. Put the equipment together and make sure that it works properly

With a pulse-dose system, the proximal end of a special nasal cannula is attached to a pressure sensor on the pulse-dose system. It senses a decrease in pressure as the patient inspires. The sensor then opens a demand valve that delivers a burst of oxygen to the cannula. See Figure 6-10. Because the nasal cannula is directly attached to the pressure sensor, a bubble-type humidifier cannot be added into the system.

Most of the units allow the respiratory therapist to work with the patient to adjust the sensor or timer to change how long the oxygen is delivered, how much is delivered, and whether the patient receives oxygen every breath or every second or third breath.

Make sure that the patient can feel a flow of gas from the cannula after he or she starts to inhale. The gas should stop during exhalation. Check the patient's pulse oximetry value at rest and during exercise to ensure that desaturation does not occur. Adjust the pressure sensor or timer to meet the patient's oxygen needs.

c. Troubleshoot any problems with the equipment

If the patient cannot feel any oxygen flowing, the following should be considered: (1) the source of oxygen might be empty, (2) the tubing might be disconnected or kinked, or (3) the sensor may not be detecting the patient's effort. The patient or therapist can switch to a second oxygen source and look for disconnections or kinks in the tubing. The therapist must adjust the nasal cannula or sensor to correct for a sensitivity problem. Do not use a system that is malfunctioning and cannot be adjusted.

4. Manipulate air compressors by order or protocol (Code: IIA9f) [Difficulty: ELE: R, Ap; WRE: An]

a. Get the necessary equipment for the procedure

b. Put the equipment together and make sure that it works properly

c. Troubleshoot any problems with the equipment

Air compressors are used whenever a high-pressure gas source other than oxygen is needed. All three systems are alike in that they use an electrically powered motor, filter the room air as it enters and exits the compressor, and have a condenser to remove water vapor as it leaves the compressor. See Figure 6-11.

1. Rotary-type compressors

Rotary-type compressors generate pressure with a rotating fan. They are used commonly in volume ventilators and in the home to power hand-held medication nebulizers. (See Figure 6-12.)

Figure 6-11 A piston-type large-volume medical air compressor. These units are used in hospitals or medical facilities. On the downstroke, the piston draws in room air that is then compressed into the reservoir tank on the upstroke. A pressure switch automatically turns the motor on and off to keep the pressure constant. As the compressed air leaves the reservoir tank, any water vapor is removed before it goes to the pressure-reducing valve. The piping system carries the air at 50 psig to any respiratory care equipment that is in use. *(From Wilkins RL, Stoller JK, Kacmarek RM, editors:* Egan's fundamentals of respiratory care, *ed 9, St Louis, 2009, Mosby.)*

2. Diaphragm-type compressors

Diaphragm-type compressors generate pressure with a diaphragm that moves up and down within a cylinder-like piston. They also are used commonly in the home to power hand-held medication nebulizers.

3. Piston-type compressors

Piston-type compressors generate pressure through piston action within a cylinder. They are much more powerful than the previous two types of compressors. Because they are designed to generate pressures of 50 psig or greater, they are used in the hospital with its piped air system. They also are used in the home setting in oxygen concentrators.

Make sure that all of these units are operational by checking that the inlet and outlet filters are cleaned. Dirty filters prevent proper airflow. Check the unit's pressure gauge to make sure that it is able to meet its manufacturer's specified pressure. Empty the water trap on the condensing unit as needed.

5. Manipulate air/oxygen proportioners (blenders) by order or protocol (ELE code: IIA9a) [Difficulty: ELE: R, Ap, An]

a. Get the necessary equipment for the procedure

Oxygen blenders are designed to change the ratio of oxygen and air to blend the specific percentage of oxygen from 21% to 100% (Figure 6-13). They are used whenever high-pressure gas is needed and the oxygen percentage may need frequent adjustment.

Figure 6-12 Photograph of a portable air compressor for home use. It is powered electrically with an on/off switch. Note the small-bore tubing that takes the compressed air to the small-volume nebulizer to aerosolize a medication. *(From Wilkins RL, Stoller JK, Kacmarek RM, editors:* Egan's fundamentals of respiratory care, *ed 9, St Louis, 2009, Mosby.)*

Figure 6-13   Example of an oxygen blender. Note the high-pressure air and oxygen hoses entering the bottom of the unit, the dial used to set the oxygen percentage (75%), and the blended oxygen outlet to the right. In this case, a Wye connector has been attached with two oxygen flowmeters. *(From Cairo JM, Pilbeam SP: Mosby's respiratory care equipment, ed 8, St Louis, 2009, Mosby.)*

b. Put the equipment together and make sure that it works properly

The oxygen and air gas sources must be pressurized to 50 psig. This can be done by taking both gases from the hospital's gas piping system or from gas cylinders. High-pressure hoses connect the gas sources with the blender. The desired oxygen percentage is set simply by adjusting the knob to the desired amount. Because the blended gases are under pressure, they must be sent directly to a mechanical ventilator or other device that uses 50 psig or through an added flowmeter.

With a blender, the oxygen percentage will remain close to the desired amount even if a small decrease in one or both line pressures occurs. Always analyze the oxygen percentage to confirm that it is correct.

c. Troubleshoot any problems with the equipment

Keep the gas inlets and outlets clear of any debris. All current units give an audible whistle if one or both of the line pressures decrease to an unsafe level (often about 30 psig). If the unit has a water trap at the compressed air inlet, keep it emptied of any condensate.

Figure 6-14   Drawing of the components of a molecular sieve oxygen concentrator. The molecular sieve beds remove nitrogen and pass oxygen through to the patient. *(Courtesy Sunrise Medical, Inc., Somerset, PA.)*

d. Independently set up or change an oxygen blender (ELE code: IIIF2d2) [Difficulty: ELE: R, Ap, An]

As mentioned previously, a blender is indicated whenever 50 psig gas is needed and frequent oxygen percentage changes are likely.

6. Manipulate oxygen concentrators (Code: IIA9c) [Difficulty: ELE: R, Ap; WRE: An] and portable oxygen concentrators (WRE code: IIA9e) [Difficulty: WRE: R, Ap, An] by order or protocol

a. Get the necessary equipment for the procedure

Two different types of oxygen concentrators (also known as oxygen enrichers) are available for the delivery of continuous low-flow oxygen in the home: molecular sieve and semipermeable plastic membrane.

1. Molecular sieve

Molecular sieve-type oxygen concentrators use an air compressor to push room air through two canisters of zeolite pellets (inorganic sodium-aluminum silicate) to remove nitrogen and water vapor. The remaining oxygen is delivered to the patient through a flowmeter (Figure 6-14). Be aware that with this unit, the oxygen percentage varies inversely with the flow that is delivered (Table 6-4).

2. Semipermeable plastic membrane

Semipermeable plastic membrane oxygen concentrators make use of a very thin plastic membrane as a filter. Room air is pulled through it by a vacuum pump. Molecular oxygen and water vapor can pass through the membrane faster than nitrogen. Any excess water vapor is removed by a simple condenser system. No need exists to add an external humidification system to the flowmeter (Figure 6-15). The oxygen percentage is fixed at 40% in these units;

Figure 6-15 Functional schematic of a semipermeable membrane oxygen concentrator. The membrane permits more oxygen and water vapor than nitrogen to pass through. *(Courtesy of the Oxygen Enrichment Company, Schenectady, NY.)*

TABLE 6-4	Comparison of Flow Rates and Oxygen Percentages in Oxygen Concentrators

Flow, L/min	Approximate Oxygen Percentage
MOLECULAR SIEVE CONCENTRATOR	
1-2	95%-92%
3-5	92%-85%
>6	<85%
SEMIPERMEABLE MEMBRANE CONCENTRATOR	
1-10	40%

however, the flow can be varied from 1 to 10 L/min, as shown in Table 6-4.

When one is deciding which type of concentrator to use, it is important to know the patient's required oxygen percentage and flow. As can be seen from Table 6-4, the molecular sieve units can deliver a higher oxygen percentage at any liter flow as compared with the semipermeable plastic membrane units.

3. Portable oxygen concentrators

Some oxygen concentrators are now small enough to be carried by the patient or can be used to fill a portable oxygen tank. The Venture HomeFill II (Invacare, North Rocks, Australia) is a home-use oxygen concentrator combined with a compressor. This allows a small portable oxygen tank to be filled, in the home, from the oxygen concentrator. The Inogen One System (Inogen, Inc., Goleta, CA) is battery powered and includes a pulse-dose nasal cannula oxygen delivery system. This unit allows the home care patient great flexibility in the home and in travel with portable oxygen delivery.

b. Put the equipment together and make sure that it works properly

c. Troubleshoot any problems with the equipment

The molecular sieve–type units deliver dry gas; therefore a humidification system is frequently added to the flowmeter. With the permeable plastic membrane–type units, the condensed water vapor must be emptied from the collection jar. In both types of oxygen concentrators, it is important to check the air-inlet filter on a monthly basis to keep it clean of dust and debris. Follow the manufacturer's requirements regarding when filters should be replaced. The delivered oxygen concentration also should be checked each month. Follow the manufacturer's guidelines for its preventative maintenance needs. The molecular sieve–type units must have the zeolite pellet canisters replaced on a scheduled basis.

Some units have a visual or audio alarm that warns when a problem occurs, such as power failure, low or high pressure, or low oxygen percentage. If the unit does not have a low oxygen percentage alarm, some home care practitioners have added an external analyzer with an alarm system. This alerts the patient to call the home care company to repair the equipment. If a patient says that he or she cannot feel any gas coming out of the cannula, have the patient place the prongs into a glass of water. If no bubbling is seen, have the patient check the tubing for any disconnections. If the concentrator is malfunctioning, have the patient turn it off and switch to oxygen from the backup oxygen cylinder until repairs can be made.

7. Manipulate portable liquid oxygen systems by order or protocol (WRE code: IIA9d) [Difficulty: WRE: R, Ap, An]

a. Get the necessary equipment for the procedure

A LOX system is used in the home when it is found to be more cost-effective than an oxygen concentrator or a battery of oxygen cylinders. An additional advantage is that the patient can carry a smaller portable unit in a shoulder bag for added mobility. Carrying it is less conspicuous than wheeling an E cylinder about. An early, widely known liquid oxygen system was the Linde Walker System (Union Carbide, Houston, TX). Figure 6-16 shows the key features of a large liquid oxygen reservoir that is kept in the patient's home. Figure 6-17 shows its smaller portable companion, which can be filled from the large reservoir.

b. Put the equipment together and make sure that it works properly

Current portable liquid oxygen systems weigh only a few pounds and can be carried over the shoulder by a strap. They can be refilled from the larger reservoir tank kept in the home. The flow rate can be adjusted to meet most patients' needs. Humidification is provided by the patient's own airway. As with any pressurized system, all fittings must be kept tight to prevent leakage.

The National Fire Protection Agency (NFPA) has established several regulations to ensure that home LOX systems are installed safely. Key safety regulations include the following:

- Stabilize the unit to prevent it from being tipped over.
- The reservoir unit should not be set up near any radiators, steam pipes, or heat ducts to reduce the rate of oxygen loss.
- No open flames or sources of ignition can be within 5 feet of the unit.
- "No smoking" signs must be posted.

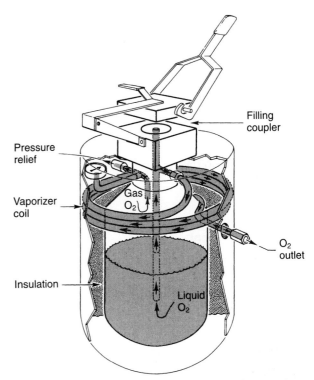

Figure 6-16 Drawing of the components of a home liquid oxygen supply unit. *(From Lampton LM: Home and outpatient oxygen therapy. In: Brashear RE, Rhodes ML, editors:* Chronic obstructive lung disease, *St Louis, 1978, Mosby.)*

Figure 6-17 Drawing of the components of a portable liquid oxygen unit. *(From Lampton LM: Home and outpatient oxygen therapy. In: Brashear RE, Rhodes ML, editors:* Chronic obstructive lung disease, *St Louis, 1978, Mosby.)*

- The patient and the family must be instructed on how to use the equipment. This includes how to fill the portable unit from the large reservoir tank. That person should wear safety goggles with side shields, loose-fitting insulated gloves, and high-top boots.
- If liquid oxygen spills and contacts skin, it can cause frostbite. Medical attention should be sought immediately.
- For at least 15 minutes, avoid contact with any equipment or the floor where liquid oxygen has spilled.

c. Troubleshoot any problems with the equipment

Check that all connections are airtight to avoid spills and minimize the loss of oxygen. Make sure that the unit is functioning at its designed working pressure. Check that the pressure relief valve operates properly and that proper oxygen flow is delivered.

d. Independently modify a liquid oxygen system (ELE code: IIIF2d3) [Difficulty: ELE: R, Ap]

A home care therapist may need to adjust the flow of oxygen, within guidelines established by the physician, to maintain patient oxygenation.

Exam Hint 6-5 (WRE)

Most past examinations have questioned the need to set up a liquid oxygen supply unit and portable unit for a home care patient or troubleshooting problems with the system. A patient may be expected to check for oxygen flowing through a cannula by placing the prongs under water to look for bubbling or by switching from the liquid oxygen system to a backup source of oxygen such as an oxygen cylinder (tank). The patient should not be expected to troubleshoot problems with the liquid oxygen (LOX) system or perform maintenance work on it. That is the home care respiratory therapist's job.

8. Manipulate helium/oxygen equipment by order or protocol (WRE code: IIA15) [Difficulty: WRE: R, Ap, An]

a. Get the necessary equipment for the procedure

Helium/oxygen (He/O_2 [heliox]) has been used historically in the management of patients with an upper airway obstruction. This may include tracheal tumor, postextubation laryngeal edema, and croup. More recently, heliox has been used with success in patients with status asthmaticus. The decreased density of a helium/oxygen mix compared with a nitrogen/oxygen mix reduces the patient's work of breathing.

Various heliox gas mixtures come in high-pressure cylinders and require the use of an American Standard System reducing valve (or regulator) designed specifically for the gas or gas mix. As is shown in Table 6-3 and Figure 6-1, a reducing valve or regulator for an E cylinder must match the appropriate pinholes on the cylinder valve face. Corresponding high-pressure hoses also may be needed. Table 6-1 shows the color codes for the various gas cylinders. Pure helium comes in a brown cylinder, whereas helium and oxygen mixes come in brown and green cylinders. Always check the cylinder label for the exact percentage of the gases within it. Heliox comes in standard mixes of 80% He/20% O_2, 70% He/30% O_2, and 60% He/40% O_2.

b. Put the equipment together and make sure that it works properly

The additional equipment needed depends on how the ordered heliox mixture is to be delivered to the patient.

1. Nonrebreather mask

In most clinical situations, a nonrebreather mask with reservoir bag is used to deliver heliox to a spontaneously breathing patient. A snugly fitting mask with one-way valves and a full reservoir bag will minimize breathing of any room air. (The next Module includes additional discussion on nonrebreather masks.) A helium flowmeter can be used to set the flow of heliox to the face mask. However, if a helium flowmeter is not available, an oxygen flowmeter can be added to the reducing valve on a heliox mix cylinder. In either case, set the gas flow high enough that the reservoir bag does not collapse on inspiration. The gas is humidified by attaching to the flowmeter a bubble humidifier with sterile water. Connect small-bore tubing between the humidifier nipple and the nonrebreather mask nipple.

If the patient is being treated for asthma, the nonrebreather mask can be modified to accept a small-volume nebulizer for bronchodilator medication delivery. (See Figure 6-18.) Care must be taken if the nebulizer is powered by the heliox mix, as shown. Some nebulizers will not operate normally. It may be necessary to increase the heliox flow by 50% to 100% from the usual rate of oxygen flow to get the unit to operate properly. Others simply choose to power the nebulizer with oxygen, as intended, for the treatment.

In the common situation where an oxygen flowmeter is being used, a calculation must be done to convert the flow seen on the oxygen flowmeter to the actual flow of heliox. This is necessary because helium is less dense than oxygen.

Often one question requires the calculation of actual flow of a heliox mixture. The heliox factor must be known to do the calculation. One possible calculation involves figuring out the heliox flow from an observed flow through an oxygen flowmeter. The other possible calculation involves setting the observed flow through an oxygen flowmeter to achieve the desired heliox flow. See the following sample calculations.

The heliox factor must be used to determine the actual flow of heliox through an oxygen flowmeter, as follows:

Helium/Oxygen Ratio	Heliox Factor
1. 80% helium/20% oxygen	1.8
2. 70% helium/30% oxygen	1.6
3. 60% helium/40% oxygen	1.4

The following examples show how the actual heliox flow can be calculated from the observed oxygen flow seen on the flowmeter:

1. When using an 80% helium and 20% oxygen mix, multiply the observed flow by the heliox factor of 1.8.
   Example: Observed oxygen flow of 10 L/min × 1.8 = 18 L/min actual heliox flow.
2. When using a 70% helium and 30% oxygen mix, multiply the observed flow by the heliox factor of 1.6.
   Example: Observed oxygen flow of 10 L/min × 1.6 = 16 L/min actual heliox flow.
3. When using a 60% helium and 40% oxygen mix, multiply the observed flow by the heliox factor of 1.4.
   Example: Observed oxygen flow of 10 L/min × 1.4 = 14 L/min actual heliox flow.

The following examples show how to set an oxygen flowmeter to deliver a needed heliox flow by dividing the desired flow by the heliox factor:

1. When using an 80% helium and 20% oxygen mix, determine the observed flowmeter setting to deliver an actual heliox flow of 10 L/min.
   Example: $\dfrac{10\,\text{L/min heliox desired}}{1.8} = 5.6\,\text{L/min set on}$
   the oxygen flowmeter.
2. When using a 70% helium and 30% oxygen mix, determine the observed flowmeter setting to deliver an actual heliox flow of 10 L/min.
   Example: $\dfrac{10\,\text{L/min heliox desired}}{1.6} = 6.3\,\text{L/min set on}$
   the oxygen flowmeter.
3. When using a 60% helium and 40% oxygen mix, determine the observed flowmeter setting to deliver an actual heliox flow of 10 L/min.
   Example: $\dfrac{10\,\text{L/min heliox desired}}{1.4} = 7.1\,\text{L/min set on}$
   the oxygen flowmeter.

Figure 6-18 A modified nonrebreathing mask and reservoir bag for delivering helium/oxygen. The Y-connector allows the heliox to be breathed from the reservoir bag while the nebulizer is aerosolizing a bronchodilator medication. A separate flowmeter is used for each component. Use enough heliox flow to keep the reservoir bag from collapsing. The nebulizer can be powered by heliox, as shown, or by oxygen. *(From Hess DR: Nonconventional respiratory therapeutics. In: Hess DR, MacIntyre NR, Mishoe SC, et al, editors: Respiratory care principles & practices, Philadelphia, 2002, WB Saunders.)*

2. Mechanical ventilator

Delivering a helium/oxygen mix through a ventilator presents several technical challenges. First, select a ventilator that has been approved by the U.S. Food and Drug Administration (FDA) to deliver a heliox mix. In many ventilators, the decreased density of helium causes flow and volume sensors (usually a flow-type pneumotachometer) to read inaccurately. If a nonapproved ventilator needs to be used, it is recommended that pressure ventilation be used rather than volume ventilation. The risk with volume ventilation is the potential delivery of a larger tidal volume than that set on the ventilator. In addition, measure the patient's exhaled tidal volume with a bellows-type spirometer rather than a pneumotachometer.

Connect the pure helium or heliox mix to the mechanical ventilator's internal air/oxygen proportioner (blender) through the high-pressure air inlet. High-pressure oxygen will go through on its side of the unit, as usual. If pure helium is mixed with pure oxygen, dial the oxygen percentage, as needed, to adjust the mix of the two gases. For example, giving the patient 35% oxygen results in the patient's also receiving 65% helium. However, if the patient is receiving a heliox mix (e.g., 70/30), more oxygen than is set on the blender will be delivered.

In any situation where a heliox mix is being used, the oxygen percentage must be measured. This is done to ascertain with certainty how much oxygen is being delivered and to ensure that the patient never receives less than 20% oxygen. Use a polarographic or galvanic fuel cell oxygen analyzer to monitor the patient's oxygen percentage.

Exam Hint 6-7 (WRE)

There is usually one question about starting heliox therapy for an asthma patient to reduce the work of breathing.

---

c. Troubleshoot any problems with the equipment

When using a nonrebreather mask, make sure that it is adjusted to give as tight a fit to the face as is practical and comfortable. All one-way valve flaps should open and close properly. Set the gas flow high enough that the reservoir bag does not collapse by more than one-third during inspiration. With a mechanical ventilator, make sure that the exhaled volume is measured accurately and that alarms are adjusted to actual patient values. With either system, it is extremely important that all connections be tight because helium easily leaks out of any openings. If the oxygen percentage is too low, be prepared to make the necessary adjustments. Clinical experience is recommended with the administration of helium/oxygen mixes.

MODULE C
Administration of oxygen therapy

1. Manipulate oxygen hoods by order or protocol (ELE code: IIA12c) [Difficulty: ELE: R, Ap]

a. Get the necessary equipment for the procedure

Oxygen hoods are used to provide a warmed aerosol, humidity, and a controlled oxygen percentage to pediatric

patients who weigh no more than 18 lb (8.2 kg). (See Figure 6-19.) Often the oxygen hood and the infant are placed inside of an incubator for better control of the environment and maintenance of body temperature. (See Chapter 8 for discussion on incubators.)

b. Put the equipment together and make sure that it works properly

When an oxygen hood is used, the following procedures should be observed:

- Use an air/oxygen proportioner with a flowmeter to control the oxygen percentage and flow to the hood. The flow should be at least 7 L/min to prevent the buildup of exhaled carbon dioxide. A flow of 10 to 15 L/min is needed to keep a stable oxygen percentage. Keeping the hood sealed as much as possible and minimizing the gap between the infant's neck and the opening to the hood also help to stabilize the oxygen percentage.
- A warmed humidifier is needed to provide a high humidity level and to warm the oxygen to the infant's body temperature. Care must be taken with infants to ensure that they are neither heated nor cooled by the gas blowing over their heads. A thermometer should be kept in the hood to note the temperature.
- An oxygen analyzer should continuously monitor how much oxygen is inside the hood. The analyzer probe should be placed at the same level as the infant's nose. This is because oxygen is heavier than air and tends to settle toward the bottom of the hood. The advantages of the hood over the oxygen tent (discussed below) are that the patient's body is accessible, and the head can be reached by lifting the top off of the hood.

c. Troubleshoot any problems with the equipment

Make sure that the oxygen and aerosol delivery systems are working properly and that the oxygen percentage can

Figure 6-19 Infant in an oxygen hood. (*Courtesy Utah Medical Products Midvale, Utah.*)

be maintained. Be aware of the noise level inside the hood to minimize damage to the infant's hearing. The sound level should be monitored and kept well below 65 dB.

2. Manipulate oxygen tents by order or protocol (ELE code: IIA12b) [Difficulty: ELE: R, Ap]

a. Get the necessary equipment for the procedure

Oxygen tents formerly were used for adults but now are used only for children who are too large and active for an oxygen hood. The tent is a clear plastic canopy used to control the environment by providing a cooled aerosol, humidity, and a controlled oxygen percentage (Figure 6-20).

b. Put the equipment together and make sure that it works properly

In addition to setup of the tent, the following must be done to make it operational:

1. Set an oxygen flowmeter to deliver 8 to 10 L/min to small tents and 12 to 15 L/min to large tents. Flows of 30 L/min or greater are needed to keep the oxygen percentage close to the 50% maximum that can be maintained reliably. (Commonly, between 35% and 50% oxygen can be kept in a tent.)
2. The oxygen should flow through a nebulizer or an ultrasonic unit to provide the needed humidity. Try to keep the relative humidity at 60% or greater to minimize any risk of a spark causing a fire inside the tent.
3. The tent must be cooled to prevent the patient from overheating the enclosed space. If the infant put into a tent has croup, the cooled air is therapeutic. A thermometer should be kept inside the tent for

continuous temperature monitoring. Be careful not to chill the infant.
4. An oxygen analyzer should continuously monitor how much oxygen is inside the tent. The analyzer probe should be placed at the same level as the infant's nose.

c. Troubleshoot any problems with the equipment

It can be difficult to maintain the ordered oxygen percentage inside the tent. Remember to close any opened ports when patient care is finished and to keep the canopy sealed with the bottom edges tucked under the mattress. Be prepared to increase or decrease the oxygen flow until the desired percentage is reached. The child should not be allowed to have any electrically powered toys inside the tent to minimize the risk of a spark and fire. Make sure the humidification and cooling systems are working properly.

3. Manipulate air entrainment devices and masks by order or protocol (ELE code: IIA1b) [Difficulty: ELE: R, Ap, An]

a. Get the necessary equipment for the procedure

Air entrainment masks are called high-flow devices because they are designed to provide the patient with a controlled oxygen percentage at a high enough flow rate to ensure that all of the patient's inspiratory flow needs are met (Figure 6-21). To ensure that this happens, the total flow through the mask must be equal to or greater

Figure 6-20   Timeter® CAM4™ Portable Child/Adult Mist Tent. *(Courtesy Allied Healthcare Products, Inc. St. Louis, Missouri).*

Figure 6-21   Adult wearing an air entrainment mask. *A*, High-velocity jet. *B*, An area of reduced lateral pressure (Bernoulli's principle). *C*, Room air entrainment. *(From White GC: Basic clinical lab competencies for respiratory care, an integrated approach, Albany, NY, 1988, Delmar.)*

TABLE 6-5	Specifications for Air Entrainment Devices and Masks				
Oxygen (%)	Approximate Air/Oxygen Ratio	Total Ratio Parts	Oxygen Flow Rate L/min*	Total Flow L/min
24	25:1	26	4	104
28	10:1	11	4	44
30	8:1	9	6	54
35	5:1	6	8	48
40	3:1	4	10	40
45	2:1	3	15	45
50	1.7:1	2.7	15	40.5

*These flow rates were selected to ensure that the minimum total flow through the system would be ≥40 L/min. The manufacturers may recommend other minimal O_2 flow rates.

than the patient's peak inspiratory flow. (The interested learner is encouraged to read about the Bernoulli principle, which regulates the mixing of fluids as the result of a decrease in pressure caused by a jet.) These masks are sometimes called Venturi masks, Venti masks, jet-mixing, and high airflow with oxygen enrichment (HAFOE) systems. See Table 6-5 for specific information on available air entrainment masks.

These masks are recommended in any clinical situation in which a known, precise oxygen percentage must be given to the patient who has a variable respiratory rate, inspiratory/expiratory (I:E) ratio, tidal volume, or minute volume. Common situations include a patient with COPD and a patient in respiratory failure who needs increasing oxygen percentages.

b. Put the equipment together and make sure that it works properly

Depending on the manufacturer, the mask my come as a completed unit, may have air entrainment adapters to add to the mask, or may have an air entrainment adapter to adjust to set the desired oxygen percentage. See Table 6-5 for the recommended starting oxygen flow rate for the different oxygen percentage masks. Because it is difficult to ensure that the patient's peak inspiratory flow is matched by the gas flow through the mask, the following guidelines are recommended:

- Make sure that the total flow through the mask is at least 40 L/min in a resting patient. More may be needed if the patient is breathing rapidly.
- Provide the patient with a total flow that is 4 to 6 times his or her measured minute volume.
- The total flow through the mask can be raised by increasing the oxygen flow. This should not significantly change the oxygen percentage because more room air is entrained to keep the same ratio.

However, to be certain, analyze the oxygen percentage inside the mask to ensure that it is as prescribed. The total flow through the mask can be calculated by adding the total of the ratio parts and multiplying by the oxygen flow rate.

Exam Hint 6-8 (ELE)

It has been necessary on past exams to calculate the needed change in the oxygen flow to increase the total gas flow to meet or exceed a patient's peak inspiratory flow. This ensures that the proper oxygen percentage is delivered.

Air Entrainment Mask Calculations

Example 1. Your patient has on a 28% air entrainment mask with an oxygen flow of 4 L/min. His condition worsens, and he increases his minute volume to 15 L/min. To ensure that he still receives his prescribed oxygen percentage, someone makes a recommendation to you to increase the oxygen liter flow to 6 L/min. The new total flow through the mask can be calculated as follows:
- a. 28% air entrainment mask has an air/oxygen ratio of 10:1.
- b. The sum of the ratio parts is 10 + 1 = 11.
- c. Total flow = 11 × 6 L/min oxygen flow = 66 L/min.
- d. This flow is more than 4 times the patient's current minute volume. He should have all of his flow needs met.
- e. Reanalyze the delivered oxygen percentage to make certain that it is as prescribed.

Example 2. Your patient is wearing a 40% air entrainment mask that has the manufacturer's suggested 8 L/min of oxygen running into it. Her peak inspiratory flow is about 48 L/min (0.75 L/sec). To what should her oxygen flow be changed to ensure that the total gas flow is greater than her peak inspiratory flow? The new oxygen flow to the mask can be calculated as follows:
- a. 40% air entrainment mask has an air/oxygen ratio of 3:1.
- b. The sum of the ratio parts is 3 + 1 = 4.
- c. Divide the sum of the ratio parts into the peak inspiratory flow: 48/4 = 12
- d. Increase the oxygen flow from 8 to 12 L/min.

Some patients may complain that the gas coming through the mask is dry. To resolve this problem, some manufacturers have designed an aerosol adapter to add at the jet. A separate bland aerosol then is added to the room air (21% oxygen that enters the jet stream). Make sure that the adapter fits properly and does not interfere with or block the jet or room air entrainment ports. Do not add a bubble-type humidifier to the jet on the mask because the high backpressure through the jet will cause the pressure relief (pop-off) valve to open, and the oxygen will leak out.

c. Troubleshoot any problems with the equipment

The two different types of air entrainment devices are based on the physical principles seen in the Bernoulli effect. It is important to know about the two different types to understand what can go wrong with them and how they can be fixed. Make sure that the correct liter flow of oxygen, jet size, and air entrainment port setting are selected to get the desired total flow and oxygen percentage.

1. Variable jet diameter

Notice that the jets have different diameters but the room air entrainment ports are the same size. You will see that the smaller the jet diameter is, the lower the oxygen percentage is. This is because as the jet becomes smaller, the lateral pressure is lower. This results in more room air being brought into the entrainment ports to dilute the oxygen and increase the total flow.

Make sure that the jets are not obstructed by mucus or anything else, or the oxygen percentage will be decreased. An obstruction downstream from the jet prevents the appropriate amount of room air from being brought into the mask. This results in the oxygen percentage increasing and the total flow decreasing.

2. Variable air entrainment ports

Notice that the jet size is fixed but the room air entrainment ports have different sizes. The smaller the entrainment ports, the higher the oxygen percentage. This is because less room air can be entrained to dilute the oxygen. The total flow is also reduced when the entrainment ports are smaller.

Make sure that the entrainment ports are not obstructed by the patient's sheet or anything else, or the oxygen percentage will increase. An obstruction downstream from the jet prevents the appropriate amount of air from being brought into the mask. This results in the oxygen percentage increasing and the total flow decreasing.

4. Manipulate a low-flow nasal cannula by order or protocol (ELE code: IIA1a) [Difficulty: ELE: R, Ap, An]

a. Get the necessary equipment for the procedure

The traditional nasal cannula is a low-flow oxygen delivery tube that has been modified with two short prongs to deliver oxygen to the nostrils (Figure 6-22). Nasal cannulas come in neonatal, pediatric, and adult sizes based on the diameter of the prongs. Care must be taken to make sure that the patient's nares are patent and are not plugged

Figure 6-22   Adult wearing a nasal cannula. (*From Wilkins RL, Stoller JK, Kacmarek RM, editors:* Egan's fundamentals of respiratory care, *ed 9, St Louis, 2009, Mosby.*)

by a common cold, a deviated septum, or another unseen problem. This simple oxygen delivery device is used very widely because it is more comfortable for many patients than an air entrainment mask or other types of face masks. Current clinical practice guidelines indicate that, in an adult, an oxygen flow of 4 L/min or less does not require additional humidification if the patient has a normal upper airway.

b. Put the equipment together and make sure that it works properly

If an adult is getting from 1 to 4 L/min of oxygen and complains of nasal dryness, or if a higher flow is given, humidification will have to be provided. Often this is a bubble-type humidifier, as discussed in Chapter 8. Make sure that it is properly filled with sterile water and that the oxygen bubbles through it. Check the high-pressure pop-off valve for pressure release and a whistling sound. Before placing the cannula on the patient, check to see that the oxygen is flowing through the tubing. If available, use a cannula with curved prongs. They direct the gas flow toward the back of the nasal passages for better natural humidification and are better for patient comfort. Take care to avoid pulling the elastic restraining band too tightly around the head. Some brands loop the oxygen tubing over the ears to be drawn up snugly under the chin. Often this type is more comfortable than the types that have an elastic band.

The problem with a nasal cannula is that the delivered oxygen percentage is unreliable. Variations in the patient's respiratory rate, I:E ratio, tidal volume, and minute volume result in different inhaled oxygen percentages. This is clearly unacceptable in an unstable patient in whom PaO_2 values are being used to help judge the changing cardiopulmonary status. Because of this clinical limi-

TABLE 6-6	Estimated Delivered Oxygen Percentage in Adults Based on the Oxygen Liter Flow Through a Nasal Cannula
Oxygen, L/min	Estimated Delivered Oxygen, %
1	24
2	28
3	32
4	36
5	40
6	44

tation, this device and the other low-flow oxygen delivery systems in the discussions that follow should be used only with stable patients. In the adult, the delivered oxygen percentage can be estimated at approximately 4% for each liter of oxygen per minute (Table 6-6). Flows usually are limited to 6 L/min to avoid excessive irritation to the nasal passages. Flows usually are limited to no more than 1 to 2 L/min in infants and 4 L/min in older children. The pulse oximetry value or PaO$_2$ level should be checked in patients of any age whenever a flow change is made or when the patient's condition changes significantly.

c. Troubleshoot any problems with the equipment

Replace a cannula that is obviously soiled or permanently obstructed. If a bubble-type humidifier is used, refill the water as needed and replace the humidifier according to protocol.

5. Manipulate an oxygen-conserving nasal cannula by order or protocol (ELE code: IIA9b) [Difficulty: ELE: R, Ap, An]

a. Get the necessary equipment for the procedure

Oxygen-conserving nasal cannulas are used for patients who need long-term, low-flow oxygen therapy and wish to reduce their costs.

b. Put the equipment together and make sure that it works properly

At least two different types of oxygen-conserving cannulas are found. Figure 6-23 shows a reservoir nasal cannula and how it operates. It has an 18-mL reservoir that fills when the patient exhales and gives up its oxygen bolus during the next inspiration. Figure 6-24 shows a pendant nasal cannula with its reservoir that hangs on the chest.

c. Troubleshoot any problems with the equipment

Both types of cannulas can have problems with tubing disconnections or kinks that can happen with any type of

Figure 6-23 Drawing of the Oximizer reservoir nasal cannula and its functions. *(Courtesy of CHAD Therapeutics, Chatsworth, CA.)*

Figure 6-24 Drawing of a patient wearing a pendant reservoir nasal cannula made by CHAD Therapeutics *(Chatsworth, CA). (From Wilkins RL, Stoller JK, Kacmarek RM, editors: Egan's fundamentals of respiratory care, ed 9, St Louis, 2009, Mosby.)*

cannula. The only problem that is unique to both of these units is failure of the diaphragm, which moves back and forth as the reservoir fills and empties. This membrane may wear out after about a week and prevent the reservoir from filling or emptying properly. Watch as the patient breathes to make sure that the diaphragm is moving properly. If not, replace the cannula.

6. Manipulate a high-flow nasal cannula by order or protocol (ELE code: IIA1c) [Difficulty: ELE: R, Ap, An]

a. Get the necessary equipment for the procedure

A high-flow nasal cannula (HFNC) is designed to provide warmed and humidified oxygen at a high enough flow rate to fully meet the patient's peak inspiratory flow needs. This type of nasal cannula is better tolerated by many severely hypoxic patients than a nonrebreather mask because it provides 100% relative humidity at body temperature (BTPS [body temperature, pressure, saturated gas] conditions), and there is no drying of the nasal mucosa. For these reasons, the HFNC has found a growing clinical application in adult and neonatal populations. Adults with congestive heart failure and pulmonary edema may be kept off of continuous positive airway pressure (CPAP) or mechanical ventilation through the use of an HFNC.

Early evidence indicates that an HFNC may be used with some premature neonates as an alternative to CPAP or mechanical ventilation. Evidence suggests that neonatal patients receiving HFNC have a positive mouth pressure of about 3 to 4 cm water, which corresponds to a similar CPAP level. However, this pressure is maintained only when the mouth is closed. There is also the risk that an HFNC will create a higher CPAP level than desired. So, the smallest possible nasal cannula should be used to allow for a leak.

Although future research will indicate the best patient populations and application methods for HFNC, currently three systems are available: Vapotherm 2000i (Vapotherm, Stevensville, MD), the Salter Labs (Arvin, CA) high-flow cannula and humidifier, and the AquinOx High Flow Humidification System (Smiths Medical ASD Inc., Kent, UK). The Vapotherm 2000i will be used in the following discussion.

b. Put the equipment together and make sure that it works properly

Figure 6-25 shows a Vapotherm 2000i that is opened to show the vapor transfer cartridge. Water is continuously supplied into the unit and is warmed before entering the cartridge to be vaporized to humidify the patient's oxygen. The temperature can be adjusted but usually is kept at body temperature. A pediatric cartridge will be used for a

Figure 6-25 The Vapotherm 2000i high-flow nasal cannula system. The vapor transfer cartridge is shown inside. It can be switched out as needed and is available in adult and pediatric sizes. *(Courtesy Vapotherm 2000i, Annapolis, MD.)*

flow of 1 to 8 L/min. An adult cartridge will be used for flows of 5 to 40 L/min. An oxygen hose is attached at the bottom of the unit and then is attached to the patient's nasal cannula. It is possible to attach the patient's nasal catheter (rarely used clinically anymore) or transtracheal oxygen catheter. The flow of oxygen is adjusted to meet the patient's clinical goal for oxygenation. The higher the oxygen flow, the higher the delivered oxygen percentage— possibly up to 100% oxygen.

c. Troubleshoot any problems with the equipment

Make sure that the proper vapor transfer cartridge is selected for the oxygen flow needed. Set the appropriate temperature. Make sure that the water supply system does not run out.

7. Manipulate oxygen masks: simple oxygen mask, partial-rebreathing mask, nonrebreathing mask, and face tent, by order or protocol (ELE code: IIA1a) [Difficulty: ELE: R, Ap, An]

a. Get the necessary equipment for the procedure

b. Put the equipment together and make sure that it works properly

c. Troubleshoot any problems with the equipment

1. Simple oxygen mask

This mask, like all others, is designed to fit over the patient's nose and mouth and act as an oxygen reservoir for the next breath (Figures 6-26 and 6-27). Various adult and pediatric sizes are available, and the patient should wear one that best fits the facial contours and size of the face. This is recommended for comfort, as well as to try to increase the inspired oxygen percentage by decreasing the amount of room air that is inspired. However, because a simple oxygen mask does not provide all of the patient's tidal volume gas, it is classified as a low-flow device. Exhaled breath escapes through the exhalation ports. The patient's breathing pattern affects the amount of room air that is breathed in through the same exhalation ports. These ports also are important in case the oxygen flow to the mask is cut off.

Because the oxygen reservoir in the mask is not large enough to meet the patient's tidal volume, the inspired oxygen percentage is unpredictable. Oxygen flows between 5 and 10 L/min should provide approximately 35% to 60% inspired oxygen. The pulse oximetry value or PaO_2 level should be checked whenever a flow change is made, or when the patient's condition changes significantly.

A bubble humidifier is often added so that the gas is not dry. Make sure that it works properly and that oxygen is flowing through the tubing before putting it on the patient. This and all other masks use an adjustable elastic strap that goes behind the head to hold it in place. Make sure that the mask fits snugly but not so tight as to cut off circulation.

2. Partial-rebreathing mask

The partial-rebreathing mask has a 500- to 1000-mL plastic bag added to the mask to act as an oxygen reservoir for the next breath (Figures 6-28, 6-29, and 6-30). Child- and adult-size masks are commonly available. When properly applied, the first third of the patient's exhaled gas from the anatomic dead space is exhaled back into this bag. This gas is close to pure oxygen and has no carbon dioxide. Exhaled breath escapes through the exhalation ports. The patient's breathing pattern affects the amount of room air that is breathed in through the same exhalation ports. Because of this room air entrainment, a partial-rebreathing mask is classified as a low-flow device. These ports also are important in case the oxygen flow to the mask is cut off; the patient will breathe in room air. The added reservoir of oxygen results in a higher percentage being given to the patient than with a simple oxygen mask. In all cases, set an oxygen flow high enough that the reservoir bag does not collapse by more than one-third on inspiration. For example, an initial oxygen flow of between 6 and 10 L/min should provide *approximately* 35% to 80% inspired oxygen.

A bubble humidifier often is added so that the gas is not dry. Make sure that it works properly, that the oxygen is flowing through the tubing, and that the reservoir bag has been filled before putting it on the patient. Adjust the flow as needed to ensure that the reservoir does not collapse by more than one-third on inspiration. This ensures

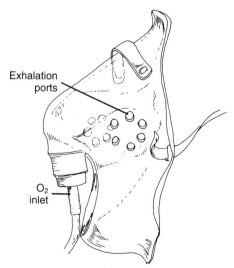

Figure 6-26   Close-up view of a simple oxygen mask. *(From McPherson SP:* Respiratory care equipment, *ed 4, St Louis, 1990, Mosby.)*

Figure 6-27   Child wearing a simple oxygen mask. *(From Gaebler G, Blodgett D: Gas administration. In Blodgett D, editor:* Manual of pediatric respiratory care procedures, *Philadelphia, 1982, Lippincott.)*

Figure 6-28 Outside view of a partial-rebreathing mask. *(From McPherson SP: Respiratory care equipment, ed 4, St Louis, 1990, Mosby.)*

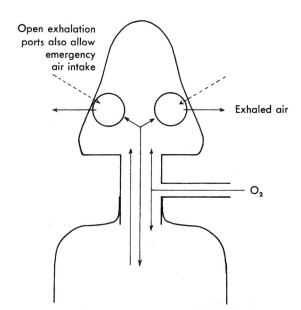

Open exhalation ports also allow emergency air intake

Exhaled air

O₂

Figure 6-29 Cutaway view of a partial-rebreathing mask showing gas flow. *(From Thalken FR: Medical gas therapy. In: Scanlan CL, Spearman CB, Sheldon RL, editors: Egan's fundamentals of respiratory care, ed 5, St Louis, 1990, Mosby.)*

Figure 6-30 Child wearing a partial-rebreathing mask. *(From Gaebler G, Blodgett D: Gas administration. In Blodgett D, editor: Manual of pediatric respiratory care procedures, Philadelphia, 1982, Lippincott.)*

that the mask and the reservoir are filled with as much oxygen as possible. A pulse oximetry value or PaO_2 level should be checked whenever a flow change is made, or when the patient's condition changes significantly.

3. Nonrebreathing mask

The nonrebreathing mask initially looks like the partial-rebreathing mask with its plastic bag added as an oxygen reservoir for the next breath (Figures 6-31 and 6-32). However, it should be noted that a one-way valve has been added between the mask and the reservoir bag. This allows the bag to be filled with pure oxygen that is available for

the next breath. No exhaled gas can enter the reservoir. Two (sometimes one) one-way valves are added to the exhalation ports on the mask. In theory, with a tight-fitting mask and a high enough oxygen flow, the patient breathes in only oxygen from the mask and reservoir and no room air. However, because of leaks between the mask and the patient's face, the nonrebreathing mask is classified as a low-flow device. Exhaled breath escapes through the exhalation ports as with the partial-rebreathing mask. Not shown is an emergency pop-in valve that allows room air to be drawn into the mask if the oxygen supply is cut off. Adult and pediatric sizes are available. The mask should be conformed to fit the patient's facial contours and size as much as possible. As mentioned earlier, this is for comfort and to try to increase the inspired oxygen percentage by decreasing the amount of room air that is inspired. In theory, it is possible to deliver 100% oxygen with this mask if the oxygen flow is high enough and the

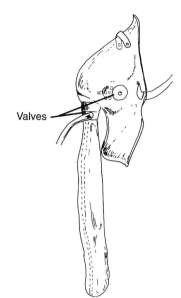

Figure 6-31 Outside view of a nonrebreathing mask. *(From McPherson SP: Respiratory care equipment, ed 4, St Louis, 1990, Mosby.)*

Valves

Figure 6-32 Cutaway view of a nonrebreathing mask showing gas flow. *(From Thalken FR: Medical gas therapy. In: Scanlan CL, Spearman CB, Sheldon RL, editors: Egan's fundamentals of respiratory care, ed 5, St Louis, 1990, Mosby.)*

Flap-valve exhalation ports; one flap may be removed for emergency air intake

Exhaled air

One-way valve

O_2

mask is airtight over the face. However, experience has shown that the disposable masks that are usually available in the hospital do not prevent room air from being drawn in. In all cases, set an oxygen flow high enough that the reservoir bag does not collapse by more than one-third on inspiration. For example, an initial oxygen flow between 8 and 10 L/min should provide approximately 60% to 80% (or more) inspired oxygen.

A bubble humidifier often is added so that the gas is not dry. Make sure that it works properly, that the oxygen is flowing through the tubing, and that the reservoir bag has been filled before putting it on the patient. Adjust the flow as needed to ensure that the reservoir does not col-

lapse by more than one-third on inspiration. This ensures that the mask and the reservoir are filled with oxygen, and that the patient's tidal volume comes completely from the reservoir bag. Try to make the mask fit as closely as possible to minimize room air entrainment. The patient's pulse oximetry value or PaO_2 level should be checked whenever a flow change is made, or when the patient's condition changes significantly.

> ### Exam Hint 6-9 (ELE, WRE)
>
> Expect to see one question dealing with the reservoir bag collapsing on inspiration. Solve the problem by increasing the flow of therapeutic gas to the mask and bag.

> ### Exam Hint 6-10 (ELE, WRE)
>
> Expect to see one question that deals with the need to switch from a low oxygen percentage mask to a nonrebreather mask to give the seriously hypoxemic patient as much oxygen as possible.

4. Face tent

These masks are designed to fit around the patient's neck, under the jaw, and around the cheeks in front of the ears. The front edge should be higher than the level of the patient's nostrils (Figure 6-33). Face tents sometimes are used to provide oxygen to a patient who cannot wear a mask or cannula because of oral and nasal trauma, burns, or surgery. The patient using a face tent should be sitting as upright as possible, because oxygen is heavier than air

Figure 6-33 Young adult wearing a face tent.

and tends to settle in the mask around the patient's nose and mouth if the fit is tight. If the patient is lying flat or if the mask fits loosely, the oxygen will simply "pour" down out of it. This makes it difficult to know with any certainty what inspired oxygen percentage is available to the patient. Flows of 5 to 10 L of oxygen per minute are commonly used with adults.

A face tent usually is ordered with the oxygen run through a humidifier or nebulizer so that the gas is not dry. Make sure that the humidifier or nebulizer is filled with sterile water, that the high-pressure pop-off works, and that gas is flowing through the tubing before the face tent is put on the patient. Try to analyze the oxygen percentage close to the patient's nose and mouth with as much accuracy as possible. A pulse oximetry value or PaO_2 level should be checked whenever a change in the oxygen percentage is made, or when the patient's condition changes significantly.

Figure 6-34 Transtracheal oxygen catheter. **A** *(top),* Photograph of a flexible, plastic transtracheal oxygen catheter. The part to the left of the flange is inserted into the patient's trachea. The part to the right of the flange is attached into standard oxygen tubing. **A** *(bottom),* The metal stylet may be used to help keep the catheter stiff during insertion and to clear the catheter of an obstruction. **B,** Drawing of a chain-link necklace keeping the external part of the catheter and flange secure. **C,** Cutaway drawing showing the catheter inserted into the trachea. *(From White GC:* Equipment theory for respiratory care, *Albany, NY, 1992, Delmar.)*

8. Manipulate a transtracheal oxygen catheter by order or protocol (ELE code: IIA1a) [Difficulty: ELE: R, Ap, An]

a. Get the necessary equipment for the procedure

The transtracheal oxygen (TTO_2) catheter is a 20-cm-long flexible, hollow plastic tube (Figure 6-34). This low-flow oxygen delivery device is inserted into the trachea via a puncture procedure at the suprasternal notch. To date, only adults with COPD have had the procedure performed. Oxygen is delivered directly into the trachea. The patient's oxygenation can be maintained at lower oxygen flows than are needed by a regular face mask or nasal cannula.

b. Put the equipment together and make sure that it works properly

The following equipment is needed:
- Transtracheal catheter of proper size (9F is the usual adult size)
- Guidewire/stylet
- Chain-link necklace to hold the catheter in place
- Regular small-bore oxygen tubing to connect to the distal end of the catheter
- Flowmeter and oxygen source
- Optional bubble humidifier with sterile water for patient comfort

Under normal working conditions, regular oxygen tubing is used to connect the oxygen source to the catheter. Oxygen flow to the catheter is set high enough to keep a satisfactory PaO_2 or SpO_2 level. Usually, this is less than is previously needed by nasal cannula. When oxygen tubing is combined with a portable LOX system or a pulse-dose oxygen delivery system, the patient has a real opportunity for increased mobility and decreased cost.

c. Troubleshoot any problems with the equipment

The patient needs to be instructed to disconnect the oxygen tubing and flush the catheter with 3 mL of sterile saline twice a day. A cleaning rod also can be pushed through the catheter to make sure that no mucus accumulates. As with any tubing system, the components can become disconnected. Make sure that all connections are tight. If the saline or cleaning rod cannot be pushed through the catheter, an obstruction is likely. The patient should come into the hospital to have the catheter removed and replaced if necessary. It is possible that the proximal catheter tip has twisted into the tracheal mucosa. This can lead to subcutaneous emphysema. The patient should be instructed on how to identify the signs of this and to turn off the oxygen to the catheter. He or she should go back to using a nasal cannula for oxygen and should call the physician for guidance.

9. Manipulate tracheostomy appliances: mask/collar and Brigg's adapter/T-piece, by order or protocol (ELE code: IIA1a) [Difficulty: ELE: R, Ap, An]

a. Get the necessary equipment for the procedure

b. Put the equipment together and make sure that it works properly

c. Troubleshoot any problems with the equipment

1. Tracheostomy mask/collar

The adult or pediatric tracheostomy mask or collar is shaped to fit over a tracheostomy tube or stoma to provide oxygen and aerosol (Figure 6-35). Because the patient's upper airway is bypassed, a nebulizer is used for humidity. It is usually an air entrainment type of device, so the oxygen percentage can be adjusted. Make sure that the nebulizer is filled with sterile water; if there is a high-pressure pop-off valve, make sure that it is working and that adequate mist is flowing through to the mask before putting it on the patient.

Because the tracheostomy mask is an open system without reservoir, it is difficult to guarantee the patient's inspired oxygen percentage. Set the gas flow high enough to make a "cloud" of aerosol around the tracheostomy. If an excess of aerosol can be seen around the tracheostomy during inspiration, it is likely that the desired oxygen percentage is being delivered. Analyze the oxygen percentage

Figure 6-35 Adult wearing a tracheostomy mask/collar.

from inside the mask to try for as much accuracy as possible. A pulse oximetry value or PaO$_2$ level should be checked whenever a flow change or oxygen percentage change is made, or when the patient's condition changes significantly.

2. Brigg's adapter/T-piece

The Brigg's adapter or T-piece is designed to provide air or supplemental oxygen and aerosol to an endotracheal or tracheostomy tube. It has one 15-mm inner diameter (ID) opening that fits over any endotracheal or tracheostomy tube adapter. The other two openings are 22 mm outer diameter (OD) so that aerosol tubing can be added (Figure 6-36). A nebulizer is commonly used for humidity because the patient's upper airway is bypassed. Make sure that the nebulizer is filled with sterile water; if there is a high-pressure pop-off valve, make sure it is working and that adequate mist is flowing through to the adapter before putting it on the patient. The nebulizer is usually an air entrainment type of device, so the oxygen percentage can be adjusted.

A length of aerosol tubing added downstream from the adapter acts as a reservoir so that the inspired oxygen percentage is ensured. A reservoir of 50 to 100 mL of aerosol tubing is commonly needed for the adult. Care must be taken to adjust the gas flow so that it is high enough to meet the patient's peak inspiratory flow rate. This can be determined by watching the aerosol flow past the adapter and reservoir. Make sure that during inspiration the aerosol is still flowing past the tracheostomy or endotracheal tube and into the reservoir. Inadequate flow could cause the patient to rebreathe gas from the reservoir. This gas has just been exhaled and is high in carbon dioxide and low in oxygen.

Figure 6-36   Child with intubated airway with a Brigg's T-piece adapter and aerosol tubing added to the endotracheal tube.

T- piece adapter

MODULE D
Specialty gas therapy

1. Changing the mode of administration (Code: IIIF2e1) [Difficulty: ELE: R, Ap; WRE: An]
2. Adjust the flow or gas concentration (Code: IIIF2e2) [Difficulty: R, Ap; WRE: An]

The indications for all of the specialty gases are listed in Box 6-1. Although none of these gases is used widely in respiratory care, all can be very beneficial when indicated.

a. He/O$_2$ (heliox) therapy

Patients who benefit from He/O$_2$ therapy can have an upper airway obstruction problem (tumor) or a lower airway obstruction problem (asthma). Because helium atoms are so much smaller than nitrogen molecules, patients find that their work of breathing is greatly

---

BOX 6-1   Indications for the Special Therapeutic Gases: He/O$_2$ (Heliox), NO (Nitric Oxide), and O$_2$/CO$_2$ (Carbogen)

HELIOX USES
Upper airway obstruction
  Tracheal tumor
  Laryngotracheobronchitis (croup)
  Postextubation stridor
Lower airway obstruction
  Status asthmaticus
  May reduce work of breathing in other conditions such as chronic obstructive pulmonary disease (COPD), bronchiolitis, or small endotracheal tube

NITRIC OXIDE USES
Treatment of term and near-term (>34 weeks) neonates with hypoxic respiratory failure associated with clinical or echocardiographic evidence of pulmonary hypertension
Possible use in acute respiratory distress syndrome (ARDS)

CARBOGEN USES
Hypoplastic left-heart syndrome (HLHS)
Carbon dioxide response curve test
Singultus (hiccup)

reduced. Normoxic patients usually are given a mix of 80% helium and 20% oxygen, whereas hypoxic patients are given 70% helium and 30% oxygen or 60% helium and 40% oxygen. If more oxygen is needed, small-bore oxygen tubing can be used to add it into the mask or reservoir bag, or a special closed system will have to be assembled from components.

Ideally any helium/oxygen delivery system should have a reservoir bag. Usually the nonrebreathing mask and the reservoir are used. The reservoir should be filled with the He/O_2 mix before the mask is placed on the patient's face. Again, the fit should be as tight as possible to minimize leaks. Adjust the flow so that the reservoir bag does not collapse by more than one-third during an inspiration. If it does, increase the flow. The flow should be increased if the patient complains of shortness of breath. Signs of increased work of breathing include agitation, increased use of accessory muscles of respiration, sweating, and increased respiratory rate, heart rate, and blood pressure.

b. Nitric oxide therapy

Because nitric oxide (NO) is a pulmonary vasodilator, it has been shown to be effective in the treatment of newborns with pulmonary hypertension (persistent pulmonary hypertension of the newborn [PPHN]). The FDA has approved the use of INOmax (0.8% nitric oxide and 99.2% nitrogen) to deliver inhaled nitric oxide to these patients. The currently recommended dosing range of inhaled NO to treat PPHN is 5 to 15 parts per million (ppm). The possible range for delivered NO is 2 to 80 ppm. Be prepared to increase the level of NO as needed, to reverse the pulmonary hypertension. When the patient improves, the NO level will need to be decreased. This usually is done by cutting the NO level in half, assessing the patient, and cutting the NO level in half again, etc., as tolerated.

To deliver the needed concentrations of nitric oxide and supplemental oxygen, the INOvent delivery system is needed. It is used to set the desired mix of INOmax to the newborn's ventilator and to monitor the levels of NO, nitrogen dioxide (NO_2), and oxygen delivered. Because NO is chemically changed in the body to toxic NO_2 and nitric acid, it is important to closely monitor the level of nitrogen dioxide. Low levels of NO_2 can cause a pneumonitis, and higher levels can cause pulmonary edema. The patient's methemoglobin level also should be monitored, as NO can cause an elevated level. Be prepared to decrease the level of NO to reduce the level of toxic NO_2.

Inhaled NO has not been approved for adult patients. However, some reports of nitric oxide administered to patients with pulmonary hypertension and acute respiratory distress syndrome (ARDS) show promising results.

Exam Hint 6-12 (WRE)

Usually one question deals with treating a patient with pulmonary hypertension. Inhaled nitric oxide in the range of 5 to 15 parts per million (ppm) is indicated. The question often includes information that shows the patient has an increased pulmonary vascular resistance (PVR), indicating pulmonary hypertension. See Chapter 5 and Box 5-2 for more information on PVR.

---

c. O_2/CO_2 (carbogen) therapy

Carbon dioxide is available in tanks of pure CO_2 or a mix of 5%:95% or 10%:90% (carbon dioxide:oxygen ratio). Carbogen is used during cardiopulmonary bypass procedures to maintain the patient's $PaCO_2$. Common clinical uses are listed in Box 6-1. Because inhaling carbon dioxide runs counter to a person's normal exhalation of CO_2, the patient's $PaCO_2$ can increase with resulting respiratory acidosis. So, the patient's arterial blood gas values, vital signs, and mental status must be monitored closely. Be prepared to decrease the carbogen percentage or stop the breathing of carbogen if the patient shows any adverse signs or symptoms.

A child with hypoplastic left-heart syndrome (HLHS) usually is being mechanically ventilated. The infant with this congenital heart defect must maintain an open foramen ovale and patent ductus arteriosus (PDA) for adequate systemic circulation (a right-to-left intracardiac shunt). Carbogen is added by small-bore tubing connecting the gas cylinder with a T-piece connected into the ventilator circuit. Usually enough carbogen flow is added to result in measurement of 1% to 4% carbon dioxide on a capnometer. Because increased carbon dioxide is a pulmonary vasoconstrictor, the PDA can be maintained. The infant's vital signs and ABG values must be closely monitored to guide the adjustment in carbogen.

The carbon dioxide response curve test is a measurement of the increase in minute volume caused by breathing different concentrations of carbon dioxide when the patient's oxygen level is normal. This pulmonary function test is performed on patients with COPD to determine whether their breathing will increase when their carbon dioxide level is increased. Depending on the method of test performed, the patient inhales between 1% and 7% carbon dioxide. The flow and concentration must be adjusted to maintain the desired carbon dioxide level as measured on a capnometer. An oxygen analyzer also should be included in the system to make sure that the patient does not inhale less than 21% oxygen.

The treatment of hiccups usually requires only that the patient rebreathe from a paper bag. If necessary, a small amount of carbon dioxide can be added to stop the hiccups.

MODULE E
Respiratory care plan

1. Analyze available information to determine the patient's pathophysiologic state (Code: IIIH1) [Difficulty: ELE: R, Ap; WRE: An]

The goal of oxygen therapy is to correct the patient's hypoxemia. Obtain an ABG sample or perform pulse oximetry, as needed, to determine the patient's oxygenation. Review the complete discussion of these subjects in Chapter 3. The specialty gases (heliox, nitric oxide, and carbogen) are needed to help manage specific clinical problems.

2. Determine the appropriateness of the prescribed therapy and goals for the identified pathophysiologic state (Code: IIIH3) [Difficulty: ELE: R, Ap; WRE: An]

Be prepared to recommend a change in the care plan depending on the patient's problem and clinical progress. Review the indications and uses of supplemental oxygen and the specialty gases.

a. Terminate the treatment or procedure based on the patient's response (Code: IIIF1) [Difficulty: ELE: R, Ap; WRE: An]

It may be necessary to stop the use of carbogen or nitric oxide if the patient has an adverse reaction to their use.

b. Recommend discontinuing the treatment or procedure based on the patient's response (Code: IIIG1i) [Difficulty: ELE: R, Ap; WRE: An]

As was discussed at the beginning of the chapter, several possible hazards occur with the use of oxygen therapy. The NBRC is most likely to ask questions related to the use of or increase or decrease in oxygen in a patient with COPD. The specialty gases can be discontinued when the clinical problem (see Box 6-1) has been corrected.

MODULE F
Respiratory care protocols

1. Develop the outcomes of respiratory care protocols (Code: IIIH6b) [Difficulty: ELE: R, Ap; WRE: An]

Many respiratory care departments have developed a protocol that relates to the use of supplemental oxygen in clinical situations such as COPD management.

2. Apply respiratory care protocols (Code: IIIH8) [Difficulty: ELE: R, Ap; WRE: An]

In many oxygen therapy protocols, it is expected that the respiratory therapist will assess the patient (vital signs, pulse oximeter results, etc.), administer oxygen, reassess the patient's response, and act accordingly.

3. Monitor the outcomes of respiratory care protocols (Code: IIIH7b) [Difficulty: ELE: R, Ap; WRE: An]

Look for signs of hypoxemia and be prepared to recommend a change in the patient's oxygen delivery system or oxygen percentage to correct the problem. Tachycardia and tachypnea are common findings in hypoxemic patients. Proper oxygen therapy should relieve the problem so that the patient's vital signs return toward normal. An abnormal heart rhythm caused by hypoxemia should return to normal with relief of the problem. Check the patient's pulse oximetry or PaO_2 value whenever a change in the inspired oxygen percentage or a significant change in the patient's clinical condition occurs.

a. Independently change the oxygen percentage (ELE code: IIIF2d1) [Difficulty: ELE: R, Ap, An]

b. Independently change the flow of oxygen (ELE code: IIIF2d1) [Difficulty: ELE: R, Ap, An]

c. Independently change the mode of administering the oxygen (ELE code: IIIF2d1) [Difficulty: R, Ap, An]

Every patient's oxygen percentage or flow must be tailored to meet the patient's clinical goals. Usually this means keeping patients who are acutely hypoxemic at a PaO_2 level between 60 and 100 torr and an SpO_2 value between 90% and 97%. Exceptions, when the blood oxygen level is kept as high as possible, include cardiopulmonary resuscitation and treatment for carbon monoxide poisoning. Another exception is the patient with COPD who is hypoxemic and hypercarbic. Usually these patients' conditions are maintained with a moderate hypoxemia. The PaO_2 level should be between 50 and 60 torr and the SpO_2 value between 85% and 90%. It is imperative to keep the oxygen in this relatively narrow range. Further hypoxemia will result in pulmonary hypertension and cor pulmonale. Cardiac dysrhythmias or arrest and death can occur if the hypoxemia is severe (<40 torr). Oxygen levels in the normal range (>60 torr) may result in blunting of the hypoxic drive. This can result in bradypnea and even greater carbon dioxide retention with corresponding acidemia. When the carbon dioxide pressure ($PaCO_2$) level exceeds 80 to 90 torr, many patients become drowsy or somnolent. The goal of treatment is to decrease the FIO_2 to reduce the PaO_2 level to 50 to 60 torr. This, in turn, stimulates the hypoxic drive so that the patient increases his or her ventilation. See Chapter 3 for a complete discussion of the interpretation of arterial blood gas values.

Exam Hint 6-13 (ELE, WRE)

Know the advantages, disadvantages, and possible oxygen ranges for the various oxygen appliances discussed earlier. Be prepared to make recommendations to change from one appliance to another or to change the oxygen percentage or flow. Expect to see one question that deals with the need to reduce the inspired oxygen percentage to a patient with chronic obstructive pulmonary disease (COPD) with hypercarbia. In addition, usually one question deals with needing to increase the inspired oxygen percentage to a patient with COPD who is too hypoxemic.

4. Communicate information relevant to coordinating patient care and discharge planning (Code: IIIA2b) [Difficulty: ELE: R, Ap; WRE: An]

The physician, respiratory therapist, nurse, and patient and the patient's family members all must understand the patient's oxygen therapy goal. This is especially important for the home care patient to ensure that the proper oxygen administration device and oxygen flow rate are used.

BIBLIOGRAPHY

AARC Clinical Practice Guideline: Oxygen therapy in the acute care hospital, *Respir Care* 36:1410-1413, 1991.

AARC Clinical Practice Guideline: Oxygen therapy in the home or extended care facility—2007 revision & update, *Respir Care* 52:1063-1068, 2007.

American Association for Respiratory Care: Clinical practice guideline: oxygen therapy for adults in the acute care facility: 2002 revision and update, *Respir Care* 47:717, 2002.

American Association for Respiratory Care: Clinical practice guideline: selection of an oxygen delivery device for neonatal and pediatric patients: 2002 revision and update, *Respir Care* 47:707, 2002.

Bageant RA: Oxygen analyzers, *Respir Care* 21:410-416, 1976.

Boggs W: High-flow nasal cannula inadequate substitute for CPAP in infants, *Respiratory Therapy Magazine* (online): www.rtmagazine.com/reuters_article.asp?id=20080114clin007.html

Burton GG, Hodgkin JE, Ward JJ, editors: *Respiratory care, a guide to clinical practice,* ed 4, Philadelphia, 1997, Lippincott-Raven.

Cairo JM: Manufacture, storage, and transport of medical gases. In: Cairo JM, Pilbeam SP: *Mosby's respiratory care equipment,* ed 8, St Louis, 2010, Mosby.

Cairo JM, Pilbeam SP: *Mosby's respiratory care equipment,* ed 8, St Louis, 2010, Mosby.

Dantzker DR, MacIntyre NR, Bakow ED, editors: *Comprehensive respiratory care,* Philadelphia, 1995, WB Saunders.

Datex-Ohmeda: INOvent delivery system, January 1, 2001: http:// www.datex-ohmeda.com Eubanks DH, Bone RC: *Comprehensive respiratory care,* ed 2, St Louis, 1990, Mosby.

Fink JB, Hunt GE, editors: *Clinical practice in respiratory care,* Philadelphia, 1999, Lippincott-Raven.

Gaebler G, Blodgett D: Gas administration. In: Blodgett D, editor: *Manual of pediatric respiratory care procedures,* Philadelphia, 1982, Lippincott.

Gluck EH, Onorato DJ, Castriotta R: Helium-oxygen mixtures in intubated patients with status asthmaticus and respiratory acidosis, *Chest* 98:693-698, 1990.

Hess DR: Nonconventional respiratory therapeutics. In: Hess DR, MacIntyre NR, Mishoe SC, et al, editors: *Respiratory care principles & practices,* Philadelphia, 2002, WB Saunders.

Hill KV: Oxygen therapy. In: Aloan CA, Hill TV, editors: *Respiratory care of the newborn and child,* ed 2, Philadelphia, 1997, Lippincott-Raven.

Hollman GA, Shen G, Zeng L, et al: Helium-oxygen improves clinical asthma scores in children with acute bronchiolitis, *Crit Care Med* 26:1731-1736, 1998.

Hunt GE: Gas therapy. In: Fink JB, Hunt GE, editors: *Clinical practice in respiratory care,* Philadelphia, 1999, Lippincott-Raven.

INOTherapeutics: Homepage, January 1, 2001: http://www.inotherapeutics.com

Kass JE, Castriotta RJ: Heliox therapy in acute severe asthma, *Chest* 107:757-760, 1995.

Kemper KJ, Ritz RH, Benson MS, Bishop MS: Helium-oxygen mixture in the treatment of postextubation stridor in pediatric trauma patients, *Crit Care Med* 19:356-359, 1991.

Kudukis TM, Manthous CA, Schmidt GA, et al: Inhaled helium-oxygen revisited: Effect of inhaled helium-oxygen during the treatment of status asthmaticus in children, *J Pediatr* 131:333-334, 1997.

McCoy R: Oxygen-conserving techniques and devices, *Respir Care* 45:95-103, 2000.

McPherson SP: *Respiratory care equipment,* ed 5, St Louis, 1995, Mosby.

Saposnick AB: Medical gases—manufacture, storage, and delivery. In Hess DR, MacIntyre NR, Mishoe SC, et al, editors: *Respiratory care principles & practices,* Philadelphia, 2002, WB Saunders.

Saposnick AB, Hess DR: Oxygen therapy: Administration and management. In Hess DR, MacIntyre NR, Mishoe SC, et al, editors: *Respiratory care principles & practices,* Philadelphia, 2002, WB Saunders.

Schaeffer EM, Pohlman A, Morgan S, Hall JB: Oxygenation in status asthmaticus improves during ventilation with helium-oxygen, *Crit Care Med* 27:2666-2670, 1999.

Shapiro BA, Harrison RA, Cane RD, et al: *Clinical application of blood gases,* ed 4, St Louis, 1989, Mosby.

Shapiro BA, Kacmarek RM, Cane RD, et al, editors: *Clinical application of respiratory care,* ed 4, St Louis, 1991, Mosby.

Tassaux D, Jolliet P, Thouret JM, et al: Calibration of seven ICU ventilators for mechanical ventilation with helium-oxygen mixtures, *Am J Respir Crit Care Med* 160:22-32, 1999.

Ward JJ: Equipment for mixed gas and oxygen therapy. In: Branson RD, Hess DR, Chatburn RL, editors: *Respiratory care equipment,* ed 2, Philadelphia, 1999, Lippincott Williams & Wilkins.

Ward JJ: Medical gas therapy. In: Burton GC, Hodgkin JE, Ward JJ, editors: *Respiratory care: a guide to clinical practice,* ed 4, Philadelphia, 1997, Lippincott-Raven.

Waugh JB, Granger WM: An evaluation of 2 new devices for nasal high-flow gas therapy. *Respir Care* 49:902-906, 2004.

Whitaker K: *Comprehensive perinatal and pediatric respiratory care,* ed 2, Albany, NY, 1997, Delmar.

White GC: *Equipment theory for respiratory care,* ed 4, Albany, NY, 2005, Delmar.

Wilkins RL, Stoller JK, Kacmarek RM, editors: *Egan's fundamentals of respiratory care,* ed 9, St Louis, 2009, Mosby.

Wojciechowski WV: *Respiratory care sciences: An integrated approach,* ed 3, Albany, NY, 2000, Delmar.

Youtsey JW: Oxygen and mixed gas therapy. In: Barnes TA, editor: *Core textbook of respiratory care practice,* ed 2, St Louis, 1994, Mosby.

SELF-STUDY QUESTIONS FOR THE ENTRY LEVEL EXAM   *See page 587 for answers*

1. Your home care patient has a problem with his O_2 concentrator and needs to change to his H-tank of O_2. If his nasal cannula is receiving a flow of 3 L/min and the tank pressure is 1300 psig, how long can the patient receive O_2?
   A. Longer than 22 hours
   B. Longer than 1300 hours
   C. 2 hours
   D. Longer than 120 hours

2. What is the most likely problem to watch for in a patient with severe COPD who is receiving supplemental O_2?
   A. Pulmonary edema from O_2 toxicity
   B. Hypoventilation
   C. Retinopathy of prematurity (ROP)
   D. Hyperventilation

3. Which of the following is the best device for giving 35% oxygen to an alert 2-year-old?
   A. Oxygen tent
   B. Nasal cannula at 3 L/min
   C. Simple mask at 3 L/min
   D. Incubator

4. You are making general rounds in the hospital when you find a patient whose reservoir tubing has fallen off his 40% T-piece. This would result in which of the following?
   A. Increased inspired O_2
   B. Increased inspired CO_2
   C. Decreased inspired CO_2
   D. Decreased inspired O_2

5. The risks of O_2 therapy include all of the following EXCEPT
   A. Pulmonary O_2 toxicity
   B. Denitrogen absorption atelectasis
   C. O_2-induced hyperventilation
   D. Retinopathy of prematurity (ROP)

6. Your patient is wearing a face tent because of recent facial surgery. It is set at 35% O_2. The nurse moves the patient from an upright to a supine position in bed. What effect will this have on her respiratory status?
   A. Increased V_T

   B. Increased inspired O_2
   C. Increased inspired CO_2
   D. Decreased inspired O_2

7. To minimize the risk of hypoxemia during a treatment or procedure, you would do which of the following?
   1. Increase the O_2 percentage by 20% above the normal setting before suctioning or changing equipment
   2. Keep the O_2 percentage the same as if the patient is not hypoxemic at this time
   3. Minimize the time that the patient would be breathing room air
   4. Increase the O_2 percentage to 100% before suctioning
   5. Make sure the replacement equipment is working properly before you place it on the patient
   A. 1, 3
   B. 3, 4, 5
   C. 2, 5
   D. 3, 4

8. Initially, the O_2 percentage found in the O_2 tent of a 2-year-old child was found to be stable at the ordered 35%. Now, less than that is found. All of the following should be tried EXCEPT
   A. Add an additional flowmeter and run them both at flush
   B. Keep the tent canopy tightly tucked under the mattress
   C. Keep the canopy flaps closed when the child is not receiving nursing care
   D. Check the analyzer for proper function

9. Your patient is wearing a partial-rebreathing mask. The reservoir bag almost totally collapses during inspiration. You would do which of the following?
   A. Tell the patient to breathe more slowly
   B. Put a nasal cannula on the patient
   C. Tell the patient to breathe more rapidly
   D. Increase the O_2 flow

10. When checking your home care patient's reservoir-type nasal cannula, you notice that the reservoir does

not fill and empty in synchrony with the patient's breathing pattern. Based on this, you would
   A. Increase the O_2 flow to deliver the intended amount
   B. Replace the cannula
   C. Decrease the O_2 flow to unstick the reservoir membrane
   D. Switch the patient to an air entrainment mask at approximately the same O_2 percentage as that given to the patient who received it by cannula

11. What O_2 delivery device would you recommend for a patient who has a variable respiratory rate, I:E ratio, and V_T?
    A. Nasal cannula
    B. Air entrainment mask
    C. Simple O_2 mask
    D. Face tent

12. The physician asks you which O_2 delivery device would be best for a patient who needs about 75% O_2. You would recommend which of the following?
    A. Nonrebreathing mask
    B. Face tent
    C. Air entrainment mask
    D. Simple O_2 mask

13. A patient has a nasal cannula and needs to be transported on a stretcher. The E-sized O_2 cylinder will have to be laid flat under the stretcher. Which flowmeter would you recommend?
    A. Backpressure-compensated Thorpe
    B. Non–backpressure-compensated Thorpe
    C. Bourdon
    D. Backpressure-compensated kinetic

14. An E-cylinder of O_2 needs to be prepared for transport of a patient. You would look for a regulator with which pinhole locations?
    A. 1 and 5
    B. 2 and 6
    C. 3 and 5
    D. 2 and 5

15. What is the duration of flow of an E-cylinder with 1700 psig that is running at 5 L/min?
    A. 0.9 hour
    B. 1.6 hours
    C. 7.7 hours
    D. 13.7 hours

16. You are called to draw an arterial blood sample from a patient who is wearing a 35% air entrainment mask. When you enter the room, you notice that his covers are drawn up over the air entrainment ports of the mask. How would this affect the function of the mask?
    A. The total flow will be increased.
    B. There will be no effect.
    C. The O_2 percentage will be increased.
    D. The O_2 percentage will be decreased.

17. You receive a call at the office from one of your home care patients. She reports that the high-pressure pop-off valve on the bubble humidifier to her transtracheal oxygen catheter is venting. In addition, she cannot flush out the catheter with saline or push the cleaning rod through it. What should you tell her to do?
    A. Remove the humidifier and double the oxygen flow rate to the catheter.
    B. Force the saline through the catheter until the obstruction is cleared.
    C. Force the cleaning rod through the catheter until the obstruction is cleared.
    D. Switch her oxygen from the transtracheal catheter to a nasal cannula.

18. A 58-year-old patient with advanced emphysema is admitted with an acute exacerbation of his condition. While breathing 2 L/min of oxygen through a transtracheal oxygen catheter, he has the following arterial blood gas results:
    pH, 7.38
    $PaCO_2$, 57 torr
    HCO_3^-, 31 mEq/L
    PaO_2, 47 torr
    SaO_2, 80%
    Based on these findings, what do you think should be done?
    A. Change the patient to 24% oxygen by an air entrainment mask.
    B. Initiate bilevel mask ventilation.
    C. Change the patient to a nonrebreathing mask with 10 L/min of oxygen.
    D. Increase the oxygen flow to the current system to 3 L/min.

19. A comatose patient is intubated and is receiving 35% O_2 with aerosol through a T-piece (Briggs adapter). While watching the patient breathe, you notice that during each inspiration, the mist disappears from the downstream end of the T-piece. What would you recommend?
    A. Add 100 mL of aerosol tubing as a reservoir on the T-adapter.
    B. Change the O_2 to 30% and increase the flow.
    C. Change the O_2 to 40% and decrease the flow.
    D. Tell the patient not to breathe so deeply.

20. A 65-year-old patient with pulmonary edema is very short of breath and hypoxic. She is ordered to have a nonrebreathing mask with 10 L/min of oxygen going to it. However, she keeps taking off her mask because of anxiety and claustrophobia. When she removes the mask, her pulse oximeter reading drops from 90% to 82%. What should be recommended to help manage the patient?
    A. Give her a nasal cannula at 10 L/min oxygen.
    B. Sedate the patient so that she will keep on her nonrebreathing mask.

C. Initiate CPAP by mask at 8 cm water and 40% oxygen.

D. Begin a high-flow nasal cannula at ≥10 L/min oxygen.

21. An 18-year-old patient with status asthmaticus is being treated in the Emergency Department. The physician has ordered him to receive a 70% helium/30% oxygen mix. What do you recommend as the best way to deliver this?

A. Partial rebreather mask with reservoir bag

B. High-flow nasal cannula

C. Nonrebreather mask with reservoir bag

D. Through a mechanical ventilator

SELF-STUDY QUESTIONS FOR THE WRITTEN REGISTRY EXAM   *See page 612 for answers*

1. A patient with COPD is going home. After a hospital exercise test is conducted, it has been determined that she will require 1 L/min of supplemental oxygen when exercising on her stationary bicycle or when she feels short of breath. Which of the following oxygen delivery systems should the respiratory therapist recommend?

A. Molecular sieve oxygen concentrator

B. Portable liquid oxygen system

C. Semipermeable membrane oxygen concentrator

D. Piston compressor

2. You are attempting to calibrate a polarographic oxygen analyzer but find that it cannot be done. Possible reasons for this include

1. The membrane is torn on the probe

2. The gas sampling capillary tube is plugged with debris

3. The electrode solution has evaporated

4. The battery needs to be replaced

5. Water has condensed on the membrane

A. 1, 3

B. 2, 3

C. 3, 4, 5

D. 1, 3, 4, 5

3. A patient has just been admitted through the Emergency Department with suspected CO poisoning. The physician wants her to receive the highest possible O_2 percentage. What would you recommend?

A. Continuous positive-airway pressure mask at 5 cm H_2O and 40% O_2

B. Simple mask at 6 L/min flow

C. Face tent at 8 L/min flow

D. Nonrebreather mask with enough flow to keep the reservoir bag at least two-thirds full

4. A newborn infant with hypoplastic left-heart syndrome (HLHS) has just been transferred to your hospital. Mechanical ventilation is being instituted. What else can be done to help improve the neonate's heart function?

A. Nitric oxide therapy

B. Carbogen therapy

C. Suture closing the patent ductus arteriosus

D. Heliox therapy

5. You are doing quality assurance on the department's flowmeters. After plugging in a backpressure-compensated Thorpe flowmeter, you set the flow at 10 L/min. The flowmeter outlet is partially and then completely obstructed. You would expect to see the following:

A. The float will stay at the 10-L/min mark.

B. The float will move upward in the flowmeter.

C. The float will move upward and then downward in the flowmeter.

D. The float will move downward and then will drop to the bottom of the flowmeter, showing zero flow.

6. You are called to evaluate a patient known to have advanced emphysema. She is wearing a nasal cannula at 6 L/min. The nurse says that she has become drowsy and less responsive since the oxygen was given to her an hour ago. Her arterial blood gas (ABG) results on the oxygen show the following:

PaO_2, 84 torr

$PaCO_2$, 65 torr

pH, 7.32

Which of the following would you recommend?

1. Leave her on the cannula.

2. Change her to 24% O_2 on an air entrainment mask and repeat the ABGs in 20 minutes.

3. Change her to a simple oxygen mask and repeat the ABGs in 20 minutes.

4. Let her rest undisturbed.

5. Monitor her closely for becoming more alert.

A. 1, 4

B. 3, 4

C. 2, 5

D. 3, 5

7. You are assisting with a bronchoscopy to obtain a biopsy of a suspicious laryngeal node on your patient. Afterward, the patient complains of shortness of breath and a "tight" throat. Which of the following recommendations could you give to the physician?

A. Give the patient a 20% oxygen and 80% helium mix to breathe.

B. Put the head of the bed down 30 degrees.

C. Give the patient a carbogen mix to breathe.

D. Do a 7-minute helium dilution test.

8. An adult patient who was rescued from a house fire is being received in the Emergency Department. He is wearing a simple oxygen mask at 5 L/min. The SpO$_2$ value by pulse oximeter is 100%, and his SaO$_2$ value from an arterial blood gas sample analyzed on a CO oximeter is 73%. What would you recommend be done at this time?
   A. Maintain the simple oxygen mask at the present flow.
   B. Change the patient to a nonrebreather mask.
   C. Decrease the oxygen flow to the simple oxygen mask to 4 L/min.
   D. Maintain present therapy and recalibrate the CO oximeter.

9. You are working with a patient who has a tracheal tumor. He is wearing a nonrebreather mask with 20% oxygen and 80% helium. The patient says that it is harder to breathe and that the mask has increased his respiratory rate. You notice that the reservoir bag has collapsed. The most appropriate action is to
   A. Decrease the flow of gas
   B. Switch to an air entrainment mask and deliver 24% oxygen
   C. Increase the flow of gas
   D. Switch to a 30% oxygen and 70% helium mix

10. An 8-year-old patient with asthma is going to be given a 30% oxygen and 70% helium mix of heliox through a nonrebreather mask and reservoir bag. The physician has ordered the child to receive 7 L/min of the gas mix. Because it will be delivered through an oxygen flowmeter, what flow should be set?
   A. 3.9 L/min
   B. 4.4 L/min
   C. 9.8 L/min
   D. 11.2 L/min

11. A 36-week gestational age neonate is hypoxic despite mechanical ventilation and has clinical evidence of persistent pulmonary hypertension of the newborn. What can be done to correct the hypoxemia?
   A. Instill intratracheal surfactant
   B. Begin nitric oxide (NO) therapy
   C. Begin 10 cm water PEEP
   D. Begin carbogen therapy

12. While you are working as the respiratory therapist assigned to the Emergency Department, a 24-year-old patient with status asthmaticus is transferred by ambulance from a small, rural hospital. The patient has been given continuous bronchodilator therapy and intravenous corticosteroids and aminophylline. She is becoming exhausted but refuses to allow intubation and mechanical ventilation. What should be recommended?
   A. Begin heliox therapy.
   B. Begin nitric oxide therapy.
   C. Intubate and ventilate the patient despite her protests.
   D. Follow the patient's wishes.

13. A neonatal patient has primary pulmonary hypertension and is receiving mechanical ventilation. After he receives 20 ppm of nitric oxide therapy, his pulmonary vascular resistance returns to the normal range. What do you recommend be done at this time?
   A. Discontinue the nitric oxide therapy.
   B. Decrease the nitric oxide to 10 ppm.
   C. Add 1% carbogen to the nitric oxide mix.
   D. Increase the nitric oxide therapy to 30 ppm.

14. A 16-year-old patient with status asthmaticus is started on a 70% helium/30% oxygen (heliox) mix through a nonrebreather mask. It is noticed that the oxygen flowmeter shows the delivery of 8 L/min of gas. What is the actual heliox gas flow?
   A. 5 L/min
   B. 8 L/min
   C. 12.8 (13) L/min
   D. 14.4 (14) L/min

15. A socially active patient with COPD requires 2 L/min of continuous oxygen. She wishes to go with her Better Breathers Club on a bus trip to shop in Chicago. What should be recommended for her in this situation?
   A. Use a portable liquid oxygen system at 2 L/min.
   B. Take a portable "E" tank of oxygen with her and run it at 2 L/min.
   C. Preposition "E" tanks of oxygen for her use in the various stores.
   D. Take a portable "E" tank of oxygen with her and run it at 1 L/min.

7 Hyperinflation Therapy

Note 1: This book is written to cover every item listed as testable on the *Entry Level Examination (ELE), Written Registry Examination (WRE),* and *Clinical Simulation Examination (CSE).*

The listed code for each item is taken from the National Board for Respiratory Care (NBRC) **Summary Content Outline for CRT (Certified Respiratory Therapist) and Written RRT (Registered Respiratory Therapist) Examinations** (http://evolve.elsevier.com/Sills/resptherapist/). For example, if an item is testable on both the ELE and the WRE, it will be shown simply as: (Code: . . .). If an item is testable only on the ELE, it will be shown as: (ELE code: . . .). If an item is testable only on the WRE, it will be shown as: (WRE code: . . .).

Following each item's code will be the difficulty level of the questions on that item on the ELE and WRE. (See the Introduction for a full explanation of the three question difficulty levels.) **Recall [R]** level questions typically expect the exam taker to recall factual information. **Application [Ap]** level questions are harder because the exam taker may have to apply factual information to a clinical situation. **Analysis [An]** level questions are the most challenging because the exam taker may have to use critical thinking to evaluate patient data to make a clinical decision.

Note 2: *A review of the most recent Entry Level Examinations (ELE) has shown that an average of two questions (1% of the exam) will cover hyperinflation therapy. A review of the most recent Written Registry Examinations (WRE) has shown that an average of two questions (out of 100), or 2% of the exam, will cover hyperinflation therapy.*

MODULE A

Perform coughing and deep-breathing procedures with the patient to help make breathing more effective.

1. Instruct the patient in deep-breathing techniques (Code: IIID1a) [Difficulty: ELE: R, Ap; WRE: An]

Explain to the patient that taking in deep breaths keeps the small air sacs in the lungs inflated and healthy. Deep breathing and coughing are indicated in patients with atelectasis, pulmonary infiltrates, or pneumonia. These exercises should help to increase secretions. It is especially important to use deep breathing and coughing to prevent or limit atelectasis and pneumonia in patients who have just had abdominal surgery such as cholecystectomy or splenectomy. Ideally, the patient is taught these techniques before surgery is performed. If not, teach them the following postoperatively:

1. To decrease the pain, minimize traction or tension on the incision by placing your or the patient's hands on both sides of the incision. Alternatively, the practitioner or the patient can hold a pillow against the incision.
2. Instruct the patient to breathe two or three times in through the nose and out through the mouth.
3. Instruct the patient to take in as deep a breath as possible and to perform a normal cough.
4. If the patient cannot cough normally because of pain, a serial cough can be performed.

Teach the following cough techniques to the patient with obstructive airways disease:

1. Avoid an ineffective, shallow, hacking cough.
2. Position the patient in a sitting position, bent slightly forward, with feet on the floor or supported. The patient who must lie in bed can be positioned on the preferred side with the legs flexed at the knees and hips.
3. Instruct the patient to perform a mid-inspiratory cough.
   a. Breathe two or three times in through the nose and out through the mouth.
   b. Breathe in to a comfortable volume larger than the tidal volume (V_T), but not as deeply as possible.
   c. Briefly hold the breath.
   d. Cough hard, or perform a serial cough at relatively low flows. This should help to raise secretions without causing airway collapse.
   e. Squeezing the knees and thighs together at the instant of coughing helps to increase the airflow and volume.

Coaching is important because patients in pain or who are suffering from chronic lung disease tend to be uncooperative and to not try hard. Give positive reinforcement when the patient does well. Correct any problems that the patient is having in trying to follow the instructions. Demonstrations often are helpful, so the patient can copy a good example.

2. Instruct the patient in inspiratory muscle training techniques (ELE code: IIID1b) [Difficulty: R, Ap]

Initially, teach the following steps to patients with obstructive airways diseases:

1. Have the patient lie in a comfortable supine position; knees can be flexed.
2. Instruct the patient to relax physically as much as possible, especially the shoulders.
3. Use soothing music, meditation, or other techniques for mental relaxation.
4. Instruct the patient to concentrate on breathing more slowly.
5. Emphasize pursed-lip breathing, wherein the patient with relaxed abdominal muscles breathes in slowly through the nose and out slowly through pursed (slightly opened) lips. Breathing with pursed lips keeps some backpressure on the airways so they stay open longer. The technique helps to improve gas exchange so the patient experiences less dyspnea.

After these first steps have been mastered, teach the following steps to patients with obstructive airways diseases:

1. The practitioner places his or her hands and the patient's hands gently over the area(s) where the patient is to concentrate the breathing effort. Usually, this is the abdominal area just below the sternum. This encourages the patient to use the diaphragm more effectively and to strengthen it. With diaphragmatic breathing, the hands move out during an inspiration.
2. The same hands-on technique can be used to aid in segmental breathing over an area that is underventilated or that has atelectasis.
3. Breathing *in* against an obstruction can also increase the strength and endurance of inspiratory muscles. A variety of devices are available. One type of device is a mouthpiece with selectable, variably sized openings at the other end (Figure 7-1). The patient breathes in through the largest opening and progresses to smaller openings as tolerated.

Increasing the strength and endurance of inspiratory muscles usually requires a training program similar to the following:

1. Plug the nose with nose clips.
2. Inspire a normal tidal volume (V_T) at a rate of 12 to 15 breaths/min through the largest opening.
3. Continue for 10 to 15 minutes per day for a total of 3 to 5 times/wk in the first week. If the patient notices shortness of breath, a noticeably increased pulse rate, or increased fatigue, the exercise should be stopped until the symptoms are gone. Resume the exercise when the patient is comfortable again.
4. Gradually increase the duration to about 30 minutes per session or two 15-minute sessions per day.

Figure 7-1   PFLEX inspiratory muscle trainer. The body of the device features a dial selector with inspiratory holes. The holes range from the 1 setting (largest opening) to the 6 setting (smallest opening). A one-way valve allows the patient to expire. The mouthpiece can be attached directly to the body, or a monitoring/oxygen adapter can be added between them. This adapter allows oxygen to be added to meet the patient's needs. An inspiratory force meter also can be added to determine the amount of negative pressure the patient is generating at each of the inspiratory hole settings. *(Courtesy of Philips Respironics, Murrysville, PA.)*

5. When this schedule can be tolerated easily 3 times/wk, switch to the next smallest hole.
6. Repeat steps **1** to **5** as tolerated. The most beneficial exercise is tiring but not exhausting. The device may be adjusted to the next larger hole setting if the patient becomes too tired. The whole process usually takes 4 to 6 weeks before positive results are seen.
7. A maintenance program necessitates that exercise be done every other day.

MODULE B
Incentive spirometry

1. Instruct the patient in incentive spirometry techniques (Code: IIID1a) [Difficulty: ELE: R, Ap; WRE: An]

Incentive spirometry (IS) is a technique whereby a patient is encouraged to breathe deeply by seeing his or her inhaled volume on the spirometry device. The patient receives positive feedback by seeing that the volume gradually increases as his or her condition improves. IS is indicated in any patient who has developed or is likely to develop atelectasis and can perform the procedure. Clinical situations and individuals in which atelectasis is likely to be seen include postoperative thoracic or upper abdominal surgery, the aged, the obese, inadequate sigh, cardiopulmonary disease, and quadriplegia and/or dysfunctional hemidiaphragm(s).

Exam Hint 7-1 (ELE, WRE)

Remember that incentive spirometry is the preferred treatment choice for atelectasis in patients who can perform it properly.

Because the goal of IS is to prevent or treat atelectasis, the patient should inhale a near-normal inspiratory capacity (IC). The patient can benefit more by holding the IC for several seconds, which is referred to as *sustained maximal inspiration (SMI)*. Before the operation, the cooperative surgical patient should have the IC measured at the bedside or calculated from a pulmonary function test in which vital capacity (VC) is measured (review Chapter 4 for IC information). The IC is measured again postoperatively.

Before you start to provide instruction, make sure that the patient is alert and cooperative enough to follow instructions. The patient's respiratory rate should be less than 25 breaths/min if the procedure is to be performed properly. Use the following steps in teaching IS:

1. Have the patient sit in semi-Fowler's position, on the edge of the bed, or up in a chair.
2. Set an initial goal of twice the patient's measured bedside V_T.
3. Tell the patient the purpose of the treatment and how to perform it properly.
4. Simulate the procedure for the patient.
5. Put the unit within easy reach, and keep it upright.
6. Have the patient exhale normally (to functional residual capacity), seal the lips around the mouthpiece, and inspire maximally through the unit. The patient must inspire in a slow, controlled effort.
7. Have the patient hold the IC for *at least* 3 seconds but no longer than 15 seconds before exhaling (the SMI).
8. Proceed to extend the patient's goal as tolerated and indicated earlier.
9. The patient should perform the deep breath at least 10 times/hr while awake. With normal breathing, a rest period should take place after each large breath.

Monitor your patient's progress in the following ways:

1. If the patient cannot meet the initial goal, reconsider whether this is the best form of treatment. Intermittent positive-pressure breathing (IPPB) might be a better choice for providing a deep breath.
2. Stop the treatment temporarily if the patient has signs of hyperventilation, such as dizziness or tingling of the fingertips. A few minutes of normal breathing should result in a normal feeling again. Have the patient take longer rest periods between maximal breaths.
3. Stop the treatment if the patient complains of acute chest pain. It is possible to cause pulmonary barotrauma by breathing in as deeply as possible. Evaluate the patient's pulmonary condition and call the physician if indicated.

2. Increase or decrease the patient's incentive spirometry goal (Code: IIIF2b) [Difficulty: ELE: R, Ap; WRE: An]

See Table 7-1 for IS guidelines. The following guidelines are also suggested:

TABLE 7-1 Guidelines for the Use of Incentive Spirometry

Postoperative Bedside Spirometry	Treatment Modality
IC >80% of the preoperative value	No treatment needed unless radiographic or clinical evidence of atelectasis exists.
IC at least 33% of the preoperative value or VC of at least 10 mL/kg	IS is indicated.
IC <33% of the preoperative value or VC <10 mL/kg	IPPB is indicated.

IC, Inspiratory capacity; *IPPB*, intermittent positive-pressure breathing; *IS*, incentive spirometry; *VC*, vital capacity.

1. Set the initial IC goal at twice the V_T.
2. Increase the goal in 200-mL increments as the patient tolerates.
3. Set a final IC goal of greater than 12 mL/kg of ideal body weight, or set a forced vital capacity (FVC) goal of greater than 15 mL/kg of ideal body weight.
4. A normal person should have an IC of about 75% of his or her FVC. For example, a predicted FVC of 5.166 L was calculated for a male patient in Chapter 4. His predicted IC would be calculated as 5.166 L × 0.75 = 3.875 L. However, because of natural variations in people, he might inhale only 80% of this (3.1 L) and still be considered within normal limits. Use this as a guideline for anticipating a patient's maximum IC, and do not expect your patient to inhale a greater IC than is physically possible.

Consider increasing the IS goal if the patient is easily able to reach the set goal, or if the patient's breath sounds are diminished in the bases. Consider decreasing the IS goal if the patient cannot reach the set goal because it is too large, if the patient is frustrated and discouraged at his or her inability to reach the set goal, or if excessive surgical site pain prevents the patient from reaching the set goal.

MODULE C
Incentive spirometry equipment

1. Manipulate incentive spirometry equipment by order or protocol (ELE code: IIA13) [Difficulty: R, Ap, An]

2. Get the necessary equipment, put it together, and make sure that it works properly

Two basic types of IS equipment exist: flow displacement and volume displacement units.

a. Flow displacement

With flow displacement units, patients breathe in a flow great enough to raise one or more plastic balls in calibrated cylinders (Figure 7-2). The patient is encouraged to try to keep the ball (or balls) suspended by breathing in more deeply. Encourage the patient to breathe in *slowly* to suspend the balls for as long as possible. Have the patient watch as the balls are held up by the inspired breath to provide positive reinforcement for doing a good job. The patient is not helped by breathing in a fast, short breath and having the balls pop up and down. Volume is calculated by multiplying the flow per second needed to suspend the balls by the number of seconds that the balls are suspended. For example, 600 cc/sec × 2 sec = 1200 cc IC. Assemble the device by attaching the flow tube to the unit and the mouthpiece to the flow tube.

b. Volume displacement units

With volume displacement units, patients breathe in a preset volume goal from the reservoir bellows (Figure 7-3). Many of these units have a whistle built into them to warn if the breath is too fast. Patients who cannot generate enough inspiratory flow to use a flow displacement unit should use a volume displacement unit instead.

Some units also have a small built-in leak so the patient must continue inspiring to keep the bellows suspended. Have the patient watch as the bellows is suspended for positive reinforcement for doing a good job. Volume is marked on the bellows container. If the unit has a built-in leak, multiply the volume inspired by the time the bellows is suspended. For example:

$$800 \text{ mL} \times 3 \text{ sec} = 2400 \text{ mL IC}$$

Assemble the device by attaching the flow tube to the unit and the mouthpiece to the flow tube.

3. Troubleshoot any problems with the equipment

In either type of incentive spirometer, an obstruction to the flow tube or mouthpiece or a built-in leak in the calibrated cylinders stops airflow. With a flow displacement unit, no balls will rise despite the patient's inspiratory effort. With a volume displacement unit, the bellows will not rise despite the patient's inspiratory effort. Clearing the obstruction or sealing the leak allows either unit to work properly.

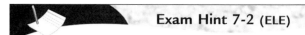

Exam Hint 7-2 (ELE)

The exam is likely to include one question that deals with selecting, adjusting, or troubleshooting IS equipment.

MODULE D
Respiratory care plan

1. Analyze the available information to determine the patient's pathophysiologic state (Code: IIIH1) [Difficulty: ELE: R, Ap; WRE: An]

Review the information in Chapter 1 that deals with the interpretation of breath sounds and chest x-ray findings. As was discussed earlier, atelectasis is the primary problem that can be treated with IS.

Figure 7-2   Triflo II incentive deep-breathing exerciser. *(From Eubanks DH, Bone RC: Comprehensive respiratory care, ed 2, St Louis, 1990, Mosby.)*

Figure 7-3   Volume incentive breathing exerciser. *(From Eubanks DH, Bone RC: Comprehensive respiratory care, ed 2, St Louis, 1990, Mosby.)*

2. Determine the appropriateness of the prescribed respiratory care plan and recommend modifications when indicated

a. Determine the appropriateness of the prescribed therapy and goals for the patient's pathophysiologic state (Code: IIIH3) [Difficulty: ELE: R, Ap; WRE: An]

IS is the easiest and least expensive way to treat atelectasis if the patient can properly perform the procedure. See Table 7-1 for guidelines on the indications for IS or IPPB.

b. Review the planned therapy to establish the therapeutic plan (Code: IIIH2a) [Difficulty: ELE: R, Ap; WRE: An]

c. Recommend changes in the therapeutic plan when indicated (Code: IIIH4) [Difficulty: ELE: R, Ap; WRE: An]

The following should be considered when the patient's response is evaluated:

- The opening of atelectatic areas would be signaled by the return of normal rather than diminished or absent breath sounds.
- Acute chest pain could be the result of a pneumothorax from barotrauma. A chest x-ray film would be needed to confirm or deny the presence of a pneumothorax. Stop the treatment if a pneumothorax is suspected.
- Be prepared to measure V_T, VC, and IC to determine the patient's goals and evaluate his or her progress.
- The patient may have an increase in sputum production if the deep-breathing exercises and IS open up atelectatic areas. The patient may have a more productive cough because of a greater VC.

d. Terminate the incentive spirometry treatment based on the patient's response to therapy (Code: IIIF1) [Difficulty: ELE: R, Ap; WRE: An]

Be prepared to stop the current treatment if the patient is having an adverse reaction to it. Usually, incentive spirometry is a safe procedure. However, some patients will hyperventilate during the procedure and will feel dizzy or light-headed. If this happens, the patient should be told to stop the treatment for a few minutes. The dizziness should go away, and the patient should be able to resume the IS procedure. Direct the patient to continue to inhale deeply but at a slower rate. If the above treatment modifications do not prevent the adverse effects, be prepared to recommend to the physician that the treatment be discontinued.

e. Recommend discontinuing the incentive spirometry treatment based on the patient's response to therapy (Code: IIIG1i) [Difficulty: ELE: R, Ap; WRE: An]

A treatment can be discontinued for one of three reasons. First, an adverse reaction to or complication of the treatment can lead to cessation of treatment. For example, stop the treatment if the patient has a serious problem, such as chest pain, that may be the result of a pneumothorax. Inform the physician if clinical evidence of this is noted. Treatment also may have to be stopped if the patient repeatedly hyperventilates during the IS procedure. Other reasons to terminate the treatment include inadequate pain control, exacerbation of bronchospasm, hypoxemia from removal of the patient's oxygen mask, and fatigue. If these problems are corrected, it may be possible to begin IS treatment again.

Second, ineffective treatment may lead to treatment discontinuation. If the patient cannot perform a proper IS treatment (unconscious, physically unable to perform, inadequate inspiratory volume), another way to treat atelectasis should be found. This could include IPPB. (See Chapter 14 for the discussion.) The physician would order this change in therapy.

Third, if the patient has recovered and no longer needs treatment, treatment can be discontinued. As the postsurgical patient recovers, walks about, and performs proper coughing and deep-breathing exercises, any atelectasis will be corrected. In many cases, IS can be stopped within a week after surgery. The physician would order that incentive spirometry be discontinued.

Exam Hint 7-3 (ELE, WRE)

Understand the indications for IS versus those for IPPB. Be prepared to recommend a change in IS volume or to change from IS to IPPB.

3. Respiratory care protocols

a. Develop the hyperinflation therapy protocol (Code: IIIH6b) [Difficulty: ELE: R; WRE: Ap, An]

b. Apply the hyperinflation therapy protocol (Code: IIIH8) [Difficulty: ELE: R, Ap; WRE: An]

c. Explain planned therapy and goals to the patient in understandable (nonmedical) terms to achieve the best results from the treatment (Code: IIIA6) [Difficulty: ELE: R, Ap; WRE: An]

d. Monitor the outcome of the hyperinflation therapy protocol (Code: IIIH7b) [Difficulty: ELE: R, Ap; WRE: An]

e. Communicate the outcome of therapy and change the treatment based on the protocol (Code: IIIA5) [Difficulty: ELE: R, Ap; WRE: An]

Review Table 7-1 for guidelines on the use of incentive spirometry. These and the previous discussion on adjusting the IS goal can be used to develop and implement a protocol and evaluate its outcomes. It may be possible to use a simpler patient care plan such as cough and deep-breathing exercises with ambulation. Or, it may be necessary to switch to IPPB.

4. Record and evaluate the patient's response to the treatment(s) or procedure(s) by doing the following:

a. Record and interpret the following: heart rate and rhythm, respiratory rate, blood pressure, body temperature, and pain level (Code: IIIA1b4) [Difficulty: ELE: R, Ap; WRE: An]

b. Record and interpret the patient's breath sounds (Code: IIIA1b3) [Difficulty: ELE: R, Ap; WRE: An]

If incentive spirometry is effective, the patient's breath sounds should improve. Areas of atelectasis, with diminished breath sounds, now should be heard as normal (vesicular).

c. Record and interpret the type of cough the patient has and the nature of the sputum (Code: IIIA1b3) [Difficulty: ELE: R, Ap; WRE: An]

If incentive spirometry is effective, the patient should be able to take in a deeper breath. This should result in a more effective cough and the ability to cough out secretions. Always note the nature of the patient's secretions.

d. Recheck any math work and make note of incorrect data (Code: IIIA1b2) [Difficulty: ELE: R, Ap; WRE: An]

Errors made in charting must be corrected by drawing a single mark through the error and writing in the correct information. Some prefer that the error be clarified further by writing in "error" next to it and adding initials. *Never erase or use any covering material over an error.*

5. Communicate information relevant to coordinating patient care and discharge planning [e.g., scheduling, avoiding conflicts, sequencing therapies] (Code: IIIA2b) [Difficulty: ELE: R, Ap; WRE: An]

Common scheduling problems involve meal times and when the patient must go to the radiology or physical therapy department.

BIBLIOGRAPHY

American Association for Respiratory Care: Clinical practice guideline: incentive spirometry, *Respir Care* 36(12):1402, 1991.

Cairo JM: Lung expansion devices. In: Cairo JM, Pilbeam SP, editors: *Mosby's respiratory care equipment*, ed 8, St Louis, 2009, Mosby.

Douce FH: Incentive spirometry and other aids to lung inflation. In: Barnes TA, editor: *Core textbook of respiratory care practice*, ed 2, St Louis, 1994, Mosby.

Eubanks DH, Bone RC: *Comprehensive respiratory care, a learning system*, ed 2, St Louis, 1990, Mosby.

Fink JB: Bronchial hygiene and lung expansion. In: Fink JB, Hunt GE, editors: *Clinical practice in respiratory care*, Philadelphia, 1999, Lippincott Williams & Wilkins.

Fink JB: Volume expansion therapy. In: Burton GG, Hodgkin JE, Ward JJ, editors: *Respiratory care: A guide to clinical practice*, Philadelphia, 1997, Lippincott-Raven.

Fink JB, Hess DR: Secretion clearance techniques. In: Hess DR, MacIntyre NR, Mishoe SC, editors: *Respiratory care principles & practice*, Philadelphia, 2002, WB Saunders.

Johnson NT, Pierson DJ: The spectrum of pulmonary atelectasis: pathophysiology, diagnosis, and therapy, *Respir Care* 31:1107, 1986.

Mang H, Obermayer A: Imposed work of breathing during sustained maximal inspiration: comparison of six incentive spirometers, *Respir Care* 34:1122, 1989.

Rutkowski JA: Hyperinflation therapy. In: Wyka KA, Mathews PJ, Clark WF, editors: *Foundations of respiratory care*, Albany, 2002, Delmar.

Scuderi J, Olsen GN: Respiratory therapy in the management of postoperative complications, *Respir Care* 34:281, 1989.

Shapiro BA, Kacmarek RM, Cane RD, et al: *Clinical application of respiratory care*, ed 4, St Louis, 1991, Mosby.

Wilkins RL: Lung expansion therapy. In: Wilkins RL, Stoller JK, Kacmarek RM, editors: *Egan's fundamentals of respiratory care*, ed 9, St Louis, 2009, Mosby.

Wojciechowski WV: Incentive spirometers, secretion evacuation devices, and inspiratory muscle training devices. In: Barnes TA, editor: *Core textbook of respiratory care practice*, ed 2, St Louis, 1994, Mosby.

SELF-STUDY QUESTIONS FOR THE ENTRY LEVEL EXAM *See page 588 for answers*

1. Your patient is quite weak and is unable to raise the ball marker on a flow displacement–type incentive spirometer to her set goal. She is becoming discouraged. What would you recommend?
   A. Have her continue trying.
   B. Recommend that she be switched to IPPB.
   C. Change her to a volume displacement–type spirometer.
   D. Discontinue the treatment because it is not effective.

2. A 16-year-old postoperative appendectomy patient has clear breath sounds and normal vital signs. What would you recommend to prevent atelectasis?
   A. CPAP at 5 cm H_2O
   B. PEP therapy
   C. IPPB
   D. IS

3. If pulmonary function results are not available, what initial IS goal should be set?
   A. The IC measured at the bedside
   B. The VC measured at the bedside
   C. Three times the V_T measured at the bedside
   D. Twice the V_T measured at the bedside

4. It is recommended that IS be performed how often while the patient is awake?
   A. At least 5 times/hr
   B. At least 10 times/hr
   C. At least 20 times/hr
   D. At least 10 times/day

5. Your patient has just performed several excellent IS efforts. She complains of tingling fingers and dizziness. Your response would be to
   A. Have her continue with additional IS maneuvers.
   B. Check her fingers and forehead for cyanosis.
   C. Call her physician to cancel the treatment order.
   D. Tell her to relax and breathe quietly until she feels normal again.

6. Your patient has a flow displacement type of IS device. She is attempting but is unable to inhale forcibly through it. What is the most likely problem?

A. The inspiratory tube is obstructed.
B. The patient is not really trying.
C. The flow resistance is set too high.
D. The bellows is in the locked-down position.

7. A patient's IS device is a flow displacement type. With good coaching, he can raise a ball with 900 cc/sec of flow. He can keep it elevated for 1.5 sec. What is his IC?
   A. 450 cc
   B. 900 cc
   C. 1350 cc
   D. 1800 cc

8. Your patient has been using an inspiratory muscle-training device. He is currently on the third largest of six settings and has been breathing comfortably through it 4 days/wk over the past 2 weeks. What would you now recommend that he do?
   A. Keep breathing through the same inspiratory hole.
   B. Breathe through the smallest hole.
   C. Breathe through the largest hole.
   D. Breathe through the next smallest hole.

9. A patient with advanced COPD is anxious and is feeling short of breath after returning from a medical procedure. What should the respiratory therapist tell the patient to do?
   A. Turn up the oxygen flow rate to his nasal cannula.
   B. Inhale through his PFLEX inspiratory muscle trainer.
   C. Use pursed-lip breathing.
   D. Exhale through his Flutter valve unit.

10. A patient is recovering from a neuromuscular disease and the physician wishes to speed up the process of strengthening his inspiratory muscles. What technique should the respiratory therapist recommend?
    A. PFLEX inspiratory muscle trainer
    B. Maximal inspiratory pressure (MIP)
    C. Maximal expiratory pressure (MEP)
    D. Trendelenburg positioning

SELF-STUDY QUESTIONS FOR THE WRITTEN REGISTRY EXAM *See page 613 for answers*

1. A previously healthy 27-year-old female had an emergency appendectomy 2 days ago. After a few minutes of incentive spirometry, she complains of tingling in her fingers and feeling dizzy. What should the respiratory therapist do?
   A. Stop the treatment and chart the patient's complaint.
   B. Have her inhale at a slower rate.

C. Reduce her IS volume goal.
D. Have her inhale a deeper volume.

2. You are the respiratory therapist assigned to teach a postoperative abdominal surgery patient about incentive spirometry. How would you explain the purpose of the treatment?
   A. It will prevent bilateral basilar microatelectasis.
   B. It will help the surgical wound heal faster.

C. It will treat pneumonia.

D. It will keep areas of the lungs from collapsing.

3. A 40-year-old cooperative female patient had her gallbladder removed 2 days ago. She is now slightly feverish and her chest x-ray shows signs of atelectasis in the right lower lobe. What should be the first treatment procedure to treat the problem?

A. Incentive spirometry

B. PEP therapy

C. Nasotracheal suctioning

D. IPPB therapy

4. As the lead respiratory therapist, you are in charge of developing an incentive spirometry protocol for an obese postoperative open heart surgery patient with bilateral atelectasis. All of the following could be outcome measures EXCEPT

A. Normal lung fields on chest x-ray

B. Increased arterial oxygen level

C. Increased cardiac output

D. Improved breath sounds

5. A 150-pound (70-kg) patient with a recent stroke has complications of atelectasis and bronchitis. His inspiratory capacity is measured at 40% of his predicted value. What therapy would be most appropriate initially?

A. Incentive spirometry with sustained maximal inspiration

B. IPPB therapy

C. Positive expiratory pressure therapy

D. Postural drainage with percussion and vibration

6. Your patient is using a flow displacement type of incentive spirometer at a rate of 20 times per minute. She is able to suspend the ball marker for 1 second at her targeted inspiratory capacity. How could the treatment be improved upon?

A. Increase her target volume by 500 mL.

B. Have her breathe at a slower rate and hold the volume longer.

C. Have her exhale more rapidly.

D. Lower her target volume by 100 mL and raise her respiratory rate to 25 times per minute.

7. You are called to evaluate a patient who has been using a volume displacement–type incentive spirometer for 2 days since her cholecystectomy procedure. She has been following a patient-directed protocol and is easily able to inspire the 1.5-liter goal set on the unit. What would you recommend?

A. Increase her goal to 3 liters.

B. Switch her to a flow displacement–type unit with a 1.5-liter goal.

C. Increase her volume goal to 2 liters.

D. Stop the protocol and begin IPPB treatments.

8. A patient with obstructive airways disease should be taught all of the following cough techniques EXCEPT

A. Take two to three breaths in and out before coughing.

B. Breathe in a volume larger than the V_T but less than the VC.

C. Perform a normal cough.

D. Perform a midinspiratory cough.

9. IS is indicated when a patient's postoperative IC is what percentage of the preoperative IC?

A. Between 30% and 50%

B. Between 50% and 80%

C. Between 80% and 90%

D. Greater than 90%

10. Your patient has an ideal body weight of 90 kg (200 lb). What would be his initial IC goal?

A. His VC

B. At least half of his VC

C. At least 1080 mL

D. At least 540 mL

11. If IS has been successful, which breath sounds can be heard in the areas where atelectasis was noted before treatment?

A. Bronchial

B. Absent

C. Normal vesicular

D. Tracheal

8 Humidity and Aerosol Therapy

Note 1: This book is written to cover every item listed as testable on the *Entry Level Examination (ELE), Written Registry Examination (WRE),* and *Clinical Simulation Examination (CSE).*

The listed code for each item is taken from the National Board for Respiratory Care (NBRC) **Summary Content Outline for CRT (Certified Respiratory Therapist) and Written RRT (Registered Respiratory Therapist) Examinations** (http://evolve.elsevier.com/Sills/resptherapist/). For example, if an item is testable on both the ELE and the WRE, it will be shown simply as: (Code: . . .). If an item is testable only on the ELE, it will be shown as: (ELE code: . . .). If an item is testable only on the WRE, it will be shown as: (WRE code: . . .).

Following each item's code will be the difficulty level of the questions on that item on the ELE and the WRE. (See the Introduction for a full explanation of the three question difficulty levels.) **Recall [R]** level questions typically expect the exam taker to recall factual information. **Application [Ap]** level questions are harder because the exam taker may have to apply factual information to a clinical situation. **Analysis [An]** level questions are the most challenging because the exam taker may have to use critical thinking to evaluate patient data to make a clinical decision.

Note 2: A review of the most recent Entry Level Examinations (ELE) has shown that an average of 7 questions (out of 140), or 5% of the exam, will cover humidity and aerosol therapy. A review of the most recent Written Registry Examinations (WRE) has shown that an average of 2 questions (out of 100), or 2% of the exam, will cover humidity and aerosol therapy. The Clinical Simulation Examination is comprehensive and may include everything that should be known by an advanced level respiratory therapist.

MODULE A

Humidity and aerosol therapy

1. Maintain adequate humidification (ELE code: IIIB8) [Difficulty: ELE: R, Ap, An]

Most patients receive supplemental humidity or aerosol delivered to their airways and lungs for one of two reasons.

First, patients with excessive pulmonary secretions benefit from the inhalation of extra humidity or an aerosol to reduce the viscosity (thickness) of their secretions. This makes it easier for the secretions to be coughed or to be suctioned out. Second, supplemental oxygen (O_2) from the central delivery system or the cylinders is absolutely dry. Adding humidity or aerosol to the O_2 prevents drying of the mucous membrane.

a. Indications for humidity therapy

1. Humidification of dry therapeutic medical gases in patients with a normal upper airway

Body humidity is the water saturation condition of the gas in the lungs. Under normal conditions with air, it is 43.9 (44) mg/L absolute humidity and 46.90 (47) mm Hg at 37° C (98.6° F). In other words, air is always warmed to body temperature and saturated with water by the time it reaches the lungs. As can be seen in Table 8-1, both water content and vapor pressure in the lungs vary with the patient's temperature.

Humidity deficit is the difference between the body humidity conditions and the room air (or other gas) conditions. Some humidity deficit is normal because the air must be warmed to body temperature and saturated by the time it reaches the lungs, and room conditions are rarely similar to those in the lung. The humidity deficit is eliminated through warming and humidifying of inhaled air by the respiratory passages.

The clinical practice guidelines of the American Association for Respiratory Care state that supplemental humidity is not needed for O_2 at flows of 4 L/min or less. This includes nasal cannulas and some air entrainment mask settings. As long as the patient has a normal upper airway and the hospital has a relative humidity (RH) of about 40%, the patient should be able to fully saturate the gas with no adverse effects. Some clinicians believe that *any* O_2 flow through a nasal cannula should be humidified to prevent the local mucosa from drying out. Usually, an unheated bubble-type humidifier is used to deliver about 40% RH at room temperature. The patient then is able to fully saturate the gas. All agree that dry O_2

TABLE 8-1	Saturated Air Values for Absolute Humidity and Vapor Pressure Under Room and Body Temperature Ranges*		
Temperature		**Absolute Humidity,**	**Vapor Pressure,**
°C	°F	mg/L	mm Hg
21	70	18.35 (18)	18.62 (19)
22	71.6	19.42 (19)	19.79 (20)
23	73	20.58 (21)	21.02 (21)
33	92	35.61 (36)	37.59 (38)
34	93	37.57 (38)	39.75 (40)
35	95	39.60 (40)	42.02 (42)
36	97	41.70 (42)	44.40 (44)
37[†]	98.6	43.90 (44)	46.90 (47)
38	100	46.19 (46)	49.51 (50)
39	102	48.59 (49)	52.26 (52)
40	104	51.10 (51)	55.13 (55)
41	106	53.70 (54)	58.14 (58)

*The warmer the air is, the more water it can hold.
[†]So-called normal body temperature; it normally varies under different conditions.

TABLE 8-2	Aerosol Particle Sizes and Their Likely Deposition Points in the Airways and Lungs
Location	**MMAD* Particle Size, μm**
Nose or mouth to larynx	10 and larger
Trachea to terminal bronchioles	9-5
Respiratory bronchioles to alveoli	5-2
Lung parenchyma (alveoli)	1-3

MMAD, Mass median aerodynamic diameter.
*MMAD is defined as the aerosol diameter around which the mass is equally divided, that is, 50% of the aerosol mass is found in particles smaller than the MMAD, and 50% of the aerosol mass is found in particles larger than the MMAD.
Note: Some controversy exists over the size of the particles that deposit in the airways and lungs. This table lists what seems to be a majority opinion. Aerosol particle diameter sizes are listed in units of micrometers, which are one-thousandth of a millimeter. As a point of clarification, most references list the symbol for a micrometer as μ; others use the international system unit of micrometer, which is symbolized as μm.

at flows of greater than 4 L/min by any device must be humidified.

2. Elimination of the humidity deficit in a patient with a bypassed upper airway

A patient with an endotracheal tube or tracheostomy tube is not able to humidify his or her inhaled gas. This creates a large humidity deficit that must be eliminated by providing a therapeutic humidity source. Failure to do so will result in drying of the mucous membrane and plugging of mucus. A heated humidifier is recommended and should be set to deliver gas at ≥33° C to provide 80% to 100% RH to the patient. In any patient situation, the humidity deficit will be eliminated if saturated air is delivered at body temperature.

3. Reduction of airway resistance

Strong evidence suggests that patients with exercise-induced and cold air–induced asthma are less likely to experience bronchospasm if they inhale warmed, humidified gas while exercising. The clinical goal in this case is to prevent an increase in airway resistance.

b. Indications for aerosol therapy
1. Humidification of dry therapeutic medical gases

Aerosol particles heated to body temperature can fully saturate inhaled carrier gas through evaporation of some of the particles. This is indicated in patients who need the

humidity *and* a medicinal aerosol. This way is not preferred for delivering just humidity to a patient, and it is possible to overhydrate the airway, especially in neonates, through long-term aerosol therapy. Aerosol particles can carry bacteria and other pathogens, whereas humidity (water vapor) alone cannot.

2. Soothing of an irritated upper airway

Two generally accepted indications exist for delivery of a bland aerosol (sterile water or normal saline solution) to soothe an irritated upper airway: (1) following extubation and (2) laryngotracheobronchitis (LTB, or pediatric croup). Generally, a cool (room temperature) aerosol is delivered to reduce airway edema.

3. Delivery of medications to the airways and lungs

Respiratory therapists give many medications to patients, and these medications obviously must reach the target area. Table 8-2 gives the particle size of each medicinal aerosol and its most likely deposition area.

4. Increased clearance of secretions

Traditionally, many patients with a mild case of bronchitis were given breathing treatments with a bland aerosol to help them mobilize secretions. The aerosol was thought to add enough liquid to the secretions to enable the patient to cough them out. The patient, as it is now understood, can cough more effectively because the aerosol irritates the airway, and the patient's own bronchial/submucosal glands pour out additional mucus. This reflex is mediated by the vagus nerve. This form of therapy probably is not indicated in most situations. It is clinically more effective to increase the patient's oral or intravenous fluids so that the bronchial/submucosal glands can produce secretions that are not thick.

5. Induced sputum production for a sputum specimen

Patients who have few, if any, secretions but from whom a sputum specimen is needed (e.g., patients with suspected tuberculosis or lung cancer) can have sputum production induced (see the mechanism of action described previously). Typically, the patient inhales an aerosol of hypertonic saline solution for about 5 to 10 minutes. Ultrasonic nebulizers are used often because they produce a dense mist of small particles.

2. Interview the patient to determine sputum production (Code: IB5c) [Difficulty: ELE: R, Ap; WRE: An]

Find out from the patient approximately how much sputum is produced in a day. Also, find out if certain times of the day are more productive or less productive than others. Try to relate this to breathing treatments, medications, activities, meals, and allergies.

3. Observe the patient's sputum production

a. Observe the patient for changes in sputum characteristics (ELE code: IIIE5) [Difficulty: ELE: R, Ap, An]

b. Use inspection to assess the patient's cough, sputum amount, and character (Code: IB1c) [Difficulty: ELE: R, Ap; WRE: An]

The patient's sputum characteristics (e.g., consistency, color, smell) and amount must be known if the effectiveness of humidity or aerosol therapy is to be assessed. Review the related discussion in Chapter 1, and see Table 1-12. Try to relate this information to breathing treatments, medications, activities, meals, and allergies.

4. Assess the patient's overall cardiopulmonary status by auscultation to determine the presence of normal or abnormal breath sounds (Code: IB4a) [Difficulty: ELE: R, Ap; WRE: An] and (Code: IIIE11) [Difficulty: ELE: R, Ap; WRE: An]

Review the discussion in Chapter 1, if necessary. The presence of expiratory crackles (also called rhonchi) would indicate airway secretions. If the patient is able to cough out the secretions, abnormal breath sounds, such as crackles, should improve. If the patient's secretions are thick (high viscosity), then aerosol therapy, as well as increased fluid intake, probably is indicated.

MODULE B

Humidity and aerosol generators and administrative devices

1. Humidity delivered through small-bore tubing

a. Manipulate bubble-type humidifiers by order or protocol (ELE code: IIA3) [Difficulty: ELE: R, Ap, An]

1. Get the necessary equipment for the procedure

Bubble-type humidifiers are used on patients with a normal upper airway who need some supplemental humidity because of the dryness of medical O_2. These devices usually are not heated and, in fact, deliver gas cooled to below room temperature. They provide around 40% RH at the delivered gas temperature. The rest of the humidity has to be made up by the patient (Figures 8-1 and 8-2). If clinically indicated, a wraparound type of heater can be added to raise the temperature of the delivered gas and reduce the patient's humidity deficit.

Figure 8-1 Comparison of humidity content by bubble-type humidifiers and various nebulizers.

Three different types of these humidifiers are designed to add some humidity to dry O_2 delivered through small-bore tubing: traditional bubble humidifiers, jet humidifiers, and underwater jet humidifiers.

a. Bubble humidifiers. Bubble humidifiers use a perforated capillary tube or a porous diffusion head to break the O_2 into small bubbles (see Figure 8-2). This allows for greater surface area contact of the O_2 with the water and raises the RH by evaporation. The water level in the reservoir must be kept within the manufacturers' specifications and, if possible, as full as possible. The lower the water level, the lower is the RH because less time exists for evaporation. The faster the O_2 flow, the lower is the RH.

b. Jet humidifiers. Jet humidifiers create an aerosol baffled out of the delivered gas flow. The RH is increased through evaporation of some of the aerosol droplets. These units deliver a higher RH than is delivered by bubble humidifiers. They have the additional advantage of delivering the same RH at higher flow levels and as the water level drops.

c. Underwater jet humidifiers. Underwater jet humidifiers create water vapor and an aerosol. The aerosol is not baffled out as it is in jet humidifiers; therefore, these units deliver the highest RH. They can deliver the same humidity level at high gas flows and as the water level drops. Aerosol particles can carry pathogens, so strict infection control standards must be met to protect the patient. Often the water and the humidifier must be changed at least every 24 hours. If the patient needs the highest-possible-delivered RH, a jet humidifier or an underwater jet humidifier would be a better choice than a bubble type.

2. Put the equipment together and make sure that it works properly

3. Troubleshoot any problems with the equipment

Many simple bubble humidifiers come prepackaged with sterile water and can be used for many short-term patients (e.g., those in the recovery room) or for a single long-term patient. When the water runs low, they are discarded. Bubble and other types of humidifiers consist of a reservoir jar for the water and a Diameter Index Safety System (DISS) O_2 connector lid that screws on. Turn on the flowmeter and make sure that O_2 flows through the delivery tube and bubbles into the water. Failure to bubble usually indicates that the lid and the jar are not screwed together tightly, or that the delivery tube is plugged. If the tube cannot be cleared, it must be replaced.

Most of the newer bubble-type units have a pop-off type of high-pressure relief valve that is released if the pressure builds up to 40 mm Hg or 2 psi. Pinch closed the small-bore tubing to build up pressure and test the pop-off valve. Feel for the gas to escape from the valve. Many valves whistle to signal a gas leak. Do not use a unit with a pop-off valve that does not open under pressure.

b. Nasal cannula

As has been discussed earlier, current guidelines state that humidity does not need to be added to these devices if the flow is 4 L/min or less. However, some patients complain of nasal dryness and discomfort if the cannula's O_2 is not humidified. The physician and the practitioner may believe that the patient's discomfort warrants the addi-

Figure 8-2 Oxygen leaving outlet of the bubble-type humidifier is cooler than room temperature because of evaporation. Some warming toward room temperature occurs as the oxygen travels through the tubing to the patient. *(From Scanlan CL: Humidity and aerosol therapy. In: Scanlan CL, Spearman CB, Sheldon RL, editors: Egan's fundamentals of respiratory care, ed 5, St Louis, 1990, Mosby.)*

tion of a bubble-type humidifier. Agreement has been reached on the addition of humidity to flows greater than 4 L/min. See Figure 8-3 for a humidified nasal cannula setup. See Chapter 6 for the discussion on a high-flow nasal cannula.

c. Oxygen masks

As has been stated, the addition of humidity to any O_2 mask with an O_2 flow of 4 L/min or less is considered unnecessary. Humidity should be added to any mask with more than 4 L/min of O_2 added. This would include simple O_2 masks at higher flows, higher O_2 percentage air entrainment masks, partial-rebreathing masks, and non-rebreathing masks.

2. Humidity delivered through large-bore tubing

Most patients who need delivery of humidity through large-bore tubing have had the upper airway bypassed by an endotracheal or tracheostomy tube; therefore, they cannot humidify inspired gas in the normal manner. In other cases, humidity is added because the patient is receiving dry medical O_2. In both situations, a heated

Figure 8-3 Adult wearing a nasal cannula that delivers oxygen humidified by a bubble-type humidifier. *(From Guidelines for disinfection of respiratory care equipment used in the home, Respir Care 33:801, 1988.)*

humidifier is recommended. It should be set to deliver gas between 31° C and 35° C to the patient and should be able to provide 80% to 100% RH in this temperature range. The following humidity- and aerosol-generating devices deliver conditioned gas to the patient through large-bore (22-mm inner diameter [ID]) tubing.

a. Manipulate large-volume humidifiers by order or protocol: cascade, wick, and passover types (ELE code: IIA3) [Difficulty: ELE: R, Ap, An]

1. Get the necessary equipment for the procedure

Cascade, wick, and passover-type humidifiers have an adjustable heater so the water in the reservoir is at or greater than body temperature. This enables them to provide up to 100% of the patient's body humidity. With all of these units, the temperature of the inspired gas near the patient must be measured. Ideally, the gas temperature is kept the same as the patient's to provide 100% relative humidity. One of these types of units is used to provide humidity when the patient's upper airway is bypassed by an endotracheal or tracheostomy tube (Figure 8-4).

The Bennett Cascade is a classic example of these types of humidifiers (Figure 8-5). It was used most commonly with a mechanical ventilator but also was used with other types of systems for delivering humidity with or without oxygen. Its basic principle of operation is an efficient bubble-type humidifier. The inspiratory gas must flow through the water before evaporation can occur. A variety of similar devices are now on the market. *Note:* Even though these units are no longer available, the NBRC refers to this basic type of device as a Cascade-type humidifier.

The wick-type heated humidifier employs a wick, often made of sponge or paper, to soak up water for evaporation (Figure 8-6). The water, wick, or both are heated so that 100% RH can be delivered. These units also are used with mechanical ventilators or other systems, including air entrainment devices, because they have very little resistance to the gas flowing through them as evaporation occurs. Some units are designed for use with a heated wire ventilator circuit and feature an automatic water feed system and a servo-controlled thermostat to keep the water and the circuit at the same temperature. This minimizes condensation.

With passover-type humidifiers, the patient's gas simply passes over the surface of a reservoir of hot water. These sometimes are called "hot pots." By themselves, these units are probably the least effective at humidifying gas. When they are used on ventilators, other features such as copper mesh in a heated inspiratory tube are used to increase the surface area for evaporation.

Figure 8-4 Gases leaving outlet of heated humidifier are hot and saturated with water vapor. As cooling occurs in the tubing, vapor condenses and absolute humidity (AH) decreases, while relative humidity (RH) remains at 100% (saturated). Note that almost half of the original vapor is "lost" to condensate in this example. *(From Wilkins RL, Stoller JK, Kacmarek RM: Egan's fundamentals of respiratory care, ed 9, St Louis, 2009, Mosby.)*

Figure 8-5 Cascade-type humidifier. *(From Scanlan CL: Humidity and aerosol therapy. In: Scanlan CL, Spearman CB, Sheldon RL, editors: Egan's fundamentals of respiratory care, ed 5, St Louis, 1990, Mosby.)*

Heated humidified
oxygen/air mixture
to patient

Dry oxygen/air
mixture from gas source
(e.g., blender)

Saturated
wick

CONCHA 1500
Prefilled, Disposable
Sterile Water Reservoir

One-way valve isolates
the reservoir from the column

Figure 8-6 Functional diagram of a wick-type humidifier with an automatic water feed system. Water automatically enters a warmed reservoir, where it is drawn up the wick. Dry gas flows past the wick, where evaporation takes place before the gas is directed to the patient. *(Redrawn from Hudson Respiratory Care, Temecula, CA. In: Cairo J, Pilbeam S: Mosby's respiratory therapy equipment, ed 8, St Louis, 2010, Mosby.)*

b. Manipulate a heat-moisture exchanger by order or protocol (ELE code: IIA3) [Difficulty: ELE: R, Ap, An]

1. Get the necessary equipment for the procedure

A heat-moisture exchanger (HME) is a passive humidifier that recycles the patient's own exhaled water vapor. The HME contains a highly absorbent material that is warmed and moistened when a patient's exhaled breath passes through it. The patient's next inspiration is warmed and humidified by the water absorbed within the HME (Figure 8-7). These units are not as efficient as the humidifiers described earlier and are not able to provide 100% of body humidity to a patient. If possible, select an HME that has these characteristics: (1) is at least 70% efficient (provides at least 30 mg/L water vapor), (2) has a low compliance if used with a ventilator circuit, (3) is lightweight, (4) has little dead space, and (5) has little flow resistance.

Many brands of HME are available for either of two clinical applications. The first clinical use involves adding an HME to the outer part of a tracheostomy tube. A 15-mm ID opening allows the HME to be attached to the tube; the other end of the HME is open to room air. This type is small and convenient to use for many patients with a permanent tracheostomy; in addition, it improves a patient's mobility. The second clinical use involves patients who require mechanical ventilation. The patient end of the HME is a 15-mm ID opening that can attach to the endotracheal or tracheostomy tube; the other end of the HME has a 22-mm ID opening so the ventilator circuit or supplemental oxygen can be attached.

2. Put the equipment together and make sure that it works properly

3. Troubleshoot any problems with the equipment

Humidifiers must be assembled properly, especially when they are used to humidify a mechanical ventilator. Any loose connections may result in an air leak and loss of tidal volume (V_T). Make sure the water level is maintained properly.

Some cooling occurs as heated gas passes through the large-bore tubing, which results in condensation (so-called "rain out") that must be drained away. Placing a water trap into the lowest point of the tubing drains the water and helps keep the tubing clear. Remember to continue to look periodically for water puffing or sloshing back and forth in the tubing. Make sure that any condensate is drained out of the tubing and thrown away. Do not drain the condensate back into the water reservoir because any microorganisms in the tubing or condensate could reproduce in the reservoir.

2. Put the equipment together and make sure that it works properly (NBRC code: IIA3) [Difficulty: R, Ap]

3. Troubleshoot any problems with the equipment (NBRC code: IIA3) [Difficulty: R, Ap]

HMEs typically come preassembled by the manufacturer. The 15-mm ID opening must be placed over the patient's endotracheal or tracheostomy tube. The other opening of the HME can be connected to the ventilator circuit or oxygen source, if needed. Follow the manufacturer's recommendation regarding how frequently the HME should be replaced—often every 24 hours. However, current guidelines indicate that they can be used safely for at least 48 hours, possibly up to a week.

Secretions coughed into the HME can obstruct the flow of gas and thus make it difficult or impossible for the patient to breathe. The HME must be removed and discarded if it becomes obstructed, and it must be replaced by a new one. An HME should *not* be used with a patient

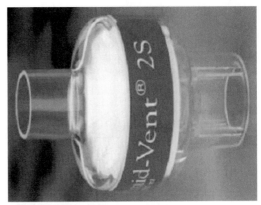

Figure 8-7   Heat-moisture exchanger (HME). **Left,** Cut-away functional drawing shows the *(left)* ventilator side and *(right)* patient side of an HME. During exhalation, the warmed and saturated air (33° C and 100% relative humidity [RH]) from the patient passes through the HME in the water-absorbing material. During inhalation, the cooler and dryer room air is warmed and becomes more saturated with water vapor as it passes through the HME to the patient. **Right,** Photograph of an HME. The opening on the left side is 15 mm inner diameter (ID) and connects to a patient's endotracheal tube. The opening on the right side is 22 mm ID and can have a ventilator circuit or T-piece attached for supplemental oxygen and aerosol. *(Courtesy Telefax Medical, Research Triangle Park, NC. In: Cairo J, Pilbeam S:* Mosby's respiratory therapy equipment, *ed 8, St Louis, 2010, Mosby.)*

known to cough out large quantities of secretions or blood.

3. Manipulate nebulizers and related delivery systems by order or protocol (ELE code: IIA4) [Difficulty: ELE: R, Ap, An]

a. Ultrasonic nebulizers

1. Get the necessary equipment for the procedure

Large-volume ultrasonic units often are chosen for delivery of bland solutions to the lower airways because of the small particle size and high output. (So-called "bland aerosols" are composed of particles of water or saline rather than medicated aerosols.) Ultrasonic nebulizers (USNs) work by converting electrical energy into high-frequency sound energy, which creates aerosol particles. The frequency is vital because it results in a stable aerosol with a mean particle size of about 3 μm in diameter. This is an ideal size for penetrating deeply into the lungs to the smallest airways. The only control on these units is used for amplitude (power), and it controls the aerosol output. The range is usually up to 3 to 6 mL/min, depending on the model. This output is greater than that possible with most pneumatic nebulizers. The aerosol can be carried to the patient via a built-in fan or by an outside O₂ source (Figure 8-8). The warm aerosol that is created minimizes the patient's humidity deficit.

Historically, ultrasonic nebulizers have not been chosen for upper airway aerosol deposition or for administration of pharmacologically active medications such as bronchodilators, mucolytics, and antibiotics. These medications may not nebulize at the same rate as the saline diluent,

Figure 8-8   Functional diagram of the ultrasonic nebulizer. **A,** Electrical current generator; **B,** cable; **C,** piezoelectric crystal; **D,** couplant chamber; **E,** solution cup; **F,** carrier gas inlet; and **G,** aerosol outlet. *(From Barnes TA, editor:* Core textbook of respiratory care practice, *ed 2, St Louis, 1994, Mosby.)*

which creates the risk that a very concentrated dose may be delivered at the end of treatment. Some medications may be mechanically broken down by the high-frequency vibration and rendered useless.

Recently, small-volume USN units have been designed to specifically nebulize medications into the circuit of a mechanical ventilator. Depending on the manufacturer, the USN can be powered electrically by the ventilator, by any electrical outlet, or by batteries. These units are designed to rapidly nebulize the small volume of medication (with or without diluent). The tidal volume breath carries the medication into the patient's airways. Be aware that even though drugs have been given this way, pharmaceutical companies have not included in their dosing information the delivery of undiluted medications.

2. Put the equipment together and make sure that it works properly

3. Troubleshoot any problems with the equipment

Always follow the manufacturer's instructions when you are setting up the delivery system. Figure 8-8 shows the common features, and Table 8-3 describes how to troubleshoot many common problems. Many clinical difficulties seem to involve keeping the proper fluid levels in the couplant chamber and the solution cup. If the sterile water in the couplant chamber is too low, the vibration cannot reach the solution cup and no aerosol will be produced. If the saline level in the solution cup is too low or too high, the vibrational energy will not focus properly on the surface of the saline solution, and no aerosol will be produced. Water should not be allowed to condense and fill low points in the large-bore tubing; if it does, ultrasonic particles will liquefy as the carrier gas is forced to pass through the condensate. The exiting gas would be humid-

TABLE 8-3 Ultrasonic Nebulizer Troubleshooting		
Symptom	**Possible Problem**	**Suggested Check**
Unit installed and connected as specified, but pilot light does not turn on when switch is turned to the "on" position	Electrical outlet defective Circuit breaker tripped Fuse blown	Check outlet with lamp or other appliance Reset the circuit breaker, or change fuse on the power switch; if the circuit breaker continues to trip or the fuse blows again, service is needed
Unit installed and connected as specified; power pilot light turns on, normal ultrasonic activity visible in nebulizer chamber, but no aerosol output occurs	Nebulizer chamber contaminated	Wash nebulizer chamber; decontaminate
Unit installed and connected as specified; power pilot light turns on, but little ultrasonic activity is visible in the nebulizer chamber, and aerosol output is low (even when on the no. 10 power setting)	Couplant water excessively aerated Nebulizer module and couplant water too cold Diaphragm distorted, permitting air bubbles to interfere with proper transmission of vibrational energy into the nebulizer chamber	Wait for deaeration Use warmer couplant water Check to see that diaphragm is properly shaped and installed; be sure that the concave (recessed) side faces the interior of the chamber Clean couplant compartment and replace couplant water
Same as symptom described previously but at a lower power setting	Power setting too low to start and establish nebulization	Turn output control knob to maximum power setting, then reduce to desired setting
Unit installed and connected as specified, and power pilot light turns on "Add couplant" light is on, and no ultrasonic activity is visible in the nebulizer chamber	Insufficient couplant water	Add water to the couplant compartment
Unit installed and connected as specified, and power pilot light turns on "Add couplant" light is off, but no ultrasonic activity is visible in the nebulizer chamber	Power supply overheated and its thermostatic control opened	The cooling air has been restricted, or cooling fins need cleaning. The switch will reset when the equipment returns to room temperature
Liquid reservoir filled and properly connected to nebulizer chamber, but chamber does not fill (for continuous-feed system only)	Foreign material or air bubbles in feed tubes Liquid level control in nebulizer chamber plugged with foreign material Air leaks at tube connection or reservoir cap	Flush the system Clean or flush the system Tighten all connections by pushing tubes into fittings

From Op't Holt T: Aerosol generators and humidifiers. In: Barnes TA, editor: *Respiratory care practice*, Chicago, 1988, Mosby.

ified through evaporation but would carry no aerosol particles. If the carrier gas is O_2 blended with air through an air entrainment system, any backpressure could result in an increase in the O_2 percentage and a decrease in the total flow. Remember to always measure the O_2 percentage near the patient.

b. Manipulate large-volume pneumatic nebulizers by order or protocol (ELE code: IIA4) [Difficulty: ELE: R, Ap, An]

1. Get the necessary equipment for the procedure

All large-volume, pneumatically powered nebulizers share the common feature of having a liquid reservoir of at least 250 mL and produce a bland aerosol. (So-called "bland aerosols" are composed of particles of water or saline rather than medicated aerosols.) These nebulizers also typically entrain room air to increase the total gas flow. They share the following common features:

- All are powered by air or O_2 that is delivered through a flowmeter. As the gas flow drops, the aerosol output decreases.
- All make use of Bernoulli's principle with a jet that is used to entrain liquid, room air, or both into the main gas flow.
- All have a capillary tube that allows the liquid to flow *up* to the jet for nebulization. (Remember that with bubble-type humidifiers, O_2 flows *down* the capillary tube.)
- All have a baffle against which the aerosol is sprayed to create a more uniform particle size.

Many, but not all, pneumatic nebulizers allow for a changeable inspired O_2 percentage. Provided that the jet is powered by O_2, the air entrainment ports can be opened up to increase air entrainment and increase total flow (lowering the inspired O_2 percentage) or closed down to decrease air entrainment and decrease total flow (raising the inspired O_2 percentage). The O_2 percentage usually can vary from 35% to 100%. Remember to always analyze the inspired O_2 percentage near the patient because both water in the aerosol tubing and backpressure decrease the entrained air and raise the O_2 percentage.

2. Put the equipment together and make sure that it works properly

3. Troubleshoot any problems with the equipment

Most pneumatic nebulizers have an appearance that is similar to that of bubble-type humidifiers. Key components include a large reservoir jar and a top with a DISS O_2 connector and a capillary tube to the jet. Make sure the nebulizer is screwed firmly onto the oxygen flowmeter and that the component parts are attached and work properly. Keep the capillary tube and jet clear of debris to keep the aerosol output from dropping. These units allow for variable O_2 percentages. Keep the air entrainment ports open so that proper gas mixing occurs and the desired O_2 percentage is provided (Figure 8-9). If water is present in the large-bore tubing or if the tubing is pinched, less room air will be entrained, and the delivered oxygen percentage will be higher than ordered. Keep the reservoir's water level at the proper level. If the water level drops to below the refill line, no water will be drawn up the capillary tube to the jet. If the water is filled to above the maximum line, the jet may not operate properly. Heating of the water, aerosol, or both is accomplished in one of the following ways:

- A heated metal rod is immersed into the reservoir water through a port in the top of the nebulizer. A dial is used to control how hot the rod gets. Water temperature varies depending on how deep it is, so as the water level drops, the remaining water gets hotter. It is very important that the gas temperature near the patient be measured, and that the water level be kept stable to prevent burning of the airway.

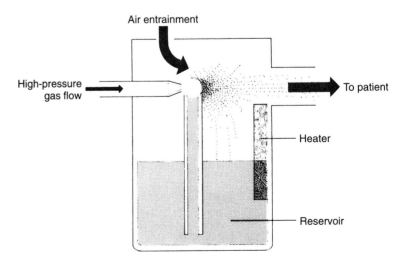

Figure 8-9 Large-volume air entrainment nebulizer. *(From Shapiro BA, Kacmarek RM, Cane RD, et al, editors:* Clinical application of respiratory care, *ed 4, St Louis, 1991, Mosby.)*

The heated rod presents the risk of burns to a practitioner who accidentally touches it. It must be disinfected between patients and changed as often as the nebulizer is changed. Because of these issues, these units are unlikely to be seen in clinical practice.

- Two other systems use variations on this idea of directly heating the water in the reservoir jar. The first heats the water as it passes through the capillary tube. The second type directly heats only a small amount of the reservoir water just before it is aerosolized. Each has the advantage of a short warm-up time compared with the heated metal rod systems. Some units have an external temperature probe for placement in the aerosol tubing. The probe acts as a servo-controller of the heating unit for better temperature regulation.

- A flexible heater is wrapped around the outside of the reservoir. A dial is used to control how hot the heater gets. The water temperature increases as the water level drops. Monitor the gas temperature near the patient for safety purposes.

- A clip-on heating base plate can be added to special reservoir jars with a metal plate. These are preferable to the previously mentioned types because they ensure a constant temperature to the aerosol as the water level drops.

Heating the water or aerosol reduces the patient's humidity deficit and usually is done if the secretions are thick. See Figure 8-1 for the location of the aerosol particles and their relationship with the dew point and with the patient's body humidity.

4. Aerosol delivery systems

Large-bore tubing (also known as *aerosol tubing* or *corrugated tubing*) is needed to connect the aerosol generator with the patient. This tubing has a 22-mm ID so it can be connected to a face mask, T-piece, etc.

c. Aerosol masks

The aerosol mask looks similar to the simple O_2 mask, except that it has larger side ports for exhalation and a 22-mm outer diameter (OD) adapter for attachment of the large-bore tubing (Figure 8-10). This often is considered to be a low-flow O_2 mask because the ports are open to room air; therefore, it is difficult to ensure that the patient receives the set O_2 percentage. If the flow is high enough that aerosol mist can be seen flowing out of the side ports during an inspiration, little or no room air is being inspired and the aerosol mask is now a high-flow device. Some clinicians have increased the total flow through an aerosol mask by using a Y adapter to combine the large-bore tubing coming from two large-volume nebulizers In any case, it is best to analyze the O_2 percentage inside the mask to be sure of what the patient is inhaling.

Flowmeter

Large-bore tubing

Aerosol mask

Large reservoir nebulizer

Figure 8-10 Adult wearing an aerosol mask who is receiving supplemental oxygen and aerosol from a heated large-volume nebulizer. As the warmed, humidified gas cools on its way to the patient, condensation will result in water draining to the lowest part of the large-bore tubing. *(From Guidelines for disinfection of respiratory care equipment used in the home,* Respir *Care 33:801, 1988.)*

Any of the previously mentioned humidity or aerosol devices can be used and powered by compressed air or O_2.

d. Face tents, tracheostomy masks, tracheostomy collars, and Brigg's adapter/T-piece

A face tent, a tracheostomy mask and collar, and Brigg's adapter (T-piece) are discussed in Chapter 6. All have a 22-mm ID adapter so that large-bore tubing can be added to them. Any of the previously mentioned humidity or aerosol devices can be used with these and are powered by compressed air or O_2.

MODULE C
Environmental control devices

1. Manipulate incubators by order or protocol (WRE code: IIA12a) [Difficulty: WRE: R, Ap]

a. Get the necessary equipment for the procedure

An incubator is indicated in the care of a sick newborn who needs an enclosed space for an isolated, controlled environment. (See Figure 8-11.) (Some practitioners may refer to an incubator as an Isolette, which is a common brand of incubator.) Most incubators are used only in neonatal or pediatric care units and are powered electrically through standard electrical outlets. However, some incubators are designed to transport an infant between

Figure 8-11 An incubator used to control an infant's environment. Typically, the incubator is made of clear Plexiglass so the infant can be seen, and it has two closeable ports on each side. These can be opened so the caregiver can work with the infant. Controls below the infant are used to adjust the temperature, humidity, and possibly oxygen percentage within the incubator. A radiant warmer may be positioned over an incubator to keep the infant in a neutral thermal environment. *(From Wilkins RL, Stoller JK, Kacmarek RM editors:* Egan's fundamentals of respiratory care, *ed 9, St Louis, 2009, Mosby.)*

hospitals or within the hospital. They can make use of a standard electrical outlet but also feature self-contained batteries and oxygen tanks.

Traditionally, an incubator has been used to do four things for the infant: (1) manage the infant's temperature, (2) manage surrounding humidity, (3) isolate the infant from the outside environment, and (4) control the infant's inspired oxygen percentage. An incubator does the first three tasks very well. However, precise oxygen delivery cannot be done easily for two reasons. First, these units have never been designed to deliver an exact oxygen percentage. Some older units have only two basic oxygen flow settings. The low-flow setting is intended to limit the infant to no more than 40% oxygen. On some older units, a red plastic "flag" must be raised to deliver a higher flow of oxygen that may provide up to 80% or more oxygen. Second, whenever the side ports on the incubator are opened for patient care, internal gases flow out, resulting in a lower oxygen percentage.

Because of these limits, it is *not* recommended that an incubator's built-in oxygen delivery system be used. Instead, it is recommended that the following components be assembled for precise oxygen delivery and humidity control: (1) an oxygen blender with flowmeter and small-bore oxygen tubing adapter (nipple); (2) small-bore oxygen tubing and an adapter to connect the flowmeter to a cascade-type or wick-type heated humidifier; (3) sterile, distilled water to fill the humidifier reservoir; (4) large-bore (aerosol) tubing to direct the heated, humidified, high-percentage oxygen; (5) an oxygen hood (also called an oxyhood) to receive the humidified oxygen (see Chapter 6 for discussion and an illustration); (6) an oxygen analyzer to check the percentage inside the oxygen hood; and (7) a temperature probe to check the temperature of the heated humidified oxygen; place this into the large-bore tubing before it enters the incubator.

b. Put the equipment together and make sure that it works properly

An incubator comes preassembled as a unit. Sterile, distilled water must be added if the built-in humidification system is used. This is not necessary if heated, humidified oxygen is given by an oxygen hood. Make sure that the temperature control, the thermometer, and other systems on the incubator are working as directed by the manufacturer. The internal temperature of the incubator usually is kept at between 36° C and 36.5° C to keep the infant in a neutral thermal environment (NTE). The desired NTE is set by the physician and is maintained by the use of a temperature sensor placed on the infant's skin. This sensor usually is placed on the abdomen and is connected to a servo-control that automatically raises or lowers the temperature inside the incubator as needed.

If an oxygen hood is being used to deliver supplemental oxygen to the infant, the components previously listed must be assembled properly. Check the temperature of the humidified oxygen and check the oxygen percentage inside the oxygen hood near the infant's nose and mouth.

c. Troubleshoot any problems with the equipment

If the incubator is not maintaining the desired internal temperature, or if the internal humidification system is not working properly, follow the manufacturer's recommendations to repair or replace the entire unit. Make sure that the oxygen hood system is assembled properly, maintaining the desired gas temperature to keep the infant's neutral thermal environment and delivering the desired oxygen percentage. Adjust the cascade-type humidifier temperature or oxygen blender settings as needed.

2. Radiant warmers

a. Get the necessary equipment for the procedure

Note: Radiant warmers are not specifically listed by the NRBC as testable. However, because many incubators include a radiant warmer, this discussion is included. A radiant warmer is used to warm an infant to maintain a neutral thermal environment (NTE). A free-standing radiant warmer can be moved, as needed, to warm an infant who must be kept out in the open for frequent medical procedures. A radiant warmer also can be attached as part of an incubator. In any clinical situation, it is important to remember that it can be dangerous to allow a newborn to become chilled.

b. Put the equipment together and make sure that it works properly

A radiant warmer comes preassembled by the manufacturer. It uses infrared light to heat the infant and the area on which the infant is laid and cared for. A temperature sensor is placed onto the infant's skin, typically on the abdomen. The sensor uses a servo-mechanism so the infant's skin temperature is used to turn the radiant warmer on or off to maintain the infant's desired NTE. This usually is between 36° C and 36.5° C.

c. Troubleshoot any problems with the equipment

If the sensor and the servo system are not calibrated properly or working, the infant may be underheated or overheated. Either situation can be dangerous because newborns are very sensitive to temperature changes. Replace a sensor or servo that is not working properly.

2. Manipulate aerosol (mist) tents by order or protocol (ELE code: IIA12b) [Difficulty: ELE: R, Ap]

a. Get the necessary equipment for the procedure

Aerosol or mist tents are essentially like the O_2 tents discussed in Chapter 6. The main difference is that no supplemental O_2 is used because the patient does not need it. The top of the canopy then can be left open for better flow-through ventilation. Aerosol tents sometimes are used to treat an active child with an upper respiratory tract problem such as laryngotracheobronchitis (LTB, or pediatric croup). The tent is used because a small, active child will not keep an aerosol mask in place. A tent is not indicated for an older child or an adult who will keep an aerosol mask in place.

b. Put the equipment together and make sure that it works properly

c. Troubleshoot any problems with the equipment

At least 10 L/min of compressed air still should be run through the nebulizer to ensure that no CO_2 builds up. The nebulizer or ultrasonic system should be cared for as described earlier to ensure that enough aerosol is available to treat the condition.

If the child has laryngotracheobronchitis, a cool aerosol is preferred over a warm aerosol to reduce airway edema. Never use so much aerosol that the child cannot be seen inside the tent. Also, be wary of fluid overloading in the young patient who is in the tent for a prolonged period.

Exam Hint 8-2 (ELE)

Typically, some examination questions cover troubleshooting of problems with aerosol delivery equipment. Examples include but are not limited to (1) water in the large-bore tubing that prevents aerosol from traveling through it, (2) a plugged capillary line in a nebulizer so that no aerosol is produced, (3) a missing baffle in a nebulizer so that no aerosol is produced, (4) an incorrect water level in an ultrasonic nebulizer so that no aerosol is produced, and (5) replacement of a heat-moisture exchanger fouled with secretions or blood. Also, it is important to remember that with an oxygen-powered jet nebulizer system, the inspired oxygen percentage increases if condensate water fills the low point of the aerosol tubing. This is because the backpressure on the jet and air entrainment ports prevents room air from being drawn into the system. (See Figure 8-10.)

MODULE D

Medication delivery systems

1. Manipulate small-volume pneumatic nebulizers by order or protocol (ELE code: IIA4) [Difficulty: ELE: R, Ap, An]

a. Get the necessary equipment for the procedure

A pneumatically powered small-volume nebulizer (SVN) is designed to hold a relatively small volume of fluid (typically 3 to 5 mL) and to nebulize liquid medications such as bronchodilators, mucolytics, or antibiotics for inhalation. Compressed air or O_2 can be used to generate the aerosol. These units operate under the same physical principles as the large-volume nebulizers described earlier.

Two different types of SVNs exist: mainstream and sidestream. *Mainstream nebulizers* are designed so the main flow of gas to the patient comes through the aerosol as it is produced. A second high-pressure gas flow is used to power the jet to create the aerosol (Figure 8-12). *Sidestream nebulizers* are designed so the aerosol is produced from the main flow of gas and is supplemented by the jet's gas flow (Figure 8-13). Many manufacturers produce disposable medication SVNs, typically sidestream, for intermittent positive-pressure breathing circuits or hand-held circuits. Select the nebulizer that produces a particle size that matches the therapeutic target.

Figure 8-14 shows a typical small-volume nebulizer circuit. The nebulizer can be powered by compressed air or O_2. Flows of 4 to 6 L/min typically are used to nebulize 3 to 5 mL of medication in about 10 minutes. The nebulizer finger control allows the patient to power the nebulizer by covering the open hole in the "T." Uncovering the hole permits the gas to exit; thus, the medication is not nebulized and wasted. The reservoir tube serves to hold O_2 and medication for the next inspiration.

Practitioners face two possible risks when they use SVNs. First, any aerosolized medications that escape into the room air may be inhaled. It is possible that the practitioner, or anyone else nearby, may have an allergic or other adverse reaction. Second, nebulized secretions from the patient's airway and lungs may be inhaled; this may place the practitioner or others at risk for acquiring a pulmonary infection from the patient. Although actual problems like these rarely occur, they are possible. If either of these situations is a concern, an SVN with one-way valves and a downstream particle filter should be used. This filter will trap any exhaled aerosol droplets (Figure 8-15). A filtered SVN is recommended when pentamidine isethionate (NebuPent) is nebulized. A filtered SVN should be used for any other antibiotic or medication that should not contaminate the room air.

b. Put the equipment together and make sure that it works properly

SVNs consist of a medication reservoir and a manifold (top piece) that contains a capillary tube and a baffle. The two pieces must be unscrewed so the liquid medication can be added, and then must be reassembled. A mouthpiece and an (optional) aerosol reservoir tube are added to the manifold. The attachment openings are of different sizes so the mouthpiece and the reservoir tube cannot be misplaced. Small-bore O_2 tubing must be connected between the SVN and the flowmeter. When the flowmeter is turned to about 4 to 6 L/min, an aerosol should be produced.

c. Troubleshoot any problems with the equipment

If an SVN fails to generate aerosol, make sure that the pieces are properly assembled, the liquid medication is at the proper depth (typically 3 to 5 mL), and the capillary tube is not plugged with debris. If the capillary tube is plugged, liquid will not be drawn up to the jet. Some-

Figure 8-12 Mainstream-type small-volume nebulizer for medications. *(From Shapiro BA, Kacmarek RM, Cane RD, et al, editors: Clinical application of respiratory care, ed 4, St Louis, 1991, Mosby.)*

Figure 8-13 Sidestream-type small-volume nebulizer for medications. *(From Shapiro BA, Kacmarek RM, Cane RD, et al, editors: Clinical application of respiratory care, ed 4, St Louis, 1991, Mosby.)*

Figure 8-14 Hand-held small-volume nebulizer with mouthpiece, reservoir tube for medication, and finger control to limit wasted medication. *(Adapted from Guidelines for disinfection of respiratory care equipment used in the home, Respir Care 33:801, 1988.)*

times, the capillary tube can be cleared by running it under water or pushing a needle through the channel. Do not use a nebulizer that does not generate an aerosol. The therapist must be sure that the patient can properly assemble, disassemble, and operate the SVN. If the patient cannot, another medication delivery system, such as a dry powder inhaler (DPI) or a metered-dose inhaler (MDI), should be recommended.

2. Manipulate metered-dose inhalers by order or protocol (ELE code: IIA23) [Difficulty: ELE: R, Ap, An]

a. Get the necessary equipment for the procedure

Metered-dose inhalers (MDIs) are designed to dispense a premeasured amount of medication into the airway. Each activation of the MDI delivers a dose of medication to the patient. Available medications include sympathomimetic and anticholinergic bronchodilators, corticosteroid drugs, and an antibiotic (see Chapter 9 for details on the medications). All MDIs operate in the same way. They contained several milliliters of medication and compressed hydrofluoroalkane (HFA) gas inside of a metal container with a built-in jet nozzle. (The older MDI units that contained the environmentally hazardous propellant chlorofluorocarbon [CFC] have been replaced by HFA gas units.)

Tipping the metering chamber over and back upright results in its filling with medication. A plastic actuator opens the jet when it is pressed into the container (Figure 8-16). The patient then can inhale the medication through the built-in mouthpiece or a spacer/holding chamber.

Figure 8-15 Diagram of the Respirgard II small-volume nebulizer system showing one-way valves and an expiratory filter to scavenge exhaust aerosol. *(From Rau JL Jr: Respiratory care pharmacology, ed 5, St Louis, 1998, Mosby.)*

Figure 8-16 The effect of a spacer on aerosol particle size and velocity coming from a metered-dose inhaler. *(From Gardenhire D: Rau's Respiratory care pharmacology, ed 7, St. Louis, 2008, Mosby.)*

b. Put the equipment together and make sure that it works properly

c. Troubleshoot any problems with the equipment

When assembling the MDI, make sure that the medication canister nozzle fits into the jet of the actuator. If they are misaligned, no medication can be released. If needed, a spacer or a holding chamber can be added to the actuator. See the following discussion. To keep the jet channel open, patients should be instructed to use warm, soapy water daily to wash out the actuator. It can air dry overnight.

Some patients (e.g., those with arthritis of the fingers) may have difficulty squeezing the canister into the actuator to dispense the medication. In these cases, it may be possible to substitute a breath-activated MDI or add an MDI holder that can be squeezed easily to push the canister into the actuator. If a patient cannot properly manipulate an MDI with or without a spacer/holding chamber, the therapist should recommend a DPI or SVN medication delivery system.

3. Manipulate spacers and holding chambers for a metered-dose inhaler by order or protocol (ELE code: IIA23) [Difficulty: ELE: R, Ap, An]

a. Get the necessary equipment for the procedure

The addition of a spacer or a holding chamber between the actuator and the patient's mouth has been shown to increase the amount of inhaled medication. These devices slow down the aerosol so that less of it impacts on the back of the throat. This should result in fewer systemic adverse effects such as the risk of oral thrush (candidiasis fungal infection) with an MDI-powered corticosteroid. Also, the patient with poor hand and breathing coordination wastes less medication.

b. Put the equipment together and make sure that it works properly

c. Troubleshoot any problems with the equipment

A spacer is a simple, open extension tube that is placed between the actuator and the patient. Its main advantage over direct inhalation from the MDI mouthpiece is that the aerosol plume expands and slows down so that more medication is inhaled (see Figure 8-16). The patient should be told to refrain from exhaling through the spacer because any remaining medication will be blown out and wasted. Some spacers are designed for use with a ventilator circuit when an MDI-based medication is to be given. The spacer should be placed into the inspiratory limb of the ventilator circuit, about 18 inches from the patient. Typically, the MDI is activated during the expiratory phase so the medication can fill the spacer and inspiratory tubing before the next inspiration.

A holding chamber holds the medication as does a spacer, but it also has valves. These holding chamber valves prevent the medicine from being exhaled out through the unit. The valves also allow the patient to inhale several times from the unit and get more medication than through a simple spacer. This is especially helpful with children or small adults with small tidal volume breaths. Some holding chambers have a built-in whistle that sounds if the patient is inhaling too quickly. Several types of spacers or holding chambers are available (Figure 8-17). Some spacers are designed to fit with only one actuator, whereas others adapt to fit with any actuator. A face mask comes attached to some holding chambers so pediatric patients or uncooperative adults can be given the medication.

Patients should be instructed that there is no need to wash out the spacer or holding chamber on a regular basis. The gradual buildup of powder inside the unit does not affect its function. If the spacer or the holding chamber becomes visibly soiled, it can be washed out with warm, soapy water. After rinsing, it can be left out to air dry.

4. Manipulate dry powder inhalers by order or protocol (ELE Code: IIA24) [Difficulty: ELE: R, Ap, An]

a. Get the necessary equipment for the procedure

Dry powder inhalers (DPIs) dispense a dry medicinal powder into the patient's airways and lungs when inhaled (Figure 8-18). The drug manufacturer sells both the medication and the dispenser to the patient. DPI inhalers that can provide the following classes of medications are now available: maintenance and fast-acting adrenergic (sympathomimetic) bronchodilators, anticholinergic (parasym-

Figure 8-17 Examples of five types of metered-dose inhaler (MDI) spacers and holding chambers. **A,** AeroChamber (Monaghan Medical Corp); **B,** MediSpacer (Allegiance Healthcare Inc); **C,** Aerosol Cloud Enhancer, ACE (DHD Inc); **D,** InspirEase (Schering Inc); and **E,** OptiHaler (Healthscan Inc). *(From Gardenhire D: Rau's respiratory care pharmacology, ed 7, St Louis, 2008, Mosby.)*

pathomimetic) bronchodilators, inhaled corticosteroids, an antiviral agent, and human insulin.

Some DPI units are designed to deliver a single dose of medication. A new gelatin capsule that contains the medication must be loaded with each treatment. Examples include the Rotahaler (albuterol [Ventolin]), the Spiriva inhaler (tiotropium), and the Aerolizer (formoterol [Foradil]). (The Spinhaler for the delivery of cromolyn sodium [Intal] is no longer available.)

Other DPI units are multidose delivery systems that contain many doses of medication within a reservoir. Examples include the Turbuhaler for formoterol (Foradil), the Turbuhaler for terbutaline (Bricanyl), and the Pulmicort Turbuhaler (for budesonide), all of which contain 200 doses; the Diskus (for salmeterol [Serevent]), the Advair Diskus (combination of salmeterol and fluticasone propionate), and the Flovent Diskus [fluticasone propio-

nate]), all of which contain 60 doses; and the Diskhaler (for zanamivir [Relenza]), which contains 4 or 8 doses. (See Chapter 9 for details on the medications.)

Note that the Turbuhaler device and the Diskus device both are being used to deliver three different types of medications. Make sure the patient knows to check the label on the unit if the same type of DPI device is being used for more than one medication.

b. Put the equipment together and make sure that it works properly

Single-use DPI units require several steps to prepare the medication before inhalation. Steps typically include the following: (1) disassemble the device, (2) properly place the first medication capsule into the device, and (3) adjust the device to pierce the capsule. With all subsequent doses, the empty capsule from the previous treatment

Mesh

Empty half of capsule

Inspiratory airflow

Powder emerging with inspiratory airflow

Detached half of capsule

B

Micronized (<5 μm) drug

Mouthpiece

Indicator window

Air inlet for optimal inspiratory resistance

Turning grip

C

Device in closed postion

Device in open postion

Mouthpiece

Drug exit port

Manifold

Strip lid peeled from pockets

Index wheel

Body

Empty strip

Contracting wheel

Base wheel

Lever

Coiled strip

Dose indicator wheel

Thumb grip

Pockets containing drug

D

Mouthpiece

Single dose blister

E

Figure 8-18 Examples of four types of dry powder inhaler (DPI). **A,** Photograph of the single-dose Rotahaler *(lower left),* the multidose Turbuhaler *(top left),* the multidose Diskus *(top right),* and the multidose Diskhaler *(lower right).* **B,** Cross section of the Rotahaler showing how it must be held horizontally when used. **C,** Internal views of the Turbuhaler showing how it dispenses a single dose from its 200-dose reservoir of medication. **D,** Operation and cross section through the Diskus. It has a strip with 60 doses of medication, which are individually opened and inhaled. **E,** Disassembled Diskhaler showing the medication wheel, which can contain four or eight doses of medication. *(From Cario J, Pilbeam S:* Mosby's respiratory therapy equipment, *ed 8, St Louis, 2010, Mosby.)*

must be removed before the new capsule can be placed. The therapist must oversee that the patient is properly performing these steps. Patients who are too young to follow directions, who cannot physically perform the steps, or who do not have the mental capacity to understand the steps should not be using one of these DPI devices.

Multiuse DPI devices are simpler to use. However, steps must be followed to properly fill the medication from the reservoir and to prepare the unit for inhalation. Both Turbuhaler and Diskus units include a counter to keep track of how many doses have been taken. When the reservoir of medication is empty, a new DPI device must be purchased. As was discussed earlier, the patient must be able to demonstrate the ability to prepare the unit before it should be used. The therapist must be ready to recommend another medication delivery system, if needed.

c. Troubleshoot any problems with the equipment

See the manufacturer's literature for proper steps to follow in using the DPI unit. Patient practice is essential to make sure that the unit is used properly. If it does not operate properly, it must be replaced. DPI units as a group have the following limits: (1) If the unit becomes wet or is used in a high-humidity environment, the powder can congeal and clog up the unit. Less medication powder will be inhaled. (2) The user must be able to rapidly inhale the powder. If the patient's peak inspiratory flow is not at least 40 to 60 L/min, less medication will be inhaled. It will not leave the dispenser, or it will impact in the back of the throat rather than being inhaled into the airways and lungs. Patients who are younger than 5 years old and patients with severe airway obstruction probably will not be able to use a DPI properly. An MDI or an SVN should be used instead to deliver the needed medications.

MODULE E
Alter the patient's breathing pattern.

1. Independently modify the patient's breathing pattern to properly deposit medication (ELE code: IIIF2c1) [Difficulty: ELE: R, Ap, An]

For medications to be deposited properly in the upper or lower airway, the patient must breathe in the correct manner. Following are recommended breathing patterns.

a. Upper airway deposition

Particles 10 μm or larger are more likely to impact the upper airway (oropharynx, larynx, trachea, and mainstem bronchi) when the patient is coached to do the following:

1. Inhale at a normal or faster speed (the flow should be greater than 30 L/min).
2. Inhale a normal V_T.
3. Breathe in a normal pattern.

b. Lower airway and alveolar deposition

Particles measuring 2 to 5 μm are more likely to deposit on the smaller airways (respiratory bronchioles) and in the alveoli when the patient is coached to do the following:

1. Inhale at a slow speed (the flow should be less than 30 L/min).
2. Inhale an inspiratory capacity (IC).
3. If possible, hold the full breath for 10 seconds before exhaling.

Obviously, not all patients can perform these techniques perfectly, but to the extent that they can, the medication is deposited where needed and the treatment is more effective.

Exam Hint 8-3 (ELE)

One question has dealt regularly with recognizing that a patient is hyperventilating during a small-volume nebulizer treatment. Signs of hyperventilation include dizziness, light-headedness, and tingling fingers. The patient should be told to breathe more slowly and less deeply.

MODULE F
Respiratory care plan

1. Analyze the available information to determine the patient's pathophysiologic state (Code: IIIH1) [Difficulty: ELE: R, Ap; WRE: An]

The patient with many secretions should be helped by the addition of a bland aerosol or mucolytic medication and should be better able to clear these medications effectively. This should cause the patient to feel better and to have improved vital signs, oxygenation, breath sounds, and spirometry values. The use of a bland aerosol therapy can cause bronchospasm in some asthmatic patients. Patients with thick, dry (inspissated) secretions can have their airways occluded if aerosol therapy causes the secretions to absorb water and swell. If the patient is not able to cough out the thinned secretions, suctioning equipment must be available to remove them.

2. Determine the appropriateness of the prescribed respiratory care plan and recommend modifications when indicated

a. Recommend changes in the therapeutic plan when indicated (Code: IIIH4) [Difficulty: ELE: R, Ap; WRE: An]

Changes in the patient's secretion volume and consistency may result in a change in the type of humidity and/or aerosol therapy needed. Be prepared to decrease humidity and/or aerosol therapy if the patient's secretions are decreased in volume and easy for the patient to cough out.

In contrast, be prepared to increase humidity and/or aerosol therapy if the patient's secretions are thick and difficult to cough out.

1. Change the type of equipment being used (ELE code: IIIF2c2) [Difficulty: ELE: R, Ap, An]

Be prepared to change the type of humidity and aerosol delivery system used from among those discussed in this chapter based on the patient's condition. Review the indications, contraindications, uses, and limitations of the various systems.

Exam Hint 8-4 (ELE)

The examination usually includes a question that deals with needing to change from one equipment item to another, based on the patient's condition. Know the indications, contraindications, uses, and limitations of the various systems.

2. Adjust the temperature of the aerosol (ELE code: IIIF2c4) [Difficulty: ELE: R, Ap, An]

In general, a cool humidity or aerosol system is used with patients with the following conditions:

- Larygotracheobronchitis (LTB, or pediatric croup)
- Upper airway irritation, such as after extubation or a bronchoscopy procedure

In general, a body temperature humidity or aerosol system is used with patients with the following conditions:

- Bypassed upper airway (endotracheal or tracheostomy tube)
- Thick secretions
- Hypothermia
- Maintenance of a neutral thermal environment for the neonate

a. Change the output of aerosol by the equipment (ELE code: IIIF2c2) [Difficulty: ELE: R, Ap, An]

Neonates are sensitive to overhydration, so long-term aerosol therapy for them should be avoided or minimized. Adult patients with heart failure or pulmonary edema also should not be given long-term aerosol therapy. Instead, a cascade-type or wick-type of humidifier can be used.

The adult patient with thick secretions may be aided by long-term aerosol therapy of a dense mist, usually by an ultrasonic nebulizer run at body temperature. Secretions often are liquefied and made easier to cough or suction out. The child with croup usually is given a dense mist of a cool bland aerosol in a mist tent. This therapy usually is needed for only a few days. Be wary of fluid overload if the mist is needed for a longer period.

1. Recommend discontinuing the treatment or procedure based on the patient's response (Code: IIIG1i) [Difficulty: ELE: R, Ap; WRE: An]

2. Terminate the treatment or procedure based on the patient's response (Code: IIIF1) [Difficulty: ELE: R, Ap; WRE: An]

Based on the previous discussion, be prepared to stop a treatment or procedure if necessary. After further evaluation, it may be possible to continue again. However, if the patient has a serious adverse reaction, the treatment or procedure should be discontinued. Usually, this would be done after consultation with the patient's physician.

1. Record and evaluate the patient's response to the treatment(s) or procedure(s), including the following:

a. Record and interpret the following: heart rate and rhythm, respiratory rate, blood pressure, body temperature, and pain level (Code: IIIA1b4) [Difficulty: ELE: R, Ap; WRE: An]

Bland aerosol therapy should not cause a significant change in the patient's vital signs.

b. Record and interpret the patient's breath sounds (Code: IIIA1b3) [Difficulty: ELE: R, Ap; WRE: An]

Hearing crackles (also called rhonchi) in the more central airways would indicate that the patient has retained secretions. Hearing normal breath sounds after humidity or aerosol therapy and a productive cough would indicate that all secretions have been removed.

The development of wheezing after aerosol therapy could indicate that the patient has bronchospastic tendencies. An aerosolized bronchodilator medication may be needed.

c. Record and interpret the type of cough the patient has and the nature of the sputum (Code: IIIAb3) [Difficulty: ELE: R, Ap; WRE: An]

Note whether the patient is able to more easily cough out any secretions after humidity or aerosol therapy. It is also important to evaluate the consistency of the secretions. Improved hydration should make the secretions more watery (less viscous).

Exam Hint 8-5 (ELE, WRE)

Past exams have had a question that deals with recognizing that the patient is having an adverse reaction. Be prepared to stop therapy if the patient has bronchospasm or becomes short of breath when swollen secretions obstruct airways.

BIBLIOGRAPHY

Adams DA: Humidity and aerosol therapy. In: Wyka KA, Mathews PJ, Clark WF, editors: *Foundations of respiratory care*, Albany, 2002, Delmar.

American Association for Respiratory Care: Aerosol consensus statement, *Respir Care* 36:916, 1991.

American Association for Respiratory Care: Clinical practice guideline: bland aerosol administration, *Respir Care* 38:1196, 1993.

American Association for Respiratory Care: Clinical practice guideline: bland aerosol administration—2003 revision & update, *Respir Care* 48:529, 2003.

American Association for Respiratory Care: Clinical practice guideline: care of the ventilator circuit and its relation to ventilator associated pneumonia, *Respir Care* 48:869, 2003.

American Association for Respiratory Care: Clinical practice guideline: delivery of aerosols to the upper airway, *Respir Care* 39:803, 1994.

American Association for Respiratory Care: Clinical practice guideline: humidification during mechanical ventilation, *Respir Care* 37:877, 1992.

American Association for Respiratory Care: Clinical practice guideline: selection of aerosol delivery device, *Respir Care* 37:891, 1992.

American Association for Respiratory Care: Clinical practice guideline: selection of aerosol delivery device for neonatal and pediatric patients, *Respir Care* 40:1325, 1995.

Barnes TA, editor: *Core textbook of respiratory care practice*, ed 2, St Louis, 1994, Mosby.

Branson RD, Hess DR, Chatburn RL, editors: *Respiratory care equipment*, ed 2, Philadelphia, 1999, Lippincott Williams & Wilkins.

Fink J: Aerosol drug therapy. In: Scanlan CL, Wilkins RL, Kacmarek, editors: *Egan's fundamentals of respiratory care*, ed 9, St Louis, 2009, Mosby.

Fink J: Humidity and aerosol therapy. In: Cairo JM, Pilbeam SP, editors: *Mosby's respiratory care equipment*, ed 8, St Louis, 2010, Mosby.

Fink J: Humidity and bland aerosol therapy. In: Wilkins RL, Stoller JK, Kacmarek RM, editors: *Egan's fundamentals of respiratory care*, ed 9, St Louis, 2009, Mosby.

Fink JB: Humidity. In: Fink JB, Hunt GE, editors: *Clinical practice in respiratory care*, Philadelphia, 1999, Lippincott-Raven.

Fink JB, Dhand R: Aerosol drug therapy. In: Fink JB, Hunt GE, editors: *Clinical practice in respiratory care*, Philadelphia, 1999, Lippincott-Raven.

Fink JB, Hess DR: Humidity and aerosol therapy. In: Hess DR, MacIntyre NR, Mishoe SC, et al, editors: *Respiratory care principles & practices*, Philadelphia, 2002, WB Saunders.

Gardenhire DS: *Rau's respiratory care pharmacology*, ed 7, St Louis, 2008, Mosby.

Hess D: Aerosol therapy. In: Dantzker DR, MacIntyre NR, Bakow ED, editors: *Comprehensive respiratory care*, Philadelphia, 1995, WB Saunders.

Hess D: The delivery of aerosolized bronchodilator to mechanically ventilated intubated adult patients, *Respir Care* 35:399, 1990.

Shapiro BA, Kacmarek RM, Cane RD, et al, editors: *Clinical application of respiratory care*, ed 4, St Louis, 1991, Mosby.

Ward JJ, Hess D, Helmholz HF Jr: Humidity and aerosol therapy. In: Burton GC, Hodgkin JE, Ward JJ, editors: *Respiratory care: a guide to clinical practice*, ed 4, Philadelphia, 1997, Lippincott-Raven.

Whitaker K: *Comprehensive perinatal & pediatric respiratory care*, ed 2, Albany, NY, 1997, Delmar.

White GC: *Equipment theory for respiratory care*, ed 3, Albany, NY, 1999, Delmar.

SELF-STUDY QUESTIONS FOR THE ENTRY LEVEL EXAM *See page 589 for answers*

1. Ten minutes into a hand-held nebulizer treatment given to deliver albuterol (Proventil), the patient complains of dizziness and tingling fingers. What should be done?
   A. Advise the patient to breathe in the same pattern.
   B. Change the medication.
   C. Tell the patient to breathe more slowly.
   D. Advise the patient to breathe deeper and faster.

2. A patient is being given a bronchodilator medication by small-volume nebulizer powered by 5 L/min of O_2. While watching the patient breathe, you notice that during each inspiration, the mist disappears from the downstream end of the SVN. What would you recommend?
   A. Add 100 mL of aerosol tubing as a reservoir.
   B. Increase the oxygen flow.
   C. Decrease the oxygen flow.
   D. Tell the patient not to breathe so deeply.

3. A 4-year-old patient with asthma is about to be discharged and needs to take an inhaled bronchodilator medication at home. What device would you recommend?
   A. MDI
   B. DPI
   C. DPI with holding chamber
   D. MDI with holding chamber

4. The physician wants more aerosol inside the mist tent of a 3-year-old child. What would be the best way to do this?
   A. Cut a hole in the top of the tent.
   B. Close the hole on the top of the tent.
   C. Lower the temperature on the refrigeration unit.
   D. Increase the gas flow to the large-volume nebulizer.

5. For an aerosolized medication to be deposited primarily in the larger airways, what breathing pattern would you recommend?
   1. Inhale a V_T.
   2. Inhale an IC.
   3. Inhale slowly.
   4. Inhale at a normal speed.
   5. Breathe in a normal pattern.
   A. 2, 3
   B. 1, 4, 5
   C. 4, 5
   D. 2, 4

6. A physician calls you to evaluate a 40-year-old patient with bronchitis and to make a recommendation for an aerosol delivery system. The patient's breath sounds indicate the presence of large airway secretions. Despite a good cough effort, the patient has difficulty in raising them. What would you recommend?
   A. Use a hand-held nebulizer with 3 cc of normal saline every 4 hours.
   B. Place the patient into a mist tent.
   C. Start a continuous ultrasonic nebulizer to an aerosol mask.
   D. Start a cascade-type humidifier to an aerosol mask.

7. A patient's humidity deficit is going to be the *smallest* under which of the following conditions?
   A. Breathing in regular hospital room air at 72° F and 40% relative humidity
   B. Breathing in outside air at 80° F and 50% relative humidity
   C. Breathing in 6 L/min of O_2 through a nasal cannula running through an unheated bubble humidifier
   D. Breathing in 40% O_2 at 95° F through a cascade-type humidifier to an aerosol mask

8. An ultrasonic nebulizer would be recommended for aerosol therapy for the following reason:
   A. It delivers a wide variety of aerosol droplets.
   B. Its aerosol droplets are between 10 and 20 μm in diameter.
   C. It delivers a uniform aerosol droplet of about 3 μm in diameter.
   D. It can be used to nebulize bland aerosols and liquid medications into an aerosol.

9. Your patient has an endotracheal tube. Which of the following devices would be the *least* effective in reducing this patient's humidity deficit?
   A. Wick-type humidifier set at 35° C
   B. Cascade-type humidifier set at 35° C
   C. Unheated bubble-type humidifier
   D. Ultrasonic nebulizer

10. An adult patient with chronic bronchitis has a normal temperature. To fully saturate the inhaled air, how much absolute humidity must be provided by the humidifier?
    A. 35° C
    B. 47 mm Hg
    C. 760 mm Hg
    D. 44 mg/L

11. Your heated humidifier unit has a water reservoir temperature of 40° C. The humidified gas is traveling through large-bore tubing to the patient. Which of the following statements are true?
    1. Condensation will occur.
    2. The gas will warm and expand as it travels to the patient.
    3. The gas will remain saturated.
    4. The relative humidity will decrease.
    5. The relative humidity will increase.
    A. 1, 3
    B. 4
    C. 2, 5
    D. 1, 4

12. The pop-off valve is whistling on your patient's bubble humidifier to a 35% O_2, air entrainment mask. What could be the problem?
    A. The reservoir jar is not screwed tightly into the top of the humidifier.
    B. The air entrainment mask should be set at 28% O_2.
    C. The small-bore tubing is pinched.
    D. The air entrainment mask should be set at 40% O_2.

13. A humidity or aerosol system delivering body temperature gas is used in all the following situations EXCEPT:
    A. Patient with a tracheostomy
    B. Twenty-month-old infant with laryngotracheobronchitis
    C. Patient with chronic obstructive pulmonary disease with thick secretions
    D. Hypothermic near-drowning victim

14. Your patient's small-volume medication nebulizer is not putting out as much aerosol as it was a short time ago. To correct the problem, you would check which of the following?
    1. Make sure the fluid level is correct.
    2. Make sure the one-way valve is patent.
    3. Make sure the jet is patent.
    4. Make sure the O_2 can flow down the capillary tube.
    5. Make sure the fluid can flow up the capillary tube.
    A. 1, 2
    B. 1, 3, 4
    C. 2, 4
    D. 1, 3, 5

15. Your patient has pneumonia and needs an inhaled antibiotic. What size particle generator would you recommend to treat the problem?
    A. 20 to 50 μm
    B. 10 to 20 μm
    C. 2 to 5 μm
    D. 1 to 3 μm

16. Your ultrasonic nebulizer has a flashing couplant indicator light. You notice that the output has decreased from what it was earlier. The most likely problem is
    A. Too much water in the solution cup
    B. Too much water in the couplant chamber
    C. Not enough water in the couplant chamber
    D. A loose electrical cable

17. You notice that water has collected at the low point of the large-bore tubing of your patient's heated aerosol system. The aerosol is "puffing" out of the end of the tubing. Your reaction should be to
    A. Add water to the reservoir jar
    B. Empty water from the reservoir jar
    C. Empty the water from the large-bore tubing into a wastewater jar
    D. Empty the water from the large-bore tubing into the reservoir jar so it is not wasted

18. The physician wants a patient with a tracheostomy to inhale room air that is fully saturated at body temperature. The device that you select must be able to meet the following criteria:
    1. Deliver 40% relative humidity
    2. Deliver 100% relative humidity
    3. Provide 47 mm Hg vapor pressure
    4. Provide 44 mm Hg vapor pressure
    5. Deliver 44 mg/L absolute humidity

A. 2, 4
B. 1, 3, 5
C. 1, 4
D. 2, 3, 5

19. It is best to coach your patient to breathe in the following pattern for particle deposition in smaller airways and alveoli:
    1. Inhale a V_T.
    2. Inhale rapidly.
    3. Inhale an IC.
    4. Hold the breath for up to 10 seconds before exhaling.
    5. Inhale at a slow speed.
    A. 1, 2
    B. 3, 4, 5
    C. 1, 5
    D. 1, 2, 4

20. When doing patient rounds, you notice that very little aerosol is going from a large-volume nebulizer to a patient's tracheostomy mask. Which of the following could be the problem?
    1. The water level is above the refill line on the nebulizer's reservoir jar.
    2. The nebulizer is not screwed tightly into the DISS connector on the flowmeter.
    3. The nebulizer jet is obstructed.
    4. The water level is below the refill line on the nebulizer's reservoir jar.
    5. The capillary tube is obstructed.
    A. 2, 3, 4, 5
    B. 1, 2
    C. 3, 4
    D. 1, 4

SELF-STUDY QUESTIONS FOR THE WRITTEN REGISTRY EXAM

See page 614 for answers

1. A 64-year-old patient with a long smoking history and a diagnosis of chronic bronchitis has been admitted again with complaints of shortness of breath and productive cough. Which of the following questions would help you gain an understanding of his problem to better guide aerosol therapy?
   1. Has the volume of your secretions changed over the past week?
   2. How many hours do you sleep a night?
   3. Are there any medications that make your breathing easier?
   4. How many flights of stairs can you climb without stopping?
   A. 1, 3
   B. 2, 4
   C. 1, 2, 3
   D. All of the above

2. The respiratory therapist is helping to care for a 1-week-old infant with pneumonia. The infant has been placed into an incubator. The physician wants to know the best way to administer high humidity and 35% oxygen to the infant. What should be recommended?
   A. Send the desired oxygen percentage to a heated cascade-type humidifier to an oxyhood.
   B. Use the incubator's humidifier and the low oxygen setting on the unit.
   C. Place a 3-L/min nasal cannula on the infant and use the incubator's humidifier.
   D. Use the incubator's humidifier and the high oxygen setting on the unit.

3. A 40-year-old patient has been sick with the flu for 8 days and was admitted to the hospital with dehydration and pneumonia. Intravenous fluids and antibiotics were started. She was given an aerosol mask with

35% oxygen and continuous aerosol of normal saline nebulized through an ultrasonic nebulizer system. An hour later, she reported worsening shortness of breath. Her breath sounds revealed crackles that were not there before this therapy was started. What is the most likely cause of these changes?

A. The dehydration is worse.

B. Her influenza is worse.

C. Her secretions have swollen.

D. She is allergic to the normal saline.

4. Current clinical guidelines indicate that an incubator can be used for all of the following situations *except* to

A. Isolate an infant

B. Provide an exact oxygen percentage

C. Control the temperature around an infant

D. Control the humidity level around an infant

5. A 14-year-old patient with severe asthma has just been given a new medication of inhaled corticosteroid by a DPI. After rapidly inhaling the medication, she begins to cough vigorously. Breath sounds reveal increased wheezing in all lung fields. What should be recommended?

A. Have her inhale rapidly through the DPI to make sure she got all of the medication.

B. Have her inhale slowly through the DPI to make sure she got all of the medication.

C. Stop taking the DPI medication.

D. Increase the dose of DPI medication until her wheezing goes away.

6. A premature infant with respiratory distress syndrome is receiving mechanical ventilation, has a nasogastric tube, and has an umbilical artery catheter. What is the best way to maintain a neutral thermal environment for the infant?

A. Place an oxygen hood over the infant's head.

B. Put the infant inside an incubator and adjust the temperature based on the infant's rectal temperature.

C. Place the infant under a radiant warmer with a skin temperature probe.

D. Place the infant inside an incubator with a skin temperature probe.

7. Complications of bland aerosol therapy include all of the following EXCEPT

A. Increased humidity deficit

B. Aerosol-induced bronchospasm

C. Fluid overload in an infant

D. Swollen secretions that may block airways

8. An alcoholic patient has been admitted with a high fever and a productive cough. A pulmonary abscess is suspected. What sputum characteristics should be evaluated to help assess the effectiveness of aerosol and other therapy?

1. Specific gravity

2. Smell

3. Consistency

4. Platelet count

5. Color

A. 2, 3

B. 4, 5

C. 1, 2, 3

D. 2, 3, 5

9 Pharmacology

Note 1: This book is written to cover every item listed as testable on the *Entry Level Examination (ELE), Written Registry Examination (WRE),* and *Clinical Simulation Examination (CSE).*

The listed code for each item is taken from the National Board for Respiratory Care's (NBRC) **Summary Content Outline for CRT (Certified Respiratory Therapist) and Written RRT (Registered Respiratory Therapist) Examinations** (http://evolve.elsevier.com/Sills/resptherapist/). For example, if an item is testable on both the ELE and the WRE, it will simply be shown as: (Code: . . .). If an item is only testable on the ELE, it will be shown as: (ELE code: . . .). If an item is only testable on the WRE, it will be shown as: (WRE code: . . .).

Following each item's code will be the difficulty level of the questions on that item on the ELE and WRE. (See the Introduction for a full explanation of the three question difficulty levels.) **Recall [R]** level questions typically expect the exam taker to recall factual information. **Application [Ap]** level questions are harder because the exam taker may have to apply factual information to a clinical situation. **Analysis [An]** level questions are the most challenging because the exam taker may have to use critical thinking to evaluate patient data to make a clinical decision.

Note 2: *A review of the most recent Entry Level Examinations (ELE) has shown an average of 11 questions (out of 140), or 8% of the exam, will cover pharmacology. A review of the most recent Written Registry Examinations (WRE) has shown an average of 6 questions (out of 100), or 6% of the exam, will cover pharmacology. The Clinical Simulation Examination is comprehensive and may include everything that should be known by an advanced level respiratory therapist.*

MODULE A

Apply computer technology to drug dispensing as a patient safety initiative (Code: IIIA4c) [Difficulty: ELE: R, Ap; WRE: An]

To try to prevent medication errors, apply safety protocols that incorporate the seven patient medication "rights." These include the following: (1) the right drug, (2) the right dose of drug, (3) the right patient, (4) the right time of drug delivery, (5) the right route of drug delivery; (6) the right technique of drug administration; (7) the right documentation. Many hospitals have incorporated these safeguards into a computer-based system that requires the practitioner to enter an access code to obtain the patient's medication. This prevents inappropriate persons from accessing medications and also tracks both the name of the person accessing a medication and the time that a medication was dispensed. A bar-code scanner can also be used to scan a medication's code and match it to the code on the patient's wrist band. If the codes do not match, the medication is not intended for the patient.

MODULE B

Recommend or administer medications

1. Administer medications

    a. Administer aerosol therapy with prescribed drugs (Code: IIIC3) [Difficulty: ELE: R, Ap; WRE: An]

    b. Administer aerosolized medications (Code: IIID5a) [Difficulty: ELE: R, Ap; WRE: An]

    c. Administer dry powder preparations (Code: IIID5b) [Difficulty: ELE: R, Ap; WRE: An]

This chapter covers the types of medications listed by the NBRC that are given to patients with pulmonary conditions. Many of the medications are administered by respiratory therapists.

    d. Administer endotracheal instillation medications (Code: IIID5c) [Difficulty: ELE: R, Ap; WRE: An]

See Chapter 7 for the discussion of cardiac and cardiovascular medications including those given via the endotracheal tube during a CPR effort.

2. Bronchodilators

The bronchodilators are medications designed to relax the bronchial smooth muscles so that the airways dilate, airway resistance is reduced, and breathing is easier. The first two classes of medications in this group are widely administered by respiratory therapists.

a. Inhaled adrenergic (sympathomimetic) agents

1. Recommend their use (ELE code: IIIG4a) [Difficulty: ELE: R, Ap, An]

A variety of names have been used to describe this group of medications, including: beta-agonists, beta-adrenergic agonists, catecholamines, sympathomimetic amines, sympathomimetic bronchodilators, and β(beta)-adrenergic bronchodilators. They have the effect of stimulating the body's sympathetic nerves, which results in bronchodilation and other effects. Be prepared to recommend the use of these types of medications in patients with asthma and chronic obstructive pulmonary disease (COPD [e.g., emphysema, chronic bronchitis]).

A brief review of the autonomic nervous system helps in understanding how these medications (and the following group of medications) work and some side effects that may occur. The autonomic nervous system is not under voluntary control. It is an automatic system designed to regulate metabolism and the vital signs. This system is made up of two branches: the sympathetic nervous system and the parasympathetic nervous system. The lungs, heart, and most other organs are innervated by both branches. The blood vessels in the mucous membranes are innervated only by the sympathetic branch. The parasympathetic nervous system is usually dominant and keeps the body functioning normally. The sympathetic nervous system is an "emergency" system that is dominant during great stress (sometimes called the "fight or flight" system). Adrenaline (or epinephrine) is released by the adrenal glands in these emergencies. Adrenaline causes a number of effects, including one that many respiratory patients need—bronchodilation. The sympathetic nervous system has the following three types of receptors that are located in different organs and are affected by adrenaline and related medications:

1. α_1-Receptors are located in the blood vessels of the mucous membranes (other tissues are not included in this discussion). Vasoconstriction results when α_1-receptors are stimulated.
2. β_1-Receptors are located in the heart. Tachycardia, increased stroke volume, and possibly arrhythmias result when β_1-receptors are stimulated.
3. β_2-Receptors are located in the airways. Bronchodilation results when β_2-receptors are stimulated.

2. Administer the prescribed medication (Code: IIIC3, IIID5a, IIID5b) [Difficulty: ELE: R, Ap; WRE: An]

Aerosolized sympathomimetic bronchodilators are usually recommended and given under one of the three following situations:

a. Acute bronchospasm with severe shortness of breath. This patient needs rapid relief. Recommend a fast-acting medication such as albuterol. The current asthma-management guidelines list albuterol and similar medications as "rescue" agents. Because these drugs tend to have a shorter duration of action they can be referred to as short-acting beta-agonist (SABA) medications. Table 9-1 lists the peak onset times and duration for the various medications. Avoid drugs with unnecessary α_1 and β_1 effects or long onset and peak times.

b. Chronic but stable bronchospasm with moderate shortness of breath. These patients need a dependable medication of longer duration such as salmeterol or formoterol. They are considered to be "controller" agents with a long onset time and a duration of up to 12 hours. Because of their longer duration they can be called long-acting beta-agonist (LABA) medications. Several newer medications also come in both oral and aerosol preparations. The oral forms are especially helpful when taken in the evening to help the patient get a good night's sleep. It is very important that the patient also have a prescription for a fast-acting drug in case of sudden bronchospasm. Table 9-1 lists information on the administration method, strength, and dosages.

c. Laryngeal edema or bleeding from a bronchoscopy biopsy site. The laryngeal edema problem requires the administration of a medication that reduces the swelling of the mucous membrane of the larynx and epiglottis. Laryngeal edema can result from a direct injury or irritation of the upper airway, such as postextubation edema or laryngotracheobronchitis (croup). In addition, if the patient has anaphylaxis from an allergic reaction, laryngeal edema and hypotension are often present. If bleeding results from a biopsy during a bronchoscopy, the cut blood vessels must be made to constrict and to form clots. In cases of laryngeal edema or biopsy bleeding, nebulized racemic epinephrine (microNefrin) is given because it stimulates α_1-receptors. This results in vasoconstriction of the mucosal and deeper blood vessels. Therefore the laryngeal edema swelling is reduced, and biopsy bleeding stops. In the case of anaphylaxis with hypotension and laryngeal edema, intravenous epinephrine is needed to treat both life-threatening problems. See Table 9-1 for information on specific medications.

Most of the medications listed in this section are chemically derived from adrenaline. They are somewhat different in their structures so that the desired effects and side (unwanted) effects vary. Box 9-1 lists the side effects of the sympathomimetic bronchodilators. Clinically, the most dangerous of these side effects are palpitations, tachycardia, and hypertension.

| TABLE 9-1 | Inhaled Adrenergic Bronchodilator Agents* |

Drug	Brand Name	Receptor Preference	Adult Dosage	Time Course (Onset, Peak, Duration)
Ultra Short Acting				
Epinephrine	Adrenalin	α, β	SVN: 0.1% solution (1 : 1000), 0.25-0.5 mL	Onset: 3-5 min
			MDI: 0.2 mg/puff, puffs as ordered or needed	Peak: 5-20 min
			(2.5-5.0 mg) qid	Duration: 1-3 hr
Isoetharine[†]	Isoetharine HCl[†]	β₂	SVN: 1% solution, 0.25-0.5 mL (2.5-5.0 mg) qid	Onset: 1-6 min
				Peak: 15-60 min
				Duration: 1-3 hr
Racemic epinephrine	microNefrin, Vaponephrine,[†] AsthmaNefrin;[†] Nephron	α, β	SVN: 2.25% solution, 0.25-0.5 mL qid	Onset: 3-5 min epinephrine Nephron,[†] S2, (5.63-11.25 mg) qid Peak: 5-20 min Duration: 0.5-2 hr
Short Acting				
Metaproterenol	Alupent,[†] Metaprel[†]	β₂	SVN: 0.4%, 0.6%, 5% solution, 0.3 mL (15 mg) tid, qid	Onset: 1-5 min
			MDI: 650 mcg/puff, 2-3 puffs tid, qid	Peak: 60 min
			Tab: 10 mg or 20 mg, tid, qid	Duration: 2-6 hr
			Syrup: 10 mg/5 mL, 2 tsp tid, qid	
Pirbuterol	Maxair Autohaler	β₂	MDI: 200 mcg/puff, 2 puffs q4-6h	Onset: 5 min
				Peak: 30 min
				Duration: 5 hr
Terbutaline[†]	Brethaire[†] Bricanyl[†] Brethine[†]	β₂	Tab: 2.5 or 5 mg, 5 mg q6h Inj: 1 mg/mL, 0.25 mg SubQ	Onset: 5-30 min Peak: 30-60 min Duration: 3-6 hr
Intermediate Acting				
Albuterol	Proventil, HFA AccuNeb	β₂	SVN: 0.5% solution, 0.5 mL (2.5 mg); 0.63 mg, Proventil HFA, 1.25 mg, and 2.5 mg unit dose, tid, qid	Onset: 15 min Peak: 30-60 min Duration: 5-8 hr
	Ventolin HFA, ProAir HFA VoSpire ER tabs		MDI: 90 mcg/puff, 2 puffs tid, qid Tab: 2 mg, 4 mg, and 8 mg, bid Syrup: 2 mg/5 mL, 1-2 tsp tid, qid	Duration: 12 hr
Levalbuterol	Xopenex Xopenex HFA Xopenex Pediatric[†]	β₂	SVN: 0.31 mg/3 mL tid; 0.63 mg/3 mL tid; 0.5 mL, tid or 1.25 mg/3 mL tid; Concentrate 1.25 mg/0.5 ml MDI: 45 mcg/puff, 2 puffs q4-6h, ≥4 yr old	Onset: 15 min Peak: 30-60 min Duration: 5-8 hr
Long Acting				
Arformoterol	Brovana	β₂	SVN: 15 mcg/2 mL unit dose, bid	Onset: 15 min Peak: 30-60 min Duration: 12 hr
Formoterol	Foradil Perforomist	β₂	DPI: 12 mcg/inhalation bid SVN: 20 mcg unit-dose vial bid	Onset: 15 min Peak: 30-60 min Duration: 12 hr
Salmeterol	Serevent evohaler HFA[†] Serevent Diskus	β₂ β₂	MDI: 25 mcg/puff, 2 puffs bid DPI: 50 mcg/blister bid	Onset: 20 min Peak: 3-5 hr Duration: 12 hr

Modified from Gardenhire DS: *Rau's Respiratory care pharmacology*, ed 7, St Louis, 2008, Mosby.
*Detailed prescribing information should be obtained from the manufacturer's package insert.
[†]At the time of this writing, these medications are only available in the United Kingdom and Canada.
bid, twice daily; *DPI*, dry powder inhaler; *MDI*, metered dose inhaler; *qid*, four times daily; *SVN*, small volume nebulizer; *tid*, three times daily; *mg*, milligram (1/1000 gram); *mcg*, microgram (1/1000 milligram-note; the abbreviation μg may be used instead of mcg.)

BOX 9-1   Clinically Observed Side Effects of Sympathomimetic Aerosolized Bronchodilators (from the Most Commonly Seen to the Least Commonly Seen)

Tremor: gentle, uncontrollable, involuntary muscle shaking

Palpitations and tachycardia: irregular heartbeats and fast heart rate

Headache

Increased blood pressure: possibly from both the α_1-adrenergic effect on blood vessels and tachycardia

Nervousness and irritability

Dizziness

Nausea

Decreased PaO_2 level from a worsening of the ventilation/perfusion ratio

---

PaO₂, partial pressure of O_2 in arterial blood.

Exam Hint 9-1 (ELE, WRE)

A fast-onset medication (albuterol [Proventil, Ventolin], levalbuterol [Xopenex]) is used to treat a patient with acute bronchospasm. A long-duration medication (salmeterol [Serevent] or formoterol [Foradil]) is used to treat a patient with chronic, stable bronchospasm. A vasoconstricting medication (racemic epinephrine [microNefrin, Nefron]) is used to treat airway edema or bleeding.

Exam Hint 9-2 (ELE, WRE)

The NBRC rarely asks questions with specific drug doses. However, the following drug doses should be known. The standard adult dose of albuterol (Proventil) for a small volume nebulizer (SVN) is 0.5 mL (2.5 mg), three or four times a day. The standard adult dose of levalbuterol (Xopenex) for an SVN is 1.25 mg, three times a day.

---

b. Inhaled anticholinergic (parasympatholytic) agents

1. Recommend their use (ELE code: IIIG4a) [Difficulty: ELE: R, Ap, An]

This group of medications works to promote bronchodilation by suppressing the action of the parasympathetic nervous system. This results in the sympathetic nervous system dominating and causing bronchial smooth muscle relaxation. The parasympatholytic (anticholinergic) group has been found to be more effective in helping patients with chronic obstructive pulmonary disease (COPD) than

in helping patients with asthma. Be prepared to recommend their use in these types of patients.

2. Administer the prescribed medication (Code: IIIC3, IIID5a, IIID5b) [Difficulty: ELE: R, Ap; WRE: An]

Many patients with COPD and asthma will be treated with nebulized medications from both the sympathomimetic and the parasympatholytic groups. Combivent and DuoNeb combine a sympathomimetic and a parasympatholytic medication. The newest drug in this group, tiotropium bromide (Spiriva), provides the patient with 24 hours of the medication's benefits. See Table 9-2 for information on the parasympatholytic medications.

c. Recommend a theophylline agent (ELE code: IIIG4a) [Difficulty: ELE: R, Ap, An]

The family of drugs called xanthines includes theophylline and caffeine. They have been used in a variety of situations. A theophylline agent (e.g., aminophylline, Elixophyllin, Theo-Dur) is sometimes used to aid the breathing of a status asthmaticus patient or a patient with moderate to severe COPD. Current guidelines indicate that theophylline agents should be given to these patients only if optimal doses of inhaled bronchodilators and corticosteroid drugs have not been able to manage the patient's problem. Then intravenous theophylline ethylenediamine (aminophylline) can be administered. However, it should be used with caution. It is very difficult to regulate the proper serum level (about 5-12 mcg/mL), and serious side effects have been associated with use of this medication.

Caffeine citrate (Cafcit) has been approved for oral or intravenous administration to a neonate with apnea of prematurity. The physician may also choose to give aminophylline for the same purpose. Both have been shown to stimulate the breathing of neonates with this condition. In most cases, as the child's central nervous system matures, breathing is properly regulated and caffeine administration can be discontinued.

3. Antiinflammatory agents

a. Inhaled corticosteroids

1. Recommend use of corticosteroids (ELE code: IIIG4b) [Difficulty: ELE: R, Ap, An]

Corticosteroids affect the respiratory system in two ways: they potentiate the effects of the sympathomimetic agents, and they stop the inflammatory response seen in the airways of asthmatic patients after exposure to an allergen. This prevents mucosal edema from developing. The patient with chronic airflow obstruction, such as asthma or asthmatic bronchitis, should be given inhaled corticosteroids. When they are used as directed, relatively little

TABLE 9-2 Inhaled Anticholinergic Bronchodilator Agents*

Drug	Brand Name	Adult Dosage	Time Course (Onset, Peak, Duration)
Ipratropium	Atrovent HFA	MDI: 17 mcg/puff, 2 puffs qid SVN: 0.02% solution (0.2 mg/mL), 500 mcg tid, qid Nasal spray: 0.03%, 0.06%; 2 sprays per nostril 2-4 times daily (dosage varies)	Onset: 15 min bromide Peak: 1-2 hr Duration: 4-6 hr
Ipratropium bromide	Combivent DuoNeb	MDI: ipratropium 18 mcg/puff and albuterol 90 mcg/puff, 2 puffs qid SVN: 3 mL: ipratropium 0.5 mg and albuterol 2.5 mg, qid	Onset: 15 min and albuterol Peak: 1-2 hr Duration: 4-6 hr
Tiotropium bromide	Spiriva HandiHaler	DPI: 18 mcg/inhalation, 1 inhalation daily (one capsule)	Onset: 30 min Peak: 3 hr Duration: 24 hr

Modified from Gardenhire DS: *Rau's Respiratory care pharmacology,* ed 7, St Louis, 2008, Mosby.
*Detailed prescribing information should be obtained from the manufacturer's package insert.
bid, twice daily; *DPI,* dry powder inhaler; *MDI,* metered dose inhaler; *qid,* four times daily; *SVN,* small volume nebulizer; *tid,* three times daily.
A holding chamber is recommended with MDI administration to prevent accidental eye exposure.

systemic (bodily) absorption occurs. However, it is best to monitor the patient, especially small children taking inhaled corticosteroids for an extended period, for any side effects. Current guidelines for asthma management classify corticosteroids as "controller" medications that are taken to prevent an asthma attack.

The patient who is diagnosed with status asthmaticus should have systemic corticosteroids promptly administered by the intravenous (IV) route. Examples of commonly used systemic corticosteroids include methylprednisolone (Medrol and Solu-Medrol), prednisone (Deltasone), prednisolone (Meticortelone and Delta-Cortef), cortisone (Cortone), and hydrocortisone (Cortef and Solu-Cortef). These drugs can be lifesavers if used properly. However, prolonged use of large oral or IV doses can lead to serious systemic complications including, but not limited to, immunosuppression, adrenal gland insufficiency, hyperglycemia, and osteoporosis. If a patient has been taking systemic corticosteroids for an extended time, he or she should be gradually weaned from them after an inhaled corticosteroid has been started. It is dangerous to suddenly stop an oral or intravenous corticosteroid that has been used for a prolonged time.

2. Administer the prescribed medication (Code: IIIC3, IIID5a, IIID5b) [Difficulty: ELE: R, Ap; WRE: An]

Table 9-3 shows specific strength and dosage information for the inhaled corticosteroids.

The patient who is using any of these medications must gargle and rinse out his or her mouth after each use. If not, the patient runs the risk of developing a fungal infection of the mouth and throat. Note that there are now two inhaled medications (Advair and Symbicort) that combine a corticosteroid and a long-acting beta agonist (LABA).

NOTE: While past Written Registry Examinations have included a question concerning nonsteroidal antiinflammatory drugs (NSAIDs), they are not included in the current detailed content outline. They are include here for the sake of completeness. There are several different types of over-the-counter medications. None is as powerful an antiinflammatory as the corticosteroid drugs. Note the other clinical uses of acetylsalicylic acid and ibuprofen:

- Acetylsalicylic acid (e.g., Bayer aspirin): antiinflammatory, mild analgesia, antipyretic, blocks platelet aggregation (clot formation)
- Ibuprofen (Advil, Motrin): antiinflammatory, mild analgesia, antipyretic
- Antihistamine (Claritin): antiinflammatory

b. Cromolyn sodium

1. Recommend the use of cromolyn sodium (ELE code: IIIG4b) [Difficulty: ELE: R, Ap, An]

Cromolyn sodium (Intal) and nedrocromil sodium (Tilade) are indicated to prevent an asthma attack. They accomplish this by coating the mast cells found in the airways so that they do not degranulate and rupture. Without pretreatment, the mast cells of asthmatic patients would rupture when exposed to immunoglobulin E (IgE) from their allergen(s). This mast cell rupture would result in the spilling of leukotriene agents, histamine, and other

TABLE 9-3	Inhaled Corticosteroids Agents*	
Drug	**Brand Name**	**Formulation and Dosage**
Beclomethasone dipropionate HFA	QVAR	MDI: 40 mcg/puff and 80 mcg/puff
		Adults ≥12 yr: 40-80 mcg twice daily,*or 40-160 mcg twice daily[†]
		Children ≥5 yr: 40-80 mcg twice daily
Budesonide	Pulmicort Turbuhaler	DPI: 200 mcg/actuation
		Adults: 200-400 mcg bid,*200-400 mcg bid,[†] 400-800 mcg bid[‡,§]
		Children ≥6 yr: 200 mcg bid
	Pulmicort Flexhaler	DPI: 90 mcg/actuation, 180 mcg/actuation
		Adults: 180-360 mcg bid usual dose range, 720 mcg bid maximum
		Children ≥6 yr: 180 mcg bid usual dose, 360 mcg bid maximum
	Pulmicort Respules	SVN: 0.25 mg/2 mL, 0.5 mg/2 mL, 1 mg/ml
		Children 1-8 yr: 0.5 mg total dose given once daily, or twice daily in divided doses;*,[†] 1 mg given as 0.5 mg bid or once daily[§]
Budesonide and formoterol fumarate HFA	Symbicort	MDI: Adults ≥12 yr: 80 mcg budesonide with 4.5 mcg formoterol/actuation, 2 puffs bid; and 160 mcg budisonide with 4.5 mcg formoterol/actuation, 2 puffs bid
		Maximum daily dose: 640 mcg budisonide and 18 mcg formoterol
Flunisolide hemihydrate HFA	Aerospan	MDI: 80 mcg/puff
		Adults ≥12 yr: 2 puffs bid, adults no more than 4 puffs daily
		Children 6-11 yr: 1 puff daily, no more than 2 puffs daily
Flunisolide	AeroBid, AeroBid-M	MDI: 250 mcg/puff
		Adults and children ≥6 yr: 2 puffs bid, adults no more than 4 puffs daily
		Children ≤15 yr: no more than 2 puffs daily
Fluticasone propionate	Flovent HFA	MDI: 44 mcg/puff, 110 mcg/puff, 220 mcg/puff
		Adults ≥12 yr: 88 mcg bid,* 88-220 mcg bid,[†] or 880 mcg bid[§]
		Children 4-11 yr: 88 mcg bid
	Flovent Diskus	DPI: 50 mcg, 100 mcg, 250 mcg
		Adults: 100 mcg bid*100-250 mcg bid,[†] 1000 mcg bid[§]
		Children 4-11 yr; 50 mcg twice daily
Fluticasone propionate/ salmeterol	Advair Diskus	DPI: 100 mcg fluticasone/50 mcg salmeterol, 250 mcg fluticasone/50 mcg propionate/salmeterol, or 500 mcg fluticasone/50 mcg salmeterol salmeterol
		Adults and children ≥12 yr: 100 mcg fluticasone/50 mcg salmeterol, 1 inhalation twice daily, about 12 hr apart (starting dose if not currently on inhaled corticosteroids)
		Maximum recommended dose 500 mcg fluticasone/50 mcg salmeterol twice daily
		Children ≥4 yr: 100 mcg fluticasone/50 mcg salmeterol, 1 inhalation twice daily, about 12 hr apart (for those who are symptomatic while taking an inhaled corticosteroid)
	Advair HFA	MDI: 45 mcg fluticasone/21 mcg salmeterol, 115 mcg fluticasone/21 mcg salmeterol, or 230 mcg fluticasone/21 mcg salmeterol salmeterol,
		Adults and children ≥12 yr: 2 inhalations twice daily, about 12 hr apart
Mometasone furoate	Asmanex Twisthaler	DPI: 220 mcg[‡] actuation, 110 mcg actuation for children 4-11
		Adults and children ≥12 yr: 220-440 mcg daily,* 220-440 mcg daily,[†] 480-880 mcg daily[§]
Triamcinolone acetonide	Azmacort	MDI: 75 mcg/puff
		Adults ≥12 yr: 2 puffs tid or qid
		Children ≥6 yr: 1-2 puffs tid or qid

Modified from Gardenhire DS: *Rau's Respiratory care pharmacology,* ed 7, St Louis, 2008, Mosby.
*Detailed prescribing information should be obtained from the manufacturer's package insert.
[†]Recommended starting dose if on bronchodilators alone.
[‡]Recommended starting dose if on inhaled corticosteroids previously.
[§]Recommended starting dose if on oral corticosteroids previously.
bid, twice daily; *qid,* four times daily; *tid,* three times daily.

chemical mediators that cause the bronchospasm, airway edema, and increased airway secretions of an asthma attack.

2. Administer the prescribed medication (Code: IIIC3, IIID5a, IIID5b) [Difficulty: ELE: R, Ap; WRE: An]

When cromolyn sodium, or nedrocromil sodium, is inhaled at least 1 week before exposure to the allergen, the asthmatic reaction is prevented or reduced. Cromolyn was first made available through a dry powder inhaler and is now only available by metered dose inhaler or small volume nebulizer (SVN). Nedrocromil sodium is similar to cromolyn in its use and effects. It is available in a metered dose inhaler. See Table 9-4 for detailed information on both medications.

It is very important to understand that both drugs are taken for prophylactic purposes to prevent an asthma attack. They are contraindicated during an asthma attack. A patient experiencing acute bronchospasm should be treated with a fast sympathomimetic bronchodilator, as previously discussed.

c. Recommend the use of leukotriene modifiers (ELE code: IIIG4b) [Difficulty: ELE: R, Ap, An]

Leukotrienes are chemicals found in mast cells that are released during an asthma attack. These released leukotriene chemicals stimulate bronchospasm, airway edema, and increased airway secretions. The leukotriene-modifier (also called leukotriene antagonists) medications work to reduce the number of leukotriene chemicals that are released or to block the effect of leukotrienes on the airways. By accomplishing this, the patient's asthma symptoms are reduced or eliminated. See Table 9-4 for detailed information on all four medications in this group.

As with cromolyn sodium or nedrocromil sodium, it is very important to understand that all of these drugs are taken for prophylactic purposes to prevent an asthma attack. They are contraindicated during an asthma attack. A patient experiencing acute bronchospasm should be treated with a fast-onset sympathomimetic bronchodilator (SABA), as previously discussed.

TABLE 9-4	Inhaled Nonsteroidal Antiasthma Agents*	
Drug	**Brand Name**	**Formulation and Dosage**
CROMOLYN-LIKE (MAST CELL STABILIZERS)		
Cromolyn sodium†	Intal	MDI: 800 mcg/actuation
		Adults and children ≥5 yr: 2 inhalations 4 times daily
		SVN: 20 mg/amp or 20 mg/vial
		Adults and children ≥2 yr: 20 mg inhaled 4 times daily
	Nasalcrom	Spray: 40 mg/mL (4%), gives 5.2 mg of drug
		Adults and children ≥2 yr: 1 spray each nostril, 3-6 times daily every 4-6 hr
Nedocromil sodium	Tilade	MDI: 1.75 mg/actuation
		Adults and children ≥6 yr: 2 inhalations 4 times daily
ANTILEUKOTRIENES		
Montelukast	Singulair	Tablets: 10 mg, 4 mg, and 5 mg cherry-flavored chewable; 4 mg packet of granules
		Adults and children ≥15 yr: one 10 mg tablet daily in evening
		Children 6-14 yr: one 5 mg chewable tablet daily
		Children 2-5 years: one 4 mg chewable tablet or one 4 mg packet of granules daily
		Children 6-23 months: one 4 mg packet of granules daily
Zafirlukast	Accolate	Tablets: 10 and 20 mg
		Adults and children ≥12 yr: 20 mg (1 tablet) twice daily, without food
		Children 5-11 yr: 10 mg twice daily
Zileuton	Zyflo	Tablets: 600 mg
	Zyflo CR	Adults and children ≥12 yr: one 600 mg tablet 4 times a day
MONOCLONAL ANTIBODY		
Omalizumab	Xolair	Adults and children ≥12 yr: subcutaneous injection every 4 weeks; dose dependent on patient's weight and serum IgE level

Modified from Gardenhire DS: *Rau's Respiratory care pharmacology,* ed 7, St Louis, 2008, Mosby.
*Detailed prescribing information should be obtained from the manufacturer's package insert.
†NOTE: Cromolyn sodium is also available in an oral concentrate giving 100 mg in 5 mL (Gastrocrom), for treatment of systemic mastocytosis, and as an ophthalmic 4% solution (Opticrom, 40 mg/mL) for treatment of vernal keratoconjunctivitis.

4. Mucolytics or proteolytic agents

a. Acetylcysteine

1. Recommend the use of acetylcysteine (ELE code: IIIG4c) [Difficulty: ELE: R, Ap, An]

N-Acetylcysteine/acetylcysteine/NAC (Mucomyst, Mucosil) is a mucolytic drug that has been widely used for many years with patients who have thick (viscous) mucus or mucus plugs. However, its use for the mycolytic effect is now controversial and some authors have advocated for the discontinuation of its clinical use. In the past, the NBRC has included questions where acetylcysteine (Mucomyst) would be indicated as a mucolytic.

Know that there are two clinical concerns with this medication. Acetylcysteine has a bad odor (rotten eggs) that may lead to nausea and vomiting in some patients. Of greater concern is the stimulation of bronchospasm in some asthmatic patients. Therefore it is wise to pretreat these patients with an aerosolized sympathomimetic bronchodilator before acetylcysteine is nebulized. Any fast-onset bronchodilator can be used in the usual dose. Because of the lack of proven clinical effectiveness and the noted hazards, acetylcysteine is no longer recommended in patients with cystic fibrosis. It is still used with chronic bronchitis patients as long as the noted precautions are taken.

2. Administer the prescribed medication (Code: IIIC3, IIID5a) [Difficulty: ELE: R, Ap; WRE: An]

Mucomyst is usually administered with a small volume nebulizer (SVN) or with intermittent positive-pressure breathing (IPPB). Most adult patients are given up to 3 to 5 mL of the 20% solution or up to 6 to 10 mL of the 10% solution. The 20% solution is often diluted with an equal volume of normal saline solution. Direct instillation of 1 to 2 mL of the drug into the trachea also helps to liquefy secretions. The manufacturer recommends that all medication in a vial be used within 96 hours or discarded. It should be stored in the refrigerator. A slightly purple color is commonly seen after the vial has been opened, but it can still be used safely. See Table 9-5 for specific information.

b. RhDNAse

1. Recommend the use of RhDNAse (ELE code: IIIG4c) [Difficulty: ELE: R, Ap, An]

Dornase alfa (Pulmozyme; the NBRC refers to this drug as recombinant human deoxyribonuclease [RhDNAse]) is a proteolytic drug that has been approved for use in the treatment of patients with cystic fibrosis. It works by breaking up strands of DNA found in the secretions of these patients with a pulmonary infection.

2. Administer the prescribed medication (Code: IIIC3, IIID5a) [Difficulty: ELE: R, Ap; WRE: An]

Usually a single daily dose of 2.5 mL of solution (containing 2.5 mg of dornase alfa) is inhaled by SVN. Store the drug in a refrigerator, and protect it from strong light. It has no serious side effects. See Table 9-5 for detailed information.

c. Hypertonic saline

1. Recommend the use of hypertonic saline (ELE code: IIIG4c) [Difficulty: ELE: R, Ap, An]

The various saline solutions (and sterile water) are known collectively as "bland" aerosols, because they have no direct pharmacologic effect on the lungs and airways. When they are inhaled as aerosols, however, a vagal nerve-mediated reflex causes the bronchial/submucosal glands

TABLE 9-5	Inhaled Mucoactive Agents*			
Drug	Brand Name	Adult Dosage		Use
Acetylcysteine 10%	Mucomyst Mucosil-10	SVN: 6-10 mL, tid, qid		Bronchitis; efficacy not proven
Acetylcysteine 20%	Mucomyst Mucosil-20	SVN: 3-5 mL, tid, qid		Bronchitis; efficacy not proven
Aqueous aerosols: water, saline (0.45%, 0.9%, 5%-10%)	N/A	SVN: 3-5 mL, as ordered USN: 3-5 mL, as ordered		Sputum induction, secretion mobilization
Dornase alfa	Pulmozyme	SVN: 2.5 mg/ampule one ampule daily*		Cystic fibrosis

Modified from Gardenhire DS: *Rau's Respiratory care pharmacology*, ed 7, St Louis, 2008, Mosby.
*Detailed prescribing information should be obtained from the manufacturer's package insert.
N/A, not applicable; *qid*, four times daily; *SVN*, small volume nebulizer; *tid*, three times daily; *USN*, ultrasonic nebulizer.
Use with an approved nebulizer system, including PARI LC Jet Plus, Hudson T Updraft II, and Marquest Acorn II.

to release more watery secretions. Therefore a saline aerosol is commonly used to help liquefy secretions and induce a patient to expel sputum. Recent clinical experience has shown hypertonic saline to be an effective mucolytic in cystic fibrosis patients.

2. Administer the prescribed medication (Code: IIIC3, IIID5a) [Difficulty: ELE: R, Ap; WRE: An]

The various saline solutions are given through an SVN or IPPB treatment or, more commonly, mixed with a bronchodilator medication. See Table 9-5 and Box 9-2 for information on the various saline solutions.

BOX 9-2   Saline Solutions Used as Mucolytics

NORMAL SALINE SOLUTION, 0.9% SALINE
Direct instillation into the airway:
- Infants may be given about 1 mL several times daily before airway suctioning.
- Adults may be given about 3-5 mL several times daily before airway suctioning.

Aerosol: Most medication nebulizers hold 3-5 mL that is nebulized several times daily.
Miscellaneous:
- Usually is well tolerated because it is isotonic to the body.
- Particle size is fairly stable as nebulized.

HYPOTONIC SALINE SOLUTION, 0.45% SALINE
Direct instillation into the airway: Same as with normal saline solution.
Aerosol: Same as with normal saline solution; many practitioners use this concentration in ultrasonic nebulizers.
Miscellaneous: Particles tend to shrink because of evaporation, which results in smaller particles than nebulized that are closer to isotonic; impaction is more likely in the smaller airways.

HYPERTONIC SALINE SOLUTION, 1.8%-10% SALINE
Aerosol: Some practitioners use a large-reservoir nebulizer with a heater to generate the aerosol. Hypertonic saline solution is most commonly used to induce a cough and sputum sample for cytologic studies (e.g., lung cancer) or for fungal or mycobacteria (e.g., tuberculosis) culture. It should not be used for a general bacterial culture because the high salt concentration inhibits the growth of most bacteria. Hypertonic saline has also been found useful as a mucolytic in cystic fibrosis patients.
Miscellaneous: Particles tend to enlarge because of the absorption of water vapor, which results in larger particles than nebulized that are closer to isotonic; impaction is more likely in the upper airway. This concentration is the most likely to cause bronchospasm in asthma patients because it is the furthest from isotonic and, therefore, the most irritating. It may be necessary to pretreat the patient with a short-acting beta-agonist (SABA) bronchodilator.

---

d. Observe the patient for signs of changes in sputum characteristics (ELE code: IIIE5a) [Difficulty: ELE: R, Ap, An]

The respiratory therapist should objectively evaluate the patient's cough and sputum production before and after a mucolytic has been administered. This will provide evidence of the medication's effectiveness. See Chapter 1 for further discussion and Table 1-13 for sputum characteristics.

5. Diuretics

a. Recommend the adjustment of fluid balance (Code: IIIG1d) [Difficulty: ELE: R, Ap; WRE: An]

A patient who is fluid overloaded or has congestive heart failure and pulmonary edema will often exhibit the following signs: peripheral edema, jugular vein distension, crackles for breath sounds, cyanosis, tachycardia, and hypotension. Arterial blood gas results will show hypoxemia. A chest radiograph will show an enlarged heart and pulmonary infiltrates. Shortness of breath is the most common symptom.

Treatment of the patient will include fluid restriction and diuresis to rapidly decrease the patient's fluid volume. Review Box 1-3 for normal fluid intake and output values.

b. Recommend use of diuretics (Code: IIIG4i) [Difficulty: ELE: R, Ap; WRE: An]

Diuretics are most commonly indicated in patients who are fluid overloaded or have hypertension. The following are examples of diuretics commonly used to treat these problems:
- Furosemide (Lasix)
- Bumetanide (Bumex)
- Torsemide (Demadex)
- Chlorothiazide (Diuril)

These are some of the most powerful diuretics in use. They produce a rapid increase in urine output. They basically prevent the kidneys from retaining sodium so that water is excreted. A side effect of their use is a loss of potassium through the kidneys.

Another category of diuretic is used in patients who have an increased intracranial pressure (ICP). The increased ICP is usually attributable to cerebral edema from a head injury. Examples of medications used to treat an increased ICP include the following:
- Mannitol (Osmitrol)
- Sterile urea (Ureaphil, Urevert)

These medications have a large molecular weight and, through osmosis, "pull" fluid from the brain into the bloodstream. Therefore they are sometimes called osmotic diuretics. The medication, after crossing into the kidney, prevents the reabsorption of water and increases urine output.

c. Recommend blood tests to measure the potassium level (Code: IIIE8) [Difficulty: ELE: R, Ap; WRE: An]

If a patient with fluid overload has been give a diuretic such as Lasix, all electrolytes, especially the serum potassium level, should be check regularly. As stated previously, Lasix and related diuretic medications cause the kidneys to excrete potassium in addition to sodium and water. The so-called potassium-sparing electrolytes (e.g., spironolactone [Aldactone], amiloride [Midamor], triamterene [Dyrenium]) can lead to an increased potassium level. (Review Table 1-2 for the normal electrolyte values.)

d. Recommend the adjustment of electrolyte therapy (Code: IIIG1e) [Difficulty: ELE: R, Ap; WRE: An]

The normal value for serum potassium (K^+) is 3.5 to 5.5 mEq/L. A potassium level of less than 3.5 mEq/L is dangerous because it increases the risk of cardiac arrhythmias. Replacement potassium is needed. It is usually given by the intravenous route because it is faster than when taken orally.

Be prepared to recommend the administration of any electrolyte that is less than the low end of the range. Conversely, be prepared to recommend withholding an electrolyte supplement if the serum level is greater than the upper end of the range.

Exam Hint 9-3 (ELE, WRE)

There will usually be at least one question that regards the use of a diuretic in a patient who is fluid overloaded, and the side effects of using a diuretic. A diuretic drug such as furosemide (Lasix) tends to cause the loss of potassium through the kidneys. Know to check the serum potassium level. Remember that the normal potassium level is 3.5 to 5.5 mEq/L. If the patient has the signs of dangerous hypokalemia (see Chapter 1), know to recommend that replacement potassium be given.

---

6. Recommend the use of sedatives (Code: IIIG4f, IIIG1c) [Difficulty: ELE: R, Ap; WRE: An]

Sedatives are medications that affect the brain to induce calming in a patient who can be either simply anxious or very agitated and uncooperative. A patient would be given a sedative in the following situations: (1) when he or she is struggling against a necessary intubation or the mechanical ventilator, thus worsening his or her condition; (2) when he or she is displaying self-destructive behavior because of a drug reaction; and (3) before a medical procedure, for so-called conscious sedation. The effects on the patient are dose related. Low to moderate doses calm the patient, and higher doses induce sleep. Three different groupings of these types of medications exist. The most widely used are the benzodiazepines, because they have fewer side effects and fewer drug interactions and are less likely to cause addiction than are the barbiturate drugs. The benzodiazepine agents can be pharmacologically reversed. The barbiturates are widely used during general anesthesia to induce sleep rapidly. Commonly used examples of the sedative agents include the following:

- Benzodiazepine minor tranquilizers: midazolam (Versed), diazepam (Valium), lorazepam (Ativan), chlordiazepoxide (Librium), alprazolam (Xanax), triazolam (Halcion), flurazepam (Dalmane)
- Nonbarbiturate sedative-hypnotics: meprobamate (Miltown), glutethimide (Doriden), chloral hydrate (Noctec)
- Barbiturate sedative-hypnotics: pentobarbital sodium (Nembutal), secobarbital sodium (Seconal), phenobarbital (Luminol), thiopental sodium (Pentothal)

The benzodiazepine antagonist drug flumazenil (Romazicon) is indicated in the reversal of benzodiazepine agents such as Valium and Librium. Unconscious patients usually awaken quickly once the proper dose of flumazenil is given. Monitor the patient for signs of seizure activity related to the rapid reversal of the benzodiazepine medication. The patient should be observed for 2 hours in case resedation occurs. In this case, flumazenil can be readministered.

7. Recommend the use of analgesics (Code: IIIG4g) [Difficulty: ELE: R, Ap; WRE: An]

Analgesics are medications that control or block pain after an injury or a surgical procedure. Morphine or similar narcotic-type analgesic drugs are indicated to control moderate to severe pain. Morphine also is indicated to treat the pain of a myocardial infarction and to produce vasodilation in the patient with pulmonary edema. Additionally, pain-relieving agents, when given in large enough doses, will sedate or induce sleep. The patient who is both in pain and agitated may be treated with a combination of an analgesic and a sedative (e.g., moderate doses of morphine and diazepam). The two drugs potentiate each other. The physician may instead decide to give the patient a larger dose of morphine rather than both drug types. Examples of commonly used analgesics include the following:

- Morphine sulfate (Duramorph) injection; Oramorph SR, tablets
- Tylenol with codeine tablets
- Oxycodone (Percocet, OxyContin)
- Hydrocodone (Vicodin)
- Hydromorphone (Dilaudid)
- Meperidine (Demerol)
- Propoxyphene (Darvon)

Patients receiving sedatives or analgesics, or both, must be closely monitored. Each type of medication can cause respiratory center depression if given in great enough doses. The patient may hypoventilate and even experience apnea and death. It is especially important to monitor a patient with COPD who is given morphine for the off-label management of dyspnea. Narcotic analgesic agents (e.g., morphine) and some other analgesic medications can become habit forming or addictive if used for a prolonged period.

The narcotic antagonist drug naloxone (Narcan) counteracts the effects of narcotic agents, such as morphine, heroin, and codeine. Narcan does not reverse benzodiazepine or barbiturate drugs. Remember that the patient who was given an accidental overdose of morphine to control pain will feel pain again when Narcan is administered.

Exam Hint 9-4 (ELE, WRE)

There is usually a question about recommending a drug for pain control. If the patient has severe pain from trauma or surgery, recommend morphine sulfate or a similar narcotic analgesic agent. Remember that too much narcotic can cause apnea. Narcan is the reversing agent for a narcotic overdose.

---

8. Recommend the use of neuromuscular blocking agents (Code: IIIG4h, IIIG1c) [Difficulty: ELE: R, Ap; WRE: An]

The NBRC may use the terms "paralytic agents" and "muscle relaxants" when describing medications that cause a medically induced paralysis. It would be more correct to call these medications neuromuscular blocking agents (NMBAs). They work by blocking nerve transmission from reaching skeletal (voluntary) muscles; and complete paralysis follows. They are most commonly used as part of balanced anesthesia before major thoracic or abdominal surgery. These drugs also are used in the intensive care unit to stop a patient from fighting against an intubation or to prevent the patient from struggling against the mechanical ventilator. All of these agents are given intravenously and act rapidly. Obviously, in all these cases, the patient stops breathing and must receive mechanical ventilation. Examples of the commonly used neuromuscular blocking agents include the following:

- Depolarizing blocker: succinylcholine chloride (Anectine, Quelicin)
- Nondepolarizing blockers: pancuronium bromide (Pavulon; preferred), vecuronium bromide (Norcuron), gallamine triethiodide (Flaxedil), atracurium besylate (Tracrium)

The nondepolarizing blockers (e.g., Pavulon) are preferred for their longer duration of action. Although all these agents induce complete paralysis of all voluntary muscles, they have little or no effect on the involuntary muscles or autonomic nervous system. Some patients may have a minor, passing change in heart rate and blood pressure. Remember that these patients are able to hear, are able to feel pain, and are completely awake and alert to their surroundings. Care must be taken to sedate the patient for anxiety and give analgesics for pain. Talk to the patient normally, and move the patient periodically to prevent pressure sores.

The nondepolarizing neuromuscular blocking agents can be reversed so that the patient can breathe and move again. These intravenous medications include neostigmine bromide (Prostigmin; preferred) and edrophonium (Tensilon). It should be noted that these reversing agents cause an outpouring of oral and bronchial secretions. Atropine is given to prevent this. The reversing agents have no effect on the depolarizing neuromuscular blocker succinylcholine chloride. Patients given this drug usually regain movement within 15 minutes after the medication is stopped.

9. Recommend the use of surfactants (Code: IIIG4j) [Difficulty: ELE: R, Ap; WRE: An]

Surfactant has been approved for the prevention or treatment of infant respiratory distress syndrome (RDS) in premature neonates. These neonates have immature lungs that lack natural surfactant. As a result, atelectasis develops. These three surfactant agents have been approved for instillation into the airways to treat this problem and are widely used:

1. Beractant (Survanta)
2. Poractant alfa (Curosurf)
3. Calfactant (Infasurf)

Dosages for all of the medications are based on the infant's weight. Once one of these medications is instilled into the neonate's airways, be prepared to make rapid changes in the mechanical ventilator settings. This is because the lungs will rapidly become more compliant. The set pressure will need to be reduced so that the neonate is not overventilated, resulting in barotrauma. In addition, the oxygen percentage can usually be rapidly reduced.

TABLE 9-6	Common Respiratory Pathogens in Approximate Order of Frequency		
	Gram Positive	**Gram Negative**	**Cell Wall Deficient**
Bacteria:	*Streptococcus pneumoniae*	*Haemophilus influenzae*	*Mycoplasma*
	*Staphylococcus aureus**	Klebsiella pneumoniae	ACID-FAST
	Streptococcus faecalis (enterococcus)	*Pseudomonas aeruginosa**	*Mycobacterium tuberculosis**
		Serratia species*	
Viruses:	Rhinovirus	Varicella virus*	
	Adenovirus	Herpes simplex virus*	
	Respiratory syncytial virus	Cytomegalovirus*	
Fungi:	*Candida albicans**	*Histoplasma capsulatum* (Ohio Valley)	
	Aspergillus species*	*Coccidioides immitis* (Southwest U.S.)	
	Pneumocystis carinii		
Protozoa:	*Toxoplasma gondii**		
	*Cryptosporidium**		

*Seen most frequently in debilitated or immunosuppressed hosts.

10. Antimicrobials

a. Recommend the use of antimicrobials (e.g., antibiotics) (Code: IIIG4e) [Difficulty: ELE: R, Ap; WRE: An]

The terms antimicrobial, antiinfective, and antibiotic refer to natural or synthetic chemicals that are toxic to bacteria and other microorganisms. Table 9-6 lists the most commonly found respiratory tract pathogens. See Table 9-7 for a summary of the most common respiratory tract pathogens and the antimicrobial agents used against them. Table 9-8 lists specific information on the four currently approved aerosolized antimicrobial agents given by respiratory therapists and likely to be tested by the NBRC. They are discussed below. Be aware that other systemic antimicrobial medications have been given by aerosol despite not having FDA approval.

b. Administer the prescribed medication (Code: IIIC3, IIID5a, IIID5b) [Difficulty: ELE: R, Ap; WRE: An]

1. Antibacterial agent: tobramycin

Tobramycin (TOBI) is used to control chronic pulmonary infection with the gram-negative bacteria *Pseudomonas aeruginosa*. It has been approved for use in children 6 years and older with cystic fibrosis. TOBI is taken through the PARI LC Plus small volume nebulizer. No other medications are to be mixed with the TOBI in the nebulizer. The currently approved treatment course involves the drug being taken for 28 days. The patient then discontinues the medication for 28 days. This treatment cycle has been shown to control the infection without antibiotic resistance developing.

2. Antiviral agent: zanamivir and ribavirin

Zanamivir (Relenza) is approved for the treatment of influenza in adults and children older than 5 years of age. To be effective, Relenza must be started within the first 2 days of symptoms and continued for 5 days. If taken early enough in the course of the infection, the patient's symptoms should be reduced and the course of the infection shortened. Relenza is available in a multidose dry powder inhaler (DPI) packet. The medication packet is loaded into the Diskhaler delivery device for inhalation (see Figure 8-18).

Ribavirin (Virazole) is most commonly used in the treatment of infants and young children who have bronchiolitis or pneumonia from the respiratory syncytial virus (RSV). Patients requiring treatment for their condition usually are very sick and have complicating factors such as prematurity or cardiopulmonary disease. They require the treatment course of 3 to 7 days of nebulization of the drug for 12 to 18 hours per day. Only the SPAG II (small particle aerosol generator) can be used for the procedure. This is because it is specifically designed to nebulize the 1- to 2-μm size particles necessary for alveoli penetration so that it can kill the virus. Virazole is also known to be effective against influenza types A and B and the herpes simplex virus. Because of the risk of side effects to health care providers, a scavenging system must be used with Vibrazole to ensure that none of the particles escape into room air.

3. Antiprotozoal agent: pentamidine isethionate

Pentamidine isethionate (NebuPent) has been approved for the prophylactic treatment of the fungal organism

TABLE 9-7	Classification of Antibiotic Agents Commonly Used Against Pulmonary Infections		
Class or Group	**Agents**	**Spectrum**	**Major Toxicity**
Aminoglycosides	Streptomycin	Primarily tuberculostatic	Vestibular, renal
	Tobramycin, TOBI	*Pseudomonas aeruginosa* lung	Auditory, renal infection in cystic fibrosis patients
	gentamicin, Garamycin	Gram-negative rods, including *Pseudomonas* and *Proteus*	Vestibular, renal
Antifungal agents	Ketoconazole, Nizoral	Major agent for systemic fungal disease	Gastrointestinal upset
	Amphotericin B	Major agent for systemic fungal disease	Renal, gastrointestinal
Antituberculosis agents	Isonicotinic acid hydrazide (INH), Isoniazid	Used for both prophylaxis and treatment	Hepatic
	Ethambutol, rifampin	Used for tuberculostatic therapy	Retinal (maculopathy), hepatic
Antiviral agents	AZT, Retrovir	Stops reproduction in retroviruses; used against HIV	Anemia
	ribavirin, Virazole	Same spectrum, used against respiratory syncytial virus; experimental against HIV	
Cephalosporin	Cephalothin, Keflin, cephalexin	Like penicillin, with antistaphylococcal effects	Renal (usually not severe)
Chloramphenicol	Chloromycetin	Broad spectrum; used for *Haemophilus* if it is ampicillin-resistant or if patient is allergic	Bone marrow
Macrolide	Erythromycin, Erythrocin	Like penicillin (used in penicillin allergy); drug of choice for *Mycoplasma*	Gastrointestinal
Penicillin	Penicillin G	Gram-positive organisms; *Staphylococcus aureus* often resistant	Allergy
Semisynthetic penicillins	Ampicillin, Omnipen Amoxicillin	Gram-positive organisms, Gram negative *Haemophilus influenzae*; variable against gram-negative rods	Diarrhea and rash, especially with viral disease (mononucleosis)
	Oxacillin, Prostaphlin	Like penicillin, with antistaphylococcal effects	Allergy
	Geopen	Like penicillin, with antipseudomonas effects	Sodium overload-congestive failure
Sulfonamides	pentamidine isethionate,	Prophylaxis against *Pneumocystis*	Impaired renal and liver function
	NebuPent, Pentam 300 trimethaprim and sulfamethoxazole, Bactrim	Used against *Pneumocystis carinii carinii allergy*	Impaired renal and liver function
Tetracyclines	tetracycline, Achromycin	Broad spectrum; useful against *Haemophilus* and *Mycoplasma* infections	Fungal overgrowth in bowel or vagina; hepatic with large IV doses

Pneumocystis carinii. Patients with impaired immune systems, such as those with acquired immunodeficiency syndrome (AIDS), are most likely to suffer from *Pneumocystis carinii* pneumonia (PCP). (NOTE: This may also be called *Pneumocystis jiroveci* pneumonia [PJP].) Currently, these patients are given a single 300-mg dose of NebuPent mixed with 6 mL of sterile water once every 4 weeks through the Respirgard II small volume nebulizer. This unit also features an expiratory scavenging filter to prevent any droplets from entering the room air (see Figure 8-15). (The AeroTech II unit may also be used to deliver NebuPent.)

Some patients must be pretreated with an inhaled bronchodilator to prevent bronchospasm before the NebuPent is inhaled. Do not mix the two medications in the Respirgard II or use the Respirgard II for any medication other than NebuPent. Mixing NebuPent with normal saline or a bronchodilator can result in a precipitation of the medications. When given by the inhalation route, there are few systemic side effects. There is also an intramuscular or intravenous form of pentamidine called Pentam 300. Bactrim (trimethoprim and sulfamethoxazole) is preferred over systemic pentamidine because there are fewer and less serious side effects.

TABLE 9-8	Inhaled Antimicrobial Agents*		
Drug	**Brand Name**	**Adult Dosage**	**Use**
Pentamidine isethionate	NebuPent	SVN:[†] 300 mg of powder in 6 mL of sterile water; once every 4 weeks	Prophylaxis against *Pneumocystis carinii* pneumonia (PCP)
Ribavirin	Vibrazole	SPAG:[‡] 6 mg of powder in 300 mL of sterile water (20 mg/mL solution); (RSV) given for 12-18 hr/day for 3-7 days	Respiratory syncytial virus
Tobramycin	TOBI	SVN:[§] 300 mg/5 mL ampule, bid, 28 days on and 28 days off drug	*Pseudomonas aeruginosa* in cystic fibrosis patient
Zanamivir	Relenza	DPI: 5 mg/inhalation Adults and children ≥5 yr for prophylaxis; ≥7 yr for treatment: 2 inhalations (one 5-mg blister per inhalation) bid about 12 hr apart for 5 days.	Influenza

Modified from Gardenhire DS: *Rau's Respiratory care pharmacology*, ed 7, St Louis, 2008, Mosby.

*Detailed prescribing information should be obtained from the manufacturer's package insert.

[†]NebuPent is only used with the Respirgard II small volume nebulizer.

[‡]Vibrazole is only used with the SPAG (small particle aerosol generator) nebulizer.

[§]TOBI is used with an approved nebulizer system, including PARI LC Jet Plus, Hudson T Updraft II, and Marquest II.

bid, twice daily; *DPI*, dry powder inhaler; *SVN*, small volume nebulizer.

Exam Hint 9-5 (ELE, WRE)

There is usually one question that considers the need for an antimicrobial medication to treat a pulmonary infection. Know these antimicrobial agents and what they are used to treat:

- Penicillin (e.g., penicillin G, ampicillin) to treat gram-positive bacteria
- Gentamicin (Garamycin) to treat gram-negative bacteria
- Aerosolized tobramycin (TOBI) to treat *Pseudomonas* pneumonia in children with cystic fibrosis
- Aerosolized pentamidine isethionate (NebuPent) for prophylactic treatment of *Pneumocystis carinii*
- Aerosolized ribavirin (Vibrazole) to treat *respiratory syncytial virus* (RSV) in young children
- Isoniazid (INH) to treat *Mycobacterium tuberculosis* (TB)

11. Recommend the use of vaccines (e.g., Pneumovax, influenza) (Code: IIIG4k) [Difficulty: ELE: R; WRE: Ap]

See Chapter 2 for the discussion on vaccination to prevent avian flu, severe acute respiratory syndrome (SARS) from the coronavirus, and *Streptococcus pneumoniae*.

12. Recommend the use of cardiovascular drugs (e.g., ACLS protocol agents) (Code: IIIG4d) [Difficulty: ELE: R, Ap; WRE: An]

See Chapter 11 for the discussion on drugs that may be used during CPR efforts.

Exam Hint 9-6 (ELE)

Expect several questions that require the respiratory therapist to recommend the use of medications in the classes discussed previously. Know the indications for these groups of medications and the main medications in each group.

MODULE C
Drug dosage calculations (math review)

Exam Hint 9-7 (ELE, WRE)

The NBRC examination content outline does not specifically list drug dosage calculations. However, previous Entry Level and Written Registry Examinations have included one calculation.

The problems are easier to solve by remembering the following:

1. One milliliter (1 mL) or 1 cubic centimeter (1 cc) of water = 1 gram (g) of mass.
2. Most drug doses are listed in milligrams instead of grams. Convert grams to milligrams by moving the decimal point three places to the right (the same as multiplying by 1000). For example, 0.5 g equals 500 mg.
3. Know how to interconvert fractions, decimal fractions, and percentages. For example: $1:100 = 1/100 = 0.01 = 1\%$.

One common way to solve any drug dosage calculation is by creating a proportional problem. The drug concentration must be converted into a fractional form. The proportional problem can then be set up to solve for the unknown *amount of active ingredient*. For example:

1. How much active ingredient would be in 0.5 mL of adrenaline?

A 1% (1:100) drug concentration means that there is 1 part of active ingredient in 100 parts of the solution, or 1 mL or 1 g of active ingredient in 100 mL or 100 g of the solution. This can be set up in the following proportion:

$$\frac{1 \text{ mL active ingredient}}{100 \text{ mL total solution}} = \frac{\text{unknown active ingredient or } x}{0.5 \text{ mL solution}} \text{(cross-multiply)}$$

$100x = 0.5$ mL (Divide both sides of the equation by 100.)

$x = 0.005$ mL $= 0.005$ g $= 5$ mg of active ingredient

2. How much active ingredient would be in 0.25 mL of Alupent? (Alupent is 5.0% active ingredient.)

A 5% drug concentration means that there are 5 parts of active ingredient in 100 parts of the solution, or 5 mL or 5 g of active ingredient in 100 mL or 100 g of the solution. This can be set up in the following proportion:

$$\frac{5 \text{ mL active ingredient}}{100 \text{ mL total solution}} = \frac{\text{unknown active ingredient or } x}{0.25 \text{ mL solution}} \text{(cross-multiply)}$$

$100x = 1.25$ mL (Divide both sides of the equation by 100.)

$x = 0.0125$ mL $= 0.0125$ g $= 12.5$ mg of active ingredient

Thus the *amount of active ingredient* can be calculated if the drug concentration is given in either a fractional or a percentage form.

The next two examples deal with calculating the *volume of medication solution* needed to deliver a desired amount of active ingredient. With these types of questions, it is necessary to convert to consistent units, usually converting grams to milligrams.

3. How much 0.5% Proventil would be needed to give a patient 2.5 mg of active ingredient by SVN?

A 0.5% (1:200) drug concentration means that there is 1 part of active ingredient in 200 parts of the solution, or 1 mL or 1 g of active ingredient in 200 mL or 200 g of the solution. This converts to 1000 mg/200 mL. Set up the following proportion:

$$\frac{1000 \text{ mg active ingredient}}{200 \text{ mL total solution}} = \frac{2.5 \text{ mg}}{x \text{ mL solution}} \text{(cross-multiply)}$$

$1000 x = 500$ mL (Divide both sides of the equation by 1000.)

$x = 0.5$ mL of Proventil should be given.

4. How much 4% Xylocaine would be needed to give a patient 100 mg of active ingredient by handheld nebulizer before a bronchoscopy?

A 4% drug concentration means that 4 parts of active ingredient are in 100 parts of the solution, or 4 mL or 4 g of active ingredient in 100 mL or 100 g of the solution. This converts to 4000 mg/100 mL. Set up the following proportion:

$$\frac{4000 \text{ mg active ingredient}}{100 \text{ mL total solution}} = \frac{100 \text{ mg}}{x \text{ mL solution}} \text{(cross-multiply)}$$

$4000x = 10{,}000$ mL (Divide both sides of the equation by 4000.)

$x = 2.5$ mL of Xylocaine should be given.

Thus the *volume of medication* solution needed to deliver a given amount of active ingredient can be calculated if the drug concentration is given in either a fractional or a percentage form.

MODULE D
Respiratory care plan

1. **Analyze the available information to determine the patient's pathophysiologic state (Code: IIIH1) [Difficulty: ELE: R, Ap; WRE: An]**

The respiratory therapist should be able to determine when the patient is having cardiopulmonary problems that could require an inhaled medication. Review, if needed, information presented in Chapters 1, 3, 4, and 5 that deals with bedside assessment, blood gases, pulmonary function tests, and advanced cardiopulmonary monitoring.

2. **Determine the appropriateness of the prescribed respiratory care plan and recommend modifications when indicated**

    a. **Determine the appropriateness of the prescribed therapy and goals for the identified pathophysiologic state (Code: IIIH3) [Difficulty: ELE: R, Ap; WRE: An]**

b. Review the planned therapy to establish the therapeutic plan (Code: IIIH2a) [Difficulty: ELE: R, Ap; WRE: An]

Patients with stable asthma or COPD will often require several inhaled medications including bronchodilators and corticosteroids. The patient with life-threatening status asthmaticus will require multiple treatment procedures. These are likely to include many of the following: admission into the intensive care unit, supplemental oxygen, monitoring of vital signs, electrocardiogram monitoring, serial arterial blood gases, continuous pulse oximetry, periodic bedside spirometry, heliox, intubation, and/or mechanical ventilation. Inhaled medications for this patient can include short-acting beta agonists (SABA) given hourly or continuously and parasympathomimetic medications. Systemic medications will likely include a corticosteroid and antileukotriene agent. Lastly, a theophylline agent may be added. The goal is to resolve the asthmatic crisis. After the patient has been stabilized, long-term care can be planned. This is likely to include long-acting beta agonists (LABA), an inhaled corticosteroid, and other preventative agents. If the patient has a pulmonary infection, the correct antimicrobial drug should be used to treat the problem.

c. Recommend changes in the therapeutic plan when indicated (Code: IIIH4) [Difficulty: ELE: R, Ap; WRE: An]

This chapter discusses medications that can be used to help treat many commonly seen cardiopulmonary conditions. When these medications are used properly for the appropriate patient condition, there is a good chance of recovery. The patient's vital signs and other clinical indicators will improve. The patient will report feeling better.

However, if the patient's signs and symptoms do not indicate improvement, be prepared to recommend a change in the medication. This may involve changing a dose or switching to another medication. Stop any medication to which the patient is having an allergic reaction. Tell the patient's physician about the problem, and ask for further orders.

d. Conduct disease management education programs (Code: IIIK4) [Difficulty: ELE: R, Ap; WRE: An]

The most recent Written Registry Exams have included questions that relate to the management and education of the patient with asthma. It also is recommended that the management and education of a patient with COPD be studied. The bibliography includes information on standard references on these two subjects.

e. Terminate the treatment or procedure based on the patient's response to therapy (Code: IIIF1) [Difficulty: ELE: R, Ap; WRE: An]

As mentioned earlier, Box 9-1 lists the side effects most often seen with adrenergic (sympathomimetic) bronchodilators. The most serious problem is tachycardia. In some cases, patients may have cardiac arrhythmias. A common clinical guideline requests the treatment be discontinued if the patient's heart rate increases by more than 20% during the treatment. The patient should be monitored to confirm that the heart rate slows. Chart the information, and notify the nurse.

> ### Exam Hint 9-8 (ELE, WRE)
>
> Expect to see a question in which the decision has to be made to stop the bronchodilator treatment because the patient's heart rate increases by *more than 20%* from the baseline. For example, stop the treatment in the following situation: The pretreatment heart rate is 100 beats/min and the heart rate during the treatment increases to greater than 120 beats/minute.

f. Recommend discontinuing the treatment or procedure based on the patient's response (Code: IIIG1i) [Difficulty: ELE: R, Ap; WRE: An]

The physician discontinues treatment for one of two reasons. First, the patient has recovered and no longer needs a medication. Some asthma patients may fully recover and not need any medications. However, it is more common to determine the right medications to control the condition so that the patient does not need to use rescue medications. Patients with emphysema or chronic bronchitis (COPD), or both, are likely to always need medications.

Second, the patient has a serious adverse reaction to the medication. As discussed earlier, Box 9-1 lists the adverse reactions to the adrenergic (sympathomimetic) bronchodilators. Repeated episodes of tachycardia or cardiac arrhythmias, or both, could lead to the physician discontinuing their use.

3. Make a recommendation to change the dosage or concentration of an aerosolized medication (Code: IIIG2b) [Difficulty: ELE: R, Ap; WRE: An]

a. Bronchodilators

Make a recommendation to increase the amount of medication if the patient's bronchospasm is not reversed and no adverse side effects are present. Bedside spirometry should be performed regularly to evaluate the patient's peak flow. An increase of at least 15% to 20% is clinically significant. Review the discussion on peak flow, percentage improvement in before and after bronchodilator therapy, and asthma zones that is found in Chapter 4.

Make a recommendation to decrease the amount of medication if the patient is having serious side effects such as tachycardia or palpitations. The current guidelines on the pharmacologic management of asthma list the medications that should be used according to the categorization of the patient's asthmatic condition. All asthmatic patients should have a rescue inhaler that is a short-acting, rapid-onset β-adrenergic bronchodilator. The medications albuterol (Proventil, Ventolin) and levalbuterol (Xopenex) are widely used for quick relief. For chronic persistent asthma, several additional medications are taken for long-term control. These include an inhaled corticosteroid (beclomethasone, triamcinolone), an inhaled long-acting β-adrenergic bronchodilator (salmeterol), and a preventive agent (cromolyn sodium or zafirlukast). Patients with the most severe persistent asthma also require a corticosteroid medication in syrup or pill form and sustained-release theophylline. It is recommended that the National Institutes of Health guidelines and others, as listed in the bibliography, be reviewed for complete information.

Exam Hint 9-9 (ELE, WRE)

A peak flow improvement of 15% to 20% after a bronchodilator treatment shows that the medication is effective. See Chapter 4 to review how to perform the calculation.

b. Mucomyst or saline solutions

Make a recommendation to increase the amount of medication if the patient's secretions are still too thick to cough or suction and if no adverse side effects to the medication exist. Make a recommendation to decrease the amount of medication if the patient's secretions are watery enough for expectoration or suctioning or if side effects to the drug (e.g., bronchospasm) exist.

4. Change the dilution of a medication used in aerosol therapy (ELE code: IIIF2c3) [Difficulty: EL: R, Ap, An]

The various saline solutions and sterile water are known collectively as bland aerosols, because they have no direct pharmacologic effect on the lungs and airways. They are used to increase the volume of liquid in an SVN after the medication has been added. Most of these nebulizers work most efficiently when they hold about 3 to 5 mL of liquid. Usually a normal saline solution (0.9% sodium chloride) is added.

Adding little or no saline to the medication results in the patient inhaling a very concentrated solution or the nebulizer not functioning properly. The nebulizer will aerosolize the medication within a few minutes, and the patient should quickly feel the beneficial effects of the treatment. However, depending on the nature of the medication, the patient might find it to be quite irritating to the airway. Coughing or bronchospasm could result. Side effects (e.g., tachycardia) should be monitored when sympathomimetic agents are administered, because the medication enters the bloodstream so quickly.

If more saline is added, the solution will be less concentrated. The nebulizer will take longer to aerosolize the medication because of the added volume, and relief of symptoms will take longer. However, it will be less likely to irritate the airway. Side effects with sympathomimetic agents could be less severe, because the drug is given over a longer period. However, remember that increasing the amount of saline makes no difference in the total amount of medication in the nebulizer for the patient. Tachycardia or other side effects may still be seen if the total amount of medication is given.

Saline-only aerosol treatments, as for induced sputum, are more effective at higher concentrations of saline. See Box 9-2 for complete information on the saline solutions.

5. Respiratory care protocols

a. Develop the outcomes of respiratory care pharmacology protocols (Code: IIIH6b) [Difficulty: ELE: R, Ap; WRE: An]

b. Apply respiratory care pharmacology protocols to patient care situations (Code: IIIH8) [Difficulty: EL: R, Ap; WRE: An]

Respiratory therapists should be familiar with the widely used respiratory disease and medication protocols.

For example, patients with asthma can be managed as described in the National Asthma Education and Prevention Program, Expert Panel Report II: *Guidelines for the Diagnosis and Management of Asthma*. Patients with emphysema and chronic bronchitis can be managed as described in Global Initiative for Chronic Obstructive Lung Disease (GOLD), Workshop Report: *Global Strategy for the Diagnosis, Management, and Prevention of COPD*. The bibliography lists the complete information on these two and other protocol documents. They are too long to list here.

The therapy guidelines for asthma and COPD rank both conditions in four categories by the severity of the illness, and medications are given based on the severity ranking.

c. Explain planned therapy and goals to the patient in understandable (nonmedical) terms to achieve the best results from the treatment or procedure (Code: IIIA6) [Difficulty: ELE: R, Ap; WRE: An]

d. Monitor the outcomes of respiratory care pharmacology protocols (Code: IIIH7b) [Difficulty: ELE: R, Ap; WRE: An]

Published guidelines list key factors to monitor for patient success. The following are common goals of therapy for the asthma patient:

- Minimal or no chronic symptoms, day or night
- Minimal or no episodes
- No limitations on activities; no school or work missed
- Peak expiratory flow greater than 80% of personal best
- Minimal use of inhaled short-acting β_2-agonist medication (fewer than one per day)
- No or minimal adverse effects from medications

The following are common goals of therapy for the COPD patient:

- Prevent disease progression
- Relieve symptoms (e.g., dyspnea, cough, fatigue)
- Improve exercise tolerance
- Improve health status
- Prevent and treat complications
- Prevent and treat exacerbations
- Reduce mortality

e. Communicate the outcomes of therapy or procedures and change the treatment based on the protocol (Code: IIIA5) [Difficulty: ELE: R, Ap; WRE: An]

Inform the patient's nurse or physician and the supervising therapist if any serious question or problem occurs with the patient. Routine communication should occur as needed between these health care personnel and any other caregiver.

6. Record and evaluate the patient's response to the treatment(s) or procedure(s), including the following:

a. Record and interpret the following: heart rate and rhythm, respiratory rate, blood pressure, body temperature, and pain level (Code: IIIA1b4) [Difficulty: ELE: R, Ap; WRE: An]

With many treatment protocols, the practitioner must count the patient's heart rate before, at least one time during, and after an aerosolized bronchodilator is given because of the risk of tachycardia. It is generally acceptable to count for 30 seconds and multiply by 2 to get a 1-minute count. Record the various heart rates and determine the heart rhythm as the pulse rate is measured. A stethoscope can be used to determine an abnormality. Treatment is usually stopped if the patient's pulse rate increases by more than 20% from the initial level.

b. Record and interpret the patient's breath sounds (Code: IIIA1b3) [Difficulty: ELE: R, Ap; WRE: An]

Listen for a reduction in wheezing after the administration of an aerosolized bronchodilator as proof of an effectively reduced bronchospasm. If the patient was given an aerosolized bronchodilator for bronchospasm, the patient's spirometry results would be expected to change toward more normal values as the bronchospasm is reduced. The two most important bedside spirometry values to monitor are the peak flow and forced expiratory volume in 1 second. Often, a 15% to 20% improvement in either one or both of these parameters after the inhalation of an aerosolized bronchodilator is used as a clinical indication that the medication works, and the patient has reversible bronchospasm. (See Chapter 4 for more specific guidelines.) A patient with stable asthma may be given a drug such as cromolyn sodium (Intal) or nedocromil sodium (Tilade) by inhalation to prevent a future asthma attack. Remember that these drugs are not to be used during an asthma attack.

c. Record and interpret the type of cough the patient has and the nature of the sputum (Code: IIIA1b) [Difficulty: ELE: R, Ap; WRE: An]

Listen for a reduction in airway secretions after a productive cough. The mucolytics should be helpful in making the secretions less thick.

d. Recheck any math work and make note of incorrect data (Code: IIIA1b2) [Difficulty: ELE: R, Ap; WRE: An]

Errors made in charting must be corrected by drawing a single mark through the error and writing the correct information. Some prefer that the error be further clarified by writing "error" or "omit" next to it and adding initials. Never erase or use any covering material over an error.

BIBLIOGRAPHY

AARC Clinical Practice Guideline: Surfactant replacement therapy, *Respir Care* 39(8):824, 1994.

Au JP, Ziment I: Drug therapy and dosage adjustment in asthma, *Respir Care* 31:415, 1986.

Bills GW, Soderberg RC: *Principles of pharmacology for respiratory care*, ed 2, Albany, NY, 1998, Delmar.

Canadian Asthma Consensus Guidelines, 2003 and Canadian Pediatric Asthma Concensus Guidelines, 2003. CMAJ 2005; 173 (6 Suppl): S1-S56.

Carter C, Solberg C: Respiratory pharmacology. In Hess DR, MacIntyre NR, Mishoe SC, et al, editors: *Respiratory care: principles and practices*, Philadelphia, 2002, WB Saunders.

Colbert BJ, Mason BJ: *Cardiopulmonary drug guide*, Upper Saddle River, NJ, 2003, Prentice Hall.

Colbert BJ, Mason BJ: *Integrated cardiopulmonary pharmacology*, ed 2, Upper Saddle River, NJ, 2008, Prentice Hall.

Colice GL: New drugs for asthma. *Respir Care* 53(6):688, 2008.

Cottrell GP, Surkin HB: *Pharmacology for respiratory care practitioners*, Philadelphia, 1995, FA Davis.

Donohue JF: Safety and efficacy of B agonists. *Respir Care* 53(5):618, 2008.

Gardenhire DS: *Rau's Respiratory care pharmacology*, ed 7, St Louis, 2008, Mosby.

Gardenhire DS: Airway pharmacology. In Wilkins RL, Stoller JK, Kacmarek RM, editors: *Egan's fundamentals of respiratory care*, ed 9, St Louis, 2009, Mosby.

Geller DE: Aerosol antibiotics in cystic fibrosis. *Respir Care* 54(5): 658, 2009.

Global Initiative for Chronic Obstructive Lung Disease (GOLD): *Workshop report: global strategy for the diagnosis, management, and prevention of COPD*, Bethesda, MD, 2000, National Heart, Lung, and Blood Institute and the World Health Organization.

Global strategy for asthma management and prevention (updated 2006): global initiative for asthma (GINA). http:www.ginasthma.org

Hill F: *Delmar's respiratory care drug reference*. Albany, NY, 1999, Delmar.

Howder CL: *Cardiopulmonary pharmacology: a handbook for respiratory practitioners and other allied health personnel*, ed 2, Baltimore, 1996, Williams & Wilkins.

Levine SR, McLaughlin AJ: *Pharmacology in respiratory care*, New York, 2001, McGraw-Hill.

Malmeister M: Pharmacology associated with respiratory care. In Fink JB, Hunt GE, editors: *Clinical practice in respiratory care*, Philadelphia, 1999, Lippincott-Raven.

Myers TR: Guidelines for asthma management: a review and comparison of 5 current guidelines. *Respir Care* 53(6):751, 2008.

McLaughlin AJ, Levine SR: *Respiratory care drug reference*, Gaithersburg, Md, 1997, Aspen.

National Asthma Education and Prevention Program, Expert Panel Report II: *Guidelines for the diagnosis and management of asthma*, Bethesda, Md, 1997, National Institutes of Health.

National Asthma Education and Prevention Program, Expert Panel Report II: *Guidelines for the diagnosis and management of asthma—update on selected topics 2002*, Bethesda, Md, June 2003, National Institutes of Health, Pub. No. 02-5074, Bethesda, Md, 1997, NIH.

National Institutes of Health: *Practical guide for the diagnosis and management of asthma*, Pub. No. 97-4053, Bethesda, Md, 1997, NIH.

Op't Hold TB: Inhaled beta agonists. *Respir Care* 52(7):820, 2007.

Physicians' desk reference, ed 60, Montvale, NJ, 2003, Thomson PDR.

Restropo RD: Use of inhaled anticholinergic agents in obstructive lung disease. *Respir Care* 52(7):833, 2007.

Rubin BK: Mucolytics, expectorants, and mucokinetic medications. *Respir Care* 52(7):859, 2007.

Sobande PO, Kercsmar CM: Inhaled cortiosteroids in asthma management. *Respir Care* 53(5):625, 2008.

Tashkin DP: Dosing strategies for bronchodilator aerosol delivery, *Respir Care* 36:977, 1991.

Witek TJ, Schachter EN: *Pharmacology and therapeutics in respiratory care*, Philadelphia, 1994, WB Saunders.

Ziment I: Drugs used in respiratory care. In Burton GG, Hodgkin JE, Ward JJ, editors: *Respiratory care: a guide to clinical practice*, ed 4, Philadelphia, 1997, Lippincott-Raven.

SELF-STUDY QUESTIONS FOR THE ENTRY LEVEL EXAM

See page 590 for answers

1. A patient with a fluid overload problem has been given a dose of furosemide (Lasix) intravenously. Following rapid diuresis in the patient, you note an arrhythmia that did not exist before the medication was given. What would you recommend?
   A. Check the patient's potassium level.
   B. Give more furosemide.
   C. Defibrillate the patient's heart.
   D. Give the patient epinephrine to reverse the allergic reaction to furosemide.

2. A 2-month-old infant has periods of apnea that result in bradycardia and cyanosis. What medication should be recommended to treat the apnea periods?
   A. Lidocaine (Xylocaine)
   B. Neostigmine (Prostigmin)
   C. Caffeine citrate (Cafcit)
   D. Isoetharine (Isoetharine HCl)

3. You are working in the emergency department when an automobile crash victim arrives by ambulance. She is conscious, screaming, and hysterical from the extreme pain of a broken lower leg. What would you recommend for sedation?
   A. Morphine sulfate (Duramorph)
   B. Ibuprofen (Advil)
   C. Succinylcholine chloride (Anectine)
   D. Ipratropium bromide (Atrovent)

4. An asthma patient is discontinuing her systemic corticosteroid. She will continue taking her aerosolized bronchodilator. The physician wants to know what you would recommend for an inhaled corticosteroid.
   A. Naloxone (Narcan)
   B. Neostigmine bromide (Prostigmin)
   C. Beclomethasone dipropionate (QVAR)
   D. Methylprednisolone (Solu-Medrol)

5. Results of your patient's pulmonary function tests show that the peak expiratory flow rate increased the most when she inhaled an aerosolized sympathomimetic drug and an aerosolized parasympatholytic

drug. The physician wants to know what you would recommend for this patient.

    A. Beclomethasone dipropionate (Vanceril) and montelukast (Singulair)
    B. Ipratropium and albuterol (Combivent)
    C. Ipratropium bromide (Atrovent) and cromolyn sodium (Intal)
    D. Salmeterol and fluticasone (Advair)

6. Your patient was extubated 30 min ago. She is hoarse and complains of "tightness in my throat"; inspiratory stridor can be heard. The drug of choice for treating this problem is

    A. Racemic epinephrine (microNefrin)
    B. Acetylcysteine (Mucomyst)
    C. Levalbuterol (Xopenex)
    D. Isoetharine (Isoetharine HCl)

7. Your patient with COPD is coughing very hard to bring up viscous, thick mucus with plugs. What drug of choice would you recommend to treat this problem?

    A. Dopamine hydrochloride (Intropin)
    B. Acetylcysteine (Mucomyst)
    C. Cromolyn sodium (Intal)
    D. Dornase alfa (Pulmozyme)

8. You receive an order to administer 5 mL of albuterol (Proventil) by handheld nebulizer. You would proceed to

    A. Confirm that the order was written and give the treatment
    B. Have the shift supervisor give the treatment
    C. Call the physician to check on the medication dose
    D. Give 0.5 mL of medication because the physician probably intended that dosage

9. You are working with a 10-year-old cystic fibrosis patient with a pulmonary infection and thick secretions. What would you recommend to help him cough out the secretions?

    A. Nebulized 0.9% (normal) saline solution
    B. Instillation of acetylcysteine (Mucomyst) into his lungs
    C. Nebulized dornase alfa (Pulmozyme)
    D. Nebulized acetylcysteine (Mucomyst)

10. How much active ingredient would be found in 0.6 mL of 2.25% racemic epinephrine (microNefrin)?

    A. 26,700 mg
    B. 0.0267 mg
    C. 13.5 g
    D. 13.5 mg

11. You are administering an aerosolized bronchodilator to your patient. Her pretreatment pulse rate was 85 beats/min. You would stop the treatment if her pulse reached

    A. 90 beats/min
    B. 100 beats/min
    C. 110 beats/min
    D. 120 beats/min

12. Your patient is being given an aerosolized adrenergic (sympathomimetic) drug for the first time. For what possible adverse effects of the medication should you monitor?

    1. Bradycardia
    2. Tremor
    3. Headache
    4. Nervousness and irritability
    5. Tachycardia
    A. 1, 2
    B. 3, 4, 5
    C. 2, 3, 4, 5
    D. 2, 4

13. Your patient is being discharged and will receive aerosolized controller-type bronchodilator therapy at home. The best medication for this chronically sick but stable patient is

    A. Arformoterol (Brovana)
    B. Metaproterenol (Alupent)
    C. Levalbuterol (Xopenex)
    D. Albuterol (Ventolin)

14. Your patient has an order for an induced sputum sample to be analyzed for tuberculosis. The best medication for this is

    A. Dornase alfa (Pulmozyme)
    B. 10% saline solution
    C. 0.9% saline solution
    D. 0.45% saline solution

15. After finishing an aerosolized dose of acetylcysteine (Mucomyst), a patient has breath sounds that reveal wheezing. These were not present at the start of treatment. What medication should be given before the next Mucomyst treatment to prevent bronchospasm?

    A. Levalbuterol (Xopenex)
    B. Sterile water
    C. Salmeterol (Serevent)
    D. 0.9% saline solution

16. You are working the night shift when a 17-year-old patient with status asthmaticus is admitted through the emergency department. She has already been given albuterol (Proventil), Combivent, and an inhaled corticosteroid medication. She has significant tachycardia. The intern on-call asks for your recommendation on what additional medication to give the patient. You would recommend

    A. Formoterol (Foradil)
    B. Terbutaline (Brethaire)
    C. Albuterol (Proventil)
    D. Theophylline ethylenediamine (aminophylline)

17. A 16-year-old patient has severe and chronic asthma. Her physician wishes to change her medications to prevent her from having asthma attacks. All of the following medications would be helpful EXCEPT

A. Zileuton (Zyflo)

B. Pirbuterol (Maxair)

C. Cromolyn sodium (Intal)

D. Zafirlukast (Accolate)

18. Your patient with COPD is being given a new inhaled adrenergic bronchodilator medication by small volume nebulizer. Within 3 min, he complains of palpitations. His pulse rate was 85 beats/minute before the treatment and is now 125 beats/minute. What should you do?

 A. Change to a different medication for the next treatment.

 B. Discontinue the order.

 C. Stop the treatment and monitor the patient.

 D. Add more saline to dilute the medication for the next ordered treatment.

19. You have finished giving your 8-year-old patient with asthma an IPPB treatment with 0.5 mL of albuterol (Proventil). You notice that her heart rate has increased 15% from before the treatment. Her breath sounds are now clear. What would you recommend to the physician for your patient's next treatment?

 A. Give her 0.5 mL of metaproterenol (Alupent).

 B. Discontinue her treatments altogether.

 C. Add more normal saline to the Proventil.

 D. Decrease the Proventil to 0.3 mL.

20. You are called to the recovery room to assist in the care of a patient who returned 2 hr ago from having a bowel resection. The patient is apneic and on a mechanical ventilator. Which medication(s) could be used to wean her from the machine?

 1. Flumazenil (Romazicon)

 2. Naloxone (Narcan)

 3. Dopamine (Intropin)

 4. Succinylcholine chloride (Anectine)

5. Diazepam (Valium)

 A. 1, 4

 B. 5

 C. 2, 3

 D. 1, 2

21. How much metaproterenol (Alupent) is needed to give the patient 20 mg of the active ingredient? Alupent contains 5% active ingredient.

 A. 1 mL

 B. 0.4 mL

 C. 40 mL

 D. 0.1 mL

22. An anxious 10-year-old asthma patient is being given a breathing treatment with levalbuterol (Xopenex). His initial heart rate of 110 breaths/minute has now increased to 120 breaths/minute. What should you do?

 A. Continue the treatment.

 B. Stop the treatment.

 C. Change to albuterol and continue the treatment.

 D. Cut the medication dose in half and continue.

23. The preliminary laboratory results of a sputum sample that was sent from your patient indicate that she has a gram-positive pulmonary infection. Which of the following medications would you recommend?

 A. Ribavirin (Virazole)

 B. Penicillin (Ampicillin)

 C. Tobramycin (TOBI)

 D. Gentamycin (Garamycin)

24. An 18-month-old infant is diagnosed with bronchiolitis from RSV. Which medication would you recommend?

 A. Ribavirin (Virazole)

 B. Pentamidine isethionate (NebuPent)

 C. Gentamycin (Garamycin)

 D. Trimethoprim and sulfamethoxazole (Bactrim)

SELF-STUDY QUESTIONS FOR THE WRITTEN REGISTRY EXAM

See page 615 for answers

1. You are called to help assess a premature neonate. The patient is having difficulty breathing, and respiratory distress syndrome is suspected. You would recommend all of the following except

 A. Flumazenil (Romazicon)

 B. Beractant (Survanta)

 C. Calfactant (Infasurf)

 D. Poractant alfa (Curosurf)

2. A 20-year-old asthmatic patient has received a standard dose of levalbuterol (Xopenex). Breath sounds reveal loud, bilateral wheezes. Over the course of the treatment, her heart rate changed from 98 to 105 beats/minute. What would you recommend?

 A. Stop the treatment and notify the physician.

 B. Repeat the treatment and monitor the patient.

 C. Switch the medication to albuterol (Ventolin).

 D. Add theophylline (aminophylline) to the intravenous line.

3. A 10-year-old patient with status asthmaticus has been admitted to the hospital. The physician plans to start her on continuous nebulization of a fast-onset "rescue" inhaled bronchodilator medication. Which of the following would you recommend as part of her care plan?

 1. Admit her to the intensive care unit.

 2. Admit her to the pediatrics floor.

 3. She should be given salmeterol (Serevent).

 4. She should be given levalbuterol (Xopenex).

 5. ECG and pulse oximeter monitoring should be done.

 6. She should be given an intravenous corticosteroid.

A. 2, 4, 6
B. 1, 2, 5, 6
C. 2, 4, 6
D. 1, 4, 5, 6

4. A mechanically ventilated patient who has been paralyzed with a neuromuscular blocking agent should be given a sedative agent for what reason?
   A. To sustain the paralysis
   B. To control pain
   C. To keep the patient synchronized with the ventilator
   D. To relieve the patient's anxiety

5. A patient had a bronchoscopy procedure and biopsy taken of a suspected lung tumor. After the biopsy, uncontrolled bleeding occurs. What should be given to control the bleeding?
   A. Instill epinephrine through the bronchoscope at the site of the bleeding.
   B. Administer heparin by intravenous line.
   C. Administer nebulized albuterol (Proventil) by small volume nebulizer.
   D. Administer lidocaine (Xylocaine) by an intravenous line.

6. Your 15-year-old patient with cystic fibrosis has large amounts of thick secretions. No sign of infection is present. What should be administered to help manage the secretion problem?
   A. Salmeterol (Serevent)
   B. 5% saline
   C. Normal (0.9%) saline
   D. Acetylcysteine (Mucomyst)

7. A home care patient with asthma has finished her standard dose of 0.25 mL of albuterol (Ventolin). After waiting 15 minutes, she performs a peak flow measurement, which shows 65% of her personal best. What should be done to improve the patient's condition?
   A. Decrease the dose of albuterol.
   B. Add an intravenous corticosteroid to the patient's medications.
   C. Maintain the present therapy.
   D. Increase the dose of albuterol.

8. A 55-year-old patient with chronic bronchitis and a pulmonary infection has many thick secretions. What should be given to help manage the secretion problem?
   A. Nebulized acetylcysteine (Mucomyst)
   B. Intravenous fluticasone (Flovent)
   C. Nebulized dornase alfa (Pulmozyme)
   D. Intravenous flumazenil (Romazicon)

9. An adult patient is panicking and fighting against the mechanical ventilator. All of the following may be used to control the patient on the ventilator EXCEPT
   A. Flumazenil (Romazicon)
   B. Pancuronium bromide (Pavulon)
   C. Succinylcholine (Anectine)
   D. Morphine sulfate (Duramorph)

10. A patient is in shock from an allergic reaction to a bee sting. In addition, she has inspiratory stridor from laryngeal edema. What is the best medication to use to help raise her blood pressure and help her breathing?
    A. Intravenous epinephrine (Adrenalin)
    B. Oral ibuprofen (Advil)
    C. Nebulized racemic epinephrine (MicroNefrin)
    D. Intravenous naloxone (Narcan)

11. A 10-year-old boy with cystic fibrosis has been having recurrent episodes of *Pseudomonas aeruginosa* pneumonia. What should be recommended to prevent further episodes?
    A. Instill pentamidine (Pentam) into the trachea by way of a suction catheter.
    B. Administer pentamidine (NebuPent) once a month by small volume nebulizer.
    C. Isonicotinic acid hydrazide (Isoniazid) should be taken twice a week for 6 months.
    D. Tobramycin (TOBI) should be taken by SVN every other month.

12. A 4-month-old pediatric patient has chronic lung disease secondary to recovering from infant respiratory distress syndrome (RDS). The patient now has pneumonia caused by respiratory syncytial virus and is on a mechanical ventilator. What can be given to improve the patient's condition?
    A. Intravenous racemic epinephrine (microNefrin)
    B. Ribavirin (Vibrazole) by SPAG II nebulizer
    C. Intratracheal beractant (Survanta)
    D. Cromolyn sodium (Intal) by small volume nebulizer

13. A 35-year-old patient has AIDS and was previously treated for *Pneumocystis carinii* pneumonia. What can be used to prevent the infection from reoccurring?
    A. Trimethoprim and sulfamethoxazole (Bactrim) by pill
    B. Pentamidine (NebuPent) by small volume nebulizer
    C. Tobramycin (TOBI) by small volume inhaler
    D. Zanamivir (Relenza) by metered dose inhaler

14. A 58-year-old patient with congestive heart failure is being treated with 40% oxygen and diuretics. Within 3 hours she has lost 1500 mL of urine and her pulse oximeter reading has improved from 84% to 90% saturation. Her electrocardiogram shows a heart rate of 110 beats/min with the new observation of premature ventricular contractions (PVCs). Her recent serum electrolyte values are within the normal range except for the potassium level of 3.4 mEq/L. What recommendation could be made in her care?
    A. Give her intravenous potassium.
    B. Decrease her oxygen to 35%.
    C. Continue her diuretic medications.
    D. Restrict her intake of potassium.

10 Bronchopulmonary Hygiene Therapy

Note 1: This book is written to cover every item listed as testable on the *Entry Level Examination (ELE), Written Registry Examination (WRE)*, and *Clinical Simulation Examination (CSE)*.

The listed code for each item is taken from the National Board for Respiratory Care's (NBRC) **Summary Content Outline for CRT (Certified Respiratory Therapist) and Written RRT (Registered Respiratory Therapist) Examinations** (http://evolve.elsevier.com/Sills/resptherapist/). For example, if an item is testable on both the ELE and the WRE, it will simply be shown as: (Code: . . .). If an item is only testable on the ELE, it will be shown as: (ELE code: . . .). If an item is only testable on the WRE, it will be shown as: (WRE code: . . .).

Following each item's code will be the difficulty level of the questions on that item on the ELE and WRE. (See the Introduction for a full explanation of the three question difficulty levels.) **Recall [R]** level questions typically expect the exam taker to recall factual information. **Application [Ap]** level questions are harder because the exam taker may have to apply factual information to a clinical situation. **Analysis [An]** level questions are the most challenging because the exam taker may have to use critical thinking to evaluate patient data to make a clinical decision.

Note 2: A review of the most recent Entry Level Examinations (ELE) has shown an average of 3 questions (out of 140), or 2% of the exam, will cover bronchopulmonary hygiene therapy. A review of the most recent Written Registry Examinations (WRE) has shown an average of 3 questions (out of 100), or 3% of the exam, will cover bronchopulmonary hygiene therapy. The Clinical Simulation Examination is comprehensive and may include everything that should be known by an advanced level respiratory therapist.

MODULE A
Bronchopulmonary hygiene therapy

The phrase bronchopulmonary hygiene is preferred by the NBRC to encompass the following cluster of related therapeutic activities: postural drainage, percussion, vibration, and directed cough. Traditionally, the phrase chest physical therapy (CPT) is used by many practitioners to include the same activities. Additionally, the terms postural drainage therapy (PDT), chest physiotherapy, and bronchopulmonary drainage have been used to describe the same therapeutic procedures.

1. **Recommend starting bronchopulmonary hygiene procedures (Code: IIIG1a) [Difficulty: ELE: R, Ap; WRE: An]**

2. **Instruct and encourage bronchopulmonary hygiene techniques (Code: IIIC4) [Difficulty: ELE: R, Ap; WRE: An]**

The directed cough is one of the simplest, yet most important bronchopulmonary hygiene procedures to teach a patient with retained secretions. Ideally, the surgical patient is taught proper coughing techniques before surgery. If not, it is necessary to teach the patient postoperatively:

1. Minimize traction or tension on the incision, to decrease the pain, by placing either your hands or the patient's hands on both sides of the incision. A pillow also can be held against the incision by the practitioner or patient.
2. Instruct the patient to breathe two or three times in through the nose and out through the mouth.
3. Instruct the patient to take in as deep a breath as possible and to perform a normal cough.
4. If the patient cannot cough normally because of pain, a serial or huff cough can be performed.

Teach the patient with chronic obstructive pulmonary disease the following cough techniques:

1. Avoid an ineffective, shallow, hacking cough.
2. Position the patient in a sitting position, bent slightly forward, with feet on the floor or supported. The patient who must lie in bed can be positioned on the preferred side with the legs flexed at the knees and hips.
3. Instruct the patient to perform a mid-inspiratory cough (also called a huff cough):
   a. Breathe two or three times in through the nose and out through the mouth.
   b. Breathe in to a comfortable volume larger than the tidal volume but not as deeply as possible.
   c. Briefly hold the breath.
   d. Cough hard or perform a serial cough at relatively low flows. This should help to raise secretions without causing airway collapse.
   e. Squeezing the knees and thighs together at the instant of coughing helps to increase the airflow and volume.

Coaching is important because patients in pain or suffering from chronic lung disease tend to be uncooperative and do not try hard. Give positive reinforcement when the patient does well. Correct any problems the patient is having following the instructions. Demonstrations are often useful so that the patient can copy a good example.

If the patient cannot cough effectively, other secretion clearance procedures will be needed. Postural drainage therapy (PDT) and other procedures follow. The American Association for Respiratory Care (AARC) *Clinical Practice Guideline* on PDT was used to help develop the following information. See Box 10-1 for indications for turning, postural drainage, percussion, and vibration. Contraindications are listed in Box 10-2, and recommended actions for problems are listed in Box 10-3. Beyond the patient assessment issues listed in Box 10-4, the following should be evaluated to determine whether PDT is needed:

- PDT is not indicated if an optimally hydrated patient is producing less than 25 mL of secretions per day with the procedure.
- A dehydrated patient should have apparently ineffective PDT continued for at least 24 hours after the patient is rehydrated. The combination of rehydration and PDT may help to mobilize previously thick secretions.
- PDT is not indicated in a patient producing more than 30 mL of secretions daily (if the PDT treatments do not increase the sputum production) because the patient is already able to expectorate the sputum effectively.

3. Perform postural drainage (Code: IIIC1a) [Difficulty: ELE: R, Ap; WRE: An]

Turning involves rotating the patient's body in the longitudinal (head-to-toe) axis to promote unilateral or bilateral lung expansion. Patients can be turned from the back to one side, side to side, or one side to back to other side, depending on their needs. The bed may be moved to any head-up or head-down position, as the patient needs and tolerates. Patients should be turned every 1 to 2 hours as tolerated. The patient can turn himself or herself, be turned by a caregiver, or be placed in a bed that is motorized and programmed to change positions in a set pattern.

Postural drainage (bronchopulmonary drainage) is performed to clear secretions or prevent the accumulation of secretions. The patient is positioned so that the bronchus of a particular segment is as vertical as possible. Gravity pulls the secretions toward a major bronchus or the trachea; the secretions are then either expectorated or suctioned. The anatomy of the pulmonary lobes with their segments and respective bronchi should be reviewed (Figure 10-1).

Note that each segment and its bronchus adjoin the right or left mainstem bronchus at a particular angle. This

---

BOX 10-1   Indications for Turning, Postural Drainage, and Percussion and Vibration

TURNING
- Patient unable to change his or her body position (e.g., the patient has a cerebral injury or neuromuscular disease, is being mechanically ventilated, or has been medicated to cause sedation or paralysis)
- Atelectasis or the potential for its development
- Hypoxemia associated with a particular position; if one-sided lung disease is present, the patient is typically turned so that the affected lung is superior
- Patient with an artificial airway

POSTURAL DRAINAGE
- Mobilize retained secretions so that they can be coughed or suctioned; patient has difficulty expectorating secretions but produces more than 25 to 30 mL/day; evidence or indications that a patient with an artificial airway has retained secretions
- Atelectasis that is known or is believed to be caused by a mucous plug
- Patient diagnosed with cystic fibrosis, bronchiectasis, or cavitating lung disease
- Foreign body in an airway
- Removal of aspirated foreign body or stomach contents

PERCUSSION AND VIBRATION
- Patient receiving postural drainage who has a large volume of thick sputum; this suggests that external manipulation of the thorax would assist gravity in its movement toward a more central airway

Based on information found in American Association for Respiratory Care: Clinical practice guideline: postural drainage therapy, *Respir Care* 36:1418, 1991.

---

critical angle determines the positioning that must be used to drain the various segments. Obviously, positioning the patient incorrectly does nothing to drain the desired segment. Auscultation, palpation, and percussion of the chest should lead the practitioner to know where the secretions are located.

Individual segments should be drained when the physician's order specifies them or when the practitioner determines that secretions are present. Individual segments are generally drained for 3 to 15 minutes. Drainage may be provided for a longer period in special situations. Postural drainage and the external manipulation of the patient's thorax (percussion and vibration) can be very strenuous or contraindicated in some patients. Watch for hypoxemia or an increase in dyspnea. If the patient normally is being administered supplemental O_2, it should be continued while in the drainage positions. Some patients need supplemental O_2 only when in certain positions, and it must be made available to them.

BOX 10-2 Contraindications for Turning/Postural Drainage and Percussion and Vibration

TURNING/POSTURAL DRAINAGE*

All positions are contraindicated for patients with the following:

1. Unstabilized head or neck injury, or both (absolute)
2. Active hemorrhage and hemodynamic instability (absolute)
3. ICP† greater than 20 mm Hg
4. Recent spinal surgery, such as a laminectomy, or acute spinal injury
5. Active hemoptysis
6. Empyema
7. Bronchopleural fistula
8. Pulmonary edema as a result of congestive heart failure
9. Large pleural effusions
10. Advanced age, anxiety, or confusion and intolerance of position changes
11. Fractured rib(s) with or without flail chest
12. Healing tissue or surgical wound

   Trendelenburg position is contraindicated in patients with the following:

1. ICP greater than 20 mm Hg
2. Sensitivity to increased ICP (e.g., neurosurgery, cerebral aneurysms, eye surgery)
3. Uncontrolled hypertension
4. Distended abdomen
5. Esophageal surgery
6. Recent gross hemoptysis (especially if associated with lung cancer that was recently treated surgically or by radiation therapy)
7. Uncontrolled airway if at risk for aspiration (recent meal or tube feeding); many authors consider < 1 hour after eating as a contraindication

Reverse Trendelenburg position is contraindicated in patients who are:

1. Hypotensive
2. Receiving a vasoactive medication

PERCUSSION AND VIBRATION

1. All of the previously listed contraindications
2. Subcutaneous emphysema (several authors list an untreated pneumothorax as an absolute contraindication)
3. Spinal anesthesia or recent epidural spinal infusion for pain control
4. Recent thoracic skin grafts or skin flaps
5. Thoracic burns, open wounds, or skin infections
6. Recently placed transvenous or subcutaneous pacemaker (especially true if a mechanical percussor/vibrator is to be used)
7. Suspicion of pulmonary tuberculosis
8. Lung contusion
9. Bronchospasm
10. Osteomyelitis of the ribs
11. Osteoporosis
12. Clotting disorder (coagulopathy)
13. Complaints of chest wall pain

   In addition, a number of authors have listed the following as contraindications to percussion and vibration:

1. Not over bare skin
2. Not over buttons, zippers, folded clothes, or seams of clothing
3. Not over female breast tissue
4. Not over the spine, sternum, or kidneys
5. Not over an area with a known lung tumor

Based on information found in American Association for Respiratory Care: Clinical practice guideline: postural drainage therapy, *Respir Care* 36:1418, 1991.

*These are relative contraindications except those marked as absolute.

ICP, intracranial pressure.

Coughing should be encouraged after each segment is drained. The patient should not cough in a head-down position, however, because of the risk of increased intracranial pressure. Have the patient sit up to cough vigorously.

a. Pulmonary drainage positions

1. Lower lobes

a. Posterior basal segment (Figure 10-2)

1. The patient lies face down on the bed. A pillow is placed beneath the hips.
2. The foot of the bed is elevated 18 inches or 30 degrees.
3. If ordered, perform percussion or vibration over the lower ribs near the spine on either or both sides, depending on whether one or both segments are to be drained. Note the shaded areas in Figure 10-2.

b. Lateral basal segment (Figure 10-3)

1. The patient is shown in a position to drain the right lateral basal segment. The left lateral basal segment would be drained by placing the patient in the same position on the opposite side.
2. The patient lies one-fourth turn up from the face-down position. A pillow may be placed in front of the patient for support or between the knees for comfort.
3. The foot of the bed is elevated 18 inches or 30 degrees.
4. If ordered, percussion or vibration would be performed over the posterolateral areas of the lower ribs. See the shaded areas in Figure 10-3.

c. Anterior basal segment (Figure 10-4)

1. The patient is shown in a position to drain the left anterior basal segment. (NOTE: This combined

---

BOX 10-3 Hazards/Complications, with Recommended Actions, and Limitations of Postural Drainage and Percussion and Vibration

HAZARDS/COMPLICATIONS

- *Hypoxemia.* The patient known to be hypoxic or prone to hypoxemia during the procedure should be given a higher inspired O_2 percentage. Administer 100% O_2 to any patient who becomes hypoxic during the procedure. Stop the treatment, return the patient to the original resting position, make sure ventilation is adequate, and consult with the physician before continuing.
- *Increased intracranial pressure or acute hypotension during the procedure.* If either of these complications occurs, stop the treatment, return the patient to the original resting position, and consult with the physician before continuing.
- *Pulmonary hemorrhage.* If this occurs, stop the treatment, return the patient to the original resting position, and call the physician immediately. Give the patient supplemental O_2 and keep an open airway until the physician responds.
- *Pain or injury to the patient's muscles, ribs, or spine.* Stop the therapy that appears to be causing the problem. Carefully move the patient to a more comfortable position, and call the physician before continuing.

- *Vomiting and aspiration.* Stop the treatment, apply suction as needed to clear the airway, give supplemental O_2, maintain a patent airway, return the patient to the original resting position, and call the physician immediately.
- *Bronchospasm.* If this develops, stop the treatment, return the patient to the original resting position, and give or increase the supplemental O_2 while calling the physician. Give the patient any aerosolized bronchodilators that the physician orders.
- *Arrhythmias.* If this occurs, stop the treatment, return the patient to the original resting position, and give or increase supplemental O_2 while calling the physician.

LIMITATIONS

- Be careful to give postural drainage therapy only to those patients who would benefit from it. Do not rely on past experiences with other patients when you judge current situations.
- Patients with ineffective coughs may be unable to clear their airways as well as desired.
- Critically ill patients are difficult to position optimally.

Based on information found in American Association for Respiratory Care: Clinical practice guideline: postural drainage therapy, *Respir Care* 36:1418, 1991.

BOX 10-4 Assessment of the Patient's Needs for Postural Drainage Therapy (PDT)*

Excessive production of sputum
Ineffectiveness of cough
Patient history of PDT that was helpful in treating past problem (e.g., bronchiectasis, cystic fibrosis, lung abscess)
Abnormal breath sounds (e.g., decreased breath sounds, crackles, or rhonchi, suggesting airway secretions)
Change in the patient's vital signs
Abnormal chest radiograph finding consistent with infiltrates, atelectasis, or mucous plug

---

Based on information found in American Association for Respiratory Care: Clinical practice guideline: postural drainage therapy, *Respir Care* 36:1418, 1991.
*These problems should be assessed together to evaluate the patient's need for PDT. Not all patients experience all of these problems. The seriousness of these problems should be assessed by the clinician in determining which patients will benefit from PDT.

segment is the anatomic equivalent of the medial basal segment and anterior basal segment of the right lung.) The right anterior basal and medial basal segments would be drained by placing the patient in the same position on the opposite side.

2. The patient lies straight up on his or her side. Pillows may be used in front or behind the patient (or both) for positioning or between the knees for comfort.

3. The foot of the bed is elevated 18 inches or 30 degrees.
4. If ordered, percussion or vibration would be performed over the lower ribs below the axilla. See the shaded areas in Figure 10-4.

d. Superior segment (Figure 10-5)
1. The patient lies face down on the bed. A pillow is placed beneath the hips.
2. The bed is flat.
3. If ordered, percussion or vibration would be performed over the middle of the back below the scapula on either or both sides of the spine, depending on whether one or both segments are to be drained. See the shaded areas in Figure 10-5.

2. Right middle lobe and left lingula

a. Right lateral and medial segments (Figure 10-6)
1. The same position is used to drain both segments.
2. The patient lies one-fourth turn up from the back-down position. A pillow may be placed in back of the patient for support or between the flexed knees for comfort.
3. The foot of the bed is elevated 14 inches or 15 degrees.
4. If ordered, percussion or vibration would be performed below the right nipple area in a male patient. See the shaded area in Figure 10-6. Percussion and vibration may not be possible on a female patient.

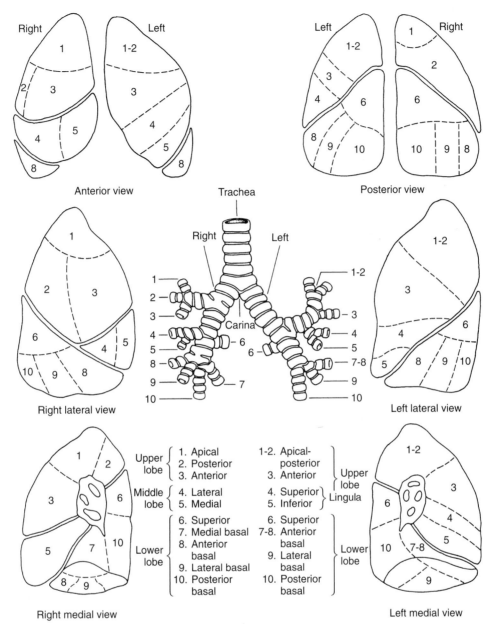

Figure 10-1 Names and locations of the lung segments and their respective bronchi. *(From Shibel EM, Moser KM, editors:* Respiratory emergencies, *St Louis, 1977, Mosby.)*

b. Left superior and inferior lingula segments (Figure 10-7)

1. The same position is used to drain both segments.
2. The patient lies one-fourth turn up from the back-down position. A pillow may be placed in back of the patient for support or between the flexed knees for comfort.
3. The foot of the bed is elevated 14 inches or 15 degrees.
4. If ordered, percussion or vibration would be performed below the left nipple area in a male patient. See the shaded area in Fig. 10-7. Percussion

and vibration may not be possible on a female patient.

3. Upper lobes

a. Posterior segment (Figure 10-8)

1. The patient leans forward 30 degrees. This can be over the back of a chair (as shown in Figure 10-8) or in bed. A pillow can be used to lean against or support the chest.
2. If ordered, percussion or vibration would be performed over the upper portion of the back on either or both sides of the spine, depending on whether

Figure 10-2 Drainage position for the posterior basal segments of both lower lobes. *(From Eubanks DH, Bone RC: Comprehensive respiratory care, ed 2, St Louis, 1990, Mosby.)*

Figure 10-4 Drainage position for the anterior basal segment of the left lower lobe. The same segment in the right lung would be drained by positioning the patient similarly on the left side. *(From Eubanks DH, Bone RC: Comprehensive respiratory care, ed 2, St Louis, 1990, Mosby.)*

Figure 10-3 Drainage position for the lateral basal segment of the right lower lobe. The same segment in the left lung would be drained by positioning the patient similarly on the right side. *(From Eubanks DH, Bone RC: Comprehensive respiratory care, ed 2, St Louis, 1990, Mosby.)*

Figure 10-5 Drainage position for the superior segments of both lower lobes. *(From Eubanks DH, Bone RC: Comprehensive respiratory care, ed 2, St Louis, 1990, Mosby.)*

one or both segments are being drained. See the shaded areas in Figure 10-8.

b. Apical segment (Figure 10-9)
1. The patient leans backward 30 degrees. This can be done in bed (as shown in Figure 10-9) or in a chair. A pillow can be leaned against to support the lower portion of the back.
2. If ordered, percussion or vibration would be performed between the clavicle and the top of the scapula on either or both sides, depending on

whether one or both segments are being drained. See the shaded areas in Figure 10-9.

c. Anterior segment (Figure 10-10)
1. The patient lies supine in bed with a pillow placed under the knees. This enables the abdominal muscles to relax so that the patient can breathe more easily.
2. If ordered, percussion or vibration would be performed between the clavicle and the nipple of a male patient on either or both sides, depending on whether one or both segments are being drained.

Figure 10-6 Drainage position for the lateral and medial segments of the right middle lobe. *(From Eubanks DH, Bone RC: Comprehensive respiratory care, ed 2, St Louis, 1990, Mosby.)*

Figure 10-8 Drainage position for the posterior segments of both upper lobes. *(From Eubanks DH, Bone RC: Comprehensive respiratory care, ed 2, St Louis, 1990, Mosby.)*

Figure 10-7 Drainage position for the superior and inferior segments of the lingula. *(From Eubanks DH, Bone RC: Comprehensive respiratory care, ed 2, St Louis, 1990, Mosby.)*

Exam Hint 10-1 (ELE, WRE)

The examination usually contains at least one question that deals with knowing the correct position to drain a particular lobe. The lower lobes are usually tested. The question may give information on an opaque area seen on the chest radiograph. The therapist is expected to know what segment or lobe needs to be drained. Review Figure 1-8 for a drawing showing areas of consolidation.

---

4. Perform percussion (Code: IIIC1a) [Difficulty: ELE: R, Ap; WRE: An]

Percussion (also known as clapping, cupping, and tapotement) is the act of rhythmically striking the adult patient's chest with cupped hands over an area with secretions. A properly cupped hand traps air against the chest and causes a popping sound. The wrists, elbows, and shoulders should be kept as loose as possible to enable the

See the shaded areas in Figure 10-10. Percussion and vibration may not be possible on a female patient.

Some authors may list slightly different positions or several additional positions. The most commonly accepted postural drainage positions have been presented. The postural drainage positions in the infant are basically the same as those in the adult. Positioning can be accomplished more easily by using pillows. Figure 10-11 shows the various segmental drainage positions.

Figure 10-9 Drainage position for the apical segments of both upper lobes. *(From Eubanks DH, Bone RC: Comprehensive respiratory care, ed 2, St Louis, 1990, Mosby.)*

Figure 10-10 Drainage position for the anterior segments of both upper lobes. *(From Eubanks DH, Bone RC: Comprehensive respiratory care, ed 2, St Louis, 1990, Mosby.)*

practitioner to keep the proper loose waving motion of the hand and minimize fatigue (Figure 10-12). Infants can be percussed by putting the index, middle, and ring fingers together into a kind of three-sided tent, or specially designed palm cups. This enables the practitioner to percuss a small area of the chest wall. Percussion is performed throughout the breathing cycle and can be done with one or both hands. Percussion should not be painful to the patient. As an added precaution, most authors recommend that the chest be covered lightly with the patient's gown or towel. Percussion should not be done over buttons or zippers or female breast tissue.

Percussion will not help to move secretions if the patient is not in the proper postural drainage position. (See the previous discussion on the drainage positions.) When the patient is properly positioned, percussion

should help to vibrate the secretions more quickly down a vertical bronchus. Percussion is recommended for 5 minutes or longer in each position. Some patients, however, may not tolerate this length of treatment; 1 minute seems to be the shortest time for some therapeutic benefit. No agreement exists on the ideal manual rate of percussion. The practitioner must vary the rate, depending on how the patient feels and what seems to produce the best clearance of secretions. Recent research indicates that the ideal percussion rate is about 13 to 15 Hz (Hertz or cycles per second). Since this is faster than humanly possible, a mechanical percussor (discussed below) can be used to percuss the patient's chest.

5. Perform vibration (Code: IIIC1a) [Difficulty: ELE: R, Ap; WRE: An]

Vibration is the gentle, rapid shaking of the chest wall directly over the lung segment that is being drained. It may be performed alone or with percussion. The practitioner places his or her hands side by side if the chest area is large enough or one on the other for a smaller chest area. The elbows are locked with the arms straight (Figure 10-13). The patient's chest is gently but effectively shaken during exhalation. The patient should exhale at least the complete tidal volume (VT) as the chest wall is vibrated. Blowing out the expiratory reserve volume should help to clear out more secretions. A vibration rate of 200 per minute (about 3 per second) has been recommended as ideal to help move secretions. The literature differs as to how the patient should exhale during the procedure. Both breathing out slowly through pursed lips and breathing out forcefully through an open mouth have been recommended. A pursed-lip exhalation pattern seems reasonable if the patient has a problem with bronchospasm and air trapping. A patient without this problem should exhale forcefully because this helps to clear more secretions.

Figure 10-11 Drainage positions in infants. **A,** Apical segment of upper lobes. **B,** Posterior segments of upper lobes. **C,** Anterior segments of upper lobes. **D-F,** Superior segments of lower lobes. **G** and **H,** Anterior basal segments of both lower lobes (*H* on right and left sides). **I,** Segments of the right middle lobe and lingula (shown). **J,** Posterior basal segments of the lower lobes. *(From Crane LD: Physical therapy for the neonate with respiratory disease. In: Irwin S, Tecklin JS, editors: Cardiopulmonary physical therapy, ed 3, St Louis, 1995, Mosby.)*

Vibration should be performed for several expiratory efforts or until it is no longer effective in helping to mobilize secretions.

6. Modify the postural drainage therapy (ELE code: IIIF2f1) [ELE difficulty: R, Ap, An]

a. Change the length of treatment time. Lung segments should generally be drained for 3 to 15 minutes. If the patient is tolerating the position, and secretions are still being cleared, the position can be held longer. Stop the treatment if the patient is showing any signs of intolerance.

The total time of the procedure is recommended to be no longer than 30 to 40 minutes if all segments are treated because the patient may become exhausted by the various position changes. If so, the practitioner must select the worst segments to be drained first. Several drainage sessions may be needed to drain all of the involved segments.

Figure 10-12 Movement of the cupped hand at the wrist during chest percussion. *(From Shapiro BA, Kacmarek RM, Cane RD, et al: Clinical application of respiratory care, ed 4, St Louis, 1991, Mosby.)*

Figure 10-13 Vibration of the chest during postural drainage therapy. *(From Eubanks DH, Bone RC: Comprehensive respiratory care, ed 2, St Louis, 1990, Mosby.)*

b. Change the treatment techniques used. Be prepared to modify the postural drainage, percussion, and vibration procedures, depending on how the patient tolerates them. For example:

- Some patients cannot tolerate certain positions, especially head down, because of pain, shortness of breath (SOB), hypoxemia, or elevated blood pressure.
- Percussion rate, pressure, and hand position may need to be modified, depending on the patient's tolerance, chest size, and secretion clearance.

- It may not be possible to percuss or vibrate female patients in the right middle lobe and left lingular positions because of breast tissue.
- Hypoxemia should be prevented with supplemental O_2 as needed. Pulse oximetry could be performed before and during the procedure to monitor the patient's O_2 saturation.
- Patients with cardiac disease should have their heart rate, heart rhythm, and blood pressure monitored. Check the heart rate before the procedure and with each position change.
- Postoperative or trauma patients may not tolerate certain positions or percussion or vibration because of pain.
- Patients with copious secretions that cannot be expectorated (e.g., those who are not alert or have a tracheostomy) should not be positioned in a compromising situation. Suctioning equipment must be available.
- Very obese patients may not tolerate any head-down positions because of increased SOB.

c. Organize the sequence of drainage positions and treatment techniques. Differences of opinion exist as to the sequence in which the segments should be drained. Some authors state that an apices-to-bases approach is better, whereas others state that a bases-to-apices pattern is preferred. It makes sense to take an apices-to-bases approach for a first treatment when all lobes are to be drained. This pattern gives the patient time to adapt to the whole procedure. It also may be safer because the practitioner can evaluate the patient through a sequence of positions that progresses from the least to the most stressful.

If the patient can tolerate all positions without any difficulties, and the lower lobes are the worst in terms of secretions, drain the lower lobes first. If time permits, work up through the middle lobe and lingula to the upper lobes.

d. Change the postural drainage therapy position based on the patient's response. During the treatment, the patient's secretions may be found to be more effectively drained if he or she is repositioned from what would seem to be the ideal angle. The patient's airway anatomy may be different from what is expected. Patients with chronic lung disease, such as cystic fibrosis or bronchiectasis, often know what positions and angles are best for draining their lungs. Follow their advice if it produces good results.

Some patients cannot tolerate being properly positioned because their underlying lung or heart disease is aggravated by the unnatural body position. This is most commonly seen in the head-down positions to drain the lower lobes. Watch for signs of hypoxemia and SOB. The patient may have to be placed in a better-tolerated but less-desirable position. As long as some downward angle to the bronchus exists, mucus will drain. Each patient must be evaluated on an individual basis.

7. Coordinate the sequence of bronchial hygiene therapies: postural drainage, percussion, vibration, and positive expiratory pressure (ELE code: IIIF2f2) [ELE difficulty: R, Ap, An]

All of the various therapeutic options should be individualized to best meet the patient's needs. Be prepared to modify the options to use on different lung segments as the patient's condition either worsens or improves. In addition, be prepared to deliver bland and therapeutic aerosols to the patient before bronchial hygiene therapy is performed.

8. Stop the treatment if the patient has an adverse reaction to it (Code: IIIF1) [Difficulty: ELE: R, Ap; WRE: An]

Be prepared to stop the treatment if the patient has an adverse reaction. Often this results when a patient is placed into a head-down position. Review Box 10-3 for hazards and complications of postural drainage, percussion, and vibration.

Exam Hint 10-2 (ELE, WRE)

Be prepared to stop the treatment if the patient becomes short of breath, becomes hypoxic, develops a headache or dizziness, or needs to cough.

---

9. Manipulate postural drainage therapy equipment by order or protocol: percussors and vibrators (ELE code: IIA14a) [Difficulty: R, Ap, An]

a. Get the necessary equipment for the procedure. The terms *percussor* and *vibrator* are sometimes used interchangeably. Several manufacturers produce either electrically or pneumatically powered percussors/vibrators. Some are large enough to be wheeled into the patient's room (Figure 10-14). Obviously, electrically powered units need a standard electrical outlet for power, and the pneumatically powered units must be plugged into a 50-psi O_2 or air source.

Handheld battery-powered pediatric units are smaller to focus accurately on the much smaller target area of the infant's chest. Some practitioners find that an electric toothbrush with padded bristles works very well. Manual percussion of infants can be aided by using soft rubber palm cups that are available in several pediatric sizes.

b. Put the equipment together and make sure that it works properly. Because various devices are powered by wall electrical output, 50-psi source gas, or batteries, check the power source if the device fails to work. Some units have different patient applicators and connectors. These must be fastened properly so that the vibrating action does not cause them to loosen or fall off. For example, the Vibramatic/Multimatic has several patient applicators that must be screwed into the percussion adapter, which is then screwed into the ring adapter (Figure 10-15).

Figure 10-14 The Vibramatic/Multimatic electrically powered mechanical percussor/vibrator. *(Courtesy General Physiotherapy, Inc., St. Louis, Mo.)*

Figure 10-15 Right-angle adapter for Vibramatic chest percussor. The percussion adapter must be tightly screwed into the ring adapter, and the various patient applicators must be tightly screwed into the percussion adapter. *(Courtesy of General Physiotherapy, Inc., St Louis, Mo.)*

Some electrically powered units use a rubber belt and different sized wheels to change gears and produce several vibration rates. Others electrically vary the motor speed to change the vibration rate. Some pneumatically driven units can have their percussion force and rate varied.

c. Troubleshoot any problems with the equipment. Pneumatically powered units would suddenly fail if the high-pressure hose to the wall gas outlet or the O_2 tank became disconnected. Electrically powered units would fail if the electrical cord was unplugged or the batteries were depleted.

MODULE B
Positive expiratory pressure therapy

Positive expiratory pressure (PEP) therapy involves having a cooperative, spontaneously breathing patient exhale against a flow-limiting orifice to create expiratory pressures between 10 and 20 cm H_2O. Since the patient's expiratory flow is limited, the faster the patient tries to exhale, the higher the airway pressure. This therapy also is called *PEP mask therapy* because many pediatric patients find it easier to exhale against a face mask rather than through a mouthpiece.

Box 10-5 lists indications for PEP therapy. In patients with air trapping because of small airways disease (asthma or COPD), PEP therapy acts like pursed-lips breathing to

---

BOX 10-5 Indications for Positive Expiratory Pressure Therapy

To reduce air trapping in patients with emphysema, bronchitis, and asthma

To prevent or reverse atelectasis

To help mobilize retained secretions in patients older than 4 years who have cystic fibrosis, chronic bronchitis, bronchiectasis, or bronchiolitis obliterans

To maximize the delivery of aerosolized medications, such as bronchodilators, to patients receiving bronchial hygiene therapy

---

BOX 10-6 Relative Contraindications to Positive Expiratory Pressure Therapy

Untreated pneumothorax

Intracranial pressure >20 mm Hg

Active hemoptysis

Recent trauma or surgery to the skull, face, mouth, or esophagus

Patient with asthma attack or acute worsening of chronic obstructive pulmonary disease who cannot tolerate increased work of breathing

Acute sinusitis or epistaxis

Tympanic membrane rupture or other known or suspected middle ear pathology

Nausea

---

keep the small airways from collapsing. This allows the trapped alveolar gas to be more completely exhaled. Patients with atelectasis, or at risk for developing atelectasis, respond well to PEP therapy if incentive spirometry is not effective. PEP seems to push air through the Kohn pores of open alveoli into adjacent areas of atelectasis to force the alveoli open. There is evidence that PEP therapy is better than incentive spirometry (IS) or intermittent positive pressure breathing (IPPB) in the treatment of patients with postoperative atelectasis.

PEP therapy has proven effective in helping patients with chronic, copious amounts of secretions, primarily children ages 4 years or older with cystic fibrosis. It also helps patients with chronic bronchitis, bronchiectasis, or bronchiolitis obliterans more effectively clear their secretions. Clinical evidence indicates that the PEP dilates the small airways so that air is able to pass obstructing secretions. This fills the alveoli and, on expiration, tends to force the secretions into the larger airways for coughing or suctioning. PEP therapy also seems to increase the effectiveness of inhaled aerosolized bronchodilators.

Box 10-6 lists relative contraindications to PEP therapy. No absolute contraindications exist. Box 10-7 lists hazards

---

BOX 10-7 Hazards or Complications of Positive Expiratory Pressure Therapy

Pulmonary barotrauma
Increased intracranial pressure
Myocardial ischemia or decreased venous return to the heart
Increased work of breathing
Air swallowing that can lead to vomiting
Discomfort from mask or skin breakdown from mask pressure
Claustrophobia

---

or complications of PEP therapy. These should be weighed against the benefits to the patient when making the recommendation to start PEP therapy. Other considerations include the patient's history of pulmonary disease and the response to CPT, ineffective cough to clear retained secretions, and breath sounds and chest radiograph findings of secretions.

PEP therapy is currently provided via two different equipment modalities. The original PEP therapy devices use a fixed-orifice resistor and are presented in Part 1. The newer PEP devices also provide airway vibrations or oscillations and are presented in Part 2.

1. Part 1: Adjustable fixed-orifice type PEP device

a. Perform positive expiratory pressure therapy (Code: IIIC1d) [Difficulty: ELE: R, Ap; WRE: An]

The patient must be old enough to understand instructions and be able to perform the procedure. Box 10-8 lists the steps in performing a proper PEP therapy treatment. Be prepared to adjust the expiratory resistance to meet the clinical goal of PEP therapy. Initially the resistance to exhalation should be kept low. As the training continues, the resistance the patient breathes against can be increased. The goal is to maintain a PEP of 10 to 20 cm H_2O with an inspiratory/expiratory (I:E) ratio of about 1:3. If the expiratory orifice is too small, the expiratory airway pressure will be too high or the expiratory time too long. The patient will likely become fatigued. If the expiratory orifice is too large, the pressure will not be high enough to be of any benefit. In any situation, the patient will probably become tired if the total treatment time lasts longer than 20 minutes.

b. Coordinate the sequence of bronchial hygiene therapies: postural drainage, percussion, vibration, and positive expiratory pressure (ELE code: IIIF2f2) [ELE difficulty: R, Ap, An]

All of the various therapeutic options should be individualized to best meet the patient's needs. Be prepared to

---

BOX 10-8 Steps in Performing Positive Expiratory Pressure (PEP) Therapy

1. Assemble the equipment as shown in Figures 10-16 and 10-17. Set the expiratory resistance to the desired setting.
2. Have the conscious patient sit up straight, rest elbows on a table, and hold the PEP mask comfortably but tightly over the nose and mouth. The patient may use a mouthpiece and nose clips if preferred.
3. The patient should inhale a deeper than normal breath, but not to total lung capacity, by using the diaphragm. The unconscious patient will inhale only a tidal volume breath.
4. The conscious patient should exhale to functional residual capacity fast enough to generate 10 to 20 cm H_2O in the manometer. Have the patient look at the pressure manometer to judge how fast to exhale. The unconscious patient will exhale passively but will still benefit from the increased baseline pressure.
5. The patient should have an expiratory time that is about three times longer than the inspiratory time (an inspiratory/expiratory ratio of 1:2 to 1:4 is acceptable). The clinician can accomplish this by changing the expiratory resistor and/or having the patient change the force of exhalation.
6. Between 10 and 20 proper PEP breaths should be performed.
7. The patient should now perform a directed cough or two or three "huff"-type coughing efforts to raise secretions.
8. Repeat steps 2 to 7 between four and eight times (for approximately 10 to 20 min) for a full PEP treatment.

Patients in the intensive care unit can perform PEP therapy as often as every hour or as rarely as every 6 hours. They should be reevaluated for treatment effectiveness every 24 hours. Patients in the acute care or home care setting can perform PEP therapy between two and four times each day. The acute care patient should be reevaluated every 72 hours; the home care patient can be evaluated at longer intervals or when a change in pulmonary status occurs.

---

modify PEP therapy and CPT as the patient's condition either worsens or improves. In addition, be prepared to deliver bland and therapeutic aerosols to the patient before or during PEP therapy.

Coordinate PEP therapy with effective directed coughing, "huff" cough techniques, CPT, or aerosolized medication delivery. As listed in Box 10-8, PEP breaths can be alternated with huff coughs to clear secretions. Huff coughs are not full, deep coughs; rather, they are performed as follows:

1. Have the patient inhale a slow, deep breath but not to total lung capacity (TLC).
2. Hold the breath for 1 to 3 seconds.
3. Perform several quick, forced exhalations with an open epiglottis.
4. Small children may be taught to say "huff" with each quick exhalation. It also may help to have the

young patient perform a "chicken breath" by flapping his or her arms against the sides of the chest during the exhalation.

CPT may be used before or after PEP therapy, or it may be alternated with PEP therapy, to help in the removal of secretions. Likewise, aerosolized medications may be inhaled before or simultaneously with PEP therapy. Bronchodilators and mucolytic agents should be very helpful with PEP therapy to mobilize secretions. Evaluate sputum for quantity, color, odor, and thickness.

c. Terminate the treatment if the patient has an adverse reaction to it (Code: IIIF1) [Difficulty: ELE: R, Ap; WRE: An]

During the treatment, ask the patient if he or she feels dyspnea, pain, or chest discomfort. Also monitor the patient's breath sounds, blood pressure, heart rate, and breathing pattern and rate. Monitor oxygenation by pulse oximetry, mental clarity, and skin color. Be prepared to stop the treatment if necessary. Review the contraindications listed in Box 10-6 and hazards listed in Box 10-7.

d. Manipulate fixed-orifice PEP therapy equipment by order or protocol (ELE code: IIA14c) [ELE difficulty: R, Ap, An]

1. Get the necessary equipment for the procedure

Currently, several positive expiratory pressure (PEP) systems are available for selection, based on the patient's needs. Figure 10-16 shows the TheraPEP device. The following basic components are included:

- Patient mouthpiece. Nose clips can be added, if needed.
- Mouthpiece adapter with hose to pressure generator.

Figure 10-16 Drawing of the DHD TheraPEP device. *1,* Patient mouthpiece. *2,* Hose to connect the mouthpiece to the pressure generator. *3,* One-way inlet valve for inspiration. *4,* Pressure generator through which the patient exhales to create positive expiratory pressure. *(From Wilkins RL, Stoller JK, Kacmarek RM, editors: Egan's fundamentals of respiratory care, ed 9, St Louis, 2009, Mosby.)*

- Inspiratory one-way valve. (Fit this into the mouthpiece if medications are not being delivered.)
- Pressure generator. Insert one of the six available fixed-orifice resistance diaphragms to suit the patient's expiratory flow goal. The pressure gauge displays the airway pressure generated during exhalation.

The following optional components are included:

- Substitute a pediatric, small adult, or regular adult face mask for the mouthpiece.
- A small volume nebulizer (SVN) or metered dose inhaler (MDI) T-piece adapter can be inserted between the mouthpiece adapter and one-way valve for medication delivery.
- Necessary adapters for the SVN or MDI are included.

Figure 10-17 shows the Resistex unit. Basic components include the following:

- Patient mouthpiece. Nose clips can be added, if needed.
- Expiratory resistor with four fixed-orifice settings.
- Pressure manometer calibrated in centimeters of water.
- Small-bore oxygen tubing to connect the expiratory resistor to the pressure manometer.

Optional components, shown in Figure 10-17, include the following:

- Substitute a pediatric, small adult, or regular adult face mask for the mouthpiece. If the patient has an endotracheal or tracheostomy tube, substitute a universal airway (elbow) adapter for the mouthpiece.
- SVN—Note that an MDI and holding chamber can be substituted for an SVN and aerosol tubing.
- T-piece and female adapter to connect the SVN to the expiratory resistor.
- Large-bore aerosol tubing to act as a medication reservoir.

Procedural accessories include a basin and tissues to collect and dispose of sputum. For infection control purposes, the respiratory therapist should have gloves, mask, goggles, and gown if indicated. With either unit, if a PEP mask is used it should be transparent, flexible, and fitted to the patient's facial contours so that no air will leak out as the pressure is increased.

2. Put the equipment together and make sure that it works properly

As described previously and shown in Figures 10-16 and 10-17, the component pieces must be gathered and properly assembled. Make sure that all connections are airtight. If a leak is present, the desired PEP goal will not be reached or maintained. In addition, an air leak may be felt or a high-pitched sound may be heard. If an SVN or MDI is added, it must be tested to ensure that it works properly. Connect the SVN (or MDI) into the system, as shown in

Figure 10-17 Positive expiratory pressure (PEP) mask components. The basic PEP assembly necessitates a transparent mask or mouthpiece, expiratory resistor (this shows the Resistex by Mercury Medical, Clearwater, Fla), and pressure manometer with connecting oxygen tubing. If a nebulized medication is added, the following also are needed: small volume nebulizer with T-piece, oxygen tubing to flowmeter, and large-bore tubing for an aerosol reservoir. *(From Malmeister MJ, Fink JB, Hoffman GL, et al: Positive-expiratory-pressure mask therapy: theoretical and practical considerations and a review of the literature,* Respir Care *36[11]:1218, 1991.)*

Figure 10-17. Add the medication and run a flow of O_2 or compressed air at 4 to 6 L/min through the nebulizer (as is customary). The slowed exhalation during PEP breathing should promote better deposition of medication into the small airways.

Be prepared to adjust the expiratory resistance to meet the clinical goal of PEP therapy. One of six small-exit diaphragms can be added to the pressure generator part of the TheraPEP device. Select the one that best meets the patient's clinical goal. The Resistex unit has four fixed-orifice settings from which to choose. The orifice interior diameters are 4, 3.5, 3, and 2.5 mm. Adjust the dial for the desired size to meet the patient's clinical goal. With either unit, the patient's treatment should begin with the largest opening for exhalation. If appropriate, smaller expiratory openings may be used to meet the patient's clinical goal.

3. Troubleshoot any problems with the equipment

Any leaks in the system will prevent the PEP goal from being reached. Tighten any loose connections. If the one-way valves in the Resistex or TheraPEP units are assembled backward, the patient will inspire against a resistance instead of exhaling against it. Observe the one-way valves in use, and ask the patient if he or she finds it easy to inhale but more difficult to exhale. Move the valves to their proper positions if incorrectly placed. If an SVN is used, check that aerosol is coming from the nebulizer. If not, check the capillary tube or baffle for an obstruction; clear it by running tap water or a sterile needle through it. See Chapter 8, if necessary, for more information on fixing problems with SVNs.

2. Part 2: Adjustable vibratory-type PEP device

a. Perform vibratory positive expiratory pressure therapy (Code: IIIC1d) [Difficulty: ELE: R, Ap; WRE: An]

The NBRC refers to this type of PEP therapy as vibratory PEP. However, since the professional literature refers to it as *oscillatory PEP* or OPEP, that terminology will be used here. OPEP has the same indications (Box 10-5), contraindications (Box 10-6), hazards (Box 10-7), and clinical benefits as PEP delivered through a fixed-orifice resistor. In theory, the airway oscillations produced with OPEP improve airway clearance better than PEP. However, this has not been proven in clinical trials. Two widely known OPEP devices will be presented here. Box 10-9 will present the basic steps in performing an OPEP treatment. Other general considerations for OPEP and related therapies are the same as those for PEP and were presented previously.

Of all the OPEP devices, the Flutter (Figure 10-18) has been used the most, primarily with cystic fibrosis patients. Because of its simplicity, both small children and adults can be instructed in its use. The Flutter is a pipe-shaped device with a steel ball nesting loosely inside the covered bowl. A perforated cap over the bowl keeps the ball from falling out but allows exhaled air to escape. The exhaled breath pushes the ball up in the bowl, air briefly escapes, and the ball falls back down again. When the ball falls back, more pressure is exerted against the patient's airway. The airway pressure generated during the exhalation varies from 5 to 35 cm H_2O, depending on how fast the patient exhales. The rate at which the ball flutters up and

---

BOX 10-9 Steps in Performing Oscillatory Positive Expiratory Pressure (OPEP) Therapy

1. Assemble the equipment shown in Figures 10-18 or 10-19.
2. Have the conscious patient sit up straight with head erect. (While not ideal, the patient may lie on either side as long as the Flutter can be held upright. The Acapella may be held in any position and work properly.)
3. The patient should inhale a deeper than normal breath, but not to total lung capacity (TLC). Hold the breath.
4. Place the Flutter or Acapella into the mouth, seal lips, and exhale actively. (Coach the patient to exhale about twice as fast as normal but not as fast as possible.)
5. Continue to actively exhale until the patient has reached functional residual capacity (FRC).
6. During the exhalation adjust the device so that the patient has the greatest sense of vibration felt within the lungs. With the Flutter, adjust the vertical tilt of the bowl. With the Acapella, adjust the dial at the distal end.
7. Repeat steps 3 to 6 while adjusting the expiratory flow rate and oscillation rate to "fine tune" the lung maximal vibrations to mobilize secretions. Perform about 10 to 20 breaths.
8. Finish with one or two maximal efforts: Inhale to TLC, hold the breath for 2 to 3 seconds, and exhale as fast as possible to FRC.
9. Perform either a maximal coughing effort or mid-inspiratory/huff-type cough to clear out any secretions.
10. Repeat steps 3 to 9 for four to eight cycles. Total treatment time should not exceed 20 minutes.

Figure 10-18 A, Patient correctly holding the Flutter for an exhalation. **B,** Cross-section drawing of the Flutter showing how the steel ball is lifted by the patient's exhaled tidal volume. When the ball drops back down into the cup, the backpressure is transmitted to the airways. *(From Fink JB, Hess DR: Secretion clearance techniques. In Hess DR, MacIntyre NR, Mishoe SC, et al, editors: Respiratory care principles and practice, Philadelphia, 2002, WB Saunders.)*

down ranges between 2 and 32 Hz (Hertz or cycles/sec) and varies with the angle of the bowl. The high-frequency oscillations of backpressure on the airway caused by the fluttering steel ball are believed to help dislodge viscous secretions. Through trial and error the patient varies the expiratory flow rate and angle of the bowl to find the best oscillation rate to mobilize secretions.

The Acapella (Figure 10-19) is available in two expiratory flow models that allow the practitioner to better match the patient's needs with the equipment. A third model, the Choice, can be disassembled for easy cleaning in the home or hospital. All models allow the user to adjust the frequency and amplitude of the oscillations. When the best expiratory flow, frequency, and amplitude of oscillations is found, the patient's secretions will be optimally mobilized. See Box 10-9 for the steps in the procedure.

b. Coordinate the sequence of bronchial hygiene therapies: postural drainage, percussion, vibration, and positive expiratory pressure (ELE code: IIIF2f2) [ELE difficulty: R, Ap, An]

If inhaled bronchodilator or mucolytic medications are ordered for the patient using the Flutter, they should be taken before the OPEP treatment. This is because it is not designed to be used with an SVN or MDI. All of the various therapeutic options should be individualized to best meet the patient's needs. Be prepared to modify OPEP therapy and CPT as the patient's condition either worsens or improves.

Coordinate OPEP therapy with effective maximal cough or "huff" cough techniques, CPT, or aerosolized medication delivery. As listed in Box 10-9, OPEP breaths should be alternated with directed coughing to clear secretions. Huff coughs are not full, deep coughs; rather, they are performed as follows:

1. Have the patient inhale a slow, deep breath but not to total lung capacity (TLC).
2. Hold the breath for 1 to 3 seconds.
3. Perform several quick, forced exhalations with an open epiglottis.
4. Small children may be taught to say "huff" with each quick exhalation. It also may help to have the

Figure 10-19 An Acapella oscillatory PEP device. This device can be a blue DM model for patients with an expiratory flow of <15 lpm, or a green DH model for patients with an expiratory flow of >15 lpm. *(Courtesy Smiths-Medical, Carlsbad, California.)*

young patient perform a "chicken breath" by flapping his or her arms against the sides of the chest during the exhalation.

CPT may be used before or after OPEP therapy, or it may be alternated with OPEP therapy, to help in the removal of secretions. Aerosolized bronchodilators and mucolytic agents should be very helpful with OPEP therapy to mobilize secretions. Evaluate sputum for quantity, color, odor, and thickness.

c. Terminate the treatment if the patient has an adverse reaction to it (Code: IIIF1) [Difficulty: ELE: R, Ap; WRE: An]

It is unlikely that a patient will have an adverse reaction from using the Flutter or Acapella device. However, it is possible that some patients will not like the feeling of increased pressure in the lungs. In this case, it may be better to stop the treatment and switch to another method of secretion management.

During the treatment, ask the patient if he or she feels dyspnea, pain, or chest discomfort. Also monitor the patient's breath sounds, blood pressure, heart rate, and breathing pattern and rate. Monitor oxygenation by pulse oximetry, mental clarity, and skin color. Be prepared to stop the treatment if necessary. Review the contraindications listed in Box 10-6 and hazards listed in Box 10-7.

d. Manipulate vibratory-type PEP therapy equipment by order or protocol (ELE code: IIA14c) [ELE difficulty: R, Ap, An]

1. Get the necessary equipment for the procedure

The Flutter (Figure 10-18) is a pipe-shaped device with a steel ball nesting loosely inside the bowl. The Flutter valve has been used with cystic fibrosis patients to help them loosen their secretions. It is believed that the high-frequency oscillations of backpressure on the airway caused by the fluttering steel ball help to dislodge thick (viscous) secretions. The Flutter valve must be kept upright during the patient's exhalation to work properly.

The Acapella devices (Figure 10-19) use an adjustable counterweighted lever and magnet to produce variable frequency and amplitude of the expiratory pressure. They have the same clinical indications as the Flutter device. The original Acapella is available with a choice of two models based on the patient's expiratory flow. The green DH model is indicated for patients with an expiratory flow >15 L/min (>0.25 L/sec). The blue MD model is indicated for patients with an expiratory flow <15 L/min (<0.25 L/sec). This allows for a better match of the unit with the patient's pulmonary function. The newer Choice model can be disassembled for easier cleaning. A possible advantage of the Acapella devices over the Flutter devices is that they can be used in any patient position.

2. Put the equipment together and make sure that it works properly

The Flutter device is preassembled by the manufacturer. A perforated cap should be over the bowl to keep the ball from falling while letting exhaled air escape. The Flutter does not have accessories for pressure monitoring or adding medications.

All Acapella models and adult mouthpiece are preassembled by the manufacturer. Each has an adjustable knob at the opposite end of the unit from the patient's mouthpiece. As the knob is rotated, a magnet is moved closer to or farther from a counterweighted lever. Rotate the knob, as needed, to set the patient's expiratory frequency and amplitude pressure. The following accessories can be added, if needed:

- A pressure port with tubing to connect to a pressure manometer can be added.
- A pediatric or adult size mask can be substituted for the mouthpiece.
- With the proper adapter, an SVN can be added for medications.

These accessories allow for the patient's airway pressure to be monitored, the unit to be fitted to the patient for better compliance, and therapeutic aerosols to be given.

3. Troubleshoot any problems with the equipment

The patient must keep the Flutter in the proper position with the perforated cap in the upright position. This keeps the patient's exhaled air blowing through the device to push up the steel ball. If a patient should cough secretions into the unit, it will become clogged. Air will not flow through it. Try clearing the obstruction from the mouthpiece with a cotton swab or by running warm water through the unit. If necessary, the cap can be unscrewed from the bowl and the steel ball and cup can be removed. Wash out any secretions and reassemble.

With the Acapella, if the adjustable knob cannot move or the frequency and amplitude pressure cannot be adjusted, the unit may be obstructed by secretions or may be defective. The DM and DH models can be washed with warm, soapy water. The Choice model can be disassembled into four parts, each of which can be washed with warm, soapy water. For disinfection purposes this model is put through a dishwasher, boiled, autoclaved, or soaked in glutaraldehyde. If after cleaning and reassembly it still does not function, it is defective and must be replaced.

Exam Hint 10-3 (WRE)

Expect to see at least one question about PEP therapy. Be prepared to recommend it in a patient with a secretion problem. PEP therapy may have to be modified to maximize secretion mobilization, or PEP therapy may be added to another treatment such as incentive spirometry, an SVN for medications, or high-frequency chest wall oscillation to help the patient mobilize and clear secretions.

MODULE C
High-frequency chest wall oscillation

1. Perform high-frequency chest wall oscillation (Code: IIIC1d) [Difficulty: ELE: R, Ap; WRE: An]

High-frequency chest wall oscillation (HFCWO) is indicated to help mobilize and clear secretions. This procedure may be used in patients with cystic fibrosis, bronchiectasis, or chronic bronchitis who do not tolerate other secretion mobilization procedures. For example, a cystic fibrosis patient may have an adverse effect when put into head-down positions for postural drainage therapy.

The patient should be instructed to sit up during the treatment, put on the inflatable vest or cuirass, and connect the air hose(s) between the vest/cuirass and the pumping unit. A general recommendation is to have the patient set whatever oscillation (chest wall compression) rate results in the greatest production of secretions. Common sense indicates that it is appropriate to start at the lowest rate and pressure and progress to a faster rate and higher pressure as the patient tolerates. However, there is laboratory evidence that an HFCWO rate of about 13 to 15 Hz (Hertz; cycles/second) is best at improving mucus movement. Treatments typically last 30 minutes and can be repeated up to six times per day. This procedure cannot be used in a patient with a chest wall injury such as broken ribs.

2. Modify high-frequency chest wall oscillation equipment by order or protocol (WRE code: IIA14b) [WRE difficulty: R, Ap]

a. Get the necessary equipment for the procedure

Currently, two HFCWO devices are available. The Vest (Figure 10-20) consists of a nonstretchable inflatable vest that covers the entire torso, an electrically powered pumping and control system, and two connecting hoses. The controls allow an adjustable air pulse rate of either 5 Hz (producing a vest pressure of 25 mm Hg) or 25 Hz (producing a vest pressure of 40 mm Hg).

The Hayek oscillator (Figure 10-21) consists of a flexible chest cuirass, an electrically powered pumping and control panel, and a connecting hose. This machine can deliver both positive and negative pressure to the patient's chest throughout the breathing cycle. Added negative pressure around the patient's chest will increase inspiration. Added positive pressure around the patient's chest will increase expiration. The therapist can adjust an oscillation rate of 8 to 999 oscillations/min, with an I:E ratio of 6:1 to 1:6, and inspiratory and expiratory pressures of up to +70 cm water.

With either unit, it is believed that the pressure on the outside of the chest is transmitted internally to increase expiratory airflow and push secretions from small to larger airways. HFCWO has been found to especially help cystic fibrosis patients mobilize retained secretions.

b. Put the equipment together and make sure that it works properly

Follow the manufacturer's guidelines to assemble the components, as shown in Figures 10-19 and 10-20.

Figure 10-20   The Vest high-frequency chest wall oscillation device. **A,** The power unit with controls for air pulse rate and vest pressure, along with two hoses to connect to the vest. **B,** The inflatable vest with two ports for the hoses from the power unit. *(Copyright © 2009 Hill-Rom Services, Inc. Reprinted with permission. All rights reserved.)*

Cuirass

Cuirass
Y-connector

Cuirass
short tubes

Wide bore tube

Pressure
sensor tubing

Keyboard/
control unit

Power unit

Figure 10-21 Drawing of the Hayek oscillator with its pumping and control unit, air hose, and patient cuirass. *(Modified from materials courtesy of Breasy Medical Equipment, Stanford, Conn.)*

c. Troubleshoot any problems with the equipment

One problem area could relate to the vest/cuirass not fitting properly. If the vest/cuirass is too large, air will leak, and the desired pressures will not be reached. Adjust the unit for a tighter fit, or place pads between the patient and the vest/cuirass to seal the leak. Too tight a vest/cuirass could rub on the skin and be uncomfortable. Loosen the vest/cuirass or add more padding over the skin. If the hose(s) loosen(s) from the vest/cuirass or the pumping unit, the air will leak out, and no pressure will be generated. Reattach the hose(s).

3. Stop the treatment if the patient has an adverse reaction to it (Code: IIIF1) [Difficulty: ELE: R, Ap; WRE: An]

In general, HFCWO seems to be well tolerated. However, be prepared to stop the treatment if the vest/cuirass is causing skin irritation. With proper fitting the treatment should be well tolerated.

MODULE D
Respiratory care plan

1. Analyze the available information to determine the patient's pathophysiologic state (Code: IIIH1) [Difficulty: ELE: R, Ap; WRE: An]

The patient's breath sounds should be auscultated before the treatment begins to determine which segments are normal or have secretions. Auscultate each segment after the treatment and after the patient has coughed. Listen for air moving into formerly silent areas or areas that are cleared of secretions.

Make a recommendation for a chest radiograph examination to find specific areas for CPT. A white shadow on a chest radiograph film over what should be normal lung may indicate areas of atelectasis or infiltrates that can be targeted for treatment. Chest radiograph examinations should be repeated to look for an improvement in the lungs. The resolution may be slow or dramatic, depending on the original problem and how it responds to the various treatments used on it.

2. Determine the appropriateness of the prescribed therapy and goals for the identified pathophysiologic state (Code: IIIH3) [Difficulty: ELE: R, Ap; WRE: An]

a. Review the planned therapy to establish the therapeutic plan (Code: IIIH2a) [Difficulty: ELE: R, Ap; WRE: An]

b. Recommend changes in the therapeutic plan when indicated (Code: IIIH4) [Difficulty: ELE: R, Ap; WRE: An]

The AARC *Clinical Practice Guideline* recommends that the following be evaluated to determine whether PDT is needed:

- CPT is usually not indicated if an optimally hydrated patient is expectorating less than 25 mL/day with the procedure.
- A dehydrated patient should have apparently ineffective CPT continued for at least 24 hours after the patient is rehydrated. The combination of rehydration and CPT may help to mobilize previously thick secretions.
- CPT is not indicated in a patient producing more than 30 mL of secretions per day if the treatments do not increase the sputum production. The patient is already able to expectorate the sputum effectively.

For any of the previously discussed procedures, be prepared to measure the patient's blood pressure, heart rate, and respiratory rate before, during, and after a change in therapy. Minor changes (less than 20%) can be expected. The patient's oxygenation should improve as secretions and mucous plugs are removed and atelectatic areas open.

The patient's breath sounds should be auscultated before and after any treatment procedure. Listen for air moving into formerly silent areas and for secretions being cleared.

Ask the patient how he or she feels before, during, and after the treatment. CPT should not be performed for at least 1 hour after a patient has eaten to minimize the chances of nausea from the head-down position.

PEP therapy has been indicated in patients who have retained secretions that are difficult to expectorate. Increase or decrease the PEP level to help the patient without causing fatigue or complications. If PEP therapy does not increase the amount of sputum produced per day in a patient who already produces more than 30 mL, PEP may not be needed. It does not make sense to continue an ineffective treatment.

c. Conduct health management education (WRE code: IIIH9) [WRE difficulty: Ap, An]

The previously discussed procedures are used primarily with cystic fibrosis or chronic bronchitis patients. All have been shown to help in the mobilization of secretions. However, each patient may find that one procedure works better than another. Teach the patient and/or family members about the ordered procedure. CPT can be performed by family members on the patient. Many patients, even older children, can be taught to self-administer PEP and OPEP therapy. Be prepared to make recommendations to change the type of procedure and the way each procedure is conducted. In addition, other respiratory care procedures (e.g., O$_2$ therapy) and inhaled bronchodilators and mucolytic medications may have to be modified as the patient's condition warrants.

3. Record and interpret the patient's breath sounds (Code: IIIA1b3) [Difficulty: ELE: R, Ap; WRE: An]

The patient's breath sounds should improve if retained secretions are expectorated.

4. Record and interpret the type of cough the patient has and the nature of the sputum (Code: IIIA1b3) [Difficulty: ELE: R, Ap; WRE: An]

All of the procedures discussed in this chapter are done to improve the patient's cough and increase sputum production. If they are ineffective, another procedure must be tried.

5. Recommend discontinuing the treatments based on the patient's response to therapy (Code: IIIG1i) [Difficulty: ELE: R, Ap; WRE: An]

Review the previous discussion for indications that the patient has recovered and no longer needs bronchopul-

monary hygiene procedures. For example, the secretions have decreased or can be easily expectorated by the patient, or both. Review Boxes 10-2 and 10-3 for contraindications and hazards/complications of postural drainage and percussion and vibration. Review Boxes 10-6 and 10-7 for contraindications and hazards/complications of PEP therapy.

BIBLIOGRAPHY

American Association for Respiratory Care: Clinical practice guideline: postural drainage therapy, *Respir Care* 36:1418, 1991.

American Association for Respiratory Care: Clinical practice guideline: use of positive airway pressure adjuncts to bronchial hygiene therapy, *Respir Care* 38(5):516, 1993.

American Association for Respiratory Care: Clinical practice guideline: directed cough, *Respir Care* 38(5):495, 1993.

Branson RD, Hess DR, Chatburn RL: *Respiratory care equipment*, ed 2, Philadelphia, 1999, Lippincott Williams & Wilkins.

Cairo JM: Lung expansion devices. In Cairo JM, Pilbeam SP, editors: *Mosby's respiratory care equipment*, ed 8, St Louis, 2009, Mosby.

Campbell TC, Ferguson N, McKinlay RGC: The use of a simple self-administered method of positive expiratory pressure (PEP) in chest physiotherapy after abdominal surgery, *Physiotherapy* 72(10):498, 1986.

Eid N, Buchheit J, Neuling M, et al: Chest physiotherapy in review, *Respir Care* 36(4):270, 1991.

Eubanks DH, Bone RC: *Comprehensive respiratory care*, ed 2, St Louis, 1990, Mosby.

Fink JB: Volume expansion therapy. In Burton GC, Hodgkin JE, Ward JJ, editors: *Respiratory care: a guide to clinical practice*, ed 4, Philadelphia, 1997, Lippincott-Raven.

Fink JB: Bronchial hygiene therapy and lung expansion. In Fink JB, Hunt GE, editors: *Clinical practice in respiratory care*, Philadelphia, 1999, Lippincott-Raven.

Fink JB, Hess DR: Secretion clearance techniques. In Hess DR, MacIntyre NR, Mishoe SC, et al, editors: *Respiratory care principals and practice*, Philadelphia, 2002, WB Saunders.

Frownfelter DL: Chest physical therapy and airway care. In Barnes TA, editor: *Core textbook of respiratory care practice*, ed 2, St Louis, 1994, Mosby.

Hess DR, Branson RD: Chest physiotherapy, incentive spirometry, intermittent positive-pressure breathing, secretion clearance, and inspiratory muscle training. In Branson RD, Hess DR, Chatburn RL, editors: *Respiratory care equipment*, ed 2, Philadelphia, 1999, Lippincott Williams & Wilkins.

Hill KV: Bronchial hygiene therapy. In Aloan CA, Hill TV, editors: *Respiratory care of the newborn and child*, ed 2, Philadelphia, 1997, Lippincott-Raven.

Hoffman GL, Cohen NH: Positive expiratory pressure therapy, *NBRC Horizons* 19(2):1, 1993.

Johnson NT, Pierson DJ: The spectrum of pulmonary atelectasis: pathophysiology, diagnosis, and therapy, *Respir Care* 31(11):1107, 1986.

Kacmarek RM, Dimas S, Mack CW: The essentials of respiratory care, ed 4, St Louis, 2005, Mosby.

Malmeister MJ, Fink JB, Hoffman GL: Positive-expiratory-pressure mask therapy: theoretical and practical considerations and a review of the literature, *Respir Care* 36(11):1218, 1991.

Myslinski MJ, Scanlan CL: Bronchial hygiene therapy. In Wilkins RL, Stoller JK, Kacmarek RM, editors: *Egan's fundamentals of respiratory care*, ed 9, St Louis, 2009, Mosby.

Myers TR: Positive expiratory pressure and oscillatory positive expiratory pressure therapies, *Respir Care* 52 (10): 1308, 2007.

Oberwaldner PT, Evans JC, Zach MS: Forced expirations against a variable resistance: a new chest physiotherapy method in cystic fibrosis, *Pediatr Pulmonol* 2(6):358, 1986.

Rutkowski JA: Pulmonary hygiene and chest physical therapy. In Wyka KA, Mathews PJ, Clark WF, editors: *Foundations of respiratory care*, Albany, NY, 2002, Delmar.

Scott AA, Koff PB: Airway care and chest physiotherapy. In Koff PB, Eitzman D, Neu J, editors: *Neonatal and pediatric respiratory care*, ed 2, St Louis, 1993, Mosby.

Shapiro BA, Kacmarek RM, Cane RD, et al, editors: *Clinical application of respiratory care*, ed 4, St Louis, 1991, Mosby.

Sobush DC, Hilling L, Southorn PA: Bronchial hygiene therapy. In Burton GC, Hodgkin JE, Ward JJ, editors: *Respiratory care: a guide to clinical practice*, ed 4, Philadelphia, 1997, Lippincott-Raven.

van der Schans CP: Conventional chest physical therapy for obstructive lung disease, *Respir Care* 52 (9): 1198, 2007.

White GC: *Equipment theory for respiratory care*, ed 4, Albany, NY, 2005, Thomson Delmar Learning.

Wilkins RL, Stoller JK, Kacmarek RM, editors: *Egan's fundamentals of respiratory care*, ed 9, St Louis, 2009, Mosby.

Wojciechowski WV: Incentive spirometers, secretion evacuation devices, and inspiratory muscle training devices. In Barnes TA, editor: *Core textbook of respiratory care practice*, ed 2, St Louis, 1994, Mosby.

SELF-STUDY QUESTIONS FOR THE ENTRY LEVEL EXAM

See page 592 for answers

1. A 15-year-old patient with cystic fibrosis has copious amounts of secretions. She cannot tolerate PDT because she gets a headache when tipped head-down. Aerosolized bronchodilators and mucolytic agents are ordered every 4 hr by SVN. What else would you recommend?
   A. Add incentive spirometry.
   B. Give the aerosolized medications by IPPB therapy.
   C. Add PEP therapy.
   D. Modify the PDT positions so that the head is not lower than the patient's body.

2. To get the best patient results, manual percussion should be performed with
   1. The hand cupped
   2. A tight, fixed-wrist position
   3. The elbows relaxed
   4. The hand flat
   5. The wrist relaxed
   A. 3, 4, 5
   B. 2, 3, 4
   C. 2, 4
   D. 1, 3, 5

3. How should manual vibration be performed as part of CPT?
   1. On inspiration
   2. At a rate of 20 to 30 cycles/sec
   3. On expiration
   4. At a rate of 3 cycles/sec
   5. Throughout the breathing cycle
   A. 2, 4
   B. 1, 4
   C. 3, 4
   D. 4, 5

4. When a patient's chart is reviewed, it is important to look for contraindications to CPT. They would include all of the following EXCEPT:

   A. Increased intracranial pressure in a patient with a recent head injury
   B. Recent stroke
   C. Small vital capacity in a bedridden patient
   D. The patient has just eaten

5. A stroke patient has been admitted and is in a coma and unable to care for himself. The physician is concerned that he may develop atelectasis and pneumonia. What would you recommend to help prevent these problems?
   A. Regular turning from side to side
   B. PEP therapy
   C. IPPB
   D. CPAP

6. You receive an order to perform postural drainage, percussion, and vibration on a patient. No segments are specified. On reviewing the chest x-ray film, you notice infiltrates in the lower right lung field. You would proceed to treat the following segments:
   1. Apical
   2. Lateral basal
   3. Superior
   4. Medial
   5. Posterior basal
   A. 2, 5
   B. 3, 4, 5
   C. 1, 4
   D. 2, 3, 5

7. A physician has ordered PEP therapy with albuterol. All of the following are needed to start the treatment EXCEPT:
   A. Variable orifice resistor
   B. Pressure manometer
   C. Bedside spirometer
   D. Nebulizer with reservoir

8. All of the following are contraindications to percussion and vibration EXCEPT:
   A. Performing the procedure over the kidneys
   B. Mobilizing large amounts of secretions
   C. Performing the procedure over bare skin
   D. Performing the procedure over or near a surgical site

9. A patient is positioned on her left side with the foot of the bed raised 18 inches. She would be draining which lung segment?
   A. Anterior basal
   B. Superior
   C. Lateral and medial lingular
   D. Posterior basal

10. Your patient has been ordered to start PEP therapy. During the initial instruction and patient practice, you notice that the pressure is 25 cm H_2O and the patient's I:E ratio is 1:5. You would proceed to
    A. Adjust the PEP device to have the patient exhale through a larger hole
    B. Have the patient continue but coach him to exhale faster
    C. Adjust the PEP device to have the patient exhale through a smaller hole
    D. Add a bronchodilator medication to the PEP device

11. When you are reviewing a patient's chart, it is important to look for indications for postural drainage. These would include all of the following EXCEPT:
    A. A patient with bronchiectasis and retained secretions
    B. A patient with cystic fibrosis who has retained secretions
    C. Draining of an empyema
    D. Removal of an aspirated foreign body

12. You receive an order to perform postural drainage, percussion, and vibration on a 23-year-old female patient. The lateral and medial segments of the right middle lobe are among those that need to be treated. You would proceed to
    A. Drain, percuss, and vibrate the segments
    B. Drain and vibrate the segments
    C. Drain but not percuss or vibrate those segments
    D. Drain and use a mechanical percussor

13. A patient is using the Flutter and coughs productively. Later, the patient tries to use the device but finds that no air will go through it. What should be done?
    A. Have the patient breathe in harder.
    B. Check for an obstruction.
    C. Remove the steel ball to reduce the backpressure.
    D. Have the patient blow out harder.

14. A patient with bilateral pneumonia is positioned for drainage of the lateral and medial segments of her right middle lobe. After 5 min in this position, the patient complains of SOB. The electrocardiogram shows the patient to be having premature ventricular contractions (PVCs). The most likely cause of this is
    A. Hypoxemia
    B. A full stomach that is causing vagal stimulation
    C. Increased intracranial pressure
    D. Increased venous return to the heart

15. You are using a pneumatically powered mechanical percussor on a patient receiving CPT. The unit is powered by an E-cylinder of O_2 because piped-in O_2 is unavailable. After a few minutes of operation, you notice that the percussor begins to slow down and then stops. What would you do?
    A. Switch to an electrically powered percussor.
    B. Make sure the cylinder is completely turned on.
    C. Check the unit's batteries.
    D. Check the electrical cord.

16. A mechanical percussor is ordered to assist with secretion clearance in a patient receiving CPT. The patient is positioned to drain the posterior basal segments of both lower lobes. The percussor is activated and applied to the patient's lower back. After 1 minute, the patient complains of skin discomfort. What should the respiratory therapist do?
    A. Have the patient sit up.
    B. Apply oxygen and check the pulse oximeter value.
    C. Increase the speed on the percussor.
    D. Change to another type of pad on the percussor.

17. A home care cystic fibrosis patient is starting HFCWO therapy. You would instruct the patient to do all of the following EXCEPT:
    A. Sit upright for the procedure.
    B. Set the controls to initially deliver the fastest rate and highest pressure.
    C. Connect the air hoses to the vest.
    D. Set the controls to initially deliver the slowest rate and lowest pressure.

1. A patient who is being instructed in positive expiratory pressure (PEP) therapy complains that it is taking too long to breathe out. What would you do?
   A. Tell the patient to blow out harder.
   B. Change the expiratory resistance to a larger diameter orifice.
   C. Change the expiratory resistance to a smaller diameter orifice.
   D. Increase the flow of oxygen to the system.

2. Your patient is 40 years old and had upper abdominal surgery 2 days ago. He is showing signs of atelectasis and retained secretions. Your instructions for a directed cough would include all of the following EXCEPT:
   A. Inhale as deep a breath as possible.
   B. Support the incision.
   C. Perform a serial cough at low air flows.
   D. Inhale and exhale several times before coughing.

3. A 56-year-old patient has been in the Trendelenburg position for 10 minutes receiving percussion and vibration. Tachycardia and dyspnea develop. Which of the following actions should be completed by the respiratory therapist?
   A. Continue for 5 minutes with gentle percussion.
   B. Turn the patient to the other side.
   C. Give the patient oxygen.
   D. Have the patient sit up.

4. A 12-year-old patient with cystic fibrosis had PEP therapy started at 5 cm water. After a few minutes of use, the patient has a strong but unproductive cough. What should be done now?
   A. Increase the PEP level to 10 cm water.
   B. Increase the PEP level to 15 cm water.
   C. Change to incentive spirometry.
   D. Discontinue the treatment.

5. After several days of receiving postural drainage and percussion therapy to all lobes in the left lung, the patient's chest radiograph shows improvement except for the lateral basal segment of the left lower lobe. In what position should he now be placed for postural drainage?
   A. Right side down with the head of the bed down 30 degrees
   B. Right side down with the bed flat
   C. Left side down with the head of the bed down 30 degrees
   D. Flat on his back with the bed flat and a pillow beneath the knees

6. For drainage of the superior and inferior lingula segments, the patient should be positioned
   1. With the foot of the bed elevated 14 inches
   2. One-fourth turn up from the front-down position on the bed
   3. One-fourth turn up from the back-down position on the bed
   4. With the foot of the bed elevated 30 degrees
   5. Flat on his or her back
   A. 1, 3
   B. 4, 5
   C. 1, 2
   D. 1, 5

7. The patient benefits from using the Flutter by which of the following?
   1. Increased transpleural pressure
   2. Airway vibrations
   3. Increased intrapleural pressure
   4. Rapid variation in airway pressure
   A. 1, 2
   B. 2, 3
   C. 3, 4
   D. 2, 4

8. A 48-year-old woman had her gallbladder removed. What is most effective in preventing postoperative atelectasis?
   A. Blow bottles
   B. PEP therapy
   C. Mechanical chest percussor
   D. Inspiratory muscle training

9. A patient is starting high-frequency chest wall oscillation (HFCWO) to help mobilize secretions. Which of the following instructions should the patient be given for the initial treatment?
   1. Lie on the side with the most secretions.
   2. Sit up straight.
   3. Set the controls at a low rate and pressure.
   4. Set the controls at a high rate and pressure.
   5. Set the unit for maximal nebulization during inspiration.
   A. 2, 3
   B. 1, 3
   C. 2, 4, 5
   D. 1, 3, 5

10. A 70-year-old patient who had a stroke has aspirated and now has a fever and pulmonary secretions. The respiratory therapist notices on the anteroposterior (AP) and right lateral chest radiographs that the posterior segment of the right upper lobe is opaque. What postural drainage position should be used with this patient?
    A. On the right side, head down 30 degrees, one-fourth turn up from face down
    B. Sitting upright and leaning forward 30 degrees
    C. Head down 15 degrees, pillow behind the right side to turn one-fourth turn up from flat
    D. Head down 15 degrees, pillow behind the left side to turn one-fourth turn up from flat

11. You are working with a patient who begins to expectorate blood after being positioned for drainage of the superior segment of the left lower lobe. Percussion was provided with a mechanical device. After the patient has expectorated 50 mL of blood, you would recommend the following as the best action:
    A. Continue the treatment because the patient has not lost a great deal of blood.
    B. Continue the treatment on only the upper and middle lobes.
    C. Stop the treatment, sit the patient up, and call the physician.
    D. Continue the treatment with manual percussion only.

12. CPT (postural drainage, percussion, and vibration) has been performed for 5 days on a cooperative patient with bronchiectasis. During that time, he has been treated with antibiotics and well-fed and hydrated. He has produced a total of 20 mL of sputum during the past 24 hr. What would you recommend?
    A. Continue the current treatment program for 48 hr and evaluate the patient again.
    B. Add ultrasonic nebulizer treatments to the CPT to better liquefy the secretions.
    C. Add nasotracheal suctioning to the CPT to remove the secretions.
    D. Discontinue the CPT and follow the patient's progress.

13. A 10-year-old patient with cystic fibrosis has large amounts of secretions. He cannot tolerate postural drainage because of nausea when he is tipped down. He is receiving aerosolized bronchodilator and mucolytic medications. To improve his condition, the respiratory therapist could recommend all of the following EXCEPT:
    A. OPEP therapy
    B. Flutter or Acapella unit
    C. High-frequency chest wall oscillation
    D. Continuous positive airway pressure (CPAP) at 10 cm water

14. Your 12-year-old patient does not tolerate postural drainage for secretion clearance. The physician wishes to consider high-frequency airway oscillation. Which of the following options would you recommend be tried first?
    A. HFCWO
    B. Acapella
    C. Intrapulmonary percussive ventilation (IPV)
    D. Autogenic drainage (AD)

11

Cardiac Monitoring and Cardiopulmonary Resuscitation

Note 1: This book is written to cover every item listed as testable on all *Entry Level Examination (ELE), Written Registry Examination (WRE),* and *Clinical Simulation Examination (CSE).*

The listed code for each item is taken from the National Board for Respiratory Care's (NBRC) **Summary Content Outline for CRT (Certified Respiratory Therapist) and Written RRT (Registered Respiratory Therapist) Examinations** (http://evolve.elsevier.com/ Sills/resptherapist/). For example, if an item is testable on both the ELE and WRE, it will simply be shown as (Code: . . .). If an item is only testable on the ELE, it will be shown as (ELE code: . . .). If an item is only testable on the WRE, it will be shown as (WRE code: . . .).

Following each item's code will be the difficulty level of the questions on that item on the ELE and WRE. (See the Introduction for a full explanation of the three question difficulty levels.) **Recall [R]** level questions typically expect the exam taker to recall factual information. **Application [Ap]** level questions are harder because the exam taker may have to apply factual information to a clinical situation. **Analysis [An]** level questions are the most challenging because the exam taker may have to use critical thinking to evaluate patient data to make a clinical decision.

Note 2: A review of the most recent Entry Level Examinations (ELE) has shown an average of six questions (out of 140), or 4% of the exam, will cover cardiac monitoring and cardiopulmonary resuscitation (CPR). A review of the most recent Written Registry Examinations (WRE) has shown an average of five questions (out of 100), or 5% of the exam, will cover cardiac monitoring and CPR. The Clinical Simulation Examination is comprehensive and may include everything that should be known by an advanced-level respiratory therapist.

MODULE A

Cardiac monitoring and diagnostic electrocardiogram

1. Manipulate electrocardiogram monitors by order or protocol (ELE code: IIA18) [Difficulty: ELE: R, Ap]

a. Get the necessary equipment for the procedure

To perform electrocardiogram (ECG) monitoring, it is necessary to select the proper cardiac electrodes and the monitoring unit. Cardiac electrodes, or leads, pick up the electrical signal from a heart contraction and conduct it to the monitor. They are usually called *chest leads* (or *chest electrodes* or *precordial leads*) and consist of four parts: (1) a conducting wire coated with an electrically neutral plastic, (2) an adapter at one end of the wire that plugs into the electrocardiograph machine, (3) a different adapter at the opposite end of the wire that attaches to a patient electrode, and (4) the patient electrode (Figure 11-1, *A*). Conducting jelly is added to the surface of the electrode to reduce the skin's resistance to the heart's electrical signal. An adhesive ring holds the electrode tightly to the skin. The conducting wire snaps or clips onto the back of the electrode. Typically, three to five of these chest leads are used for a period of hours or days for basic rhythm monitoring or Holter monitoring. Typically, three or four chest leads are used for rhythm monitoring. Holter monitoring typically involves using five chest leads.

One of the following monitoring units must be selected, based on the patient's situation:

1. Basic bedside rhythm monitoring

A bedside rhythm monitoring unit usually receives input from three or four chest leads (Figure 11-1, *B*). That collective signal is sent to an oscilloscope (video display terminal) for a real-time display of the patient's rhythm. These ECG machines have several additional features. They continuously display the patient's heart rate. High and low heart rate alarm settings can be set. If the high or low setting is reached, an audible and visual alarm is triggered. The patient's heart rhythm can be recorded on ECG paper manually by pushing a record button or automatically when an alarm setting is reached. These units are often seen mounted at the patient's bedside in the intensive care unit.

2. Cardiopulmonary resuscitation cart

Cardiopulmonary resuscitation (CPR) "crash" carts have electrocardiographs and oscilloscopes mounted on them. These are connected to the defibrillator to allow synchronous defibrillation (cardioversion) or asynchronous defibrillation. Typically, three or four chest leads are used for rhythm monitoring (Figure 11-1, *B*). Crash carts have other features that are similar to those seen on bedside

Figure 11-1 **A,** Close-up of the features of a prepackaged monitoring electrode or lead. **B,** Standard electrode placements for lead II monitoring. This results in the traditional-looking electrocardiogram waveform with upright P, QRS, and T waves. (Note: The electrodes are often labeled as right arm [RA] instead of negative pole, left arm [LA] instead of ground electrode, and left leg [LL] instead of positive electrode.) *(From Eubanks DH, Bone RC: Comprehensive respiratory care, ed 2, St Louis, 1990, Mosby.)*

Figure 11-2 Holter monitoring system for ambulatory electrocardiography. *(From Pagana K, Pagana TJ: Mosby's manual of diagnostic and laboratory tests, ed 3, St Louis, 2006, Mosby.)*

rhythm monitoring units. Portable versions of these units are used when the patient must be transported. A portable unit operates by battery power when unplugged from the wall electrical outlet.

3. Holter monitoring

Holter monitoring involves recording a patient's complete ECG for 1 to 3 days through the use of a portable, battery-powered monitor. In addition, the patient keeps a diary of any episodes of chest pain, dyspnea, and so forth. The whole system includes the recording device for the patient's ECG, a set of chest leads, a carrying bag for the recording device, and a patient activity diary (Figure 11-2).

a. Put the equipment together and make sure that it works properly. Connect the patient's chest leads cable into the proper monitor. Turn on the monitor, and select the desired electrical signal from the heart (usually lead II). Confirm that the electrical signal is displayed on the monitor, and set any alarm limits.

b. Troubleshoot any problems with the equipment. Successful ECG monitoring requires that the right electrodes be chosen, put together properly, attached to the patient as indicated, and connected to the correct ECG machine. Any errors will result in an electrical signal that is distorted or absent. Recheck all patient electrodes and wire connections if a problem is seen.

2. Manipulate diagnostic electrocardiogram machines by order or protocol (ELE code: IIA19) [Difficulty: ELE: R, Ap]

a. Get the necessary equipment for the procedure

To perform a diagnostic (also called *12-lead*) ECG, get the proper cardiac electrodes and recording electrocardiogram machine. These electrodes will only be use for a few minutes as the recording of the heart's activity is being done. They come in two sets, one for the limbs and one for the chest.

A 12-lead ECG test requires a machine capable of receiving electrical input from the four limb leads and six precordial leads (see Figures 11-3 and 11-4). The operator

Figure 11-3   Limb electrodes or leads properly placed on all four of the patient's limbs. Make sure that the right leg lead is placed on the right leg, the right arm lead is placed on the right arm, and so forth. The electrode cables are then plugged into the electrocardiograph machine to record the ECG tracings. *(From Eubanks DH, Bone RC: Comprehensive respiratory care, ed 2, St Louis, 1990, Mosby.)*

Figure 11-4   Proper placement of the six precordial leads. (See Table 10-1 for a description of the locations.) *(From Eubanks DH, Bone RC: Comprehensive respiratory care, ed 2, St Louis, 1990, Mosby.)*

can manually select the lead combinations needed to get the 12 different combinations for a 12-lead ECG tracing. However, modern units do this automatically when the operator turns them on. The various ECG combinations are printed out on ECG paper. Modern units also store the patient's information on a self-contained computer.

b. Put the equipment together and make sure that it works properly

The limb leads come as a group of four with one for each arm and leg (Figure 11-3). Precordial leads came in a group of six and are placed on the chest in the positions

shown in Figure 11-4. A conducting and adhesive jelly is used to reduce the skin's resistance and to hold the lead in place. The limb leads are longer, and they may need to be held in place by a rubber strap.

c. Troubleshoot any problems with the equipment

Successful ECG monitoring requires that the right electrodes be chosen, put together properly, attached to the patient as indicated, and connected to the correct ECG machine. Any errors will result in an electrical signal that is distorted or absent. With all types of cardiac leads, bad skin contact, dried conducting jelly, or a disconnected wire results in a distorted or absent electrical signal. Recheck all patient electrodes and wire connections if a problem is seen.

3. Cardiac monitoring

a. Review cardiac monitoring data in the patient record (Code: IIB8) [Difficulty: ELE: R; WRE: Ap]

Review the chart of any patient admitted with a significant cardiopulmonary problem for a record of previous cardiac monitoring. Look for a record of rhythm disturbances.

b. Recommend cardiac monitoring (Code: IC9) [Difficulty: ELE: R, Ap; WRE: An]

Recommend cardiac monitoring in any patient with a significant cardiopulmonary problem. This could include, but is not limited to, congestive heart failure, previous myocardial infarction, suspicion of current myocardial infarction, pulmonary embolism, pneumonia, or other problem that could result in serious hypoxemia.

c. Monitor the cardiac rhythm to evaluate the patient's response to respiratory care (Code: IIIE6) [Difficulty: ELE: R, Ap; WRE: An]

Many hospitalized patients have serious cardiopulmonary problems. The patient may receive supplemental oxygen or inhaled bronchodilator medications. If a possibility exists that the patient will experience significant changes in heart rate or rhythm, he or she should be continuously monitored. This could include patients with serious cardiopulmonary problems, as listed previously. In addition, it could be a patient with an electrolyte disturbance or who is receiving replacement electrolytes intravenously, especially potassium. A bedside rhythm monitoring unit should have an oscilloscope for viewing the rhythm and additional features for counting the heart rate, setting high and low heart rate alarms, and recording the rhythm on standard ECG paper for a permanent record.

The most common chest electrode pattern used for rhythm monitoring is called *lead II*. The three chest electrodes are placed as shown in Figure 11-1, B. The negative (right arm, RA) electrode is on the right upper chest. The positive (left leg, LL) electrode is placed on the left lateral chest. The ground (left arm, LA) electrode is placed on the left upper chest. With this electrode configuration, known as the Einthoven triangle, the heart's electrical signal is followed as it flows from the right atrium to the left ventricle. This results in the so-called normal ECG tracing with upright P, R, and T waves, as shown in Figures 11-5 and 11-6. Table 11-1 shows the sequential electrical events

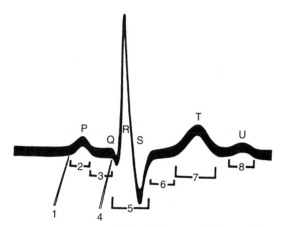

Figure 11-5 Sequence of electrical events of the cardiac cycle during normal sinus rhythm. (See Table 10-2 for the description of each event.) *(From Phillips RE, Feeney MK: The cardiac rhythms: a systematic approach to interpretation, ed 3, Philadelphia, 1990, Saunders.)*

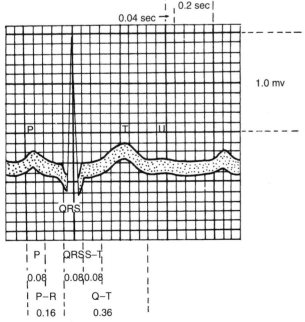

Figure 11-6 Timing of the electrical events of the cardiac cycle during normal sinus rhythm. *(From Spearman CB, Sheldon RL, Egan DF: Egan's fundamentals of respiratory therapy, ed 4, St Louis, 1982, Mosby.)*

of the normal cardiac rhythm that correspond with those in Figure 11-5.

Holter monitoring is done to evaluate noncritical, home care patients with a suspected cardiac problem. Because the patient will be mobile for at least 1 day, the limb leads are placed on the upper and lower chest area. Precordial leads are placed normally. The patient wears a tight-fitting undershirt or netlike dressing to keep the leads in place. The patient cannot bathe while the leads are on.

4. Diagnostic electrocardiogram

a. Review electrocardiogram data in the patient record (Code: IB8) [Difficulty: ELE: R; WRE: Ap]

Review the chart of any patient admitted with a significant cardiac problem for a record of a previous electrocardiogram. Look for a record of rhythm disturbances or diagnosis of the problem.

b. Recommend an electrocardiogram to obtain additional data (Code: IC9) [Difficulty: ELE: R, Ap; WRE: An]

A diagnostic electrocardiogram (also called a *12-lead ECG*) test is indicated if the patient is suspected of having cardiac problems. Symptoms such as syncope, angina pectoris, sudden crushing chest pain, shortness of breath, or unstable heart rate and blood pressure point to a heart

TABLE 11-1	Electrophysiologic Events Represented by the Electrocardiogram Sequential Electrical Events Electrocardiographic of the Cardiac Cycle Representation
1. Impulse from the sinus node	Not visible
2. Depolarization of the atria	P wave
3. Depolarization of the atrio-ventricular node	Isoelectric
4. Repolarization of the atria	Usually obscured by the QRS complex
5. Depolarization of the ventricles	QRS complex
a. Intraventricular septum	a. Initial portion
b. Right and left ventricles	b. Central and terminal portions
6. Quiescent state of the ventricles immediately after depolarization	ST segment: isoelectric
7. Repolarization of the ventricles	T wave
8. Afterpotentials following repolarization of the ventricles	U wave

From Phillips RE, Feeney MK: *The cardiac rhythms: a systematic approach to interpretation*, ed 3, Philadelphia, 1990, WB Saunders.

problem. Growing evidence indicates that men and women have different signs and symptoms during an acute myocardial infarction (AMI or MI). Men tend to have crushing central chest pain that may radiate down the left arm or the left side of the neck, diaphoresis, cold extremities, shortness of breath, and a feeling of impending doom. Women tend to experience pain in the lower back and the abdominal area. A diagnostic ECG is indicated to document the nature of the cardiac problem or rule out the heart as a source of the symptoms.

c. Perform a diagnostic electrocardiogram (Code: IB9a) [Difficulty: ELE: R, WRE: Ap, An]

The 12-lead ECG involves the use of an electrocardiograph machine with heat-sensitive ECG recording paper, four limb leads, and six precordial leads (see Figures 11-3 and 11-4). Table 11-2 describes the locations of the precordial leads and the positive and negative electrode combinations that are used to record the heart's electrical

signal through the 12 different leads. Each lead individually records the heart's electrical activity, but it does so from a different position in relation to the heart. These 12 leads give the physician a three-dimensional impression of how the cardiac conduction system and the myocardium are functioning. Abnormal functioning can be diagnosed. Review the normal anatomy and physiology of the heart and its conduction system, if necessary.

Clinical experience is important in performing a diagnostic ECG. Improper placement of the precordial or limb leads can easily result in a misleading ECG tracing and a misdiagnosis. For example, reversing the arm leads causes the QRS to be reversed in lead I. Technical errors in grounding the patient and not keeping the patient still during the ECG also result in useless tracings because of electrical interference and an unstable baseline.

TABLE 11-2   Standard Electrocardiogram Leads

	Leads	Positive Electrode	Negative Electrode
Bipolar	1. I	Left arm	and Right arm
	2. II	Left leg	and Right arm
	3. III	Left leg	and Left arm
Unipolar	4. aV_R	Right arm	Central terminal*
	5. aV_L	Left arm	
	6. aV_F	Left leg	
Precordial	7. V_1	Right of sternum in 4th intercostal space (4th ICS)	Central terminal*
	8. V_2	Left of sternum in 4th ICS	
	9. V_3	Midway between V_2 and V_4	
	10. V_4	Midclavicular line in 5th ICS	
	11. V_5	Midway between V_4 and V_6	
	12. V_6	Lateral chest in 5th ICS	

*The *central terminal* is a combination of electrode potentials, producing a summation effect. This serves as the single negative or *indifferent* electrode. The specific combination of electrodes for each lead is automatically determined in the lead selector switch.
aV, augmented voltage; *ICS*, intercostal space.
From Phillips RE, Feeney MK: *The cardiac rhythms: a systematic approach to interpretation*, ed 3, Philadelphia, 1990, WB Saunders.

Exam Hint 11-1 (ELE)

The NBRC does not specifically list cardiac electrodes on it content outlines. However, recent exams have had questions about troubleshooting problems with electrodes and artifacts when performing an electrocardiogram (ECG).

Exam Hint 11-2 (ELE, WRE)

Usually one or two questions require the respiratory therapist to recognize possible signs of a myocardial infarction and recommend either ECG monitoring or the performance of a diagnostic 12-lead ECG.

MODULE B
Cardiopulmonary resuscitation equipment

1. Manipulate a manual resuscitator (bag-valve or bag-mask by order or protocol (ELE code: IIA5) [Difficulty: ELE: R, Ap, An]

a. Get the necessary equipment for the procedure

The first consideration when deciding which manual resuscitator to select is the size of the patient. Although the volume of the reservoir bag and the tidal volume expelled from it vary among the types of bags, three basic sizes are available. An infant or newborn unit typically has a reservoir bag volume of about 250 mL. A pediatric unit usually has a reservoir bag volume of about 250 to 500 mL, and an adult unit typically has a reservoir bag volume of 1500 to 2000 mL. In addition to all of these reusable units, a number of disposable units are thrown away after one patient use. They also come in comparable infant, pediatric, and adult reservoir bag volumes.

Any unit should deliver 100% oxygen at the flow rate of 15 L/min. An oxygen reservoir system must be added to the basic unit to achieve these oxygen percentages. The valve to the patient must be clearable within 20 seconds if it becomes fouled by vomitus, sputum, or blood.

Neonatal and pediatric units must have a pressure release (pop-off) valve that opens at 40 cm H₂O pressure. The pressure may be adjustable. If an adult unit has a pressure release valve, it must have an override system that is easy to operate.

b. Put the equipment together and make sure that it works properly

Figure 11-7 shows line drawings of a complete set of Laerdal infant, pediatric, and adult manual resuscitators. The following steps should be taken when the function of a manual resuscitator is evaluated:

1. Squeeze and release the bag to see if the nonrebreathing valve and air/oxygen reservoir intake valve open and close properly.
2. Feel the air leave the outlet port of the nonrebreathing valve when the bag is squeezed.
3. Occlude the outlet port, and squeeze the bag. No gas should leak out. If present, the pop-off valve should open at the correct pressure.
4. The face mask should fit onto the 22-mm outer diameter (OD) fitting and have its cushion properly inflated. The mask is selected based on the size of the patient's face. As Figure 11-7 shows, the masks come in pediatric, infant, and adult sizes.

c. Troubleshoot any problems with the equipment

Check for a reversed or improperly seated one-way valve (spring-loaded, duckbill, or leaf type) if the gas does not enter or exit the unit as it should. In clinical use, mucus,

Figure 11-7 **A,** Cutaway drawings of a resuscitation bag showing its features and how the one-way valves open and close during exhalation and inhalation. Note that during exhalation, the patient's breath is vented to the room and supplemental oxygen is drawn from the reservoir bag into the main bag. To deliver a breath to the patient, the operator squeezes the main bag. This opens the valve to the patient and closes the valve from the reservoir bag. **B,** Photograph showing an adult, child, and infant resuscitation bag with attached face mask and oxygen reservoir bag. These features are found on all modern units: a self-filling main bag, exhalation valve that does not jam at an oxygen flow of 15 L/min or in subfreezing temperatures (it must be clearable of debris within 20 seconds), intake valve for adding draw room air or supplemental oxygen into the reservoir bag, transparent mask that easily conforms to the patient's face, pressure relief (pop-off) valve that is set to open at 40 cm water, standard 15-mm inner diameter/22-mm outer diameter connector for the endotracheal tube or face mask, and an oxygen enrichment/reservoir system. In addition, some units have an adjustable positive end-expiratory pressure valve (not shown) attached to the exhalation valve. (**A** from Cairo JM, Pilbeam SP: Mosby's respiratory care equipment, ed 8, St Louis, 2010, Mosby. **B** courtesy Laerdal Medical, Wappingers Falls, NY.)

vomitus, and blood can foul the expiratory one-way valve system. By regulation, the valve must be clearable within 20 seconds. Do this by disconnecting the unit from the patient, aiming the adapter into a neutral area, and squeezing the bag to blow out the obstruction. Replace a unit that cannot be promptly cleared of any debris.

2. Manipulate a mouth-to-valve mask resuscitator (ELE code: IIA5) [Difficulty: ELE: R, Ap, An]

a. Get the necessary equipment for the procedure

The following are important considerations when selecting the best mouth-to-valve device (also called a mouth-to-mask device or pocket mask) for the victim:

- The mask must fit the victim's face so that no air leak is present. Infant, child, and adult sizes should be available.
- The mouthpiece should be designed so that it fits only one way into the mask. Some units include a short length of aerosol tubing between the mouthpiece and mask for greater flexibility.
- The one-way (nonrebreathing) valve should be designed to ensure that all of the rescuer's breath is directed into the victim and the victim's exhaled breath is vented to room air rather than back at the rescuer. Some units include a bacteria filter in the one-way valve between the rescuer and victim.
- It should be possible to add supplemental oxygen through a T-piece or nipple on the mask. This is important for hospital or ambulance use. If a T-piece is added, it must be designed to easily fit between the mouthpiece and face mask. An oxygen administration nipple should have a cap over it when not in use to prevent any leakage of the delivered breath.

b. Put the equipment together and make sure that it works properly

Mouth-to-valve resuscitators are relatively simple devices. Most have only two or three pieces: a face mask, a mouthpiece with a one-way valve, and possibly an oxygen T-piece (Figure 11-8). The "male" and "female" connections are designed to fit together in only one way. When they are properly assembled, no air should leak out when the breath is delivered to the victim.

c. Troubleshoot any problems with the equipment

If the breath cannot be delivered, check the one-way valve to make sure that it has not been put together backward. Reverse it, if necessary, and ventilate the victim's airway. Keep the oxygen nipple on the mask or T-piece capped off if it is not being used. Air will leak out during the delivered breath if the cap is left off the nipple.

Figure 11-8 Proper positioning to use a mouth-to-valve mask resuscitator. The top rescuer has added supplemental oxygen to the device. The bottom rescuer is ventilating without the use of added oxygen. *(Courtesy Laerdal Medical Corporation, Wappingers Falls, NY.)*

Exam Hint 11-3 (ELE)

Usually an exam question deals with a malfunctioning manual resuscitator or mouth-to-valve resuscitator. Often the question involves identifying that the patient's chest does not rise despite the ventilating device being used to deliver a breath. Fixing the problem can involve clearing an obstruction or properly assembling a one-way valve. If the unit cannot be quickly repaired, it should be replaced.

Exam Hint 11-4 (ELE)

An endotracheal tube should be inserted into the patient as soon as possible during a CPR attempt. If an endotracheal tube cannot be placed, a laryngeal mask airway (LMA) or Combitube can be inserted. Then, a manual resuscitation bag with 100% oxygen should be used to ventilate the patient. Less effective ventilation methods include a mouth-to-mask valve or bag-mask system. A gas-powered pneumatic (demand valve) resuscitator should not be used because the delivered tidal volume is unpredictable and too large a volume can cause barotrauma.

MODULE C

Perform cardiopulmonary resuscitation and related functions

1. Basic cardiac life support (ELE code: III I1a) [Difficulty: ELE: R, Ap, An]

The key steps of basic cardiac life support (BCLS) include the following:

a. Establish that the patient is unresponsive and needs cardiopulmonary resuscitation

Observing a patient who *appears* to be dead does not prove that the patient needs CPR. Clinical death must be proved before CPR is begun. Adults should be tapped or gently shaken while you shout, "Are you okay?" Infants should have the bottom of their feet gently slapped while you shout, "Wake up!" The rescuer also can clap his or her hands together loudly to wake a sleeping infant. CPR should never be started on a person who does not need it.

b. Call out for help

Call out for help if the victim does not respond to any attempts at arousal. The second rescuer should be told to call in the cardiac arrest team. Many hospitals have a cardiac arrest button in each patient's room. If this is the case, the first rescuer can push the button while calling out for help. Dial 911 if the victim is found at home.

c. Open the airway

The head-tilt/chin-lift maneuver is the procedure of choice for opening the airways of all victims except those with a known or suspected cervical (neck) spine injury. The victim is gently positioned on his or her back. In an adult, the head is firmly pushed back with one hand, and the jaw is pulled upward with the fingers of the other hand (Figure 11-9). In an infant, it is not necessary to tilt the

head back beyond a neutral position. Children may need to have the head pushed back slightly beyond neutral.

The jaw-thrust maneuver is the procedure of choice for opening the airway of all victims with a known or suspected cervical spine injury. The rescuer's elbows are rested on the ground, and the hands are placed on either side of the victim's jaw. Lifting of the jaw usually opens the airway and eliminates the need to tilt the head back. See Figure 11-10 for the adult maneuver.

Any obstruction that can be seen in the mouth or throat should be removed. The cross-finger technique can be used to open the mouth wide enough so that a finger or suction device can be inserted to remove a blockage (Figure 11-11). An oral airway should be used only in an unconscious patient to keep the tongue from falling back and blocking the airway.

d. Determine that the patient is not breathing

The rescuer places his or her face close to the victim's face to *look* for rising and falling of the chest, *listen* for victim's

Figure 11-10   Opening the adult's airway by the jaw-thrust method. *(From Watson MA: Cardiopulmonary resuscitation. In: Barnes TA, editor: Respiratory care practice, St Louis, 1988, Mosby.)*

Figure 11-9   Opening the adult's airway. *Top,* Airway obstruction produced by the tongue and epiglottis. *Bottom,* Relief by head-tilt/chin-lift method. *(From Standards and guidelines for cardiopulmonary resuscitation [CPR] and emergency cardiac care [ECC], JAMA 268:2186, 1992.) Copyright © 1992, American Medical Association. All rights reserved.*

Figure 11-11   The cross-finger method of opening the victim's mouth to look for an obstruction. *(From Watson MA: Cardiopulmonary resuscitation. In: Barnes TA, editor: Respiratory care practice, St Louis, 1988, Mosby.)*

air movement, and *feel* any air movement from the victim's breathing (Figure 11-12). The entire procedure should not take longer than 10 seconds.

e. Ventilate the patient
1. Mouth-to-mouth breathing

The first rescuer should begin mouth-to-mouth breathing as soon as possible if no spontaneous breathing by the victim occurs once the airway is opened. No matter the age of the victim, an effective seal must be present between the rescuer and the victim. The adult victim's nose must be pinched closed; often the rescuer's cheek can block the infant's nose. The rescuer's mouth can cover both the nose and mouth of an infant. Alternative methods include mouth-to-nose and mouth-to-stoma ventilation (Figure 11-13).

In an adult, two breaths large enough to raise the victim's chest should be given. An adequate volume of 500 to 600 mL may be given. Blow into the victim's mouth for more than 1 second. This is to ensure a large enough volume without having to use much pressure. Keeping the ventilating pressure as low as possible minimizes the risk of forcing air into the stomach. Ensure that the victim exhales completely by watching the chest fall and feeling the air escape against your cheek. Rescue breathing should be performed at a rate of 10 to 12 times per minute (every 4 to 5 seconds) if the victim has a pulse but is apneic.

A child should be given two breaths large enough to raise the victim's chest. A child obviously needs less

A

B

Figure 11-12 Determining breathlessness by looking, listening, and feeling. *(From Standards and guidelines for cardiopulmonary resuscitation [CPR] and emergency cardiac care [ECC], JAMA 268:2187, 1992.) Copyright © 1992, American Medical Association. All rights reserved.*

C

Figure 11-13 **A,** Adult mouth-to-mouth, mouth-to-nose (**B**), and mouth-to-stoma (**C**) ventilation. *(From Standards and guidelines for cardiopulmonary resuscitation [CPR] and emergency cardiac care [ECC], JAMA 268:2188, 1992.) Copyright © 1992, American Medical Association. All rights reserved.*

volume than an adult. All of the same considerations apply as for the adult. Rescue breathing should be performed at a rate of 12 to 20 per minute (every 3 to 5 seconds) in an infant and a child. A newly born infant should be ventilated at a rate of 40 to 60 per minute.

If the victim's airway cannot be ventilated, reposition the head and attempt to ventilate again. Failure to ventilate a second time means that the victim has an obstructed airway. The following steps should be taken:

a. **Unconscious adult obstructed airway maneuvers**

1. *Position.* Place the victim on his or her back.

2. *Heimlich maneuver.* Perform the Heimlich maneuver (also known as abdominal thrusts) several times, if needed, by kneeling astride the victim, placing the heel of one hand midline on the abdomen slightly above the navel, but well below the xiphoid process. The other hand is placed on top, and both are quickly thrust upward toward the chest (Figure 11-14). The rescuer can also perform chest thrusts on the markedly obese or obviously pregnant victim. The rescuer's hands should be placed on the lower half of the sternum as with cardiac compressions. Several compressions should be performed slowly but similarly to a cardiac compression.

3. *Finger sweep.* Attempt to clear out any foreign body with a finger sweep. Only attempt this when solid material can be seen in the throat of an unconscious patient. First, grasp the victim's tongue and jaw between your thumb and fingers, and lift the jaw open. Next, insert the index

Figure 11-14 Administering the Heimlich maneuver to an unconscious adult victim of an airway obstruction. *(From Standards and guidelines for cardiopulmonary resuscitation [CPR] and emergency cardiac care [ECC], JAMA 268:2193, 1992.) Copyright © 1992, American Medical Association. All rights reserved.*

finger of the other hand along the inside of the victim's cheek and down the back of the throat so as to hook and remove food, gum, dentures, and so on.

b. **Unconscious child (1 year old and older) obstructed airway maneuvers**

1. *Position.* Same as the adult position previously described.

2. *Heimlich maneuver.* Same as the adult maneuver but with up to five thrusts performed if needed. Chest thrusts are not used.

3. *Finger sweep.* Only attempt this when solid material can be seen in the throat of an unconscious patient. Remember that blindly inserting the index finger may push a foreign body farther down the throat.

c. **Unconscious infant obstructed airway maneuver**

1. *Position.* The infant is straddled over the rescuer's forearm. The infant's jaw and head are held by the rescuer's hand. The infant's head should be lower than the body. Five firm back blows are delivered between the shoulder blades with the heel of the rescuer's other hand (Figure 11-15).

2. *Heimlich maneuver.* The infant is sandwiched by the rescuer's other arm, and the head and body are supported and turned to a supine position. The head should remain lower than the body. Five chest thrusts are performed in the same location and manner as cardiac compressions but at a slower rate. These steps can be done by placing the infant on the rescuer's lap.

3. *Finger sweep.* Same as finger sweep in the unconscious child, mentioned previously.

2. Manual resuscitator (bag-valve)

A manual resuscitator should be used during hospital-based CPR as soon as one is available. The resuscitation mask must be held to the victim's face so that no air leak occurs during the forced inspiration (Figure 11-16). An assistant can hold the mask tightly to the face so that the rescuer who is pumping the resuscitation bag can use both hands. This has been shown to produce a larger tidal volume. If the victim's airway contains an endotracheal tube or tracheostomy tube, the expiratory valve adapter fits directly over the tube adapter. Rescue breathing continues with the previously mentioned considerations for volume and rate. After an adult victim has had an endotracheal tube placed, the tidal volume goal is 500 to 600 mL over a 1-second period to produce a visible chest rise.

3. Mouth-to-valve mask ventilation

A mouth-to-valve mask device (or *pocket mask*) combines a resuscitation mask with a one-way valve mouthpiece. It is used to ventilate an apneic patient rather than perform mouth-to-mouth breathing. Concerns about protecting the rescuer from patient infections such as acquired immunodeficiency syndrome (AIDS) and hepatitis have

A

Figure 11-16 Ventilation of an adult with a manual resuscitation bag and mask. *(From Eubanks DH, Bone RC: Comprehensive respiratory care, ed 2, St Louis, 1990, Mosby.)*

B

Figure 11-15 Administering **(A)** back blows and **(B)** chest thrusts to an infant victim of an obstructed airway. *(From Standards and guidelines for cardiopulmonary resuscitation [CPR] and emergency cardiac care [ECC], JAMA 268:2258, 1992.) Copyright © 1992, American Medical Association. All rights reserved.*

led to their widespread acceptance. As shown in Figure 11-8, the patient's neck is hyperextended, the mask is applied over the mouth and nose to get an airtight seal, and the rescuer breathes into the mouthpiece. It is best if the rescuer is positioned at the victim's head so that the chest can be seen to rise with each delivered breath. The one-way valve is designed so that the victim's exhaled gas is vented out to the room air. Some units have a nipple adapter so that supplemental oxygen can be added to the delivered breath. Simply attach oxygen tubing between the nipple and oxygen flowmeter, and turn the flowmeter

on to the manufacturer's recommended flow. When this type of device is used with an adult victim, the tidal volume goal is 500 to 600 mL over a 1-second period to produce a visible chest rise. These devices should be replaced by a manual resuscitator as soon as possible.

f. Add supplemental oxygen (ELE code: IIID6) [Difficulty: ELE: R, Ap, An]

The victim should be given 100% oxygen as soon as possible. There is no contraindication for giving pure oxygen during a resuscitation effort. This can be done easily if a manual resuscitator is used to ventilate the victim. All modern units are capable of delivering 100% oxygen when receiving an oxygen flow of at least 10 to 12 liters/minute and a reservoir is added.

g. Determine pulselessness

The carotid pulse is felt for in all victims except children younger than 1 year. The carotid pulse is found by gently feeling with two or three fingers in the groove between the larynx and the sternocleidomastoid muscle on either side of the neck (Figure 11-17). Check for 5 to 10 seconds to be sure that the victim is pulseless and not just brady-cardic. In addition, check for other signs of circulation such as spontaneous breathing, coughing, and move-ment. An infant younger than 1 year should have the pulse felt in the brachial artery; the carotid artery is dif-ficult to find in such young children because they have short, chubby necks.

The femoral pulse can be felt for as an alternative site in victims in the hospital who are wearing few clothes. Once the CPR team has arrived and two-person CPR is instituted, the femoral pulse may be most accessible for monitoring the pulse and the effectiveness of the chest compressions.

Figure 11-17 Determining pulselessness by checking the carotid pulse of an adult. *(From Standards and guidelines for cardiopulmonary resuscitation [CPR] and emergency cardiac care [ECC], JAMA 268:2189, 1992.)*

h. Perform external chest compressions

The absence of a palpable pulse confirms a cardiac arrest. Blood must be pumped by external chest compressions of the heart. The victim must be supine on a hard surface. A CPR backboard is placed behind a victim who is in bed.

In adults and large children or those older than 8 years, the heel of the rescuer's hand is placed over the lower half of the sternum. This is found by placing the middle finger of one hand in the notch where the ribs meet the sternum, placing the index finger next to it, and placing the other hand next to the finger. The first hand is placed over it, the elbows are locked, and the shoulders are directly over the hands. This creates the most efficient pumping action (Figure 11-18). The rescuer pivots from the hips, with half of the time spent pumping down and half of the time releasing pressure. The hands should always touch the victim's chest. The sternum must be compressed 4 to 5 cm (1.5 to 2.0 inches) in an adult at a rate of 100 compressions per minute for an actual rate of more than 80 per minute.

In a child 8 years old or younger, hand position is found as in the adult. The child's sternum must be compressed with *one* hand to a depth of 2.5 to 4 cm (1 to 1.5 inches). Half of the time should be spent on compression and half on relaxation. The rate should be 100 compressions per minute for a rate of more than 80 per minute between ventilations.

In newly born infants and older infants, the preferred method of chest compressions is called the two thumbs–encircling hands technique (Figure 11-19). This method works best when a second rescuer can ventilate the infant. It also is acceptable to compress with two or three fingers placed over the middle of the sternum one finger's width below an imaginary line drawn between the nipples

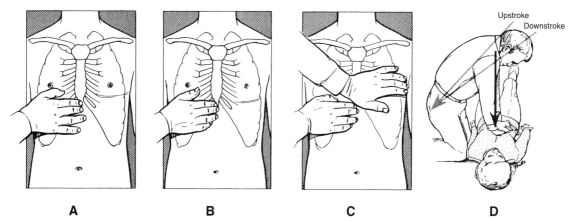

A   B   C   D

Figure 11-18 Cardiac compression of an adult. **A,** Locate tip of xiphoid process. **B,** Place two fingertips at xiphoid process. **C,** Place palm of other hand on sternum next to fingers. **D,** Arm and body positions for cardiac compression. *(From Barnes TA, editor: Respiratory care practice, St Louis, 1988, Mosby.)*

Figure 11-19 The preferred way to provide chest compressions on a newly born neonate is called two thumbs-encircling hands. This method is best when one rescuer can provide chest compressions and another can ventilate the patient. The two thumbs are placed over the sternum and below an imaginary line between the nipples. If the newborn is very small, the two thumbs can overlap. *(From Wilkins RL, Stoller JK, Kacmarek RM: Egan's fundamentals of respiratory care, ed 9, St. Louis, 2009, Mosby.)*

Figure 11-20 Locating the proper finger position for chest compressions on an infant. *(From Standards and guidelines for cardiopulmonary resuscitation [CPR] and emergency cardiac care [ECC], JAMA 268:2256, 1992.) Copyright © 1992, American Medical Association. All rights reserved.)*

(Figure 11-20). This method is easier when one rescuer must provide ventilations and compressions. In either case, the child's sternum must be compressed to a depth of 1.3 to 2.5 cm (0.5 to 1 in.). Half the time should be spent on compression and half the time on relaxation. A newly born infant should have a rate of at least 120 compressions per minute to achieve an actual rate of 90 per minute.

The steps for one- and two-person hospital-based CPR follow.

1. Adult one-rescuer CPR

1. Assess the victim's need for CPR.
2. Call out for help.
3. Open the airway.
4. Assess the victim's lack of breathing.
5. Give two rescue breaths.
6. Assess the victim's lack of a pulse.
7. Perform 30 chest compressions at a rate of 100 compressions per minute.
8. Reopen the airway, and give two breaths of more than 1-second duration to produce visible chest rise.
9. Repeat this cycle (30:2 ratio) a total of five times.
10. Check the victim's carotid pulse for less than 10 seconds. If it has not returned, give two breaths, and continue with compressions.
11. If the pulse has returned, check on the return of breathing. If it has not returned, give 10 to 12 breaths per minute.
12. If CPR is continued, check for the return of a heartbeat and breathing after five cycles.

2. Adult two-rescuer CPR

1. Perform steps 1 to 6, as previously described, for adult one-rescuer CPR.
2. If the victim has not been intubated, the compression/ventilation ratio should be 30:2.
3. After the victim has had an endotracheal tube inserted (or laryngeal mask airway or Combitube), the compression/ventilation ratio changes. The compressing rescuer delivers continuous chest compressions at a rate of 100 per minute without pausing for ventilation.
4. The second rescuer gives 8 to 10 breaths per minute (about every 6 seconds). A manual resuscitator with 100% oxygen is used to ventilate the victim.
5. Provide breathing, circulation, or both, as needed. If CPR is continued, check for the return of a heartbeat and breathing every few minutes.
6. Switch positions whenever one rescuer becomes tired, about every 2 minutes. Make the switch at the end of a cycle, check the victim for a return of pulse or breathing, and continue as needed.

3. Infant and child one- and two-rescuer CPR

1. Perform steps 1 to 6, as described for adult one-rescuer CPR.
2. If the victim has not been intubated, the compression/ventilation ratio should be 15:2.
3. After the victim has had an endotracheal tube inserted (or laryngeal mask airway or Combitube), the compression/ventilation ratio changes. The compressing rescuer

delivers continuous chest compressions at a rate of 100 per minute without pausing for ventilation.

4. The second rescuer gives 8 to 10 breaths per minute (about every 6 seconds). A manual resuscitator with 100% oxygen is used to ventilate the victim.

5. Provide breathing and circulation or both as needed. If CPR is continued, check for the return of a heartbeat and breathing every few minutes.

6. Switch positions whenever one rescuer becomes tired; about every 2 minutes. Make the switch at the end of a cycle, check the victim for a return of pulse or breathing, and continue as needed.

4. Neonatal one and two-rescuer CPR

1. Perform steps 1 to 4 as described for adult one-rescuer CPR.

2. If the patient is apneic or if breathing is inadequate, provide ventilations at a rate of 40 to 60 per minute. In the hospital setting, provide bag-mask ventilation with 100% oxygen.

3. Check the pulse.

4. Begin chest compressions if the heart rate is less than 60 beats per minute despite assisted ventilation with supplemental oxygen for 30 seconds.

5. The ratio of chest compressions to ventilations is 3:1. These are delivered at a rate of 90 compressions per minute and 30 breaths per minute.

6. Assess the patient's heart rate, respirations, and color about every 30 seconds.

7. Continue CPR efforts until the spontaneous heart rate is at least 60 beats per minute.

8. Continue assisted ventilation with oxygen at a rate of 40 to 60 per minute, if needed.

Exam Hint 11-5 (ELE, WRE)

Past exam questions have focused on adult basic cardiac life support (BCLS) procedures. This information is now listed as exclusively testable on the Entry-Level Exam. ACLS level questions will be found primarily on the Written Registry Exam.

Exam Hint 11-6 (ELE, WRE)

There is usually at least one CPR-related question that may include an ECG tracing. Usually it is of *ventricular tachycardia* or *ventricular fibrillation*. The question usually involves the patient being pulseless or without a blood pressure. The therapist must realize that the situation is life threatening and requires CPR or defibrillation.

---

2. Advanced cardiac life support (Code: III I1b) [Difficulty: ELE: R, Ap; WRE: An]

It is beyond the scope of this text to present advanced cardiac life support (ACLS) in detail. The following items relate to procedures that are important in the care of adult, pediatric, and neonatal patients needing advanced resuscitation.

a. Interpret the results of a diagnostic electrocardiogram (Code: IB10a) [Difficulty: ELE: R, Ap; WRE: An]

1. ECG paper

Before discussing 12-lead ECG interpretation, it is important to understand how ECG paper is designed so that the heart's electrical signal traced on it can be understood. This special paper is heat sensitive and, after exiting the ECG machine, shows a black line from the heated stylus. Figure 11-21 shows the grid markings on the paper and how to interpret the ECG tracing for voltage and time. Each large square box is 5 mm in height and represents 0.5 millivolts (mV) of the heart's electrical force. The large square box is divided into five smaller boxes that are 1 mm in height and represent 0.1 mV. Timing of the ECG tracing is determined by the speed with which the paper passes under the heated stylus. Normally, this is 25 mm/sec. At this speed, each large square box is 20 seconds, and each of the five small boxes is 0.04 seconds; 300 large boxes compose 1 minute's time (0.20 seconds ¥ 300 = 60 seconds).

Figure 11-21 ECG paper with added details on how to interpret time and voltage. *(From Patel JM, McGowan SG, Moody LA:* Arrhythmias: detection, treatment, and cardiac drugs, *Philadelphia, 1989, Saunders.)*

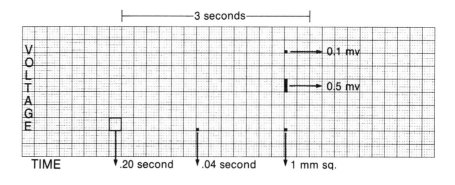

The following 10 features should be examined and time interval measured in every ECG:

1. Heart rate
2. Rhythm
3. P wave
4. PR interval
5. QRS interval
6. QRS complex
7. ST segment
8. T wave
9. QT interval
10. U wave

The systematic evaluation of these factors usually results in a clear understanding of the patient's cardiac function. All of these factors are discussed and illustrated in this chapter. Before evaluating the ECG paper tracing for possible cardiac arrhythmias, first rule out any artifacts and determine the patient's heart rate.

2. Artifacts

An ECG *artifact* is an artificially made electrical signal that does not relate to the patient's heart activity. An artifact can usually fall into one of three causes. First, the ECG electrodes are not in good contact with the skin or placed in the wrong area. For example, a chest lead has come off or the limb leads are reversed. Second, wires from another monitoring system are in contact with the ECG leads and there is electrical interference. Third, unusual electrical activity is coming from the patient. For example, the patient is shivering, having muscle tremors, or seizures. The respiratory therapist can cause an artifact by performing chest percussion over a patient's chest ECG lead. In many cases, artifacts can be eliminated by the filtering systems built into the recording unit. In other cases, the underlying problem will have to be corrected in order to get an accurate electrical signal showing cardiac activity.

3. Heart rate

The *heart rate* can be most accurately found by counting it for 1 minute; however, this time-consuming method is not always practical. An approximate heart rate can be quickly found. First, find a heartbeat tracing in which the R wave is on a heavy vertical line. Then count the number of large boxes between this first R wave and the next R wave. Approximate heart rates can be estimated as follows:

- Two large boxes = 150 beats/min (300 divided by 2)
- Three large boxes = 100 beats/min (300 divided by 3)
- Four large boxes = 75 beats/min (300 divided by 4)
- Five large boxes = 60 beats/min (300 divided by 5)
- Six large boxes = 50 beats/min (300 divided by 6)

For example, in Figure 11-22, during inspiration there are three large boxes between R waves for a heart rate of about 100/minute. During exhalation there are four large boxes between R waves for a heart rate of about 75/minute.

a. Normal sinus rhythm. Obviously, the normal cardiac rhythm must be understood to distinguish it from the abnormal rhythms. The normal adult's cardiac rhythm is usually called normal sinus rhythm (NSR) and has these characteristics:

- Heart rate between 60 and 100 beats/min while at rest
- Rhythm that varies by no more than ± 10% between QRS complexes
- P wave before every QRS complex and upright in lead II
- A QRS complex follows every P wave
- Proper timing of the components of the ECG rhythm Figure 11-6 shows the timing of the components of a normal sinus rhythm.

b. Abnormal cardiac rhythms. The following list of abnormal cardiac rhythms (usually called arrhythmias or dysrhythmias) includes many of those that are commonly encountered in clinical practice. It is beyond the scope of this text to discuss all possible arrhythmias. Instead, those that are either frequently seen or dangerous are described. Each of the following cardiac irregularities is (1) defined, (2) exemplified, (3) described, (4) discussed in terms of its clinical significance, and (e) accompanied by a treatment (if any) description.

1. Arrhythmias with a sinoatrial node origin. The following three arrhythmias all originate from the sinoatrial (SA) node. The electrical signal follows the normal pathway and results in contraction of both atria and

Figure 11-22 Sinus arrhythmia showing slightly increased heart rate during inspiration and slightly decreased heart rate during exhalation. *(From Goldberger AL: Clinical electrocardiography: a simplified approach, ed 7, St Louis, 2006, Mosby.)*

ventricles, as expected. They are distinguished from NSR by the differences in rate and regularity of the impulses.

a. Sinus arrhythmia. This arrhythmia is characterized by normal complexes but is a heart rate that varies with the respiratory cycle (see Figure 11-22 for an example). Notice how the QRS complexes are closer together on inspiration than on expiration. This is because the increased venous return to the heart during inspiration causes the heart to fill more quickly, so that the pulse rate quickens. The opposite rhythm effect is sometimes seen with a patient on a mechanical ventilator. No cardiac treatment is needed. Every attempt should be made to lower the intrathoracic pressure in the mechanically ventilated patient.

b. Sinus tachycardia. Sinus tachycardia in the adult is defined as a heart rate of more than 100 beats/min while at rest. All complexes are normal, and the rate is seldom more than 140 (see Figure 11-23 for an example). Causes include caffeine, anxiety, fever, pain, or hypotension. Correction of the problem results in the heart rate decreasing to the normal range. Cardiac drugs are not needed.

c. Sinus bradycardia. Sinus bradycardia is defined as a heart rate of less than 60 beats/min while at rest (Figure 11-24). All complexes remain normal. This is commonly seen in well-trained athletes during rest and in patients receiving digitalis or morphine. Cardiac drugs are not needed.

If sinus bradycardia is associated with a myocardial infarct, it may result in fainting or congestive heart failure (pulmonary edema). The patient must be treated not only for the heart attack but also to increase the heart rate.

Atropine is the first medication given to speed the heart rate. A pacemaker is needed if the patient does not respond to medications and continues to have symptoms.

2. Arrhythmias with an abnormal atrial origin. The following three arrhythmias originate in either one or both atria from a source other than the SA node. The electrical signal travels through the atria, which contracts them. It then moves on to the atrioventricular (AV) node and the ventricles, which contract normally. All of these arrhythmias result in faster than normal atrial contraction and often in a faster than normal ventricular contraction.

a. Paroxysmal atrial tachycardia. Paroxysmal atrial tachycardia (PAT) (also known as paroxysmal supraventricular tachycardia [PSVT]) is a series of three or more premature atrial contractions. It is characterized by a heart rate between 140 and 250 beats/min with an average rate of 180. The ECG tracing will show a normal QRS complex after each P wave (Figure 11-25). Notice the abnormal origin of the P wave seen during the PAT episode. The recommended term for any abnormal origin to a heartbeat is *focus*. The term *foci* refers to more than one abnormal site to a heartbeat.

Patients with long runs of PAT usually complain of a sudden onset of pounding or fluttering in the chest. This is often associated with breathlessness, weakness, and angina pectoris in patients with coronary artery disease. Because of these problems, long runs of PAT must be treated. Treatment usually progresses in the following sequence: (1) give a sedative, (2) stimulate the vagus nerve by rubbing the carotid sinus (Figure 11-26), (3) give propranolol (Inderal) or a similar medication, and (4) perform

Figure 11-23 Sinus tachycardia. *(From Goldberger AL: Clinical electrocardiography: a simplified approach, ed 7, St Louis, 2006, Mosby.)*

Figure 11-24 Sinus bradycardia. *(From Golderberger AL: Clinical electrocardiography: a simplified approach, ed 7, St Louis, 2006, Mosby.)*

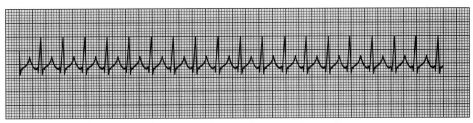

Figure 11-25   A short run of paroxysmal trial tachycardia (PAT). Although a short run is probably not dangerous, a long run should be treated. *(From Wilkins RL, Dexter JR, Heuer AJ: Clinical assessment in respiratory care, ed 6, St Louis, 2010, Mosby.)*

Atrial Flutter

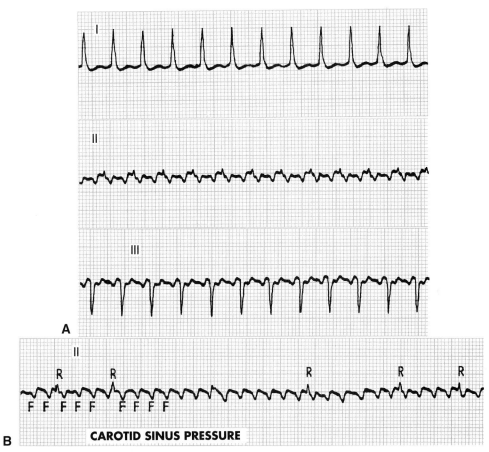

Figure 11-26   Two examples of atrial flutter. **A,** Note the variable appearance of the flutter waves in different leads. This example shows a 2 : 1 ratio between atrial contractions and ventricular contractions. **B,** This shows how the ventricular rate is decreased after carotid sinus pressure is applied. The "F" letterings show flutter waves from a single focus. The "R" letterings mark R waves when the electrical signal traveled through the atrioventricular node to stimulate the ventricles. *(From Goldberger AL: Clinical electrocardiography: a simplified approach, ed 7, St Louis, 2006, Mosby.)*

synchronized cardioversion. (This last procedure is described in Chapter 18.) Obviously, if the patient responds to one treatment method, no need exists to go on to the next.

b. Atrial flutter. Atrial flutter is characterized by a single, fast, abnormal atrial focus that fires at a rate of about 250 to 350 beats/min. This rate is so fast that the AV node does not pass all of them along to the ventricles. On an ECG, a ratio between the fast flutter waves and the QRS complex is seen. Usually this ratio is 2 : 1, but it may be 3 : 1, 4 : 1, or more. (See Figure 11-26 for several example ECG tracings of atrial flutter.) As with PAT, the fast ventricular rate found in atrial flutter is not well tolerated. An attempt must be made to suppress the abnormally fast atrial focus. Carotid sinus pressure, digoxin (Lanoxin), and synchronized cardioversion are the preferred treatments to slow the heart rate.

c. Atrial fibrillation. This condition is identified by the variably shaped fibrillation waves and the irregular spacings between the QRS complexes. Each focus is seen on the ECG as a separately shaped wave. As with atrial flutter, the AV node does not pass the electrical current from each fibrillation wave through to the ventricles. However, with atrial fibrillation, the ratio is not set, and variable spacing is seen between the QRS complexes and an inconsistent rate (Figure 11-27). Patients with atrial fibrillation do not completely empty their atria. Often this results in the formation of blood clots that become pulmonary or cerebral emboli. Digitalis and synchronized cardioversion usually are effective treatments. Heparin or Coumadin may be added to prolong the blood-clotting time.

3. Arrhythmias with an atrioventricular node origin. Both of the following arrhythmias originate in an AV node. The patient may or may not have a normal SA node, atria, and ventricles.

a. Atrioventricular block. AV block is most commonly caused by digitalis toxicity, arteriosclerosis, or myocardial infarction. The latter two may result in scarring, inflammation, or edema. These slow or prevent the transmission of the electrical signal from the SA node through the AV node and to the ventricles. *First-degree* AV block is seen with an increased PR interval of at least 0.20 seconds. Each P wave is followed by a normal QRS complex (Figure 11-28). It does not require any treatment. *Second-degree* AV block results in some P waves being blocked out completely with no ventricular response. This more serious condition comes in two different variations. Wenckebach (also known as Mobitz type I) is characterized by a progressively longer PR interval until a P wave is not conducted through at all. Then the cycle starts over again and continues to repeat itself. (See Figure 11-29 for examples.) Medications such as atropine or isoproterenol may be used to increase the heart rate. Mobitz type II is seen on the ECG as a rhythm in which the PR interval is normal for those that result in a QRS complex, but some P waves are completely blocked (Figure 11-30). The ratio between

Figure 11-27   Atrial fibrillation. Note the variable shapes to the fibrillation waves, indicating their different origins. Also note how the distances between the R waves change considerably. This depends on when an electrical signal from the atria passes through the atrioventricular node to the ventricles. *(From Wilkins RL, Dexter JR, Heuer AJ: Clinical assessment in respiratory care, ed 6, St Louis, 2010, Mosby.)*

Figure 11-28   First-degree atrioventricular block results in a PR interval that is longer than the normal interval of five small blocks or 20 seconds. **ECG strip A** shows a PR interval of 0.30 seconds. **ECG strip B** shows a PR interval of 0.24 seconds. *(A From Conover MB: Understanding electrocardiography, arrhythmias, and the 12-lead ECG, ed 4, St Louis, 1984, Mosby. B From Conover MB: Understanding electrocardiography, ed 8, St Louis, 2003, Mosby.)*

Mobitz Type I (Wenckebach) Second-Degree AV Block

A

Mobitz Type I (Wenckebach) Second-Degree AV Block

B

Figure 11-29 Two examples of Wenckebach (Mobitz type I) second-degree atrioventricular block. Note how the PR interval progressively lengthens with each beat until one P wave is not conducted through at all. The cycle then repeats itself. *(From Goldberger AL:* Clinical electrocardiography: a simplified approach, *ed 7, St Louis, 2006, Mosby.)*

Figure 11-30 Mobitz type II second-degree heart block. Note how some P waves are conducted through the atrioventricular node with a resulting QRS complex, and other P waves are not conducted. *(From Aehlert B:* ECGs made easy, *ed 3, St Louis, 2006, Mosby.)*

those P waves that conduct and those that are blocked off may be 2:1, 3:1, or 4:1. Mobitz type II is a sign of severe conduction-system disease. The usual treatment is to place a cardiac pacemaker into the patient. *Third-degree* AV block also is known as complete heart block (Figure 11-31). No P waves are conducted through to the ventricles. The ventricles beat about 40 times per minute based on the intrinsic rate of the bundle of His and Purkinje fibers. Obviously, a heartbeat this slow is not normal or healthy. Patients have no stamina and frequently faint. A cardiac pacemaker must be placed into these patients.

b. Junctional premature beats. A junctional premature beat is also known as a premature AV nodal contraction (PNC), nodal beat, or junctional beat (Figure 11-32). This arrhythmia involves the AV node sending out a premature electrical signal and becoming the primary pacemaker instead of the SA node. The ventricles contract normally with the expected QRS complex.

4. Arrhythmias with a ventricular origin myocardial infarction. A myocardial infarction (MI) or acute myocardial infarction (AMI), commonly known as a heart attack, is an occlusion of a coronary artery that results in the death of some segment of the heart muscle. Often the patient with partial or complete coronary artery occlusion has symptoms of shortness of breath, central chest pain, pain that radiates down the left arm or up the left side of the neck, or a feeling of stomach upset. If an ECG is performed, it may show ST-segment depression as a sign of myocardial hypoxia (Figure 11-33). If the patient is properly treated, an MI may be prevented by opening the blocked artery.

Often, however, the patient comes to the hospital too late, and an MI with heart damage is present. If the damaged area is large enough, the heart fails to pump adequately, and the patient dies. A smaller infarct weakens the heart. In addition, the damaged or dying tissue acts as an abnormal focus for the arrhythmias discussed next. The ECG changes that occur during the acute stage of an MI and as the heart heals are shown in Figure 11-34 and are listed here:

THIRD-DEGREE (COMPLETE) AV BLOCK

THIRD-DEGREE (COMPLETE) AV BLOCK

Figure 11-31   Two examples of third-degree (complete) heart block. Both show P waves that have no relation with the QRS complexes. The top example has QRS complexes of the normal width, indicating that the atrioventricular (AV) junction is acting as the pacemaker. The bottom example has QRS complexes that are wider than normal because the ventricles are being paced from below the AV junction. Instead, an idioventricular pacemaker is determining the patient's heart rate. *(From Goldberger AL: Clinical electrocardiography: a simplified approach, ed 7, St Louis, 2006, Mosby.)*

JUNCTIONAL PREMATURE BEAT

JUNCTIONAL PREMATURE BEAT

Figure 11-32   Two electrocardiogram tracings of junctional premature beats. They are from the same patient but from different leads. Arrows, Retrograde P waves of opposite polarity from normal. *(From Goldberger AL, Goldberger E: Clinical electrocardiography, St Louis, 1981, Mosby.)*

Figure 11-33   An electrocardiogram tracing showing ST segment depression. This is usually caused by myocardial hypoxia and can lead to a myocardial infarction if not promptly treated. *(From Wilkins RL, Dexter JR, Heuer AJ: Clinical assessment in respiratory care, ed 6, St Louis, 2010, Mosby.)*

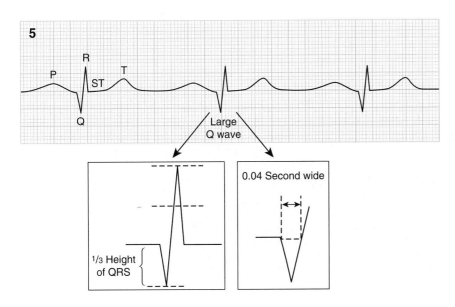

Figure 11-34 The sequence of electrocardiogram rhythms commonly seen after a myocardial infarction. See the text for a description of each step in the sequence.

- The initial ECG may be normal. This happens about 15% of the time. The patient should be admitted for observation and cardiac enzyme studies if symptoms are present.
- The first sign of an MI is an elevated ST segment. This occurs within a few hours of the injury.
- Next the T wave inverts. This happens within hours to days of the infarct.
- The ST segment returns to the normal baseline position within days to weeks.
- After a period of weeks to months, the T wave becomes upright again. A lasting ECG change is an enlarged Q wave as shown.

a. Premature ventricular contraction. A premature ventricular contraction (PVC) is an abnormal, fast contraction of the ventricles that originates from a focus below the AV node (Figure 11-35). This is usually a sign of a diseased or hypoxic ventricle. Pathologic causes include arteriosclerotic heart disease or MI. An example of an isolated PVC is shown in Figure 11-36 and has these traits:

- It is premature and happens before the normal heartbeat.
- No P wave is present.
- The QRS complex is bizarre looking and more than 0.12 seconds wide.

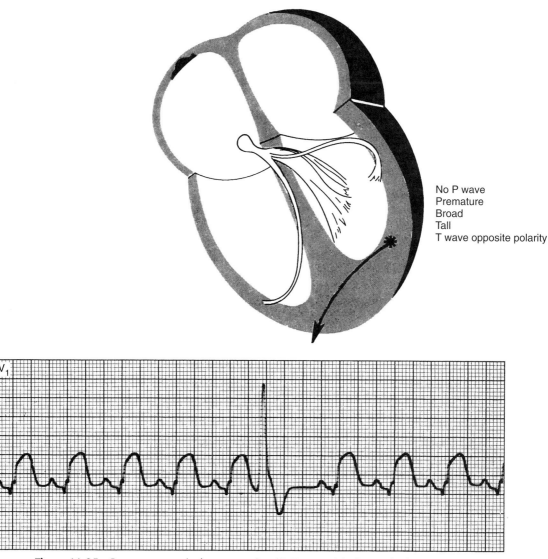

No P wave
Premature
Broad
Tall
T wave opposite polarity

Figure 11-35 Premature ventricular contraction (PVC; arrow) is detected when an impulse is propagated from a ventricular focus before the next normal beat is due. The QRS complex is commonly widened and not preceded by a P wave. A longer than usual (compensatory) pause follows. Retrograde activation of the atria may occur after a premature contraction, or the normal sinus P waves may continue. The sinus P waves after the PVC are blocked by conduction-system refractoriness. *(From Conover MB: Understanding electrocardiography, ed 8, St Louis, 2003, Mosby.)*

- The T wave is inverted.
- Usually, a fully compensatory pause occurs before the next normal heartbeat.

A single PVC is not dangerous unless it originates during the T wave, when the heart is especially vulnerable

R₁-R₂
520 msec

R₃-R₄
1040 msec

Figure 11-36 Premature ventricular contractions (PVCs) cause a fully compensatory pause. Note that the interval between the two sinus beats that surround the PVC (R₃ and R₄ in this case) is exactly two times the normal interval between the sinus beats R₁ and R₂. Notice that the P waves come on time, except that the third P wave is interrupted by the PVC and therefore does not conduct normally through the atrioventricular junction. The next (fourth) P wave also comes on time. The fact that the sinus node continues to pace despite the PVC results in the fully compensatory pause. *(From Goldberger AL: Clinical electrocardiography: a simplified approach, ed 7, St Louis, 2006, Mosby.)*

to electrical stimulation (Figure 11-37). Then, it can cause ventricular fibrillation.

If all PVCs look the same, they originate from the same area (focus) and are called *unifocal.* All patients with PVCs should be watched more closely and probably treated when their PVCs are seen more frequently than 1 in 10 beats, seen in groups of two or three, or seen in multiple configurations. For example, two different-looking PVCs mean that two different ventricular foci are firing prematurely (Figure 11-38). These different looking PVCs would be called *multifocal. Bigeminy* occurs when every second beat is a PVC; *trigeminy* is when every third beat is a PVC. These dangerous situations must be rapidly treated. Lidocaine (Xylocaine) is given intravenously if the heart rate is more than 60 beats/min. If that does not work, procainamide hydrochloride (Pronestyl) is added. Additionally, the patient is given supplemental oxygen to improve oxygenation to the irritable heart.

b. Ventricular tachycardia. Ventricular tachycardia (VT or V tach) is a serious consequence of untreated premature ventricular contractions. VT is defined as a series of three or more consecutive PVCs. Runs of VT may be fairly short or prolonged. The rate counted during VT is between 110 and 250 beats/min. Cardiac output decreases dramatically during this arrhythmia. If the patient has a stable blood pressure, VT is treated with lidocaine as an antiarrhythmic. Synchronized cardioversion is needed if

Figure 11-37 An electrocardiogram tracing showing multifocal premature ventricular contractions (PVCs). Counting from the left, after the normal beat, note that the next beat and sixth beat are PVCs. Because they look different, they do not originate at the same abnormal focus. Therefore the patient has multifocal PVCs. This dangerous situation should be quickly corrected. *(From Wilkins RL, Dexter JR, Heuer AJ: Clinical assessment in respiratory care, ed 6, St Louis, 2010, Mosby.)*

Figure 11-38 Electrocardiogram tracing showing normal sinus rhythm that suddenly converts to ventricular tachycardia. This can happen if a premature ventricular contraction occurs early in the heart's repolarization process and is called the R-on-T phenomenon. If ventricular tachycardia is not treated promptly, it will deteriorate into ventricular flutter or ventricular fibrillation. *(From Wilkins RL, Dexter JR, Heuer AJ: Clinical assessment in respiratory care, ed 6, St Louis, 2010, Mosby.)*

Figure 11-39   Example of an electrocardiogram showing ventricular flutter. If this arrhythmia is not treated promptly, it will deteriorate into ventricular fibrillation. *(From Kacmarek RM, Mack CW, Dimas S: The essentials of respiratory care, ed 3, St Louis, 1990, Mosby.)*

the lidocaine is ineffective. If the VT is sustained and the patient is unresponsive, pulseless, hypotensive, or, in pulmonary edema, defibrillation (also called unsynchronous cardioversion) is necessary. The medication amiodarone HCl (Pacerone) may also be used to help stop ventricular tachycardia. If left untreated, VT usually progresses to either ventricular flutter (Figure 11-39) or ventricular fibrillation (discussed next). Ventricular flutter looks similar on the ECG to VT except that the rate is usually faster and the rhythm less regular. Its treatment is the same as that for VT and, if left untreated, it will progress to ventricular fibrillation. Both of these arrhythmias originate from a single fast ventricular focus, as shown in Figure 11-35.

c. Ventricular fibrillation. Ventricular fibrillation (VF or V fib) is caused when multiple, fast ventricular foci are firing (see Figure 11-40 for the electrical pathways). When several ventricular foci are firing in an uncoordinated manner, the rhythm is chaotic and without any pattern. Virtually no cardiac output occurs. The patient is pulseless and without any blood pressure. This is a true medical emergency. If it is not treated immediately, brain death will occur within minutes. CPR must be started to provide oxygen to the brain. The treatment of choice for VF is defibrillation as quickly as possible. No attempt is made to synchronize the electrical shock. Figure 11-41 shows the usual position of the defibrillator paddles. It is hoped that with prompt CPR efforts and electrical defibrillation, the patient's heartbeat will return to a normal sinus rhythm (see Figure 11-5).

d. Ventricular asystole. Ventricular asystole (or asystole) occurs when no cardiac electrical signal and no myocardial activity are present. The ECG tracing shows a flat line, indicating the absence of cardiac electrical activity. The presence of this arrhythmia is ominous. When seen after a full attempt at CPR, it indicates a nonfunctioning heart. The patient will almost assuredly die. Some physicians may elect to defibrillate the patient in asystole in an attempt to generate some sort of rhythm. Because of the dire consequences of ventricular asystole, it is wise to double-check all the equipment. This includes the ECG leads or defibrillator paddles being used to check the rhythm, all electrical connections, and the functioning of

Figure 11-40   Multiple disorganized contractions of the ventricles characterize ventricular fibrillation and represent cardiac arrest. It may be of sudden onset or may follow premature ventricular contractions, ventricular tachycardia, or ventricular flutter. *(From Stein E: Clinical electrocardiography: a self-study course, Philadelphia, 1987, Lea & Febiger.)*

the ECG monitor to be sure that no technical error can be found.

b. Draw an arterial blood gas sample (Code: IB9f, IIIE2a) [Difficulty: ELE: R, Ap; WRE: An]

Blood for arterial blood gas (ABG) determination is usually drawn in any hospital-based CPR effort. It should not be done at the expense of time that should be spent starting effective ventilations and chest compressions or defibrillating the heart. The blood gas values give important information on the patient's oxygenation and helps to determine whether the patient is acidotic. Changes in the ventilation efforts and medications such as bicarbonate are based on information from the ABGs. See Chapter 3 for the discussion on arterial blood sampling.

Event documentation

Battery pack

Module   Tape

Patient cables
and defibrillation
electrodes

Monitor/
Command
display

Automatic mode
override by

Keyboard

Shock
Energy
Analysis
Power

Module   Key

Figure 11-41 Schematic drawing of automated external defibrillator and its attachment to the patient. *(Modified from Cummins RO: Advanced cardiac life support, Dallas, Tex., 1994, American Heart Association.)*

The femoral site is usually the best to draw from in a CPR situation because it is the largest artery and the easiest to hit. It is far enough from the chest that blood can be drawn without interfering in the chest compression efforts.

c. Interpret the results of arterial blood gas analysis (ELE code: IIIE4a) [Difficulty: ELE: R, Ap, An]

The full discussion of ABG interpretation is presented in Chapter 3. During a CPR attempt, the key things to look for are the patient's PaO_2 and $PaCO_2$, because they relate to the adequacy of ventilations and chest compressions. If the patient has an acidotic pH and a normal or low $PaCO_2$, the patient has an uncorrected metabolic acidosis. Intravenous (IV) sodium bicarbonate is indicated.

d. Perform endotracheal intubation (Code: IIIB3) [Difficulty: ELE: R, Ap; WRE: An]

Oral endotracheal intubation is usually performed during a CPR attempt. See Chapter 12 for a complete discussion of endotracheal tubes, intubation equipment, and the process of performing intubation. Current CPR guidelines indicate that if an endotracheal tube cannot be placed into a patient, a laryngeal mask airway (LMA) or Combitube may be inserted to provide a secure airway.

e. Make the recommendation to defibrillate the patient

Defibrillation sends a specific amount of direct electrical current (DC) through the patient's chest wall and heart. Its purpose is to stimulate the entire cardiac muscle and electrical system so that the source of an abnormal signal

will be suppressed. The SA node usually then takes over as the normal pacemaker. Chapter 18 includes a table listing the stepped progression of power used in defibrillation.

Synchronized defibrillation (cardioversion) (see Chapter 18) should be performed under the following circumstances: atrial flutter, PAT, atrial fibrillation, and ventricular tachycardia unless the patient is pulseless, unresponsive, hypotensive, or in pulmonary edema.

Unsynchronized defibrillation should be performed as soon as possible under the following circumstances: ventricular fibrillation or ventricular tachycardia when the patient is pulseless, unresponsive, hypotensive, or in pulmonary edema.

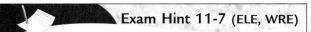

Exam Hint 11-7 (ELE, WRE)

Usually one question requires the therapist to identify the indications for defibrillation and recommend the procedure.

f. Recommend ACLS protocol agents (Code: IIIG4d) [Difficulty: ELE: R, Ap; WRE: An]

1. Cardiotonic (positive inotropic) drugs

Positive inotropic agents are used to increase the contractility of the heart muscle. Two classes of drugs do this, and both are used in patients who have a weak or damaged myocardium. They increase the patient's myocardial contractility. This results in increased cardiac output, increased blood pressure, and increased urine output. The best-known, older group consists of cardiac glycosides and is commonly referred to as "digitalis." The cardiac glycosides increase the level of intramuscular sodium and calcium to increase the contraction of the heart muscle. Of these, Lanoxin (digoxin) is the preferred medication for a patient with congestive heart failure.

The newer group includes synthetic catecholamine agents. The catecholamine agents are similar to adrenaline and stimulate b receptors in the heart. Dobutamine hydrochloride (Dobutrex) is used as a short-term agent in adult patients who have organic heart disease or who have had heart surgery. Its use results in an increase in contraction with only a minor increase in heart rate. Epinephrine (Adrenaline) is used during a cardiac arrest to increase heart rate and contractility.

2. Antiarrhythmic drugs

Bradycardia is defined as a heart rate of less than 60 beats/min in an adult at rest. If the patient has symptoms such as light-headedness or low blood pressure, the heart rate should be increased. Common medications that increase the heart rate include atropine (atropine sulfate), isoproterenol (Isuprel), and epinephrine (Adrenaline chloride).

Tachycardia (a resting adult heart rate of greater than 100 beats/min) and abnormal, fast heartbeats originating from the atria or ventricles are potentially very dangerous. Fast tachycardia and dangerous arrhythmias must be controlled with medications that slow the heart's conduction system or suppress the generation of abnormal electrical signals. Common medications that do this include propranolol (Inderal), lidocaine (Xylocaine), and procainamide (Pronestyl).

3. Vasoconstricting drugs

Vasoconstrictors are medications that cause the peripheral blood vessels to constrict so that blood flow is reduced through them. Many medications do this by stimulating the alpha-1 (α1 receptors on the vessels. They are chiefly used in a hypotensive patient. Hypotension is usually defined as a systemic blood pressure of less than 80 mm Hg in an adult and less than 70 mm Hg in a child. A pressure of less than this does not adequately perfuse the kidneys. Urine output decreases dramatically or stops altogether. Cerebral blood flow also is greatly reduced. When hypotension is caused by vasodilation, as in allergic anaphylaxis or sepsis, it usually has to be treated by inducing vasoconstriction. Hypotension from heart failure or an MI often also must be treated with a vasoconstrictor. Common examples of medications that cause vasoconstriction to increase blood pressure include dopamine hydrochloride (Intropin) and norepinephrine (Levophed, Levarterenol).

The effects of dopamine are dose related. At relatively low doses, an increase in renal blood flow is noted, and urine output increases, with no change in blood pressure. At medium doses, an increase in myocardial contractility and a progressive peripheral vasoconstriction is found. These effects increase the blood pressure without decreasing renal blood flow. At high doses, the total systemic vascular resistance further increases. However, renal blood flow and urine output both decrease. Current practice indicates that dopamine works best in patients with moderate hypotension. A patient who does not respond to dopamine probably needs norepinephrine (Levophed or Levarterenol) to increase the blood pressure. Any time a hypotensive patient is given a vasoconstricting agent, the blood pressure, peripheral blood flow, and urine output must be watched closely. The prognosis is grim for patients who do not respond to these medications or for attempts to correct the underlying condition.

4. Vasodilating drugs

Hypertension in the adult is defined as a blood pressure of greater than 140 to 150/90 mm Hg. The higher the blood pressure, the greater the strain on the heart. It also increases the risk of vessel rupture and stroke.

A wide variety of medications in a number of drug categories are used to reduce blood pressure. They range from diuretics to reduce blood volume, to calcium and sympathomimetic blockers that reduce heart rate and vasodilate, to angiotensin-converting enzyme (ACE) inhibitors. Medications in these categories are used to treat moderate, chronic hypertension.

The patient in a hypertensive crisis (blood pressure greater than 200/120 mm Hg) must be treated quickly and effectively. The following medications are commonly given by the IV route to control severe hypertension:
- Nitroprusside (Nipride)
- Diazoxide (Hyperstat)
- Trimethaphan (Arfonad)

Nitroprusside also is given to reduce the afterload in a patient with left ventricular failure after an MI. Any patient who is receiving a powerful vasodilator must have frequent blood pressure monitoring.

5. Bicarbonate (sodium bicarbonate)

According to the most recent guidelines, bicarbonate (sodium bicarbonate) should be used, if at all, only after all other CPR procedures have been instituted. Bicarbonate may then be used if a diagnosis has been made and arterial blood gas results document that the patient has a metabolic acidosis. Additionally, bicarbonate is given to help treat the patient with hyperkalemia, or tricyclic or phenobarbital overdose. Bicarbonate also may be beneficial if the patient has been in prolonged arrest or if CPR has been performed for an extended time.

When used, bicarbonate should be given initially at a dose of 1 mEq/kg; a half dose is then given every 10 minutes. If available from ABG results, use the calculated base deficit or bicarbonate concentration as a guideline for giving more bicarbonate. Do not completely correct the base deficit to avoid accidentally making the patient alkalotic.

g. Administer ACLS protocol medications by endotracheal installation (Code: IIID5c) [Difficulty: ELE: R, Ap; WRE: An]

Cardiac medications may be instilled down the endotracheal tube when a resuscitation attempt is under way and the patient does not have a functional central or peripheral IV line. The following medications may be instilled into adult patients: naloxone (Narcan), atropine, vasopressin (Arginine), epinephrine, and lidocaine (Xylocaine). (Hint: Use "NAVEL," from the first letters of the generic name of these medications, to help remember them.) Naloxone should only be given intravenously to a newborn infant. The dose of any medication is based on the patient's size and may be larger than that given intravenously. This is because the medication is diluted through the airways and must be absorbed through the mucous membrane. Previous adult guidelines indicated that the endotracheal dose should be 2 to 2.5 times greater than the normal IV amount. The medication should be diluted by adding 10 mL of normal saline or distilled water. '

The following steps for instillation are recommended:

1. Disconnect the manual resuscitator from the endotracheal tube, and stop the chest compressions.
2. (Optional) Pass a suction catheter or feeding tube past the distal tip of the endotracheal tube.
3. Quickly inject the drug solution down the endotracheal tube or catheter.
4. If used, withdraw the suction catheter.
5. Reconnect the manual resuscitator to the endotracheal tube and give the patient several deep breaths. This helps to force the medication down to the alveolar level or causes aerosolization so that faster absorption occurs.
6. Resume chest compressions and ventilation.

Exam Hint 11-8 (ELE, WRE)

Epinephrine (Adrenaline) is a first-line drug used in a CPR attempt. It is used during bradycardia, asystole, and ventricular fibrillation because it increases the heart rate, stroke volume, and vasoconstriction to raise blood pressure. (In addition, it is a bronchodilator.)

h. Observe the size of the patient's pupils and their reaction to light

Normally the pupils constrict when a light being shined into them. The pupils dilate within 30 to 40 seconds after cardiac arrest and do not constrict normally when the brain is hypoxic. If CPR is being done properly to deliver oxygen to the brain, the pupils should constrict normally. Fixed (nonreactive) and dilated pupils are ominous signs. Even if the heart can be restarted, the brain has probably had irreversible damage.

In several conditions, the pupils do not react as expected. The pupils remain constricted if the victim has received morphine sulfate or other opiates. The pupils are dilated if the victim has received atropine, quinidine, or epinephrine. Hypothermia also causes the pupils to dilate.

i. Recommend (Code: IC10) [Difficulty: ELE: R, Ap; WRE: An] and perform capnography or exhaled carbon dioxide measurement (Code: IB9c) [Difficulty: ELE: R; WRE: Ap, An] to evaluate the adequacy of resuscitation

The general discussion of capnography was presented in Chapter 5, and exhaled carbon dioxide monitoring was presented in Chapter 12. Either can be used to help confirm that the endotracheal tube is properly located within the trachea and the patient is exhaling carbon dioxide. It also is helpful if the patient is being trans-

ported or the endotracheal tube is being repositioned. In addition, clinical evidence suggests that monitoring the exhaled carbon dioxide level during a CPR attempt is helpful in evaluating the patient's metabolic response. In general, if chest compressions and assisted ventilation are effective, carbon dioxide will be removed from the tissues and circulated to the lungs for exhalation. If the CPR efforts are ineffective, little exhaled carbon dioxide is measured. The absence of exhaled carbon dioxide, despite a proper CPR effort, is a grave sign.

Exam Hint 11-9 (WRE)

The Written Registry Exam usually has one ACLS-level question. Review the advanced COR procedures such as life-threatening arrhythmia recognition, intubation, and defibrillation.

3. Pediatric advanced life support (Code: III I1c) [Difficulty: ELE: R, Ap; WRE: An]

The general steps and procedures related to pediatric advanced life support (PALS) are covered in this chapter and Chapter 12.

4. Neonatal resuscitation program (Code: III I1d) [Difficulty: ELE: R, Ap; WRE: An]

A neonatal resuscitation program (NRP) provides training in resuscitating a newborn at birth in the delivery room. In addition to the basic and advanced CPR steps discussed in this chapter and Chapter 12, the person trained in NRP is prepared to perform the following:

1. Dry the newborn and keep it warm.
2. Suction the airway to remove amniotic fluid and meconium.
3. Evaluate the newborn to determine the need for 100% oxygen, bag-mask ventilation, intubation, and chest compressions.

It is beyond the scope of this text to cover all aspects of ACLS, PALS, and NRP training. The bibliography lists helpful sources of information.

Exam Hint 11-10 (ELE, WRE)

The Written Registry Exam usually includes one question relates to PALS or NRP. Realize that if a newborn has a low Apgar score, is apneic, has bradycardia, or has hypotension, action must be taken. A child who is apneic, has bradycardia, or has hypotension also must be treated quickly. Past questions have required the therapist to begin bag-mask ventilation with oxygen.

MODULE D
Respiratory care plan

1. Analyze available information to determine the patient's pathophysiologic state (Code code: IIIH1) [Difficulty: ELE: R, Ap; WRE: An]

It is critical for the respiratory therapist to be able to recognize the need to start CPR procedures. Discussion in this chapter should be helpful in preparing for this possibility.

2. Determine the appropriateness of the prescribed therapy and goals for the identified pathophysiologic state (Code: IIIH3) [Difficulty: ELE: R, Ap; WRE: An]

BCLS, ACLS, PALS, and NRP are all CPR-related protocols. CPR should be started, adjusted, and terminated based on these protocols and the patient's recovery.

a. Terminate the treatment or procedure based on the patient response (Code: IIIF1) [Difficulty: ELE: R, Ap; WRE: An]

The practitioner should make a recommendation to the physician to stop a procedure being performed as an adjunct to CPR if the patient is having an adverse reaction to it. For example, bag and mask ventilation may force air into the stomach; recommend intubation. Always notify the physician of any change in the patient's condition or if a complication to any CPR-related procedure is seen.

b. Recommend discontinuing treatment based on the patient's response (Code: IIIG1i) [Difficulty: ELE: R, Ap; WRE: An]

The physician will make the decision to stop futile CPR activities that are taking place in the hospital.

BIBLIOGRAPHY

2005 American Heart Association Guidelines for Cardiopulmonary Resuscitation and Emergency Cardiac Care: Part 4: Adult basic life support. *Circulation 2005*; 112: IV-19-IV-34, Nov. 28, 2005.

2005 American Heart Association Guidelines for Cardiopulmonary Resuscitation and Emergency Cardiac Care: Part 7.1: Adjuncts for airway control and ventilation. *Circulation 2005*; 112: IV-51-IV-75, Nov. 28, 2005.

2005 American Heart Association Guidelines for Cardiopulmonary Resuscitation and Emergency Cardiac Care: Part 11: Pediatric basis life support. *Circulation 2005*; 112: IV-156-IV-166, Nov. 28, 2005.

2005 American Heart Association Guidelines for Cardiopulmonary Resuscitation and Emergency Cardiac Care: Part 12: Pediatric advanced life support. *Circulation 2005*; 112: IV-167-IV-187, Nov. 28, 2005.

2005 American Heart Association Guidelines for Cardiopulmonary Resuscitation and Emergency Cardiac Care: Part 13: Neonatal resuscitation guideline. *Circulation 2005*; 112: IV-188-IV-195, Nov. 28, 2005.

Abedin Z, Conner RP: 12-Lead ECG interpretation: the self-assessment approach, Philadelphia, 1989, WB Saunders.

Aloan CA, Hill TV, editors: *Respiratory care of the newborn and child,* ed 2, Philadelphia, 1997, Lippincott-Raven.

American Association for Respiratory Care: Clinical practice guideline: capnography/capnometry during mechanical ventilation—2-3 revision & update, *Respir Care* 48(5):534, 2003.

American Association for Respiratory Care: Clinical practice guideline: defibrillation during resuscitation, *Respir Care* 40(7):744, 1995.

American Association for Respiratory Care: Clinical practice guideline: resuscitation and defibrillation in the health care setting: 2004 revision and update, *Respir Care* 49(9):1085, 2004.

American Association for Respiratory Care: Clinical practice guideline: management of airway emergencies, *Respir Care* 40(7):749, 1995.

American Association for Respiratory Care: Clinical practice guideline: resuscitation in acute care hospitals, *Respir Care* 38(11):1179, 1993.

American Heart Association: ACLS provider manual, Dallas, Tex, 2001, American Heart Association.

American Heart Association: PALS provider manual, Dallas, Tex, 2002, American Heart Association.

American Heart Association, Part 4: Adult basic life support. Circulation 112:IV18-IV34, 2004.

American Heart Association, Part 11: Pediatric basic life support. Circulation 112:IV156-IV166, 2005.

American Heart Association, Part 13: Neonatal resuscitation guidelines. Circulation 112:IV188-IV195, 2005.

Barnes TA: Emergency cardiovascular life support. In: Wilkins RL, Stoller JK, Kacmarek RM, editors: *Egan's fundamentals of respiratory care,* ed 9, St Louis, 2009, Mosby.

Barnes TA, editor: *Core textbook of respiratory care practice,* ed 2, St Louis, 1994, Mosby.

Barnes TA, Boudin KM: Cardiopulmonary resuscitation. In: Burton GG, Hodgkin JE, Ward JJ, editors: *Respiratory care: a guide to clinical practice,* ed 4, Philadelphia, 1997, Lippincott-Raven.

Barnes TA, Hess DR: Cardiopulmonary resuscitation. In: Hess DR, MacIntyre NR, Mishoe SC, editors: *Respiratory care principles and practice,* Philadelphia, 2002, WB Saunders.

Barnhart SL, Czervinske MP: *Perinatal and pediatric respiratory care,* Philadelphia, 1995, WB Saunders.

Branson RD, Hess DR, Chatburn RL, editors: *Respiratory care equipment,* ed 2, Philadelphia, 1999, Lippincott Williams & Wilkins.

Burton GC, Hodgkin JE, Ward JJ, editors: *Respiratory care: a guide to clinical practice,* ed 4, Philadelphia, 1997, Lippincott-Raven.

Butler HH: How to read an ECG, *RN* 36(1):35, 1973.

Butler HH: How to read an ECG, *RN* 36(2):49, 1973.

Butler HH: How to read an ECG, *RN* 36(3):50, 1973.

Cairo JM: Assessment of cardiovascular function. In: Cairo JM, Pilbeam SP, editors: *Mosby's respiratory care equipment,* ed 8, St Louis, 2010, Mosby.

Davis D: *Differential diagnosis of arrhythmias,* Philadelphia, 1991, WB Saunders.

Durbin CG: Airway management. In: Cairo JM, Pilbeam SP, editors: *Mosby's respiratory care equipment,* ed 7, St Louis, 2004, Mosby.

Eubanks DH, Bone RC: *Comprehensive respiratory care,* ed 2, St Louis, 1990, Mosby.

Fink JB, Hunt GE, editors: *Clinical practice in respiratory care,* Philadelphia, 1999, Lippincott-Raven.

Fluck RR: Emergency medicine. In: Wyka KA, Mathews PJ, Clark WF, editors: *Foundations of respiratory care,* Albany, NY, 2002, Delmar.

Goldberger AL, Goldberger E: *Clinical electrocardiography,* St Louis, 1981, Mosby.

Harwood R: *Exam review and study guide for perinatal/pediatric respiratory care,* Philadelphia, 1999, FA Davis.

Hess D, Goff G, Johnson K: The effect of hand size, resuscitator brand, and use of two hands on volumes delivered during adult bag-valve ventilation, *Respir Care* 34:805, 1989.

Kacmarek RM, Mack CW, Dimas S: *The essentials of respiratory care,* ed 3, St Louis, 1990, Mosby.

Madama VC: Safe mouth-to-mouth resuscitation requires adjunct equipment, caution, Occup *Health Saf* 60(1):56, 1991.

Marriott HJL: *Practical electrocardiography,* ed 7, Baltimore, 1983, Williams & Wilkins.

Marshak AB: Emergency life support. In: Wilkins RL, Stoller JK, Scanlan CL, editors: *Egan's fundamentals of respiratory therapy,* ed 8, St Louis, 2003, Mosby.

Pagana K, Pagana TJ: *Mosby's diagnostic and laboratory test reference,* ed 9, St Louis, 2009, Mosby.

Patel JM, McGowan SG, Moody LA: *Arrhythmias: detection, treatment, and cardiac drugs,* Philadelphia, 1989, WB Saunders.

Phillips RE, Feeney MK: *The cardiac rhythms: a systematic approach to interpretation,* ed 3, Philadelphia, 1990, WB Saunders.

Physicians' desk reference, ed 60, Montvale, NJ, 2006, Thomson PDR.

Shapiro BA, Kacmarek RM, Cane RD, et al, editors: *Clinical application of respiratory care,* ed 4, St Louis, 1991, Mosby.

Simmons KF, Scanlan CL: Airway management. In: Wilkins RL, Stoller JK, Kacmarek RM, editors: *Egan's fundamentals of respiratory care,* ed 9, St Louis, 2009, Mosby.

Sorensen KA, Wilkins RL: Interpretation of the electrocardiogram. In: Wilkins RL, Stoller JK, Kacmarek RM, editors: *Egan's fundamentals of respiratory care,* ed 9, St Louis, 2009, Mosby.

Stein E: *Clinical electrocardiography: a self-study course,* Philadelphia, 1987, Lea & Febiger.

Sweetwood HM: *Clinical electrocardiography for nurses,* Rockville, Md, 1983, Aspen Systems.

Whitaker K: *Comprehensive perinatal and pediatric respiratory care,* ed 2, Albany, NY, 1997, Delmar.

White GC: *Equipment theory for respiratory care,* ed 4, Albany, NY, 2005, Delmar.

Wilkins RL, Heuer AJ: Interpretation of electrocardiogram tracings. In: Wilkins RL, Dexter JR, Heuer AJ, editors: *Clinical assessment in respiratory care,* ed 6, St Louis, 2010, Mosby.

Wilkins RL, Stoller JK, Kacmarek RM, editors: *Egan's fundamentals of respiratory care,* ed 9, St Louis, 2009, Mosby.

SELF-STUDY QUESTIONS FOR THE ENTRY LEVEL EXAM

See page 593 for answers

1. A fully compensatory pause is seen after which type of heartbeat?
   A. Normal sinus rhythm
   B. PVC
   C. Paroxysmal atrial tachycardia
   D. VT

2. All the following are acceptable ways to ventilate a patient during CPR EXCEPT:
   A. Endotracheal tube
   B. Pneumatic (demand-valve) resuscitator
   C. Mouth-to-valve resuscitator
   D. Manual resuscitator

3. A patient comes into the Emergency Department appearing ashen gray and complaining of sudden, severe pain beneath his sternum and shortness of breath. He says this began after he exercised vigorously for 45 minutes. After putting an O_2 mask on the patient, what should you do?
   A. Start ECG monitoring.
   B. Recommend that he begin a supervised exercise program at the hospital.
   C. Perform a peak flow test to check on exercise-induced asthma.
   D. Immediately draw an ABG sample.

4. The nurse calls you into a patient's room. You notice from the ECG monitor that the patient is in ventricular tachycardia. You cannot find a carotid pulse, and the nurse says that he cannot find a blood pressure. What would you recommend?
   A. Check the other arm for a blood pressure.
   B. Defibrillate the patient.
   C. Intubate the patient and start her on a ventilator.
   D. Initiate synchronized cardioversion of the patient.

5. Counting from the left, the first and sixth rhythms on the ECG strip shown here represent:
   A. Atrial flutter
   B. Second-degree heart block
   C. Unifocal PVCs
   D. Multifocal PVCs

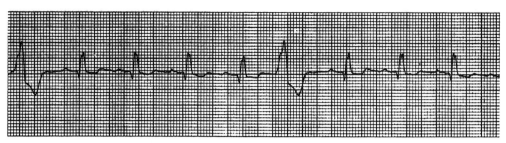

From Patel JM, McGowan SG, Moody, LA: *Arrhythmias: detection, treatment and cardiac drugs,* Philadelphia, 1989, Saunders.

6. A 65-year-old patient has been successfully resuscitated in the Emergency Department after suffering an MI. He is still unstable with frequent PVCs. He needs to be transported to the cardiac care unit for management. Which of the following would be most important for monitoring him during the transportation?
   A. Pulse oximeter
   B. Portable capnography unit
   C. Portable ECG machine with defibrillator
   D. 12-lead ECG unit to record any arrhythmias

7. You are performing chest compressions during a resuscitation attempt while another therapist is manually ventilating the intubated patient. The nurse and physician are both unable to start an IV line to give medications. What would you recommend?
   A. Instill the medications down the endotracheal tube.
   B. Keep trying new sites from which to start the IV line.
   C. Nebulize the medications.
   D. Give the medications by subcutaneous injection.

8. You are doing O_2 rounds on patients in the coronary care unit. You notice that the patient whose 28% venturi mask you are checking is unresponsive to your questions. Looking up, you see the ECG rhythm strip shown here. What would you recommend as a first reaction?
   A. Check the calibration on the ECG machine.
   B. Replace the ECG leads.
   C. Increase the O_2 percentage because the patient is hypoxic.
   D. Defibrillate the patient.

From Patel JM, McGowan SG, Moody, LA: *Arrhythmias: detection, treatment and cardiac drugs,* Philadelphia, 1989, Saunders.

9. You notice during a diagnostic ECG that the QRS complex is inverted on lead II. What would most likely cause this?
   A. An electrode is loose.
   B. The patient is shivering.
   C. The arm electrodes are reversed.
   D. The unit is out of calibration.

10. You enter a patient's room to check on her nasal cannula. She is slumped over in her chair and appears cyanotic. Your first reaction would be to:
    A. Open the airway.
    B. Determine whether the patient is responsive.
    C. Begin mouth-to-mouth ventilation.
    D. Check for a pulse.

11. You are working in the Emergency Department when an automobile accident victim is brought in. You suspect that the driver has a cervical spine injury. What is the best way to open the airway?
    A. Tracheostomy
    B. Head-tilt/chin-lift maneuver
    C. Jaw-thrust maneuver
    D. Nasal intubation

12. To determine breathlessness, it is best to:
    1. Feel for air movement with your cheek by the victim's mouth.
    2. Feel the chest rise and fall with your hand.
    3. Listen for air movement with your ear by the victim's mouth.
    4. Look at the victim's chest for a rising and falling movement.
    5. Look at the victim's face for nasal flaring.

A. 1, 2
B. 3, 5
C. 1, 3, 4
D. 4, 5

13. The best way to determine pulselessness in a 10-month-old infant is by checking:
    A. Brachial pulse for 5 to 10 sec
    B. Carotid pulse for 3 to 5 sec
    C. Femoral pulse for 3 to 5 sec
    D. Brachial pulse for 3 to 5 sec

14. While doing O_2 equipment rounds, you come upon a cyanotic patient who is not breathing. As you reposition the patient and hyperextend his neck, you notice that he has open lip ulcers. What would be the best way to ventilate this patient?
    A. Perform mouth-to-mouth ventilation.
    B. Use a mouth-to-valve device stored in the room for this purpose.
    C. Run to the CPR crash cart and get a manual resuscitation bag and mask.
    D. Wait for the anesthesiologist to intubate the patient's airway, then use a manual resuscitation bag.

15. When one rescuer is performing CPR on an unintubated adult, what chest compression:ventilation ratio should be used?
    A. 5:1
    B. 5:2
    C. 15:2
    D. 30:2

16. To ensure that a manual ventilator is ready for use, you would:
    1. Make sure that no gas escapes through the outlet port when it is closed off and the bag is squeezed.
    2. Squeeze the bag, and make sure that the air/O_2 reservoir intake valve closes properly.
    3. Squeeze the bag, and make sure the nonrebreathing valve opens properly.
    4. Feel for air leaving the outlet port when the bag is squeezed.
    5. Squeeze the bag, and make sure that the air/O_2 reservoir intake valve opens properly.
    A. 1, 2, 3, 4
    B. 1, 2, 5
    C. 4, 5
    D. 2, 3

17. Blood for an ABG measurement needs to be drawn during a CPR attempt. Which site would you recommend for this?
    A. Carotid
    B. Radial
    C. Brachial
    D. Femoral

18. A mouth-to-valve resuscitation device is being used on an apneic patient. The respiratory therapist delivers a breath, but the patient's chest does not rise. What should be done next?
    A. Begin chest compressions.
    B. Request a lateral neck radiograph.
    C. Check the valve for proper position.
    D. Perform abdominal thrusts.

19. After a 10-year-old child has been intubated, what compression:ventilation ratio should the two rescuers use?
    A. 3:1
    B. 5:1
    C. 30 compressions: 2 ventilations per minute
    D. 100 compressions: 8 to 10 ventilations per minute

SELF-STUDY QUESTIONS FOR THE WRITTEN REGISTRY EXAM   *See page 618 for answers*

1. A normal sinus rhythm can be identified by:
   1. A resting rate of 60 to 100 beats/min in an adult
   2. A P wave before every QRS complex
   3. A regular rhythm
   4. A QRS complex after every P wave
   5. An upright T wave in lead II
   A. 2, 4
   B. 2, 3, 4
   C. 1, 2, 3, 5
   D. All of the above

2. Your ventilator-dependent patient is set up for routine ECG monitoring. Because of refractory hypoxemia, the physician orders 10 cm water of positive end-expiratory pressure (PEEP). Shortly after the PEEP therapy is added, you notice that sinus arrhythmia has developed. Which of the following is the best course of action to follow?
   A. Recommend the administration of atropine.
   B. Recommend synchronized cardioversion.
   C. Recommend decreasing the PEEP from 10 to 5 cm water.
   D. Make a record of the rhythm, and inform the nurse and physician of your observation.

3. Electrocardiogram monitoring is justified with a patient in the intensive care unit in all of the following situations EXCEPT:
   A. If it is used to evaluate peripheral perfusion.
   B. The patient has an electrolyte disturbance.
   C. The patient has a history of arrhythmias.

D. The patient is being given a rapid infusion of potassium.

4. After an exercise routine, a 59-year-old man experiences sudden chest pain with shortness of breath. ECG monitoring in the Emergency Department reveals the following rhythm strip. What should the respiratory therapist recommend?
   1. Synchronized cardioversion
   2. 12-lead ECG
   3. Defibrillation
   4. Administer oxygen
   5. Angioplasty
   A. 1, 5
   B. 2, 4
   C. 2, 3, 4
   D. All of the above

(Wilkins RL, Krider SJ, Sheldon RL: Clinical assessment in respiratory care, *ed 4, St Louis, 2000, Mosby.)*

5. As the respiratory therapist assisting with the delivery of a high-risk infant, you are providing bag-mask ventilation with 100% oxygen. The nurse finds the newborn's heart rate to be 55/minute. What should be done?
   A. Add 5 cm PEEP to the bag mask.
   B. Apply a pulse oximeter to check the saturation.
   C. Begin chest compressions.
   D. Stimulate the infant to increase its vital signs.

6. Which of the following medications can be administered down the endotracheal tube during a CPR attempt on an adult?
   1. Epinephrine
   2. Potassium chloride
   3. Atropine
   4. Lidocaine
   A. 1
   B. 2, 3
   C. 1, 4
   D. 1, 3, 4

7. Two respiratory therapists respond to a cardiopulmonary-arrest call and begin CPR procedures on an adult patient. On looking at the ECG monitor, the following rhythm strip is seen. What should be recommended in this situation?
   A. Defibrillate the patient.
   B. Increase the oxygen flow to the manual resuscitation bag and mask.
   C. Change ventilation and chest compression duties.
   D. Intubate the patient.

(Goldberger AL, Goldberger E: Clinical electrocardiography, *ed 4, St Louis, Mosby.)*

8. CPR steps have been under way for 15 minutes when an arterial blood gas sample is drawn and sent off for analysis. The following results are obtained with 100% oxygen being used to ventilate the patient:
   pH, 6.97
   PaCO$_2$, 30 torr
   PaO$_2$, 210 torr
   HCO$_3^-$, 8 mEq/L

What should the therapist recommend at this time?
   A. Decrease the oxygen percentage.
   B. Decrease the respiratory rate.
   C. Administer intravenous sodium bicarbonate.
   D. Add mechanical dead space to the manual resuscitator.

9. During a CPR attempt on a 50-year-old patient, the respiratory therapist successfully intubates the patient

and begins ventilating with a manual resuscitator. The physician is unable to start an IV line. How should the CPR drugs be given?

- A. Intraosseous injection
- B. Endotracheal instillation
- C. Intracardiac injection
- D. Nasal spray

10. A 59-year-old patient is brought to the hospital with a complaint of sudden, severe substernal chest pain and dyspnea. What initial thing should the respiratory therapist recommend?

- A. Begin ECG monitoring.
- B. Draw an ABG sample.
- C. Get a chest radiograph.
- D. Get a capnometer value.

11. Defibrillation should be done immediately in which of the following patient situations?

- A. Second-degree heart block
- B. Atrial flutter
- C. Pulseless ventricular tachycardia
- D. Sinus tachycardia

12. You are the respiratory therapist attending the delivery of a preterm neonate. His vital signs are:

Respiratory rate, 12 per minute
Heart rate, 70 beats/min

In addition, he has peripheral cyanosis and is responding minimally to stimulation. What should be done?

- A. Direct supplemental oxygen to his face.
- B. Begin chest compressions.
- C. Begin manual ventilation with 100% oxygen.
- D. Continue to stimulate the newborn to breathe more deeply.

13. An infant has just been delivered by cesarean section to an anesthetized mother. Because the infant is not breathing adequately, it has been intubated. What can be done to improve the infant's condition and get it to breathe?

- A. Give intravenous epinephrine.
- B. Give intravenous naloxone (Narcan).
- C. Begin bag-mask ventilation with oxygen.
- D. Give endotracheal atropine (atropine sulfate).

14. Bag-mask ventilation with oxygen is being provided to a 57-year-old adult at a rate of 12/minute. His other vital signs include heart rate of 52/minute and blood pressure 95/55 mm Hg. What can be done to improve his vital signs?

- A. Administer endotracheal lidocaine (Xylocaine).
- B. Begin chest compressions.
- C. Intubate the patient.
- D. Administer intravenous epinephrine (Adrenaline).

12 Airway Management

Note 1: This book is written to cover every item listed as testable on the *Entry Level Examination (ELE), Written Registry Examination (WRE),* and *Clinical Simulation Examination (CSE).*

The listed code for each item is taken from the National Board for Respiratory Care's (NBRC) **Summary Content Outline for CRT (Certified Respiratory Therapist) and Written RRT (Registered Respiratory Therapist) Examinations** (http://evolve.elsevier.com/Sills/resptherapist/). For example, if an item is testable on both the ELE and the WRE, it will simply be shown as: (Code: . . .). If an item is only testable on the ELE, it will be shown as: (ELE code: . . .). If an item is only testable on the WRE, it will be shown as: (WRE code: . . .).

Following each item's code will be the difficulty level of the questions on that item on the ELE and WRE. (See the Introduction for a full explanation of the three question difficulty levels.) **Recall [R]** level questions typically expect the exam taker to recall factual information. **Application [Ap]** level questions are harder because the exam taker may have to apply factual information to a clinical situation. **Analysis [An]** level questions are the most challenging because the exam taker may have to use critical thinking to evaluate patient data to make a clinical decision.

Note 2: A review of the most recent Entry Level Examinations (ELE) has shown an average of 9 questions (out of 140), or 7% of the exam, that cover airway management. A review of the most recent Written Registry Examinations (WRE) has shown an average of 6 questions (out of 100), or 6% of the exam, that cover airway management. The Clinical Simulation Examination is comprehensive and may include everything that should be known by an advanced level respiratory therapist.

MODULE A

General airway management topics

1. Assess the patient's airway by inspection

a. Inspect the patient's face to identify the presence of macroglossia (Code: IB1b) [Difficulty: ELE: R, Ap; WRE: An]

Macroglossia is an excessively large tongue that is often seen to protrude out of the mouth (Figure 12-1). It can partially obstruct the neonate's upper airway and may be associated with inspiratory stridor. Macroglossia is associated with Down syndrome, Beckwith-Wiedemann syndrome, and several metabolic disorders. Immediate treatment may require (1) manually moving the mandible forward to pull the large tongue out of the airway, (2) inserting an oropharyngeal airway or nasopharyngeal airway, (3) placing the infant in the prone position. If the infant has life-threatening airway obstruction that is not corrected by these procedures, an endotracheal tube or tracheostomy tube must be inserted. Long-term management may require a tracheostomy or corrective facial surgery.

b. Assess for limits in neck range of motion (Code: IB1b) [Difficulty: ELE: R, Ap; WRE: An]

It is standard practice for emergency medical personnel to place a neck brace on a trauma victim (for example, an automobile crash) to prevent a cervical spine injury. In some cases, the patient is strapped on a body board in addition to wearing a neck brace. Usually the neck brace is not removed until after neck radiographs are taken and a physical exam is performed to disprove a cervical spine injury.

Other people with limited neck range of motion include a patient who has recently had cervical spine surgery and is being weaned from a neck brace or a patient with kyphoscoliosis who is wearing a supportive brace. If a patient wearing a neck brace has an upper airway obstruction, it may be possible to insert an oropharyngeal airway or nasopharyngeal airway to push the tongue forward to ease breathing. If these devices are not effective, and the neck cannot be hyperextended to open the airway, an emergency airway is needed. It is possible that a laryngeal mask airway (LMA) or Combitube could be inserted by an emergency medical technician, paramedic, or respiratory therapist. If these devices are not able to provide a secure airway, a physician will need to perform nasotracheal intubation or a tracheostomy (see Chapter 18).

Figure 12-1 Close-up photograph of an infant with macroglossia. Note the larger than normal tongue that can obstruct the upper airway. *(From Zitelli and Davis, 1992; courtesy Dr. Christine L. Williams, New York Medical College.)*

2. Properly position the patient

a. Recommend a change in the patient's position (Code: IIIG2a) [Difficulty: ELE: R, Ap; WRE: An]

A patient who is hypoxic may have oxygenation improved by a change in position that better matches ventilation and perfusion. A patient with unilateral lung disease is usually placed flat in bed and rolled onto the side of the unaffected lung. It has been found that some patients with acute respiratory distress syndrome (ARDS) have improved oxygenation when placed in the prone position. The Trendelenburg position should not be used in a patient with head trauma and increased intracranial pressure. Lowering the patient's head could increase the pressure on the brain.

b. Properly position the patient to maintain a patent airway (Code: IIIB1) [Difficulty: ELE: R, Ap; WRE: An]

Positioning of the head to open the airway is discussed in Chapter 11. Briefly, use the head tilt-chin lift maneuver to hyperextend the neck of an adult, and slightly extend the neck of a child to open the airway. You can place a small pad behind the neck and head to put the patient in the "sniff position." Always keep the head in line with the body. If the patient has a known or suspected cervical spine injury, the neck cannot be hyperextended. Instead, open the airway with the jaw-thrust maneuver. Keep the head in line with the body.

The patient may be supine during the airway-opening procedures just mentioned. Frequently, however, the patient is positioned with the head and body elevated. An unconscious patient is less likely to vomit and aspirate in either Fowler's or semi-Fowler's position. The combination of either of these body positions with the head and neck hyperextended into the sniff position will probably keep the airway open and minimize the risk of aspiration of vomitus. Turning the patient's head to one side may also reduce the risk of aspiration. Placing the patient into either Fowler's or semi-Fowler's position will also minimize the patient's work of breathing (WOB) and help to reduce hypoxemia.

3. Recommend the insertion of an artificial airway or a change in the type of artificial airway (Code: IIIG1f) [Difficulty: ELE: R, Ap; WRE: An]

An artificial airway is indicated in any patient who cannot protect his or her airway. The patient may be at risk of upper airway obstruction from the tongue falling back, may have facial trauma or be undergoing surgery, may be at risk of vomiting and aspirating, or may need mechanical ventilation for assisted breathing. A number of possible airways are available; select the best one based on the patient's needs. These airways are presented in the remainder of this chapter.

> **Exam Hint 12-1** (ELE, WRE)
>
> Identify that the patient has an airway problem. Know the uses, advantages, and disadvantages of the various airway devices. Be prepared to make a recommendation for which device to use or when to change to a different airway device, as necessary.

4. Humidify an artificial airway

a. Maintain adequate humidification to the patient's airway (ELE code: IIIB8) [Difficulty: ELE: R, Ap, An]

b. Independently change the type of humidification equipment (ELE code: IIIF2g1) [Difficulty: ELE: R, Ap, An]

Patients with an oropharyngeal or nasopharyngeal airway may also be given supplemental humidity by a simple aerosol mask to help prevent drying of secretions. If a patient is given more than 4 L/min of oxygen, supplemental humidity should be provided. Patients with an endotracheal or tracheostomy tube in place should ideally be provided 100% relative humidity at body temperature. If not, secretions in the airway may dry and result in mucous plugs. Depending on the patient situation, a heat-moisture exchanger (HME) or heated humidifier may be used. However, it may be necessary to change from a heat-moisture exchanger to a cascade-type or wick-type humidifier if the patient has thick secretions that are difficult to remove by coughing or suctioning. Humidification is discussed with the various oxygen delivery systems.

See Chapter 8 for a complete discussion of humidity and aerosol therapy and administrative devices.

MODULE B
Oropharyngeal airways

1. Recommend the insertion of an artificial airway or a change in the type of artificial airway (Code: IIIG1f) [Difficulty: ELE: R, Ap; WRE: An]

An oropharyngeal airway is typically used in one of the three following situations: (1) in an unconscious patient at risk of obstructing the airway with his or her tongue; (2) in an unconscious seizure patient who may bite his or her tongue during another seizure; (3) in an orally intubated patient to prevent the endotracheal tube from being bitten. An oropharyngeal airway should not be used in a conscious patient because it may cause gagging.

2. Manipulate oropharyngeal airways by order or protocol (ELE code: IIA7a) [Difficulty: ELE: R, Ap, An]

a. Get the necessary equipment

The oropharyngeal airway (or *bite block*) is made of plastic that is hard enough to withstand any patient's biting force. A properly sized and placed oropharyngeal airway lifts the tongue forward from the posterior portion of the oropharynx to keep a patent airway and make suctioning oral secretions easier. An oropharyngeal airway is poorly tolerated in a conscious patient and can cause gagging and even vomiting. Oropharyngeal airways are available in a variety of sizes that fit infants or adults. The proper size is found by holding the airway against the patient's face with the flange against the lips. The end of the airway should reach the angle of the jaw (Figure 12-2). Too large an airway can block the oropharynx by extending past the

Figure 12-2   Procedure for measuring the proper size of the oropharyngeal airway. *(From Eubanks DH, Bone RC: Comprehensive respiratory care, ed 2, St Louis, 1990, Mosby.)*

tongue. An airway that is too small can push the tongue back into the oropharynx rather than pulling the tongue forward, as intended. Figure 12-3 shows a properly placed and sized oropharyngeal airway.

A number of manufacturers make oropharyngeal airways, which fall into two basic types: hollow center and I-beam (Figure 12-4).

1. Hollow center

Hollow center types (Guedel is a common brand) have an oval or rectangular shape in cross section and are hollow in the center. A suction catheter can be easily placed through the hollow center so that the back of the throat can be cleared of secretions. Some types have an outer tube that can be attached by a practitioner to provide a mouthpiece for rescue breathing. If rescue breathing must be performed, it is probably more effective to ventilate with a mask and manual resuscitator when one becomes available.

2. I-beam

I-beam types (Berman is a common brand) are shaped like an I-beam in cross section. A suction catheter can easily be guided along the groove on either side of the I-beam to the back of the throat so that secretions can be removed.

b. Put the equipment together and make sure that it works properly

Most oropharyngeal airways are single units. There is nothing to assemble. There are some hollow-center types that have an attachable outer part. The outer part is snapped onto the oropharyngeal airway when the practitioner must perform rescue breathing. It has a wide flange so that the lips can be covered and sealed to prevent a leak.

c. Troubleshoot any problems with the equipment

Make sure that the channel in the hollow-center types is patent. If a unit is plugged by secretions, blood, or a foreign substance, the patient cannot breathe through the opening. A suction catheter cannot be passed through either. Remove an airway that is not patent.

d. Insert the correct oropharyngeal airway (ELE Code: IIIB2) [Difficulty: ELE: R, Ap, An]

There are three widely used methods to insert an oropharyngeal airway.

1. First method

a. Open the patient's mouth with the cross-finger technique. Insert the airway upside down into the patient's mouth until it reaches the palate. Some authors recommend inserting it past the uvula.

Figure 12-3 Three different possible procedures for inserting an oropharyngeal airway. **A,** Airway is placed with the tip pointing toward the palate. Then it is rotated 180 degrees to support the tongue. **B,** A tongue depressor is used to move the tongue toward the jaw. The airway is then slid behind the tongue to support it, and the tongue depressor is removed. **C,** A cheek is gently pulled aside to make room to place the airway behind the tongue. *(From Shilling A, Durbin CG: Airway management devices. In Cairo JM, Pilbeam SP, editors:* Mosby's respiratory care equipment, *ed 8, St Louis, 2010, Mosby, Inc.)*

Figure 12-4 Close-ups of hollow and I-beam types of oropharyngeal airways.

b. Twist the airway 180 degrees, and insert it the rest of the way until the tongue is supported by the curved body.

c. The flange should rest at the lips (Figure 12-3, *A*).

2. Second method

a. Insert a tongue blade into the mouth and push the tongue toward the jaw.

b. The curved body of the airway is directed into the mouth to support the tongue.

c. The flange should rest at the lips (Figure 12-3, *B*).

3. Third method

a. Open the patient's mouth with the cross-finger technique. Insert the airway into the mouth with the curved body rotated toward a cheek.

b. Twist the airway 90 degrees, and insert it the rest of the way so that the tongue is supported by the curved body.

c. The flange should rest at the lips (Figure 12-3, *C*).

MODULE C
Nasopharyngeal airways

1. Recommend the insertion of an artificial airway or a change in the type of artificial airway (Code: IIIG1f) [Difficulty: ELE: R, Ap; WRE: An]

A nasopharyngeal airway has three indications. First, it is used to keep the tongue from blocking the airway when an oropharyngeal airway cannot be used. This would include conscious supine patients or patients with oral trauma or jaw surgery. Second, it is also used as a guide to pass a catheter for tracheal suctioning or to pass a flexible fiberoptic bronchoscope. The nasopharyngeal airway protects the patient's mucous membranes from the trauma of repeatedly passed catheters. Third, a nasopharyngeal airway is used in a patient currently seizuring with a tightly closed jaw. In this case, an oropharyngeal airway cannot be used. The nasopharyngeal airway can be passed into the patient's oropharynx to push the tongue forward and maintain an airway. The nasopharyngeal airway is probably not as effective in keeping the tongue forward as the oropharyngeal airway. However, it is better tolerated in a semiconscious or alert patient.

2. Manipulate nasopharyngeal airways by order or protocol (ELE code: IIA7a) [Difficulty: ELE: R, Ap, An]

a. Get the necessary equipment

Nasopharyngeal airways (also known as *nasal airways, nasal trumpets,* or *nasal stents*) are made of a relatively soft and pliable plastic or rubber. This decreases the chances of damaging the delicate mucous membranes of the nasal turbinate opening as it passes through the nasopharynx.

Several manufacturers make the two basic types of nasopharyngeal airways—the *blunt tip* and the *beveled tip.* The beveled-tip types are available with right-sided and left-sided cut bevels. If possible, open the airway with the bevel cut opening toward the patient's oropharynx (toward the nasal septum). For example, if the airway is going to be inserted into the left naris, the bevel should be cut on the right side of the tube so that it is open to the patient's oropharynx. If you were inserting the tube into the right nostril, you would want the bevel cut on the left side of the tube.

See Figure 12-5 for a close-up of a nasopharyngeal airway. All nasopharyngeal airways have a flange that fits close to the patient's nostril. This prevents the entire tube from being pushed into the patient. All nasopharyngeal airways have a cannula with a channel for breathing or suctioning. Nasopharyngeal airways are available in a variety of sizes for adults. They can be properly sized by measuring from the tip of the nose to the tragus of the ear and adding 2 to 3 cm (Figure 12-6).

b. Put the equipment together and make sure that it works properly

All nasopharyngeal airways are made up of a single piece. There is nothing to assemble.

c. Troubleshoot any problems with the equipment

Make sure that the tube is not plugged by dried secretions, blood, or a foreign body. If plugged, the patient cannot

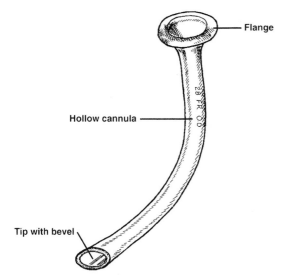

Figure 12-5 Typical nasopharyngeal airway.

Figure 12-6 Procedure for measuring the proper size of the nasopharyngeal airway. *(From Eubanks DH, Bone RC: Comprehensive respiratory care, ed 2, St Louis, 1990, Mosby.)*

breathe through it, and a suction catheter cannot be passed through it. Remove a plugged nasopharyngeal airway.

d. Insert the correct nasopharyngeal airway (ELE Code: IIIB2) [Difficulty: ELE: R, Ap, An]

The following steps are taken to insert a nasopharyngeal airway:

1. Select the most patent nostril. Check the patient's chart for a history of a broken nose, deviated septum, or current head cold. Interview the conscious patient to determine whether one nostril is more open than the other. Place your finger in front of the patient's nostrils to feel which one has greater airflow. Avoid forcing the airway into a nostril and nasal passage that may be damaged by the procedure.

Figure 12-7 Proper position of the nasopharyngeal airway behind the tongue can be determined by looking into the mouth. The tube is also secured by placing a safety pin through the flange and taping it to the cheek.

2. Lubricate the properly sized airway with a sterile, water-soluble lubricant such as K-Y jelly. Place the lubricant on a sterile, 4 × 4 inch gauze pad, and then smear it over the length of the airway.
3. Tell the patient what you are going to do.
4. Gently place the airway into the nostril. It should be directed straight back parallel to the hard palate. Stop if you feel any resistance. Try a different angle if resistance is felt. Do not force the airway. Try the other nostril if necessary.
5. Secure the airway by sticking a safety pin through the flange and taping the pin to the bridge of the patient's nose or cheek (see Figure 12-7). This helps prevent the airway from being accidentally dislodged or inserted further.
6. Rotate the airway to the other nostril, if possible, on a regular basis. This helps prevent ulceration of the mucous membrane. Some authors recommend rotation at least every 48 hours, whereas others recommend rotation at much shorter time intervals.

e. Assess the nasopharyngeal tube placement (ELE code: IIIB5) [Difficulty: ELE: R, Ap, An]

Check the placement by looking into the patient's mouth with a flashlight and tongue depressor. A properly placed nasopharyngeal airway can be seen in the oropharynx and extends behind the tongue (Figures 12-7 and 12-8). The placement should be checked each time a tube is replaced or moved from one nostril to the other. If a nasopharyn-

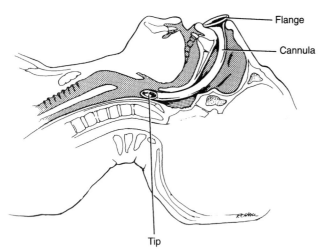

Figure 12-8 Cross section of the head showing the proper position of the nasopharyngeal airway. *(From Ellis PD, Billings DM: Cardiopulmonary resuscitation: procedures for basic and advanced life support, St Louis, 1980, Mosby.)*

geal tube is inserted too deeply, it can block the glottis opening into the trachea.

MODULE D

Laryngeal mask airways

1. Recommend the insertion of an artificial airway or a change in the type of artificial airway (Code: IIIG1f) [Difficulty: ELE: R, Ap; WRE: An]

A laryngeal mask airway (LMA) is composed of a modified endotracheal tube with a standard 15-mm-outer diameter (OD) adapter (for attaching a resuscitation bag or ventilator circuit) at the proximal end and a silicone laryngeal mask at the distal end. The mask is inflated by attaching a syringe to the one-way valve and pilot balloon on an inflation tube, in the same manner as an endotracheal tube cuff (Figure 12-9). When the mask is inflated it surrounds and seals the larynx. LMAs were first used in the operating room by anesthesiologists. Their use has been expanded; today, emergency medical personnel and respiratory therapists use LMAs as an alternative to endotracheal tubes or Combitubes in patients with a difficult airway or during a CPR effort. Experience has shown that an LMA can be easily and quickly inserted without any additional equipment. Patients with asthma or irritable airways will have less coughing or bronchospasm than if an endotracheal tube were inserted. It has been shown that ventilating a patient with a resuscitation bag to an LMA is as effective or better than bag-mask ventilation. See Box 12-1 for indications, contraindications, and limits to an LMA.

Remember that an LMA does not provide as secure an airway as an endotracheal tube. There are two limitations

Figure 12-9 Laryngeal mask airway (LMA). It features an inflatable mask that creates a seal around the patient's larynx. A syringe is attached to the one-way valve to deflate and inflate the mask. The proximal end of the tube can be connected to a resuscitation bag, anesthesia machine, or mechanical ventilator. *(From Intavent International SA, Henley-on-Thames, England.)*

BOX 12-1   Indications, Contraindications, and Limits of a Laryngeal Mask Airway

INDICATIONS

Patient has undergone CPR effort or has a difficult airway and cannot have an endotracheal tube or Combitube.

Patient needs a patent airway and cannot have his/her neck hyperextended for endotracheal intubation.

A channel is needed through which to pass an endotracheal tube into the trachea.

CONTRAINDICATIONS

Patient is conscious or resists placement of the LMA.

Patient is known to have or might have food in the stomach.

Patient will require high pressure to ventilate (because of low lung compliance and/or high airway resistance).

Patient has severe gastroesophageal reflux disease (GERD).

LIMITS

Aspiration is possible if the patient's stomach is not empty or has GERD.

There is tidal volume leakage out of the mouth or into stomach if the ventilating pressure is >20 cm H_2O.

---

to using an LMA. First, the LMA does not absolutely protect against aspiration. Second, tidal volume gas can leak if mechanical ventilation pressures are greater than 20 cm H_2O. This can lead to a smaller than desired tidal volume and/or gas being forced into the stomach. Excessive air in the stomach can cause vomiting. If either of these possibilities is of paramount clinical concern, the patient should have an endotracheal tube inserted rather than an LMA.

2. Manipulate laryngeal mask airways by order or protocol (Code: IIA7f) [Difficulty: ELE: R, Ap; WRE: An]

a. Get the necessary equipment

The LMA is available in eight sizes for insertion into patients ranging in weight from a small child to a large adult. Selected sizes include mask size 1 for a neonate or child up to 5 kg (up to 11 pounds); mask size $2\frac{1}{2}$ for children weighing between 20 and 30 kg (44 and 66 pounds); mask size 4 for adults weighing 50 to 70 kg (110 to 154 pounds); and mask size 5 for large adults weighing 70 to 100 kg (154 to 220 pounds). Other mask sizes are available for patients within these weight ranges or for very large adults.

Several manufacturers make standard LMAs like that shown in Figure 12-9. In addition, there are two commonly seen modifications. The first is an LMA that facilitates tracheal intubation by easily allowing an endotracheal tube to slide through its lumen. The second is an LMA that includes a port for gastric suction to vent any air in the stomach. Adjunct supplies include a water-soluble lubricant for the laryngeal mask, syringe to inflate the mask, and protective gear for the practitioner, such as a face mask and gloves.

b. Put the equipment together and make sure that it works properly

Make sure that the proximal end has a 15-mm-OD adapter attached. Check the laryngeal mask to be sure it is functioning. Inflate the cuff with a syringe, disconnect the syringe to make sure the one-way valve works, reattach the syringe, and deflate the mask.

c. Troubleshoot any problems with the equipment

Do not use an LMA that does not have a proximal adapter or if the mask will not inflate properly.

3. Assess the placement of the LMA (ELE code: IIIB5) [Difficulty: ELE: R, Ap, An]

While the NBRC does not list the insertion of an LMA as a testable item, proper placement is needed to ensure that it can be correctly maintained in the airway. Figure 12-10 shows the procedure for inserting an LMA and how the inflated mask covers the laryngeal inlet (glottis opening into the trachea). When the properly sized LMA is being placed, it is gently advanced until resistance is felt. (If the LMA is too small, no resistance will be felt since it will slide into the esophagus.) The distal tip of the mask will stop at the upper esophageal sphincter. The cuff is then inflated to cover the tracheal opening and seal off the esophagus. (Later, the cuff pressure can be measured; it should not exceed 60 cm H_2O.) Manually ventilate the patient's lungs with a resuscitation bag. The following steps should be taken to ensure that the LMA is properly placed to cover the opening to the trachea: (1) when the LMA mask is inflated, the tube will move out of the mouth about 1 to 2 cm; (2) auscultate for equal, bilateral breath sounds; (3) auscultate for the absence of sounds over the stomach; (4) an end-tidal carbon dioxide monitor should show exhaled CO_2.

4. Maintain the proper position and appropriate cuff inflation of a laryngeal mask airway (Code: IIIB4a) [Difficulty: ELE: R, Ap; WRE: An]

Once the LMA is properly located, it needs to be stabilized. This is usually done by taping the tube to the patient's upper lip or using a manufactured tube-holding device. Observe that the black line that runs the length of the tube, and marks its center, is not twisted. If the tube is twisted, the tracheal mask may not cover the glottis. This would cause a leak and loss of tidal volume. A standard cuff measuring device (like the Cufflator) can be used to measure the mask pressure. It should not be greater than 60 cm H_2O to seal the airway. (See the later discussion on managing an endotracheal tube for more information on securing the tube and measuring cuff pressure.)

MODULE E

Esophageal obturator airway: Combitube

1. Recommend the insertion of an artificial airway or a change in the type of artificial airway (Code: IIIG1f) [Difficulty: ELE: R, Ap; WRE: An]

The Combitube (also known as the esophageal-tracheal Combitube or ETC) is a double-lumen tube that can be used to ventilate a patient whether the tube is placed into the esophagus (as intended) or trachea (Figure 12-11). The Combitube is one version of a series of tubes called esophageal obturator airways (EOAs) that are designed to be placed into the esophagus of an unconscious adult patient. Clinical experience has shown that a Combitube provides a reasonably secure airway in emergency situations, such as when performing CPR. It can be used as an alternative to an LMA. At the time this book was being published, there were five different types of EOA that

Figure 12-10   Steps to insert an LMA to make sure that it seals the patient's larynx. **A,** The lubricated mask is deflated and manually inserted into the mouth. **B,** The mask should easily slide behind the tongue into the oral pharynx. **C,** The mask is gently advanced until resistance is felt as the mask lodges at the opening of the larynx. **D,** The syringe is attached to the one-way valve and air is pumped into the mask to seal the larynx. Attach a resuscitation bag to the proximal end of the tube and inflate the patient's lungs. Listen for bilateral breath sounds. See the inset for the anatomic structures related to the larynx, glottis, and esophagus. *(Redrawn from Gensia Automedics, San Diego, Calif. In Cairo JM, Pilbeam SP, editors:* Mosby's respiratory care equipment, *ed 8, St Louis, 2010, Mosby, Inc.)*

Figure 12-11 Combitube with its component features. Note that the Combitube has two lumens and two cuffs. The lumen with the distal cuff is inserted into the patient's esophagus (or occasionally the trachea). The proximal cuff is inserted into the patient's pharynx. Each cuff has its own inflating tube with one-way valve. There are perforations in the esophageal tube between the two cuffs that allow ventilation through the esophageal port. The proximal end of both tubes has a standard 15-mm-OD adapter for attachment of a resuscitation bag. Depending on the placement of the Combitube in the esophagus (as intended) or trachea, the patient's lungs can be ventilated through the esophageal or tracheal port when both cuffs are inflated. *(From Blosser SA, Stauffer JL:* Clin Chest Med *17:355-378, 1996.)*

provide the same two functions: ensure a stable airway for artificial ventilation and prevent vomiting and aspiration. Clinical experience with the various types of esophageal obturator airways is highly recommended because they do not appear or operate like standard endotracheal tubes. See Box 12-2 for a comparison of a Combitube with an endotracheal tube.

2. Manipulate a Combitube by order or protocol (Code: IIA7g) [Difficulty: ELE: R, Ap; WRE: An]

a. Get the necessary equipment

The Combitube is available in two sizes. The longer, larger size (41Fr) version is used for patients who are more than 16 years old and more than 60 inches (5 feet) in height. The Combitube SA is smaller (37Fr) and intended for smaller patients. Neither size is intended for small pediatric patients. Both Combitube types are included in a kit with a 140-mL syringe to inflate the larger, proximal cuff in the patient's oral pharynx and a 20-mL syringe to inflate the smaller, distal cuff in the patient's esophagus (or trachea). The practitioner should have protective gear such as a face mask and gloves.

b. Put the equipment together and make sure that it works properly

Before placing either Combitube version into the patient, check that each cuff will inflate, hold air, and deflate

properly. Each of the tubes should have a standard 15-mm-OD ventilator adapter inserted into its proximal end.

c. Troubleshoot any problems with the equipment

Do use a unit that has a defective cuff(s) or missing adapters. If a cuff should fail during patient use, the Combitube should be removed. It can be replaced by another unit, another type of secure airway can be inserted, or bag-mask ventilation can be performed.

3. Assess the placement of the Combitube (ELE code: IIIB5) [Difficulty: ELE: R, Ap, An]

While the NBRC does not list the insertion of the Combitube as a testable item, proper placement is needed to ensure that it can be correctly maintained in the airway. Figure 12-12 shows the procedure for inserting a Combitube. When the tube enters the esophagus as intended, both cuffs are inflated, and the patient is ventilated through the longer, colored tube, bilateral breath sounds will be heard (see Figure 12-12, C). Continue to ventilate the patient's lungs and tape the tube in place. If breath sounds are not heard, the tube has accidentally entered the patient's trachea. Now, ventilate through the shorter, clear tube and listen for bilateral breath sounds. If they

---

BOX 12-2   Indications, Contraindications, Advantages, and Disadvantages of the Combitube

GENERAL INDICATIONS

Emergency personnel are not trained in endotracheal intubation.

Attempted endotracheal intubation has not been successful.

Patient is apneic, without reflexes, and unconscious.

GENERAL CONTRAINDICATIONS

Endotracheal intubation can be performed.

Patient is responsive with an intact gag reflex.

Patient is too small for the Combitube.

Esophageal obturator device would be needed for more than 1 to 2 hours.

Patient is known to have esophageal trauma, pathology, or to have ingested a corrosive substance.

ADVANTAGES

Rapidly controls the airway.

Can be inserted into the patient in an awkward position without the head or neck being hyperextended.

Prevents the insufflation of gas into the stomach during bag-mask ventilation.

Prevents the movement of stomach contents into the pharynx.

Has esophageal gastric tube airway (EGTA) advantages.

The stomach can be emptied by passing a Levin tube through the esophageal tube.

The patient's lungs can be ventilated whether the tube is placed into the esophagus (as intended) or trachea.

Prevents aspiration of blood from the upper airway.

DISADVANTAGES

Accidental and unrecognized tracheal intubation is possible.

The possibility of upper airway tear and hemorrhage during tube insertion exists.

Incomplete cuff seals result in air leak during ventilation.

The airway cannot be reliably kept open.

---

are heard, continue to ventilate and tape the tube in place (see Figure 12-12, *D*).

4. Maintain the proper position and appropriate cuff inflation of a Combitube (Code: IIIB4b) [Difficulty: ELE: R, Ap; WRE: An]

Tape can be used to secure the tube to the patient's upper lip. Follow the manufacturer's recommendation for cuff volumes. With the original Combitube, the large, pharyngeal cuff is designed to hold 100 mL of air; the smaller cuff is designed to hold 15 mL of air. Use enough air in the cuffs so that there is no air leak when manual resuscitation is performed.

MODULE F
Tracheostomy tubes

1. Recommend the insertion of an artificial airway or a change in the type of artificial airway (Code: IIIG1f) [Difficulty: ELE: R, Ap; WRE: An]

The tracheostomy tube offers the same uses as the endotracheal tube, such as maintaining a secure airway, providing a direct suctioning route to the lungs, preventing aspiration, and assuring a safe route to provide mechanical ventilation. In addition, it is placed in the patient who has an upper airway obstruction or facial trauma that makes intubation impossible. A tracheostomy tube is often placed in a patient who requires long-term mechanical ventilation. Some patients with a permanent neurologic problem that limits their breathing will have a tracheostomy performed. By not breathing through the upper airway, their anatomic dead space is reduced. In the long term, a tracheostomy is said to be more comfortable than an endotracheal tube, even though it requires a surgical procedure for its placement. An additional advantage of a tracheostomy tube over an endotracheal tube is that it allows the patient to eat and drink.

2. Manipulate standard and fenestrated tracheostomy tubes by order or protocol (ELE code: IIA7c) [Difficulty: ELE: R. Ap, An]

a. Get the necessary equipment

These tubes are available in a variety of sizes for patients of all ages from neonate to adult. See Table 12-1 for tracheostomy tube sizes (this also applies to tracheostomy buttons and endotracheal tubes) based on patient age. It is common practice to refer to the needed tube size by its inner diameter (ID). For example, a tracheostomy tube for an adult female would be 7.5- or 8.0-mm ID.

Most modern tracheostomy tubes are constructed of a hard polyvinyl chloride (PVC) plastic and have a high-volume, low-pressure cuff. Some specialty tubes are made of silver, rubber, or latex. The older, silver tubes may not have a cuff or the cuff may be removed. A syringe is needed to inflate the tube cuff. The practitioner should wear gloves and a mask when working with a patient's tracheostomy tube and stoma.

b. Put the equipment together and make sure that it works properly

The following are commonly seen examples of tracheostomy tube styles:

1. Standard tracheostomy tube

After the tracheostomy procedure is completed, the majority of patients have a standard tube placed into the stoma.

Figure 12-12 Steps in the insertion of a Combitube to make sure that it seals the patient's airway. **A,** One hand is used to grasp the jaw and pull it forward. With both cuffs deflated and the patient's head in a neutral position, the Combitube is inserted into the center of the mouth. **B,** Outer view of the Combitube after it has been gently inserted until the black rings on the tube are at the teeth. **C,** Inner view of the *usual* location of the tube in the patient's esophagus. Both cuffs are inflated. The resuscitation bag is attached to the longer, colored esophageal tube and the patient's lungs are ventilated. Listen for bilateral breath sounds. **D,** Inner view of the *occasional* location of the tube in the patient's trachea. Both cuffs are inflated. The resuscitation bag is attached to the shorter, clear tracheal tube and the patient's lungs are ventilated. Listen for bilateral breath sounds. *(From Cairo JM, Pilbeam SP:* Mosby's respiratory care equipment, *ed 8, St Louis, 2010, Mosby, Inc.)*

Refer to Figure 12-13 for these features of a typical tracheostomy tube:

   a. The cannula is the airway through which the patient breathes. The proximal end is outside of the patient's stoma and attached to an adjustable flange. The angle of the flange can be adjusted so that the distal end of the cannula fits properly into the patient's trachea. Soft, cloth tracheostomy tie strings are attached to the ends of the flange. The loose ends are tied behind the patient's neck to hold the tube in place. The distal end of the cannula has a small area where radiopaque material is imbedded. As with an endotracheal tube, this allows the end of the cannula to be seen on a chest radiograph. The cuff is a high residual volume, low-pressure type. Air is inserted and withdrawn from the cuff by an inflation tube with a pilot balloon and one-way valve.

Age	ID (mm)	Approximate OD (mm)	Fr size (OD)
NEWBORN			
<1000 g	2.5	4.0	12
1000-2000 g	3.0	5.0	14
2000-3000 g	3.5	5.5	16-18
3000 g to 6 mo old	3.5-4.0		
PEDIATRIC			
18 mo	4.0	6.0	18
3 yr	4.5	6.5	20
5 yr	5.0	7.0	22
6 yr	5.5	8.0	24
8 yr	6.0	9.0	26
ADULT			
16 yr	7.0	10.0	30
Normal sized woman	7.5-8.0	11.0	32-34
Normal sized man	8.0-8.5	12.0	34-36
Large adult	9.0-10.0	13.0-14.0	38-42

TABLE 12-1 Endotracheal and Tracheostomy Tube Sizes Based on Patient Age*

*Two notes: First, it is important to always use the largest tube that can be placed into the patient without causing any harm during the intubation. This is because the larger the ID of the tube, the less airway resistance it causes. Be prepared to insert a tube that is one size larger or smaller than anticipated based on individual variances. Second, the mathematical relationship between the OD in millimeters and Fr size can be easily calculated. The Fr size is determined by multiplying the OD in millimeters by 3. The OD in millimeters is found by dividing the Fr size by 3.

Fr, French; *ID*, internal diameter; *OD*, outer diameter.

Figure 12-13 Typical tracheostomy tube with its component parts and features.

Figure 12-14 Fenestrated tracheostomy tube with its component parts and features. *(From Eubanks DH, Bone RC: Comprehensive respiratory care, ed 2, St Louis, 1990, Mosby.)*

b. The obturator is slid into the outer cannula's opening before it is inserted into the patient's stoma. The obturator has a rounded end that protrudes from the end of the cannula. This prevents any tissue trauma during the insertion. The obturator is removed as soon as the cannula is in place.

c. An inner cannula is slid into the outer cannula's opening and locked into place with a clockwise twist. This completes the airway. The proximal end has a standard 15-mm outer diameter (OD) adapter so that all respiratory care equipment fits onto it. The distal end is flush with the end of the outer cannula. Some practitioners believe that the inner cannula should be periodically removed and cleaned so that secretions do not accumulate. Other practitioners believe that this is unnecessary if the airway is properly humidified and suctioning is performed as needed.

2. Fenestrated tracheostomy tube

A fenestrated tube is often placed in a patient who can breathe spontaneously and who is being considered for a complete removal of the tracheostomy tube. If the patient does well with this tube, it can probably be removed safely. If the patient has difficulty, the plug can be removed, the inner cannula can be replaced, and the patient's airway can be suctioned or mechanically ventilated.

Refer to Figure 12-14 when reviewing these features of the fenestrated tracheostomy tube:

a. The outer cannula has an opening called the fenestration (Dutch for window). The rest of the cannula, cuff, inflation tube, and flange are the same as already discussed.

b. The inner cannula functions as discussed earlier. When it is in place, the tube functions in the same manner as the standard model.

c. The outer cannula plug is used to prevent the patient from breathing through the proximal end of the tube. The plug does not cover the fenestration; therefore the patient is able to breathe through the upper airway. The patient can now talk and expectorate any secretions.

Exam Hint 12-2 (ELE, WRE)

A standard tracheostomy tube should be replaced with a fenestrated tube when a patient is improving and can breathe spontaneously (off of the ventilator) for an extended time. Remove the inner cannula and deflate the cuff so that the patient can breathe through the upper airway. Replace the inner cannula and inflate the cuff when mechanical ventilation is resumed.

---

c. Troubleshoot any problems with the equipment

Before a tracheostomy (or endotracheal) tube is inserted into a patient, the cuff must be tested. Do this by attaching a syringe to the one-way valve and inflating the cuff. Remove the syringe. The cuff must stay inflated to show that it and the one-way valve work properly. Then reattach the syringe and deflate the cuff. Do not use a tube with a leaking cuff or leaking one-way valve. Make sure that the obturator, inner cannula, and plug all fit properly into the outer cannula. They all should easily snap into place and be easily removable. Check this before inserting the tube into the patient.

Secretions, blood, or foreign matter can plug the lumen of the tube. Suction to remove any obstruction. It is also possible for the cuff to herniate and cover the end of the tube. If the catheter cannot be inserted beyond the tube and the patient is having respiratory distress, the tube will have to be removed. Replace the defective tracheostomy tube with another as soon as possible.

Exam Hint 12-3 (ELE)

The following factors can contribute to obstruction of the lumen of the cannula: (1) secretions or foreign matter; (2) a cuff that has herniated or slipped over the end of the tube; (3) placement of the tip of the tube into the subcutaneous tissues. Initially, attempt to suction to remove any obstruction. If the catheter cannot be inserted beyond the tube and the patient is having respiratory distress, the tube must be removed and replaced.

---

3. Assess the placement of a tracheostomy tube (ELE code: IIIB5) [Difficulty: ELE: R, Ap, An]

The first step in assessing tube placement is knowing that it was properly inserted. With the cuff deflated and the obturator inserted into the cannula, the tube should be gently slid through the stoma. The natural curvature of the tube should result in the distal tip being placed within the trachea and the flange being against the neck of the patient. Forcing should be avoided as this may indicate that the tip of the tube is entering the surrounding tissues. Also, the proper size tube will not need to be forced through the stoma. Inflate the cuff. All of the patient's breathing should pass through the tube. Auscultate for equal and bilateral breath sounds. No breath sounds should be heard over the patient's stomach area. An exhaled carbon dioxide monitor can also be attached to the proximal end of the tube to measure the concentration of carbon dioxide being exhaled by the patient. Lastly, the physician may want to have an upper airway or chest radiograph taken. Ensure that the distal tip of the tube is within the center of the trachea.

4. Maintain the proper position and appropriate cuff inflation of a tracheostomy tube (Code: IIIB4d) [Difficulty: ELE: R, Ap; WRE: An]

After being assured that the tracheostomy tube is properly located, wrap the tie strings behind the patient's neck and tie them with a bowknot or fasten the Velcro straps. Tying the strings should help to prevent the tube from being misplaced or pulled out. The cuff pressure should be measured on a regular basis to make sure that it is being kept at a safe level. In most patients, a safe cuff pressure is no more than 20 to 25 mm Hg (25 to 35 cm H_2O). (A more complete discussion of cuff pressure measurement follows in the discussion on endotracheal tubes.)

If the patient experiences a sudden partial or complete airway obstruction, it is possible that the tube has become twisted or partially pulled out and forced into the soft tissues around the trachea. However, first eliminate other possible causes. Quickly deflate the cuff to rule it out as a cause of the obstruction. If the obstruction is still present, attempt to pass a suction catheter. If it can be passed though the tube, perform suctioning to remove any mucous plug. If the tube has an inner cannula and the catheter cannot be passed, remove the inner cannula. If it is plugged with mucus, either remove the mucus or replace the inner cannula. If none of these procedures opens the patient's airway, it is likely that the distal tip of the tracheostomy tube is misplaced into the soft tissues. Withdraw the tube and let the patient breathe through the stoma. As quickly as possible, replace the tube through the stoma and into the trachea. Inflate the cuff and check that the patient can breathe normally.

5. Change the tracheostomy tube (ELE code: IIIB7) [Difficulty: R, Ap, An]

A tracheostomy tube may have to be changed because of a ruptured cuff or because of another problem. In addition, patients with a permanent tracheostomy have the tube changed on a routine schedule as part of tracheostomy care. These two different situations are discussed separately.

a. Emergency tube change

Several factors can cause the clinical emergency of obstruction, such as the cuff herniating over the end of the tube, a mucous plug blocking the lumen, or the end of the tube being forced into the tracheal tissues. Unfortunately, these problems cannot be seen from the outside. If the patient is in acute respiratory distress and an obstruction is suspected, attempt to pass a suction catheter. Failure to pass it beyond the end of the tube confirms the obstruction. A rapid clinical decision has to be made to choose the best action. The tube should be removed if the obstruction is complete and the patient cannot breathe. A spontaneously breathing patient can continue to breathe through the stoma. An apneic patient must be temporarily ventilated with mouth-to-stoma breaths. As rapidly and carefully as possible another tracheostomy tube should be inserted. This usually results in a patent airway. If loose tracheal mucosa is blocking the airway, an endotracheal tube must be inserted past the tissue and deeper into the trachea. Call the physician as soon as possible to evaluate the patient's condition.

b. Routine tube change

If possible, the tube should not be changed until 7 to 10 days after a fresh tracheostomy procedure. This allows time for the stoma site to form granulomatous tissue as it begins to heal. The site is then less likely to bleed as the tube is changed. When the tracheostomy tube is changed, it is usually part of tracheostomy wound care. The following are typical steps in changing the tracheostomy tube:

1. Gather the necessary equipment: a new tracheostomy tube of the same size and the next size smaller, its inner cannula, its obturator, tracheostomy tie strings to secure the tube in the patient (see Figure 12-10), a sterile tracheostomy dressing pad (4 × 4 inches for an adult), sterile scissors, a 10-mL syringe to inflate the cuff, sterile water-soluble lubricant, sterile gloves, and goggles. Make sure the cuff inflates and deflates properly.
2. Put on the gloves and goggles.
3. Maintaining sterile technique, make sure the obturator easily fits into and can be withdrawn from the tracheostomy tube.
4. Open the tracheostomy dressing pad (it has a slit into the center of the gauze pad).
5. Apply some lubricant to the tip of the tracheostomy tube.
6. Tell the patient what you are going to do.
7. Remove the oxygen and/or aerosol from the patient.
8. Suction the patient's trachea. Reoxygenate the patient.
9. Untie the tracheostomy strings or separate the Velcro straps.
10. Deflate the cuff.
11. Remove the current tracheostomy dressing pad.
12. Remove the tracheostomy tube by pulling it in a curved motion toward the patient's chest.
13. Inspect the tracheostomy opening for signs of infection such as redness, pus, or swelling. Report signs of infection to the nurse or physician.
14. Carefully insert the new tracheostomy tube with obturator into the stoma. The motion should be opposite that used to remove the original tube. Make sure not to force the tube into the tissues of the trachea.
15. Remove the obturator and insert the inner cannula. Lock it in place.
16. Give the patient oxygen and/or aerosol as before the tube change.
17. Inflate the cuff to a safe pressure.
18. Listen for bilateral breath sounds.
19. Slide the new tracheostomy dressing pad around the tube so that the slit fits around it.
20. Tie the tracheostomy tie strings or fasten the Velcro straps behind the patient's neck.

6. Independently perform tracheostomy care (Code: IIIF2g5) [Difficulty: ELE: R, Ap; WRE: An] (ELE code: IIIB6) [Difficulty: ELE: R, Ap, An]

Routine tracheostomy care generally includes the steps previously described, except the removal of the tracheostomy tube. While performing tracheostomy care, inspect the stoma for possible signs of infection, clean the stoma site, apply a topical antibiotic, if indicated, and replace the 4 × 4 inch tracheostomy dressing pad.

7. Extubate the patient

a. Recommend extubation (Code: IIIG1h) [Difficulty: ELE: R, Ap; WRE: An]

Extubation should only be performed after correction of the causes that led to insertion of the tracheostomy tube. If the patient has required mechanical ventilation, review the discussion in Chapter 15 that relates to weaning the patient and extubation.

b. Perform extubation (Code: IIIB9) [Difficulty: ELE: R, Ap; WRE: An]

Extubation should be performed only by trained personnel and under the proper conditions to ensure the patient's safety. See Box 12-3 for a list of complications that can occur after extubation. The generally recommended steps in extubation include the following:

1. Evaluate the patient's cardiopulmonary status. The reason(s) for the tube being placed should be corrected. The most recent blood gas results should be acceptable. Tracheal secretions should be minimal and not so thick that they cannot be expectorated by the patient. Bedside spirometry results should show an acceptable tidal volume, vital capacity, and maximal inspiratory pressure.
2. Inform the patient about the removal of the tube and the follow-up care that is needed.
3. The patient's inspired oxygen percentage may be kept the same or increased before the extubation. If increased, it should be done at least 5 to 10 minutes before the tube is removed.
4. Suction the trachea until all secretions are removed.
5. Suction the oral pharynx to remove all saliva. Be prepared to suction additional oral secretions and mucus after extubation.
6. In rapid succession:
   a. Give a deep sigh breath.
   b. Deflate the cuff. Cut the inflation tube to the cuff to ensure its collapse.
   c. Pull out the tube when the lungs are full.
   Alternatively, in rapid succession:
   a. Give a deep sigh breath.
   b. Place a suction catheter through the tube into the trachea. This works best with a self-contained catheter and sheath system.
   c. Deflate the cuff. Cut the inflation tube to the cuff to ensure its collapse.
   d. Pull out the tube when the lungs are full.
   e. Apply suction as the tube is withdrawn.
7. Have the patient cough vigorously to remove any secretions.
8. Depending on the physician's order, do one of the following:
   • Apply a bland aerosol by tracheostomy mask to the stoma site with the previous amount of oxygen.
   • Cover the stoma site with a sterile 4 × 4 inch dressing. Tape it in place. Apply a bland aerosol by face mask with the previous amount of oxygen.
9. Monitor and evaluate the patient every 30 minutes for several hours. Encourage deep breathing and coughing. Check the vital signs and breath sounds. Be prepared to reintubate the patient if necessary. Measure pulse oximetry continuously or arterial blood gases after 10 to 20 minutes.

Routine stoma care to ensure healing usually includes the following each shift:

1. Remove the dressing. Inspect the stoma for signs of infection such as pus, redness, and swelling.
2. Clean the stoma site with hydrogen peroxide on a sterile gauze pad.
3. Apply antibiotic ointment to the stoma site, if indicated
4. Reapply a sterile dressing.

BOX 12-3 Complications after Extubation

TRACHEOSTOMY TUBE REMOVAL
Difficult tube removal from a tight stoma
Granuloma or scar at the stoma
Unhealed, open stoma
Hypoxemia and/or hypercapnia secondary to hypoventilation

ENDOTRACHEAL TUBE REMOVAL
Reflex laryngospasm
Bronchospasm
Regurgitation and aspiration of stomach contents
Aspiration of oral secretions
Sore throat
Dysphagia
Postintubation laryngeal edema (croup)
Hoarseness from vocal cord edema or paralysis
Hypoxemia and/or hypercapnia secondary to hypoventilation

CUFF-RELATED COMPLICATIONS
Granuloma
Tracheomalacia
Tracheal stenosis
Tracheal web formation
Tracheoesophageal fistula
Tracheoinnominate artery fistula

MODULE G
Tracheostomy buttons

1. Recommend the insertion of an artificial airway or a change in the type of artificial airway (Code: IIIG1f) [Difficulty: ELE: R, Ap; WRE: An]

A tracheostomy button is a hard plastic tube that is placed into the patient's stoma to keep it open after the tracheostomy tube has been removed (Figure 12-15). A button is inserted because the physician has determined that the stoma must be kept open in case the tracheostomy tube must be reinserted. Advantages of the button include the patient being able to eat, talk, and cough normally. Yet, in case the patient has difficulty or needs

Figure 12-15 Typical tracheostomy button properly positioned in patient. The insert shows its component parts.

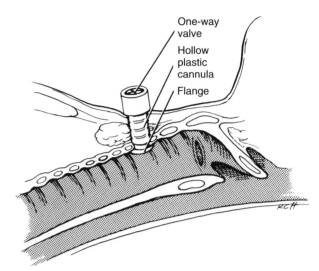

Figure 12-16 Kistner tracheostomy button. *(From Eubanks DH, Bone RC: Comprehensive respiratory care, ed 2, St Louis, 1990, Mosby.)*

a breathing treatment, a secure airway can be quickly reestablished.

2. Manipulate a tracheostomy button by order or protocol (ELE code: IIA7c) [Difficulty: ELE: R, Ap, An]

a. Get the necessary equipment

In general, the patient sizes for tracheostomy buttons match the sizes for tracheostomy tubes listed in Table 12-1.

b. Put the equipment together and make sure that it works properly

Refer to Figure 12-15 when reviewing these features of the tracheostomy button and accessories:

- The hollow outer cannula has a slightly flared proximal end. This keeps the button from slipping entirely into the patient. The distal end is flanged and split into several flexible "grippers."
- A closure plug fits into the outer cannula and snaps into the flexible grippers on the end of the outer cannula. This seals the button so that the patient breathes through the upper airway.
- A hollow inner cannula can be inserted into the outer cannula instead of the plug. This inner cannula has a standard 15-mm OD so that a T-piece/Briggs adapter or other respiratory care equipment can be attached if needed. The patient's secretions can also be suctioned.

- Spacers of various widths are used to make sure that the inner cannula is placed at the right depth. The end of the tube should enter the trachea but not obstruct it. See the airway picture in Figure 12-15 for the proper position.

A one-way valve may be added to the button. This would be used for patients who must not inspire through their upper airway but may exhale through it. In patients with a very small tidal volume, inhaling through one of these valves reduces the patient's upper airway anatomic dead space. Since expiration is through the upper airway, the patient can speak normally. Refer to Figure 12-16 when reviewing these features of the Kistner tracheostomy tube with an attached one-way valve:

- The hollow plastic cannula keeps the stoma open. The distal end is flanged so that it is not likely to be pulled out of the trachea accidentally.
- The proximal end of the cannula is capped with a one-way valve. The valve allows the patient to inhale room air or an oxygen- and aerosol-enriched gas source. Expiration is through the upper airway. The patient can talk, eat, and cough normally.

c. Troubleshoot any problems with the equipment

Make sure that all component pieces of these tracheostomy buttons fit together properly and can be easily disconnected if necessary. The cannula must be kept clear of any secretions, blood, or foreign debris. A suction catheter should be passable through the hollow opening in the cannula. If the button is obstructed and the patient is having trouble breathing through the upper airway, the button should be removed and replaced with another button or a tracheostomy tube.

3. Assess the placement of a tracheostomy button (ELE code: IIIB5) [Difficulty: ELE: R, Ap, An]

After the physician removes the tracheostomy tube, the depth of the stoma is measured. Based on that depth, spacers are added to the cannula to obtain the appropriate depth. Once the button is placed, the patient should not have any added resistance to breathing. If the button becomes misplaced and the patient has difficulty breathing, the button should be removed. A tracheostomy tube can then be inserted.

MODULE H
Speaking tubes and valves

1. Recommend the insertion of an artificial airway or a change in the type of artificial airway (Code: IIIG1f) [Difficulty: ELE: R, Ap; WRE: An]

A speaking tracheostomy tube is indicated in a patient who requires support on a mechanical ventilator but is conscious and wishes to speak. Some speaking valves can be added to a standard tracheostomy tube in a ventilator-dependent patient. In this situation, the cuff must be deflated for the exhaled tidal volume gas to pass through the vocal cords for speaking. Remember to reset the ventilator's exhaled low tidal volume alarm because no exhaled gas will return through the ventilator circuit.

Usually, a speaking valve is added to a tracheostomy button in a patient who is not ventilator-dependent. This patient cannot or should not be inhaling through the nose or mouth but can exhale through the natural upper airway. Commonly, these are patients with a neuromuscular disease. Their condition causes them to have a small tidal volume, which results in a large percentage of dead space ventilation. Placing a tracheostomy tube or button into these patients improves their dead space to tidal volume ratio and improves their blood gas values.

2. Manipulate a speaking tube or valve by order or protocol (ELE code: IIA7d) [Difficulty: ELE: R, Ap, An]

a. Get the necessary equipment

Table 12-1 lists the standard sizes of tracheostomy tubes. A speaking tracheostomy tube should match the same size as the current tracheostomy tube or button, if it is available.

Speaking tracheostomy tubes are only available in adult sizes. See Figure 12-17 for the features of a speaking tracheostomy tube (Pitt and Vocalaid have versions). The

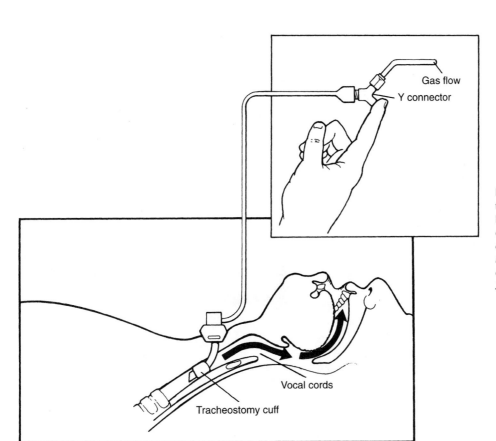

Figure 12-17 Pitt tracheostomy tube permits the patient to speak. Note its special feature that directs outside gas flow past the vocal cords. *(From Wilkins RL, Stoller JK, Kacmarek, RM: Egan's fundamentals of respiratory care, ed 9, St Louis, 2010, Mosby.)*

cannula is the standard type except that an additional tube has been added to carry a compressed gas through a hole in the back of the cannula. This gas flows through the vocal cords and allows the patient to speak. The voice is not as strong as normal but should be understandable. Improved communication ability is a great help to the patient's psychologic well-being. Patients can still be mechanically ventilated and have their secretions suctioned, and can eat and drink as usual.

Passy-Muir (Figure 12-18) and Kistner (see Figure 12-16) are common types of speaking valves that can be attached to a tracheostomy tube or tracheostomy button. All feature a one-way valve that opens when the patient inspires to allow room air or supplemental oxygen to be inhaled. When the patient exhales, the valve closes. This causes all of the exhaled tidal volume to pass through the vocal cords for speech. Aerosol therapy may be provided either by a tracheostomy mask over the valve or by a T-piece attached to it. (See Chapter 6 for a discussion of these aerosol/oxygen delivery systems.) As an alternative, the Trach-Talk combines an elbow adapter to the tracheostomy tube and a T-piece with a one-way valve (Figure 12-19). This device provides the patient with aerosol and/or oxygen with humidity through the one-way valve during inspiration. On exhalation, the valve closes and the patient exhales through the vocal cords for speech.

b. Put the equipment together and make sure that it works properly

With a speaking tracheostomy tube, a Y-connector is added to the compressed gas tube. Usually about 4 to 6 L/min of compressed air or oxygen are set by a flowmeter to run to the Y. Closing off the other opening in the Y with a finger diverts the gas into the patient's larynx for speaking. A little experimentation with flows helps the patient

find the flow that works best for speaking (see Figure 12-17). If the patient cannot speak at all, check that the gas is turned on and that the tubing is properly connected.

All speaking valves are available in a standard size to fit onto a 15-mm-OD tracheostomy tube. Passy-Muir makes a variety of valves. Whether the patient is breathing spontaneously or is ventilator-dependent, the one-way valve directs the tidal volume into the patient. The valve closes on exhalation so that gas passes through the vocal cords for speaking. Be aware that for this system to work with a ventilator-dependent patient, the cuff must be deflated. This will result in some loss of delivered tidal volume. Make sure that the patient can tolerate this. Also adjust the ventilator's alarm settings accordingly. If the patient is breathing spontaneously and needs low-flow supplemental oxygen, use the valve that includes a small-bore oxygen tubing nipple (see Figure 12-18).

c. Troubleshoot any problems with the equipment

For a speaking tracheostomy tube, see the preceding discussion on care of standard or fenestrated tracheostomy tubes. The same problems can occur with speaking tracheostomy tubes. Assess the patient's ability to speak in an understandable way. Enough compressed gas must pass through the vocal cords for this to happen. Yet, too high

Figure 12-18 Photograph of a variety of speaking valves made by Passy-Muir. When the one-way valve is attached to a tracheostomy tube, the patient breaths in through the valve and exhales through the upper airway for speech. *(Courtesy Passy-Muir, Inc., Irvine, Calif.)*

Figure 12-19 A patient with a tracheostomy tube and attached Olympic Trach-Talk speaking device. It features a one-way valve so that the patient breaths in through the valve and exhales through the upper airway for speech. *(From Cairo JM, Pilbeam SP: Mosby's respiratory care equipment, ed 8, St Louis, 2010, Mosby.)*

a gas flow can cause some resistance to the patient's tidal volume exhalation.

With a speaking valve, make sure that the one-way valve opens and closes properly. If a spontaneously breathing patient's valve was to become plugged with secretions, the patient would have to inhale through the natural upper airway rather than the valve.

3. Assess the placement of a speaking tube (ELE code: IIIB5) [Difficulty: ELE: R, Ap, An]

The assessment of the placement of a speaking tracheostomy tube would be the same as discussed previously with standard tracheostomy tubes.

MODULE I
Endotracheal tubes and intubation equipment

1. Recommend the insertion of an artificial airway or a change in the type of artificial airway (Code: IIIG1f) [Difficulty: ELE: R, Ap; WRE: An]

An endotracheal tube is indicated when a secure, patent airway is required for endotracheal suctioning or mechanical ventilation. Aspiration is also prevented when the cuff is inflated. It is generally accepted that an endotracheal tube provides for a more secure airway than a laryngeal mask airway or Combitube. In most emergency situations an oral endotracheal tube is indicated over a nasal endotracheal tube because the oral route is faster and easier. A nasal endotracheal tube is indicated when the patient has oral trauma or when a cervical spine injury prevents the neck from being hyperextended for placing the oral tube.

2. Manipulate oral and nasal endotracheal tubes by order or protocol (ELE code: IIA7b) [Difficulty: ELE: R, Ap, An]

a. Get the necessary equipment

An endotracheal tube is the best emergency device for maintaining a secure airway. It also provides a direct suctioning route to the lungs and prevents aspiration. Mechanical ventilation can easily be provided through it. See Table 12-1 for a list of endotracheal tube sizes (this also applies to tracheostomy tubes and buttons) based upon the patient's age. It is common practice to refer to the needed tube size by its inner diameter (ID). For example, a tracheostomy tube for an adult male would be 8.0- or 8.5-mm ID.

An endotracheal tube is meant to be a temporary airway; however, it can stay in patients for weeks if necessary. Virtually all endotracheal tubes used clinically now are made of pliable plastic. Always select a tube that has a large residual volume and low-pressure cuff unless there is a specific contraindication. For the most part, oral and nasal endotracheal tubes can be used interchangeably. The nasal endotracheal tube is longer and more curved than an oral endotracheal tube. The greater curve of the nasal tube should result in less pressure on the nasal mucosa. An anesthesiologist requests a nasal tube if he or she is going to place it by the nasal route. Oral tubes are used in the majority of patients.

The tubes are available in sizes from 4-mm OD through 14-mm OD so that patients of all ages and sizes can be intubated. The OD size increments are 0.5 mm. The thickness of the outer wall of the tube varies from 0.5 to 1 mm, which results in a reduction of the inner diameter (ID) of the tube by about 1 to 2 mm. Table 12-1 lists the approximate ID of an endotracheal tube to place into a patient based on age. It is common practice to refer to the size of endotracheal tube (or tracheostomy tube) needed by its ID. Once the tube is properly placed into the patient, the excess tube, beyond 3 to 4 cm past the teeth, should be removed. This reduces the airway resistance and mechanical dead space.

Most endotracheal tubes have the standard features shown in Figure 12-20. There are a number of specialty endotracheal tubes that can be found in limited use. They all share the same characteristics except for some special feature. These tubes are worth considering if available.

1. Pediatric endotracheal tubes

Pediatric endotracheal tubes are available in two basic types. One type has a constant diameter. During intuba-

Figure 12-20 Typical, modern endotracheal tube with its component parts. The insert shows important features found at the distal end of the tube.

tion, the tube should be inserted until the black mark about 2 cm from the tip is at the vocal cords. The second type has a body with a relatively wide proximal part that narrows at the distal end. The design is supposed to allow the smaller diameter tip to be passed through the vocal cords but prevent the wide "shoulder" from passing into the trachea. The distal ends of both types of tube have a single opening with a bevel cut (Figure 12-21). It is recommended that children less than 8 years of age have a tube without a cuff.

2. Wire-reinforced tubes

Wire-reinforced (also called armored) tubes have a steel spring coiled through them (Figure 12-22). An advantage of these tubes over regular tubes is that they are more resistant to collapse if the patient bites on them. Furthermore, the tube may be bent for shape and does not kink

Figure 12-21 Comparison of the two different types of pediatric endotracheal tubes. The top type of tube is made by several manufacturers and has a uniform diameter. The bottom tube is made by Cole and features a narrowing of the distal tip to pass through the vocal cords. Note that neither has a cuff. *(From Burgess WR, Chernick V: Respiratory therapy in newborn infants and children, ed 2, New York, 1986, Thieme.)*

if the patient's head is turned at an angle that might kink an ordinary tube.

3. Preformed tubes

Preformed tubes have been preshaped for surgical procedures on the head and neck. One style has a forward bend so that the tube can be taped to the chin (Figure 12-23). This shape keeps the tube and anesthesia circuit away from the patient's nose, eyes, and top of the head. There are also tubes with a backward bend so that it can be taped to the forehead (Figure 12-24). This shape keeps the tube and anesthesia circuit away from the patient's throat area.

4. Guidable (trigger) tubes

Guidable tubes have a string embedded within the wall of the tube (Figure 12-25). When the ring at the proximal end is pulled, the distal tip is flexed up to shorten the radius of the curve. This allows the tube to be directed into the anterior trachea. Guidable trigger tubes make it easier to intubate a patient with an anterior larynx or to perform a blind nasal intubation.

5. Double-lumen endotracheal tubes

Double-lumen endotracheal tubes are used to allow independent lung ventilation. A double-lumen tube is also used during special procedures performed on one lung such as bronchoscopy, bronchoalveolar lavage, lobectomy, and pneumonectomy. The other lung may be mechanically ventilated to maintain the patient's blood gas values (Figure 12-26). An adapter can be added to join the two proximal ends of the channels so that a single ventilator can be used to ventilate both lungs. The Carlens tube is used to preferentially intubate the left bronchus. The White tube is used to preferentially intubate the right

Figure 12-22 Photograph of a spiral wire–reinforced (also called an armored) endotracheal tube. *(From Cairo JM, Pilbeam SP: Mosby's respiratory care equipment, ed 8, St Louis, 2010, Mosby, Inc.)*

Figure 12-24 Photograph of cuffed SAE endotracheal tubes with a posterior bend to allow access to the patient's neck area. *(From Cairo JM, Pilbeam SP: Mosby's respiratory care equipment, ed 8, St Louis, 2010, Mosby, Inc.)*

Figure 12-23 Photograph of cuffed and uncuffed SAE endotracheal tubes with an anterior bend to allow access to the upper part of the patient's face and head. *(From Cairo JM, Pilbeam SP: Mosby's respiratory care equipment, ed 8, St Louis, 2010, Mosby, Inc.)*

Figure 12-25 Photograph of an Endotrol guidable (trigger) endotracheal tube. A wire is embedded within the wall of the tube. When the ring at the proximal end is pulled, the distal tip is flexed up to shorten the radius of the curve. This allows the tube to be directed into the anterior trachea. *(From Cairo JM, Pilbeam SP: Mosby's respiratory care equipment, ed 8, St Louis, 2010, Mosby, Inc.)*

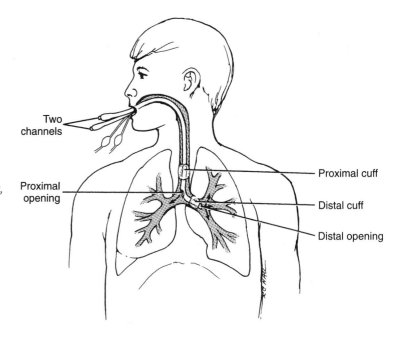

Figure 12-26 Double-lumen endotracheal tube properly positioned in patient so that both lungs can be independently ventilated or suctioned, or have special procedures performed. *(From Eubanks DH, Bone RC: Comprehensive respiratory care, ed 2, St Louis, 1990, Mosby-Year Book.)*

Figure 12-27 Two types of double-lumen endotracheal tubes. **A,** Carlens tube; its distal end enters the left mainstem bronchus. **B,** White tube; its distal end enters the right mainstem bronchus. Note how both tubes have a cuff that seals the trachea and a cuff that seals a bronchus. Each has its own inflation tube, pilot balloon, and one-way valve. *(From Miller RD, editor: Anesthesia, New York, 1981, Churchill Livingstone.)*

bronchus (see Figure 12-27 for both). Robertshaw makes tubes for either right or left bronchial intubation.

Several limitations are inherent in all double-lumen tubes. First, they can be used only on adults because the smallest size is 8-mm OD. Second, the small internal diameter of the two lumens results in a high airway resistance. Third, a much smaller than normal suction catheter must be used to remove any tracheal secretions.

6. Tubes for high-frequency jet ventilation

These special purpose tubes have a main lumen for a standard ventilator and an additional lumen to which a jet

ventilator is attached. See Chapter 15 for more discussion and a photograph.

7. Oropharyngeal suctioning tubes

In response to the concern about oropharyngeal secretions leaking around the endotracheal tube cuff and causing ventilator-associated pneumonia, an endotracheal tube with a built-in suctioning catheter has been invented (Figure 12-28). The catheter runs down the outer curve of the tube to just above the cuff. When vacuum is applied to the catheter, any secretions that have accumulated above the cuff are suctioned out of the area. It functions like a standard, cuffed endotracheal tube in all other aspects.

Exam Hint 12-4 (ELE)

Know the proper size of endotracheal or tracheostomy tube to use with an adult man or woman (about 8-mm ID) and a small neonate (about 3-mm ID).

Exam Hint 12-5 (ELE)

Know the indications, features, and any uses for the various types of endotracheal tubes.

---

b. Put the equipment together and make sure that it works properly

Refer to Figure 12-20 for these components of a standard endotracheal tube:

- The hollow curved body is the main part of the tube through which the patient can breathe, or a suction

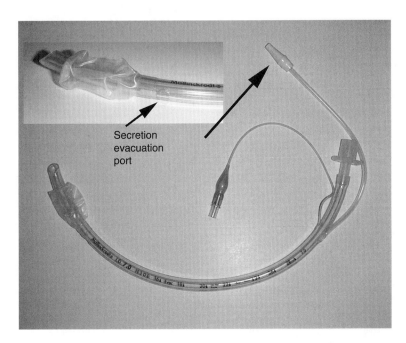

Secretion
evacuation
port

Figure 12-28 Photographs of a Hi-Low Evac endotracheal tube that has an added channel to suction oral secretions from the subglottic area. The removal of these secretions should help to reduce the possibility of the patient developing ventilator-associated pneumonia. *(From Cairo JM, Pilbeam SP: Mosby's respiratory care equipment, ed 8, St Louis, 2010, Mosby, Inc.)*

catheter can be placed. The OD and ID sizes are printed on the side of the tube. Make sure that the central channel is not plugged by dried secretions, blood, or foreign debris.

- The proximal end is left outside of the patient's nose or mouth. An adapter with a 15-mm-OD equipment connector is inserted into the tube. The other end of the adapter narrows and is individually sized to fit snugly into the ID of the endotracheal tube. The adapters cannot be cross-fitted to different sizes of endotracheal tubes.
- The distal end is inserted into the patient's trachea. The tip is cut with either a right- or left-sided bevel. The bevel cut creates an oval-shaped opening that is less likely to become plugged with secretions than is a round opening. An extra hole (the Murphy eye) is cut in the tube on the opposite side of the bevel.
- A line of radiopaque material is imbedded in the tube from the tip back to the cuff. It is seen as a white line on the chest radiograph, showing the location of the tube's tip in the trachea (see the insert in Figure 12-20).
- A cuff (balloon) is located a few centimeters from the tip of the tube. It is inflated with air to seal the trachea so that mechanical ventilation can be performed and aspiration is prevented. Most modern tubes have a large residual volume, low-pressure cuff.
- NOTE: Most tubes that are 4.0-mm ID/6.0-mm OD or larger have cuffs. However, there are cuffless tubes larger than this for pediatric patients. Pediatric and neonatal tubes smaller than 4.0-mm ID/6.0-mm OD will not have a cuff.

- A cuff-filling inflation tube is connected about halfway down the tube. The proximal end is left out of the patient's mouth, and the distal end goes to the cuff so that it can be inflated and deflated. A pilot balloon that inflates and deflates with the cuff is found in the middle of the capillary tube or connected with the one-way valve at the distal end. The one-way valve has an end that connects to any syringe. When the syringe is disconnected, the one-way valve seals to prevent the air in the cuff from escaping.
- With a double-lumen endotracheal tube, each lumen has its own 15-mm adapter, cuff, one-way valve, pilot balloon, and inflation tube to inflate the cuff. As with traditional endotracheal tubes, both cuffs should be test-inflated. They should hold the air without a leak and then be easily deflated. One additional piece of equipment, a plastic Y, can be used with a double-lumen tube. The plastic Y can be used to connect the proximal ends of both tubes. Both 15-mm adapters are removed and one branch of the Y is inserted into each of the proximal ends of the tubes. The open end of the Y has a 15-mm adapter so that it can be connected to a ventilator or oxygen source.

c. Troubleshoot any problems with the equipment

The cuff(s) should be inflated and the syringe should be disconnected from the one-way valve before the tube is placed in the patient. This ensures that the system works properly. The cuff(s) should hold the air. Do not use any tube with a leaking cuff or leaking one-way valve. Deflate the cuff before placing the tube into the patient.

3. Manipulate intubation equipment: laryngoscope and blades, by order or protocol (WRE Code: IIA7d) [Difficulty: An]

a. Get the necessary equipment

The laryngoscope is made up of two basic parts: a handle and a blade. The most commonly seen handle is made of stainless steel; some newer units are made of plastic. The handle contains two C-cell batteries to power the light source in the blade. They all have a common base with a hooking bar so that the blades can be attached (Figures 12-29 and 12-30).

Blades are available in a variety of sizes from pediatric to adult. They all have a common hook so that they can be snapped and locked in place on the handle. The stainless-steel handles use stainless-steel blades. The newer plastic handles use plastic blades. The two different sets of handles and blades are not interchangeable. The blades are available in two different shapes. The Miller blades are straight and the MacIntosh blades are curved (see Figure

12-30). The person performing the intubation may specify a particular style of blade as well as blade size.

b. Put the equipment together and make sure that it works properly

See Figure 12-29 for the steps in fastening the blade to the handle:

1. Hold the handle in the left hand and the blade in the right hand.
2. Place the hook on the blade over the hooking bar on the base of the handle.
3. Pull the blade down so that it snaps into place on the handle. The handle and blade should fit together at a 90-degree angle.
4. Make sure that the light bulb in the stainless-steel blade is tight.

c. Troubleshoot any problems with the equipment

The light source shines when the handle and blade are properly connected because an electrical circuit has been completed. Failure of the light source to shine may result from any of the following problems:

- The handle and blade are not properly connected and snapped into place. Disconnect them by performing the opposite motions and reconnect them properly.
- There are cross-connected stainless-steel and plastic components. Stainless-steel handles go only with stainless-steel blades, and plastic handles go with plastic blades.

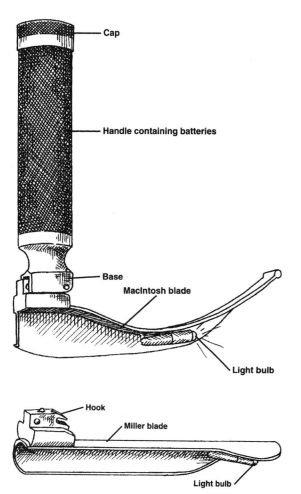

Figure 12-29 Laryngoscope handle with a MacIntosh (curved) blade attached. A Miller (straight) blade is shown below for comparison. Note component parts and features.

Figure 12-30 Motions to attach a laryngoscope to a handle.

- The batteries are low, as shown by the bulb failing to glow or glowing with a yellow instead of a white light. Unscrew the cap from the handle. Replace the old batteries with two new C-cell batteries. When reassembled, the bulb should glow with a white light.
- The batteries are not placed properly. It does not matter if a positive or negative pole touches the base of the handle. Be sure that a positive pole touches a negative pole or vice versa so that electrical current will flow properly. When reassembled, the bulb should glow with a white light.
- The light bulb in the stainless-steel blade is loose or defective. Tighten the light bulb by turning it clockwise. It should glow if it was just loose. Unscrew and throw away a defective light bulb. Replace it with a light bulb of the same size. When reassembled, the bulb should glow with a white light. The newer plastic laryngoscopes use a fiberoptic bundle as the light source. There is no light bulb to tighten or replace.

Besides the laryngoscope handle and blades, there are a number of additional items that are typically needed to ensure a smooth, safe intubation procedure. These are listed in Box 12-4.

Exam Hint 12-6 (ELE)

Know how to troubleshoot and repair a malfunctioning laryngoscope and blade.

---

4. Manipulate intubation equipment: fiberoptic devices, by order or protocol (ELE code: IIA7e) [Difficulty: ELE: R, Ap, An]

a. Get the necessary equipment

A physician may use a fiberoptic laryngoscope (Figure 12-31) or bronchoscope (see Figure 18-3) to visualize the larynx and trachea during a difficult intubation. Either can be used during a nasal or oral endotracheal intubation procedure.

A fiberoptic lighted stylet or lightwand (Figure 12-32) can be placed through the lumen of the endotracheal tube

---

BOX 12-4   Equipment for Oral and Nasal Intubation

Pediatric and adult laryngoscope handles with batteries
Straight and curved pediatric and adult laryngoscope blades
Variety of nasal and oral endotracheal tubes
Water-soluble, sterile lubricant
Metal stylet
Magill forceps for nasal intubation
Hemostat
Tongue depressors
Oropharyngeal airways
Bite block
Nasopharyngeal airways
10-mL syringe with three-way stopcock
Manometer to measure intracuff pressure
Tape or tube-restraining device
Yankauer or other oral suction device
Sterile suction catheter for tracheal suctioning
Stethoscope for listening to breath sounds

Figure 12-31 A fiberoptic laryngoscope that is being used to insert an endotracheal tube through the nasal passage. *(From Wilkins RL, Stoller JK, Kacmarek RM: Egan's fundamentals of respiratory care, ed 9, St Louis, 2010, Mosby.)*

Figure 12-32 Photograph of a lightwand inserted through the lumen of an endotracheal tube. The lightwand's light will shine through the laryngeal structures to show that the tip of the tube has entered the patient's trachea. *(From Cairo JM, Pilbeam SP: Mosby's respiratory care equipment, ed 8, St Louis, 2010, Mosby, Inc.)*

so that the lighted distal tip is at the end of the tube. When the room is darkened and the tube enters the trachea, a bright light will shine though the tissues over the throat.

Recently, a closed-circuit system has been developed that employs a laryngoscope handle and blade with a tiny camera at the tip of the blade. A fiberoptic bundle carries the image of the patient's larynx from the blade to a monitor for viewing. This could be used to replace direct visualization of the larynx by the person performing the intubation.

b. Put the equipment together and make sure that it works properly

See the following section.

c. Troubleshoot any problems with the equipment

Review the discussion on bronchoscopy in Chapter 18 for the details on the equipment. The fiberoptic tube should be lubricated so that it will easily slide through the lumen of the endotracheal tube (see Figure 12-31). After the physician has confirmed that the distal end of the fiberoptic tube has entered the trachea, the endotracheal tube is gently pushed into the trachea. The fiberoptic tube is then withdrawn, the cuff is inflated, and the endotracheal tube is secured. If the endotracheal tube will not slide into the patient's trachea, it is either too large or there is not enough lubricant on the fiberoptic tube. It may be necessary to withdraw them, correct the problem, and start over again.

The lightwand needs functioning batteries in the proximal handle in order to glow. Replace any nonfunctioning batteries. The unit should have a water-soluble lubricant added so that it easily passes in and out of the endotracheal tube's channel.

The closed-circuit laryngoscope handle and monitor need to plugged into an electrical outlet and properly assembled. Each laryngoscope blade is disposed of after single-patient use.

BOX 12-5 Indications and Contraindications for Oral Endotracheal Intubation

GENERAL INDICATIONS FOR ENDOTRACHEAL INTUBATION
Provides a secure, patent airway.
Provides a route for mechanical ventilation.
Prevents aspiration of stomach or mouth contents.
Provides a route for suctioning the lungs.
Uses a general anesthetic.

INDICATIONS FOR ORAL INTUBATION
Is fastest, easiest method to secure the airway.
Simpler, less invasive method cannot ensure an open airway.

CONTRAINDICATIONS FOR ORAL INTUBATION
Cervical spine injury such that the patient's neck cannot be hyperextended
Lower facial injury
Oral surgery

MODULE J
Endotracheal intubation and tube management

1. Perform endotracheal intubation (Code: IIIB3) [Difficulty: ELE: R, Ap; WRE: An]

Oral endotracheal intubation is the recommended procedure for securing the airway during an emergency such as a CPR attempt. In uncomplicated cases, the patient can be quickly intubated with an apneic period of no more than 20 seconds. This procedure is explained for a team of two respiratory therapists. It is difficult, if not impossible, for a single therapist to perform this important task without placing the patient at great risk. Usually the therapist who intubates is considered the leader and the other therapist acts as the assistant. Therapists must feel comfortable in both roles. See Box 12-5 for a list of indications and contraindications for oral intubation and Box 12-6 for a list of complications.

Steps in an emergency oral endotracheal intubation include the following:
1. Prepare the patient. The assistant should:
   a. Place the head and neck in the sniff position.
   b. Ventilate the patient's lungs with 100% oxygen by a face mask and manual resuscitator or demand valve.
2. The intubator should put on a surgical mask, goggles, and clean gloves on both hands, and then perform the following.
3. Prepare the endotracheal tube.
   a. Select the proper endotracheal tube. (See Table 12-1 for the recommended tube sizes based on the patient's age. It is common practice to select the tube size based on its inner diameter [ID]. For example, a premature neonate would need a 2.5-

BOX 12-6 Complications of Endotracheal Intubation

GENERAL COMPLICATIONS

Reflex laryngospasm

Perforation of the esophagus or pharynx

Esophageal intubation

Bronchial intubation

Reflex bradycardia

Tachycardia or other arrhythmias from hypoxemia

Hypotension

Bronchospasm

Aspiration of tooth, blood, gastric contents, laryngoscope bulb

Laceration of pharynx or larynx

Nosocomial infection

Vocal cord injury

Laryngeal or tracheal injury from the tube or excessive cuff pressure

COMPLICATIONS OF THE ORAL ROUTE

Cervical spine injury

Tooth trauma from the blade being pulled back

Eye trauma from the handle or the operator's hand

COMPLICATIONS OF THE NASAL ROUTE

Bleeding

Ulceration

Sinusitis

Figure 12-33 Stylet with stopper properly placed in standard endotracheal tube to maintain its curved shape. *(From Eubanks DH, Bone RC: Comprehensive respiratory care, ed 2, St Louis, 1990, Mosby.)*

mm-ID tube.) If time permits, the next smaller and larger tube sizes should also be selected.

   b. Inflate the cuff using a 10- or 20-mL syringe. Remove the syringe from the one-way valve. Make sure that it holds the air and then deflate the cuff completely.

   c. Lubricate the last few centimeters of the endotracheal tube with a water-soluble lubricant.

   d. (Optional step) Lubricate a stylet with the sterile water-soluble lubricant. Place the stylet into the tube so that the natural curve of the tube is maintained. The tip of the stylet should not go past the end of the tube (Figure 12-33). Some practitioners may prefer not to use a stylet. Many believe that the stylet offers the advantage of being able to bend the tube to match the patient's anatomy if a second attempt is needed.

4. Prepare the laryngoscope and blade.

   a. Select a laryngoscope handle.

   b. Select a laryngoscope blade. The blades are available in several sizes from pediatric to adult. There are two main classes of blades: straight and curved (see Figure 12-29). The straight blades (Miller is a common brand) are designed to lift the epiglottis to expose the tracheal opening. The curved blades (MacIntosh is a common brand) are designed to fit into the vallecula (between the base of the tongue and the epiglottis). As the blade is lifted, the epiglottis is raised and the tracheal opening can be seen. Personal experience and training leads the practitioner to select between the two styles.

   c. Attach the blade to the handle (see Figure 12-30). Make sure that the light bulb shines brightly.

5. The intubator should tell the assistant to stop ventilating the patient and stand clear so that an intubation can be attempted. The assistant should check his or her watch to silently count off 20 seconds. The intubator should be told when 20 seconds has passed so that the patient can be reventilated if the intubation is proving to be difficult.

6. Open the victim's mouth as widely as possible without using force. Remove any dentures or foreign material. Suction any saliva, blood, or vomitus.

7. Grasp the laryngoscope handle in the left hand. Carefully advance the blade between the teeth or gums along the right side of the mouth. Move the tongue to the left side of the mouth to allow a clear view of the oropharynx (Figure 12-34). Advance the blade along the base of the tongue until the epiglottis is seen.

8. With a *straight* blade:

   a. Advance the blade so that it barely passes the epiglottis.

   b. Do not advance the blade too far or it will enter the esophagus or trachea.

   With a *curved* blade:

   a. Advance the blade tip into the vallecula.

   b. Lift the blade tip into this space.

9. With either blade, lift the laryngoscope handle and blade toward the patient's chest at a 45-degree angle (Figure 12-35). The straight blade lifts the epiglottis. The curved blade lifts the soft tissues of the vallecula

and the epiglottis lifts with them. Do *not* pull back on the patient's upper teeth.

10. The vocal cords and glottis should be clearly seen (Figure 12-36). If needed, tell the assistant to put gentle, downward pressure on the patient's larynx. This may help to bring the glottis into better view.

11. Tell the assistant to place the endotracheal tube into your right hand.

12. Place the tube into the right side of the patient's mouth and direct it into the trachea. (The assistant may feel over the larynx as the tube enters the trachea. If necessary, the assistant may need to apply gentle pressure over the larynx to move it more posterior.) In the adult, advance the tube until the proximal end of the cuff is 3 to 4 cm past the vocal cords (Figure 12-37). In children less than 6 months of age, with an uncuffed endotracheal tube, advance the tube until the tip is about 1 cm past the vocal cords.

13. Hold the tube in place.

14. Withdraw the laryngoscope blade.

15. Tell the assistant to inflate the cuff. Place about 10 mL of air into the cuff (of an adult's tube; less in a pediatric tube) so that some resistance can be felt. The cuff pressure can be measured and adjusted later.

Figure 12-34   Proper placement of the laryngoscope blade to move the patient's tongue. **A,** Proper placement of the laryngoscope blade to the right of the patient's tongue to move it to the left. This should give a clear view of the glottis. **B,** Tongue partially obstructs the view if it is not moved to the left. *(From Shapiro BA et al: Clinical application of respiratory care, ed 4, St Louis, 1991, Mosby.)*

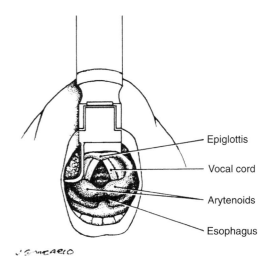

Figure 12-36   Major anatomic features that can be seen when epiglottis is lifted. Opening to trachea can be seen between vocal cords. *(From Shapiro BA et al: Clinical application of respiratory care, ed 4, St Louis, 1991, Mosby.)*

Figure 12-35   Proper use of the laryngoscope blade to expose the larynx by lifting the glottic structures. Note how the lifting is at a 45-degree angle toward the patient's chest. *Never* pull back on the blade against the teeth. **A,** A straight blade is used to lift the epiglottis to expose the trachea. **B,** A curved blade is used to lift soft tissues of the vallecula to expose the trachea. *(From Shapiro BA et al: Clinical application of respiratory care, ed 4, St Louis, 1991, Mosby.)*

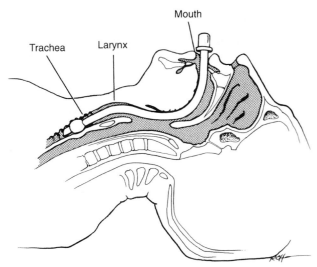

Figure 12-37   Oral endotracheal tube properly positioned within the trachea. *(From Eubanks DH, Bone RC:* Comprehensive respiratory care, *ed 2, St Louis, 1990, Mosby.)*

16. Pull out the stylet (if used).
17. The assistant should ventilate the patient's lungs with the manual resuscitator bag or a demand valve.
18. The intubator should listen to both lung fields in the upper lobes and bases. Bilateral breath sounds should be heard.
19. If the breath sounds are equal and bilateral, the assistant can secure the tube in place with tape or a tube holder. If the breath sounds are unequal or absent on one side, the tube has been placed into a bronchus (usually the right mainstem). The cuff should be deflated and the tube then withdrawn 1 to 2 cm in an adult, less in a child. The cuff should be reinflated and breath sounds assessed again. When the breath sounds are equal, the tube can be secured.
20. If no breath sounds are heard, listen over the stomach area. If air is heard bubbling into the stomach, the tube has been placed into the esophagus. Immediately remove the tube. Ventilate the patient's lungs and prepare to attempt reintubation with a new endotracheal tube.

The practitioner should only perform those procedures for which he or she has been trained. If the patient cannot be intubated with the standard equipment and procedure, an anesthesiologist or trained physician should be requested. Be prepared to assist as necessary.

2. Assess the placement of an endotracheal tube (ELE code: IIIB5) [Difficulty: ELE: R, Ap, An]

Clinical experience has shown that there is no single foolproof procedure that can confirm that the endotracheal tube is within the trachea. Current guidelines recommend that several of the following procedures be done to confirm proper tube placement within the trachea.

3. Palpate the patient to determine asymmetric chest movements, crepitus, and/or tracheal deviation (Code: IB2b) [Difficulty: ELE: R, Ap; WRE: An]

As discussed previously, the first step to confirm tube placement during the intubation procedure is to palpate it passing through the larynx and entering the trachea. Most often the endotracheal tube can be palpated in an infant as it is being inserted. This is because the laryngeal structures are so pliable. Feeling the tube being inserted through the larynx indicates that it is properly located within the trachea. If the tube cannot be palpated through the larynx, it has probably been inserted into the esophagus. It is more difficult to use this technique with confidence in adults because their laryngeal structures are stiffer.

If the tube is advanced and cannot be palpated within the trachea, there are two other possible locations. First, the endotracheal tube could have been placed into the esophagus. Breath sounds will be heard over the epigastric area rather than the lungs. Deflate the cuff, withdraw the tube, and bag-mask ventilate the patient's lungs. Second, the tube could have entered the trachea but deviated through the tracheal wall to enter one or the other lung field. Assess the patient for a possible pneumothorax, including findings of asymmetric chest movements, crepitus, and/or tracheal deviation. Withdraw the tube and begin bag-mask ventilation. Call a physician for help.

4. Auscultate the patient's breath sounds and interpret any changes (Code: IB4a) [Difficulty: ELE: R, Ap; WRE: An]

Respiratory efforts without breath sounds indicate that a complete obstruction exists in the patient's airway. Inspiratory stridor or wheezing indicates that a partial obstruction exists in the patient's airway. Listen for stridor over the larynx and wheezing over the major airways. The restoration of the normal airway should result in the return of normal breath sounds over all areas of both lung fields (unless there is another, unrelated problem).

After intubation, deliver a breath and listen over the epigastric area to rule out tube placement in the esophagus. After ruling out esophageal placement, check for bilateral breath sounds. Confirm equal bilateral breath sounds by first listening over the apical areas and then the lateral areas. If the tube has been inserted too far, it usually enters the right mainstem bronchus because it separates from the trachea at a less acute angle than the left mainstem bronchus. No breath sounds will be heard over the left lung field. If both lung fields cannot be auscultated, at least listen to the right apical area. This one site can be checked because the segmental bronchus to the right upper lobe separates from the right mainstem bronchus in such a way that if the right mainstem bronchus is intubated, the upper lobe segmental bronchus will be blocked.

While listening to the patient's breath sounds, look at the endotracheal tube. The condensation of moisture on the inside of the tube during exhalation would also confirm that the tube is in the trachea (or a bronchus) instead of the esophagus.

a. Esophageal detection device

The esophageal detection device (EDD) is able to show that the endotracheal tube has been placed within an airway by pulling a small sample of gas from the patient's lungs. If the endotracheal tube has been accidentally put into the esophagus, the deflated bulb will stay collapsed (Figure 12-38). A limitation of the EDD is that it inflates whether the endotracheal tube is placed into the trachea or either mainstem bronchus. Remember to auscultate for bilateral breath sounds.

Figure 12-38 Esophageal detection device (EDD). This squeeze bulb device is attached to the proximal end of the patient's endotracheal tube and air is squeezed out. **A,** Shows reinflation of bulb with air from patient's lungs when the endotracheal tube has been properly placed. **B,** Shows that the bulb fails to reinflate when the endotracheal tube has been accidentally placed into the patient's esophagus. *(From Scanlan C, Simmons K: Airway management. In Scanlan CL, Wilkins RL, Stoller JK, editors: Egan's fundamentals of respiratory care, ed 7, St Louis, 1999, Mosby.)*

5. Detect exhaled carbon dioxide

a. Recommend capnography to obtain additional data (Code: IC10) [Difficulty: ELE: R, Ap; WRE: An]

It is now common clinical practice to check for the presence of exhaled carbon dioxide to confirm endotracheal intubation. In the operating room the anesthesiologist will attach a capnography system to a patient's endotracheal tube or add one into a ventilator circuit. In most other intubation situations, a simple, inexpensive colorimeter device is used. With either device, if the patient is not in cardiopulmonary arrest and the tube is within the trachea or a major bronchus, exhaled CO_2 will be found. If none is detected, the tube has been placed into the esophagus. Deflate the cuff, remove the tube, and begin bag-mask ventilation. Both units are discussed in the following sections.

b. Manipulate intubation equipment: exhaled carbon dioxide detectors, by order or protocol (ELE code: IIA7e) [Difficulty: ELE: R, Ap, An]

1. Get the necessary equipment

Most exhaled carbon dioxide detectors are inexpensive, single-patient use, disposable devices. They are called colorimetric units because they change color when exhaled carbon dioxide passes through the sensitive material within the capsule (Figure 12-39). The units are placed onto an endotracheal tube's 15-mm-OD adapter to monitor the proper placement of the endotracheal tube.

Figure 12-39 Easy Cap E_TCO_2 detector. This disposable device is available in adult and pediatric sizes and is able to detect exhaled carbon dioxide. Color change from dark purple to yellow indicates exhaled CO_2 to confirm tracheal placement of endotracheal tube or effective efforts at cardiopulmonary resuscitation. *(Courtesy Nellcor Puritan Bennett, Pleasanton Calif, part of Covidien [formerly Tyco Healthcare].)*

This is often done if a patient is being transported and there is a possibility that the tube could be dislodged. Exhaled carbon dioxide detectors are also used during CPR attempts to help determine if resuscitation attempts are being performed on a viable patient. If the patient is not producing exhaled CO_2, there is no metabolic activity. The physician may then decide to stop CPR efforts.

Currently available disposable units include the Easy Cap, the A.C.E. STAT-Check CO_2 Indicator, and the unit produced by Resuscitation ACE Inc. The Easy Cap end-tidal CO_2 detector (Figure 12-39) is the original unit and quite widely used. It is available in a neonatal/pediatric size for infants weighing less than 15 kg and in a standard size for larger children and adults. Its carbon dioxide indicator changes color from dark purple to yellow when CO_2 is exhaled through it. The other two disposable units also indicate the presence of exhaled CO_2 by an indicator turning purple.

One choice for an intubation capnograph is the MiniCAP III CO_2 detector. It is a reusable item that has a mainstream type of infrared carbon dioxide detector. The unit is powered by a battery pack. Its light-emitting diode signals the presence of carbon dioxide with each exhalation. A capnograph should be selected if it is necessary to obtain a more accurate CO_2 reading. Remember that capnography cannot confirm that the tube is properly placed in the trachea rather than a bronchus. Check for equal, bilateral breath sounds. See Chapter 5 for a full discussion on capnometry.

2. Put the equipment together and make sure that it works properly

The Easy Cap is a single unit within a sealed foil container. Remove the unit from the container and compare the initial purple color of the indicator with the purple color labeled CHECK on the product dome. Do *not* use an Easy Cap unit whose color is not the same or darker than that on the product dome. Attach the Easy Cap to the patient's endotracheal tube by its 15-mm-ID connector port. The Easy Cap's 15-mm-OD circuit end is connected to the manual resuscitator to ventilate the patient's lungs. If a heat and moisture exchanger is used, it should be placed between the patient's endotracheal tube and the Easy Cap and manual resuscitator. The Easy Cap should not be used with a heated humidifier or nebulizer because too much humidity affects its accuracy. The unit is not intended to be used for more than 2 hours because the color change will fade.

The MiniCAP III has a disposable adapter that connects the mainstream CO_2 detector to the patient's endotracheal tube. The adapter has a 15-mm-ID end for attachment to the endotracheal tube and a 15-mm-OD end to which the manual resuscitator can be attached. The assembly and operation of a capnograph are discussed in Chapter 5. Review this material if necessary.

3. Troubleshoot any problems with the equipment

Because the Easy Cap is a self-contained single-piece unit, there is nothing to repair. The following items can contaminate the Easy Cap and cause a patchy yellow or white discoloration of the indicator: stomach contents, mucus, pulmonary edema fluid, and intratracheal epinephrine. If the color does not change with the breathing cycle, the Easy Cap unit should be discarded. The 15-mm-ID patient connector port fits only over the endotracheal tube adapter. The 15-mm-OD circuit connector port fits only into the manual resuscitator or demand-valve adapter.

The adapter is the only removable part in the MiniCAP III. It fits only in one direction into the CO_2 detection unit. The other end of the adapter fits only into a manual resuscitator outlet. Some limitations exist in the use of an Easy Cap carbon dioxide detector. It should not be used during mouth-to-mouth resuscitation, to detect right mainstem bronchus intubation, to detect hypercarbia, or to determine the placement of an esophageal obturator airway.

Troubleshooting with a capnograph was presented in Chapter 5.

6. Recommend a chest radiograph to help determine the patient's condition and review the chest radiograph (Code: IC2 and IIIE1) [Difficulty: ELE: R, Ap; WRE: An]

A chest radiograph should always be taken to confirm the location of a newly placed endotracheal or tracheostomy tube. The chest radiograph should be repeated if there has been a significant change in the patient's condition or if the tube has been pulled back or pushed deeper into the trachea. Ideally the tip of the tube is in the middle of the trachea. In the adult this would be several centimeters above the carina.

A chest radiograph also confirms the presence and location of an opaque foreign body in the airway. Metallic objects, stones, and coins can be clearly seen. Less radiopaque objects can be barely seen, if at all. The chest radiograph also detects a pneumothorax related to the tracheostomy procedure or other pulmonary conditions. If needed, an upper airway radiographic examination can be performed to look for a foreign body or to check the position of the tracheostomy tube.

7. Review the upper airway or chest radiograph to see the position of the endotracheal or tracheostomy tube (Code: IB7b) [Difficulty: ELE: R, Ap; WRE: An]

All modern endotracheal and tracheostomy tubes contain a strip of radiopaque material near the distal tip of the tube. This is easily noticed as the white line s een on the chest radiograph and confirms the location of the tip of the tube in the airway (see Figure 12-20). The ideal location of the tip of the endotracheal tube is the middle third of the trachea. When the tube is positioned properly, it is less likely for the tip to be pushed into the carina when the patient bends his or her head forward or for the cuff to hit the vocal cords if the patient's head is bent back. Both endotracheal and tracheostomy tubes should be positioned midline within the trachea. They should not be twisted laterally because the tip can cause damage to the tracheal wall.

Exam Hint 12-7 (ELE)

Be prepared to determine the proper placement of the endotracheal tube by any of the following: (1) palpation of the larynx and neck, (2) auscultation of bilateral breath sounds, (3) determination of moisture condensation within the tube during exhalation, (4) detection of exhaled carbon dioxide, (5) observation of bilateral symmetric chest movement on inspiration, (6) visualization of the tip of the tube on a chest radiograph, or (7) observation that the 24-cm mark on the tube will be at an adult's front teeth (incisors).

8. Maintain the proper position of an endotracheal tube (Code: IIIB4c) [Difficulty: ELE: R, Ap; WRE: An]

As mentioned earlier, an endotracheal tube is ideally located within the middle third of the trachea. Check the chest radiograph for positioning. If the tube is too high within the trachea, it may be pulled up through the vocal cords if the patient's head is hyperextended. An air leak may be heard at the larynx if the patient is using a mechanical ventilator. In this case, the cuff should be deflated and the tube inserted deeper into the trachea.

Conversely, if the tip of the tube is inserted too deeply into the trachea, it may be pushed into a mainstem bronchus if the patient's head is moved toward the chest. In this situation no breath sounds would be heard in the opposite lung (usually the left). The cuff should be deflated and the tube pulled up into the middle third of the trachea. Reinflate the cuff after the tube is repositioned. A chest radiograph should be taken to confirm the tube's position after it has been moved.

The endotracheal tube body has centimeter marks inscribed on it, starting at the distal end and finishing at the proximal end. Check and record the centimeter mark present at the patient's teeth or gums. The average adult's distance from the midtrachea to the teeth is about 23 to 25 cm. The practitioner can determine if the tube has been accidentally pulled out a little or pushed further into the patient by looking at the current centimeter mark. If the tube is intentionally adjusted, the new centimeter mark should be checked and recorded.

A wide variety of handmade, as well as manufactured, devices are available to secure the endotracheal tube in the correct position. Figure 12-40 shows one way to make a tube holder from adhesive tape. This is flexible when the patient moves and is inexpensive. Tincture of benzoin can be applied to the patient's cheeks to make the tape hold more securely without tearing the skin. An oropharyngeal airway may or may not be needed.

The manufactured tube holders are made of plastic with cloth ties and usually include a built-in bite block. Make sure that it is sized properly to the patient's mouth. Too large a bite block can injure the tongue, lips, and mouth. Watch for a gag reflex. This type of holder is useful in the patient who is prone to seizures.

A tracheostomy tube should be positioned so that the flange is snug against the base of the neck and the outer cannula is within the trachea. If pulled out too far, the cuff may be seen at the stoma. An air leak may be heard or secretions may be seen to bubble out of the stoma. Correct the problem by deflating the cuff, inserting the tube so that the flange is against the base of the neck, and reinflating the cuff.

Exam Hint 12-8 (ELE, WRE)

There is usually a question that addresses understanding that the lack of breath sounds over the left lung indicates that the endotracheal tube has been placed into the right mainstem bronchus. Deflate the cuff and withdraw the tube into the trachea. Note the 24-cm mark on the tube is at the adult patient's front teeth (incisors).

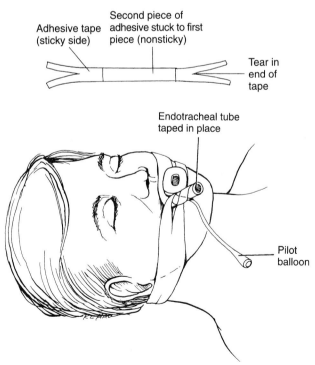

Figure 12-40 Taping the endotracheal tube to secure it in the airway. *(From Eubanks DH, Bone RC: Comprehensive respiratory care, ed 2, St Louis, 1990, Mosby.)*

9. Maintain the appropriate cuff inflation of an endotracheal tube or tracheostomy tube (Code: IIIB4c, 4d) [Difficulty: ELE: R, Ap; WRE: An]

All of the adult and larger pediatric endotracheal and tracheostomy tubes have a cuff for sealing the airway. Most brands of modern tubes have cuffs that are designed to have a relatively large reservoir volume that fills at a relatively low pressure. The soft, flexible balloon seals the airway by having a large surface area that conforms to the shape of the trachea.

a. Determine tracheal tube cuff pressure and/or volume (Code: IB9r) [Difficulty: ELE: R, Ap; WRE: An]

There are two slightly different ways to inflate the cuff and maintain a safe cuff pressure. Both methods can be used only with patients on a positive-pressure ventilator.

1. Minimal leak

1. Connect the cuff pressure measuring device (see next discussion) to the one-way valve on the cuff inflating tube.
2. Listen with a stethoscope over the patient's larynx.
3. Inflate or deflate the cuff as necessary while listening for an air leak.
4. Stop changing the air volume when a minimal leak is heard at the peak airway pressure in the breathing cycle. The tidal volume should still be delivered except for this minor leak.
5. Note the cuff pressure when the minimal leak was heard. Note the cuff volume, if possible.
6. Disconnect the cuff pressure measuring device.
7. It may be necessary to add more volume and pressure to the cuff if the leak gets worse when the peak airway pressure increases.

2. Minimal occluding volume

The purpose is to find the cuff pressure that results in *no leak* at the cuff when the patient's airway pressure is greatest. The following are the steps in the procedure:

1. Connect the cuff pressure measuring device (see next discussion) to the one-way valve on the cuff inflating tube.
2. Listen with a stethoscope over the patient's larynx.
3. Inflate or deflate the cuff as necessary while listening for an air leak.
4. Stop changing the air volume when no leak is heard at the peak airway pressure in the breathing cycle.
5. Note the cuff pressure when the seal was heard. Note the cuff volume, if possible.
6. Disconnect the cuff pressure measuring device.

7. It may be necessary to add more volume and pressure to the cuff if a leak results when the peak airway pressure increases.

This discussion relates only to those tubes that must be actively filled with air and have variable intracuff pressures. Several manufacturers have developed endotracheal and tracheostomy tubes that have built-in cuff pressure limitations. Follow the manufacturer's guidelines when inflating these cuffs. This discussion would not be complete without mentioning the recent manufacture of systems designed to raise the cuff pressure to match the peak airway pressure of a patient using a mechanical ventilator. A tube connects the inspiratory circuit to the one-way valve on the cuff inflating tube. As a positive-pressure breath is delivered, the pressure in the circuit is also applied to the patient's cuff. There should be no loss of tidal volume. When the patient exhales and the airway pressure drops to normal, the cuff pressure also drops back to its normal level.

3. Select a cuff pressure and/or volume measuring system

A cuff pressure manometer is needed to measure the air pressure within an endotracheal or tracheostomy tube cuff. When a tracheal tube is first inserted, the volume of air that is injected into the cuff should be measured and charted. The pressure within the cuff should also be noted. After that, if more air is inserted or any air is removed from the cuff it should be measured and recorded in the chart. The resulting final cuff pressure must also be recorded. A number of manufactured units are available for measuring cuff pressure. The Cufflator (Figure 12-41) is discussed here because it is widely used. This system consists of a pressure gauge calibrated in centimeters of water, a hand-pumped reservoir, an internal one-way valve, a pressure release valve, and an adapter to fit into the one-way valve on the cuff inflating tube. A three-way stopcock can be added to the one-way valve adapter. This

Figure 12-41 Cufflator device used to measure cuff pressure with its component parts.

can be used to prepressurize the system before attaching it to the patient's one-way valve on the cuff inflating tube. The pressure in the cuff can be measured as air is added by squeezing the hand pump or as air is removed by the pressure release valve. The volume of air added or removed cannot be measured.

A second system can be "homemade," although it is also commercially available. It consists of a 5- to 10-mL syringe, a three-way stopcock, and a pressure gauge (either millimeters of mercury or centimeters of water). The syringe and pressure gauge are attached to two of the ports on the stopcock. The third port on the stopcock is connected to the one-way valve on the cuff inflating tube. When the stopcock handle is opened to all three ports, the pressures throughout the system and the cuff are the same. Air can be added or removed with the syringe. The pressure gauge shows the system and cuff pressure as the air volume is adjusted (Figure 12-42). One advantage of this system over the Cufflator is that the volume of air that is added or subtracted can be measured. This system can also be prepressurized so that its pressure matches the pressure anticipated in the cuff. With any of these systems, it is necessary to keep airtight connections. If the pressure drops unexpectedly, an air leak will be noticed. Tighten the connections to create a seal so that the pressure is maintained.

It is commonly recommended that the cuff pressure be monitored at least every 8 hours or whenever air is injected or withdrawn from the cuff.

b. Interpret the tracheal tube cuff volume and/or pressure (Code: IB10r) [Difficulty: ELE: R, Ap; WRE: An]

All manufacturers (except Kamen-Wilkenson) have designed cuffs that must be actively filled with air by way

Pressure manometer

Syringe

Three-way stopcock

Cuff

Figure 12-42 Cuff measuring device made from pressure manometer, three-way stopcock, and 10-mL syringe.

of a one-way valve and syringe. These cuffs have greater than atmospheric pressure within them. That pressure is placed against the wall of the trachea. The greater the pressure on the wall of the trachea, the greater the disruption of normal lymphatic and blood flow. Shapiro and colleagues (1991) stated that a patient with a normal blood pressure (120/80 mm Hg) has the following effects at these cuff pressures:

- Lymphatic flow blockage occurs at cuff pressures greater than 5 mm Hg (8 cm H_2O). Edema of the tracheal mucosa results.
- Capillary blood flow blockage occurs at cuff pressures greater than 18 mm Hg (24 cm H_2O). (Hess [1999] states that the capillary perfusion pressure ranges between 25 and 30 mm Hg.) Venous (and lymphatic) drainage stops as a result.
- Arterial blood flow blockage occurs at cuff pressures greater than 30 mm Hg (42 cm H_2O). Arterial (and lymphatic and capillary) flow stops as a result.

In general, the clinical goal is to keep the cuff pressure as low as possible to make sure that the circulation through the tracheal wall is normal. Based on the information from Shapiro and colleagues and Hess, it seems reasonable to try to keep the *cuff pressure no greater than 20 to 25 mm Hg (25 to 35 cm H_2O)*. This is true for all normotensive patients. Hypertensive patients may be able to tolerate higher cuff pressures than normotensive patients before blood flow to the tracheal tissues is stopped. Hypotensive patients suffer from the loss of blood flow to the tracheal wall at lower cuff pressures than those previously listed.

c. Inflate and/or deflate the cuff (ELE code: IIIF2g4) [Difficulty: ELE: R, Ap, An]

A spontaneously breathing patient must have the cuff inflated to prevent the aspiration of oral secretions into the lungs. In general, keep the pressure at about 20 mm Hg (25 cm H_2O), as discussed earlier. It may be necessary to keep a higher cuff pressure in a mechanically ventilated patient. However, Shapiro and associates recommend that if the cuff pressure must be greater than 20 mm Hg, the endotracheal or tracheostomy tube is too small. Ideally, the tube should be replaced with a larger one. However, some patients are too unstable to tolerate reintubation of their airways and must simply have the cuff pressure increased temporarily.

It is clear that a cuff pressure greater than the patient's mucosa capillary pressure prevents the flow of blood through the area covered by the cuff. Tissue ischemia (hypoxemia) results. If the ischemia is severe enough, tissue necrosis follows. The higher the cuff pressure and the longer the high cuff pressure is maintained, the greater the likelihood of tissue necrosis. If the necrosis is circumferential (all the way around) to the trachea, tracheal stenosis may occur. Tracheal stenosis is found when the diameter of the trachea is narrowed because of scar tissue buildup after the normal mucosa and underlying tissues have died. The patient's airway is permanently narrowed and, if serious, must be surgically corrected. Another severe complication of high cuff pressures and tracheal necrosis is the development of a tracheoesophageal fistula. This is an opening between the trachea and esophagus. This is more likely when the patient also has a nasogastric tube in place. The fistula permits food to pass into the airway and lungs, causing pneumonia. Mechanical ventilation is more difficult because of the air leak from the lungs to the esophagus. Surgical repair of the fistula is required.

Exam Hint 12-9 (ELE, WRE)

There is usually a question that either addresses adjusting a cuff pressure to a safe level of no more than 20 to 25 mm Hg (25 to 35 cm H_2O) or involves recommending replacement of a tracheal tube that is too small and requires too high a cuff pressure with a larger tube. A small endotracheal tube should also be replaced with a larger one if a patient cannot wean from the ventilator because of the high airway resistance created by the smaller tube.

MODULE K
Endotracheal extubation

1. Recommend the insertion of an artificial airway or a change in the type of artificial airway (Code: IIIG1f) [Difficulty: ELE: R, Ap; WRE: An]

There are usually only two reasons to replace a patient's endotracheal tube. First, the tube should be changed if it is too small and the cuff must be overfilled to seal the airway. Excessive pressure results in damage to the tracheal wall as previously discussed.

Second, the tube should be replaced if the cuff is leaking or ruptured and the airway cannot be sealed. The patient may be reintubated by the procedure described earlier. Alternatively, a tube-changing stylet may be used (Figure 12-43). The stylet is a hollow, flexible plastic tube that can be bent and holds its shape. It has a center mark and 1-cm markings counting out to each end. These are to help keep the proper depth for inserting the replacement endotracheal tube. It can be used on an endotracheal tube that is at least 7.5-mm inner diameter. The procedure for changing the endotracheal tube with a tube-changing stylet includes the following:

1. Obtain the needed equipment: replacement endotracheal tube and one that is a size smaller, 10-mL

Figure 12-43 Endotracheal tube changer (guide) inserted through an endotracheal tube. The JEM 400 unit can be inserted through a tube that is 7.5-mm ID or larger. The tube changer is used to aid in replacement of an esophageal obturator airway or a defective endotracheal tube with a functional endotracheal tube. See text for how to use the tube changer instead of traditional intubation equipment. *(Modified from Heffner JE: Respir Manage 19(3):53, 1989.)*

syringe to inflate the cuff, sterile gloves, goggles, and sterile water-soluble lubricant. Make sure the cuff inflates and deflates properly.
2. Tell the patient what you are going to do. Put on the gloves, goggles, and mask.
3. Remove the patient's oxygen equipment.
4. Suction the secretions from the patient's trachea and oral pharynx.
5. Reoxygenate and ventilate the patient's lungs.
6. Place some lubricant on the outside of the stylet.
7. Remove the oxygen equipment and pass the stylet through the endotracheal tube into the patient's trachea.
8. Insert it to about the same depth as marked on the distal end of the endotracheal tube. For example, if the distal end of the endotracheal tube is 22 cm, insert the tube changer to 22 cm.
9. Deflate the cuff on the endotracheal tube.
10. While holding the distal tip of the tube changer in place, pull the defective endotracheal tube over the tube changer and out of the patient.
11. Advance the new endotracheal tube over the stylet. Hold the distal end of the stylet and push the new tube into the patient to the same depth mark on the stylet as the old tube had been positioned.
12. Hold the endotracheal tube in place and remove the stylet.
13. Ensure that the tube has been placed into the trachea to the proper depth by listening for bilateral breath sounds.

14. Inflate the cuff to a safe pressure.
15. Secure the tube in place and note the depth marking at the patient's teeth or gums.
16. Obtain a chest radiograph.

A defective one-way valve or severed cuff inflating tube may not necessarily lead to a reintubation; often it can be bypassed. This is done by slipping a small-diameter blunt needle (usually about 21 gauge) into the inflating tube, attaching a three-way stopcock to the hub of the needle, and screwing a 10-mL syringe into one of the stopcock ports (Figure 12-44). The cuff pressure can be measured by attaching a pressure manometer to the other port on the stopcock. Air can be added by the 10-mL syringe and the pressure measured simultaneously (Figure 12-45). There is now a commercially available system to bypass a severed cuff inflating tube.

Figure 12-44 Emergency system for inflating the cuff when the one-way valve and inflating tube are severed. *(From Sills JR: Respir Care 31:199-201, 1986.)*

Figure 12-45 Measuring intracuff pressure as the cuff is reinflated with an emergency system. The stethoscope is used to listen for the presence of a leak at the larynx. *(From Sills JR: Respir Care 31:199-201, 1986.)*

2. Extubation

a. Recommend extubation (Code: IIIG1h) [Difficulty: ELE: R, Ap; WRE: An]

Extubation should only be considered after it has been determined that the original problem(s) that necessitated the endotracheal tube has (have) been corrected. It should be reasonably anticipated that once the endotracheal tube has been removed it will not have to be replaced. The patient should be able to sustain a patent airway, expectorate secretions effectively, and maintain acceptable arterial blood gas values. Supplemental oxygen may be needed. Also see the discussion in Chapter 15 that relates to weaning from mechanical ventilation and readiness for extubation. (The only exception to the preceding general guidelines would be when terminal extubation is performed. In this situation, it has been determined that further medical intervention is futile and the patient and/or family want extubation.)

If extubation is planned, make sure that all needed personnel, supplies, and equipment are available in case the patient needs to be reintubated. This includes, but is not limited to, someone trained to perform intubation, intubation equipment and endotracheal tubes, alternative airways such as a laryngeal mask airway, suctioning equipment, bag-mask resuscitator, ECG monitor, and pulse oximeter.

b. Perform extubation (Code: IIIB9) [Difficulty: ELE: R, Ap; WRE: An]

Extubation should be performed only by trained personnel and under the proper conditions to ensure the patient's safety. See Box 12-3 for a list of complications that can occur after extubation. The generally recommended steps in extubation include the following:

1. Evaluate the patient's cardiopulmonary status. The reason(s) for the tube being placed should be corrected. The most recent blood gas results should be acceptable. Tracheal secretions should be minimal and not so thick that they cannot be expectorated by the patient. Bedside spirometry results should show an acceptable tidal volume, vital capacity, and maximal inspiratory pressure.
2. Inform the patient about the removal of the tube and the follow-up care that is needed.
3. The patient's inspired oxygen percentage may be kept the same or increased before the extubation. If increased, it should be done at least 5 to 10 minutes before the tube is removed.
4. Suction the trachea until all secretions are removed.
5. Suction the oral pharynx to remove all saliva. Be prepared to suction additional oral secretions and mucus after extubation.
6. In rapid succession:

a. Give a deep sigh breath from the ventilator or resuscitation bag.

b. Deflate the cuff. Cut the inflation tube to the cuff to ensure its collapse.

c. Pull out the tube following its natural curve when the lungs are full.

Alternatively, in rapid succession:

a. Give a deep sigh breath from the ventilator or resuscitation bag.

b. Place a suction catheter through the tube into the trachea. This works best with a self-contained catheter and sheath system.

c. Deflate the cuff. Cut the inflation tube to the cuff to ensure its collapse.

d. Pull out the tube when the lungs are full.

e. Apply suction as the tube is withdrawn.

7. Have the patient cough vigorously to remove any secretions.

8. Apply a cool, bland aerosol by face mask with the previous amount of oxygen.

9. Monitor and evaluate the patient every 30 minutes for several hours. Encourage deep breathing and coughing.

10. Check the vital signs.

11. Measure pulse oximetry or arterial blood gases after 20 minutes.

12. Listen to the breath sounds and larynx. Inspiratory stridor is a sign of laryngeal edema.

Exam Hint 12-10 (ELE, WRE)

Inspiratory stridor after endotracheal extubation is a sign of serious laryngeal edema. Administer oxygen and nebulize 2.25% racemic epinephrine (microNephrin, Nephron) as a topical vasoconstrictor. Be prepared to intubate a patient who does not respond.

MODULE L
Respiratory care plan

1. Analyze available information to determine the patient's pathophysiologic state (Code: IIIH1) [Difficulty: ELE: R, Ap; WRE: An]

Be able to recognize an airway obstruction problem in a patient and recommend or place the proper airway device to correct the problem. A chest x-ray film should always be taken to confirm the location of a newly placed endotracheal or tracheostomy tube. All modern endotracheal and tracheostomy tubes contain a strip of radiopaque

material near the distal tip of the tube. This is easily noticed as the white line seen on the chest x-ray film and confirms the location of the tip of the tube in the airway (see Figure 12-20). The chest x-ray examination should be repeated if a significant change has occurred in the patient's condition, or if the tube has been pulled back or pushed more deeply into the trachea. The chest x-ray film would also show a pneumothorax related to the tracheostomy procedure or other pulmonary condition.

2. Independently initiate suctioning to manage an artificial airway (ELE code: IIIF2g3) [Difficulty: ELE: R, Ap, An]

Be prepared to suction the patient's endotracheal tube or tracheostomy tube, as needed, to remove secretions. The procedure is described in Chapter 13.

3. Determine the appropriateness of the prescribed therapy and goals for the patient's pathophysiologic state (Code: IIIH3) [Difficulty: ELE: R, Ap, An]

4. Recommend changes in the therapeutic plan when indicated (Code: IIIH4) [Difficulty: ELE: R, Ap; WRE: An]

The indications or uses for the various airways are listed with the information on that airway. In general, the airway should be removed when it is no longer needed. Typically, an oropharyngeal airway should be removed from a patient who has regained consciousness. A nasopharyngeal airway should be removed if the patient no longer needs it as an airway or for a suctioning route. If a laryngeal mask airway (LMA) is employed in the operating room it is typically removed when the patient has recovered from the anesthesia. If an LMA or Combitube is used as a temporary emergency airway, they are typically removed when the patient has recovered. Or, if a longer duration and more secure airway is needed, these tubes are replaced with an endotracheal tube. Endotracheal and tracheostomy tubes can be removed when the patient does not need mechanical ventilation or a suctioning route, is no longer in danger of aspiration, or does not need a permanent artificial airway.

Effective communication is important for good patient care. The conscious patient with an endotracheal tube or tracheostomy is unable to speak. Alternative ways to communicate must be provided. A speaking tracheostomy tube or valve may be tried. Other examples of communication adjuncts include alphabet boards and picture boards for pointing, and pencil and paper for notes. Head nods for yes and no and lip reading are often used. It is important that questions are worded so that they can be answered with a *yes* or *no*. Avoid questions that require a lengthy written answer unless the patient seems ready and willing to do so.

It is not possible to predict how a patient may react to the placement of an artificial airway or its prolonged need. Some patients react with relief and relax when the WOB is reduced. Others may become angry at the limitations imposed on them. Still others may become depressed. Be prepared to deal with these reactions or changes in the patient's emotional response to this very stressful situation.

5. Terminate the treatment or procedure based on the patient's response (Code: IIIF1) [Difficulty: ELE: R, Ap; WRE: An]

6. Recommend discontinuing the treatment or procedure based on the patient's response (Code: IIIG1i) [Difficulty: ELE: R, Ap; WRE: An]

Be prepared to stop or recommend the discontinuation of a particular airway and initiate the use of another, as needed. The indications for each type of airway have been presented earlier in the chapter.

7. Record and evaluate the patient's response to the treatment(s) or procedure(s), including the following:

a. Record and interpret the following: heart rate and rhythm, respiratory rate, blood pressure, body temperature, and pain level (Code: IIIA1b4) [Difficulty: ELE: R, Ap; WRE: An]

b. Record and interpret the patient's breath sounds (Code: IIIA1b3) [Difficulty: ELE: R, Ap; WRE: An]

The vital signs and breath sounds must be documented after an artificial airway is established to document the patient's response.

BIBLIOGRAPHY

American Association for Respiratory Care: Clinical practice guideline: management of airway emergencies, *Respir Care* 40(7):749, 1995.

American Association for Respiratory Care: Clinical practice guideline: removal of the endotracheal tube, *Respir Care* 44(1):85, 1999.

American Association for Respiratory Care: Clinical practice guideline: removal of the endotracheal tube—2007 revision & update, *Respir Care* 52(1):81, 2007.

American Heart Association, Emergency Cardiac Care Committee and Subcommittees: Guidelines for cardiopulmonary resuscitation and emergency cardiac care: adult advanced cardiac life support, *JAMA* 268(16):2199, 1992.

Anesthesia: Practice guidelines for management of the difficult airway, V 98, No 5, pages 1269-1277, May 2003.

Cario, J and Pilbeam S: Mosby's Respiratory Therapy Equipment, 8e, St. Louis, 2010, Mosby

Circulation 2005: Adjuncts for airway control and ventilation, 112; IV-51-IV-51; originally published online Nov 28, 2005.

Desai TR, Statter MB, Aresnman RM, Surgical management of the airway. In Goldsmith JP, Karotkin EH, editors: Assisted ventilation of the neonate, ed 3, Philadelphia, W. B. Saunders Company, 1996.

Eubanks DH, Bone RC: *Comprehensive respiratory care*, ed 2, St Louis, 1990, Mosby.

Frownfelter DL: Chest physical therapy and airway care. In Barnes TA, editor: *Core textbook of respiratory care practice*, ed 2, St Louis, 1994, Mosby.

Gorback MS: Airway management. In Dantzker DR, MacIntyre NR, Bakow ED, editors: *Comprehensive respiratory care*. Philadelphia, 1995, W. B. Saunders Company.

Heffner JE: Managing difficult intubations in critically ill patients, *Respir Management* 19(3):53, 1989.

Hess DR, Branson RD, Airway and suction equipment. In Branson RD, Hess DR, Chatburn RL, editors: *Respiratory care equipment*, ed 2, Philadelphia, 1999, Lippincott Williams & Wilkins.

JEM 400 Endotracheal Tube Changer (Guide), product literature, Instrumentation Industries Inc, Bethel Park, Penn.

Kovac AL: Dilemmas and controversies in intubation, *Respir Management* 21(4):77, 1991.

Kurth CD, Goodwin SR, Obstructive airway diseases in infants and children. In Koff PB, Eitzman D, Neu J, editors: Neonatal and pediatric respiratory care, ed 2, St. Louis, Mosby-Year Book, Inc., 1993.

Levitzky MG, Cairo JM, Hall SM: *Introduction to respiratory care*, Philadelphia, 1990, WB Saunders.

Lewis RM: Airway care. In Fink JB, Hunt GE, editors: *Clinical practice in respiratory care*, Philadelphia, 1999, Lippincott-Raven.

May RA, Bortner PL: Airway management. In Hess DR, MacIntyre NR, Mishoe SC, et. al., editors: *Respiratory Care Principles & Practice*. Philadelphia, 2002, W.B. Saunders Company.

McIntyre D: Airway management. In Wyka KA, Mathews PJ, Clark WF, editors: *Foundations of respiratory care*. Albany, 2002, Delmar.

Part 4: Adult basic life support. *Circulation* 112:IV18-IV34, 2005.

Plevak DJ, Ward JJ: Airway management. In Burton GC, Hodgkin JE, Ward JJ, editors: *Respiratory care: a guide to clinical practice*, ed 4, Philadelphia, 1997, Lippincott-Raven.

PressureEasy Cuff Pressure Controller, ReviveEasy PtL Airway, and Endotracheal/Trach Tube Pilot Tube Repair Kit, product literature, Respironics, Monroeville, Penn.

Roth P: Airway care. In Aloan CA, Hill TV, editors: *Respiratory care of the newborn and child*, ed 2, Philadelphia, 1997, Lippincott-Raven.

Shapiro BA, Kacmarek RM, Cane RD, et al, editors: *Clinical application of respiratory care*, ed 4, St Louis, 1991, Mosby.

Shilling A, Durbin CG, Airway management devices. In Cairo JM, Pilbeam SP, editors: *Mosby's respiratory care equipment*, ed 8, St Louis, 2010, Mosby, Inc.

Sills JR: An emergency cuff inflation technique, *Respir Care* 31(3):199, 1986.

Simmons KF, Scanlan CL: Airway management. In Wilkins RL, Stoller JK, and Scanlan CL, editors: *Egan's fundamentals of respiratory care*, ed 8, St Louis, 2003, Mosby, Inc.

Simmons KF, Scanlan CL: Airway management. In Wilkins RL, Stoller JK, Kacmarek RM, editors: *Egan's fundamentals of respiratory care,* ed 9, St Louis, 2009, Mosby, Inc.

Whitaker K: *Comprehensive perinatal & pediatric respiratory care,* ed 2, Albany, NY, 1997, Delmar.

White GC: *Equipment theory for respiratory care,* ed 4, Albany, NY, 2005, Delmar.

Wilkins RL, Stoller JK, and Scanlan CL, editors: *Egan's fundamentals of respiratory care,* ed 8, St Louis, 2003, Mosby, Inc

---

SELF-STUDY QUESTIONS FOR THE ENTRY LEVEL EXAM   *See page 594 for answers*

1. You are preparing a stainless-steel–type laryngoscope handle and blade for an anesthesiologist. The light does not shine. Which of the following would you do to fix the problem?
   1. Get a smaller blade to fit the handle.
   2. Get a larger blade to fit the handle.
   3. Tighten the light bulb.
   4. Replace the handle with a plastic one.
   5. Check the batteries and replace them if necessary.
   A. 1, 4
   B. 2
   C. 3, 5
   D. 4

2. An oropharyngeal airway would be indicated under which of the following conditions?
   1. To maintain an airway before performing a tracheostomy
   2. Seizure activity is expected or present
   3. To treat an unconscious patient in the supine position with a soft-tissue upper airway obstruction
   4. To stabilize the mouth in a patient with a traumatic jaw injury
   5. An orally intubated patient is biting the tube
   A. 3, 5
   B. 4, 5
   C. 1, 4
   D. 2, 3, 5

3. You have just assisted with the intubation of a normotensive adult patient. To minimize the risk of soft-tissue injury to the trachea, what is the highest endotracheal tube cuff pressure that should be employed?
   A. Less than 15 cm H_2O
   B. Less than 25 cm H_2O
   C. Less than 35 cm H_2O
   D. Less than 45 cm H_2O

4. All of the following may be used to help determine the position of an endotracheal tube:
   1. End-tidal carbon dioxide monitoring
   2. An esophageal detection device (EDD)
   3. Laryngeal palpation during tube insertion
   4. Neck and chest radiographs
   5. Observation of bilateral chest movement
   A. 1, 3, 4
   B. 2, 4, 5
   C. 1, 2, 3, 4
   D. All of the above

5. A respiratory therapist replaces a patient's tracheostomy tube with another one of the same size and inflates the cuff with 5 mL of air as was previously. Immediately, the patient has difficulty breathing and no air can be felt coming from the tube. What could be the problem?
   A. The tip of the tube has been placed into the subcutaneous tissues.
   B. The patient has closed her epiglottis over the trachea.
   C. More air must be added to the cuff to form a seal.
   D. The tube has accidentally been placed into the esophagus.

6. While assisting with a CPR attempt, the anesthesiologist asks you to get a properly sized endotracheal tube so that the patient's airway can be quickly intubated. The patient is a large, physically fit man. What tube would you obtain?
   A. A 7.0-mm-ID oral endotracheal tube
   B. A 10.0-mm-ID nasal endotracheal tube
   C. An 8.0-mm-ID nasal endotracheal tube
   D. A 9.0-mm-ID oral endotracheal tube

7. You have just measured a tracheostomy tube's cuff pressure with a blood pressure–type mercury manometer. The pressure was 17 mm Hg. What would you recommend?
   A. Leaving the cuff pressure as it is and charting the measured value
   B. Increasing the cuff pressure to 20 mm Hg
   C. Rechecking the cuff pressure with a Cufflator device
   D. Replacing the tube with a larger one

8. A 45-year-old female patient is brought into the emergency department from an automobile accident. She has facial trauma, including a broken nose and jaw. Because of heavy bleeding into her mouth, she is having difficulty breathing. Which of the following would you recommend to ensure a safe, effective airway?
   A. Place an oral airway.
   B. Place a tracheostomy tube.

C. Place a nasopharyngeal airway.

D. Place a nasal endotracheal tube.

9. While working in the neonatal intensive care unit, you are called to assist in the care of a newborn. The neonatologist asks you to get the proper endotracheal tube size for a premature newborn. What size tube would you obtain?

A. 1.5-mm ID

B. 2.5-mm ID

C. 3.5-mm ID

D. 4.0-mm ID

10. A 59-kg (130-lb) woman must be intubated to initiate mechanical ventilation. What size tube should be used?

A. 6.0-mm ID

B. 6.5-mm ID

C. 7.5-mm ID

D. 9.0-mm ID

11. You are going to assist in the ambulance transport of a 25-year-old patient. The patient has an oral endotracheal tube, and you are going to manually ventilate his lungs during the trip. Which of the following would you choose to help you be sure that the endotracheal tube stays properly placed within the trachea?

A. Pulse oximeter

B. Capnograph

C. Disposable exhaled-CO_2 detector

D. Electrocardiogram

12. All of the following should be monitored after a patient returns from having a tracheostomy tube placed EXCEPT

A. Cuff pressure

B. Bowel sounds

C. Bilateral breath sounds

D. Excessive bleeding

13. Auscultation of a recently intubated patient in respiratory failure reveals absent breath sounds on the left side of the chest. The most likely cause of this finding is

A. Placement of the endotracheal tube into the right mainstem bronchus

B. Placement of the endotracheal tube into the left mainstem bronchus

C. Placement of the endotracheal tube into the esophagus

D. A pneumothorax on the right side

14. While working the night shift, you are called to intubate an apneic patient. Which of the following would you need for an emergency oral intubation?

1. **Laryngoscope handle**

2. **Stylet**

3. **Proper laryngoscope blade**

4. **10-mL syringe**

5. **Magill forceps**

A. 1, 2

B. 1, 2, 5

C. 1, 2, 3, 4

D. 2, 4, 5

15. You are assisting with the extubation of an adult patient. At what point in the procedure should the tube be removed?

A. At the end of a peak inspiratory effort

B. At the end of a normal exhalation

C. At the start of a peak inspiratory effort

D. During a forced vital capacity effort

16. A patient with a tracheostomy has just returned from a series of x-ray procedures. Suddenly, she develops respiratory distress and cannot breathe. Your attempt to pass a suction catheter through the tracheostomy tube does not work. You should proceed to

A. Attempt to pass a smaller suction catheter

B. Remove the tracheostomy tube

C. Attempt to ventilate the patient's lungs with a manual resuscitator

D. Insert an endotracheal tube

17. After a successful CPR attempt, a patient with an oral endotracheal tube is placed on a mechanical ventilator in the intensive care unit. The respiratory therapist notices that the exhaled CO_2 monitor is appropriately changing color with each breath cycle. The patient's breath sounds are present on the right side but diminished on the left side. What is the most likely cause of this situation?

A. Left-sided pneumothorax

B. Right bronchial intubation

C. Malfunctioning exhaled CO_2 monitor

D. Delivered tidal volume is too small

18. Your patient is an 18-year-old woman who was found unconscious from a drug overdose. She has severe atelectasis of the left lung caused by lying on her left side for 2 days. Her right lung is normal. She is going to require mechanical ventilation to open the atelectatic areas. What endotracheal tube would you suggest should be used to properly treat the abnormal lung?

A. Double-lumen

B. Standard

C. Fenestrated tracheostomy

D. Wire-reinforced

19. Your patient has epilepsy and has been having unpredictable seizure activity. What oral endotracheal tube would you suggest should be used to provide a secure airway?

A. Double-lumen

B. Preformed

C. Wire-reinforced

D. Guidable

20. A conscious patient is recovering from Guillain-Barré syndrome and is able to breathe spontaneously off of

the mechanical ventilator for several hours. She currently has a standard 7.5-mm-ID tracheostomy tube. To help her weaning process but to enable her to be ventilated at night, what should be done?

A. Remove the tracheostomy tube when she is off of the ventilator.

B. Substitute a speaking-type tracheostomy tube.

C. Replace the current tracheostomy tube with one that is 6.0-mm ID.

D. Substitute a fenestrated tracheostomy tube.

21. A semiconscious patient with many tracheal secretions will need frequent nasotracheal suctioning. What can be done to minimize trauma from the procedure?

A. Insert a tracheostomy button with a speaking valve.

B. Insert a nasopharyngeal airway.

C. Sedate the patient and insert an oropharyngeal airway.

D. Suction through a fenestrated tracheostomy tube.

22. Your patient who has a tracheostomy button with attached speaking valve is complaining that it is difficult to breathe. You find that a 12Fr suction catheter cannot be passed through the button. What should be done?

A. Place a transtracheal oxygen catheter through the tracheostomy button.

B. Force a larger suction catheter through the button.

C. Remove the button and orally intubate the patient.

D. Remove the speaking valve and assess the patient.

23. During a surgical procedure, the anesthesiologist wishes to protect the patient's airway and provide mechanical ventilation, but does not want to place an endotracheal tube. What airway should be used?

A. Combitube

B. Laryngeal mask airway

C. Oropharyngeal airway

D. Nasopharyngeal airway in each nostril

24. You are called to the delivery room to assist in the care of a newborn diagnosed with macroglossia. What should a respiratory therapist be prepared to do in this situation?

A. Maintain a patent upper airway.

B. Instill surfactant.

C. Initiate mechanical ventilation.

D. Provide supplemental oxygen.

25. After assisting in an emergency oral intubation procedure of an adult patient, you assess his breath sounds and find them absent in the left lung area. The tube depth marking shows it is at the 29-cm mark at the patient's front teeth. What do you recommend be done?

A. Check the chest radiograph results for the tube's placement.

B. Pull the tube back to the 24-cm mark.

C. Push the tube down to the 32-cm mark.

D. Listen for inspiratory sounds over the stomach area.

26. An unconscious 17-year-old patient has arrived in the emergency department. She was involved in an automobile accident, has a neck injury, and is wearing a neck brace. If she were to show signs of an upper airway obstruction, all of the following could be easily used to maintain the airway EXCEPT

A. Oral endotracheal tube

B. Nasopharyngeal airway

C. Laryngeal mask airway

D. Oropharyngeal airway

SELF-STUDY QUESTIONS FOR THE WRITTEN REGISTRY EXAM *See page 619 for answers*

1. Immediate complications of an oral intubation include all of the following EXCEPT

A. Tooth trauma

B. Esophageal intubation

C. Tracheoesophageal fistula

D. Bronchial intubation

2. A hospitalized patient rapidly develops ventilatory failure because of an accidental overdose of morphine sulfate for pain control. The preferred way to quickly provide a safe, secure airway is to

A. Place an oropharyngeal airway

B. Hyperextend the patient's neck into the sniff position

C. Place a nasal endotracheal tube

D. Place an oral endotracheal tube

3. Indications for oral intubation include all the following EXCEPT

A. The patient requires mechanical ventilation

B. The patient has a cervical spine injury

C. The patient requires frequent tracheal suctioning

D. The patient is at risk for vomiting and aspirating

4. A 2-year-old child admitted with severe croup has just been extubated after 2 days with an oral endotracheal tube. The child is given oxygen and aerosolized water through a heated large-volume nebulizer. Thirty minutes later, mild inspiratory stridor is heard over the child's throat area. What should be done *first*?

A. Deliver nebulized racemic epinephrine.

B. Reintubate the child.

C. Perform a cricothyrotomy.

D. Perform a tracheostomy.

5. A 55-year-old, 77-kg (170-lb) male patient with a tracheostomy tube has been returned from the operating room after a gastric procedure. The respiratory therapist determines the cuff pressure on the 6.0-mm-ID tracheostomy tube to be 35 mm Hg. The ventilator is delivering a tidal volume of 750 mL and returning a tidal volume of 650 mL, and a leak can be heard at the tracheostomy site. What should be done?

    A. Increase the tidal volume by 100 mL.

    B. Increase the cuff pressure to seal the trachea to stop the tidal volume leak.

    C. Replace the tracheostomy tube with one that is 8.5-mm ID.

    D. Deflate the cuff enough to reduce the cuff pressure to 15 mm Hg.

6. An intubated and mechanically ventilated adult patient has been returned to the long-term care unit after being transported to the radiology department for an abdominal radiograph examination. The respiratory therapist observes that the patient's trachea is midline. However, the patient's left chest area does not rise with inspiration as much as the right chest area. The endotracheal tube is at the 28-cm mark at the patient's teeth. What should be done now?

    A. Check the abdominal radiograph for signs of vomiting and aspiration.

    B. Pull the endotracheal tube back about 4 cm.

    C. Check the patient's end-tidal carbon dioxide level.

    D. Deliver a larger tidal volume breath to inflate the left lung better.

7. A patient is about to have an oral endotracheal tube inserted. What can be done during and/or after the procedure to determine its position within the trachea?

    1. Get a chest radiograph.

    2. Palpate the larynx during insertion.

    3. Auscultate bilateral breath sounds.

    4. Attach an esophageal detection device (EDD) after the tube is placed.

    5. Check for exhaled carbon dioxide.

    A. 1, 4

    B. 2, 3

    C. 1, 3, 5

    D. 1, 2, 3, 4, 5

8. A patient who suffered facial burns and smoke inhalation has recovered enough to be extubated. Although the patient is receiving 40% oxygen with a bland aerosol, significant inspiratory stridor is noticed within 15 minutes. Following the inhalation of a vasoconstricting medication the patient's breath sounds are improved. Thirty minutes later the patient's SpO$_2$ level is 80% and the inspiratory stridor is more serious. The patient is very anxious and is pulling off the oxygen mask. What should the respiratory therapist recommend to best manage the patient's problem?

    A. Draw an arterial blood gas sample for measurement.

    B. Increase the patient's oxygen to 50%.

    C. Intubate the patient.

    D. Administer a sedative medication.

9. During a CPR attempt, a pediatric patient had an oral endotracheal tube placed. To ensure that the endotracheal tube is placed properly, you would recommend all of the following EXCEPT:

    A. Listen to the right upper lobe if the left lung field is inaccessible

    B. Listen for bilateral lung sounds

    C. Have a lateral neck x-ray film taken

    D. Have a chest x-ray film taken

10. While checking the tracheostomy tube cuff pressure on a patient in the recovery room, you find that the pressure is 33 mm Hg. This cuff pressure will likely cause which of the following?

    1. **Loss of capillary flow through the tracheal soft tissues**

    2. **Loss of lymphatic flow through the tracheal soft tissues**

    3. **Tracheal wall damage**

    4. **Protection of the vocal cords from damage caused by the tracheostomy tube**

    5. **Loss of venous flow through the tracheal soft tissues**

    A. 1, 2, 3, 5

    B. 2, 4

    C. 3, 5

    D. 1, 2

11. A Combitube is used to

    1. **Intubate the trachea orally**

    2. **Intubate the trachea nasally**

    3. **Prevent vomiting**

    4. **Maintain the airway**

    A. 1

    B. 1, 3

    C. 2, 4

    D. 3, 4

12. A newborn child with macroglossia is having moderate airway obstruction episodes. What could be done to help manage the current situation?

    1. **Place a nasopharyngeal airway.**

    2. **Place a tracheostomy button.**

    3. **Place the newborn in the prone position.**

    4. **Place an oral endotracheal tube.**

    A. 2

    B. 1, 3

    C. 3, 4

    D. 1, 2, 4

13. A 28-year-old patient is brought into the emergency department. She has a cervical spine injury from a diving accident and is wearing a neck brace.   T h e patient is unconscious and inspiratory stridor can be heard. Arterial blood gases on 40% oxygen show the following: PaO_2 57 mm Hg, $PaCO_2$ 56 mm Hg, and pH 7.30. The physician has decided to establish a secure airway. What device would you recommend be used?
    A. 7.0-mm nasotracheal tube
    B. Berman oral airway
    C. 8.5-mm Carlens orotracheal tube
    D. 9.0-mm nasotracheal tube

14. An adult patient is recovering from her neuromuscular disease. She has a standard tracheostomy tube and only requires mechanical ventilation during the night when sleeping. The physician asks for your recommendation about what can be done to enable her to communicate during the day but be put on the ventilator at night. What would you recommend?
    A. Change her to a fenestrated tracheostomy tube.
    B. Put a tracheostomy button into her during the day.
    C. Put an uncuffed tracheostomy tube into her.
    D. Put the obturator into her current tracheostomy tube during the day.

15. The Combitube has advantages over the standard laryngeal mask airway (LMA) because
    1. It can be placed nasally
    2. A gastric tube can be placed through it to empty the stomach
    3. It is available in small pediatric sizes

    4. The patient can be ventilated whether it is placed into the esophagus or the trachea
    A. 2, 4
    B. 1, 2
    C. 3, 4
    D. 1, 4

16. Your patient is being mechanically ventilated. Despite 30 mm Hg pressure in the cuff, there is still a significant tidal volume leak. Which of the following is the best way to correct the problem?
    A. Insert a larger diameter endotracheal tube with a high-volume, low-pressure cuff and inflate the cuff to a safe pressure.
    B. Leave the cuff inflated to 30 mm Hg.
    C. Inflate the cuff to whatever pressure is needed to seal the trachea.
    D. Deflate the cuff to 20 mm Hg and increase the respiratory rate to compensate for the leak.

17. Immediate complications of the oral intubation procedure include all of the following EXCEPT
    A. Tooth trauma
    B. Laceration of the pharynx
    C. Esophageal intubation
    D. Tracheoesophageal fistula

18. After extubation, a patient develops signs of severe respiratory distress with marked inspiratory stridor. It would be best at this time to
    A. Administer a vasoconstrictor drug
    B. Administer an IPPB treatment with a bronchodilator
    C. Administer a cool aerosol with 40% oxygen
    D. Reintubate the patient

13 Suctioning the Airway

Note 1: This book is written to cover every item listed as testable on the *Entry Level Examination (ELE), Written Registry Examination (WRE),* and *Clinical Simulation Examination (CSE).*

The listed code for each item is taken from the National Board for Respiratory Care's (NBRC) **Summary Content Outline for CRT (Certified Respiratory Therapist) and Written RRT (Registered Respiratory Therapist) Examinations** (http://evolve.elsevier.com/Sills/resptherapist/). For example, if an item is testable on both the ELE and WRE, it is shown simply as (Code: . . .). If an item is testable only on the ELE, it is shown as (ELE code: . . .). If an item is testable only on the WRE, it is shown as (WRE code: . . .).

Following each item's code, the difficulty level is indicated for the questions on that item on the ELE and WRE. (See the Introduction for a full explanation of the three difficulty levels.) **Recall [R]** level questions typically expect the exam taker to recall factual information. **Application [Ap]** level questions are more difficult, because the exam taker may have to apply factual information to a clinical situation. **Analysis [An]** level questions are the most challenging, because the exam taker may have to use critical thinking to evaluate patient data to make a clinical decision.

Note 2: A review of the most recent versions of the Entry Level Examination (ELE) has shown that an average of 4 questions (out of 140), or 3% of the exam, will cover suctioning of the airway. A review of the most recent versions of the Written Registry Examination (WRE) has shown that an average of 3 questions (out of 100), or 3% of the exam, will cover suctioning of the airway. The Clinical Simulation Examination (CSE) is comprehensive and may include everything that an advanced respiratory therapist should know.

MODULE A
Oropharyngeal suction devices

1. Manipulate suctioning devices by order or protocol (ELE code: IIA8) [ELE Difficulty: R, Ap, An]

a. Get the necessary equipment for the procedure

Oropharyngeal suctioning is considered a clean (not sterile) procedure. The suctioning device is often origi-

nally packaged sterile but may be used more than once. The Yankauer suction catheter is widely used, although several types are available. The Yankauer suction catheter is made of hard plastic and is angled to reach into the back of the mouth. One large opening or several medium-sized openings may be found at the tip of the catheter. The openings are large enough to permit easy suctioning of saliva, food, or vomit. Some handles include a thumb control valve so that suction can be applied to the tip only when wanted. Covering the opening with a thumb creates a vacuum at the tip for suctioning the patient's mouth (Figure 13-1). The Yankauer may be discarded when no longer needed or sterilized for use with another patient.

A flexible plastic or rubber catheter also can be used. It should be the largest diameter possible to reduce the chance of its becoming plugged. The opening at the catheter tip should be cut straight (perpendicular) across instead of at an angle. No side openings should be present (Figure 13-2). The catheter is discarded when no longer needed.

b. Put the equipment together and make sure that it works properly

The catheters just mentioned are single pieces with nothing to assemble. They must be attached to a vacuum source by a length of soft rubber tubing. With clean gloves on both hands, attach the Yankauer, plastic, or rubber catheter to the vacuum tubing. The vacuum must be applied to the tip of the catheter for oral secretions to be removed. Check for a vacuum at the tip by any of the following methods:

- Listen for the sound of air being drawn into the tip.
- Put the tip into a container of sterile water. Close the thumb control opening. The water must be drawn up the catheter.
- Place a clean-gloved hand over the tip if no water is available. Close the thumb control opening. The glove should be sucked onto the catheter.

c. Troubleshoot any problems with the equipment

If no vacuum is felt at the catheter tip, several causes are possible and must be investigated.

Tip

Catheter

Thumb-control valve

Handle

Large openings at tip

Connector for vacuum

Vacuum tubing

Figure 13-1 Features of the Yankauer suction catheter.

Thumb-control valve

Connector for vacuum

Catheter

Vacuum tubing

Tip with a single opening

Figure 13-2 Features of a suction catheter with a cross-cut tip.

1. The vacuum is not turned on.

Check the following:
- a. Some centralized vacuum systems have a single dial that turns the system off and on and sets the vacuum level. Other centralized vacuum systems have an ON and OFF switch and a dial for the vacuum level.
- b. Freestanding vacuum systems must be plugged into a working electrical outlet. The ON and OFF switch must be turned on. The simpler systems have a preset vacuum level. Variable vacuum levels can be set with a dial in the more sophisticated systems.

2. The system is not sealed, and the vacuum is lost to the atmosphere.

Check the following:
- a. Make sure the rubber vacuum tubing fits tightly over the connectors on the catheter and on the vacuum system.
- b. Make sure the catheter and vacuum tubing are not cracked or cut. Replace a Yankauer, plastic, or rubber catheter or vacuum tubing that is defective.
- c. Close the thumb control if it has been left open.
- d. Check the central or freestanding vacuum system to make sure the secretion collection bottle is sealed properly.

3. The system is blocked, and no vacuum can get through to the tip.

Check the following:
- a. Check for a pinch in the vacuum tubing or soft catheter.
- b. Check for a blockage in the catheter or vacuum tubing. Try to suction some sterile water to clear the blockage into the secretion collection bottle. Replace the catheter or vacuum tubing, or both, if the blockage cannot be cleared.
- c. Empty a full collection bottle.

2. Suction catheters

Suctioning catheters are used to remove secretions and foreign material from the trachea. They come sterile and individually packaged. It is highly recommended that the outer diameter (OD) of the catheter be no more than one-half the inner diameter (ID) of the airway that it is passing through. This guideline is intended to minimize obstruction of the airway, so that the patient is able to breathe around the catheter.

Exam Hint 13-1 (ELE, WRE)

Remember that the outer diameter of the suction catheter should be no more than one half the inner diameter of the endotracheal or tracheostomy tube.

Table 13-1 presents the recommended suction catheter sizes for the various endotracheal or tracheostomy tubes. The practitioner also can easily compare the relative sizes of the tube and suction catheter at the bedside before suctioning. Suction catheters are sized by the French (Fr) scale of the OD. Endotracheal and tracheostomy tubes are sized by ID and OD in millimeters and often by OD in French. Review Table 12-1 if necessary.

	Tube Internal	Size of Suction
Age	Diameter (mm)	Catheter (Fr)
NEWBORN		
1,000 g	2.5	5
1,000-2,000 g	3	6
2,000-3,000	3.5	8
3,000 g to 6 mo	3.5-4	8
PEDIATRIC		
18 mo	4	8
3 yr	4.5	8
5 yr	5	10
6 yr	5.5	10
8 yr	6	10
ADULT		
16 yr	7	10
Normal-size woman	7.5-8	12
Normal-size man	8-8.5	14
Large adult	9-10	16

TABLE 13-1 Recommended Suction Catheter French Sizes for Endotracheal and Tracheostomy Tubes*

*For suctioning of endotracheal tubes (ET) and tracheostomy tubes (TT), the suction catheter's outer diameter should be no more than one half the inner diameter of the ET or TT.

a. Calculations related to catheter size (math review)

The following formula can be used to calculate the OD of any suction catheter to determine the endotracheal or tracheostomy tube size with which the suction catheter may be used:

$$\text{Suction catheter size (Fr)} \times 0.33 = \text{OD (mm) of suction catheter}$$

EXAMPLE 1

Calculate the OD of a 12 Fr suction catheter:

$$12 \text{ Fr} \times 0.33 = 3.96 \text{ (about 4) mm OD}$$

This size catheter, therefore, could be used with an 8-mm ID endotracheal tube. Figure 13-3 shows the relative sizes of this endotracheal tube and catheter.

Use the following formula to estimate the maximum French size suction catheter for the ID of an endotracheal or tracheostomy tube:

$$\frac{\text{ID of endotracheal tube} \times 3}{2}$$
$$= \text{Maximum diameter (Fr) of catheter}$$

EXAMPLE 2

Calculate the largest suction catheter that should be used with a size 8 (ID) endotracheal tube:

Figure 13-3 A 12 Fr suction catheter inside an endotracheal tube with an 8-mm internal diameter (ID). The outer diameter (OD) of the suction catheter should be no more than one half the ID of the tube so that the patient can breathe around it.

$$\frac{8 \times 3}{2} = \frac{24}{2} = 12 \text{ Fr suction catheter}$$

Therefore, a 12 Fr suction catheter could be used with an 8-mm ID endotracheal (or tracheostomy) tube (see Figure 13-3).

Knowing the ID of a suction catheter is helpful because it relates to the maximum particle size that can pass through it. The following formula can be used to interconvert from French OD to millimeters ID:

$$\text{mm} = \frac{\text{Fr} - 2}{4}$$

EXAMPLE 3

What is the ID in millimeters of a 12 Fr suction catheter?

$$\text{mm} = \frac{12 - 2}{4}$$

$$\text{mm} = \frac{10}{4}$$

$$\text{mm} = 2.5 \text{ (see Figure 13-3)}$$

Therefore, a 12 Fr suction catheter (with a 4-mm OD) can be used to suction particles up to 2.5 mm in diameter.

b. Get the necessary equipment for the procedure

The term *open-airway suctioning* is used here to refer to a suctioning procedure on a patient who is spontaneously breathing room air after being disconnected from the source of supplemental oxygen. For example, in a patient with a normal upper airway, the oxygen mask is removed for nasotracheal suctioning. Also, in a patient with an endotracheal or a tracheostomy tube, the aerosol T-piece (Briggs adapter) or ventilator circuit is removed to allow suctioning.

These types of catheters have been in use for many years. The two basic types are shown in Figure 13-4. Closing the thumb control, as shown in Figure 13-5, allows the vacuum to be selectively applied to the secretions when desired. The tips of the catheters can vary

greatly. A considerable amount of effort has been spent trying to develop a catheter tip that most effectively removes secretions without damaging the tracheal mucosa. Figure 13-6 shows some of the catheter tips that have been developed to minimize mucosal damage. Note that all feature at least one opening in the catheter that is back from the opening at the tip. Compare this with the single end opening found on the oral suction catheter (see Figure 13-2). The side openings are designed to prevent the vacuum from being applied to the tip when it makes contact with the mucosa.

Notice in Figures 13-4 and 13-6 that most catheters are straight throughout their length. All of these catheters tend to enter the right mainstem bronchus during deep suctioning. This is because the right mainstem bronchus's angle off of the trachea is less acute than that of the left mainstem bronchus. Therefore, it is difficult, if not impossible, to use any of these catheters to suction the left mainstem bronchus. The Coudé catheter has an angled tip to make it easier to guide into the left (or right) mainstem bronchus (see Figure 13-6, C). When these catheters are used, the direction of the thumb control valve can help determine the angle of the bent tip.

Use of these traditional types of catheters during open-airway suctioning always results in some level of hypoxemia. The newer, insufflating suction catheter is designed to provide alternatively oxygen through the catheter or vacuum for suctioning. The thumb control end of the catheter is modified with two male-type tubing connectors and a way to switch the lumen of the catheter between them. The thumb control is set to direct the oxygen through the catheter and into the patient as the catheter is advanced. After the catheter has been deeply placed into the trachea for suctioning, the thumb control is switched from delivering oxygen to applying suction.

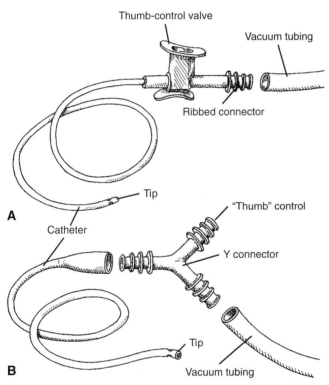

Figure 13-4 Features of two types of suction catheters with angle-cut tips and side holes. **A,** This catheter has its own thumb control valve. **B,** This catheter must have a thumb control valve constructed from a Y-connector.

Figure 13-5 Close-up of a thumb control valve showing how room air is drawn into vacuum tubing when the valve is left open. Closing the valve creates a vacuum at the catheter tip, allowing secretions to be suctioned.

Figure 13-6 Close-ups of the ends of three suction catheters. **A,** Bevel-cut tip with two offset side holes. **B,** Ring tip with several side holes around it. **C,** Coudé (curved-tip) catheter; the curve may help guide the catheter into either the left or right mainstem bronchus. *(From Rarey KP, Youtsey JW:* Respiratory patient care, *Englewood Cliffs, NJ, 1981, Prentice-Hall.)*

c. Get the necessary equipment for the procedure

The term *closed-airway suctioning* is used here to refer to a suctioning procedure in which the patient remains connected to the original source of oxygen. This may be done through a special aerosol T-piece or, more commonly, for an intubated patient receiving mechanical ventilation with positive end-expiratory pressure (PEEP). In addition, closed-airway suctioning may reduce the risk of ventilator-associated pneumonia (VAP). This suctioning method is preferred in patients who are likely to become hypoxic when disconnected from their oxygen source.

In closed-airway suctioning systems, a flexible, clear plastic sheath covers the catheter to maintain its sterility (Figure 13-7). The practitioner does not need gloves. When used for patients who need frequent suctioning, self-contained systems have a financial advantage over the traditional catheter and gloves suctioning method, because they can be reused. Closed-system suction catheters come with either the traditional straight tip or the Coudé tip for selective bronchial suctioning.

Another device used to create a sealed system for endotracheal tube suctioning consists of an elbow adapter that has an inner plastic sleeve or diaphragm. As the traditional catheter is inserted into the opening on the elbow adapter, the sleeve or diaphragm conforms to the catheter so that no air leakage occurs (Figure 13-8). This ensures that the ventilator-delivered volumes and pressures are not lost through a leak.

d. Put the equipment together and make sure that it works properly

Figure 13-4 shows the attachment of an open-airway suction catheter to the vacuum tubing, and Figure 13-7 shows the attachment of a closed-airway suction catheter to the vacuum tubing. The other end of the vacuum tubing is attached to the vacuum regulator system.

With open-airway suctioning, only a hand covered by a sterile glove can be allowed to touch the area of the catheter that enters the patient's trachea. The practitioner's other hand also should be gloved. A clean glove is acceptable for that hand, because it does not touch the part of the catheter that will enter the patient's trachea.

While holding the body of the catheter, the thumb control valve, and the vacuum connector with the sterile-gloved hand and the vacuum tubing with the clean-gloved hand, slip the vacuum tubing over the catheter's vacuum connector. The seal should be tight so that no vacuum leak occurs. From now on, only the sterile-gloved hand may touch the part of the catheter that makes contact with the patient. The clean-gloved hand may touch only the thumb control valve and vacuum tubing. If the catheter is contaminated, it must be discarded.

Figure 13-7 Self-contained catheter and sheath suctioning system for closed-airway suctioning (based on the Kimberly-Clark/Ballard Trach Care closed endotracheal suction device).

Figure 13-8 Features and placement of a special elbow adapter, which allows closed-airway suctioning without loss of tidal volume or pressure during mechanical ventilation.

The catheter can be tested for patency and vacuum at the tip by the three methods described earlier in the discussion on oropharyngeal suction devices. Note that only a *sterile* glove may be touched against the tip of the suction catheter to check for a vacuum.

The practitioner does not need gloves when a self-contained catheter is used for closed-airway suctioning, because the sheath covers the catheter to prevent contamination.

Exam Hint 13-2 (ELE, WRE)

Remember that endotracheal suctioning is a sterile procedure. Gloves or a catheter that has become contaminated must be replaced with sterile equipment.

---

e. Troubleshoot any problems with the equipment

The three common causes of an equipment failure and how to troubleshoot them are described in the earlier discussion on oropharyngeal suction devices. Remember to withdraw the closed-airway suctioning catheter completely from the endotracheal tube into the sheath, or it will partially obstruct the tube.

3. Specimen collectors

a. Get the necessary equipment

A variety of specimen collectors (commonly called *Lukens traps*) are available. They are packaged as sterile so that no contamination of the sputum sample occurs with nonpatient organisms. Figures 13-9 through 13-12 show the key features and functions of several sputum sample collectors. The sputum sample is obtained through a suction catheter or bronchoscope.

The specimen jar has volume markings. It screws into either a special lid used to suction the specimen or a regular lid. The regular lid is used for shipment to the laboratory. The special lids used in the systems featured in Figures 13-9 and 13-10 must be connected to a sterile catheter. Figure 13-11 shows a system with its own catheter. The vacuum source is provided to these specimen collectors by a length of vacuum tubing, as in the previously described suction catheter systems. Figure 13-12 shows a DeLee system, which is sometimes used in the delivery room. The physician, nurse, or practitioner uses mouth suction to remove secretions from the newborn. In all of these examples, after the sample has been collected, the special lid is unscrewed and replaced with the regular specimen jar lid.

b. Put the equipment together and make sure that it works properly

A properly working specimen collection system provides a vacuum to the tip of the suction catheter when the thumb control valve or mouthpiece is sealed and vacuum is applied. This is tested by dipping the catheter tip into a container of sterile water or saline solution. The liquid is drawn up the catheter and deposited in the specimen jar. (The water can be discarded from the jar.)

Figure 13-9 Features of a collection system for sputum specimens that includes a thumb control valve.

Figure 13-10 Features of a collection system for sputum specimens that does not have a thumb control valve.

Figure 13-11 Features of a collection system for sputum specimens that has a thumb control valve built into catheter.

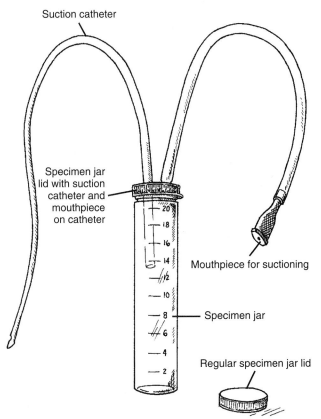

Suction catheter

Specimen jar lid with suction catheter and mouthpiece on catheter

Mouthpiece for suctioning

Specimen jar

Regular specimen jar lid

Figure 13-12 Features of the DeLee collection system for sputum specimens, showing the mouthpiece through which the practitioner can apply suction.

Figure 13-13 Portable suction machine, showing the electrically powered motor, collection bottle and cap, and connecting tubing. *(Courtesy Allied Health Care Products, St Louis, Mo.)*

c. Troubleshoot any problems with the equipment

Failure to have a vacuum at the tip of the suction catheter may be caused by any of the previously mentioned possibilities. They can be checked and corrected by the methods listed earlier. Two causes of an inability to suction secretions are common. One cause is that the jar is not screwed tightly into the special lid, allowing room air to be drawn in. Simply screw the lid in tightly. The second cause is that the secretion channel is plugged. Discard it and replace it with a new specimen collector.

MODULE B
Vacuum regulator systems

1. Manipulate vacuum regulator systems by order or protocol (ELE Code: IIA21) [ELE Difficulty: R, Ap, An]

2. Get the necessary vacuum regulator system: vacuum pump, regulator, and collection bottle

3. Put the equipment together and make sure that it works properly

Vacuum regulators are preassembled by the manufacturer. The two basic types are described here. Components must be added to make them fully functional.

a. Portable vacuum systems

Portable units are designed to be moved with the patient. They may be mounted on a small platform (Figure 13-13) or on a wheeled cart. The portable systems generally include an electrically powered vacuum pump with an ON/OFF switch and a collection bottle. Some units have a control valve for adjusting the level of negative pressure. A negative-pressure gauge is used to determine how much vacuum is being applied. A length of rubber vacuum tubing is used to pass the negative pressure from the pump to the collection bottle. Another length of vacuum tubing is used to pass the vacuum through to the suction catheter. Portable systems are not as powerful as central vacuum systems. They are not very effective at suctioning out large amounts of thick secretions.

In general, the following steps are followed to make the units operational:

1. Plug the vacuum pump into a working electrical outlet. Battery-operated units should have fully charged batteries.
2. Place a clean, empty collection bottle into its holder on the cart. The bottle should be able to hold at least 500 mL of fluid.
3. Slip the rubber lid onto the open top of the collection bottle. Both vacuum tubing connectors on the lid must be patent.
4. Slip one end of a short length of vacuum tubing over the connector on the vacuum pump and the other end over one of the tubing connectors on the collection bottle lid.

5. Slip one end of a length of vacuum tubing over the other tubing connector on the collection bottle lid. The vacuum tubing should be no more than 3 feet long. The other end of the vacuum tubing is connected to the suction catheter when needed.

6. Turn on the unit and determine the negative pressure as follows:
   • Pinch closed the long vacuum tubing
   • Turn on the vacuum pump
   • Observe the pressure on the negative-pressure gauge

7. If the unit has a fixed vacuum level, the observed negative pressure should match that listed by the manufacturer.

8. If the unit has a variable vacuum level, adjust the vacuum control knob to the desired level.

b. Central vacuum systems

Central (wall) vacuum systems usually are available at each patient's bedside in all special care units. Each of the wall outlets is connected through a hospital-wide piping system to a large, electrically powered vacuum pump. It is capable of generating a negative pressure far greater than that needed in most patient care situations. A regulator is used to reduce the vacuum to the desired clinical level (Figure 13-14). Either a Quick Connect or a Diameter Index Safety System (DISS) connector is used to attach the regulator to the central vacuum system.

Most regulators have a selector knob that allows the user to turn the vacuum off (OFF setting) or to switch between full vacuum (FULL setting) and a regulated level of vacuum (REG setting). The FULL setting opens the unit to the maximum level of vacuum available from the central pump. The REG setting allows the user to adjust the vacuum level through a wide range.

In general, the following steps are followed to make the units operational:

1. Connect the regulator to a working suction outlet.

2. Screw a clean, empty collection bottle onto its connector on the regulator. The bottle must be able to hold at least 500 mL of fluid.

3. Slip one end of a length of vacuum tubing over the tubing connector on the collection bottle. The vacuum tubing should be no more than 3 feet long. The other end of the vacuum tubing is connected to the suction catheter when needed.

4. Determine the negative pressure as follows:
   • Pinch closed the vacuum tubing (Figure 13-15)
   • Turn the selector knob to REG
   • Observe the pressure on the negative-pressure gauge

5. Adjust the vacuum control knob to the desired level. If the secretions are too thick to be drawn up by the suction catheter, the negative pressure must be increased.

Figure 13-14 Features of the Ohmeda central vacuum regulator with a three-position selector knob. *(Courtesy Ohmeda Medical, Columbia, Md.)*

c. Troubleshoot any problems with the equipment

1. Portable vacuum systems

With a portable vacuum system, check the following when trying to determine the cause of a loss of vacuum:
   • The vacuum pump is plugged into a working electrical outlet.
   • The vacuum pump is turned on.
   • The vacuum control valve is set at the desired negative pressure.
   • The lid to the collection bottle is tightly sealed.
   • The vacuum tubing tightly connects the pump to the collection bottle and the collection bottle to the suction catheter.
   • No knots or obstructions are present in the vacuum tubing or catheter.
   • The collection bottle is not filled above its maximum level.

Correct any potential problems. Do not use a portable vacuum system that will not generate the negative pressure it is supposed to generate.

Figure 13-15 The negative pressure level is set on the Ohmeda central vacuum regulator by pinching the vacuum tubing and adjusting the vacuum control knob. The vacuum pressure is displayed on the pressure gauge. *(Courtesy Ohmeda Medical, Columbia, Md.)*

2. Central vacuum systems

With a central vacuum system, check the following when trying to determine the cause of a loss of vacuum:

- The regulator is plugged into a working vacuum outlet.
- The vacuum control valve is set at the desired negative pressure.
- The collection bottle is tightly screwed onto the suction-regulator outlet.
- The vacuum tubing tightly connects the collection bottle to the suction catheter.
- No knots or obstructions are present in the vacuum tubing or catheter.
- The collection bottle is not filled above its maximum level.

Correct any potential problems. Do not use a central vacuum system outlet that will not generate the negative pressure it should generate. Occasionally, less negative pressure is found than expected when the central vacuum system is being heavily used. No problem exists with the

regulator or tubing, and the vacuum pressure will increase when fewer people are using it.

Exam Hint 13-3 (ELE)

The exam usually includes a question about setting up, adjusting, or fixing suctioning equipment.

MODULE C

Initiate suctioning procedures to remove tracheal and oral secretions

Tracheal or oral secretions must be actively removed by suctioning whenever the patient cannot clear them out and there is a risk of airway obstruction. Suctioning may be needed in patients who are unconscious and lack swallowing or coughing reflexes or in patients who may be too weak to cough effectively to remove tracheal secretions. Often the physician writes a standing order to suction the patient on a regular basis or as needed. However, in many institutions, a protocol exists to suction any patient who is at risk of obstruction of the airway. For example, a comatose patient who vomits should have the mouth suctioned out even if no specific physician's order is written.

Suctioning secretions from a patient's trachea, by any method, places the patient at risk. The following two factors must be understood, identified when they occur, and prevented or corrected.

1. Prevent hypoxemia during the suctioning procedure (ELE code: IIID9) [ELE Difficulty: R, Ap, An]

Suctioning the trachea removes air (including oxygen), as well as secretions, from the lungs. However, hypoxemia can be minimized by hyperoxygenating the patient for 1 to 2 minutes before suctioning. It is generally recommended that the patient receive 100% oxygen, if possible. Infants younger than 6 months should be given a fractional concentration of inspired oxygen (F_1O_2) only 10% to 20% greater than their base level to minimize the risk of retinopathy of prematurity (ROP), also known as *retrolental fibroplasia*.

Before beginning the procedure, check the patient's arterial blood gas results or SpO_2 to see whether the patient is hypoxic. The SpO_2 also can be monitored throughout the suctioning procedure to see how low the saturation drops (review the chapter for guidelines on oxygenation and limiting hypoxemia). After suctioning, give the patient supplemental oxygen until the SpO_2 reaches at least 90%. The patient's chart also should be checked for any history of cardiac problems. Sudden hypoxemia from suctioning can result in life-threatening dysrhythmias, such as premature ventricular contractions (PVCs). Check the patient's pulse rate and rhythm before and after suctioning. If the patient is using a cardiac monitor, it should be watched for rate and rhythm changes that are related to the suctioning procedure. Tachycardia is frequently seen with hypoxemia. Check the blood pressure of any patient who has suctioning-related dysrhythmias. The patient's vital signs should return to normal when oxygenation is restored.

Any modern mechanical ventilator can be set to deliver 100% oxygen. The most current ventilators have a 100% oxygen button designed just for this purpose. Pushing it results in the patient receiving pure oxygen for 1 to 2 minutes (depending on the manufacturer). Several sigh breaths also can be delivered. A closed-airway suction catheter can be used with the ventilator, as discussed earlier, to minimize hypoxemia.

For a spontaneously breathing patient, a nonrebreathing mask can be applied and set to deliver close to 100% oxygen. If a nonrebreathing mask is not available, turn up the oxygen flow or percentage on whatever appliance the patient is using. A spontaneously breathing patient with an endotracheal or tracheostomy tube can have 100% oxygen delivered through a Brigg adapter/aerosol T-piece. A manual resuscitation bag also can be used to give the patient several sigh breaths.

All patients must be reoxygenated before another attempt at suctioning is made. Giving 100% oxygen after the suctioning episode helps the patient to reoxygenate faster. Giving several sigh breaths also helps reoxygenation to occur faster than normal tidal volume breathing does.

a. Vagus or vagal nerve stimulation

Vagal nerve endings are found in the hypopharynx and trachea. When they are mechanically stimulated by a suction catheter, any of the following may be seen:
- The patient may have an induced bronchospasm.
- The patient may become bradycardic.
- The patient's blood pressure may decrease because of the bradycardia.

Listen to the patient's breath sounds before and after suctioning to determine whether an increase in wheezing is present, which shows bronchospasm. Check the heart rate and rhythm by palpation or cardiac monitor to determine whether the patient is becoming bradycardic. The blood pressure also can be measured to check for hypotension.

Further suctioning should be delayed, if possible, until the patient's wheezing and vital signs have returned to normal. It may be necessary to modify the suctioning procedure by not going as deeply and striking the carina, not twisting the catheter, or not suctioning for as long to reduce the risk of vagal stimulation. A local anesthetic, such as lidocaine (Xylocaine), can be nebulized (with a physician's order) to reduce the local reaction to the catheter.

Exam Hint 13-4 (ELE, WRE)

Understand the importance of hyperoxygenating a patient before and after a tracheal suctioning procedure. Hypoxemia can result in unstable vital signs, and vagal stimulation can cause bronchospasm. Be prepared to stop suctioning, give extra oxygen, or get help.

---

2. Perform endotracheal or tracheostomy tube suctioning on the patient (Code: IIIC2) [Difficulty: ELE: R, Ap; WRE: An]

The American Association for Respiratory Care (AARC) Clinical Practice Guidelines listed at the end of the chapter present all the suctioning indications. Key indications include:
- Removing accumulated secretions, blood, or other debris from the breathing tube or the patient's airways
- Obtaining a sputum sample for microbiology or cytology examination
- Stimulating the patient's cough to help mobilize pulmonary secretions
- Clinical indications of retained secretions, such as breath sounds demonstrating rhonchi (crackles), increased tactile fremitus, worsening oxygenation, or worsening mechanical ventilation parameters (e.g., increased peak inspiratory pressure and/or decreased tidal volume)

The procedure for endotracheal or tracheostomy tube suctioning is the same for both types of tubes, except that the catheter does not need to be inserted as far into the tracheostomy tube before hitting the carina. The generally accepted steps in the procedure are as follows:
1. Check the chart for specific orders, an order to suction as needed, or any special patient considerations, such as unstable vital signs, cardiopulmonary conditions, oxygenation, and the types and amounts of secretions.
2. Gather the necessary equipment:
   - Suction catheter no larger than one-half the ID of the patient's endotracheal or tracheostomy tube
   - Two sterile gloves or one sterile glove and one clean glove (this may be skipped if a closed-airway, self-contained system is used)
   - Specimen collector if ordered
   - Vacuum system and vacuum tubing
   - Sterile water or normal saline in a sterile basin
3. Tell the patient what to expect during the procedure.

4. If possible, place the patient in the semi-Fowler and sniff positions.

5. Give the patient 100% O_2 for at least 30 seconds before suctioning and for at least 1 minute afterward until the patient is no longer hypoxemic. (For an infant younger than 6 months, increase the F_1O_2 by 10% to 20%.)

6. Get help if necessary.

7. Wash your hands.

8. Using sterile technique, put on the gloves, get the catheter out of its packaging, and connect the vacuum tubing to the catheter.

9. The AARC Clinical Practice Guidelines suggest that the vacuum be set at the lowest possible level that still effectively removes secretions. The following ranges for vacuum are appropriate:
   - Adults: −100 to −150 mm Hg
   - Children: −100 to −120 mm Hg
   - Infants: −80 to −100 mm Hg
   - Neonates: −60 to −80 mm Hg

   To prevent tissue trauma, hypoxemia, and atelectasis, negative pressures greater than −150 mm Hg should not be used.

10. Test that the vacuum is reaching the tip of the catheter.

11. Disconnect the ventilator circuit or O_2 appliance from the tube (except with a closed-airway suctioning system).

12. Suction the tube:
    (1) Without any vacuum, quickly and gently pass the catheter down the tube until an obstruction is felt. Withdraw the catheter 2 cm.
    (2) In an adult, the entire procedure of disconnection of the O_2, suctioning, reconnection of the O_2, and normal breathing should take no longer than 10 to 15 seconds. In an infant, the entire procedure should take no longer than 10 seconds.
    (3) Withdraw the catheter with a twisting motion while suctioning intermittently. Suction to clear out any secretions. Typically, in an adult, suctioning may be applied for 5 to 10 seconds. In an infant, suctioning may be applied for no longer than 5 seconds.
    (4) Turning the patient's head to the right might help direct the catheter down the left mainstem bronchus. The catheter tends to enter the right mainstem bronchus if the head is in a neutral position or twisted to the left.

13. Reoxygenate the patient for at least 1 minute before suctioning again. Giving 100% O_2 (or 10% to 20% more than the base level in an infant) and several sigh breaths helps accomplish this faster.

14. Monitor the patient's vital signs, O_2 level, and breath sounds before suctioning again. Suction again, if needed, when the patient is stable.

15. Normal saline solution may be instilled into the tube if the secretions are too thick to be suctioned out easily. The saline solution may help to loosen the secretions. The patient also is likely to cough vigorously. The amount of saline solution to be instilled varies with the size of the patient and the thickness of the secretions. The general guidelines for instillation of normal saline solution are as follows:
    - Neonates: A few drops to 0.33 mL at a time
    - Adults: 5 to 10 mL at a time or in divided doses
    - A physician's order may be needed to instill saline solution.

16. Dispose of the catheter and glove by pulling the glove inside out over the catheter. If a self-contained system is part of the ventilator circuit, it would be replace when the circuit is replaced. Current guidelines recommend replacement when obviously soiled or malfunctioning.

17. Rinse water or saline through the vacuum tubing to clear it of secretions.

18. Turn off the suction unit.

Box 13-1 presents the hazards and complications of endotracheal suctioning.

3. Perform nasotracheal suctioning on the patient (Code: IIIC1b) [Difficulty: ELE: R, Ap; WRE: An]

See the AARC Clinical Practice Guidelines listed at the end of the chapter for all of the suctioning indications. Key indications include:
- Removing accumulated secretions, blood, or other debris from the patient's airways
- Obtaining a sputum sample for microbiology or cytology examination

---

BOX 13-1 Hazards and Complications of Endotracheal Suctioning

Cardiac arrest
Respiratory arrest
Hypoxemia
Cardiac dysrhythmias
Bronchospasm
Increased intracranial pressure
Hypertension
Hypotension
Apnea from interruption of mechanical ventilation
Pulmonary hemorrhage
Mechanical trauma to tracheal and bronchial mucosa
Infection of and/or from the patient and respiratory care practitioner
Atelectasis

- Stimulating the patient's cough to help mobilize pulmonary secretions
- Clinical indications of retained secretions, such as breath sounds demonstrating rhonchi (crackles), increased tactile fremitus, or worsening oxygenation

The nasotracheal suctioning (NTS) procedure is performed on a patient who does not have an endotracheal tube or tracheostomy tube. Significant clinical practice is needed to become proficient.

The generally accepted steps in the procedure are as follows:

1. Check the chart for specific orders, an order to suction as needed, or any special patient considerations, such as a deviated nasal septum, unstable vital signs, cardiopulmonary conditions, oxygenation, and type and amount of secretions.
2. Gather the needed equipment:
   - Suction catheter no larger than one-half the diameter of the patient's nostril
   - Appropriate size and type of nasopharyngeal airway to minimize nasal mucosal damage (see Chapter 12 for information on nasopharyngeal airways and their insertion)
   - Sterile, water-soluble lubricant jelly
   - Sterile 4 × 4-inch gauze pad
   - Two sterile gloves or one sterile glove and one clean glove
   - Specimen collector if ordered
   - Vacuum system and vacuum tubing
   - Sterile water or normal saline in a sterile basin
3. Prepare the patient for the procedure:
   - Tell the patient what to expect during the procedure.
   - Put lubricating jelly on the nasopharyngeal airway and insert it into the selected nostril.
   - If possible, place the patient in the semi-Fowler and sniff positions.
4. Give the patient 100% O_2 for at least 30 seconds before suctioning and for at least 1 minute afterward until the patient is no longer hypoxemic. (For an infant younger than 6 months, increase the FiO_2 by 10% to 20%.)
5. Get help if necessary.
6. Wash your hands. (This may be skipped in an emergency.)
7. Using sterile technique, put on the gloves, get the catheter out of its packaging, apply lubricant jelly to the catheter tip, and connect the vacuum tubing to the catheter.
8. The AARC Clinical Practice Guidelines suggest that the vacuum be set at the lowest possible level that still effectively removes secretions. The following ranges for vacuum are appropriate:
   - Adults: −100 to −150 mm Hg
   - Children: −100 to −120 mm Hg

- Infants: −80 to −100 mm Hg
- Neonates: −60 to −80 mm Hg

To prevent tissue trauma, hypoxemia, and atelectasis, negative pressures greater than −150 mm Hg should not be used.

9. Test that the vacuum is reaching the tip of the catheter.
10. If the patient is wearing an O_2 appliance, remove it so that the nose can be reached. If supplemental oxygen was being used, directing the end of the O_2 tubing or nasal cannula prongs toward the patient's mouth may help to prevent hypoxemia.
11. Suction the trachea:
    (1) Without any vacuum, advance the catheter into the nasopharyngeal airway. If no nasopharyngeal airway is available, without any vacuum, advance the catheter into the most open nasal passage. The catheter should be advanced parallel to the turbinates to minimize tissue trauma. Never force the catheter. (The most patent nasal passage can be determined by checking the chart for a history of deviated septum, asking the patient if one side feels more open, or feeling which nostril has more airflow through it.)
    (2) Have a cooperative patient stick out the tongue. With an uncooperative patient, the practitioner or assistant can grasp the tongue with a 4 × 4-inch gauze pad or gloved hand.
    (3) Advance the catheter as the patient inspires. The epiglottis and vocal cords are open at this time, and it is easiest to slip the catheter into the trachea. A cooperative patient should be told to inhale slowly and deeply. Some practitioners find it helpful to disconnect the catheter from the vacuum tubing and listen to the end of the catheter for the sound of air movement. The patient will cough vigorously when the catheter is in the trachea (Figure 13-16).
    (4) Advance the catheter until an obstruction is felt. Then pull the catheter back about 2 cm.
    (5) Withdraw the catheter with a twisting motion while suctioning intermittently. Suction to clear out any secretions. Typically, in an adult, suctioning may be applied for 5 to 10 seconds. Suctioning in an infant should be applied for no longer than 5 seconds. If the secretions are cleared, the catheter is pulled out. Practitioners disagree on whether the catheter should be withdrawn or left in place if the patient still has secretions. Some prefer to withdraw the catheter, let the patient rest and reoxygenate, and reinsert the catheter for more suctioning. Others prefer to leave the catheter in place to minimize tissue trauma from a reinsertion, let the patient rest and reoxygenate, and then suction again.

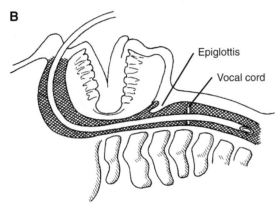

Figure 13-16   Cross section through the airway showing nasotracheal suctioning. **A,** The patient's head may be kept in a neutral position as the catheter is advanced through a nostril to the back of the throat. **B,** The patient's head is carefully moved to the sniff position. During inspiration, the catheter is advanced into the trachea. The patient will cough, and secretions can be suctioned out.

BOX 13-2   Contraindications, Hazards, and Complications of Nasotracheal Suctioning

CONTRAINDICATIONS

Absolute

Epiglottitis

Laryngotracheobronchitis (croup)

Relative

Blocked nasal passages

Nasal bleeding

Acute facial, neck, or head injury

Bleeding disorder

Upper respiratory tract infection

Irritable airway

Laryngospasm

HAZARDS AND COMPLICATIONS

Cardiac arrest

Respiratory arrest

Hypoxemia

Cardiac dysrhythmias

Bronchospasm

Increased intracranial pressure

Hypertension

Hypotension

Pulmonary hemorrhage

Infection of and/or from patient and respiratory therapist

Atelectasis

Pain

Catheter misdirected into esophagus

Gagging and/or vomiting

Uncontrolled coughing

Mechanical trauma (nasal turbinates, perforation of pharynx, nasal bleeding, bleeding of the tracheal and bronchial mucosa)

---

(6) The entire procedure usually takes longer than 20 seconds, therefore the O_2 tubing must be kept directed toward the patient's mouth.

(7) Turning the patient's head to the right may help direct the catheter down the left mainstem bronchus. The catheter will tend to enter the right mainstem bronchus if the head is in a neutral position or twisted to the left.

12. Reoxygenate the patient for at least 1 minute before suctioning again. Giving 100% O_2 (or 10% to 20% more than the base level in an infant) helps accomplish this faster.

13. Monitor the patient's vital signs, O_2 level, and breath sounds before suctioning again. Suction again, if needed, when the patient is stable.

14. Normal saline solution may be instilled down the suction catheter by pulling off the vacuum tubing, inserting the tip of the syringe (not needle) into the end of the catheter, covering the thumb control valve, and squirting the saline solution into the catheter. The other considerations listed earlier would apply here.

15. Dispose of the catheter and glove by pulling the gloves inside out over the catheter.

16. Rinse water or saline through the vacuum tubing to clear it of secretions.

17. Turn off the suction unit.

Box 13-2 presents the contraindications, hazards, and complications of nasotracheal suctioning.

4. Perform oropharyngeal suctioning on the patient (Code: IIIC1c) [Difficulty: ELE: R, Ap; WRE: An]

If a patient is unable to swallow saliva or food properly or has vomitus in the mouth, it must be removed. Signs of improper swallowing may include drooling, gagging, retching, and coughing. Oropharyngeal suctioning is performed on intubated and unintubated patients. In many institutions, the suctioning device may be used more than once.

The generally accepted steps for oropharyngeal suctioning of an unintubated patient are as follows:

1. Check the chart for specific orders, an order to suction as needed, or any special patient considerations.
2. Gather the needed equipment:
   - Yankauer or regular suction catheter
   - Two clean gloves
   - Vacuum system
   - Water or normal saline solution in a basin
3. Tell the patient what to expect during the procedure.
4. If possible, place the patient in the semi-Fowler and sniff positions.
5. If the patient is not using supplemental oxygen, it is probably not necessary to give it. Keep a nasal cannula in place during the procedure. Remove an oxygen mask only long enough to perform the suctioning procedure and then replace the mask.
6. Get help if necessary.
7. Wash your hands. (This may be skipped in an emergency.)
8. Using clean technique, put on the gloves, get the catheter out of its packaging, and connect the vacuum tubing to the catheter.
9. The AARC Clinical Practice Guidelines suggest that the vacuum be set at the lowest possible level that still effectively removes secretions. The following ranges for vacuum are appropriate:
   - Adults: −100 to −150 mm Hg
   - Children: −100 to −120 mm Hg
   - Infants: −80 to −100 mm Hg
   - Neonates: −60 to −80 mm Hg

   To prevent tissue trauma, hypoxemia, and atelectasis, negative pressures greater than −150 mm Hg should not be used.
10. Test that the vacuum is reaching the tip of the suctioning device.
11. If the patient is wearing an O_2 mask, it must be removed so that the mouth may be reached. If necessary, an assistant may be able to direct the end of the O_2 tubing toward the patient's mouth to help prevent hypoxemia.
12. Suction the oropharynx:
    (1) Gently insert the Yankauer or catheter along one side of the mouth between the cheek and tongue and advance it toward the throat. Apply vacuum to remove any secretions, vomitus, or food. Repeat the procedure on the other side of the mouth.
    (2) A spontaneously breathing patient should be able to tolerate several seconds of suctioning.
    (3) Try to avoid stimulating the patient's gag reflex by not striking the oropharynx. Retching,

gagging, and vomiting can result from a stimulated gag reflex. An unintubated patient would be at risk of aspirating vomitus.
    (4) After suctioning, allow the patient to recover. Replace the oxygen mask if it was removed.
    (5) Monitor the patient's vital signs and oxygenation.
    (6) Open the patient's mouth and look for additional secretions that need to be removed.
    (7) If necessary, repeat the oral suctioning procedure and re-evaluate the patient.
13. Pull the gloves inside out over each other and dispose of them.
14. Suction some water or saline through the device and vacuum tubing to rinse the secretions clear.
15. Turn off the suction unit.

MODULE D
Respiratory care plan

1. Analyze available information to determine the patient's pathophysiologic state (Code: IIIH1) [Difficulty: ELE: R, Ap; WRE: An]

Coarse, intermittent expiratory sounds (crackles, or rhonchi) indicate that secretions are in the airway. Tracheal suctioning should clear these secretions and result in the return of normal breath sounds (or at least an improvement). Pneumonia and bronchitis result in chest radiograph changes that show areas of infiltrate. Disease involvement of the right or left lung (or both), individual lobes, and segments can be determined. As the patient's condition improves, the chest radiograph should show clearing of infiltrates.

2. Determine the appropriateness of the prescribed therapy and goals for the identified pathophysiologic state (Code: IIIH3) [Difficulty: ELE: R, Ap; WRE: An]

The standard physician's order for suctioning states that suctioning should be done as needed (PRN). The respiratory therapist or the nurse, or both, should be able to evaluate the patient and perform suctioning when it is justified. The physician should not suction the patient on a set schedule (e.g., every hour). This could result in the patient being suctioned when it is not needed. Also, the therapist and nurse could not suction the patient more often. The respiratory care plan should allow the therapist to make the following changes.

a. Make a change in the size and type of suction catheter (ELE code: IIIF2h2) [ELE Difficulty: R, Ap, An]

As discussed earlier, the OD of the suction catheter should be no more than one-half the ID of the patient's endotracheal tube. If the secretions are easy to suction out, a smaller catheter may be used. A spontaneously breathing patient is less likely to become hypoxic if the tube is less obstructed.

A catheter with a Coudé tip should be used if the catheter must be directed into one or the other mainstem bronchus (usually the left). Closed-airway catheters, such as those made by Ballard Medical Products, offer two advantages over single-use catheters. First, they are more economical if the patient needs frequent suctioning. Second, a patient using a mechanical ventilator continues to be ventilated and oxygenated and to have PEEP maintained during the suctioning episode. The newer catheters that offer intermittent or continuous insufflation of oxygen may reduce the hypoxemia that many patients experience during the suctioning procedure. However, they can be difficult to use and costly.

b. Change the level of vacuum used when suctioning (ELE code: IIIF2h3) [ELE Difficulty: R, Ap, An]

In general, the lowest possible vacuum level should be used that adequately removes secretions. The AARC Clinical Practice Guidelines on suctioning list appropriate negative pressure ranges for patients based on their age. These are listed in the suctioning procedures given earlier. Be prepared to reduce the suctioning pressure if the patient's secretions are watery and easy to remove. Conversely, be prepared to increase the suctioning pressure if the patient's secretions are thick and difficult to remove.

c. Instill an irrigating solution into the trachea (ELE code: IIIF2h4) [ELE Difficulty: R, Ap, An]

Sterile normal saline solution (0.9%) is widely accepted as useful for instilling into the trachea to dilute and mobilize pulmonary secretions. It should be used whenever secretions are difficult to suction out. Because the secretions are easier to remove, the respiratory therapist also can use a lower vacuum level. In adults, about 5 to 10 mL is instilled into the trachea and then suctioned out with any secretions. Less is used with children, but no universal guidelines are available. Neonates reportedly have been given amounts ranging from a few drops to 0.33 mL.

d. Change the frequency of suctioning (ELE code: IIIF2h1) [ELE Difficulty: R, Ap, An]

Secretions obstruct the airways and should be removed if possible. Often this requires more than one suctioning episode. The patient is unlikely to be harmed with repeated suctioning as long as proper technique is followed and the patient is reoxygenated between sessions. Watch for any of the complications listed in Boxes 13-1 and 13-2. Listen to the patient's breath sounds for crackles (rhonchi) or palpate the chest for secretions (tactile fremitus) between suctioning efforts. Stop suctioning when it is no longer needed.

e. Change the duration of suctioning (ELE code: IIIF2h1) [ELE Difficulty: R, Ap, An]

The entire procedure should take 10 to 15 seconds. Actual suctioning generally takes 5 to 10 seconds. However, some patients may not be able to tolerate it this long because of hypoxemia or unstable vital signs. Be prepared to suction for a shorter period. It is safer to suction repeatedly than to increase the suctioning time.

f. Terminate the procedure based on the patient's response (Code: IIIF1) [Difficulty: ELE: R, Ap; WRE: An]

Stop the procedure if the patient becomes hypoxic or has tachycardia, bradycardia, arrhythmias, hypotension, bronchospasm, or any of the other hazards or complications listed in Boxes 13-1 and 13-2. Bloody secretions indicate possible mucosal damage and justify stopping the procedure. Hypoxemia can cause unstable vital signs, and vagal stimulation can cause bradycardia and bronchospasm. Be prepared to stop suctioning, give extra oxygen, or get help.

Conscious patients should be able to report how they feel after the suctioning of secretions. Hopefully, a patient's feeling of dyspnea will have improved. Inform the patient's nurse or physician and the supervising therapist if the patient has any serious questions or problems. Routine communication should occur as needed between these people and any other caregiver.

g. Recommend discontinuation of the procedure based on the patient's response (Code: IIIG1i) [Difficulty: ELE: R, Ap; WRE: An]

When hypoxemia, tachycardia, bradycardia, arrhythmias, hypotension, bronchospasm, pneumothorax, or pulmonary hemorrhage occur during endotracheal suctioning, the patient's life is in danger. If any of these problems arise repeatedly, cancellation of the suctioning order is justified. Once the underlying problem has been corrected and safe suctioning can be performed, the order may be reinstated.

Suctioning should be discontinued when the patient has recovered to the point where it is no longer needed. Either the patient's secretions have decreased in volume, or the patient now is able to cough them out.

Exam Hint 13-5 (ELE)

Be prepared to adjust the suctioning equipment as needed for the secretions or to adjust the procedure based on the patient's reaction to it.

MODULE E

Record in conventional terminology any procedure(s) performed, including the date, time, frequency of therapy, medication, and ventilatory data

1. Record and evaluate the patient's response to the procedure or procedures.

a. Record and interpret the following: heart rate and rhythm, respiratory rate, blood pressure, body temperature, and pain level (Code: IIIA1b4) [Difficulty: ELE: R, Ap; WRE: An]

See the discussion on these topics in Chapter 1 or earlier in this chapter.

b. Record and interpret the patient's breath sounds (Code: IIIAb3) [Difficulty: ELE: R, Ap; WRE: An]

If suctioning is effective, the patient's breath sounds will improve. The crackles (rhonchi) that were heard before suctioning should now be absent. Normal breath sounds should be heard.

c. Record and interpret the type of cough the patient has and the nature of the sputum (Code: IIIAb3) [Difficulty: ELE: R, Ap; WRE: An]

The amount and consistency of sputum a patient produces depends on the lung problem and whether it is worsening or improving. For example, if pneumonia or bronchitis is worsening, secretion production is increased. If the patient is dehydrated, the sputum contains less water than normal. The patient may complain that the secretions are thicker and harder to cough out. Airway suction may be needed to remove the secretions. As the patient's condition improves, a return to normal sputum consistency should occur, and less should be produced. The patient should be able to cough it out effectively.

BIBLIOGRAPHY

American Association for Respiratory Care (AARC) Clinical Practice Guideline: Endotracheal suctioning of mechanically ventilated adults and children with artificial airways, *Respir Care* 38:500, 1993.

American Association for Respiratory Care (AARC) Clinical Practice Guideline: Nasotracheal suctioning: 2004 revision and update, *Respir Care* 49:1080, 2004.

American Association for Respiratory Care (AARC) Clinical Practice Guideline: Nasotracheal suctioning, *Respir Care* 37:898, 1992.

American Association for Respiratory Care (AARC) Clinical Practice Guideline: Suctioning of the patient in the home, *Respir Care* 44:99, 1999.

American Association for Respiratory Therapy: Guidelines for the prevention of nosocomial infections, *AAR Times* 7(9):49-52, 1983.

Burton GG: Patient assessment procedures. In Barnes TA, editor: *Respiratory care practice*, St Louis, 1998, Mosby.

Cairo JM, Pilbeam SP, editors: *Mosby's respiratory care equipment*, ed 8, St Louis, 2009, Mosby.

Caldwell SL, Sullivan KN: Suctioning protocol. In Burton GG, Hodgkin JE, editors: *Respiratory care*, ed 2, Philadelphia, 1984, Lippincott.

Durbin CG: Airway management. In Cairo JM, Pilbeam SP, editors: *Mosby's respiratory care equipment*, ed 7, St Louis, 2004, Mosby.

Eubanks DH, Bone RC: *Comprehensive respiratory care*, ed 2, St Louis, 1990, Mosby.

Fink JB, Hess DR: Secretion clearance techniques. In Hess DR, MacIntyre NR, Mishoe SC, et al, editors: Respiratory care principles and practice, Philadelphia, 2002, WB Saunders.

Hess DR, Branson RD: Airway and suctioning equipment. In Branson RD, Hess DR, Chatburn RL, editors: *Respiratory care equipment*, ed 2, Philadelphia, 1999, Lippincott Williams & Wilkins.

Lewis RM: Airway care. In Fink JB, Hunt GE, editors: *Clinical practice in respiratory care*, Philadelphia, 1999, Lippincott Williams & Wilkins.

May RA, Bortner PL: Airway management. In Hess DR, MacIntyre NR, et al, editors: *Respiratory care: principles and practice*, Philadelphia, 2002, WB Saunders.

McIntyre D: Airway management. In Wyka KA, Mathews PJ, Clark WF: *Foundations of respiratory care*, Albany, NY, 2002, Delmar.

Pettignano MM, Pettignano R: Airway management. In Barnhart SL, Czervinske MP, editors: *Perinatal and pediatric respiratory care*, Philadelphia, 1995, WB Saunders.

Plevak DJ, Ward JJ: Airway management. In Burton GG, Hodgkin JE, Ward JJ, editors: *Respiratory care*, ed 4, Philadelphia, 1997, Lippincott-Raven.

Rarey KP, Youtsey JW: *Respiratory patient care*, Englewood Cliffs, NJ, 1981, Prentice-Hall.

Roth P: Airway care. In Aloan CA, Hill TV, editors: *Respiratory care of the newborn and child*, ed 2, Philadelphia, 1997, Lippincott.

Scott AA, Koff PB: Airway care and chest physiotherapy. In Koff PB, Eitzmann DV, Neu J, editors: *Neonatal and pediatric respiratory care*, ed 2, St Louis, 1993, Mosby.

Shapiro BA, Kacmarek RM, Cane RD, et al: *Clinical application of respiratory care*, ed 4, St Louis, 1991, Mosby.

Simmons KF, Scanlan CL: Airway management. In Wilkins RL, Stoller JK, Kacmarek RM, editors: *Egan's fundamentals of respiratory care*, ed 9, St Louis, 2009, Mosby.

White GC: *Equipment theory for respiratory care*, ed 4, Clifton Park, NY, 2005, Thomson Delmar Learning.

Wilkins RL, Stoller JK, Kacmarek RM, editors: *Egan's fundamentals of respiratory care*, ed 9, St Louis, 2009, Mosby.

Wilkins RL, Specht L: Fundamentals of physical examination. In Wilkins RL, Krider SJ, Krider SJ, editors: *Clinical assessment in respiratory care*, ed 5, St Louis, 2005, Mosby.

Wilkins RL, Hodgkin JE, Lopez B: *Lung sounds: a practical guide*, St Louis, 1988, Mosby.

Wojciechowski WV: Incentive spirometers and secretion evacuation devices and inspiratory muscle training devices. In Barnes TA, editor: *Core textbook of respiratory care practice*, ed 2, St Louis, 1994, Mosby.

1. All of the following statements about the use of a Lukens trap are true EXCEPT:
   A. A vacuum source is needed.
   B. All connections must be tight for it to work properly.
   C. Either a suction catheter or a bronchoscope is also needed.
   D. It is used to collect a sputum sample from a patient with a strong, productive cough.

2. Your patient is being mechanically ventilated with 60% oxygen and 8 cm H_2O of PEEP. Twice her SpO_2 and blood pressure have decreased when she was removed from the ventilator for suctioning. What should be recommended to prevent this from happening again?
   A. Switch to a smaller suction catheter
   B. Switch to a larger suction catheter
   C. Increase the PEEP to 10 cm H_2O before and after suctioning
   D. Use a closed-system suction catheter

3. The proper-size suction catheter should be no larger than what fraction of the endotracheal tube's ID?
   A. $^1/_4$
   B. $^1/_2$
   C. $^2/_3$
   D. $^3/_4$

4. Removing the tracheal secretions from your adult patient is difficult when you use −60 mm Hg of vacuum pressure. What should you do?
   A. Suction for 20 seconds
   B. Suction more frequently
   C. Increase the vacuum pressure to −80 mm Hg
   D. Change from the central vacuum system to a portable one

5. If your patient has a room air arterial O_2 pressure of 65 mm Hg, the most important step to take to prevent hypoxemia during suctioning is to
   A. Give the patient 100% O_2 before and after the procedure
   B. Use a large catheter to remove the secretions quickly
   C. Hyperextend the patient's neck and head
   D. Use a small catheter so that the patient can breathe around it

6. The best positions in which to place a patient before nasotracheal suctioning are
   1. Supine
   2. Trendelenburg's position
   3. Sniff position (neck and head hyperextended)
   4. Semi-Fowler position
   A. 1, 4
   B. 1, 3

C. 2, 3
D. 3, 4

7. Making sure a central vacuum system is working properly includes all of the following steps EXCEPT:
   A. Setting the vacuum control to FULL
   B. Screwing a 500-mL collection bottle tightly onto the vacuum connector
   C. Attaching 3 feet of vacuum tubing to the tubing connector on the collection jar
   D. Pinching closed the vacuum tubing when the vacuum is turned on to measure the vacuum level

8. Your 40-year-old patient has pneumonia in her left lower lobe with a large amount of secretions. What would you recommend to be able to suction her better?
   A. Use the largest diameter suction catheter available
   B. Use a suction catheter with a Coudé tip
   C. Use the longest suction catheter available
   D. Suction for a longer period

9. You notice that a Yankauer suction catheter you are using is cracked. The best thing to do is
   A. Continue to use it
   B. Tape over the crack
   C. Put lubricating jelly in the crack to seal it
   D. Replace the catheter

10. You are preparing to suction a patient for a mucus sample when you notice that the vacuum is not reaching the end of the catheter. All of the following are possible causes of this problem EXCEPT:
    A. The vacuum is not turned on to the proper level.
    B. The vacuum tubing, specimen collector, and catheter system are connected so that they are airtight.
    C. The catheter is plugged with foreign matter.
    D. The specimen jar is not screwed tightly into the special lid.

11. Your patient is receiving mechanical ventilation through an 8-mm oral endotracheal tube. Over the course of the shift, the patient is seen to have more tracheal secretions. What is the best course of action?
    A. Suction more often
    B. Suction for longer periods
    C. Change to a closed-airway suction catheter
    D. Administer nebulized atropine

12. You are suctioning your patient when the vacuum is lost. You should do all of the following EXCEPT:
    A. Make sure the vacuum system is working
    B. Make sure a tight connection exists between the suction catheter and the vacuum tubing

C. Check the catheter to make sure it is not obstructed

D. Get a larger suction catheter

13. A ventilator-dependent patient required a vacuum pressure of −120 mm Hg to remove her thick secretions. After treatment with a mucolytic drug, her secretions are much easier to remove. What would you recommend?

A. Reduce the vacuum pressure to −100 mm Hg and monitor the ease of secretion removal

B. Maintain the present vacuum level and suction less often

C. Increase the vacuum pressure to −140 mm Hg and suction less often

D. Reduce the vacuum pressure to −60 mm Hg and suction more often

14. A conscious patient requires nasotracheal suctioning. During the procedure, the patient's blood pressure decreases to 100/60 mm Hg, and the heart rate decreases from 110 to 60 beats/min. What should be done?

A. Change to a catheter with a larger diameter

B. Shorten the suctioning time

C. Insert an oropharyngeal airway before suctioning

D. Squirt 5 mL of saline down the suction catheter into the patient's trachea

15. The respiratory therapist is called to set up a suctioning system for a new patient in the intensive care unit. To measure the vacuum pressure, what should be done?

A. Check the manometer while occluding the catheter tip

B. Set the vacuum control to maximum.

C. Close the thumb control valve on the catheter

D. Check the manometer while pinching off the connecting tubing

16. An intubated patient has pneumonia, and a sputum sample must be sent to the laboratory for culture and sensitivity testing. What is the most appropriate way to obtain a sample?

A. Place a Lukens trap between the suction catheter and the vacuum tubing

B. Suction the oropharynx with a sterile Yankauer suction catheter

C. Place a Lukens trap between the vacuum tubing and the collection bottle.

D. Suction the patient and place the catheter inside the Lukens trap

SELF-STUDY QUESTIONS FOR THE WRITTEN REGISTRY EXAM

See page 621 for answers

1. Before a patient with an intubated airway is suctioned for the first time, the chart must be checked for
   1. A history of cardiac disease or arrhythmia
   2. A written order
   3. A history of a strong gag reflex
   4. Blood gas or SpO_2 results
   5. A history of asthma or bronchospasm
   A. 2, 3
   B. 4, 5
   C. 1, 2, 4, 5
   D. 3, 4

2. Placing a suction catheter into your patient's trachea and applying vacuum pressure cause
   1. Transient hypoxemia
   2. Removal of secretions
   3. Stopping of the hypoxic drive because of vagal stimulation
   4. Removal of air from the lungs
   A. 3, 4
   B. 3
   C. 2, 4
   D. 1, 2, 4

3. When a catheter OD is selected for suctioning through a fenestrated tracheostomy tube, it is important that the OD be

A. No more than one fourth the ID of the tube

B. No less than one half the ID of the tube

C. No less than three fourths the ID of the tube

D. No more than one half the ID of the tube

4. During nasotracheal suctioning, it is important to
   A. Lubricate the catheter with sterile water
   B. Lubricate the catheter tip with a sterile, water-soluble lubricant jelly
   C. Place the catheter in the refrigerator to make it firmer and easier to pass
   D. Lubricate the catheter with a sterile, normal saline solution

5. While connecting the suction catheter to the vacuum tubing, you accidentally touch the tip of the catheter with your clean-gloved hand. You would proceed to
   A. Discard the clean glove and start over
   B. Suction the patient
   C. Put a sterile glove over the clean glove and suction the patient
   D. Discard the catheter and start over

6. A 17-year-old patient with an oral endotracheal tube has just had open-airway suctioning performed. The respiratory therapist notes that bright red blood is removed, along with some clear secretions. What should be done?

    A. Stop the suctioning procedure and monitor the patient

    B. Change to a closed-airway suctioning system

    C. Instill 5 mL of normal saline and suction again to remove the saline and blood

    D. Change to a nasal endotracheal tube and suction normally

7. A 67-year-old woman who suffered a stroke is having difficulty swallowing her oral secretions. An order is written to perform oropharyngeal suctioning. Are any risks or hazards associated with this procedure?

    A. Bradycardia from vagal stimulation

    B. Gagging

    C. Hypoxemia if preoxygenation is not performed

    D. Tachycardia from adrenergic stimulation

8. A 16-year-old young woman is receiving mechanical ventilation via a 7-mm endotracheal tube. After she is suctioned with a 14 Fr catheter, the electrocardiograph monitor shows that she is bradycardic. What should be recommended?

    A. Administer 10 cm H_2O PEEP

    B. Limit suctioning to twice a shift

    C. Change to a 10 Fr catheter

    D. Use a catheter with a Coudé tip

9. An adult patient receiving mechanical ventilation with 80% oxygen and 10 cm H_2O PEEP experiences hypoxemia, tachycardia, and hypotension every time open-airway suctioning is performed. What should the respiratory therapist recommend to the physician?

    A. Increase the PEEP level to 15 cm H_2O before suctioning

    B. Reduce the duration of suctioning but do it more often

    C. Discontinue suctioning until a closed-airway suctioning system can be set up

    D. Turn up the oxygen level to 100% before the patient is suctioned

10. A 47-year-old woman with COPD and pneumonia has copious amounts of thick secretions. Nasotracheal suctioning is being initiated because of her weak, ineffective cough. What is the maximum suctioning pressure that may be used?

    A. −80 mm Hg

    B. −100 mm Hg

    C. −120 mm Hg

    D. −150 mm Hg

14 Intermittent Positive-Pressure Breathing

Note 1: This book is written to cover every item listed as testable on the *Entry Level Examination (ELE), Written Registry Examination (WRE),* and *Clinical Simulation Examination (CSE).*

The listed code for each item is taken from the National Board for Respiratory Care's (NBRC) **Summary Content Outline for CRT (Certified Respiratory Therapist) and Written RRT (Registered Respiratory Therapist) Examinations** (http://evolve.elsevier.com/Sills/resptherapist/). For example, if an item is testable on both the ELE and the WRE, it will simply be shown as: (Code: . . .). If an item is only testable on the ELE, it will be shown as: (ELE code: . . .). If an item is only testable on the WRE, it will be shown as: (WRE code: . . .).

Following each item's code will be the difficulty level of the questions on that item on the ELE and WRE. (See the Introduction for a full explanation of the three question difficulty levels.) **Recall [R]** level questions typically expect the exam taker to recall factual information. **Application [Ap]** level questions are harder because the exam taker may have to apply factual information to a clinical situation. **Analysis [An]** level questions are the most challenging because the exam taker may have to use critical thinking to evaluate patient data to make a clinical decision.

Note 2: A review of the most recent Entry Level Examinations (ELE) has shown an average of 3 questions (out of 140), or 2% of the exam, that cover intermittent positive-pressure breathing (IPPB). A review of the most recent Written Registry Examinations (WRE) has shown an average of 2 questions (out of 100), or 2% of the exam, that cover IPPB. The Clinical Simulation Examination is comprehensive and may include everything that should be known by an advanced level respiratory therapist.

MODULE A

Initiate and adjust intermittent positive-pressure breathing (IPPB) therapy to achieve adequate respiratory support (Code: IIID2a) [Difficulty: ELE: R, Ap; WRE: An]

1. Description

The Respiratory Care Committee of the American Thoracic Society published the following definition in its 1980 *Guidelines for the Use of Intermittent Positive Pressure Breathing (IPPB):* "'IPPB treatments' refers to the use of a pressure-limited respirator to deliver a gas with humidity and/or aerosol to a spontaneously breathing patient for periods of time that are generally no greater than 15 to 20 minutes each."

A pressure-limited respirator may be powered by compressed gas or electricity. The patient's tidal volume (V_T) should be greater than normal when enhanced by IPPB. This greater-than-normal V_T is caused by the use of positive pressure against the lungs. Pressure is also directed against the airways and, through contact with the airways and lungs, the entire chest. The patient's exhalation is usually passive but can be slowed through modification of the exhalation valve.

Shapiro and associates (1991) list the following as the physiologic effects of IPPB:

a. Increased mean airway pressure

By definition of IPPB, the patient is receiving a positive airway pressure instead of generating a negative intrathoracic pressure to create the V_T. Most authors recommend that patients with heart disease be monitored closely for the effects of increased mean airway pressure. Decreasing the normal return of venous blood to the heart, thereby decreasing the cardiac output, is possible. Shapiro and associates (1991) recommend an expiratory time that is long enough to allow for normal venous return before the next positive-pressure breath is given. The patient's heart rate and blood pressure can be monitored to ensure that they stay in the normal range.

Pulmonary barotrauma is the second concern raised by the use of positive airway pressure. It is possible for patients with small airways disease to trap air in the alveoli. This can lead to the rupture of a bleb, thus causing a pneumothorax. Care must be taken with the patient with bullous emphysema to ensure that the V_T is exhaled completely.

b. Increased tidal volume

The primary goal of IPPB is to increase the patient's assisted V_T to greater than the spontaneous V_T. Indeed, if the spontaneous V_T is greater than the assisted V_T, IPPB is not needed for lung expansion.

c. Decreased work of breathing

A properly coached passive treatment with the controls set to meet the patient's inspiratory needs causes a decrease in the work of breathing (WOB). This necessitates considerable skill on the part of the practitioner. Sensitivity, inspiratory flow, and peak pressure must be frequently adjusted to minimize the patient's work. The patient must be asked if the control adjustments make it easier or harder to inhale. Failure to tailor the breathing treatment to the patient's needs may actually increase the WOB.

d. Alteration of the inspiratory/expiratory ratio

Patients with high airway resistance or low lung compliance often change their breathing patterns to reduce the WOB (see Chapter 1). These new breathing patterns may lead to worsening of the patient's condition. Alteration of normal ventilation and perfusion ratios in the lungs may worsen hypoxemia. Properly administered and coached IPPB can be used to adjust the inspiratory/expiratory (I:E) ratio to the benefit of the patient. The patient can be taught how to breathe in a more physiologically normal pattern.

2. Indications

The following indications and guidelines are listed in the American Association for Respiratory Care (AARC) *Clinical Practice Guidelines* (1991, 2003) on IPPB:

a. To treat atelectasis when other deep breathing methods are ineffective

Patients who are uncooperative, unconscious, or physically incapable of being coached in deep-breathing and coughing techniques or in performing incentive spirometry (IS) may be helped by IPPB. An inspiratory pause at the end of the IPPB breath helps to better distribute the gas to open areas of atelectasis. As has been discussed in Chapter 7, a patient would benefit from IPPB rather than IS if any of the following apply:

- Inspiratory capacity (IC) of less than 12 mL/kg
- Vital capacity (VC) of less than 15 mL/kg
- Postoperative IC less than 33% of the predicted value (predicted IC = $\frac{1}{3}$ [i.e., 0.33] × 50 mL/kg of ideal body weight)

The AARC guidelines on IPPB list the following poor pulmonary function values as supporting the need for IPPB because the patient would have an ineffective cough:

- Vital capacity (VC) less than 70% of predicted or less than 10 mL/kg
- Forced expiratory volume in 1 second (FEV_1) less than 65% of predicted
- Maximum voluntary ventilation (MVV) less than 50% of predicted

---

Exam Hint 14-1 (ELE)

It is important to understand the indications of IPPB versus incentive spirometry (IS) in the treatment of a patient with atelectasis. In general, IPPB would be indicated in a patient who could not properly perform IS.

---

b. To more effectively deliver aerosolized medications

If the patient cannot coordinate his or her breathing pattern to make use of a metered dose inhaler or handheld nebulizer, IPPB may be used. Examples of when IPPB is preferable include any situation in which the patient is unconscious, uncooperative, or physically incapable. These patients are physically unable to make effective use of simpler methods of lung inflation (incentive spirometry) or to take an aerosolized medication (metered dose inhaler or handheld nebulizer). Examples of these types of patients include the elderly, the chronically debilitated, patients with neuromuscular diseases, and patients with kyphoscoliosis. It may also be used to provide temporary support to home care patients.

c. To enhance the patient's cough effort and sputum clearance

The combination of aerosolized saline, with or without a bronchodilator or mucolytic, and deeper tidal volumes may help the patient to cough more productively. The practitioner must stop the treatment periodically to coach the patient's cough effort.

The following additional indications were listed in the *Guidelines for the Use of Intermittent Positive Pressure Breathing (IPPB)* published by the Respiratory Care Committee of the American Thoracic Society (1980).

d. To treat impending ventilatory failure as seen by an increased arterial carbon dioxide partial pressure ($PaCO_2$)

It may be possible to delay or avoid intubation and mechanical ventilation in the deteriorating chronic obstructive pulmonary disease (COPD) patient. The patient is able to relax and reduce the work of breathing (WOB) during a passive IPPB treatment. It may be necessary to give IPPB for 5 to 10 minutes as often as every 30 minutes to 1 hour. The treatment should also be given with the intention of helping the patient's cough and sputum clearance. (An alternative to frequent IPPB treatments is noninvasive positive-pressure ventilation. This is discussed in Chapter 15.)

e. To help manage the patient with acute pulmonary edema

IPPB can help in the management of this patient by temporarily increasing mean airway pressure. This reduces the venous return to the heart, which may reduce pulmonary edema. The IPPB procedure does not correct the underlying cardiac problem, which must be treated by other means.

f. To induce a sputum sample for culture and sensitivity or other diagnostic studies

Inducing a sputum sample by IPPB is indicated only if simpler methods have failed.

g. To deliver medications for special purposes when simpler methods are ineffective

IPPB should be used to deliver medication when simpler methods fail, for example, to deliver a local anesthetic such as lidocaine (Xylocaine) before a bronchoscopy procedure.

3. Contraindications

a. An untreated pneumothorax is listed by all authors and the AARC guidelines as an absolute contraindication. An increased intrathoracic pressure converts a simple pneumothorax into a tension pneumothorax. The consequences can be fatal. Once a chest tube has been inserted into the pleural space and a pleural drainage system set up, IPPB can be administered. There may be an increase in the air leak, but it will not be life-threatening.

The AARC guidelines list the following as relative contraindications. Any patient with one of the following contraindications should be evaluated carefully before a decision about the clinical use of IPPB is made:

b. Active hemoptysis

Expectoration of blood indicates that a tear has occurred in the airway or lung tissues. The IPPB treatment should be stopped if there is a large amount of hemoptysis. Certainly massive hemoptysis (defined as greater than 600 mL of blood expectorated in a 16-hour period) contraindicates IPPB.

c. Hemodynamic instability

d Intracranial pressure greater than 15 mm Hg

e. Chest radiograph that shows a bleb

f. Tracheoesophageal fistula

g. Recent surgery on the esophagus, skull, face, or mouth

h. Untreated, active tuberculosis (hazard to the practitioner)

i. Nausea, air swallowing, or hiccups (singultation)

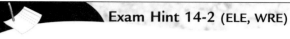

Exam Hint 14-2 (ELE, WRE)

Past examinations have included questions about the contraindications for IPPB, especially untreated pneumothorax or hemoptysis.

4. Hazards and precautions

The AARC guidelines list the following hazards and precautions for IPPB therapy:

  a. Pneumothorax

  b. Barotrauma

  c. Increased airway resistance from a bronchospastic reaction to the positive pressure or an adverse reaction to a medication. This can result in alveolar overdistension and air trapping.

  d. Hyperoxia when 100% oxygen is delivered to the patient. Some COPD patients who are hypercarbic and breathing on hypoxic drive may hypoventilate as a result.

  e. Secretions that may become impacted when the inhaled gas is not humidified adequately

  f. Nosocomial infection

  g. Decreased venous return

  h. Increased ventilation-to-perfusion mismatch. This may worsen any hypoxemia.

  i. Hyperventilation

  j. Psychologic dependence. This may be seen in the long-term home care patient who does not want to switch to another method of taking inhaled medications.

  k. Hypocarbia

  l. Hemoptysis

  m. Gastric distension

  n. Air trapping, auto-PEEP, or overdistended alveoli

5. Initiation of therapy

a. Steps in the basic procedure

1. Check for a complete and proper order specifying the patient, oxygen percentage, frequency of treatment, medication, and any special considerations.

2. Gather the necessary equipment, medication, and so on.

3. Assemble the equipment outside of the patient's room.

4. Introduce yourself and the department you represent, and state your purpose to the patient.

5. Confirm the patient's identity.

6. Have the patient sit up in bed or in a chair; an obese patient may stand.

7. Interview the patient.

8. Assess the patient's vital signs.

9. Assess the patient's breath sounds.

10. Prepare the IPPB unit for operation:
    A. If the unit is electrical, plug it into a working outlet.
    B. If the unit is pneumatic, plug it into either a compressed air or an oxygen outlet as ordered.
    C. Set the following controls:
       i. Set sensitivity at −1 cm H_2O pressure.
       ii. If a Bennett PR-2 is being used, set the nebulizer to run on inspiration only.
       iii. Adjust the flow as necessary.
       iv. Set the peak pressure at about 10 to 15 cm H_2O.
    D. Test the nebulizer by turning on the machine.
    E. Cover the mouthpiece with a clean tissue to ensure that it cycles off at the preset pressure.
11. Instruct the patient to sip on the mouthpiece like a straw to turn the machine on. Have the patient relax and let the machine fill his or her lungs with air. The patient should hold his or her breath in for 2 to 3 seconds and exhale slowly.

b. Giving a passive treatment

Most authors describe the patient taking a passive treatment. In a passive treatment, the patient relaxes and lets the machine fill the lungs until the preset pressure is reached. As mentioned earlier, the patient is then told to hold in his or her breath before exhaling passively. This treatment is given with the intent of minimizing the patient's WOB. As slow a flow rate as possible is used so that any nebulized medication is deposited deeply into the small airways and lungs.

c. Giving an active treatment

Several authors advocate having the patient take an active treatment in which he or she interacts with the IPPB machine to obtain as deep a breath as possible.

Welch and colleagues (1980) have found that the patient's posttreatment IC is greatest when the practitioner (1) uses as high a peak pressure as the patient can tolerate and (2) coaches the patient to inhale as deeply as possible with the IPPB machine. They and others believe that this is the best way to treat or prevent atelectasis. Monitor the patient for signs of barotrauma/volutrauma.

6. Initial settings on the Bird Mark 7

The older version of the Mark 7 is used as the model respirator of the Bird series. The current Mark 8 has similar features. Other Bird units have slightly different controls and features. Refer to Figure 14-1 for the following:

- Adjust the *air-mix* knob to the desired gas mix.
- Sensitivity should be set so that the patient has to generate about −1 cm H_2O pressure to cycle the unit on. Set the *sensitivity* control (on the left-hand side of the unit when facing it) to the reference number 15. This is at approximately the 2 o'clock position.

Turning the control lever counterclockwise makes the unit more sensitive. Push in the hand timer rod to note that the unit cycles on easily.
- Flow should be set so that the patient feels comfortable with the inspiratory time. Set the *flow rate* knob so that the reference number 15 is at the 12 o'clock position; the *off* sign will be at the 8 o'clock position. Turning the *flow rate* knob counterclockwise increases the flow.
- Peak pressure should be set at about 10 to 15 cm H_2O pressure. Set the *pressure* control (on the right-hand side of the unit when facing it) to the reference number 15. This is at approximately the 10 o'clock position. Turning the control lever more clockwise increases the peak pressure. Hold a clean tissue against the patient's mouthpiece to see that the unit cycles off at the desired peak pressure.

7. Initial settings on the Bennett PR-2

The PR-2 is used as the model respirator of the Bennett series. (Although the PR-2 is no longer being manufactured, many are still in clinical use.) Other Bennett units have slightly different controls and features. Refer to Figures 14-2 and 14-3 for the following:

- Adjust the *air dilution* knob to the desired gas mix.
- Sensitivity should be set so that the patient has to generate about −1 cm H_2O pressure to cycle the unit on. Turning the control lever counterclockwise makes the unit more sensitive. Push up on the Bennett valve strut to note that the unit cycles on easily.
- Flow should be set so that the patient feels comfortable with the inspiratory time. The Bennett valve is designed to automatically open and close itself to allow the patient as much flow as desired. Set the *peak flow* control knob as counterclockwise as possible so that it is at the maximum setting. Turning the *peak flow* knob more clockwise will decrease the patient's peak flow.
- Peak pressure should be set at about 10 to 15 cm H_2O pressure. Dial the *pressure* control clockwise until the *control pressure* gauge shows the desired peak pressure. Hold a clean tissue against the patient's mouthpiece to see that when the unit cycles off the *system pressure* gauge reads the same as the *control pressure* gauge.
- Turn the *inspiration nebulization* control counterclockwise for medication to be nebulized only during an inspiration. Some practitioners believe that the *expiration nebulization* control should be turned on slightly so that the mouthpiece and circuit dead space are filled with medication before the next breath. Others are opposed to this because it wastes medication when the patient stops the treatment.

Figure 14-1 Controls and features of the Bird Mark 7 IPPB unit.

- A small leak in the circuit, mouthpiece, or face mask can be overcome by adding some additional flow by turning on the *terminal flow* control. It is normally left off. Turn the control counterclockwise to add as much additional flow as necessary to overcome the leak.

Details on the design and control specifications for the various Bird and Bennett models can be found in the manufacturers' literature and books on respiratory therapy equipment.

MODULE B

Independently modify IPPB based on the patient's response to therapy (Code: IIIF2a) [Difficulty: ELE: R, Ap; WRE: An]

1. Change the patient-machine interface

a. Mouthpiece

A conscious, cooperative patient can take a treatment with a mouthpiece. He or she must be instructed to place the mouthpiece between the teeth (or gums) and seal the lips

Figure 14-2 Front controls and features of the Bennett PR-II IPPB unit.

around it so that there is no leak. Instruct the patient to sip gently on it to turn on the IPPB machine. As long as the lips are sealed and there are no other leaks, the positive-pressure breath will stop when the preset pressure is reached. Nose clips are often helpful to prevent a leak through the nose as the patient is learning how to take the treatment. The nose clips can be removed after the patient has learned how to seal the nasopharynx with the soft palate.

A variety of mouthpieces are available. All share two common features: a raised edge so that the teeth do not slip off; and a 22-mm outer diameter (OD) connector end to insert into the IPPB circuit (Figure 14-4).

b. Mouth seal (Bennett seal)

An unconscious, uncooperative, or aged patient who cannot seal his or her lips can be aided by placing a soft rubber seal around the mouthpiece. The practitioner gently holds the seal around the patient's lips to seal the airway so that the patient can trigger the breath and cycle the machine off (Figure 14-5). Nose clips are also commonly needed.

c. Face mask

The face mask can be used if the mouth seal does not provide an airtight seal. This might be because of the patient's facial structure or lack of teeth. Mouth trauma, surgery, or lip sores are other reasons to use a face mask.

Figure 14-3 Right-side controls and features of the Bennett PR-II IPPB unit.

Figure 14-4   Universal IPPB mouthpiece with a tapered 22- to 18-mm machine connector.

Figure 14-6   Giving an IPPB treatment with the use of a face mask.

Figure 14-5   *Top,* Bennett or mouth flange seal. *Bottom,* IPPB mouthpiece inserted into the seal.

The mask should be clear and properly sized to fit comfortably over the patient's nose and mouth. The practitioner should be able to get a seal with a minimum amount of hand pressure (Figure 14-6). The equipment connection opening in the mask has a 22-mm inner diameter (ID) so that it connects directly to the IPPB circuit. A 22-mm-OD male adapter and short length of aerosol tubing can be added for flexibility and patient comfort. The clear mask is important so that the practitioner can see whether the patient has vomited or has a large amount of secretions or saliva in his or her mouth. The mask should never be strapped to the patient's face so that the practitioner can attend to another patient.

This is the least effective patient attachment device if the therapeutic goal is to deliver an aerosolized medication. Much of the medication drains out on the patient's face or in the nasal passages if he or she is a nose breather.

d. Tracheostomy/endotracheal tube (elbow) adapter

The elbow adapter is designed to connect the patient's tracheostomy or endotracheal tube to the IPPB circuit (or other respiratory care equipment). The IPPB end has a 22-mm-ID connector. The tracheostomy/endotracheal tube end has a 15-mm-ID connector (Figure 14-7). If the tube's cuff has been deflated, it must be reinflated to seal the airway. An unsealed cuff results in an air leak, and the gas flow will not turn off.

2. Improve patient synchrony (Code: IIIG3a) [Difficulty: ELE: R, Ap; WRE: An]

Synchrony refers to the patient breathing in a coordinated pattern with the IPPB unit. Because the patient has to interact with the unit, some practice is required. The respiratory therapist must coach the patient to alter his or her breathing pattern as well as adjust the controls on the IPPB unit. Usually this involves adjusting sensitivity and flow.

a. Adjust the sensitivity

The sensitivity of the IPPB unit refers to how much effort or work the patient must perform to turn the unit on for a breath. Commonly, the sensitivity is set so that the patient has to generate a negative pressure of only about −1 cm H_2O pressure to begin an inspiration. This can be seen by the needle deflecting into the negative range on the pressure manometer. Ask the patient whether the machine can be easily turned on to get a breath. The IPPB

Figure 14-7 Giving an IPPB treatment with the use of a tracheostomy/endotracheal tube adapter.

Tracheostomy/endotracheal tube adapter

Flex tube with connectors

IPPB nebulizer

unit should not be set at a level so sensitive that it self-cycles.

The sensitivity range on the Bird series is −0.01 to −5 cm H₂O. Turning the *sensitivity/starting effort* adjustment lever counterclockwise toward the smaller reference numbers makes the unit more sensitive. The sensitivity range on the Bennett series is −0.5 to −1 cm H₂O. Turning the *sensitivity* control counterclockwise makes the unit easier to turn on.

b. Adjust the flow

The patient should initially feel comfortable with the flow rate and the inspiratory time. Ideally, the flow should result in a smooth, steady rise in the pressure up to the preset maximum pressure. Reduce the flow if the pressure rises too quickly. Increase the flow if the pressure wavers higher and lower; this indicates the patient is breathing in faster than the gas is being delivered. Ask the patient a simple question such as, "Is the breath coming too fast or too slow?" He or she can give you a short answer or even a hand gesture in response. As the treatment progresses, the practitioner may be able to adjust the flow to modify the patient's breathing pattern to better achieve the therapeutic goal, for example:

- Anxious patients may initially need a fast flow. As they are coached to relax and become accustomed to the treatment, the practitioner should try to reduce the flow.

- Slower flows result in medications being deposited deeper into the lungs. This is important if the patient is having a bronchodilator, mucolytic, or antibiotic nebulized.
- Faster flows result in the deposition of medications in the upper airways. This is important if the patient is receiving racemic epinephrine for laryngeal edema or lidocaine for a local anesthetic of the upper airway before bronchoscopy.

Turning the *inspiratory time/flow rate* control counterclockwise increases the flow rate on the Bird series. Pulling the *air-mix* knob out from the center body increases the total flow by allowing room air to be entrained along with the source gas. Flow rate in the PR-II is determined by the patient's inspiratory effort and the degree to which the Bennett valve is open. Flow can be decreased somewhat by turning the *peak flow* control clockwise. Flow is not affected by the position of the *air dilution* knob.

3. Adjust the fractional concentration of inspired oxygen

Compressed air or oxygen can power both the Bird and Bennett units. The patient's condition determines the oxygen percentage administered. The physician may include the oxygen percentage in the treatment order. Some departments have oxygen protocols in their treatment procedure. Generally, compressed air (21% oxygen) should be used whenever the patient does not need supplemental oxygen.

A patient with COPD who is retaining carbon dioxide and breathing on hypoxic drive should also be given room air via the IPPB unit. The patient may be allowed to keep wearing a nasal cannula with oxygen during the treatment so that the blood oxygen level is kept normal. The unavailability of piped-in compressed air should not be an excuse to give a patient a high oxygen percentage when it may be harmful. IPPB can be given through a gas-powered unit driven by a compressed air cylinder or through an electrically powered unit.

Supplemental oxygen is given if either unit is powered by oxygen and the *air-mix/air dilution* knobs are set to dilute the source gas with room air. This is appropriate for patients who require supplemental oxygen and are not at risk of stopping their spontaneous ventilation. Most practitioners use this method of giving IPPB because piped oxygen is usually available in all patient rooms.

Pure oxygen should be given to the patient who is severely hypoxemic. Examples include acute pulmonary edema, respiratory failure, and carbon monoxide poisoning. The *air-mix/air dilution* knobs must be set so that only the source gas (oxygen) is delivered to the patient.

For varying oxygen percentages on the Mark 7, note the following guidelines:

- Pushing the *air-mix* knob into the center body results in pure source gas. This can be either air or oxygen.
- Pulling the *air-mix* knob out of the center body results in a dilution of the source gas with room air. If oxygen is the source gas, the room air will dilute the delivered gas to between 60% and 90% (or more) oxygen.

For varying oxygen percentages on the PR-II, note the following guidelines:

- Pulling the *air dilution* knob out of the body results in pure source gas. This can be either air or oxygen.
- Pushing the *air dilution* knob into the body results in a dilution of the source gas with room air. If oxygen is the source gas, the room air will dilute the delivered gas to between 40% and 80% oxygen.
- Turning on the *terminal flow* control results in the dilution of source gas with room air. This dilutes the final percentage if the source gas is oxygen.

4. Adjust the volume, pressure, or both

A review of the current respiratory care textbooks reveals that all authors agree that the basic goal of IPPB is to increase how deeply the patient inspires. Unfortunately, there is considerable difference about what inspiratory volume is being measured or by how much that breath should be increased for therapeutic goals to be achieved. The AARC has released the following guidelines on the subject:

- The *AARC Clinical Practice Guideline* (1991) on incentive spirometry: IPPB, rather than incentive spirometry, is indicated to treat atelectasis if (a) the patient's IC is less than 33% of the preoperative value or (b) the patient's VC is less than 10 mL/kg of ideal body weight.
- Therefore IPPB would only be indicated when the patient cannot perform incentive spirometry or is unable to reach the above clinical goals.
- The *AARC Clinical Practice Guideline* (1993) on IPPB: The tidal volume delivered during an IPPB-assisted breath should be at least 25% greater than the patient's spontaneous breaths.

EXAMPLE

Calculate the minimum IPPB-delivered tidal volume goal for a 35-year-old 150-pound ideal body weight male with pneumonia. He has a spontaneous tidal volume of 500 mL. Steps in the calculation include:

Minimum IPPB-assisted tidal volume
$$= \text{spontaneous tidal volume} \times 1.25$$

Minimum IPPB-assisted tidal volume $= 500 \text{ mL} \times 1.25 = 625 \text{ mL}$

- The 2003 revision and update of the 1993 *AARC Clinical Practice Guideline* on IPPB states that the tidal volume delivered during an IPPB-assisted breath should be at least one third (0.33) of the patient's predicted inspiratory capacity (IC).

EXAMPLE

Calculate the minimum IPPB-delivered tidal volume goal for a 35-year-old 150-pound ideal body weight male with pneumonia. He has a spontaneous tidal volume of 500 mL. Steps in the calculation include:

1. Convert the patient's body weight in pounds (lb) to kilograms (kg):

$$\frac{150 \text{ lb}}{2.2 \text{ lb/kg}} = 68.18 \text{ kg (use 68 kg for this calculation)}$$

2. Calculate the patient's predicted inspiratory capacity:

$$\text{Predicted IC} = 50 \text{ mL} \times \text{kg of ideal body weight}$$

$$\text{Therefore predicted IC} = 50 \text{ mL} \times 68 \text{ kg} = 3400 \text{ mL}$$

3. Calculate the patient's minimum IPPB-assisted tidal volume goal:

$$\begin{aligned} \text{Minimum IPPB goal} &= 0.33 \times \text{predicted IC} \\ &= 0.33 \times 3400 \text{ mL} = 1122 \text{ mL} \end{aligned}$$

Therefore the patient should receive an IPPB-assisted tidal volume of at least 1122 mL.

If the therapeutic goal is to prevent or treat atelectasis, having the patient inspire a deeper than spontaneous tidal volume breath should help. It seems reasonable to follow the AARC guidelines as clinical goals. Following the 2003 updated guidelines would provide the patient with a larger IPPB-assisted tidal volume. However, depending on the patient's tolerance, it may be necessary to begin with a smaller initial tidal volume goal (1993 guidelines) and then increase the goal as tolerated.

Because all of the current IPPB units are pressure cycled, the only way to increase the inspired volume during a passive treatment is to increase the peak pressure. Coaching the patient during an active treatment results in a larger volume without the need for as great a peak pressure. Decrease the peak pressure if the patient complains of discomfort or cannot hold that much pressure without losing the lip seal.

5. Reduce auto-PEEP (Code: IIIG3l) [Difficulty: ELE: R, Ap; WRE: An]

Positive end-expiratory pressure (PEEP) is pressure added through a mechanical ventilator at the end of an exhalation to prevent the patient from exhaling fully. PEEP keeps the patient's airway pressure greater than atmospheric (commonly given as the baseline pressure of zero). The clinical effect of PEEP is to increase a patient's residual volume (RV) and functional residual capacity (FRC) to improve oxygenation. It is used when the patient has a clinical condition, such as atelectasis or acute respiratory distress syndrome (ARDS), that results in small lung volumes. Auto-PEEP is end-expiratory pressure in the lungs that cannot be seen on the IPPB unit's (or ventilator's) pressure manometer. Auto-PEEP is caused by air trapping because the patient does not have enough time to exhale completely. In other words, the patient starts another inspiration before the previous breath was completely exhaled. This problem is most commonly seen in patients with small airways disease such as asthma and COPD.

Over the course of an IPPB treatment, patients who have small airways disease can develop air trapping. This can lead to an increased RV and FRC, which is seen as auto-PEEP. This unwelcome lung overinflation increases the risk of pulmonary barotrauma. If auto-PEEP is known or suspected during an IPPB treatment, *expiratory retard* can be added to help ensure a complete exhalation. Adding expiratory retard to the treatment increases back-pressure on the airways and has the same effect as pursed-lip breathing. The clinical effect of adding some back-pressure on the smallest airways is to keep them open longer so that the more distal air can be exhaled.

The following two procedures can be used to help identify the presence of auto-PEEP:

1. Measure the exhaled volumes during the treatment and monitor the patient's response to the inspired breath. If the patient is exhaling less tidal volume with succeeding breaths or the patient complains of fullness, it is likely that air trapping is taking place.
2. Listen to the patient's breath sounds for a pause at the end of exhalation before the next inspiration begins. If there is no end-expiratory pause before the next breath, it is likely that the patient is air trapping.

If auto-PEEP is identified, expiratory retard can be added to reduce it. Too little retard results in some air trapping and an incompletely exhaled tidal volume. Too much retard results in an uncomfortably long expiratory time and additional air trapping. This would cause an increased mean intrathoracic pressure. The proper amount of expiratory retard should result in the patient feeling comfortable with the breathing cycle and being able to completely exhale the delivered tidal volume. Listen to the patient's breath sounds for a silent pause at the end of exhalation. If wheezing is present, it should be minimized when the proper amount of retard is added. This is because the back-pressure is properly adjusted to minimize small airway collapse and distal gas is fully exhaled.

Bird makes a retard cap that fits over the exhalation valve port on their permanent circuit. The cap has a series of different size holes through which the exhaled gas can pass (Figure 14-8). By rotating the cap progressively from the largest to the smallest opening and evaluating the patient at each setting, the proper size opening and amount of retard can be determined. The largest hole results in the least expiratory retard, while the smallest hole results in the greatest retard.

Bennett makes a retard exhalation valve that can be substituted for the regular exhalation valve on their permanent circuit (Figure 14-9). The valve consists of a spring attached to a nut and a diaphragm. As the nut is turned counterclockwise the spring pushes the diaphragm closer to the exhalation valve opening. This causes resistance to the exhalation of the tidal volume and a

Figure 14-8 Bird retard cap for providing adjustable expiratory resistance. *(From McPherson SP: Respiratory therapy equipment, ed 5, St Louis, 1995, Mosby.)*

Figure 14-9 Bennett retard exhalation valve for providing adjustable expiratory resistance. *(From McPherson SP: Respiratory therapy equipment, ed 5, St Louis, 1995, Mosby.)*

back-pressure is created against the airways. Start with the least amount of expiratory retard and evaluate the patient before increasing the amount of expiratory retard. Be aware that if too much pressure is placed against the exhalation valve opening, the patient will not be able to exhale back to atmospheric pressure. This would create PEEP and should not be done without an order from the physician.

Be sure to ask the patient's opinion about the use of expiratory retard. The conscious, cooperative patient can tell you if he or she feels like more air is getting out by the use of the retard or if the lungs feel more full because too much retard is being used. Too much retard may also make the expiratory time uncomfortably long.

Exam Hint 14-3 (ELE, WRE)

There is usually a question that requires the therapist to modify the treatment. Increase the pressure to give a larger tidal volume; decrease the pressure to give a smaller tidal volume. If the patient wants a faster breath, increase the flow.

MODULE C

Manipulate IPPB equipment by order or protocol (ELE code: IIA11b) [ELE difficulty: R, Ap, An]

1. Get the proper IPPB circuit for the patient's treatment

The two most widely used IPPB machines are the Bird Mark 7/8 (or a variation of it found in the series) and the Bennett PR-2. Both are pneumatically powered and found in most hospitals. Each unit requires a circuit that is designed specifically for it. See Figure 14-10 for a drawing of a permanent (reusable after cleaning) and disposable circuit for a Bird machine. See Figure 14-11 for a drawing of a permanent (reusable after cleaning) and disposable circuit for a Bennett machine.

2. Put the IPPB circuit together and make sure that it works properly

See Figure 14-10 for the Bird setup and Figure 14-11 for the Bennett setup.

a. General setup procedures

1. Check for plentiful source gas. Make sure that the oxygen or air tank has the proper regulator. Check the pressure in the gas cylinder.

Figure 14-10 Features of permanent and disposable Bird IPPB circuits.

High-pressure hose
Gas inlet

BENNETT PERMANENT CIRCUIT

Optional inline bacteria filter
Nebulizer hose
Exhalation valve hose
Exhalation valve
To patient
Nebulizer
Mainstream hose

BENNETT DISPOSABLE CIRCUIT

Optional inline bacteria filter
Nebulizer hose
Exhalation valve hose
Exhalation valve
To patient
Measure exhaled volume here
Nebulizer

Figure 14-11   Features of permanent and disposable Bennett IPPB circuits.

2. Attach the high-pressure hose to the source gas and the IPPB unit at the gas inlet. Make sure that the connections are tight.
3. Bacteria filters are optional. They are inserted between the IPPB unit gas outlets and the mainstream and nebulizer hoses.
4. A cascade-type humidifier is optional. Some practitioners prefer to warm and humidify the mainstream gas before it reaches the patient.
5. Check to see that the IPPB circuit is assembled properly and that all of the connections are tight.
6. Set the initial treatment parameters for sensitivity, flow, and peak pressure. Manually cycle the unit on. Cover the mouthpiece to see that the unit cycles off at the preset pressure.
7. Add any medication to the nebulizer. Check to see that the nebulizer is producing a mist.

b. Bird setup

1. One end of the mainstream (large-bore) hose is connected to the mainstream breathing hose connector on the right side of the unit. The other end is connected to the nebulizer.
2. One end of the nebulizer (small-bore) hose is connected to the small nipple on the right-hand side of

the unit. The other end is connected to a T-piece at the nebulizer.
3. A piece of small-bore hose is used to connect one limb of the T-piece and the exhalation valve. Gas flowing through this hose powers both the nebulizer and the exhalation valve.

c. Bennett setup

1. One end of the mainstream (large-bore) hose is connected to the mainstream breathing hose connector on the underside of the unit. The other end is connected to the nebulizer.
2. One end of the nebulizer (medium-bore) hose is connected to the larger of two nipples on the underside of the unit. The other end is connected to the nebulizer nipple.
3. One end of the exhalation (small-bore) hose is connected to the smaller of two nipples on the underside of the unit. The other end is connected to the exhalation valve nipple.

3. Troubleshoot any problems with the equipment

Fixing a problem is only possible after the problem has been identified. The practitioner should be familiar with both permanent and disposable types of Bird and Bennett circuits. Leaks of any sort in the circuit prevent the unit from cycling off so that the patient can exhale. Tighten any friction-fit or screw-type connections to stop the leak. A leak at the source gas connection or high-pressure hose gas inlet connection results in a rather loud hissing sound. When connections are tightened properly, the hissing and leak will stop.

Debris such as mucus or blood can plug the nebulizer capillary tube and prevent any mist from being formed. Disassemble the nebulizer and rinse it under running water to try to clear the capillary tube. Replace the nebulizer if necessary.

Exam Hint 14-4 (ELE)

Past examinations have included questions regarding the reasons that an IPPB machine would fail to cycle off. Identify the following leaks and know how to seal them: around the patient's mouthpiece (use a Bennett seal or face mask), within the circuit (tighten all connections), cuff on a tracheostomy or endotracheal tube (inflate the cuff), defective exhalation valve (replace the circuit).

MODULE D
Respiratory care plan

1. Analyze available information to determine the patient's pathophysiologic state (Code: IIIH1) [Difficulty: ELE: R, Ap; WRE: An]

Atelectasis is determined by characteristic chest radiograph findings and decreased or absent breath sounds over the affected area. Wheezing breath sounds is a finding indicating bronchospasm. Pulmonary edema has characteristic chest radiograph findings and cardiovascular indicators. Review the discussion on these conditions and their findings in Chapters 1 and 5. IPPB has been used in the management of patients with these conditions if other methods are not effective.

2. Determine the appropriateness of the prescribed respiratory care plan and recommend modifications when indicated

a. Determine the appropriateness of the prescribed therapy and goals for the patient's pathophysiologic state (Code: IIIH3) [Difficulty: ELE: R, Ap; WRE: An]

IPPB should be used for hyperinflation therapy only when less expensive options (such as incentive spirometry) are shown to be impractical. One of the goals of IPPB is to give the patient larger tidal volumes than normal. The

larger tidal volumes should result in breath sounds being heard more clearly at the bases of the lungs. Additional secretions may be heard in the airways if the larger tidal volumes result in their mobilization. However, if deeper breaths enable the patient to cough more effectively, additional secretions should be expectorated. Wheezing should be diminished if a bronchodilator medication is nebulized to a patient with bronchospasm.

Ask about the patient's feelings about the treatment, and write them in the chart. Note any significant comments made by the patient. Note the patient's preferred flow and pressure or volume settings.

b. Review the planned therapy to establish the therapeutic plan (Code: IIIH2a) [Difficulty: ELE: R, Ap; WRE: An]

c. Recommend changes in the therapeutic plan when indicated (Code: IIIH4) [Difficulty: ELE: R, Ap; WRE: An]

In order for the patient to receive the best care possible, the respiratory therapist must know the indications, contraindications, complications, and hazards of the respiratory care procedures the patient will receive. The patient must be assessed before, during, and after the treatment or procedure to determine if it was effective. The key goal of an appropriate care plan is that the patient's condition be treated in the best way possible. Modifications to the care plan must be made, as needed, as the patient's condition changes.

The respiratory therapist should be a member of the patient care team of the physician, nurse, and others in deciding how best to care for the patient. The following steps are necessary in developing the respiratory care plan for any patient:

1. Determine an expected outcome or goal(s).
2. Develop a plan to achieve success.
3. Decide how to measure if the goal(s) have been achieved.
4. Plan a timeline to measure the patient's progress.
5. Document the patient's response to care and the final outcome.

The patient should be fully cooperative to make the best use of IPPB. It may be counterproductive to try to force an IPPB treatment on a combative or uncooperative patient. A patient who has a neuromuscular deficit may need assistance in holding the IPPB circuit or keeping a good mouth seal. A mouth seal or face mask treatment may have to be given. Be prepared to make a recommendation to have a patient use either incentive spirometry, short-term continuous positive airway pressure (CPAP), or IPPB for hyperinflation therapy. Also be prepared to make a recommendation for a patient to use either a metered dose inhaler, small volume nebulizer, or IPPB for the delivery of an aerosolized medication.

d. Terminate the IPPB treatment if the patient has an adverse reaction to it (Code: IIIF1) [Difficulty: ELE: R, Ap; WRE: An]

Patient safety should always be an important consideration during the treatment. The respiratory therapist should know the complications and hazards of any patient care activity that is performed. Be prepared to stop the treatment if the patient has a sudden adverse reaction to it (for example, hemoptysis or signs and symptoms of a pneumothorax). Additionally, be prepared to recommend to the physician that the treatment be discontinued if it is likely to result in additional serious adverse reactions.

However, some adverse reaction may only require a pause or adjustment in the IPPB treatment. For example:

- If a patient hyperventilates and feels nauseated or faint, a short pause for normal breathing will help the patient feel normal again. Then IPPB can be restarted but with a slower respiratory rate or smaller tidal volume.
- The general treatment length of 15 to 20 minutes may cause fatigue. This is often seen in aged or debilitated patients. Provide a shorter but still effective treatment.
- Stop the treatment if the patient has a pulse rate change of 20% per minute or more. It is most common to see the pulse rate increase because of a nebulized bronchodilator drug. Wait for the heart rate to drop to normal before resuming the treatment. If tachycardia occurs again, discuss with the physician decreasing the medication dose.
- IPPB may cause a decreased venous return to the heart that may be shown by an increased heart rate or drop in blood pressure. Stop the treatment and monitor the patient's vital signs. If they return to normal, give the IPPB treatment with a lower peak pressure and smaller tidal volume.

e. Recommend discontinuing treatment based on the patient's response (WRE code: IIIG1i) [Difficulty: ELE: R, Ap; WRE: An]

The contraindications, hazards, and precautions to IPPB were discussed earlier in Module A under the sections "Contraindications" and "Hazards and precautions." The treatment should be discontinued if the patient has an untreated pneumothorax or massive hemoptysis. Other serious problems also justify the cancellation of the order.

The IPPB treatments can be discontinued if the patient's atelectasis is resolved. Or, IPPB can be discontinued if another, less expensive treatment, such as incentive spirometry, can be properly performed by the patient.

3. Respiratory care protocols

a. Develop the IPPB protocol (Code: IIIH6b) [Difficulty: ELE: R; WRE: Ap, An]

b. Apply IPPB protocol (Code: IIIH8) [Difficulty: ELE: R, Ap; WRE: Ap]

The respiratory therapist may be involved in developing an individualized patient treatment plan utilizing IPPB. Review the previously listed indications and tidal volume targeting information.

c. Explain planned therapy and goals to the patient in understandable (nonmedical) terms to achieve the best results from the treatment (Code: IIIA6) [Difficulty: ELE: R, Ap; WRE: An]

Because IPPB involves the patient interacting with the unit and the therapist making adjustments to the unit based on the patient's responses, clear and simple explanations are paramount. Be prepared to make adjustments to sensitivity, flow, and pressure and coach/teach the patient to get the best results.

d. Monitor the outcomes of IPPB protocol (Code: IIIH7b) [Difficulty: ELE: R, Ap; WRE: An]

The goal of all protocols is to restore the patient's condition to as close to normal as possible. When it is not possible to restore normal conditions, acceptable conditions must be listed as the target for care. The patient must be evaluated before, during, and after a protocol is used to determine if improvement has occurred. Based on the results of the patient assessment, the care can be upregulated (increased) or downregulated (decreased).

IPPB should be used only for hyperinflation therapy when less expensive options (such as incentive spirometry) are not practical. One of the goals of IPPB is to give the patient larger tidal volumes than normal. Bedside spirometry should confirm that IPPB is indicated and that the patient's IPPB breath is at least 25% greater than spontaneous breaths. Breath sounds should be heard more clearly to the bases of the lungs. More secretions may be heard in the airways if the larger tidal volumes result in their mobilization. However, if the deeper breaths enable the patient to cough more effectively, more secretions should be expectorated. Wheezing should be diminished if a bronchodilator medication is nebulized to a patient with bronchospasm.

e. Communicate the outcomes of therapy and change the therapy based on the protocol (Code: IIIA5) [Difficulty: ELE: R, Ap; WRE: An]

Inform the patient's nurse or physician and the supervising therapist if any serious question or problem occurs with the patient. Routine communication should occur as needed between these people and any other caregiver.

4. Record and evaluate the patient's response to the treatment, including the following:

a. Record and interpret the following: heart rate and rhythm, respiratory rate, blood pressure, body temperature, and pain level (Code: IIIA1b4) [Difficulty: ELE: R, Ap; WRE: An]

Monitor the patient's vital signs before, during, and after the treatment. Ask about the patient's feelings about the treatment. Note the vital signs in the chart and add any significant comments made by the patient. Note the patient's preferred flow and pressure or volume settings.

b. Record and interpret the patient's breath sounds (Code: IIIA1b3) [Difficulty: ELE: R, Ap; WRE: An]

If atelectatic areas have been opened, normal breath sounds should be heard there. If a nebulized bronchodilator medication has been effective, wheezing will be diminished or absent.

c. Record and interpret the type of cough the patient has and the nature of the sputum (Code: IIIA1b3) [Difficulty: ELE: R, Ap; WRE: An]

If IPPB helps to deliver a larger tidal volume to the patient, the cough may be more effective. If IPPB has been used to deliver a nebulized mucolytic drug, the patient's sputum may be easier to expectorate.

d. Recheck any math work and make note of incorrect data (Code: IIIA1b2) [Difficulty: ELE: R, Ap; WRE: An]

Make sure that the patient's IPPB tidal volume goal is properly calculated.

5. Communicate information relevant to coordinating patient care and discharge planning (e.g., scheduling, avoiding conflicts, and sequencing of therapies) (Code: IIIA2b) [Difficulty: ELE: R, Ap; WRE: An]

Common scheduling problems include meal times and prearranged procedures or therapies, such as radiology or physical therapy. Some procedures, such as giving an IPPB treatment with aerosolized medications and performing chest physiotherapy, should be performed before eating.

BIBLIOGRAPHY

AARC Clinical Practice Guideline: Incentive spirometry, *Respir Care* 30:1402, 1991.

AARC Clinical Practice Guideline: Intermittent positive pressure ventilation, *Respir Care* 38:1189, 1993.

AARC Clinical Practice Guideline: Intermittent positive pressure ventilation—2003 revision & update, *Respir Care* 48: 540, 2003.

Branson RD, Hess DR, Chatburn RL, editors: *Respiratory care equipment*, ed 2, Philadelphia, 1999, Lippincott Williams & Wilkins.

Cairo JM: Lung expansion devices. In Cairo JM, Pilbeam SP: *Mosby's respiratory care equipment*, ed 9, St. Louis, 2010, Mosby.

Eubanks DH, Bone RC: *Comprehensive respiratory care*, ed 2, St Louis, 1990, Mosby.

Fink JB: Volume expansion therapy. In Burton GG, Hodgkin JE, Ward JJ, editors: *Respiratory care*, ed 4, Philadelphia, 1997, Lippincott.

Fink JB: Bronchial hygiene and lung expansion. In Fink JB, Hunt GE, editors: *Clinical practice in respiratory care*, Philadelphia, 1999, Lippincott Williams & Wilkins.

Fink JB: Volume expansion therapy. In Burton GG, Hodgkin JE, Ward JJ, editors: *Respiratory care*, ed 4, Philadelphia, 1997, Lippincott.

Fink JB: Hess DR: Secretion clearance techniques. In Hess DR, MacIntyre NR, Mishoe SC: *Respiratory care principles & practices*, Philadelphia, 2002, WB Saunders.

Fluck RJ Jr: Intermittent positive-pressure breathing devices and transport ventilators. In Barnes TA, editor: *Respiratory care practice*, ed 2, St Louis, 1994, Mosby.

McPherson SP: *Respiratory care equipment*, ed 5, St Louis, 1995, Mosby.

Miller WF: Intermittent positive pressure breathing (IPPB). In Kacmarek RM, Stoller JK, editors: *Current respiratory care*, Philadelphia, 1988, BC Decker.

Respiratory Care Committee of the American Thoracic Society: Guidelines for the use of intermittent positive pressure breathing (IPPB), *Respir Care* 25:365, 1980.

Shapiro BA, Kacmarek RM, Cne RD, et al: *Clinical application of respiratory care*, ed 4, St Louis, 1991, Mosby.

Weizalis CP: Intermittent positive-pressure breathing. In Barnes TA, editor: *Respiratory care practice*, ed 2, St. Louis, 1994, Mosby.

Welch MA et al: Methods of intermittent positive pressure breathing, *Chest* 78:463, 1980.

White GC: *Equipment theory for respiratory care*, ed 4, Albany, NY, 2005, Delmar.

Wilkins RL: Lung expansion therapy. In Wilkins RL, Stoller CL, Kacmarek RM, editors: *Egan's fundamentals of respiratory care*, ed 9, St. Louis, 2009, Mosby.

1. Your patient complains of difficulty in starting the IPPB treatment. You would adjust which of the following controls?
   A. Pressure
   B. Flow
   C. Sensitivity
   D. Terminal flow

2. Your patient is having difficulty keeping a tight seal around the mouthpiece. He complains that the breath is too long and takes out the mouthpiece. To help cycle off the PR-2, you would adjust which of the following?
   A. Pressure
   B. Flow
   C. Terminal flow
   D. Expiratory retard

3. Your patient is progressing to pulmonary edema. She has crackles in both lung fields, has cyanotic lips and nail beds, and is coughing up pink, frothy sputum. What O_2 percentage would you recommend for her IPPB treatment?
   A. 21%
   B. 40%
   C. 80%
   D. 100%

4. All of the following indicate the need for IPPB EXCEPT
   A. Delivery of medications to a patient who cannot coordinate the use of an MDI or a handheld nebulizer
   B. Treatment of a comatose patient with atelectasis
   C. The need for an IS substitute in a patient with an IC that is 30% of predicted
   D. Treatment of a cooperative patient with atelectasis

5. You are ordered to give an IPPB treatment to a comatose patient who has lip ulcers. What patient-machine connection would you use?
   A. Mouthpiece
   B. Face mask
   C. Bennett seal with mouthpiece
   D. Endotracheal tube adapter for intubation

6. The sensitivity control should be set at what level at the start of IPPB treatment?
   A. 0 cm H_2O
   B. −1 cm H_2O
   C. −3 cm H_2O
   D. −5 cm H_2O

7. While coaching an active IPPB treatment, you notice that the needle on the pressure manometer "bounces" around as the pressure increases. To better adjust

treatment to the patient's needs, you would do which of the following?
   A. Increase the flow.
   B. Decrease the flow.
   C. Increase the peak pressure.
   D. Decrease the expiratory retard.

8. You are giving an IPPB treatment on a Bird Mark 7 unit. To give the patient 100% O_2, you push in the air-mix control knob. What effect does this adjustment have on the flow rate to the patient?
   A. Decreases the flow of gas
   B. Increases the flow of gas
   C. No effect
   D. Increases the sensitivity

9. In the emergency department, you are giving an IPPB treatment with albuterol (Ventolin) to an asthmatic patient. During a break in the treatment, the patient complains that his lungs feel too full and he does not feel like all the IPPB volume is getting out. What would you recommend?
   A. Increase the flow.
   B. Add expiratory retard.
   C. Increase the system pressure.
   D. Change to 100% oxygen.

10. While giving an IPPB treatment, a hissing sound is heard and the patient complains that the inspiratory time is too long. What is the most likely problem?
   A. The nebulizer hose is attached to the exhalation valve.
   B. The nebulizer medication jar is loose.
   C. The bacteria filter is missing.
   D. The inspiratory and expiratory hoses are reversed.

11. A patient who was initially anxious about taking an IPPB treatment and needing a fast breath is now breathing in a more relaxed manner. What adjustment should be made to allow for a longer inspiratory time?
   A. Decrease the peak pressure.
   B. Increase the sensitivity.
   C. Set the air-mix knob to allow room air to be entrained.
   D. Decrease the flow.

12. A patient you are evaluating has a spontaneous V_T of 400 mL and has been diagnosed with atelectasis after bowel surgery. IPPB has been ordered. What would you recommend as the minimal volume goal?
   A. 300 mL
   B. 400 mL
   C. 500 mL
   D. 800 mL

13. After 10 min of being given an IPPB treatment, the patient complains of a sharp chest pain. After a few

more deep breaths, he says he is short of breath. You notice that his breath sounds are now diminished on the left side. What would you recommend?

    A. Continue the treatment for the next 5 min to finish the ordered time.

    B. Decrease the peak pressure and complete the ordered treatment.

    C. Stop the treatment and notify the physician of the patient's complaints.

    D. Monitor the patient closely for the duration of the treatment, and notify the nurse of the patient's complaints.

SELF-STUDY QUESTIONS FOR THE WRITTEN REGISTRY EXAM

See page 622 for answers

1. You would stop an IPPB treatment under which of the following conditions?

    1. You suspect that the patient has just developed a pneumothorax.

    2. The patient has a difficult time keeping his lips sealed.

    3. The patient feels faint and dizzy.

    4. The patient coughs up a large amount of blood.

    A. 1, 2

    B. 3, 4

    C. 2, 4

    D. 1, 3, 4

2. A patient with emphysema has been changed from a handheld nebulizer to IPPB for bronchodilator therapy. While evaluating the patient during treatment, you note that her exhaled tidal volume is decreasing. She says, "I feel full; like I can't get all of my air out." What would you recommend?

    A. Decrease the flow.

    B. Add expiratory retard.

    C. Increase the system pressure.

    D. Pull out the air-mix knob.

3. You are delivering an IPPB treatment to an elderly patient without teeth or dentures. He has difficulty keeping his lips tight around the mouthpiece and pressure fails to rise enough to cycle off the breath. What should be done?

    A. Switch the mouthpiece to a mask.

    B. Increase the inspiratory flow.

    C. Place nose clips on the patient.

    D. Change from IPPB to incentive spirometry.

4. You are about to give an asthmatic 16-year-old patient her second IPPB treatment with a bronchodilator medication. When checking the equipment you notice that it is set with a rather fast inspiratory flow. Her chart had a note that she was very anxious when first admitted. She seems calmer now. How would you start the treatment?

    A. Increase the pressure setting to deliver a larger breath.

    B. Keep the flow the same to deliver a larger breath.

    C. Make the machine as sensitive as possible to easily trigger it.

    D. Decrease the flow on the machine.

5. Your 45-year-old female 50-kg (110-pound) patient is recovering after abdominal surgery. The physician has ordered IPPB to help correct her atelectasis after incentive spirometry was found to be ineffective. Her spontaneous tidal volume is 350 mL. Based on this information, at what level should her minimum initial IPPB tidal volume be set?

    A. 350 mL

    B. 450 mL

    C. 700 mL

    D. 900 mL

6. Atelectasis has been diagnosed by chest radiograph in a patient who had recent open heart surgery. His best bedside spirometry inspiratory capacity (IC) value is 25% of his predicted. What should be recommended to treat his atelectasis problem?

    A. IPPB

    B. Incentive spirometry

    C. Nasotracheal suctioning

    D. Flutter

7. Your patient with COPD has been receiving IPPB treatments on a Bird Mark 7 for 5 days. Expiratory retard was added 4 days ago. Because the retard has not been evaluated since then, the physician asks you to do so. You proceeded to make the following adjustments in the retard cap settings and make the following observations:

Retard Cap Setting	Exhaled Tidal Volume (mL)	Wheezing	Patient's Impression
1 (smallest)	850	None	Exhalation too long
2	825	Some in bases	Exhalation too long
3	800	Some in bases	Comfortable
4	700	All lobes	Lungs feel full

Based on this information, which retard cap setting would you recommend?

A. 1

B. 2

C. 3

D. 4

8. A 13-year-old patient with cystic fibrosis is receiving IPPB to deliver an aerosolized bronchodilator and mucolytic. You notice that the pressure gauge needle is bouncing higher and lower as she takes a breath. What should you do?

A. Increase the target pressure.

B. Increase the sensitivity setting.

C. Increase the flow.

D. Tell the patient to inhale more quickly.

9. Your patient has an IPPB tidal volume goal of 900 mL but is only exhaling 700 mL. What would you do to deliver a larger volume?

A. Increase the delivered pressure.

B. Decrease the flow.

C. Add expiratory retard.

D. Have the patient inhale more forcefully.

10. An 82-kg (180-pound) male is recovering after an accidental drug overdose. Because of hypoventilation and being semicomatose, he has developed bilateral atelectasis. Calculate the ideal minimum IPPB delivered tidal volume goal for him. His spontaneous tidal volume is 600 mL.

A. 700 mL

B. 900 mL

C. 1400 mL

D. 3000 mL

15

Mechanical Ventilation of the Adult

Note 1: This book is written to cover every item listed as testable on the *Entry Level Examination (ELE), Written Registry Examination (WRE),* and *Clinical Simulation Examination (CSE).*

The listed code for each item is taken from the National Board for Respiratory Care (NBRC) **Summary Content Outline for CRT (Certified Respiratory Therapist) and Written RRT (Registered Respiratory Therapist) Examinations** (http://evolve.elsevier.com/Sills/resptherapist/). For example, if an item is testable on both the ELE and the WRE, it will be shown simply as: (Code: . . .). If an item is testable only on the ELE, it will be shown as: (ELE code: . . .). If an item is testable only on the WRE, it will be shown as: (WRE code: . . .).

Following each item's code will be the difficulty level of the questions on that item on the ELE and the WRE. (See the Introduction for a full explanation of the three question difficulty levels.) **Recall [R]** level questions typically expect the exam taker to recall factual information. **Application [Ap]** level questions are harder because the exam taker may have to apply factual information to a clinical situation. **Analysis [An]** level questions are the most challenging because the exam taker may have to use critical thinking to evaluate patient data to make a clinical decision.

Note 2: A review of the most recent ELEs has shown that an average of 43 questions (out of 140), or 31% of the exam, cover mechanical ventilation of the adult. A review of the most recent WRE has shown that an average of 23 questions (out of 100), or 23% of the exam, cover mechanical ventilation of the adult. The CSE is comprehensive and may include everything that should be known by an advanced level respiratory therapist.

MODULE A

Review the patient's chart for the following data and recommend and perform the following diagnostic procedures.

1. Ventilator flow, volume, and pressure waveforms

a. Review the patient's chart for information on airway graphics (Code: IA7c) [Difficulty: ELE: R; WRE: Ap]

A patient who has been intubated and placed on a modern mechanical ventilator with a microprocessor and graphics software can have ventilator flow, volume, and pressure waveforms visualized on the monitor, stored in memory, or printed out. Look for this information and compare it with the patient's current situation. See Figure 15-1 for examples of pressure, volume, and flow tracings. See Figure 15-2 for key points of information available from a flow vs. time graph.

b. Perform the procedure to measure ventilator pressure/volume and flow/volume loops (WRE Code: IB9o) [Difficulty: WRE: R, Ap, An]

Follow the ventilator manufacturer's steps to direct the unit to create flow, volume, and pressure waveforms. The patient can be instructed, based on the breathing test, to perform a breathing maneuver actively or to lie passively as the ventilator delivers a breath.

c. Select ventilator graphics (Code: IIID3) [Difficulty: ELE: R, Ap; WRE: An]

The operator typically can select any two of the following for display on the monitor: time, flow, pressure, and/or volume. Certain combinations are selected to best present the needed information. For example, air trapping is best shown by comparing flow vs. time (Figure 15-3) peak and plateau pressures are best shown by comparing pressure vs. time (Figure 15-4), and lung inflection points are best shown by comparing volume vs. pressure (discussed later). Note examples of ventilator graphics throughout this chapter.

d. Interpret ventilator pressure/volume and flow/volume loops (WRE code: IB10o) [Difficulty: WRE: R, Ap, An]

A number of flow, volume, and pressure waveforms have been included in this chapter for practice. In addition, review Figures 4-1 and 4-10 for examples of pulmonary function test waveform tracings. The examples in this chapter include common clinical situations and are accompanied explanations to help with interpretation.

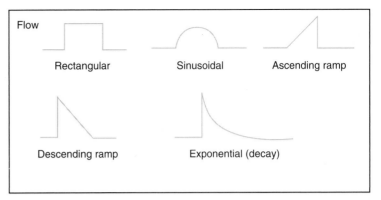

Figure 15-1 Examples of waveforms for pressure, flow, and volume that can be seen on the graphics monitor of a microprocessor-type ventilator. The practitioner can select from these and other options to display needed graphs to help guide patient care. See examples throughout the chapter. *(From Pilbeam SP: Ventilator graphics. In: Pilbeam SP, Cairo JM (editors): Mechanical Ventilation: Physiologic and clinical applications, ed 4, St Louis, 2006, Mosby.)*

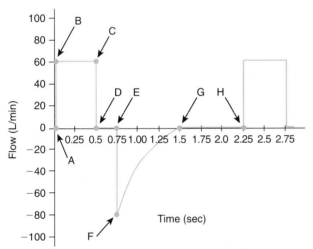

Figure 15-2 Analysis of key points in a flow/time graph. Shown is the inspiratory rectangular waveform during volume ventilation and exhalation of the tidal volume. *A,* Start of inspiratory flow. *B,* Peak inspiratory flow of 60 L/min (1 L/sec). *C,* End of inspiratory flow. Total inspiratory flow time is found between points *B* and *C* (0.5 sec) when the tidal volume is delivered. The tidal volume can be calculated at 500 mL. (1 L/sec of flow × 0.5 sec of inspiratory time = .5 L [500 mL] tidal volume.) *D* and *E,* Inspiratory hold (inflation hold) of 0.25 second after the end of inspiration. Without inspiratory hold, the patient would begin exhalation at point *D.* Total inspiratory time is 0.75 second (0.5 sec inspiratory flow time + 0.25 inspiratory hold time = 0.75 second). *F,* Peak expiratory flow of −80 L/min (−1.33 L/sec). *G,* End of expiratory flow. Expiratory flow time is 0.75 second. *H,* Start of the next inspiration. *G* and *H,* 0.75 second of zero flow time. Total expiratory time is 1.5 second (0.75 sec expiratory flow time + 0.75 sec zero flow time). Inspiratory/expiratory (I:E) ratio is 1:2 (0.75 sec of total inspiratory time/1.5 sec of total expiratory time). *(Modified from Pilbeam SP: Ventilator graphics. In: Pilbeam SP, Cairo JM (editors): Mechanical ventilation: physiologic and clinical applications, ed 4, St Louis, 2006, Mosby.)*

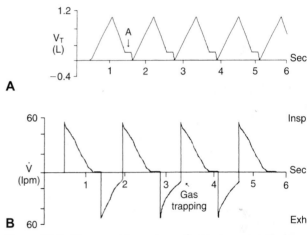

Figure 15-3 Two graphic tracings of expiratory air trapping. *Top,* Volume vs. time. *A* shows that the exhaled tidal volume tracing does not reach the baseline. Inspiratory tidal volume is greater than expiratory tidal volume, indicating air trapping. *Bottom,* Flow vs. time. Inspiratory flow is the tracing above the horizontal baseline of zero flow. Expiratory flow is the tracing below the horizontal baseline. The patient's expiratory flow does not return to zero; this indicates air trapping. The higher the flow rate, the more air trapping is present. Air trapping leads to auto-positive end-expiratory pressure. It can be minimized by increasing expiratory time, giving an aerosolized bronchodilator to treat bronchospasm, or suctioning out any secretions. *(Reprinted by permission of Nellcor Puritan Bennett LLC, Boulder, CO, part of Covidien.)*

Figure 15-4   Decreased dynamic compliance *(Cdyn)* with a stable static compliance *(Cst)*. **A,** Original pressure manometer reading and pressure/volume curve. **B,** Altered pressure manometer reading and pressure/volume curve.

Exam Hint 15-1 (WRE)

Expect to see at least one examination question that describes a waveform or shows a waveform that must be analyzed.

---

2. Review the patient's chart for information on the work of breathing (Code: IA7d) [Difficulty: ELE: R; WRE: Ap]

Work of breathing (WOB) normally refers to how much energy the patient has to expend to inhale. Patients with stiff lungs or high airway resistance or both have an increased WOB. Exhalation normally is passive and requires no work. However, some patients with high airway resistance have to work to exhale. Look in the patient's chart for information on patient complaints of shortness of breath and easy tiring as signs of increased WOB.

A patient who has been intubated and placed on a modern mechanical ventilator with a microprocessor and graphics software can have WOB measured. See Figure 15-5 for a pressure/volume loop tracing that shows a patient's WOB. WOB is minimized when the ventilator is set to minimize the negative pressure and inspiratory flow the patient has to generate.

If the breathing of an intubated and ventilated patient appears to be unsynchronized with the ventilator, his or her WOB should be evaluated. Ask the conscious patient

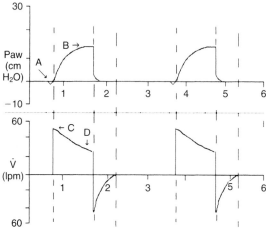

Figure 15-5   Two graphic tracings of pressure support ventilation. *Top graphic* shows pressure/volume loop of a patient triggering a breath. *A,* Amount of work patient has to provide. *Shaded area on right side* indicates how much work was provided by ventilator. *Bottom graphic* shows pressure (Paw) vs. time and flow (V̇) vs. time tracings. *A,* Where patient initiated a breath. *B,* Where ventilator cycled off when pressure support level of 15 cm water was reached. *C,* High peak flow at start of the breath. *D,* How flow rate decreases as pressure support level is reached. *(Reprinted by permission of Nellcor Puritan Bennett Inc LLC, Boulder CO, part of Covidien.)*

simple questions to try to determine what the problem is. Observe the patient for use of accessory muscles as a sign of increased WOB. If the ventilator is capable, program it to perform a pressure/volume loop of the patient's WOB. Be prepared to adjust parameters such as the machine's sensitivity and inspiratory flow to minimize the patient's workload.

3. Airway resistance

a. Review the patient's chart for information on airway resistance (Code: IA7d) [Difficulty: ELE: R; WRE: Ap]

Airway resistance (Raw) may have been measured earlier in the pulmonary function laboratory or on the ventilator.

Compare any earlier values with new measurements. This is important for understanding the patient's trends toward an improving or worsening pulmonary condition.

Airway resistance is measured in units of centimeters of water per liter per second at a standard flow rate of 0.5 L/sec (30 L/min). The normal spontaneously breathing adult's Raw is 0.6 to 2.4 cm water/L/sec; the normal 3-kg infant's Raw is 30 cm water/L/sec. Do not forget that this procedure is being performed on a patient with an intubated airway on a ventilator. The endotracheal tube adds to the patient's total Raw. The smaller the tube, the greater is the resistance that it offers to gas flowing through it. Altering inspiratory flow has an influence on the peak pressure measured for the calculation. As flow is reduced, gas turbulence is reduced and peak pressure is reduced. Conversely, a higher flow creates more turbulence and a higher peak pressure is seen.

b. Recommend measurement of the patient's airway resistance (Code: IC7) [Difficulty: ELE: R, Ap; WRE: An]

This calculation is important because it provides valuable information on the patient's pulmonary condition. The Raw value indicates how difficult it is to move the tidal volume through the patient's airways and whether aerosolized bronchodilating medications are effective.

It is reasonable to recommend an airway resistance measurement on any patient who has an increased airway resistance problem such as chronic obstructive pulmonary disease (COPD), asthma, bronchospasm, or wheezing breath sounds. It also is reasonable to measure airway resistance before and after a bronchodilator medication is given to determine whether it had any benefit.

c. Determine the patient's airway resistance (Code: IB9n) [Difficulty: ELE: R, Ap; WRE: An]

Most of the microprocessor ventilators offer software for calculating all of these values. However, in other situations, they must be calculated manually.

1. Procedure for calculating airway resistance

1. Cycle a tidal volume. The patient should be breathing passively; fighting the breath will result in an erroneously high peak pressure, and assisting with the breath will result in an erroneously low peak pressure.
2. Note the peak airway pressure on the manometer.
3. Briefly prevent the tidal volume from being exhaled. No air should be moving. Note that the pressure manometer shows a peak pressure and then a static or plateau pressure that is stable as long as the tidal volume is held in the lungs. Record the plateau pressure.

4. Calculate the flow in liters per second by taking the flow in liters per minute and dividing it by 60 seconds.
5. Place the peak airway pressure, plateau pressure, and flow into the following formula and solve for airway resistance:

$$Raw = \frac{\text{Peak airway pressure} - \text{Plateau pressure}}{\text{Flow in L/sec}}$$

Exam Hint 15-2 (ELE)

The airway resistance calculation has been tested on previous examinations, so review the math.

EXAMPLE

A mechanically ventilated patient has a peak airway pressure of 30 cm water and a plateau pressure of 20 cm water. The peak flow is set at 60 L/min.

Calculate peak flow in liters per second:

$$\frac{60\,\text{L/min}}{60\,\text{sec}} = 1\,\text{L/sec}$$

Calculate airway resistance:

$$Raw = \frac{\text{Peak airway pressure} - \text{Plateau pressure}}{\text{Flow in L/sec}}$$

$$Raw = \frac{30\,\text{cm H}_2\text{O} - 20\,\text{cm H}_2\text{O}}{1\,\text{L/sec}} = 10\,\text{cm H}_2\text{O/L/sec}$$

This value is greater than normal for a patient who is breathing spontaneously. However, remember that the patient's airway is intubated. This results in a smaller airway diameter and greater resistance. Some practitioners use the calculated airway resistance as the basis for setting the pressure support ventilation (PSV) level (discussed later). Increased airway resistance may indicate bronchospasm or secretions in the airways. Delivering an aerosolized bronchodilator or suctioning should result in the return of resistance to the original level.

4. Auto-PEEP detection

a. Perform the procedure to detect auto-PEEP (WRE code: IB9w) [Difficulty: WRE: R, Ap, An]

Auto-PEEP is positive end-expiratory pressure in the lungs that cannot be seen on the ventilator's pressure manometer. (The terms *inadvertent PEEP* and *intrinsic PEEP* also are used.) Auto-PEEP is caused by air trapping resulting from an inadequate expiratory time. It becomes more likely when the inspiratory time is increased or the expiratory time is decreased, or in patients with long time constants of ventilation. Simply put, the next breath is delivered before the patient has exhaled completely (see Figure 15-3). This problem is seen frequently in patients with status asthmaticus or COPD because of early small airway closure. In patients with acute respiratory distress syndrome (ARDS) who are receiving pressure-controlled inverse ratio ventilation (PCIRV), the long inspiratory times used increase the risk of expiratory air trapping. Auto-PEEP is more likely to be found when the inspiratory/expiratory (I:E) ratio becomes 2:1 or greater.

The level of auto-PEEP can be determined in different ways, depending on the type of ventilator that is being used. It can be measured on the pressure manometer of most ventilators. The trapped expiratory gas also can be seen on the graphic display of all current generation microprocessor-type ventilators. The following procedure can be followed for determining the presence or level of auto-PEEP:

1. Note the delivery of a tidal volume.
2. Watch the pressure gauge as it decreases to zero (or the level of therapeutic PEEP) at the end of exhalation. Make sure that the patient is exhaling passively to obtain an accurate reading.
3. Reduce the rate control to delay the next breath.
4. Occlude the expiratory tubing (or push the expiratory hold button or add inflation hold on other ventilators) to prevent any further exhalation for about 3 to 5 seconds. See Figure 15-6.
5. If the pressure gauge is being monitored, note any pressure increase above the baseline pressure, or, if the ventilator has a graphics monitor, note the failure of the exhaled tidal volume or expiratory flow to return to baseline to confirm the presence and amount of auto-PEEP (see Figure 15-4).
6. Listen to the patient's breath sounds during a standard breath and during the prolonged exhalation. It is likely that during the standard breath, expiratory sounds will be heard until inspiratory sounds begin. During prolonged exhalation, the expiratory sounds continue for a longer time and then end with silence. This silent pause time indicates that no more expiratory airflow is occurring.

It is important to add any auto-PEEP to the amount of therapeutic PEEP the patient has. This should be recorded as the total PEEP. For example, the patient has 5 cm of therapeutic PEEP and 2 cm of auto-PEEP for 7 cm of total PEEP. It may be thought that the total PEEP level places the patient at risk for volutrauma or decreased venous return and lowered cardiac output. The amount of auto-PEEP can be reduced by decreasing the inspiratory time, increasing the expiratory time, or decreasing the tidal volume. Lack of auto-PEEP can be confirmed by this procedure. If the auto-PEEP cannot be eliminated, therapeutic PEEP can be added to match it. By increasing the baseline pressure, the patient can more easily trigger an

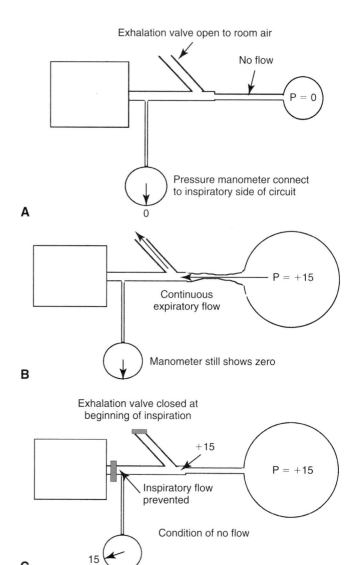

Figure 15-6 Identification of auto–positive end-expiratory pressure (PEEP) from air trapping. **A,** A normal patient will completely exhale before the next tidal volume breath is delivered. The manometer shows a pressure of zero (ambient, atmospheric pressure), which matches the patient's airway and lung pressures. **B,** A patient with increased airway resistance (asthma or chronic obstructive pulmonary disease [COPD]) who is not able to exhale completely before the next breath is started. Even though the manometer shows zero pressure, pressure from the trapped gas is increased within the airways and lungs. **C,** Auto-PEEP can be measured by closing the exhalation valve at the end of inspiration and stopping the next tidal volume breath. During this prolonged expiratory time, flow and pressure equilibrate. The manometer pressure now shows the actual increased pressure with the patient's airways and lungs. Reduce auto-PEEP by reducing airway resistance and increasing the expiratory time. *(Redrawn from PePe PE, Marini JJ: Am Rev Respir Dis 126:166, 1982, in Pilbeam S, Cairo J [editors]: Mechanical ventilation, ed 4, St Louis, 2009, Mosby.)*

assisted or synchronous intermittent mandatory ventilation (SIMV) breath. It is especially important to decrease auto-PEEP and therapeutic PEEP levels as the patient's lung compliance improves and airway resistance returns to normal.

b. Interpret ventilator graphics to detect auto-PEEP (WRE code: IB10w) [Difficulty: WRE: R, Ap, An]

Figure 15-3 demonstrates two ways that air trapping on exhalation can be identified as auto-PEEP (unintended positive end-expiratory pressure). Note in Figure 15-3 (bottom) that the patient's expiratory flow does not reach baseline pressure before another breath is delivered. This proves that air trapping has occurred. The larger the gap between the pressure at the end of expiration and at baseline, the greater is the air trapping.

5. Determine the patient's plateau pressure (Code: IB9n) [Difficulty: ELE: R, Ap; WRE: An]

The plateau pressure on the ventilator is determined for evaluation of the patient's lung compliance (C_{LT}). A change in the patient's lung compliance will correlate with changes in the patient's lung condition. The following two areas of discussion cover lung compliance, performing the lung compliance procedure, and interpreting the results.

There are two ways to determine the plateau pressure. First, have the patient lie passively and set the ventilator to prevent a delivered tidal volume from being exhaled (inflation hold). Second, have the patient lie passively, and manually cover the end of the expiratory tubing to prevent a delivered tidal volume from being exhaled.

The hold should be held for about 2 seconds so that the pressure manometer value is stable. Note the pressure as the plateau pressure (see Figure 15-4, *A*). After the plateau pressure has been determined, the patient must exhale completely. It may be necessary to delay the next timed ventilator tidal volume breath to avoid "stacking" a new breath when the first has not yet been exhaled. It is recommended that the plateau pressure procedure be repeated to ensure that the measured pressure is accurate.

6. Lung compliance

a. Review the patient's chart for information on lung compliance (Code: IA7d) [Difficulty: ELE: R; WRE: Ap]

This value may have been measured earlier in the pulmonary function laboratory or on the ventilator. Compare any earlier values with new values. This is important for determining the patient's trends toward an improving or worsening pulmonary condition.

The compliance values indicate how easily the tidal volume can be delivered into the lungs. Static compliance (Cst) is the measurement of work required to overcome the elastic resistance to ventilation. It is a measurement of the compliance of the lungs and thorax (C_{LT}). Static compliance is measured in units of milliliters per centimeters of water pressure. The normal adult's static compliance is 100 mL/cm water; the normal 3-kg infant's static compliance is 5 mL/cm water.

Dynamic compliance (Cdyn), sometimes called *dynamic characteristic,* is the measurement of the combination of the patient's static compliance and airway resistance. As was discussed previously, airway resistance is the pressure required to move a tidal volume through the airways. It also is known as *nonelastic resistance to ventilation.*

b. Recommend measurement of the patient's lung compliance (Code: IC7) [Difficulty: ELE: R, Ap; WRE: An]

It is reasonable to recommend that lung compliance should be measured on any patient who has clinical evidence of a significant change in lung compliance. This may occur in conditions such as ARDS, pneumonia, pulmonary edema, or pulmonary fibrosis. Compliance can be measured to document worsening of the patient's condition or to determine whether compliance is improving with treatment.

c. Determine the patient's plateau pressure and lung compliance (Code: IB9n) [Difficulty: ELE: R, Ap; WRE: An]

Most microprocessor ventilators offer software that can be used for calculating all of these values. However, in other situations, they must be calculated manually, as follows.

1. Procedure for calculating the tubing compliance factor

Before the actual calculation of the patient's static and dynamic compliance can be performed, the compliance of the breathing circuit should be determined. During positive-pressure ventilation, some of the set tidal volume never reaches the patient because it is "lost" in the circuit. Remember that when a positive-pressure breath is delivered, the ventilator circuit will be expanded and the gas within the tubing will be compressed. The term *compressed volume* is commonly used to describe this lost volume. Subtract the compressed volume from the exhaled volume coming from the ventilator to determine the patient's actual tidal volume. (Some of the current generation of microprocessor ventilators will calculate the compressed volume. The therapist can have the ventilator compensate for the lost volume and deliver a tidal volume that meets the set volume on the ventilator.)

For greatest accuracy in the calculation of static and dynamic compliance and the calculation of actual tidal and sigh volumes, any lost volume must be subtracted from the exhaled tidal volume to find the actual tidal volume. The tubing compliance factor is used in the calculation to determine the compressed volume, through the following procedure:

1. Remove the patient from the ventilator and manually ventilate him or her during this procedure.
2. Set the pressure limit as high as possible.
3. Block the breathing circuit at the patient connector. Make sure there are no leaks.
4. Cycle a tidal volume. If possible, set inflation hold for 2 seconds to see a stable pressure.
5. Perform either of the following: (a) note the pressure developed in the circuit as the tidal volume stretches out the circuit; or (b) if the ventilator's peak pressure hits the pressure limit, note the delivered tidal volume and the pressure limit. In both cases, measure the exhaled tidal volume.

   Note: If the patient is receiving PEEP therapy, subtract the PEEP level from the measured pressure to find the true pressure.
6. The compliance factor is found by dividing the exhaled tidal volume by the pressure.
7. Return the patient to the ventilator.

EXAMPLE

The patient has a set tidal volume of 600 mL. By using step 5b, the pressure is found to be 80 cm water, and the measured tidal volume is found to be 320 mL.

$$\text{Compliance factor} = \frac{320\,\text{mL}}{80\,\text{cm}} = 4\,\text{mL/cm water}$$

The compressed volume is found by multiplying the compliance factor by either the peak or the plateau pressure when a tidal volume is delivered. The compressed volume is then subtracted from the exhaled tidal volume to determine the patient's actual tidal volume.

 Exam Hint 15-3 (ELE, WRE)

Commonly, examinations have had a question requiring the calculation of static compliance or dynamic compliance or both. Be able to perform the following calculations.

2. Procedure for calculating static compliance

1. Determine the compliance factor of the breathing circuit (as described previously).

2. Reattach the patient to the ventilator. Reset all controls to their ordered or preset positions.
3. Cycle a tidal volume. The patient should be breathing passively; fighting the breath will result in an erroneously high peak pressure, and assisting with the breath will result in an erroneously low peak pressure.
4. Briefly prevent the tidal volume from being exhaled. No air should be moving. Note that the pressure manometer shows a peak pressure and then a static or plateau pressure that is stable as long as the tidal volume is held in the lungs. Note the *plateau* pressure.
5. Calculate the Cst by using this formula:

$$Cst = \frac{\text{Exhaled tidal volume} - \text{Compressed volume}}{\text{Plateau pressure} - \text{PEEP}}$$

in which compressed volume is Compliance factor × Plateau pressure.

3. Procedure for calculating dynamic compliance

1. Determine the compliance factor of the breathing circuit (as described previously).
2. Reattach the patient to the ventilator. Reset all controls to their ordered or preset positions.
3. Cycle a tidal volume. The patient should be breathing passively; fighting the breath will result in an erroneously high peak pressure, and assisting with the breath will result in an erroneously low peak pressure.
4. Note the *peak pressure* on the manometer. If the pressure at the end of inspiration is less than the peak pressure, the pressure at the end of inspiration should be used in the calculation.
5. Calculate the dynamic compliance (Cdyn) by using this formula:

$$Cdyn = \frac{\text{Exhaled tidal volume} - \text{Compressed volume}}{\text{Peak pressure} - \text{PEEP}}$$

in which compressed volume is Compliance factor × Peak pressure.

EXAMPLE

Calculate the static and dynamic compliance on a ventilated patient *without PEEP* therapy.

The patient has an exhaled tidal volume of 600 mL. The peak pressure is 30 cm water, and the static or plateau pressure is 20 cm water. The compliance factor has been determined to be 4 mL/cm water. The compressed volume at the plateau pressure is determined to be 80 mL (4 mL/cm compliance factor × 20 cm). The compressed volume at the peak pressure is determined to be 120 mL (4 mL/cm compliance factor × 30 cm).

$$Cst = \frac{600\ mL - 80\ mL}{20\ cm - 0}$$
$$= \frac{520\ mL}{20\ cm}$$
$$= 26\ mL/cm\ water$$

$$Cdyn = \frac{600\ mL - 120\ mL}{30\ cm - 0}$$
$$= \frac{480\ mL}{30\ cm}$$
$$= 16\ mL/cm\ water$$

EXAMPLE

Calculate the static and dynamic compliance on a ventilated patient *with PEEP* therapy.

The same patient has an exhaled tidal volume of 600 mL. Because of refractory hypoxemia, 10 cm of PEEP therapy is started. The peak pressure is now 36 cm water, and the static or plateau pressure is now 25 cm water. The compliance factor has been determined to be 4 mL/cm water. The compressed volume at the plateau pressure is determined to be 60 mL [4 mL/cm compliance factor × 15 cm (25 cm − 10 cm PEEP)]. The compressed volume at the peak pressure is determined to be 104 mL [4 mL/cm compliance factor × 26 cm (36 cm − 10 cm PEEP)].

$$Cst = \frac{600\ mL - 60\ mL}{25\ cm - 10\ cm}$$
$$= \frac{540\ mL}{15\ cm}$$
$$= 36\ mL/cm\ water$$

$$Cdyn = \frac{600\ mL - 104\ mL}{36\ cm - 10\ cm}$$
$$= \frac{496\ mL}{26\ cm}$$
$$= 19\ mL/cm\ water$$

7. Interpret the patient's lung mechanics results: plateau pressure, airway resistance, dynamic lung compliance, and static lung compliance values on the ventilator (Code: IB10n) [Difficulty: ELE: R, Ap; WRE: An]

Exam Hint 15-4 (ELE, WRE)

Every examination has had questions that deal with the interpretation of increasing or decreasing peak pressure (changing airway resistance) or increasing or decreasing plateau pressure (changing lung compliance). Be able to identify a clinical change, possible causes of the change, and corrective actions.

Any increase in airway resistance or decrease in lung compliance or both creates an increase in the patient's WOB. Examples of conditions or situations in which an increased airway resistance is found include bronchospasm, secretions, mucosal edema, airway tumor, placement of a small endotracheal tube, and biting or kinking of the endotracheal tube. Lung compliance is decreased by pneumonia, pulmonary edema, ARDS, pulmonary fibrosis, atelectasis, consolidation, hemothorax, pleural effusion, air trapping, pneumomediastinum, and pneumothorax. Examples of chest wall and abdominal conditions that reduce compliance include various chest wall deformities, circumferential chest or abdominal burns, enlarged liver, pneumoperitoneum, peritonitis, abdominal bleeding, herniation, and advanced pregnancy. Correction of the problem should return the patient's ventilator pressure(s) to baseline and normalize the patient's WOB.

Six possible combinations of increasing or decreasing static and dynamic lung compliance exist. Each has its own possible causes and is discussed in turn. The patient must be passive on the ventilator for the measured values to be accurate. Check two or three breaths for increased accuracy. Let the patient have a normal breath or two between each of the peak and plateau pressure measurement breaths.

a. Decreased dynamic compliance with stable static compliance

Decreased dynamic compliance with stable static compliance is noticed as an *increase* in the peak pressure with an unchanged plateau pressure (see Figure 15-4). It is caused by increased airway resistance (bronchospasm, secretions, water in the circuit, kinked circuit, or endotracheal tube). Correction of the underlying problem results in return of the peak pressure to the original level.

Note that the inspiratory resistance has doubled from the original 10 to 20 cm, while the plateau pressure has not changed. This confirms that the problem originates in the airway or breathing circuit. The patient's lung compliance has not changed.

b. Increased dynamic compliance with stable static compliance

Increased dynamic compliance with stable static compliance is noticed as a *decrease* in peak pressure with an unchanged plateau pressure (Figure 15-7). This represents an improvement in the patient's airway resistance from the original condition. Secretions can be diminished, mucus plugs cleared, bronchospasm corrected, and so forth.

Note that the inspiratory resistance has decreased from the original level of 20 cm to just 5 cm. This confirms that the patient's airway resistance has decreased. The patient's lung compliance has not changed.

c. False decreased dynamic compliance with true decreased static compliance

False decreased dynamic compliance with true decreased static compliance is noticed as an *increase* in *both* peak and

Figure 15-7   Increased dynamic compliance *(Cdyn)* with a stable static compliance *(Cst)*. **A,** Original pressure manometer reading and pressure/volume curve. **B,** Altered pressure manometer reading and pressure/volume curve.

Figure 15-8   False decreased dynamic compliance *(Cdyn)* with true decreased static compliance *(Cst)*. **A,** Original pressure manometer reading and pressure/volume curve. **B,** Altered pressure manometer reading and pressure/volume curve.

plateau pressures (Figure 15-8). This is seen when the patient's lung/thoracic compliance worsens. The plateau pressure is elevated, and the static compliance is decreased.

As an artifact of the stiffer lungs, the peak pressure also is elevated and the dynamic compliance is decreased. However, the difference between peak and plateau pres-

Figure 15-9   True decreased dynamic compliance *(Cdyn)* with true decreased static compliance *(Cst)*. **A,** Original pressure manometer reading and pressure/volume curve. **B,** Altered pressure manometer reading and pressure/volume curve.

sures remains the same. This demonstrates that no real increase in the patient's airway resistance has occurred.

d. True decreased dynamic compliance with true decreased static compliance

True decreased dynamic compliance with true decreased static compliance also is noticed as an *increase* in *both* peak and plateau pressures (Figure 15-9). This is seen with the combination of decreased lung compliance and increased airway resistance. Causes of both of these problems were discussed earlier.

e. False increased dynamic compliance with true increased static compliance

False increased dynamic compliance with true increased static compliance is noticed as a *decrease* in *both* peak and plateau pressures (Figure 15-10). This is seen when the patient's lung/thoracic compliance improves. The plateau pressure decreases, and, as an artifact, the peak pressure also decreases. Notice that the difference between peak and plateau pressures remains the same. This indicates that the patient's airway resistance is unchanged.

f. True increased dynamic compliance with true increased static compliance

True increased dynamic compliance with true increased static compliance also is noticed as a *decrease* in *both* peak and plateau pressures (Figure 15-11). This is seen when the patient's airway resistance and his or her lung/thoracic compliance improve. Notice that the plateau pressure has decreased, thus indicating more compliant lungs.

Figure 15-10 False increased dynamic compliance *(Cdyn)* with true increased static compliance *(Cst)*. **A,** Original pressure manometer reading and pressure/volume curve. **B,** Altered pressure manometer reading and pressure/volume curve.

Figure 15-11 True increased dynamic compliance *(Cdyn)* with true increased static compliance *(Cst)*. **A,** Original pressure manometer reading and pressure/volume curve. **B,** Altered pressure manometer reading and pressure/volume curve.

Also notice that the difference between peak and plateau pressures has decreased. This demonstrates that the airway resistance also has decreased.

All six examples of increasing or decreasing static or dynamic lung compliance or both make use of a single tidal volume that is analyzed for peak and plateau pres-

sures. Some practitioners advocate using several different tidal volumes (e.g., 8, 10, and 12 mL/kg of ideal body weight) when measuring dynamic and static pressures. The measured values are plotted on a graph to find the patient's optimal tidal volume that results in the highest static compliance value. Figure 15-12 shows a series of these graphs. The curves for diseased lungs and airways are quite different from those of a normal person or a patient with a pulmonary embolism. Because of this, a pulmonary embolism should be considered if the patient's condition deteriorates rapidly and no change in dynamic or static compliance values is observed.

MODULE B

Provide conventional mechanical ventilation to adequately oxygenate and ventilate the patient.

Conventional mechanical ventilation is defined here as the use of a single ventilator that can provide the customary modes and options needed by the large majority of patients. This ventilatory support is provided through an endotracheal tube or a tracheostomy tube. Several physiologic criteria have been compiled to help the clinician determine when a patient is in respiratory or ventilatory failure (Box 15-1) and needs ventilatory support. Remember that the patient may not fail each and every criterion; however, the patient often will fail one or more criteria in each category.

BOX 15-1   Indications for Ventilatory Support

VENTILATION
Apnea
$PaCO_2$ ≥55 torr in a patient who is not ordinarily hypercapneic
Dead space: tidal volume (V_D/V_T ratio) of >0.55-0.6 (55%-60%)

OXYGENATION
PaO_2 <80 torr on 50% oxygen or more
$P(A-a)O_2$ <300-350 torr on 100% oxygen
Intrapulmonary shunt >5%-20%

PULMONARY MECHANICS
Spontaneous tidal volume 3-4 mL/lb or 7-9 mL/kg of ideal body weight
Vital capacity <10-15 mL/kg
Maximum inspiratory pressure (MIP) <−20 to −25 cm water pressure
Forced expiratory volume in 1 second (FEV_1) <10 mL/kg
Respiratory rate <12 breaths/min or >35 breaths/min in an adult
Rapid, shallow breathing index (breaths/minute divided by tidal volume in liters) >105

MISCELLANEOUS
Unconscious patient
Unstable and unacceptable vital signs
Unstable cardiac rhythm caused by hypoxemia and/or acidosis
Worsening cardiopulmonary or other major organ system

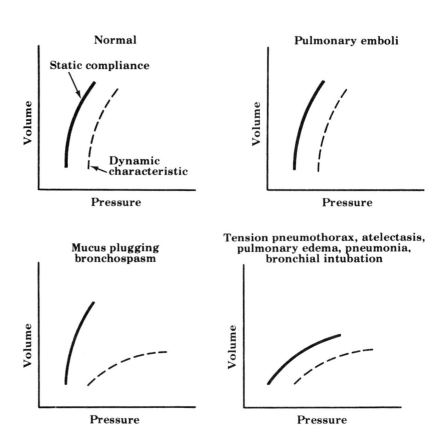

Figure 15-12 Pressure/volume curves for normal airways and lungs, pulmonary embolism (no change in airway resistance or lung compliance), increased airway resistance, and decreased lung compliance. *(From Bone RC: Respir Care 28[5]:597, 1983.)*

1. Perform the following procedures to make sure that the patient is adequately oxygenated

a. Minimize hypoxemia by positioning the patient properly (WRE code: IIID7) [Difficulty: Ap, An]

Most patients who receive mechanical ventilation will be in the supine position. However, if a patient is short of breath when lying supine, he/she should be repositioned to sit more upright in a Fowler's or semi-Fowler's position. This seems to work best in patients with bilateral pulmonary problems such as congestive heart failure or pneumonia. If the patient cannot sit up and the lung problem is one-sided, roll the patient so that the more functional lung is *down*. The good lung should be positioned *up* in the following exceptions:

- Undrained pulmonary abscess that should not be drained into the good lung
- Neonatal congenital diaphragmatic hernia in which the good lung should not be compressed by the bowel in the chest cavity
- Pulmonary interstitial emphysema in which, by lying on the bad lung, the air leak and the functional residual capacity can be reduced.

In either case, always ask the patient whether the new position helps to make breathing easier. If not, reposition the patient until breathing is more comfortable with less shortness of breath. In general, Trendelenburg is not well tolerated. A patient with a closed head injury and brain edema should not be put into the Trendelenburg position. Recent research has shown that some patients with ARDS will be better oxygenated when placed in the prone position.

b. Administer oxygen, as needed, to prevent hypoxemia (ELE code: IIID6) [Difficulty: ELE: R, Ap, An]

Oxygen administration and adjustment were discussed in Chapter 6. In brief, the goal of oxygen administration is to keep the PaO_2 level of most patients between 60 and 90 torr and the SpO_2 level greater than 90%. Exceptions are the patient with COPD who is breathing on hypoxic drive and the patient who is in a cardiac arrest situation. The following formula can be used to help guide the use of supplemental oxygen in most stable patients:

$$\text{Desired } FIO_2 = \frac{\text{Desired } PaO_2 \times \text{Current } FIO_2}{\text{Current } PaO_2}$$

EXAMPLE

Your patient has a PaO_2 level of 55 mm Hg on 30% oxygen. The clinical goal is a PaO_2 level of 90 mm Hg. What oxygen percentage should the patient have?

$$\text{Desired } F_{I}O_2 = \frac{\text{Desired } Pa_{O_2} \times \text{Current } F_{I}O_2}{\text{Current } Pa_{O_2}}$$

$$\text{Desired } F_{I}O_2 = \frac{90 \text{ mm Hg} \times 0.3}{55 \text{ mm Hg}}$$

$$\text{Desired } F_{I}O_2 = \frac{27}{55}$$

$$\text{Desired } F_{I}O_2 = 0.49 \text{ or } 49\% \text{ oxygen}$$

Those patients who have refractory hypoxemia (e.g., ARDS) will not respond with a normal increase in Pa_{O_2} level as the oxygen percentage is increased. In the short term, use whatever oxygen percentage is needed to achieve the clinical goal. The risk of oxygen toxicity increases when the $F_{I}O_2$ is greater than 0.5 for periods of longer than 48 hours. Always recheck the patient's arterial oxygen level after a change in the $F_{I}O_2$ has been made.

Either of the following formulas can be used in the special situation of determining the flows of air and oxygen into a "bleed-in" type of intermittent mandatory ventilation (IMV) or continuous positive airway pressure (CPAP) system to obtain an ordered $F_{I}O_2$. Either version can be used for determining gas flows, total flow, and oxygen/air ratio through an air entrainment (Venturi) mask.

The first formula follows:

$$(\text{L/min air} \times F_{I}O_2 \text{ of air}) + (\text{L/min } O_2 \times F_{I}O_2 \text{ pure } O_2) = \text{Total flow} \times \text{Unknown } F_{I}O_2$$

The second formula follows:

$$F_1 C_1 + F_2 C_2 = F_T C_T$$

in which F_1 is the flow of first gas (oxygen), C_1 is the concentration of oxygen in the first gas (1.0 for pure oxygen), F_2 is the flow of second gas (air), C_2 is the concentration of oxygen in the second gas (0.21 for air), F_T is the total flow of both gases, and C_T is the concentration of oxygen in the mix of both gases. Use algebraic manipulation to solve for the unknown.

EXAMPLE

Determine the oxygen percentage through a bleed-in system that has an oxygen flow of 10 L/min and an airflow of 15 L/min. Determine the total flow through the system. Determine the ratio of oxygen to air.

$$(\text{L/min air} \times F_{I}O_2 \text{ of air}) +$$
$$(\text{L/min } O_2 \times F_{I}O_2 \text{ pure } O_2) = \text{Total flow} \times \text{Unknown } F_{I}O_2$$
$$(15 \times 0.21) + (10 \times 1.0) = (15 + 10) \times \text{Unknown } F_{I}O_2$$
$$(3.15) + (10) = (25) \times \text{Unknown } F_{I}O_2$$
$$13.15 = 25 \, F_{I}O_2$$

(Divide both sides by 25.)

$$0.526 \text{ or } 52.6\% = F_{I}O_2$$

$$\text{Total flow} = 15 + 10 = 25 \text{ L/min}$$

$$\text{Ratio} = \frac{10 \text{ L/min oxygen}}{15 \text{ L/min air}}$$

c. Adequately oxygenate the patient to prevent accidental hypoxemia before and after suctioning, changing the ventilator circuit, or performing other procedures in which the patient is disconnected from the ventilator (ELE code: IIID9) [Difficulty: ELE: R, Ap, An]

Ensuring adequate oxygenation during suctioning is discussed in Chapter 13. In brief, remember to give the adult patient 100% oxygen for at least 30 seconds before suctioning. Perform the task as quickly and safely as possible to minimize time off the ventilator. Leave the patient on 100% oxygen for at least 1 minute after the procedure is completed, or until he or she returns to a stable condition as before the procedure. Children younger than 6 months can have the $F_{I}O_2$ increased by 10% for the procedure.

In an adult, it is acceptable to increase the inspired oxygen up to 100% before and after a procedure that requires disconnection from the ventilator. The goal is to prevent hypoxemia. The patient should be ventilated manually with a resuscitation bag if indicated. Always remember to return the patient to the original oxygen percentage when clinically indicated.

2. Initiate and adjust continuous mechanical ventilation settings (Code: IIID2b) [Difficulty: ELE: R, Ap; WRE:An]

a. Sensitivity

Sensitivity is the term used to describe the amount of work or effort the patient must perform to trigger the ventilator to deliver a tidal volume breath. Many ventilators require the patient to generate a *negative pressure* to trigger the unit. The term *pressure triggering* is used often to describe this type of sensitivity. With these machines, the sensitivity usually is set at about −1 to −2 cm water pressure.

Several of the newer ventilators also have an option in which the patient generates an *inspiratory flow* to trigger a ventilator tidal volume breath. The term *flow-triggering* often is used to describe this sensitivity option on the ventilator. With a ventilator using flow triggering sensitivity, the patient initiates a tidal volume when his or her inspiratory flow is about 2 L/min (33 mL/sec) less than the set baseline flow through the circuit. Very weak patients find that it requires less effort with flow sensitivity than with pressure sensitivity to initiate a ventilator breath.

b. Flow

Flow is adjusted to set the inspiratory time and the I:E ratio. In addition, flow is set to meet the patient's needs.

Inspiratory flow should be great enough to minimize the WOB. Increase flow if the patient has signs of greater demand, such as using accessory muscles of inspiration or lack of synchrony with the ventilator, or if the pressure manometer deflects greatly below the baseline pressure or shows a low initial increase in inspiratory pressure.

In addition, most current generation ventilators offer more than one inspiratory flow pattern (see Figure 15-1). The sine wave is most physiologically like a normal, spontaneous inspiration. The other waveforms can be compared with the sine wave to determine which one best meets the patient's needs. Ideally, the best flow pattern is one in which the patient's peak and mean airway pressures are lowest, exhalation is complete, breath sounds are improved bilaterally, heart rate and blood pressure are stable, and the patient feels most comfortable.

c. I:E ratio

The I:E ratio is adjusted to ensure that the patient can inhale in as physiologically appropriate a manner as possible and completely exhale the inspired tidal volume. Typically, the I:E ratio should be 1:2 or more. Incomplete exhalation will cause air trapping and auto-PEEP (see Figure 15-3).

Exam Hint 15-5 (ELE, WRE)

Usually two questions are related to modifying the inspiratory flow to meet the patient's need for a faster breath or modifying the inspiratory/expiratory (I:E) ratio. Remember that if the patient has auto-positive end-expiratory pressure (PEEP), the expiratory time must be increased to allow a more complete exhalation.

---

d. Alarms

Alarm systems are different for each type of ventilator. Generally speaking, they are set with a safety margin of ±10% from the patient's normal ventilator settings. A variation of greater than 10% results in an audible or visual alarm condition. Most ventilators alarm if the I:E ratio is 1:1 or less.

e. Gas temperature

The goal for most patients is to minimize their humidity deficit by using gas that is humidified and warmed to near body temperature. This can be accomplished by a cascade- or wick-type humidifier or by a heat-moisture exchanger (HME). It is common to see the gas warmed to 90° F to 95° F (31° C to 35° C). This decreases the patient's humidity deficit to a minuscule level and reduces the "rain out" of water vapor condensing in the ventilator circuit. A temperature probe should be placed in the inspiratory tubing as close to the patient as possible to monitor the inspired gas temperature.

f. Modes of ventilation

The following modes of ventilation are delivered through most types of electrically powered and microprocessor-type volume-cycled ventilators.

1. Control

Control (C) is the simplest method of providing ventilatory support and is used on an apneic patient. The ventilator is set with a mandatory respiratory rate and tidal volume. The machine is incapable of allowing any patient interaction. For example, the ventilator might be set to deliver a tidal volume of 700 mL at a rate of 14 times/min. Because of this limitation, it is rarely, if ever, used in modern medicine except when the patient must be kept sedated or pharmacologically paralyzed (Figure 15-13, A shows the pressure/time curve).

2. Assist/control

The assist/control (A/C) mode has a set backup respiratory rate but allows the patient to trigger additional machine-delivered breaths. A sensitivity control is adjusted to allow the patient to start a breath easily as needed. All tidal volumes are the same (Figure 15-13, B shows the pressure/time curve).

3. Intermittent mandatory ventilation

IMV was used in older ventilators before there was a way to synchronize the patient and ventilator breaths. With IMV, a set backup respiratory rate and tidal volume are delivered to the patient. In addition, between mandatory breaths, the patient can breathe spontaneously as frequently as desired. The patient also can take in as large a spontaneous tidal volume as needed. The sensitivity control is set so that the patient cannot trigger any extra ventilator tidal volume breaths (Figure 15-13, C shows the pressure/time curve). The IMV mode has been replaced in modern ventilators with the SIMV mode, as discussed below.

4. Synchronous intermittent mandatory ventilation

SIMV is similar to IMV except that the sensitivity control is functional. The patient can trigger a machine-delivered tidal volume during a preset time interval. The timing of the backup rate is such that the patient can get only as many ventilator breaths as are set. Spontaneous tidal volumes vary with the patient's efforts. For example, the ventilator might be set to deliver a 700-mL tidal volume 8 times/min. Let us say that the patient breathes spontaneously 10 more times and has an average tidal volume of 400 mL. The total rate is counted at 18. The total minute volume is the combination of the machine's minute

Figure 15-13   Pressure vs. time waveforms for various modes of mechanical ventilation. **A,** Control (C) mode shows no patient effort and consistent inspiration/expiration ratios. **B,** Assist/control (A/C) mode shows that patient's initial effort triggers machine tidal volume breath. **C,** Intermittent mandatory ventilation (IMV) mode shows spontaneous tidal volume breaths occurring between predetermined machine tidal volume breaths. Note "stacked" breaths that happen when patient takes in a breath that then is supplemented by a machine breath. **D,** Synchronous intermittent mandatory ventilation (SIMV) mode shows that a patient effort within a time window results in delivery of machine tidal volume. Any other patient efforts within the time window result in a spontaneous tidal volume. If no patient efforts occur within the time window, machine tidal volume will be delivered automatically. **E,** Pressure support ventilation (PSV) mode shows how patient must initiate all breaths that then are supported to the predetermined airway pressure. Stable tidal volumes are seen if the patient inhales passively. Variably larger tidal volumes result if the patient inhales more actively. **F,** Positive end-expiratory pressure (PEEP) therapy can be added to A/C mode (as shown) or any other mode. The elevated baseline pressure prevents alveolar collapse. The sensitivity control must be set at −1 to −2 cm water so that the patient is able to trigger a breath without undue effort. **G,** Continuous positive airway pressure (CPAP) shows that the patient takes spontaneous tidal volumes while exhaling against an elevated baseline pressure.

volume and the patient's minute volume (Figure 15-13, *D* shows the pressure/time curve).

5. Pressure support ventilation

Pressure support ventilation (PS or PSV) is similar to intermittent positive-pressure ventilation (IPPV) in that when the patient initiates a ventilator breath, a preset pressure is delivered to the airway. The patient has the flexibility to determine the respiratory rate. The physician orders a PSV level for one of two reasons, depending on the clinical goal. First, enough PS is ordered to overcome the patient's calculated airway resistance. This

usually is done when the patient has an increased work of breathing from a smaller than ideal endotrachal tube. Second, PS is ordered to deliver a targeted tidal volume. In most cases, the tidal volume will be stable if the patient passively takes the PSV breath, or it can be larger if the patient interacts actively with the pressure that is delivered (Figures 15-5 and 15-13, *E* show the pressure/time curve).

Because PS utilizes a set delivered pressure, the patient's tidal volume can vary with changing lung compliance and/or airway resistance. To bring stability to the tidal volume under changing patient conditions, several ventilator manufacturers have developed automatic compensation systems. They are designed to provide additional volume if the patient's lung compliance and/or airway resistance should worsen. Conversely, they will reduce automatically the set pressure when the patient is easier to ventilate, so that too large a tidal volume will not be delivered. All manufacturers have their own name for this compensation system and have developed different ways to accomplish the goal of a stable tidal volume. Examples include *pressure augmentation* on the Bear 1000, *volume-assured pressure support* on the Bird 8400, *dual-control pressure ventilation* on the Puritan Bennett 840, *volume support* on the Servo-i, and *AutoFlow* on the Dräger Evita 4. It is beyond the scope of this text to cover each of these. However, the practitioner is encouraged to understand their essential features and to know that they are added to the pressure support mode to ensure a stable, ordered tidal volume.

6. Pressure control ventilation

Pressure control ventilation (PC or PCV) involves the delivery of tidal volume breaths that are pressure limited and time cycled. A set ventilator rate can be set and the patient can trigger additional breaths. Because the pressure is limited, tidal volumes may vary. This must be monitored closely in patients with frequently changing lung compliance and airway resistance. As the inspiratory time is increased, it can become longer than the expiratory time. This results in pressure control inverse ratio ventilation (PCIRV). Figure 15-14 shows the volume, flow, and pressure tracings.

As was discussed earlier with the PS mode, the patient's delivered tidal volume can vary with the PC mode when lung compliance and/or airway resistance is changing. Review the previous discussion on PS for the automatic compensation systems that manufacturers have added to their ventilators. Use of these ensures that the delivered tidal volume is stable in the PC mode despite changing patient conditions.

7. Airway pressure release ventilation

Several ventilator manufacturers offer the airway pressure release ventilation (APRV) mode (as well as other modes). These ventilators are microprocessor controlled and include a monitor for patient data and graphics. The APRV mode has been used with success in patients with ARDS who have not responded well to constant volume ventilation. APRV can be described simply as a mode in which the patient can breathe spontaneously at two different levels of CPAP. A difference from conventional CPAP is that the two levels are held for set periods. The ventilator options for this mode are simple. The practitioner sets the low pressure (P_{low}), the high pressure (P_{high}), and the times that the patient will be at those pressure levels. Low pressure sometimes is referred to as CPAP and high pressure as *release pressure*. The timing changes from low pressure to high pressure and back to low pressure effectively deliver a tidal volume. (See Figure 15-15 for a pressure/time tracing.)

When APRV is compared with other modes of ventilation, several similarities are evident between it and PCIRV

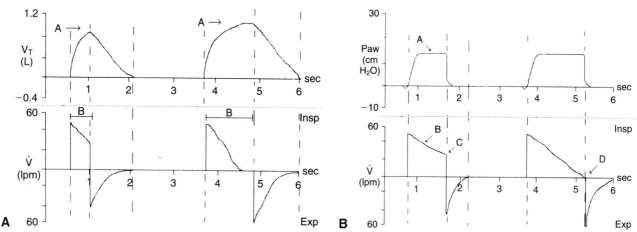

Figure 15-14   Two sets of graphic tracings of pressure control ventilation. **A,** Two tracings show volume (V_T) vs. time and flow (V̇) vs. time. *A* shows tidal volume; *B* shows inspiratory flow. Note how tidal volume increases as inspiratory time is increased. However, as is shown in the lower right tracing, as flow decreases to zero, no more volume is delivered. **B,** Two tracings show pressure vs. time and flow vs. time. *A* shows the pressure control level being reached with an inspiratory plateau or "square wave" appearance. *B* shows declining inspiratory flow. *C* shows final flow when inspiration is time cycled off and exhalation begins. This graphic can be used to help adjust a longer inspiratory time. If pressure control inverse ratio ventilation (PCIRV) were being optimally adjusted, the inspiration time could be increased until inspiratory flow reached zero (indicated by *D*). *(Image used by permission from Nellcore Puritan Bennett, LLC, Boulder CO, part of Covidien.)*

Figure 15-15 Airway pressure release ventilation (APRV) involves spontaneous breathing under one or two elevated baseline pressures. In the *top graph,* the patient can breathe during ambient pressure and during continuous positive airway pressure (CPAP). In the *bottom graph,* the patient breathes during a lower CPAP level and a higher CPAP level. In both situations, the patient breathes spontaneously at a high pressure level for a prolonged, adjustable length of time. Then, for a short, adjustable time, the higher pressure drops to the lower pressure level. This allows the patient to exhale a larger than usual volume. The higher pressure then is restored. This causes a large tidal volume to be inhaled. *(From Dupuis Y: Ventilators: theory and clinical applications, ed 2, St Louis, 1992, Mosby.)*

Figure 15-16 Pressure/volume loop showing lower and upper inflection points in a patient with acute respiratory distress syndrome (ARDS). *A,* Lower inflection point during inspiration that indicates the opening pressure of alveoli (15 cm water). This is the minimum positive end-expiratory pressure level needed to maintain a patient's functional residual capacity. *B,* Upper inflection point during inspiration that indicates that the lungs are being overstretched (40 cm water). This should be the upper limit of peak airway pressure to avoid overdistention and volutrauma. Flattening of the pressure/volume loop to the right of point *B* shows that little volume is delivered despite increased pressure. *C,* Upper inflection point of expiration (20 cm water). As the airway pressure drops below this point, alveolar collapse can occur.

with PEEP and bilevel ventilation. All have an elevated baseline pressure that allows the patient to breathe spontaneously. All have variable inspiratory times for the higher pressure level. None delivers a set tidal volume to the patient. The only real difference seems to be that the patient can breathe spontaneously at the higher pressure level only with APRV. If the patient does not make any respiratory efforts, APRV functions like PCV or bilevel ventilation.

A set of blood gases, vital signs, pulmonary artery catheter values, and so forth should be obtained on the current constant volume ventilator settings as a baseline before APRV is started. The following suggestions for initiating APRV are similar to those listed earlier for starting PCIRV:

1. Set the high pressure (release pressure) at the patient's optimal PEEP/CPAP level. Often this is in a range between the patient's static lung compliance pressure and peak pressure (Figure 15-16). The clinical goal is to maximize safely the patient's functional residual capacity (FRC).

2. Set the low pressure (CPAP) at the level of PEEP that was used on the constant volume ventilator. This is done to maintain the patient's FRC. See point *A* of Figure 15-16.

3. Set the inspired oxygen in the same way as before. Some may prefer to set it at 100%, as with PCIRV, until blood gas results show that it can be lowered.

4. Set the timing of the high pressure and low pressure values so that more time is spent at the high pressure than at the low pressure. Often the low pressure time is limited to 1 to 1.5 seconds. Keep the same respiratory rate as before. Even if the patient is apneic, as the ventilator switches from high pressure to low pressure, the patient exhales a tidal volume to blow off carbon dioxide.

Monitor the patient's ventilator delivered and spontaneous tidal volumes and rates. Check vital signs. Get an arterial blood gas (ABG) sample in about 15 minutes.

If the patient's initial blood gas results on APRV show hypoxemia, the following options are available: (1) increase the inspired oxygen percentage if it is not already at 100%, (2) increase the low pressure level, (3) increase the high pressure level, or (4) increase the time the patient is kept at the high pressure level. Reducing any or all of these options will decrease the patient's PaO_2 if it is too high.

If the blood gas results show hypoventilation, the following options are available: (1) increase the high pressure level, or (2) decrease the time at the high pressure level to increase the respiratory rate. Do the opposite to increase the $PaCO_2$ if the patient is being hyperventilated.

As with the previous ventilator modalities, the patient should be monitored closely and should have an ABG drawn for evaluation of every change.

Exam Hint 15-6 (ELE, WRE)

The NBRC examinations have used a variety of terms and phrases to describe modes or modifications of modes of ventilation, including the following:

Terms related to delivering a set tidal volume include volume ventilation; volume-cycled mechanical ventilation; volume-controlled ventilation; volume-preset ventilation; volume-controlled, flow-limited ventilation; volume-controlled, pressure-limited ventilation; volume-controlled with synchronous intermittent mandatory ventilation (SIMV), assist/control (A/C), or control (C); and volume-controlled with continuous flow intermittent mandatory ventilation (IMV) circuit added.

Terms related to not delivering a set tidal volume include pressure-cycled ventilation; pressure control; pressure-controlled, pressure-limited, time-cycled ventilation; pressure-controlled with constant inspiratory time; pressure-limited; and any previous term with inverse ratio ventilation.

BOX 15-2   Indications of Intermittent Mandatory Ventilation (IMV)/Synchronous Intermittent Mandatory Ventilation (SIMV) Tolerance

INDICATIONS THAT IMV/SIMV IS BEING WELL TOLERATED

Stable spontaneous respiratory rate
Stable heart rate
Stable spontaneous tidal volume
Stable vital capacity, minimal inspiratory pressure (MIP), and/or forced expiratory volume in 1 second (FEV_1)
No use or stable use of accessory muscles of ventilation
Patient indicates that he or she is comfortable
Stable blood gases

INDICATIONS THAT IMV/SIMV IS NOT BEING WELL TOLERATED

Increased spontaneous respiratory rate
Tachycardia or dysrhythmias such as premature ventricular contractions
Decrease in spontaneous tidal volume
Decrease in vital capacity, MIP, and/or FEV_1
Beginning or increased use of accessory muscles of ventilation
Patient complaints of dyspnea
Deterioration of blood gases as seen by a falling PaO_2 or SpO_2 and a rapidly falling or rising $PaCO_2$

---

3. Begin and modify combinations of ventilatory techniques to oxygenate the patient adequately: synchronous intermittent mandatory ventilation, pressure support ventilation, pressure control ventilation, and positive end-expiratory pressure (Code: IIID2b) [Difficulty: ELE: R, Ap; WRE: An]

The current generation of mechanical ventilators offers the physician and the practitioner a number of options for how best to tailor ventilatory support to meet the patient's needs. The following should be considered when one is deciding what modes to use and combine.

a. Increased work of breathing

Patients who show increased WOB may have a very high airway resistance, as in status asthmaticus, or may have a very low lung/thoracic compliance, as in ARDS. Some practitioners believe that the C or A/C mode, when applied properly to a sedated patient, is best for these problems because the patient's breathing efforts are almost eliminated. Other practitioners believe that IMV and SIMV are physiologically superior modes of ventilation. More recently, PSV has been shown to be beneficial to patients with increased efforts at breathing from the high airway resistance caused by a small-diameter endotracheal tube.

b. Hypercapnia

A patient may have hypercapnia (a high carbon dioxide level) because of sedation from a morphine or heroin overdose or may have COPD with worsening of the chronic

hypercapnia. In either case, the patient becomes progressively more hypoxemic (unless given supplemental oxygen) as the carbon dioxide level increases. Control or A/C modes are best for setting a minimum minute volume to determine the maximum carbon dioxide level. As the patient recovers, SIMV or PSV allows the gradual reduction of ventilatory support. See Box 15-2 for indications of SIMV tolerance.

c. Hypoxemia

If hypoxemia is secondary to a decreased FRC, as in ARDS or atelectasis, the treatment of choice for hypoxemia is CPAP on a free-standing system or PEEP on a conventional volume-cycled ventilator. If the problem results from an increased intrapulmonary shunt, the patient may need PEEP or CPAP, as well as up to 100% oxygen. See Box 15-3 for patient monitoring during PEEP and CPAP. PCIRV and high-frequency ventilation (HFV) have been used with success in hypoxemic patients with a pulmonary air leak for whom conventional volume ventilation has failed.

Often, when a patient has more than one problem, more than one solution will be needed. The following are combinations of modes from which to choose.

1. Mandatory minute ventilation

Mandatory minute ventilation (MMV) is a relatively new variation on the SIMV mode. It has been used as a weaning

BOX 15-3   Patient Monitoring During Therapy

GOOD TOLERANCE OF CPAP/PEEP THERAPY

Increased PaO_2
Increased static lung compliance
Stable cardiac output as shown by the following:
   Stable heart rate without rhythm disturbances
   Stable blood pressure
   The following can be measured only through a pulmonary
      artery/Swan-Ganz catheter:
   Stable or increased $Pv-O_2$ (mixed venous oxygen)
   Stable cardiac output
   Decreased pulmonary vascular resistance
   Decreased intrapulmonary shunt

POOR TOLERANCE OF CPAP/PEEP THERAPY

Increased PaO_2 (This can be deceiving if it is the only information
   observed.)
Decreased static lung compliance
Decreased cardiac output as shown by the following:
   Increased heart rate or rhythm disturbances
   Decreased blood pressure
   The following can be measured only through a pulmonary
      artery/Swan-Ganz catheter:
   Decreased $Pv-O_2$ (mixed venous oxygen)
   Decreased cardiac output
   Increased pulmonary vascular resistance
   Increased intrapulmonary shunt

---

mode that limits the increase in carbon dioxide if the patient should tire. With MMV, the patient is assured of a preset minute volume regardless of his or her spontaneous breathing. It has been proposed as an effective way to ventilate and wean patients who can breathe spontaneously but who have an unreliable respiratory drive and unstable tidal volume. Examples include patients who have received narcotic, sedative, anesthetic, or neuromuscular blocking medications. Patient conditions for which MMV is indicated include encephalopathy and cerebral disorders such as stroke. In addition, MMV may be used during the recovery period of a neuromuscular disease. Ventilators that include the MMV mode all are controlled by a microprocessor that monitors the ventilator's and the patient's tidal volume and rate. The following guidelines have been recommended for the initiation of MMV:

1. Set the ventilator tidal volume according to established guidelines (10 to 15 mL/kg of ideal body weight).
2. Spontaneous breaths may be taken through a demand valve or may be pressure supported.
3. Determine the minimum minute volume according to the patient's preexisting condition and the clinical goals:

The patient who has been on SIMV should have the MMV set at 90% of the SIMV-delivered minute volume. For example, the patient has an SIMV rate of 5 breaths/min and a tidal volume of 800 mL. Therefore the ventilator is delivering 4 L of minute volume (5 × 800 mL), and the MMV would be set at 3600 mL (90% of 4 L).

The patient who has been on A/C should have the mandatory minute volume set at 80% of the A/C-delivered minute volume. For example, the patient has an A/C rate of 10 breaths/min and a tidal volume of 1000 mL. Therefore the ventilator is delivering 10 L of minute volume (10 × 1000 mL), and the MMV would be set at 8 L (80% of 10 L).

Ideally MMV establishes a minimum safe volume of ventilation. If the patient inhales less than this volume, the ventilator delivers as many breaths as necessary at the preestablished tidal volume to make up the difference. Be aware that a patient who is breathing rapidly with a small tidal volume may move enough gas to exceed the minimum minute volume. Because of this risk, it is important to set a low tidal volume alarm or a high respiratory rate alarm or both to give warning. Do not let the programming of an MMV create a false sense of security with these patients.

2. Pressure control/pressure control inverse ratio ventilation, synchronous intermittent mandatory ventilation, and positive end-expiratory pressure

PCV or, if necessary, PCIRV has been used with success in patients with low compliance (ARDS) or a pulmonary air leak. When the peak pressure is limited, less air seems to leak out and the tissues are more likely to heal. Therapeutic PEEP is applied to increase the patient's FRC to correct hypoxemia. The SIMV feature is added to let the patient breathe spontaneously if desired and to stay more synchronized with the ventilator. With lung healing, the PEEP level is decreased and the inspiratory time is shortened. SIMV with a constant tidal volume may be used during the weaning phase. Figure 15-17 shows pressure and flow tracings during PCV.

3. Synchronous intermittent mandatory ventilation with pressure support ventilation and positive end-expiratory pressure

SIMV is used to give the patient a controlled number of deep tidal volume breaths. The patient can breathe as often as desired between the mandatory breaths. The patient's total minute volume can be determined by adding the combination of SIMV and pressure-supported breaths. A maximum acceptable $PaCO_2$ can be established with the proper combination of SIMV breaths and pres-

Figure 15-17 Modification of combinations of intermittent mandatory ventilation (IMV)/synchronous intermittent mandatory ventilation (SIMV), pressure support ventilation (PSV), and positive end-expiratory pressure (PEEP). **A,** IMV/ SIMV with PSV and PEEP. **B,** IMV/SIMV with PEEP. **C,** IMV/ SIMV with PSV. **D,** PSV with PEEP. See text for descriptions of various combinations and their clinical applications.

sure support (PS) level. A PS level of more than 10 cm water may be needed. In addition, the PS ensures that the airway resistance of the endotracheal tube is overcome. (See the airway resistance calculation earlier in the chapter.) PEEP therapy is applied to the level necessary to obtain a clinically safe PaO_2 at the lowest possible FIO_2. Figure 15-17, A shows the pressure/time curve.

Patients who have both a ventilation problem and an oxygenation problem benefit from these modes of ventilation. They have the desire to breathe on their own but a very limited ability to do so. All three modes can be adjusted independently for more or less support, as indicated by the patient's clinical condition and blood gas results.

4. Synchronous intermittent mandatory ventilation with positive end-expiratory pressure

IMV/SIMV and PEEP therapy are applied as indicated. Pressure support is not needed if the patient is strong

enough to overcome the airway resistance of the endotracheal tube and breathe with a clinically acceptable tidal volume. Figure 15-17, B shows the pressure/time curve.

5. Synchronous intermittent mandatory ventilation with pressure support ventilation

SIMV and PS levels are increased or decreased on the basis of the factors discussed earlier. This patient has the ability to provide some, but not all, of his or her own ventilation. The PaO_2 is clinically acceptable at an oxygen percentage probably no higher than 40%.

A fairly common clinical situation is seen in which the recovering patient does well on a gradually decreasing number of SIMV breaths until he or she can go no lower. The barrier seems to be the airway resistance of the endotracheal tube. (See the airway resistance calculation earlier in this chapter.) The addition of some PS overcomes that resistance so that the SIMV level can be reduced further. When the SIMV frequency is down to four or less, the patient is providing almost all of his or her minute volume. The greatest barrier to breathing is likely to be the resistance of the endotracheal tube. The decision then can be made to extubate the patient. Figure 15-17, C shows the pressure/time curve.

6. Pressure support ventilation with positive end-expiratory pressure

PSV and PEEP are applied as discussed earlier. This patient has the drive to breathe on his or her own; however, he or she has some limitation in the ability to overcome the resistance of the endotracheal tube or to generate a consistently large enough tidal volume. (See the airway resistance calculation earlier in the chapter.) In addition, the patient has a significant oxygenation problem and needs some PEEP therapy. With recovery, both PS and PEEP can be reduced. They may be reduced individually or simultaneously as the patient's strength and/or oxygenation improves. Figure 15-17, D shows the pressure/time curve.

Exam Hint 15-7 (ELE, WRE)

Usually several questions require the therapist to evaluate a patient and make a change in the mode of ventilation. Select "Assist/control" if the patient needs full support. Select "SIMV" if the patient needs to be partially supported. Frequently, one of the questions deals with identifying the need to increase the pressure support (PS) level to overcome the resistance of the endotracheal tube.

4. Choose and adjust the tidal volume for mechanical ventilation

A spontaneously breathing person exhales a large enough tidal volume (at the necessary respiratory rate) to remove carbon dioxide as fast as it is produced by his/her metabolism. This results in a normal carbon dioxide level and acid-base balance. Obviously, a person's tidal volume and respiratory rate will vary considerably with activity level. A 70-kg (154-lb) adult with normal lungs and metabolism needs a tidal volume of about 7 mL/kg (3 mL/lb) of ideal body weight to remove carbon dioxide adequately. So, this person would have a spontaneous tidal volume of about 500 mL (70 kg × 7 mL/kg). The Radford nomogram can be used for predicting normal spontaneous tidal volumes and rates on the basis of body weight (Figure 15-18). It can be used to help establish an initial target for the ventila-

tor tidal volume for many patients with normal lungs. However, because compressed volume within the ventilator circuit causes some of the set tidal volume to not reach the patient's lungs, a larger set tidal volume usually is needed. (Review "Procedure for calculating the tubing compliance factor" earlier in the chapter.) In addition, patients with lung problems will have different tidal volume requirements. Following are the current tidal volume recommendations based on the patient's pulmonary condition:

- **Normal lungs:** *Set* ventilator tidal volume of *10 to 12 mL/kg* of ideal body weight (IBW).

This might be a patient with a normal cardiopulmonary system who is receiving mechanical ventilation because of a neurologic problem. For example, the previously mentioned 70-kg (154-lb) adult with normal lungs needs a *set* mechanical ventilator tidal volume in the following range:

Figure 15-18 Radford nomogram. To use the nomogram, place the left edge of a ruler on the patient's estimated body weight and move the right edge to the patient's breathing frequency. The predicted basal tidal volume now can be found. For example, a 150-pound male who is breathing 12 times per minute will have a predicted tidal volume of 500 cc (mL). *(From Radford EP Jr: Ventilation standards for use in artificial respiration. J Appl Physiol 7[4]:451, 1955.)*

Corrections of predicted basal tidal volumes.
    For patients not in coma: add 10%
    Fever: add 5% for each °F above 99 (rectal)
            add 9% for each °C above 37 (rectal)
    Altitude: add 5% for each 2000 feet above sea level
            add 8% for each 1000 meters above sea level
    Intubation: subtract volume equal to one-half body weight in pounds
            subtract 1 cc/kg of body weight
    Dead space: add equipment dead space

$$10 \text{ mL} \times 70 \text{ kg} = 700 \text{ mL}$$

$$12 \text{ mL} \times 70 \text{ kg} = 840 \text{ mL}$$

- **Restrictive lung disease:** *Set* ventilator tidal volume of *4 to 8 mL/kg* of ideal body weight (IBW).

This might be a patient with ARDS who is at risk for pulmonary barotrauma/volutrauma. For example, the previously mentioned 70-kg (154-lb) adult with stiff lungs needs a *set* mechanical ventilator tidal volume in the following range:

$$4 \text{ mL} \times 70 \text{ kg} = 280 \text{ mL}$$

$$8 \text{ mL} \times 70 \text{ kg} = 560 \text{ mL}$$

- **Obstructive lung disease:** *Set* ventilator tidal volume of *8 to 10 mL/kg* of ideal body weight (IBW).

This might be a patient with COPD or status asthmaticus who is at risk for air trapping on exhalation. For example, the previously mentioned 70-kg (154-lb) adult with overstretched lungs needs a *set* mechanical ventilator tidal volume in the following range:

$$8 \text{ mL} \times 70 \text{ kg} = 560 \text{ mL}$$

$$10 \text{ mL} \times 70 \text{ kg} = 700 \text{ mL}$$

Remember that the set tidal volume and measured exhaled tidal volume are *greater* than the patient's actual tidal volume that reaches the lungs. This is because the compressed volume is lost in the circuit and does not go into the patient. So, in all of the above examples, the set tidal volumes are greater than the patient's actual tidal volume.

It is common practice to get a set of ABG values after the patient is stable on the ventilator. The tidal volume can be adjusted within the range depending on whether the patient's arterial CO_2 pressure ($PaCO_2$) value is too high or too low for the therapeutic goal. The most direct way to change alveolar ventilation is to modify the delivered tidal volume. If everything else remains the same, a larger tidal volume results in a lower $PaCO_2$ value. Conversely, although everything else remains the same, a smaller tidal volume results in a higher $PaCO_2$ value.

The following formula can be used to help predict what *tidal volume* produces a *desired $PaCO_2$* value:

$$(V_T - [VD_{anat} + VD_{mech}]) \times f \times PaCO_2 =$$
$$(V_T' - [VD_{anat} + VD_{mech}]) \times f \times PaCO_2'$$

in which

- V_T = current tidal volume
- VD_{anat} = anatomic dead space (This is calculated at 1 mL/lb or 2.2 mL/kg of ideal body weight.)
- VD_{mech} = added mechanical dead space
- f = respiratory (ventilator) rate

- $PaCO_2$ = actual patient $PaCO_2$ value
- V_T' = desired tidal volume
- $PaCO_2'$ = desired patient $PaCO_2$ value

Note that other, simpler formulas are available for calculating a change in minute volume or tidal volume. This one is presented because it takes into account more factors and can be used to calculate a change in tidal volume, rate, or mechanical dead space.

EXAMPLE

The patient is a 70-kg (154-lb) man who is being ventilated on the control mode (he is apneic). His ventilator settings are tidal volume of 1000 mL, rate of 12 times/min, fractional inspired oxygen concentration (FIO_2) of 0.3, and no added mechanical dead space. His ABG values are arterial oxygen pressure (PaO_2) of 90 torr, $PaCO_2$ of 30 torr, pH of 7.48, SaO_2 of 95%, and base excess (BE) of 0. The clinical goal is to adjust the patient's tidal volume as needed to produce a $PaCO_2$ value of 40 torr. In summary,

- V_T = 1000 mL current tidal volume
- VD_{anat} = 154 mL of anatomic dead space (This is calculated at 1 mL/lb or 2.2 mL/kg of ideal body weight.)
- VD_{mech} = no added mechanical dead space
- f = 12 times/min for the ventilator rate
- $PaCO_2$ = 30 torr actual patient $PaCO_2$ value
- V_T' = desired tidal volume
- $PaCO_2'$ = 40 torr desired patient $PaCO_2$ value

Placing the data and goal into the formula results in the following:

$$(V_T - [VD_{anat} + VD_{mech}]) \times f \times PaCO_2 =$$
$$(V_T' - [VD_{anat} + VD_{mech}]) \times f \times PaCO_2'$$

$$(1000 - [154 + 0]) \times 12 \times 30 = (V_T' - [154 + 0]) \times 12 \times 40$$

Simplifying produces the following:

$$(846) \times 12 \times 30 = (V_T' - 154) \times 480$$

Exam Hint 15-8 (ELE, WRE)

Every available NBRC examination has had several problems that require the test taker to determine an original ventilator tidal volume or a new tidal volume to correct for overventilating (low carbon dioxide level) or underventilating (high carbon dioxide level) a patient. Start with a set tidal volume of 10 mL/kg of body weight. Increase or decrease the tidal volume, as needed, from this starting point. A patient with ARDS or COPD may have a smaller tidal volume. Often the patient's height and weight are given. Be careful to not overventilate a patient who is obese.

$$304,560 = 480 \, V_T' - 73,920$$

$$378,480 = 480 \, V_T'$$

$$788 \text{ mL} = V_T'$$

The solution is to reduce the patient's tidal volume from 1000 to 788 mL.

5. Choose and adjust the rate for mechanical ventilation

See Table 1-2 for a listing of the normal resting respiratory frequencies based on age. If the patient is apneic and has a normal temperature and an appropriately set tidal volume, respiratory rates in the indicated ranges will produce a normal $PaCO_2$ level. This must be confirmed by ABG measurements. If the tidal volume cannot be changed, adjusting the respiratory rate will modify alveolar ventilation. A higher respiratory rate, with everything else remaining the same, will result in a lower $PaCO_2$ level. Conversely, a lower respiratory rate, with everything else remaining the same, will result in a higher $PaCO_2$ level.

See Figure 15-18 for the Radford nomogram for use in predicting a normal respiratory rate and tidal volume based on weight. It can be used to establish an initial rate for most patients. As was mentioned earlier, chronically hypercapneic patients must be ventilated with some caution. Giving this type of patient a higher ventilator-delivered rate and a larger tidal volume may result in blowing off too much carbon dioxide and may cause a respiratory alkalosis. Adult patients with severe chronic restrictive lung disease or those who have had a pneumonectomy may need respiratory rates of 20 to 30 per minute or greater to meet their minute volume needs because their delivered tidal volume must be smaller than normal owing to their condition.

The same formula that was used to predict a tidal volume change can be used to help predict what *respiratory rate* will produce a desired $PaCO_2$ value:

$$(V_T - [V_{D_{anat}} + V_{D_{mech}}]) \times f \times PaCO_2 = \\ (V_T - [V_{D_{anat}} + V_{D_{mech}}]) \times f' \times PaCO_2'$$

EXAMPLE

The patient is the same 70-kg (154-lb) man who is being ventilated on the control mode (he is apneic). His ventilator settings are tidal volume of 1000 mL, rate of 12 times/min, FIO_2 of 0.3, and no added mechanical dead space. His ABG values are arterial oxygen pressure (PaO_2) of 90 torr, $PaCO_2$ of 30 torr, pH of 7.48, SaO_2 of 95%, and BE of 0. The clinical goal is to adjust the patient's rate as needed to produce a $PaCO_2$ value of 40 torr. In summary,

- $V_T = 1000$ mL current tidal volume
- $V_{D_{anat}} = 154$ mL of anatomic dead space (This is calculated at 1 mL/lb or 2.2 mL/kg of ideal body weight.)

- $V_{D_{mech}} =$ no added mechanical dead space
- $f = 12$ times/min for the ventilator rate
- $f' =$ desired ventilator rate
- $PaCO_2 = 30$ torr actual patient $PaCO_2$ value
- $PaCO_2' = 40$ torr desired patient $PaCO_2$ value

Placing the data and goal into the formula results in the following:

$$(V_T - [V_{D_{anat}} + V_{D_{mech}}]) \times f \times PaCO_2 = \\ (V_T - [V_{D_{anat}} + V_{D_{mech}}]) \times f' \times PaCO_2'$$

$$(1000 - [154 + 0]) \times 12 \times 30 = (1000 - [154 + 0]) \times f' \times 40$$

$$[846] \times 12 \times 30 = [846] \times f' \times 40$$

$$304,560 = 33,840 \, f'$$

$$9 = f'$$

The solution is to reduce the patient's respiratory rate from 12 to 9 breaths/min.

> ### Exam Hint 15-9 (ELE, WRE)
>
> **E**very available NBRC examination has had several problems that require the test taker to determine an original ventilator respiratory rate or a new respiratory rate to correct for overventilating (low carbon dioxide level) or underventilating (high carbon dioxide level) a patient. Typically start with a respiratory rate of 10 to 14 in an adult. Increase or decrease the rate as needed from this starting point.

6. Choose and adjust the minute ventilation for mechanical ventilation

The subjects of minute ventilation and alveolar minute ventilation were covered in Chapter 4. Review the calculations as needed. Blood gases must always be evaluated for the $PaCO_2$ level to tell whether the patient's minute ventilation is adequate. A high carbon dioxide level indicates a need to increase the tidal volume, respiratory rate, or both. A low carbon dioxide level indicates a need to decrease the tidal volume, respiratory rate, or both. In both cases, the key to modifying the carbon dioxide level is to modify the alveolar ventilation. This is best accomplished by changing the tidal volume rather than the rate. The following formula can be used to calculate a change in the minute volume:

$$\dot{V}_E' = \frac{PaCO_2 \times \dot{V}_E}{PaCO_2'}$$

in which

$$\dot{V}_E' = desired \text{ minute volume}$$

$\dot{V}_E$ = current minute volume

Pa_{CO_2} = current carbon dioxide level

Pa_{CO_2}' = *desired* carbon dioxide level

EXAMPLE

The patient is the same 70-kg (154-lb) man who is being ventilated on the control mode (he is apneic). His ventilator settings are tidal volume of 1000 mL, rate of 12 times/min, Fi_{O_2} of 0.3, and no added mechanical dead space. His ABG values are Pa_{O_2} of 90 torr, Pa_{CO_2} of 30 torr, pH of 7.48, Sa_{O_2} of 95%, and BE of 0. The clinical goal is to adjust the patient's minute volume as needed to produce a Pa_{CO_2} value of 40 torr. Placing the data and the goal into the formula results in the following:

$$\dot{V}_E' = \frac{Pa_{CO_2} \times V_E}{Pa_{CO_2}}$$

$$\dot{V}_E' = \frac{30 \times 12,000}{40 \, \dot{V}_E'}$$

$$\dot{V}_E' = \frac{360,000}{40 \, \dot{V}_E'}$$

$$\dot{V}_E' = 9000 \text{ mL}$$

The goal can be accomplished by reducing the minute volume from 12,000 to 9000 mL. As was mentioned earlier, this is best done by reducing the tidal volume. Remember that the tidal volume must be kept at no less than 10 mL/kg of ideal body weight to avoid the development of atelectasis. The respiratory rate may be decreased, if necessary, to provide this reduced minute volume.

7. Initiate and adjust positive end-expiratory pressure therapy (Code: IIID2d) [Difficulty: ELE: R, Ap; WRE: An]

Positive end-expiratory pressure (PEEP) is a mechanically elevated baseline pressure. In other words, the patient's end-expiratory pressure is above atmospheric. PEEP is administered through a mechanical ventilator and is not a mode by itself. Rather, it is used in conjunction with any of the previously mentioned modes.

PEEP generally is indicated in any acute, bilateral, generalized pulmonary condition in which the FRC is decreased. When the FRC is decreased, shunt is increased, and the patient has refractory hypoxemia. Examples of small FRC conditions helped by PEEP include generalized atelectasis, pulmonary edema, ARDS, and infant respiratory distress syndrome (RDS). All of these patients show decreased lung compliance as measured by their static compliance (Cst). The higher the level of PEEP, the more progressively the patient's FRC is increased. The therapeutic goal of this is to increase the patient's arterial oxygen pressure (Pa_{O_2}). (Figure 15-13, *F* shows the pressure/time curve.) Patients with chronically small FRC, such as those with pulmonary fibrosis and kyphoscoliosis, are not helped by the application of PEEP.

Specific indications for PEEP include the following:

- Intrapulmonary shunt >15%
- Refractory hypoxemia (Pa_{O_2} <60 mm Hg despite an Fi_{O_2} of up to 0.8 to 1.0)
- The patient has had an Fi_{O_2} >0.5 for 48 to 72 hours and shows no indication of a rapidly improving Pa_{O_2}. PEEP is added so that the Fi_{O_2} can be lowered to a safer level.

Before PEEP is begun, the patient should be monitored carefully to establish the baseline condition. The same parameters should be monitored after each change in the PEEP level to determine how the patient is tolerating it. The best or optimal level of PEEP is the level that results in the best delivery of oxygen to the tissues (not necessarily the arterial blood). Often, a secondary goal is to reduce the inspired oxygen to a safe level. The patient is at risk for oxygen toxicity if more than 50% oxygen is inhaled for longer than 48 to 72 hours. See Box 15-3 for recommendations on what to monitor during the application of PEEP and how to evaluate the data.

The application of PEEP has risks. Clinically, these risks must be weighed against the potential benefit to the patient. In the profoundly hypoxic patient, PEEP can be lifesaving. Some clinicians use low levels of PEEP (up to 5 cm water) in patients with normal lungs or overly compliant lungs (emphysema) to maintain the baseline level of FRC. Hazards of PEEP include the following:

- Pulmonary barotrauma: pneumothorax, tension pneumothorax, mediastinal emphysema, pulmonary interstitial emphysema (PIE) in the neonate, subcutaneous emphysema
- Decreased venous return to the heart, causing decreased cardiac output and tachycardia, decreased blood pressure, decreased tissue perfusion as measured by a decreased mixed venous oxygen ($P\bar{v}_{O_2}$) level, decreased urine output

a. Increasing PEEP

PEEP therapy usually is begun at initial levels of 2 to 5 cm water. After the patient's response has been determined, 2 to 5 cm more PEEP may be applied. The patient is reevaluated. This process goes on until the desired clinical benefit is reached. See Figure 15-19 for a number of physiologic parameters that can be measured and evaluated.

Different approaches to the application of PEEP are used to find the best level. One approach could be called minimum PEEP. It involves the application of PEEP to the minimum level that allows the inspired oxygen percentage to be lowered to a safer level. A clinical goal is to minimize the risk of oxygen toxicity. In this approach, PEEP is raised until the Pa_{O_2} is greater than 60 torr or the Sp_{O_2} is greater than 90% on 60% oxygen or less. Usually no more than 10 to 15 cm water of PEEP is needed.

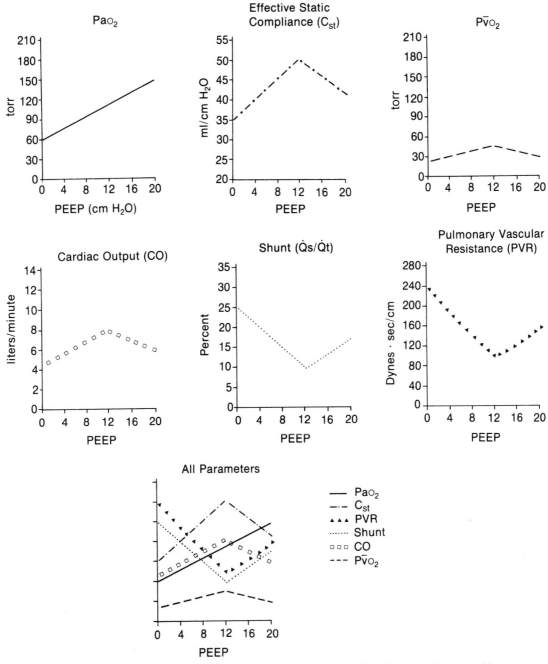

Figure 15-19 Optimal or best positive end-expiratory pressure (PEEP) level is determined by monitoring some or all of the following parameters: PaO₂, effective static compliance (Cst), pressure of mixed venous oxygen (Pv-O₂), cardiac output (CO), shunt (Q̇s/Q̇t), and pulmonary vascular resistance (PVR). Ideally, as functional residual capacity (FRC) is increased by PEEP, lung compliance is improved, and ventilation and perfusion are better matched. Cardiac output should remain stable. It can be measured by the use of a pulmonary artery (Swan-Ganz) catheter or indirectly followed by monitoring the patient's heart rate and blood pressure. As can be seen, the optimal PEEP is found at 12 cm water pressure. Excessive PEEP is seen by the resulting decrease in static compliance and cardiac output.

Another approach could be called *best PEEP* or *optimum PEEP*. This approach has the clinical goal of reducing the patient's shunt fraction to less than 15%. Often this requires more pressure than the minimal PEEP approach. Because this higher pressure level is more likely to cause

hemodynamic problems, the patient should have a pulmonary artery catheter inserted. With it, the patient's cardiac output, mixed venous oxygen level, pulmonary capillary wedge pressure, and pulmonary vascular resistance can be measured (see Figure 15-19). In addition, the patient may need increased intravenous fluids, dopamine (Intropin), and digitalis (Digoxin) for cardiovascular support. The higher PEEP levels increase the risk of pulmonary barotrauma. Therefore the patient must be watched closely for signs of a pneumothorax.

b. Decreasing PEEP

As the patient begins to recover, the PEEP level may be reduced in steps of 2 to 5 cm water. Again, the patient is evaluated after every change in the PEEP level. If the patient's cardiovascular status is normal, the following are recommendations for how to decrease PEEP and oxygen levels:

- Decrease PEEP first if the PaO_2 level is greater than 60 torr and the FIO_2 is less than 0.5.
- Decrease oxygen first if the PaO_2 level is greater than 60 torr and the FIO_2 is greater than 0.5.

If the patient is showing an adverse reaction to the PEEP level, such as decreased cardiac output or barotrauma, the PEEP level should be decreased before the oxygen percentage. Clinical judgment must be used to decide whether a high oxygen percentage or a high PEEP level is a greater danger to the patient. Minimize or remove the element that puts the patient at greater risk.

Exam Hint 15-10 (ELE, WRE)

Typically, several questions deal with the clinical application and modification of PEEP. Know to increase PEEP if the patient is hypoxic, is receiving a high oxygen percentage, and is hemodynamically stable. Know to decrease PEEP if the patient is well oxygenated and is receiving a moderate oxygen percentage, is not hemodynamically stable, or has a PEEP-related complication. A decrease in the patient's cardiac output is a key indicator of excessive PEEP causing hemodynamic problems.

MODULE C
Provide unconventional mechanical ventilation to adequately oxygenate and ventilate the patient.

Unconventional mechanical ventilation is defined here as the use of specialized ventilators that can provide unique modes and options needed by special populations of patients. This ventilatory support may or may not be provided through an endotracheal tube or a tracheostomy tube.

1. Initiate high-frequency ventilation and select appropriate settings

High-frequency ventilation (HFV) is needed whenever the patient's condition calls for a higher respiratory rate or a smaller tidal volume than usually is delivered on a conventional volume-cycled ventilator. A high-frequency ventilator can deliver a respiratory rate far higher than the limit of 150/min set by the U.S. Food and Drug Administration (FDA) on all conventional adult and neonatal/pediatric ventilators.

The FDA has approved HFV for use on adults during bronchoscopy and laryngoscopy procedures and when a patient with a bronchopleural fistula cannot be managed on a conventional ventilator. Although patients with ARDS have not been officially approved for HFV, the procedure has been used when a patient is hypoxic despite maximum settings on a conventional ventilator. (Box 16-5 lists clinical uses for HFV with infants and children.)

Currently HFV can be delivered in three different ways. The first involves the use of a conventional ventilator set at a rate of up to the FDA maximum of 150/min. This method is called high-frequency positive-pressure ventilation (HFPPV). With it, the set tidal volume is decreased to something less than standard (<10 mL/kg). The second involves the use of high-frequency jet ventilation (HFJV) and a special endotracheal tube with a standard lumen and an additional small-diameter air entrainment lumen (Figure 15-20). The HFJV unit is connected to the air entrainment lumen. Gas from the HFJV unit entrains other gas through the main lumen to create the patient's tidal volume. HFJV units can deliver a small tidal volume several hundred times per minute. The third method involves a high-frequency oscillation (HFO) ventilator. HFO makes use of a conventional endotracheal tube (as

Figure 15-20 A HiLo Jet endotracheal tube. This special purpose endotracheal tube features four lumina. *A,* Pilot line to the cuff. *B,* Jet catheter used to deliver small bursts of tidal volume gas from a high-frequency jet ventilator. It opens within the endotracheal tube above the cuff. *C,* Catheter for measuring proximal airway pressure within endotracheal tube near its tip. The main lumen of the endotracheal tube is used for suctioning and adding entrained, humidified gas from a conventional volume-cycled ventilator. *(From Cardinal Health Respiratory Care Products and Services, McGaw Park, IL.)*

does HFPPV). However, the delivered tidal volume is the smallest, and the respiratory rate can be the fastest of all three methods. Table 16-2 presents a comparison of all three methods. The equipment used for HFJV and for HFO is described later in this chapter. Table 15-1 lists considerations for the initial settings and for adjustment of HFV delivered to infants and adults by a jet ventilator or an oscillator ventilator.

Current clinical experience is recommended for any HFV method. Although adult patients have been treated successfully with HFV, far greater use of these techniques has occurred with infants and children. Therefore, Chapter 16 provides further discussion.

2. Independent (differential) lung ventilation

Independent lung ventilation (ILV) involves the use of a separate mechanical ventilator for each lung. A double-lumen endotracheal tube must be placed into the patient to allow this procedure. (See Figures 12-36 and 12-37 and the related discussion.) Box 15-4 lists indications for double-lumen endotracheal tubes and ILV. In all cases, the patient has one normal lung and one abnormal lung. Overriding concerns with ILV are to ventilate the patient adequately through the normal lung and to allow the injured lung to heal.

A common initial approach is to select two identical ventilators that allow synchronization of the patient's respiratory rate. The Servo and Dräger ventilators are suited for this. They allow one unit to be designated the "primary" ventilator to set the respiratory rate for it and the "secondary" unit. Each unit then can have the same mode and I:E ratio. This synchronized ILV method still allows the independent setting of tidal volume, oxygen percentage, and PEEP for each lung.

For example, an 80-kg adult man normally receives an initial tidal volume of about 800 mL (10 mL × 80 kg). If both lungs functioned normally, each would receive 400 mL. However, with unilateral lung disease, the bad lung receives little tidal volume and the normal lung receives too much and becomes overdistended. It is therefore important to set the initial tidal volume to the good lung at *half* the normal volume for both lungs. For this patient example, the normal lung's initial tidal volume should be set at 400 mL (5 mL × 80 kg). To avoid changing too many parameters at once, the same oxygen percentage and PEEP level as originally set are kept. The abnormal lung is ventilated on the basis of its pathologic condition or may be left unventilated.

After 15 minutes, check the patient's ABG values. Depending on the results, adjust the ventilator settings for the good lung as would be done typically to remove carbon dioxide and maintain oxygenation. The ventilator settings for the diseased lung must be adjusted carefully to allow healing and prevent complications such as atelectasis and pneumonia.

When the patient has a bronchopulmonary fistula, the air leak through the bad lung can be so great that an HFV must be used rather than a conventional ventilator. In this

TABLE 15-1 High-Frequency Ventilation Operational Considerations				
	Infant Jets	**Adult Jets**	**Infant Oscillators**	**Adult Oscillators**
Initial recommended frequency	7 Hz (IMV background rate of 2)	5 Hz	15 Hz	3-5 Hz
Initial tidal volume and pressures	Jet-drive pressure to produce 90% of CV peak pressure; 1 time 0.02 sec	Jet drive pressure of 25-35 psi; 1:E = 1:2-1.1	Amplitude to create chest vibration visually; I:E = 1:1 Mean pressure = CV mean + 5 cm H_2O	Amplitude to create chest vibration visually; I:E = 1:2-1.1 Mean pressure = CV mean + 5 cm H_2O
To change effective V_A	Alter drive pressure*; alter inspiratory time†; alter frequency‡	Alter drive pressure*; alter inspiratory time†; alter frequency‡	Alter pressure amplitudes*; alter inspiratory time†; alter frequency‡	Alter pressure amplitudes*; alter inspiratory time†; alter frequency‡
To change mean Paw (for $\dot{V}/\dot{Q}$ effects on PaO_2)	Alter applied PEEP; alter inspiratory time†	Alter applied PEEP (if available); alter inspiratory time	Alter bias flow; alter outflow resistor; alter inspiratory time†	Alter bias flow: alter outflow resistor; alter inspiratory time†

CV, Conventional ventilation; *I*, inspiratory; *I:E*, inspiratory:expiratory ratio; *IMV*, intermittent mandatory ventilation; *PaO₂*, arterial oxygen pressure; *Paw*, airway pressure; *PEEP*, positive end-expiratory pressure; V_A, alveolar ventilation; *VT*, tidal volume; $\dot{V}/\dot{Q}$, ventilation-perfusion ratio.

*↑pressure = ↑tidal volume = ↑V_A.

†↑Inspiratory time = ↑ tidal volume = ↑ V_A *unless* air trapping develops, in which case, tidal volume may ↓.

‡Frequency response may be variable: ↑ frequency may increase total ventilation *but* ↑ frequency can ↓ tidal volume through shorter inspiratory time and pulse attenuation through narrow endotracheal tubes.

From MacIntyre NR: High-frequency ventilation. In: MacIntyre NR, Branson RD, editors: *Mechanical ventilation*, ed 2, St Louis, 2009, Saunders.

BOX 15-4   Indications for Double-Lumen Endotracheal Tubes and Independent Lung Ventilation

Thoracic surgery
   Pneumonectomy
   Some lobectomies
   Thoracic aortic surgery
   Thoracoscopy
   Some esophageal surgery
Selective airway protection
   Secretions (tuberculosis, bronchiectasis, or abscess)
   Whole-lung lavage
   Massive hemoptysis
Bronchopleural fistula
Unilateral lung disease
   Unilateral parenchymal injury
   Aspiration
   Pulmonary contusion
   Pneumonia
   Massive pulmonary embolism
   Reperfusion edema
   Asymmetric ARDS
   Asymmetric pulmonary edema
   Atelectasis
Unilateral airflow obstruction
   Single-lung transplant for chronic airflow obstruction
   Unilateral bronchospasm
Severe bilateral lung disease
   ARDS
   Aspiration
   Pneumonia

ARDS, Acute respiratory distress syndrome.
From Tuxen D: Independent lung ventilation. In: Tobin MJ, editor: *Principles and practice of mechanical ventilation,* New York, 1994, McGraw-Hill, pp 571-588.

Figure 15-21   Patient in chest cuirass (LifeCare). Note control box on right that contains a vacuum motor. Hose connects vacuum motor to patient inside chest shell. *(From Hill NS: Clinical application of body ventilators,* Chest 90[6]:897, 1986.)

situation, no synchronization of rate or any other parameters can be set. The good lung is ventilated conventionally to maintain the patient's blood gas values. The HFV is set to provide some support with a small tidal volume and low ventilating pressures. The clinical goal is to prevent excessive lung pressure so that the lung tear heals.

The patient can be converted back to breathing through one conventional ventilator when normal functioning returns to the injured lung. This can be done when the peak pressure, plateau pressure, and mean airway pressure for both lungs are about the same. When these values match or are close, similar lung compliance and airway resistance values are indicated. The first step in converting from ILV to conventional ventilation involves combining the proximal ends of the double-lumen endotracheal tube with a Y adapter. When this is done, one ventilator can deliver tidal volume breaths to each lung. It is suggested that the PC mode be used so that excessive pressure is not applied to the healing lung. Set the peak pressure at or just below the previous peak pressure used with the healing lung. Set the PEEP level at the previous pressure used with the healing lung. Check the patient's ABG values after 15 minutes. Be prepared to adjust the conventional ventilator as needed to get the desired blood gas values. Watch for problems with the healing lung, and be prepared to go back to independent lung ventilation if necessary. When it appears certain that the patient is tolerating conventional ventilation, the double-lumen endotracheal tube should be removed and replaced with an appropriate single-lumen tube. This allows better suctioning and results in less airway resistance through the tube. Wean and extubate the patient when appropriate.

3. External negative-pressure ventilation

These ventilators have proved useful in patients with the following characteristics: (1) normal, intact upper airway, (2) ability to swallow, (3) normal airway resistance, (4) normal lung/thoracic compliance, and (5) ability to ventilate until respiratory muscle fatigue becomes too great.

Patients with the following disease conditions have been ventilated successfully by a negative-pressure ventilator: (1) neuromuscular defects such as poliomyelitis, postpolio syndrome, muscular dystrophy, and high spinal cord injury; (2) kyphoscoliosis with resulting restrictive lung disease; and (3) COPD during an acute worsening.

Negative-pressure ventilators work by creating negative pressure around the patient's whole body or over the anterior chest and abdomen. The negative pressure expands the thorax, and a tidal volume is inhaled. If the patient needs supplemental oxygen, it must be given by nasal cannula or face mask. Three basic types of external negative-pressure ventilators are available: Drinker body respirator (so-called "iron lung"), body wrap, and chest cuirass (Figure 15-21).

The following steps are used to initiate ventilation:
1. Select a ventilator rate that meets the patient's needs. This can be about 5 to 10 breaths less than the patient's own rate in a patient with some breathing ability. In an apneic patient, the rate can be varied between 14 and 24 per minute.

2. Gradually increase the negative pressure until the patient cannot speak during the inspiratory phase. A pressure of −7 to −15 cm water is enough for most patients. A maximum pressure of −35 cm water often can be achieved. It is possible to create a positive pressure during exhalation, if needed, by closing a valve. This usually is limited to times when an assisted cough is called for.

3. Use a hand-held spirometer to measure the patient's tidal volume.

4. After a few minutes, ask the patient, "Does the breath feel deep enough, too deep, or not enough? Do you have tingling fingers or feel dizzy (signs of hyperventilation)?"

5. Adjust the negativity or rate or both to meet the patient's needs.

6. Draw an ABG sample after about 15 minutes. Speed is important because the unit must be opened for collection of the sample. Interpret the ABG results as usual.

7. If the carbon dioxide level is higher than desired, increase the rate or set a more negative pressure to increase the minute volume. Do the opposite if the patient is being hyperventilated. If the patient is hypoxic, provide supplemental oxygen by nasal cannula or face mask.

4. Initiate and adjust noninvasive ventilation (Code: IIID2c) [Difficulty: ELE: R, Ap; WRE: An]

Noninvasive ventilation (NIV) is also known as noninvasive positive-pressure ventilation (NPPV). These patients will be ventilated without the use of an endotracheal tube. Most of the time, patients receiving NIV are ventilated with the aid of a nasal mask similar to that used to deliver mask CPAP. A full face mask often is needed if the patient leaks through the mouth with a nasal mask.

Most patients who are candidates for NIV are fairly stable, are not intubated, can do some spontaneous breathing, and will need only short-term ventilator support. Examples include patients with the following conditions:

- COPD or asthma and an elevated carbon dioxide level
- Congestive heart failure with pulmonary edema and moderate hypoxemia despite supplemental oxygen
- Neuromuscular disease with chronic ventilatory muscle dysfunction
- Sleep apnea from upper airway obstruction

If the patient is critically ill, is unstable, must be intubated to secure the airway for secretion removal, needs a high level of therapeutic PEEP to maintain the FRC, or experiences a combination of these, he or she should be placed on a standard volume-cycled ventilator.

Often patients receiving NPPV are ventilated with two different levels of positive pressure. This is referred to as *bilevel ventilation*. The baseline pressure is greater than zero for setting a CPAP or PEEP level. The peak pressure is set to deliver a desired tidal volume (similar to PS ventilation). Both levels can be adjusted independently. If only the baseline pressure is elevated, the patient is receiving CPAP. If only the peak pressure is elevated, the patient is receiving PS ventilation. Respironics (Carlsbad, CA) has pioneered the development of ventilators for conventional ventilation or noninvasive bilevel ventilation.

As was stated above, the patient must have a properly fitting nasal or face mask to receive noninvasive ventilation. These ventilation masks are similar to CPAP masks and are referred to as such. CPAP masks are available in different sizes for children older than 3 years and for adults. Nasal masks are designed to cover only the nose. They allow the patient to eat, drink, speak, and use the mouth as a second airway for breathing in case a malfunction of the CPAP system occurs. The mouth also acts as a pressure relief route should the CPAP pressure become too great. Pressures of up to 10 to 15 cm water usually can be maintained (Figure 15-22). Usually, the mask is made of a transparent plastic. Face masks are designed to cover the nose and mouth. They are similar in design to the masks used during bag/mask ventilation and also are made of a transparent plastic. The face mask must be used if the patient has persistent mouth breathing and cannot use a nose mask. With a good seal, pressures of greater than 15 cm water can be maintained.

In recent years, a wide variety of NIV mask systems have been developed (Figure 15-23). In any situation, the clinical goal is to find a CPAP/NIV mask with a soft, very compliant seal that closely fits the contours of the patient's face. A strapping system is needed to hold the mask in place. Too large a mask will not seal and will allow gas to leak and pressure to decrease. The patient may show increased snoring or airway obstruction with periods of apnea. A mask that is too small or misfitting can cause an uneven distribution of pressure on the face. This can lead to abrasions or pressure sores and ulcers on the face.

The bilevel settings must be determined at the bedside by asking for the patient's subjective opinion, listening to breath sounds, checking vital signs, and evaluating ABG values. If supplemental oxygen is needed, it can be added at a port on the patient's mask, at the humidifier, or at the outlet from the BiPAP unit. Up to 15 L/min can be added without affecting the performance of the BiPAP system. It is not possible to know the delivered oxygen percentage until after the bilevel ventilation settings have been determined. The oxygen flow then should be increased gradually while the patient's SpO_2 value increases to the desired saturation level.

Figure 15-22 Effects of nasal continuous positive airway pressure (CPAP) mask. **A,** Normal upper airway remains patent during sleep. **B,** Abnormal upper airway of patient with obstructive apnea collapses on inspiration during sleep. **C,** Pressure from nasal CPAP mask keeps abnormal upper airway patent during sleep. *(Modified from Scanlan CL, Spearman CB, Sheldon RL, editors:* Egan's fundamentals of respiratory care, *ed 5, St Louis, 1990, Mosby.)*

Nasal CPAP mask

Figure 15-23 Examples of types of masks used to deliver continuous positive airway pressure or noninvasive positive-pressure ventilation. **A,** Nasal mask designed to cover the entire nose. **B,** Full face mask (oronasal mask) designed to cover the nose and mouth. **C,** Nasal pillows that fit into the nostrils. **D,** Total face mask that covers the entire facial area. The key elements to consider in deciding which mask to use are patient fit without leaks and comfort. *(A, C, and D from Hess DR, Kacmarek RM:* Essentials of mechanical ventilation, *ed 2, New York, 2002, McGraw-Hill.* **B** *from Hill NS:* Complications of noninvasive positive pressure ventilation, Respir Care *42(12):432-442, 1997.)*

The function of the Respironics Esprit system is reviewed briefly. The operator can choose from two modes of operation and can select from the following:

- Expiratory positive airway pressure (EPAP) for an elevated baseline pressure. This is functionally similar to CPAP.
- Inspiratory positive airway pressure (IPAP) to deliver a tidal volume. This is functionally similar to setting the peak pressure on a pressure-cycled ventilator.
- Spontaneous ventilation mode (SPONT) requires the patient to initiate each assisted breath. The therapist can set IPAP and EPAP levels. This delivers bilevel ventilation.
- Spontaneous/timed ventilation mode (SPONT/T) allows the patient to breathe spontaneously while having a time-cycled minimum respiratory rate set by the therapist. IPAP and EPAP levels also are set to deliver bilevel ventilation.

When bilevel ventilation is started, set the EPAP level, if needed, to elevate the patient's baseline pressure. The EPAP level establishes the patient's functional residual capacity (FRC) to improve oxygenation. Increase or decrease EPAP as you would adjust PEEP or CPAP. Review Box 15-3 for patient monitoring with EPAP. Next, set the IPAP level to achieve the desired tidal volume.

With bilevel ventilation, the difference between IPAP and EPAP is called *pressure boost* and delivers the tidal volume. If a larger tidal volume is needed, increase the IPAP level. Conversely, decrease the IPAP level to obtain a smaller tidal volume. It is important to remember that the delivered tidal volume varies depending on changes in the patient's airway resistance and lung/thoracic compliance, as well as in the machine settings.

5. Initiate and adjust continuous positive airway pressure (Code: IIID2d) [Difficulty: ELE: R, Ap; WRE: An]

CPAP is a pressure above atmospheric that is maintained at the airway opening throughout the respiratory cycle during spontaneous breathing. CPAP is similar to PEEP in purpose and effect. Remember that with CPAP, the patient does not receive any ventilator-delivered tidal volume breaths. The patient must be capable of providing *all* ventilation for carbon dioxide removal. Although CPAP usually is delivered through the mechanical ventilator, the respiratory rate is turned off. However, alarm systems still are functioning for patient safety. Some hospitals will make use of a free-standing system for delivering CPAP. This system is discussed below (Figure 15-13, *G* shows the pressure/time curve for CPAP).

Before a patient receives CPAP therapy, the practitioner and the physician must be assured that the patient has the ability to breathe adequately to eliminate carbon dioxide. CPAP is contraindicated in an apneic patient or in one who may become apneic. (This patient must be fully supported on the ventilator.) The patient must have an adequate respiratory rate, tidal volume, and minute volume. The heart rate and blood pressure should be stable. Maximum inspiratory pressure and vital capacity values may be acceptable or low. Blood gas analysis typically shows refractory hypoxemia but a normal or low $PaCO_2$ level. This shows that the patient would benefit from an elevated baseline pressure to increase the FRC but is capable of ventilating.

CPAP involves the same indications, hazards, and patient evaluation processes as were discussed earlier in PEEP therapy. One possible physiologic benefit of CPAP over PEEP is that less reduction in venous return to the heart is seen. This occurs because with CPAP, the patient is breathing spontaneously. Therefore patients treated with CPAP may be able to tolerate higher pressure levels than those being ventilated with PEEP therapy.

CPAP usually is increased and decreased in steps with 2 to 5 cm water. As with PEEP, the patient is evaluated before CPAP is begun and again after each pressure change is made. See Box 15-3 for recommendations on what to monitor during the application of CPAP and how to evaluate the data.

The patient must be monitored carefully for fatigue because the patient is providing all of the minute ventila-

tion. Signs of fatigue include increasing respiratory rate, decreasing tidal volume or vital capacity, decreasing maximum inspiratory pressure, and tachycardia. Blood gas measurement may show a stable or decreasing PaO_2 value. An increasing $PaCO_2$ level is a definite sign of fatigue. The patient may complain of dyspnea. The practitioner may notice that the patient is working harder than normal to breathe, as shown by increased use of the accessory muscles of ventilation and heavy perspiration. When these signs occur, CPAP therapy should be discontinued and mechanical ventilation instituted in a mode that best fits the patient's needs.

Exam Hint 15-11 (WRE)

Recent exams have focused on delivery of mechanical ventilation through conventional modes or combinations of modes. Typically only one or two questions deal with rarely used modes such as high-frequency ventilation, independent lung ventilation, or negative-pressure ventilation.

Exam Hint 15-12 (ELE, WRE)

Know that CPAP can be used and increased if the patient's carbon dioxide level is normal and hypoxemia is present. Increase or decrease CPAP by following the same parameters used to evaluate a change in PEEP. Know to switch to mechanical ventilation when (1) the maximum level of CPAP is being used and the patient is still hypoxemic, or (2) the patient is hypoventilating.

MODULE D
Mechanical ventilation equipment

Note: The literature produced by the manufacturers and the descriptions used in many standard texts break down the various ventilators into more categories than are used by the NBRC. To avoid confusion, this text uses the more simplified terminology of the NBRC.

A *pneumatically powered ventilator* is defined here as a ventilator powered by compressed gas. Older units operate without any electrically powered control systems (electrically powered alarm systems may or may not be added). More recent units will also have electrically powered controls and alarm systems. An *electrically powered ventilator* is defined here as a ventilator that is electrically powered or controlled. Most volume-cycled ventilators fall into this category. *Microprocessor ventilators* are electrically powered but are controlled by one or more microprocessors (computers). Many of the most current volume-cycled ventilators have microprocessors to control their functions. *Fluidic ventilators* typically make use of electrical circuits with flip-flops to respond to changes in gas flow and pressure throughout the system. Fluidic ventilators are powered by compressed gas. *Noninvasive ventilators* are designed for home use or short-term hospital use and are electrically powered and controlled. They have fewer controls and alarms than hospital-based critical care ventilators. A nasal or full face mask, rather than an endotracheal tube, is used to attach the ventilator to the patient. *High-frequency ventilators* are used in a limited population of critically ill patients who are doing poorly despite all attempts at conventional mechanical ventilation. These units are designed to deliver very rapid respiratory rates and very small tidal volumes.

1. Manipulate pneumatic ventilators by order or protocol (Code: IIA6a) [Difficulty: ELE: R, Ap; WRE: An]

a. Get the necessary equipment for the procedure

Historically, the most commonly used pneumatically powered ventilators include the Bird series and the Bennett PR-2. A control or backup rate can be set on these units in case the patient is apneic. All other controls and functions are the same as those discussed in Chapter 14. The following equipment and procedures are necessary:

- Bennett PR-2 or Bird ventilator with an air/oxygen blender and hoses
- Bennett or Bird breathing circuit
- Bacteria filters
- Proper humidification system: a passover- or cascade-type humidifier or an HME (discussed later). Put sterile, distilled water into the passover- or cascade-type humidifier.
- One or two water traps for condensation from the circuit
- Add an alarm system(s) such as a low-volume bellows spirometer or a low-pressure/disconnection alarm.
- If a low-volume bellows spirometer alarm is used, a length of large bore tubing is needed to connect the exhalation valve to the bellows.

Most modern pneumatically powered ventilators require electricity by battery or wall outlet to operate properly. They are used for patient transportation within or between hospitals or at the scene of a disaster. The Impact Uni-Vent 750 is an example. It has been included in the Strategic National Stockpile for rapid shipment to the site of a natural disaster or terrorist attack.

b. Put the equipment together and make sure that it works properly

Refer to Figures 14-10 and 14-11 in Chapter 14 for the IPPB circuits. The ventilator and circuits are similar

to those used in IPPB therapy with the following exceptions:

- Set the ordered oxygen percentage on the blender; set the Bird *air mix* and Bennett *air dilution* selection controls to pure source gas from the blender. Analyze the FIO_2 through a port in the inspiratory limb of the circuit.
- If a passover or cascade humidifier is used, a short length of large bore tubing is connected between the outlet of the mainstream in-line bacteria filter and the inlet of the humidifier. The inspiratory limb of the circuit is connected to the outlet of the humidifier. If a heat-moisture exchanger (HME) is used, it is added between the circuit and the tracheostomy/endotracheal tube adapter (Figure 15-24).
- A tracheostomy/endotracheal tube adapter is always used to connect the circuit to the patient.
- Add at least one disconnection alarm to the circuit. It could be a low-pressure or disconnection alarm added into the inspiratory limb of the circuit with a Briggs adapter/T-piece.
- Water traps are placed in the lowest part of the inspiratory and expiratory limbs of the circuit to hold any condensed water vapor.

c. Troubleshoot any problems with the equipment

Both of these types of ventilators send gas through the circuit during an inspiration and do not cycle off until the preset pressure is reached. Test the tightness of the circuit, backup rate, and delivered tidal volume by placing a test lung on the patient connection of the circuit. Set the controls to deliver the prescribed order. Be prepared to make final adjustments once either unit has been placed on the patient. The patient's airway resistance and lung compliance greatly affect the functioning of both units.

Troubleshooting problems with these units were discussed in Chapter 14. Make sure that all connections are tight; more are available now with the addition of the humidification system and expiratory limb to the spirometer.

A defective exhalation valve will allow gas to pass through the circuit rather than go to the patient. A pressure-cycled ventilator will not cycle to exhalation.

2. Manipulate electrical ventilators by order or protocol (Code: IIA6a) [Difficulty: ELE: R, Ap; WRE: An]

a. Get the necessary equipment for the procedure

Many mechanical ventilators are powered or controlled electrically. They function primarily as volume-cycled units, meaning that a preset volume is delivered from the ventilator with each breath regardless of the patient's con-

Figure 15-24 The basic components of the two main types of patient breathing circuits for continuous mechanical ventilation. **A,** This circuit contains an *external exhalation valve* and is used on a limited number of pressure-type ventilators. Note that when gas is sent through the expiratory valve line, the exhalation valve balloon inflates to seal the circuit. **B,** This circuit is used on most current ventilators and does not contain its own exhalation valve. Instead, the exhalation valve is part of the ventilator. This is called an *internal exhalation valve. (From Cairo JM, Pilbeam SP:* Mosby's respiratory care equipment, *ed 8, St Louis, 2010, Mosby.)*

dition. Each ventilator is unique in its abilities, modes, and so forth. It is beyond the scope of this book to discuss each and every volume-cycled ventilator. They are presented in a generic manner. The learner should become familiar with the function of the Maquet Servo-*i* (Maquet Inc., Wayne, NJ) and other widely used machines.

b. Put the equipment together and make sure that it works properly (WRE code: IIA6a) [Difficulty: An]

Each ventilator must be learned for its specifics. Generally speaking, the following steps should be taken to ensure that the ventilator is functioning properly:

1. Select the proper ventilator for the physician's orders and the patient's needs.
2. Attach the circuit properly, and make sure that all connections are tight (see Figure 15-24).
3. Select the appropriate humidification device: a passover type, cascade type, or HME. Put sterile, distilled water into the passover or cascade unit.

4. Preset all of the physician-ordered parameters and any other settings that are needed to make the ventilator fully functional.
5. Place a test lung on the circuit at the patient connection.
6. Make sure that the ventilator delivers the preset rate, volume, oxygen percentage, I : E ratio, and so forth.

c. Troubleshoot any problems with the equipment

A low volume can be caused by a leak; check all connections, and tighten them as needed. The volume can be measured directly as it leaves the ventilator and at the exhalation valve to help determine the source of the wrong volume. If the unit shows a volume entering the exhalation valve and spirometer instead of the test lung during inspiration, the exhalation valve is broken. All alarms must be working properly. Batteries must be replaced when discharged.

3. Manipulate microprocessor ventilators by order or protocol (Code: IIA6a) [Difficulty: ELE: R, Ap; WRE: An]

a. Get the necessary equipment for the procedure

The microprocessor ventilators (e.g., Maquet Servo-*i* [Maquet Inc.], Hamilton GALILEO [Hamilton Medical AG, Reno, NV], Dräger E-4 [Draeger Medical Inc., Telford, PA]) are the most advanced generation of mechanical ventilators. They are powered electrically but are controlled by one or more microprocessors (computers). They offer all commonly found modes of ventilation. In addition, many of these machines offer computer software for measuring bedside spirometry for weaning, work of breathing, and other parameters that give the clinician much valuable information. Airway resistance and static and dynamic lung compliance can be calculated automatically. Flow, volume, and pressure tracings are displayed graphically on the computer screen. Auto-PEEP can be documented and measured. These units offer the greatest quantity of patient data and the best clinical flexibility of all currently available ventilators. The most challenging patients probably can be best cared for on one of these machines.

b. Put the equipment together and make sure that it works properly

c. Troubleshoot any problems with the equipment

All of the previous general discussion on electrically powered ventilators applies to the microprocessor ventilators as well. An additional advantage of these units is that they self-diagnose most problems and display the problem for you. If a microprocessor should fail, the unit should be removed from the patient. The biomedical department or manufacturer has to replace the computer chip.

4. Manipulate fluidic ventilators by order or protocol (Code: IIA6a) [Difficulty: ELE: R, Ap; WRE: An]

a. Get the necessary equipment for the procedure

An example of a commonly available fluidic ventilator is the Bio-Med MVP-10 (Bio-Med Devices, Guilford, CT). It is a neonatal/pediatric unit that can be used in the hospital or for patient transport.

b. Put the equipment together and make sure that it works properly

Make sure that high-pressure gas hoses between the unit and wall outlets are connected tightly to prevent leaks.

The patient circuit and humidification system must be installed properly and must be operating.

c. Troubleshoot any problems with the equipment

Typically, fluidic ventilators are powered pneumatically and have fluidic controls. Make sure that the oxygen and air sources are up to the required pressure (usually 50 psig). Fluidic controls are very sensitive to any obstruction and to changes in other settings. Make sure that gas inlet and outlet filters are kept clear of obstructions.

5. Manipulate noninvasive positive-pressure ventilators by order or protocol (Code: IIA6b) [Difficulty: ELE: R, Ap; WRE: An]

a. Get the necessary equipment for the procedure

A noninvasive ventilator is intended for an adult patient who is capable of some spontaneous breathing for a limited period. The unit typically is used for a short period with a patient who is having breathing difficulty but does not require intubation and full ventilatory support. Current ventilators include the Respironics Esprit (Respironics, Philips Healthcare, Carlsbad, CA) and the Puritan-Bennett GoodKnight 425 (Covidien-Puritan Bennett, Boulder, CO).

b. Put the equipment together and make sure that it works properly

c. Troubleshoot any problems with the equipment

Follow the manufacturer's guidelines for putting the circuit on the unit and adding a humidifier, if needed. A nasal or full face mask of proper size is needed to attach the circuit to the patient. Check carefully for any leakage between the mask and the patient's face.

6. Manipulate high-frequency ventilators by order or protocol (WRE code: IIA6c) [Difficulty: WRE: R, Ap]

a. High-frequency jet ventilators (HFJVs)

1. Get the necessary equipment for the procedure

The Bunnell Life Pulse High-Frequency Jet Ventilator (Bunnell Inc., Salt Lake City, UT) is designed for use with neonatal patients with infant respiratory distress syndrome (RDS) who have failed with conventional ventilation. The ventilator is unique in that it must be used in conjunction with a conventional ventilator that is placed in the CPAP or SIMV mode during use of the jet.

In addition, a special endotracheal tube must be placed into the patient before HFJV can be initiated. Ideally, the patient is intubated with a triple-lumen Hi-Lo Jet tube (see Figure 15-20). If the neonate has already had a standard endotracheal tube inserted, the Bunnell LifePort Endotracheal Tube Adapter (Bunnell Inc.) can be substituted for the standard adapter (Figure 15-25). Both tubes now allow the jetted gas from the Bunnell ventilator to go to the patient. The traditional ventilator is attached to the main lumen of the endotracheal tube. Based on the physical principles that govern jets, additional gas is entrained

Figure 15-25 Special airways needed for high-frequency ventilation. **A,** A multiple-channel endotracheal tube needed for high-frequency jet ventilation. The jet gas enters the patient through the jet line. The pressure-sensing line is used to monitor pressures at the end of the endotracheal tube. The main channel is used to entrain additional tidal volume gas and to perform suctioning. **B,** If the patient is already intubated, the standard endotracheal tube adapter is replaced by the jet cannula adapter. Jet gas enters through the jet connection. The main channel is used to entrain additional tidal volume gas and to perform suctioning. *(From Cairo JM, Pilbeam SP: Mosby's respiratory care equipment, ed 8, St Louis, 2010, Mosby.)*

through the main lumen. This entrained gas should be humidified if the jet gas is dry. All exhaled gas passes out through this main lumen, where it can be measured through the traditional ventilator's spirometry system. This ventilator's alarm systems also can be used, and SIMV breaths and PEEP can be added if needed.

2. Put the equipment together and make sure that it works properly

Figure 15-26 shows a schematic drawing of an HFJV. Also select a companion neonatal/pediatric ventilator and make sure it is operating properly. The following are general considerations with setting up the HFJV system:

- 50 psig source gas(es) of oxygen or oxygen and air are needed to generate a driving pressure.
- A patient circuit is specifically suited to the jet ventilator.
- A drive pressure control lets the operator set the peak pressure of the jet.
- An inspiratory time control sets the I:E ratio.
- Rate can be varied within the limits set by the unit.
- The inspired oxygen percentage can be dialed on the unit itself or on an external air/oxygen blender before going into the unit.
- Humidification must be provided by the Bunnell ventilator and the conventional ventilator.
- Both ventilators must be attached to the special endotracheal tube.

3. Troubleshoot any problems with the equipment

As with any ventilator, make sure that all connections are tight. Leaks are a particular problem because of the high pressures leaving the unit and the small tidal volumes that are delivered.

b. High-frequency oscillator ventilators (HFOVs)

1. Get the necessary equipment for the procedure

The SensorMedics 3100A (Viasys Healthcare, Yorba Linda, CA) is used with neonates and children, and the SensorMedics 3100B (Viasys Healthcare) is used with adults. Both units require a special circuit.

2. Put the equipment together and make sure that it works properly (WRE code: IIA6c) [Difficulty: R, Ap, An]

3. Troubleshoot any problems with the equipment (WRE code: IIA6c) [Difficulty: R, Ap, An]

Experience with the equipment is recommended for assembly of the specific circuit, as needed. Any humidifica-

Figure 15-26 Schematic diagram of a high-frequency jet ventilator concept. *(From MacIntyre NR: Jet ventilation in the adult with breathing rates up to 150 bpm, Riverside, CA, 1985, Bear Medical Systems. Courtesy of Viasys Respiratory Care Inc.)*

tion system can be added. Both ventilators' circuits are designed to combine two separate flows of gas for the patient's tidal volume. As with any circuit, make sure that all connections are tight.

7. Manipulate continuous mechanical ventilation and noninvasive ventilation breathing circuits by order or protocol (ELE code: IIA11a and IIA11d) [Difficulty: Ap, An]

a. Get the necessary equipment for the procedure

A permanent or a disposable circuit may be selected, based on the type of ventilator on which it must be placed. A circuit with an external exhalation valve must be used with older ventilators such as the Bennett MA-1 (Covidien-Puritan Bennett) and the Bear 2 (Cardinal Health, Viasys Bear Medical Systems, Palm Springs, CA). In addition, if a Bird-series unit is used as a ventilator, its circuit has an external exhalation valve (see Figure 15-24, *A*). All modern electrical and microprocessor ventilators feature an internal exhalation valve and do not need one included in the circuit (see Figure 15-24, *B*). If the patient must receive aerosolized medications, the circuit should include a nebulizer or should be able to accept one. If not included, the nebulizer or metered-dose inhaler adapter must be added into the inspiratory limb of the circuit (Figure 15-27).

Also consider whether it is better to use an unheated or heated circuit. Usually the circuit is unheated. With these, a cascade-type humidifier or an HME is used to warm and humidify the inspired gas. However, some practitioners prefer to use a heated circuit for the care of neonates. These circuits may have heated wires loosely

running through the lumen of the tubing or may have a wire embedded within the tubing itself. A heated-wire circuit offers finer control over the temperature of the inspired gas and minimizes condensation. Follow the manufacturer's guidelines to make sure that the system can adequately humidify the minute volume that is being used.

Noninvasive ventilators, such as the Respironics series, have specific circuits designed only for the unit. Traditional ventilator circuits cannot be placed on a noninvasive ventilator.

b. Put the equipment together and make sure that it works properly

Assemble the circuit with the features needed to manage the patient. Common, but not universal, features of the inspiratory limb of the circuit include a water trap, a humidification system, a nebulizer, a thermometer or temperature probe, a pressure-monitoring port, and an oxygen-monitoring port. Common, but not universal, features of the expiratory limb of the circuit include an exhalation valve and a water trap.

The heated-wire circuits must be used only with the humidifier with which they are specifically designed to work. The humidifier has a thermostat that regulates warming of the humidifier water and heated wires to the same temperature. Never cover a heated-wire circuit with a patient's sheets or blanket or any other material. Do not rest the circuit on anything such as the bed rail, patient's body, or medical equipment. These circuits should always be supported on a boom arm or tube-tree.

Noninvasive ventilator circuits must be set up as specified for the ventilator. Depending on the unit, an HME or cascade-type humidifier is added to add moisture to the patient's tidal volume gas.

Figure 15-27   The CircuVent™ adapter allows the medication aerosol from a small-volume nebulizer to bypass a heat-moisture exchanger (HME). After treatment, remember to reset the adapter so that the patient's tidal volume passes though the HME normally. The HME is located properly between the Y of the ventilator circuit and the patient's endotracheal tube. Try to select an HME that has the smallest internal volume to minimize mechanical dead space and rebreathed carbon dioxide. Mechanical dead space in this system includes all tubing between the Y of the circuit and the endotracheal tube. This includes the CircuVent adapter and its bypass tubing when used, or the HME and its large-bore tubing during normal breathing. *(From DHD Healthcare, Wampsville, NY.)*

All circuits use a Y-connector to tie the inspiratory and expiratory limbs together and attach the circuit to the patient. See Figure 15-25 for examples of a generic ventilator circuit. Make sure that the water level is maintained properly in the humidifier.

c. Troubleshoot any problems with the continuous ventilation circuit

Check the circuit and connections for leaks if the volume returned from the patient is less than what was set or delivered. The set volume should be measured with a hand-held spirometer as it exits the ventilator, at connection points through the circuit, and at the exhalation valve or ventilator spirometer or both. The volume control or ventilator spirometer may be out of calibration. If the unit shows a volume entering the spirometer instead of the test lung during inspiration, the exhalation valve is broken. Replace a circuit with a leak or a defective exhalation valve that cannot be fixed.

d. Independently change the patient's ventilator circuit as needed (ELE code: IIIF2i10) [Difficulty: R, Ap, An]

A circuit must be replaced if it is damaged in a way that prevents the patient from being ventilated. This is seen most commonly in circuits with external exhalation valves (see Figure 15-24A). If the balloon-type valve is damaged and will not close, the tidal volume will leak out rather than enter the patient. The circuit must be replaced. If the expiratory valve line is pulled off at the ventilator or exhalation valve, it must be replaced or the valve will not close.

The American Association for Respiratory Care (AARC) Clinical Practice Guideline on ventilator circuit changes (1994) included the following recommendations:

- The circuit should be changed every 24 hours if a nebulizer is used for humidification.
- The circuit may be used for up to 5 days if a cascade- or wick-type humidifier is used for humidification.
- If an HME is used, it should be changed every 24 hours.

More recently, the AARC Clinical Practice Guideline on care of the ventilator circuit and its relation to ventilator-associated pneumonia (2003) included the following guidelines:

- The circuit should not be changed routinely for infection control purposes.
- Change the circuit when it is obviously soiled (e.g., blood, sputum).
- Passive humidifiers (HMEs) do not need to be changed daily.
- An HME can be used for at least 48 hours, and possibly for up to a week.
- Change an HME when it is obviously soiled (e.g., blood, sputum).

It is reasonable to expect the 2003 guidelines to be tested by the NRBC.

8. Manipulate ventilator breathing circuits: PEEP valve assembly, by order or protocol (ELE code: IIA11c) [Difficulty: ELE: R, Ap, An]

a. Get the necessary equipment for the procedure

A variety of PEEP systems can be added to a ventilator or CPAP circuit. Consult an equipment book for the details of their operation. Many of the newer ventilators have internal exhalation valves and PEEP-generating Venturi systems with nothing to assemble at the bedside. Failure to generate PEEP indicates that the exhalation valve or the PEEP-generating Venturi system has failed in some manner (see Figure 15-24, *B*).

Most older ventilators (Bird-series, Bennett MA-1, and Bear 2) use a balloon-like exhalation valve. A direct relationship exists between the volume of gas that is kept in the balloon, the pressure and resistance that it creates, and the PEEP level that is generated (see Figure 15-24, *A*).

b. Put the equipment together and make sure that it works properly

The key thing to check with any PEEP-generating system is that the proper level of PEEP is generated and maintained. Once the ordered PEEP level is set, it should be seen as stable on the pressure manometer throughout the respiratory cycle. Sensitivity should be set at no more than −1 to −2 cm water. That way, the PEEP level is maintained at close to the ordered level even during an assisted breath. For example, PEEP is set at 10 cm, and the sensitivity is set at −1 cm. When the patient triggers a breath, it will occur at 9 cm PEEP.

c. Troubleshoot any problems with the equipment

Malfunctioning internal exhalation valves or PEEP-generation Venturi systems cannot be repaired easily at the bedside. The ventilator must be replaced. Balloon-type exhalation valves (see Figure 15-24, *A*) are prone to the following two problems:

1. The small-bore tube carrying gas from the ventilator to the balloon valve is pulled off. Reconnect the tubing to the ventilator nipple connection or to the exhalation valve nipple connection.
2. The balloon is torn, and the gas leaks out. This can be confirmed by disassembling the exhalation valve assembly. If possible, replace the balloon, and reassemble the exhalation valve. If the balloon cannot be repaired, replace the entire circuit with a new exhalation valve.

Both of these problems are exhibited when the inspiratory tidal volume flows past the patient and directly into the exhaled tidal volume spirometer. Little or no airway pressure is generated. The patient is poorly ventilated, if at all. This problem must be corrected immediately while the patient is ventilated manually.

9. Manipulate continuous positive airway pressure (CPAP) systems: breathing circuits, by order or protocol (ELE code: IIA11c) [Difficulty: ELE: R, Ap, An]

a. Get the necessary equipment for the procedure

Most current generation ventilators have a built-in CPAP mode. No additional circuitry is needed. After switching to the CPAP mode, set the desired level by adjusting the PEEP/CPAP dial and watching the reading on the pressure manometer.

Several manufacturers make CPAP systems for home use in the treatment of patients with obstructive sleep apnea. These CPAP systems typically include an air pump to generate flow to the patient, a CPAP generating device, a circuit designed to work with the system, patient mask(s), and an alarm system.

Free-standing CPAP breathing circuits used in hospitals vary considerably. No manufacturer has developed a system that dominates the marketplace. Most commonly, each respiratory care department develops its own breathing circuit to meet its own needs.

b. Put the equipment together and make sure that it works properly

Figure 15-28 shows the typical components used in a freestanding CPAP breathing circuit. Components include the following:

- Air/oxygen blender
- Pediatric or adult flowmeter on the blender
- Cascade-type humidifier
- Inspiratory circuit of large-bore or aerosol tubing with the following additions: water trap, one-way valve, and thermometer
- Y connector to connect the inspiratory and expiratory limbs of the circuit
- Patient connector (elbow adapter) to endotracheal or tracheostomy tube, CPAP prongs, or CPAP mask
- Expiratory circuit of large bore or aerosol tubing with the following additions: water trap, high-pressure pop-off valve (not shown), pressure manometer for measuring the CPAP level, low-pressure or disconnection audible alarm, anesthesia bag as a reservoir, variable resistance clamp on the tail of the anesthesia bag, Briggs adapters/T-pieces for connecting the various features, emergency pop-in valve in case gas flow is stopped, and CPAP device.

Figure 15-28 Sample free-standing patient breathing circuit for CPAP. Note the components that are commonly added into the circuit.

The CPAP level is adjusted by means of a variety of devices collectively called *threshold resistors,* which include the following:

- A column of water with a length of expiratory tubing inserted the needed depth below the surface (so-called "bubble CPAP").
- A vertically mounted ball bearing. It creates a resistance as gas flows up past it. These ball-bearing resistors come in weights of 2.5, 5, and 10 cm water.
- A spring-loaded resistor that is adjusted to apply the desired CPAP level against the airway.
- A free-standing Venturi PEEP system. Gas from the Venturi jet creates backpressure against the escaping patient tidal volume.

Air exits through each of these devices when it is working properly. All CPAP systems must be adjusted by

checking the pressure level on the manometer. Set the low pressure or disconnection audible alarm to sound at a few centimeters below the CPAP level. For example, if 10 cm CPAP is ordered, set the alarm to sound if the pressure drops below 8 cm of CPAP.

c. Troubleshoot any problems with the equipment

Flow through the CPAP breathing circuit must be sufficient to meet the patient's needs. Adjust the flowmeter setting and clamp on the anesthesia bag so that it is somewhat inflated, with excess air escaping out past the clamp. With all of the devices, gas escapes through the path of least resistance. All or some may escape through the anesthesia bag, the CPAP device, or both. The bag should collapse somewhat during the patient's inspiration and expand somewhat during the expiration. The CPAP level should not decrease by more than 1 or 2 cm from baseline during an inspiration.

Make sure that the water level is maintained properly in the humidifier. Fill it with sterile, distilled water as often as necessary.

A sudden decrease in the CPAP level to zero indicates a disconnection at the patient or somewhere in the breathing circuit. Check all connections, and reassemble the break. The patient may have to be ventilated manually while the problem is corrected.

If the CPAP level decreases by more than 2 cm water during an inspiration, the flow is inadequate and should be increased. Flow also is inadequate if the patient shows increased use of accessory muscles of respiration or complains of increased WOB. Too high a flow is seen by an inadvertently high level of CPAP or the patient complaining of difficulty exhaling.

Water column systems must be monitored frequently because of water loss caused by evaporation. The actual CPAP level is progressively less than desired as the water is lost gradually. This system must have water added to it regularly or must have the expiratory tubing inserted deeper to keep the desired CPAP level.

The ball-bearing resistor system must be mounted vertically for gravity to keep the desired weight against the circuit. If it falls over and is horizontal, the CPAP pressure will be lost.

10. Manipulate CPAP systems: masks, nasal, and bilevel, by order or protocol (Code: IIA2) [Difficulty: ELE: R, Ap; WRE: An]

a. Get the necessary equipment for the procedure

A CPAP mask and breathing circuit are used primarily for patients who have obstructive sleep apnea. CPAP, by means of the mask, forces soft tissues open to the point that the airway is never obstructed (see Figure 15-22). The patient now is able to sleep normally and remain oxygenated. The patient should have the CPAP mask, breathing circuit, and proper CPAP level determined by a sleep study in the hospital. The patient can use the system at home once it is set up properly and he or she has been trained in its use.

In recent years, a CPAP mask has been used with a noninvasive mechanical ventilator to assist temporarily in the breathing of a patient with respiratory distress. The hope is to support the patient's breathing long enough to treat the underlying problem(s). If this is successful, the patient does not need to be intubated. These patients require careful assessment and monitoring.

The two main categories of CPAP masks come in different sizes for children older than 3 years to adults. (See Figure 15-23 for examples.) Nasal mask and pillow systems are designed to cover only the nose. These allow the patient to speak and offer the mouth as a second airway for breathing in case a malfunction of the CPAP system occurs. The mouth also acts as a pressure relief route if the CPAP pressure should become too great. Pressures of up to 15 cm water usually can be maintained in an adult. Pressures of up to 10 cm water usually can be maintained in a child.

Full face mask and total face mask systems are designed to cover the nose and mouth. These are transparent and are similar to the mask used during bag/mask ventilation. The face mask must be used if the patient has persistent mouth breathing and cannot use a nose mask. With a good seal, pressures of greater than 15 cm water can be maintained.

All types of CPAP masks have a soft, very compliant seal to closely fit the contours of the face. Straps are needed to hold the mask in place. It is imperative that the mask properly fit the patient's face.

b. Put the equipment together and make sure that it works properly

Several companies manufacture mask CPAP systems for home care. These are relatively simple circuits that do not have a humidification system or the other attachments seen in the hospital. Check the manufacturer's literature for specific directions on their application to the patient. As is shown in Figure 15-23, the straps must be tight enough to seal the mask to the face but not so tight as to cut off circulation to the skin. Any mask CPAP system must be able to generate enough flow to meet the patient's minute volume and peak flow needs. The CPAP level must be stable throughout the breathing cycle.

c. Troubleshoot any problems with the equipment

Too large a mask does not seal and allows gas to leak out. This is seen as decreased CPAP pressure on the manometer. The patient may show increased snoring or airway obstruction with periods of apnea. A mask that is too small or misfitting can cause an uneven distribution of pressure on the face. This can lead to abrasions or pressure sores and ulcers on the face.

A sudden decrease in the CPAP level to zero indicates a disconnection at the patient or somewhere in the breathing circuit. Check all connections, and reassemble the break. If the CPAP level decreases by more than 2 cm water during an inspiration, the flow is inadequate and should be increased. Flow also is inadequate if the patient shows increased use of accessory muscles of respiration or complains of increased WOB. Too high a flow is seen by an inadvertently high level of CPAP or by the patient's complaining of difficulty exhaling.

Exam Hint 15-13 (ELE)

Two or more questions usually relate to troubleshooting equipment problems. Expect a question that involves a leak with the loss of delivered tidal volume. If the source of the leak is a loose CPAP or NIV mask, it must be adjusted or replaced. Be prepared to troubleshoot problems with a leak in the circuit tubing or the exhalation valve. Change a ventilator circuit that is obviously fouled with blood or secretions.

---

11. Manipulate humidifiers by order or protocol (ELE code: IIA3) [Difficulty: ELE: R, Ap, An]

a. Get the necessary equipment for the procedure

A cascade-type, wick-type, etc. humidifier is indicated in these situations:

- The patient has thick or copious secretions. An increase in the amount or thickness of secretions or a change from white to yellow or green justifies the switch to a cascade-type humidifier.
- The patient probably will require mechanical ventilation for longer than 96 hours.
- The patient cannot have mechanical dead space added to the breathing circuit. If the patient's (especially a child's) tidal volume is smaller than the HME dead space, the HME should not be used. SIMV systems typically are set up without mechanical dead space, so an HME should not be used.
- An HME should not be used for a patient receiving very large tidal volumes because the filter's ability to hold moisture is exceeded, and the patient will breathe in some dry air. Check the manufacturer's literature for the maximum recommended tidal volume.
- If the patient has a large air leak, as seen with a deflated cuff or bronchopleural fistula, an HME should not be used. With a large air leak, more air is inspired than expired, and the exchanger will not be able to fully humidify the inspired tidal volume.

b. Put the equipment together and make sure that it works properly

A general discussion of this equipment was presented in Chapter 8. (See Figure 15-28 for a setup in a CPAP breathing circuit.) The selected humidifier must be capable of providing 100% relative humidity. Passover-type systems are preferred with neonates.

The humidifier's temperature usually is maintained at between 31° C and 35° C. Normally, the temperature at the patient's airway should never be greater than 37° C.

An exception to this rule is the hypothermic patient. Inhaled gas that is warmed to a few degrees above normal body temperature speeds the rewarming process.

Typically, a temperature probe is added into the inspiratory limb of the circuit near the Y. If a heated-wire circuit is being used with an infant, the temperature probe should be outside of the incubator and away from a radiant warmer's direct heat. The humidifier should provide at least 30 mg/L of water vapor.

Make sure that the water level is kept in the recommended range to humidify the gas properly. Avoid being sprayed with any circuit water during disconnections from the patient. It is considered contaminated and should be disposed of similarly to any other contaminated fluid from the patient.

An AARC Clinical Practice Guideline on ventilator circuit changes (1994) recommends that a cascade- or wick-type humidifier and the patient circuit be changed at least every 5 days for infection control purposes. The guideline also recommends that a nebulizer used for humidification purposes and the patient circuit should be changed every 24 hours for infection control purposes.

More recently, the AARC Clinical Practice Guideline on care of the ventilator circuit and its relation to ventilator-associated pneumonia (2003) included the following guidelines:

- The circuit should not be changed routinely for infection control purposes.
- Change the circuit when it is obviously soiled (e.g., blood, sputum).
- Passive humidifiers (HMEs) do not need to be changed daily.
- An HME can be used for at least 48 hours, and possibly for up to a week.
- Change an HME when it is obviously soiled (e.g., blood, sputum).

c. Troubleshoot any problems with the equipment

A loose connection at the humidifier (or anywhere else in the circuit) results in loss of volume or pressure or both to the patient. Check the entire circuit. When the leak is fixed, the volume and pressure are restored. The humidifier should warm to the desired temperature. Do not use a humidifier that does not warm properly.

12. Manipulate heat and moisture exchangers by order or protocol (ELE code: IIA3) [Difficulty: ELE: R, Ap, An]

a. Get the necessary equipment for the procedure

A heat-moisture exchanger (HME) is designed to be warmed by the patient's exhaled breath and to absorb the water vapor from the gas. The next inspired volume then is warmed and humidified by evaporation. The key element in the exchanger is a hygroscopic filter medium. Under ideal conditions, the units can achieve up to 70% to 90% body humidity. They should provide minimally 30 mg/L of water at 30° C. A general discussion of this equipment was presented in Chapter 8. See Figure 15-25 for a setup in a ventilator breathing circuit.

An HME is indicated in the following situations:
- The patient has few, if any, secretions.
- The patient probably will be weaned from the ventilator within 96 hours.
- The patient is being transported on mechanical ventilation.

An HME is contraindicated in the following situations:
- The patient has thick, bloody, or large amounts of secretions.
- The patient has a large air leak such that the exhaled volume is less than 70% of the inhaled tidal volume. This results in a relatively dry hygroscopic filter. (Patients with uncuffed or torn cuffs on their endotracheal tubes or large bronchopleurocutaneous fistulas have large tidal volume leaks.)
- The patient's temperature is less than 32° C.
- The patient's spontaneous minute volume is greater than 10 L/min.

Consider the following when selecting an HME:
- Select a unit with the smallest possible dead space volume. Watch for an increase in the patient's $PaCO_2$ if the HME adds too much dead space or the patient's tidal volume is too small.
- Pick the unit that provides the greatest percentage of body humidity. Do not use one that cannot meet these minimum standards.
- If the patient has a known pulmonary infection, select an HME that is also a bacteria filter.
- Should the unit be disposable or reusable? Staffing, infection control, and equipment processing considerations make a difference in unit selection.

Remember to always remove or bypass the HME when delivering nebulized medications through the circuit. If not, the HME will trap all of the nebulized medication and none will be delivered to the patient.

b. Put the equipment together and make sure that it works properly

Most of these units are preassembled by the manufacturer, with nothing to add. It may be necessary to attach a length of large-bore or aerosol tubing or an elbow adapter to make the unit fit onto the Y or endotracheal tube. All come with standard 15- or 22-mm connector ends. Air should flow easily through them with little resistance.

An AARC Clinical Practice Guideline on circuit changes (1994) states that HMEs can be used for up to 4 days if the patient does not have a major secretion problem. Each individual HME can be used for at least 24 hours unless it is obviously fouled. The whole patient circuit should be changed at least every 5 days for infection control purposes. The AARC Clinical Practice Guideline on care of the ventilator circuit and its relation to ventilator-associated pneumonia (2003) included the following guidelines:
- Passive humidifiers (HMEs) do not need to be changed daily.
- An HME can be used for at least 48 hours, and possibly for up to a week.
- Change an HME when it is obviously soiled (e.g., blood, sputum).

c. Troubleshoot any problems with the equipment

Any disconnections can be easily noticed and reconnected. Replace any unit that has a mucous plug or other debris obstructing the channel. This might be demonstrated by a sudden increase in the patient's peak airway pressure.

Exam Hint 15-14 (ELE)

When secretions are coughed into a HME, it becomes obstructed. This is demonstrated by a rapid increase in the peak pressure during an inspiration. Remove the obstructed HME. Replace it or change to a cascade-type humidifier.

---

13. Perform quality control procedures on mechanical ventilators (Code: IIC5) [Difficulty: ELE: R, Ap; WRE: An]

Follow the manufacturer's guidelines for quality control procedures on a mechanical ventilator. Microprocessor ventilators usually have a software package that performs self-diagnostic tests on the unit. Obviously, the ventilator should deliver the volume, flow, and pressure that are set on the controls. Do not use a unit that fails a quality control check.

MODULE E
Evaluate and monitor the patient's response to mechanical ventilation.

1. Observe the patient for signs of patient-ventilator dyssynchrony (Code: IIIE5b) [Difficulty: ELE: R, Ap; WRE: An]

Signs that the patient is breathing out of phase with the ventilator (dyssynchrony) include the following:

- The use of inspiratory accessory muscles (see Figures 1-16 and 1-21)
- Chest and abdominal wall not moving at the same time (see Figure 1-26)
- Nasal flaring (see Figure 1-20)
- Distressed look on the patient's face
- Tachycardia and increased respiratory rate
- Insensitivity to trigger a ventilator breath. This can cause increased work of breathing (WOB) and is noted on the ventilator's pressure/volume loop graphic display (see Figure 15-5).

Because a patient with an intubated airway cannot speak, it is necessary to communicate about the patient's feelings by asking simple questions that can be answered by a *yes* nod or *no* shake of the head. Other methods of communication include a pad of paper and pencil and picture boards.

It is not possible to predict how a patient will react to the initiation of mechanical ventilation or its prolonged need. Some patients react with relief and relax when the WOB is reduced. Others may become angry at the limitations imposed on them. Still others may become depressed. The issue of a patient's emotional reaction to illness is discussed in detail in Chapter 1.

2. Monitor airway pressures (ELE code: IIIE9) [Difficulty: ELE: R, Ap, An].

a. Sensitivity

If pressure sensitivity is used, it should be set so that the patient has to generate only −1 to −2 cm water pressure to trigger a ventilator breath. If the ventilator is insensitive to the patient's needs, WOB will be increased (see Figure 15-5).

b. Peak pressure (or P_{peak})

The peak pressure reached during delivery of a tidal volume is the pressure required to push the gas through the circuit, the endotracheal tube, and the patient's airways, and to expand the lungs. The sigh volume requires greater pressure because it is a larger volume. These pressures should be recorded regularly whenever the patient and the machine are checked. The importance of peak pressure in calculating dynamic compliance was discussed earlier in the chapter.

c. Plateau pressure (or P_{plat})

The plateau pressure is found when the tidal volume has been delivered to the lungs and is held within them temporarily. The importance of plateau pressure in calculating static compliance was discussed earlier in the chapter.

d. Baseline pressure

The baseline pressure is the pressure measured at the end of exhalation. Normally it is seen as zero on the ventila-

tor's pressure manometer. (Remember that in this case, zero is actually local barometric pressure.) If the patient has therapeutic PEEP or CPAP, the baseline pressure will be greater than zero.

e. Mean airway pressure (Paw)

Paw is the average pressure over an entire breathing cycle. Most of the newer ventilators display a mean airway pressure. This pressure results from changes in the patient's peak and baseline pressures plus the I:E ratio.

3. Perform and interpret the patient's lung compliance and airway resistance (Code: IIIE7b) [Difficulty: ELE: R, Ap; WRE: An]

Check the patient's airway resistance if there is clinical evidence of a change. For example, increased wheezing may indicate bronchospasm. Check the patient's lung compliance if there is clinical evidence of a change. For example, the recent development of crackles may indicate atelectasis or fluid in the lungs. These measurements and their interpretations are presented earlier in this chapter.

4. Recommend radiographic and other imaging studies to obtain additional data (Code: IC2) [Difficulty: ELE: R, Ap; WRE: An]

A chest radiograph should be taken after the patient is intubated and if there has been a significant change in condition, for example, if a pneumothorax is suspected. Review the discussion on chest radiographs in Chapter 1.

5. Recommend blood gas analysis, pulse oximetry, and transcutaneous monitoring to obtain additional data (Code: IC2) [Difficulty: ELE: R, Ap; WRE: An]

An arterial blood sample should be taken for analysis in the following situations: (1) after the patient is first established on the ventilator, (2) when there is a significant change in ventilator settings (inspired oxygen percentage, rate, tidal volume, PEEP level), and (3) when the patient's condition changes significantly. Pulse oximetry or transcutaneous monitoring values are monitored routinely for oxygenation. Chapter 3 provides a complete discussion of these topics.

6. Interpret results of arterial blood gases (ELE code: IIIE4a) [Difficulty: ELE: R, Ap, An]

Interpretation of the ABG results will provide vital information to guide additional ventilator changes. Chapter 3 provides a complete discussion on interpretation.

7. Measure the patient's inspired oxygen percentage (WRE code: IIIE10) [Difficulty: Ap, An]

Most ventilators have very accurate oxygen delivery systems. However, standard practice requires the use of a calibrated, external oxygen analyzer to confirm the oxygen percentage. It is vital to know the patient's inspired oxygen percent to correctly assess oxygenation.

Exam Hint 15-15 (ELE, WRE)

Expect to see many ABG values incorporated into questions about adjusting the ventilator. Review Chapter 3, if necessary, for interpretation guidelines. Hypoxemia should be treated by increasing the oxygen percentage or increasing the PEEP level. As the patient improves, these can be reduced. If the patient's carbon dioxide level is too high, increase the rate or the tidal volume. If too much carbon dioxide is being blown off, decrease the rate or the tidal volume.

8. Recommend capnography to obtain additional data (Code: IC10) [Difficulty: ELE: R, Ap; WRE: An]

Capnography is used to evaluate the patient's ability to exhale carbon dioxide and to evaluate certain conditions in which dead space can change. Changes in tidal volume, rate, and mechanical dead space will affect carbon dioxide removal. See the capnography discussion in Chapter 5.

9. Interpret results of capnography (Code: IIIE4e) [Difficulty: ELE: R, Ap; WRE: An]

See Chapter 5 for a discussion of interpretation and examples of exhaled carbon dioxide waveforms that indicate clinical problems.

10. Auscultate the patient's chest and interpret changes in breath sounds (Code: IIIE11) [Difficulty: ELE: R, Ap; WRE: An]

Check for equal, bilateral breath sounds after a patient has been intubated. Also, auscultate the patient's breath sounds after any significant change in the ventilator or in the patient's condition. Review the discussion on breath sounds in Chapter 1, if necessary.

11. Perform and interpret spirometry (Code: IIIE7a) [Difficulty: ELE: R, Ap; WRE: An]

When the patient is breathing in the SIMV or PSV mode, the machine-delivered and spontaneous tidal volumes

---

BOX 15-5   Indications That the Patient Probably Can Be Weaned From the Ventilator

OXYGENATION

PaO_2 ≥80 torr or SpO_2 >90% on 50% oxygen or less
$P(A-a)O_2$ <300-350 torr on 100% oxygen
Intrapulmonary shunt of <15%

VENTILATION

$PaCO_2$ <55 torr in a patient who is not ordinarily hypercapneic
Dead space/tidal volume ($V_D : V_T$) ratio <0.55-0.6 (55%-60%)
Rapid, shallow breathing index (breaths/minute divided by tidal volume in liters) <105

PULMONARY MECHANICS

Spontaneous tidal volume of 3-4 mL/lb or 7-9 mL/kg of ideal body weight
Vital capacity of ≥10-15 mL/kg
Maximum inspiratory pressure (MIP) more than −20 to −25 cm water pressure
Forced expiratory volume in 1 second (FEV_1) >10 mL/kg
Respiratory rate of 12-35/min (adult)

MISCELLANEOUS

Conscious and cooperative patient who wants to breathe spontaneously
Stable and acceptable normal blood pressure and temperature
Stable cardiac rhythm; heart rate should not increase by >15% to 20%
Corrected underlying problem that led to ventilatory support
Normal fluid balance and electrolyte values
Proper nutritional status

---

must be measured and recorded. Evaluate any significant change in the patient's tidal volume and respiratory rate.

The recovering patient who is being considered for weaning must have his or her respiratory rate, spontaneous tidal volume, vital capacity, and maximum inspiratory pressure measured. Review the discussion in Chapter 4 on these bedside spirometry parameters. These and other factors are used to judge weanability. See Box 15-5 for more information. A full discussion on weaning is provided later.

12. Monitor the ventilator alarm systems and adjust them as needed (ELE code: IIIE9) [Difficulty: ELE: R, Ap, An]

All alarm systems must function properly. Test all audible and visual alarms. The practitioner should be familiar with the most widely used adult and infant ventilators and their alarm systems. It is common practice to set most alarms at ± 10% of the set value. For example,

- The tidal volume is 1000 mL. Set the low-volume alarm at 900 mL and the high-volume alarm at 1100 mL.

- The minute volume is 10,000 mL. Set the high-volume alarm at 11,000 mL and the low-volume alarm at 9000 mL.
- The oxygen percentage is set at 40%. Set the high-percentage alarm at 45% and the low-percentage alarm at 35%.
- The low-pressure or disconnection alarm is set to sound if the ventilator-delivered pressure is about 5 cm water below the peak pressure. For example, if the peak pressure has been at about 40 cm water, the low-pressure or disconnection alarm should be set at 35 cm water. If a leak or disconnection occurs, the alarm sounds when the peak pressure does not reach 35 cm water. If the patient is on a CPAP system, the low-pressure or disconnection alarm should be set to sound if the pressure decreases about 2 to 3 cm water below the set level. For example, if the patient is on 10 cm water CPAP, the alarm should be set at 8 cm water.

Many types of alarms have a timer that can be set to delay when the alarm sounds. If the alarm is on a ventilator, the delay should be set for about 3 to 5 seconds longer than the cycling time. For example, if the patient has a backup rate of 10 times/min, the cycling time between mandatory breaths is 6 seconds. Set the timer to delay the alarm sounding for about 10 seconds. If the patient is disconnected from the ventilator and the peak pressure does not reach 35 cm water, the alarm will sound in 10 seconds. If the patient is on a CPAP system, the timer may be set for no delay or for a short delay. Adjust all the alarms to fit the clinical setting and the patient's condition. Some may need tighter limits, and others may need wider limits than those just discussed.

Exam Hint 15-16 (ELE)

Be able to troubleshoot an alarm situation, correct the problem, and reset the alarms settings as needed. For example, the high pressure alarm will go off if the peak pressure hits the alarm setting because of an increase in airway resistance or a decrease in lung compliance.

---

13. Maintain the position of the endotracheal tube or tracheostomy tube and appropriate cuff inflation (ELE code: IIIB4c and d) [Difficulty: ELE: R, Ap; WRE: An]

After a patient has been intubated, always confirm the location of the tube within the trachea through two or more procedures, for example, breath sounds and capnometry. Review the complete discussion in Chapter 12, if necessary.

MODULE F

Recommend modifications in mechanical ventilation based on the patient's response.

1. Change the mechanical ventilator

a. Recommend a change in the type of mechanical ventilator (Code: IIIG3i) [Difficulty: ELE; R, Ap; WRE: An]

Selection among types of mechanical ventilators was discussed earlier in this chapter. In brief, a pressure-cycled unit can be used with a patient without cardiopulmonary disease. Most patients with conditions that cause abnormal Raw or C_{LT} should be placed on electrically powered, volume-cycled units. Microprocessor ventilators offer increased ventilating options and monitoring of clinical information; they are best for the most critical patients. Noninvasive ventilation and negative-pressure ventilation are used with patients who do not need intubation and who have some ability to breathe for themselves.

b. Independently change the type of ventilator (Code: IIIF2i9) [Difficulty: ELE: R, Ap; WRE: An]

Be prepared to change from one type of ventilator to another as the patient's condition warrants. A malfunctioning ventilator should be replaced with one that is capable of providing the same level of ventilatory support.

2. Change the ventilator circuit

a. Recommend a change in the ventilator circuit (ELE code: IIIG3j) [Difficulty: ELE: R, Ap, An]

b. Independently change the ventilator circuit (ELE code: IIIF2i10) [Difficulty: ELE: R, Ap, An]

Changing circuits was discussed earlier in this chapter. In brief, change a circuit that has a leak or is obviously soiled by blood or sputum.

3. Humidification equipment

a. Maintain humidification equipment (ELE code: IIIB8) [Difficulty: ELE: R, Ap, An]

b. Independently change the type of humidification equipment (ELE code: IIIF2g2) [Difficulty: ELE: R, Ap, An]

An HME is indicated in the following situations:
- The patient has few, if any, secretions.
- The patient probably will be weaned from the ventilator within 96 hours.
- The patient is being transported on mechanical ventilation.

An HME is contraindicated in the following situations:

- The patient has thick, bloody, or copious secretions.
- The patient has a large air leak such that the exhaled volume is less than 70% of the inhaled V_T. This causes a relatively dry hygroscopic filter. (Patients with uncuffed or torn cuffs on their endotracheal tubes or large bronchopleural fistulas would have large V_T leaks.)
- The patient's temperature is less than 32° C.
- The patient's spontaneous minute volume ($\dot{V}_E$) is greater than 10 L/min.

A cascade-type bubble humidifier is indicated in these situations:

- The patient has thick or copious secretions. An increase in the amount or thickness of secretions or a change from white to yellow or green justifies the switch to a cascade-type humidifier.
- The patient probably will require mechanical ventilation for longer than 96 hours.
- The patient cannot have mechanical dead space added to the breathing circuit. If the patient's V_T (especially a child's) is smaller than the HME dead space, it should not be used. IMV systems typically are set up without mechanical dead space, so an HME should not be used.
- An HME should not be used with a patient receiving very large V_Ts because the filter's ability to hold moisture will be exceeded, and the patient will breathe in some dry air. Check the manufacturer's literature for the maximum recommended V_T.
- If the patient has a large air leak, as may be seen with a deflated cuff or a bronchopleural fistula, an HME should not be used. With a large air leak, more air is inspired than expired, and the exchanger cannot fully humidify the inspired V_T.

4. Change the oxygen percentage

a. Make a recommendation to change the oxygen percentage (ELE code: IIIG2c) [Difficulty: ELE: R, Ap, An]

b. Independently change the oxygen percentage (ELE code: IIIF2d1) [Difficulty: ELE: R, Ap, An]

As was discussed earlier, the goal of O_2 administration is to keep the PaO_2 level of most patients at between 60 and 90 torr and the SpO_2 level at greater than 90%. Exceptions are patients who are breathing on hypoxic drive and who are in a cardiac arrest situation. The patient with COPD who has a chronically low PaO_2 level and a chronically high $PaCO_2$ level may be allowed to have a PaO_2 value as low as 50 to 55 torr and an SpO_2 value as low as 85%. The patient who is extremely hypoxic must be given up to 100% O_2. Those patients who have refractory hypoxemia (e.g., ARDS) do not respond with a normal increase in the PaO_2 level as the O_2 percentage is increased.

5. Use graphics to guide ventilator adjustments

a. Recommend the adjustment of ventilator settings based on ventilator graphics (Code: IIIG3h) [Difficulty: ELE: R, Ap; WRE: An]

b. Independently adjust ventilator settings based on ventilator graphics (Code: IIIF2i8) [Difficulty: ELE: R, Ap; WRE: An]

Watch for signs that the patient's condition is changing. These may include, but are not limited to, air trapping, increasing or decreasing airway resistance, and increasing or decreasing lung compliance. See the previous discussion and example figures.

6. Improve alveolar ventilation

a. Recommend changes in mechanical ventilation to improve alveolar ventilation (Code: IIIG3c) [Difficulty: ELE: R, Ap; WRE: An]

b. Independently change mechanical ventilation to improve alveolar ventilation (Code: IIIF2i3) [Difficulty: ELE: R, Ap; WRE: An]

c. Tidal volume

The specific V_T to select, based on the patient's condition, was discussed earlier in this chapter. When an adult has essentially normal lungs, the NBRC uses the lower level for a set V_T as 10 mL/kg of ideal body weight. The upper end for a set V_T in an adult is 12 to 15 mL/kg of ideal body weight. Conditions in which the V_T should be increased include atelectasis, consolidation, and conditions in which the present V_T is at the small end of the normal range and the patient has an elevated CO_2 level.

Conditions in which the initial V_T should be smaller than specified in the normal guidelines include the following:

- ARDS when the lung protective strategy is being employed
- Chronic restrictive lung disease such as pulmonary fibrosis
- Surgically reduced lung structure such as lobectomy or pneumonectomy
- COPD or asthma when air trapping is present and/or hyperinflated lungs are seen on the chest radiograph film by wide intercostal margins or flattened hemidiaphragms
- When the present V_T is at the large end of the recommended range and the patient has a decreased CO_2 level

d. Sigh volume

An additional consideration is whether to give the patient a sigh breath, which is a volume larger than the normal V_T. People normally sigh every few minutes. It serves the purpose of opening up atelectatic alveoli and reorienting the surfactant in the alveoli so that they are stable. It is controversial to add sighs to a patient who is receiving mechanical ventilation.

Historically, many patients who are being ventilated in the A/C mode received a ventilator sigh volume just as they did a V_T. A sigh volume is typically 1.5 to 2 times the V_T if the V_T is in the low range. If the patient has a problem of atelectasis or consolidation, a sigh volume may be indicated. The patient may not need a sigh volume if the set V_T is at the middle to upper limit. When a sigh is given, compare the inspired and expired volumes to ensure that no air trapping occurs. Most current ventilators allow the clinician to tailor the sigh frequency to best meet the patient's clinical needs. The sigh frequency should be increased in patients with atelectasis or consolidation. The sigh frequency may have to be decreased or eliminated in patients who are air trapping the V_T or sigh volume. Sighs usually are not given in any mode other than A/C.

A patient with COPD or asthma, pneumothorax, or cardiac status that is sensitive to high peak pressures may be contraindicated for a sigh volume. The patient with air trapping of the V_T should have a smaller (possibly no) sigh volume. Sighs are not recommended when a patient is receiving a tidal volume at the upper end of the normal range and the plateau pressure is >30 cm water. This patient is at risk for barotrauma/volutrauma.

e. Respiratory rate

Respiratory rate was discussed earlier in this section. Increase the backup rate on the ventilator if the patient has an elevated CO_2 level and the V_T is at the high end of the normal range. Decrease the backup rate on the ventilator if the patient has a decreased CO_2 level and the V_T is at the low end of the normal range.

7. Improve patient synchrony

a. Make a recommendation to improve patient synchrony (Code: IIIG3a) [Difficulty: An]

b. Independently improve patient synchrony (Code: IIIF2i1) [Difficulty: ELE: R, Ap; WRE: An]

Sensitivity was discussed earlier in this chapter. If the patient seems to be working too hard to trigger a ventilator breath, make a recommendation to increase the sensitivity. Be careful not to make the ventilator so sensitive that it self-cycles.

8. Monitor and adjust the alarm settings

a. Recommend changes in mechanical ventilation to monitor and adjust alarm settings (ELE code: IIIG3g) [Difficulty: ELE: R, Ap, An]

b. Independently monitor and adjust alarm settings (ELE code: IIIF2i7) [Difficulty: ELE: R, Ap, An]

Alarm settings were discussed earlier in this chapter. Be prepared to adjust the alarm settings according to the patient's clinical situation.

9. Mechanical dead space

a. Make a recommendation to change the mechanical dead space (WRE code: IIIG3k) [Difficulty: Ap, An]

Mechanical dead space (VD_{mech}) should be recommended when the mechanically ventilated patient is hyperventilating and attempts to reduce the tidal volume and/or rate have not increased the $PaCO_2$ to the desired goal.

b. Independently change the mechanical dead space (Code: IIIF2i11) [Difficulty: ELE: R, Ap; WRE: An]

Mechanical dead space is added to increase the patient's $PaCO_2$ level. This is done by having the patient rebreathe gas from his or her anatomic dead space. This high-CO_2 gas then is inhaled back to the alveolar level and increases the patient's $PaCO_2$ level. The more dead space tubing there is, the more carbon dioxide is retained. It is important to realize that this same rebreathed volume of gas is lower in oxygen because of its diffusion into the patient's pulmonary circulation. If a large amount of mechanical dead space is added, it will be necessary to increase the FIO_2 to keep the ordered level. Measure the oxygen percentage between the dead space and the endotracheal or tracheostomy tube adapter.

Mechanical dead space is used only in the C and A/C modes. It should not be used in SIMV, pressure support, or CPAP mode. Typically, a length of large-bore or aerosol tubing is added into the breathing circuit between the Y and the patient's endotracheal or tracheostomy tube (see Figure 15-29).

The following formula can be used to predict what amount of *mechanical dead space* (VD_{mech}') will produce the desired $PaCO_2$ level. It can be used to calculate how much dead space should be added or subtracted.

$$([V_T - VD_{anat}] - VD_{mech}) \times f \times PaCO_2 = \\ ([V_T - VD_{anat}] - VD_{mech}') \times f \times PaCO_2'$$

in which

V_T = current tidal volume

$V_{D_{anat}}$ = anatomic dead space. This is calculated at 1 mL/lb or 2.2 mL/kg of ideal body weight.

$V_{D_{mech}}$ = current mechanical dead space

f = ventilator rate

Pa_{CO_2} = actual patient Pa_{CO_2} value

$V_{D_{mech}}{}'$ = *desired mechanical dead space*

$Pa_{CO_2}{}'$ = desired patient Pa_{CO_2} value

EXAMPLE

Your patient is a 70-kg (154-lb) man who is being ventilated on the control mode (he is apneic). His ventilator settings are tidal volume of 1000 mL, rate of 12/min, FIO_2 of 0.3, and no added mechanical dead space. His ABGs are Pa_{O_2} of 90 torr, Pa_{CO_2} of 30 torr, pH of 7.48, Sa_{O_2} of 95%, and BE of 0. The clinical goal is to adjust the patient's mechanical dead space as needed to produce a Pa_{CO_2} of 40 torr. In summary,

V_T = 1000 mL current tidal volume

$V_{D_{anat}}$ = 154 mL anatomic dead space. This is calculated at 1 mL/lb or 2.2 mL/kg of ideal body weight.

$V_{D_{mech}}$ = no added mechanical dead space

f = 12 for ventilator rate

Pa_{CO_2} = 30 torr actual patient Pa_{CO_2} value

$V_{D_{mech}}{}'$ = *the desired amount of mechanical dead space*

$Pa_{CO_2}{}'$ = 40 torr desired patient Pa_{CO_2} value

Placing the data and the goal into the formula results in the following equation:

$$([V_T - V_{D_{anat}}] - V_{D_{mech}}) \times f \times Pa_{CO_2} = [[V_T - V_{D_{anat}}] - V_{D_{mech}}{}'] \times f \times Pa_{CO_2}{}'$$

$$([1000 - 154] - 0) \times 12 \times 30 = ([1000 - 154] - V_{D_{mech}}{}') \times 12 \times 40$$

Simplifying produces the following equation:

$$(846) \times 12 \times 30 = (846 - V_{D_{mech}}{}') \times 480$$

$$304,560 = (846 \times 480) - (V_{D_{mech}}{}' \times 480)$$

$$304,560 = 406,080 - 480\,V_{D_{mech}}{}'$$

$$-101,520 = -480\,V_{D_{mech}}{}'$$

$$211.5\ \text{mL} = V_{D_{mech}}{}'$$

The solution is to increase the patient's mechanical dead space from 0 to 212 mL.

10. Modify ventilator techniques

a. Make a recommendation to modify ventilator techniques (Code: IIIG3e) [Difficulty: ELE: R, Ap; WRE: An]

b. Independently modify ventilator techniques (Code: IIIF2i5) [Difficulty: ELE: R, Ap; WRE: An]

Changing the mode of ventilation was discussed earlier in this chapter. Be prepared to change the mode as the patient's condition varies. A patient who is apneic can be placed on the A/C mode. A patient with an acceptable spontaneous tidal volume can be placed on the SIMV mode. The following two modes are finding increasing clinical acceptance in a wide variety of patient situations.

1. Recommend a change in the pressure support level

When the PSV level is adjusted to deliver a V_T, this is called maximum PSV (PSV_{max}). The clinical guidelines for PSV_{max} are as follows:

- Use enough pressure to deliver a V_T of 10 to 12 mL/kg of ideal body weight.
- The patient should not have to assist the ventilator at a rate greater than 20 times/min to achieve acceptable ABG values.

PSV_{max} has been used in patients with resolving acute respiratory failure. Usually these patients have been maintained on the A/C mode for several days to minimize their WOB while they are undergoing treatment for their condition. PSV_{max} is considered ideal for reconditioning the diaphragm and other respiratory muscles. Reconditioning occurs when the assist or "trigger" pressure for the breath is kept as low as possible (−1 to −2 cm H_2O pressure) and the V_T is kept large. This pattern results in a low respiratory muscle workload. As the patient continues to improve, the PSV level is reduced. The patient's V_T is stable as long as the patient passively takes in the PSV-supported breath; the V_T can be larger if the patient interacts actively with the delivered pressure. See Figure 15-5, *B* for a pressure/flow curve, and Figure 15-13, *E* for a pressure/time curve.

The PSV level also has been used to overcome the Raw caused by the patient's endotracheal tube. (See the example calculated earlier in the chapter.) Too small an endotracheal tube may prevent some patients from successfully weaning by the SIMV mode. The addition of enough PSV to overcome the additional WOB caused by the tube enables the patient to wean successfully and the airway to be extubated.

The PSV level is reduced, as tolerated, when the patient's C_{LT} or Raw improves. As both return to normal, the only barrier to extubation is the resistance offered by the endotracheal tube. Some practitioners advocate extubation when the PSV level is 10 cm H_2O or less, which is probably the pressure level needed to overcome the tube's resistance. Thus the patient should tolerate extubation without any increase in WOB.

2. Recommend a change in the pressure control ventilation level

PCV involves the delivery of V_T breaths that are pressure limited and time cycled. It has been advocated for patients with bilateral low-compliance conditions (e.g., ARDS) and patients with a pneumothorax secondary to volutrauma/barotrauma.

The PCV level is set as low as possible to achieve an adequate V_T for gas exchange. The exhaled volume must be monitored continuously because the V_T will decrease if the patient's C_{LT} or Raw worsens. If either or both improve, the V_T will increase. The patient with a pulmonary air leak loses variable amounts of V_T from the chest tube, depending on changes in compliance and resistance. An ABG sample must be evaluated with a change in the PCV level or V_T. The PCV mode is well tolerated by many patients because of the freedom they have to set the rate, inspiratory flow through the demand valve, and $\dot{V}_E$. PCV also may be combined with SIMV and PSV as the clinical situation indicates. Following are some suggestions for initial PCV settings:

1. Set the PEEP to the same level used on the constant volume ventilator to maintain the patient's FRC.
2. Set the PCV level at the patient's static lung compliance pressure. Be prepared to increase this pressure. The clinical goal is to give a V_T close to that delivered previously.
3. Set the rate the same as before.
4. Set the inspired O_2 the same as before. Some may prefer to set it at 100% until blood gas results show that it can be lowered.
5. Set the inspiratory time under pressure control so that the I:E ratio is the same as before.

Check the patient's vital signs for tolerance, and get an ABG sample in about 15 minutes. If the Raw or C_{LT} worsens, the PCV level must be increased to maintain or increase the V_T. Obviously, as the patient's Raw and C_{LT} improve (or pulmonary air leak decreases), the PCV level must be decreased to maintain the desired V_T.

11. Enhance oxygenation

a. Recommend changes in mechanical ventilation to enhance oxygenation (Code: IIIG3b) [Difficulty: ELE: R, Ap; WRE: An]

Each patient should have an oxygenation goal set. Review the discussion in Chapter 3, as needed. The first step in improving oxygenation usually involves increasing the oxygen percentage. If doing this does not result in the desired PaO_2, it is likely that the patient will need an elevated baseline pressure.

b. Independently modify mechanical ventilation to enhance oxygenation (Code: IIIF2i2) [Difficulty: ELE: R, Ap; WRE: An]

The most effective way to enhance oxygenation is to increase the patient's baseline pressure above atmospheric. This could involve the use of PEEP or CPAP. PEEP therapy was discussed earlier in this chapter. Remember that therapeutic PEEP is indicated for situations in which the patient has bilaterally small lungs with a reduced FRC. This causes hypoxemia. The proper level of PEEP restores the FRC and improves oxygenation. Watch for side effects of barotrauma or decreased cardiac output from too much pressure. The patient should be monitored carefully with blood gas analysis and vital sign checks before PEEP is started and after each change.

CPAP therapy was discussed earlier. In brief, all of the considerations for PEEP apply to CPAP except that the patient must be able to breathe adequately to maintain a normal CO_2 level.

12. Recommend a change in the ventilator to reduce the inspiratory plateau pressure (Code: IIIG3m) [Difficulty: ELE: R, Ap; WRE: An]

Inspiratory hold (also known as *inflation hold*) is a technique whereby the patient is prevented temporarily from exhaling the ventilator-delivered V_T. Figure 15-29 shows the pressure/time waveform. The pressure found during the

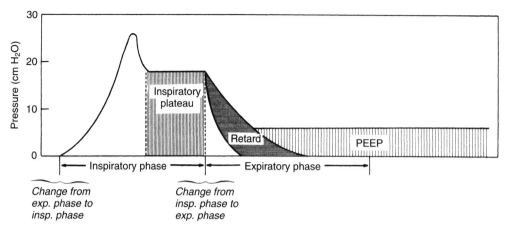

Figure 15-29 Pressure/time waveform showing how exhalation can be modified. Inspiratory plateau (inflation hold) is seen when the tidal volume is held within the lungs for a period of time. With expiratory retard, the gas is exhaled more slowly than during a passive breath. These two modifications of exhalation may or may not be combined with positive end-expiratory pressure. *(From Kirby RR, Smith RA, Desautels DA: Modes of mechanical ventilation. In: Burton GG, Hodgkin JE, editors: Respiratory care: a guide to clinical practice, ed 2, Philadelphia, 1984, Lippincott.)*

inspiratory hold period is called the *inspiratory plateau* or *plateau pressure*. Inspiratory hold is added therapeutically to improve distribution of the V_T. Patients with ARDS and pulmonary edema can benefit from it. Oxygenation should improve in direct proportion to the duration of the inspiratory plateau. The duration of inspiratory plateau is measured in different ways, depending on the ventilator. For example, some ventilators add inspiratory hold in steps of 0.1 second up to several seconds total. Other ventilators add it as a variable percentage of the total duration of the breathing cycle.

Notice that the use of an inspiratory plateau increases the inspiratory phase of the breathing cycle. For example, adding 0.5 second of inspiratory hold to 1 second of inspiratory time results in a total inspiratory phase of 1.5 seconds. This will cause a shorter expiratory time if the rate is kept the same (or the rate must be reduced to keep the same I:E ratio). Because of the shortened expiratory time, it is very important to make sure that the V_T is exhaled completely. If the expiratory time is too short, the patient will have air trapping and auto-PEEP (see Figure 15-3). The patient's condition should be monitored closely to determine whether the level of inspiratory plateau is appropriate. The inspiratory plateau must be reduced as the patient's ventilation and C_{LT} improve. Patients with normal ventilation and compliance should not receive any inspiratory plateau.

Nontherapeutic inspiratory plateau is added temporarily to determine the plateau pressure on the ventilator. This is considered to be the pressure needed to deliver the V_T. With this information, the patient's effective Cst can be calculated. Its calculation and interpretation were discussed earlier in this chapter. An inspiratory plateau of 1.0

second usually is long enough to find the plateau pressure. Remember to turn off the inspiratory plateau afterward.

Expiratory retard also is shown in the Figure 15-29 pressure/time waveform. Some ventilators have a control that adjusts both inspiratory hold and expiratory retard, so care must be taken when a change is made in either. As was discussed in Chapter 14, expiratory retard is indicated in any patient who is air trapping and is not exhaling completely. It functions similarly to pursed-lip breathing in the spontaneously breathing patient. The backpressure prevents the collapse of the smallest airways. Expiratory retard may be indicated in a patient with an air-trapping condition such as asthma, emphysema, or bronchitis. It is important with these types of patients to measure the inspiratory and expiratory V_T. Air trapping is confirmed when the expiratory volume is less than the inspiratory volume. When one is listening to the patient's breath sounds, it will be noted that no pause occurs at the end of exhalation before the next inspiration is started. In extreme cases, the pressure manometer does not return to the baseline level. These patients should be checked for the presence and level of auto-PEEP. The proper level of expiratory retard is determined by trial and error. The following parameters should be monitored to find the proper amount:

- Inspiratory and expiratory V_Ts should be the same.
- The patient's breath sounds should reveal wheezing to be absent or minimal and a silent pause should be noted at the end of exhalation before the next V_T is delivered.
- Auto-PEEP should not occur.
- The patient should feel subjectively that he or she has exhaled completely before the next breath is given.

The patient must be monitored frequently when expiratory retard is being used. As the patient is treated with bronchodilating medications, the bronchospasm should diminish. Expiratory retard should not be necessary when the airway resistance has returned to normal.

13. Inspiratory-to-expiratory ratio

a. Recommend changes in mechanical ventilation to adjust the inspiratory/expiratory settings (Code: IIIG3d) [Difficulty: ELE: R, Ap; WRE: An]

b. Independently adjust the inspiratory/expiratory ratio settings (Code: IIIF2i4) [Difficulty: ELE: R, Ap; WRE: An]

A general discussion of I:E ratio was presented earlier. If the ventilator does not display the I:E ratio, it can be calculated from the inspiratory time and expiratory time. See Table 15-2 for the calculation of time variables in mechanical ventilation.

Increasing expiratory time to eliminate auto-PEEP is discussed in the next section. This discussion will focus on the need to increase the inspiratory time. This is done to improve oxygenation by holding the tidal volume in the lungs for longer than normal. When the inspiratory time is longer than the expiratory time (e.g., 2:1), the patient is said to have an *inverse I:E ratio* and *inverse ratio ventilation* (IRV). This technique has been used successfully in low lung compliance adult patients who do not respond to PCV. Increased inspiratory time and decreased expiratory time should be used in any condition in which the patient has a small time constant of ventilation (T_C) ($T_C = C_{LT} \times$ Raw). This would be observed clinically as a normal Raw but a low C_{LT} in such conditions as ARDS, pulmonary edema, pneumonia, or an enlarged abdomen. Increasing the inspiratory time to create an inverse I:E ratio keeps the alveoli inflated longer to provide more time for O_2 to diffuse, prevent atelectasis, and maintain the FRC. Typi-

cally patients being considered for IRV are already being ventilated in the PC mode. Therefore the merging of the two modes is called *pressure controlled inverse ratio ventilation* (PCIRV). The following have been recommended as initial PCIRV settings:

1. If the patient is being switched from volume-cycled ventilation to PCIRV, set the PCV level at the patient's static lung compliance pressure. However, if the patient was already on PCV at a higher pressure, keep this higher pressure.
2. Set the O_2 at 100%.
3. Keep the current respiratory rate.
4. Keep the I:E ratio at 1:1 for now.
5. PEEP should be removed if it is currently less than 8 cm H_2O. Cut the PEEP level in half if it is currently more than 8 cm H_2O. As the I:E ratio is made inverse, air trapping increases the patient's FRC.

Draw a set of ABGs after 15 minutes on PCIRV, and check the patient's vital signs. Monitor the exhaled V_T for a decrease. If the ventilator gives a real-time graph of pressure, volume, and flow, these should be monitored for air trapping (auto-PEEP). (See Figure 15-3 for an auto-PEEP flow/time tracing.)

If the initial set of blood gases on PCIRV does not show adequate oxygenation, the inspiratory time will have to be increased. The inspiratory time must be increased progressively and expiratory time decreased if the patient's C_{LT} worsens. It is also possible to alternate a 2- to 3-cm H_2O increase in PCV level with small increases in inspiratory time. Blood gases must be analyzed with each increase in inspiratory time, decrease in expiratory time, or increase in PCV. Once an acceptable PaO_2 is established, it usually is not necessary to make additional increases in inspiratory time if the patient's pulmonary condition does not worsen. Look for an increase in $PaCO_2$ or end-tidal CO_2 as a sign of inadequate V_T. It may be necessary to increase the PCV level to increase the V_T. Also monitor the patient's vital signs and cardiac output, if possible, to look for a decrease in cardiac output. PCIRV ratios as inverse as 3:1 or 4:1 have been reported. When this happens, the pressure/volume curve takes on a characteristic "square wave" shape, as is shown in Figure 15-14, *B*. The I:E ratio must be returned to normal as the patient's C_{LT} improves through a gradual decrease in inspiratory time or increase in expiratory time. The patient's blood gas result should be evaluated with each step to be sure that oxygenation is maintained at a safe level.

14. Recommend changes in mechanical ventilation to reduce auto-PEEP (Code: IIIG3l) [Difficulty: ELE: R, Ap; WRE: An]

If a patient has auto-PEEP (see Figure 15-3), every attempt should be made to determine why the patient is air trapping. Although the basic problem is an expiratory time that is too short for full exhalation of the tidal volume, a

TABLE 15-2	Time Variables in Mechanical Ventilation	
Term	**Symbol**	**Formula for Calculation**
Frequency (rate)	f	Count breaths/min or $60/t_I + t_E$
Cycle time	$t_I + t_E$	Add $t_I + t_E$ or $60/f$
Inspiratory time	$t_I(I)$	$t_I = 60/f - t_E$ or $t_I = \%t_I \times (t_I + t_E)$
Expiratory time	$t_E(E)$	$t_E = 60/f - t_I$
Inspiratory/expiratory ratio	I:E or t_I/t_E	I:E $= t_I t_E$, usually numerator
Percentage inspiratory time	$\%t_I$	$\%t_I = t_I t_I + t_E \times 100$

TABLE 15-3	Reasons/Solutions for Air Trapping and Auto-PEEP
Problem	**Solution(s)**
a. Bronchospasm causing slow expiratory flow	Administer a bronchodilator medication. Increase expiratory time. Add expiratory retard.
b. Secretions causing slow expiratory flow	Suction the patient's airway.
c. Large tidal volume that is not fully exhaled	Reduce the tidal volume. Increase the expiratory time.

PEEP, Positive end-expiratory pressure.

Figure 15-30   Pressure/time tracing showing mean airway pressure (Paw). PEEP, Positive end-expiratory pressure; PIP, peak inspiratory pressure; T_E, expiratory time; T_I, inspiratory time. *(From Chatburn RL: Classification of mechanical ventilators, Respir Care 36(6):569, 1991.)*

more specific reason should be found, and then a solution can be found. Table 15-3 shows possible reasons for air trapping and auto-PEEP and solutions.

Not every possible solution can be used. The patient's situation must be considered. For example, increasing the expiratory time will reduce the inspiratory time if the same rate is to be kept. Increasing the expiratory time and keeping the same inspiratory time will reduce the patient's respiratory rate. This will reduce the minute volume and will increase the patient's carbon dioxide level. Additionally, reducing the tidal volume will reduce the minute volume and will increase the patient's carbon dioxide level.

15. Noninvasive positive-pressure ventilation

a. Recommend changes in mechanical ventilation to modify noninvasive positive-pressure ventilation (Code: IIIG3f) [Difficulty: ELE: R, Ap; WRE: An]

b. Independently modify mechanical ventilation to adjust noninvasive positive-pressure ventilation (Code: IIIF2i5) [Difficulty: ELE: R, Ap; WRE: An]

Noninvasive ventilation (NIV) was discussed earlier in this chapter. In brief, if the patient's V_T needs to be increased, the level of positive pressure must be increased. Lowering the level of positive pressure decreases the V_T. Blood gases and vital signs should always be monitored after any change is made.

16. Monitor airway pressures to determine the patient's response to respiratory care (ELE code: IIIE9) [Difficulty: ELE: R, Ap, An]

Modern microprocessor-type ventilators allow the operator to monitor the patient's sensitivity pressure, peak pressure, plateau pressure, and mean airway pressure. Because the first three of these pressures have been presented

earlier, this discussion will be limited to mean airway pressure.

Mean airway pressure (Paw or MAP) is the average pressure over an entire breathing cycle. A number of current neonatal and adult ventilators are able to calculate the value (see Figure 15-30). MAP is influenced by the patient's lung/thoracic compliance (C_{LT}), airway resistance (Raw), and ventilator settings. If a volume-cycled ventilator is being used, a decrease in compliance or an increase in resistance results in an increase in the MAP because it takes more pressure to deliver the tidal volume; a higher peak pressure is seen. Conversely, if the patient's compliance increases or his resistance decreases, the MAP decreases. It is important to evaluate the patient further when a change in MAP is noticed. This is because the new pressure, by itself, does not clarify whether a change in compliance, resistance, or both has occurred. Any treatments that improve lung compliance and reduce airway resistance result in reduced MAP. It is important to calculate both dynamic and static compliance (discussed earlier) when trying to determine how the patient's condition has changed.

In general, an increase in MAP increases the patient's oxygenation because the alveoli are kept open longer, allowing more time for diffusion and preventing alveolar collapse. (Figure 16-11 shows how several ventilator adjustments can change the mean airway pressure. See the related discussion in Chapter 16.) If alveolar ventilation is improved, the $PaCO_2$ also may be reduced.

If the MAP is too high, risk of pulmonary barotrauma is increased and cardiac output is decreased. This is especially true if PEEP is increased to raise the MAP. Watch the patient closely whenever a ventilator change is made that increases the MAP. A sudden deterioration in cardiopulmonary function may be caused by a pneumothorax. Reduced urine output, increased heart rate, and decreased blood pressure often are seen when cardiac output is reduced. The MAP should be reduced if any of these situations is seen. To prevent these complications, it is necessary to reduce the MAP whenever the patient's pulmonary condition improves. As compliance increases toward normal, it is not necessary to use as high an MAP to maintain acceptable blood gases.

17. Recommend the use of sedatives or muscle relaxants (paralyzing agents) as needed (Code: IIIG1c) [Difficulty: ELE: R, Ap; WRE: An]

An adult who is attempting to inhale or exhale out of sequence with the ventilator is considered to be "bucking" or "fighting" the ventilator. This problem is seen most commonly in the control and A/C modes. If the asynchrony between the patient's efforts and the ventilator is too great, the risks of hypoxemia, air trapping, and pneumothorax are increased. Carefully evaluate the patient to determine whether he or she is breathing rapidly because of pain, anxiety, or improper adjustment of the ventilator. Make sure that the settings (inspiratory flow, respiratory rate, pressure limit, etc.) are set correctly for the patient's condition. Sedation or paralysis should be considered only after all other causes of asynchrony have been ruled out. The following patient questions and conditions must be considered before a medication is selected to control the patient's breathing efforts:

- *Is the patient in pain?* If so, an opiate analgesic such as morphine sulfate is commonly administered intravenously for fast onset. Morphine has the additional effects of reducing anxiety and inducing sleep. The synthetic opioid fentanyl citrate (Sublimaze) is given intravenously and is preferred in patients with renal insufficiency or hemodynamic instability. Because all opiates are central nervous system depressants, make sure that the ventilator alarm systems are functioning properly in case the patient becomes disconnected.
- *Is the patient agitated?* Asynchrony with the ventilator for no known physical reason often can be attributed to anxiety or fear. Benzodiazepines, including diazepam (Valium) and midazolam (Versed), are the drugs of choice for the treatment of agitation. They have a sedating effect within minutes when given intravenously.
- *Does the patient need to be paralyzed?* If total muscular relaxation along with apnea is necessary, a skeletal muscle–paralyzing agent should be used. Usually a short-term, depolarizing neuromuscular blocker such as succinylcholine (Anectine) is used during a difficult intubation. A single intravenous dose paralyzes a combative patient for about 10 minutes. For paralysis during mechanical ventilation, one of the following long-term, nondepolarizing neuromuscular blocking agents is used commonly: pancuronium (Pavulon), atracurium (Tracrium), or vecuronium (Norcuron). These are given intravenously and cause paralysis that lasts 2 to 4 hours.

Remember that these paralyzing agents have no effect on the patient's ability to feel pain or on fear of what is happening. Pain medications such as morphine must be given as necessary. A sedating agent such as Valium is also given to counteract the emotional stress of being awake but unable to move. Review related medication discussions in Chapter 9, if needed.

Exam Hint 15-19 (ELE, WRE)

Expect to see questions requiring the therapist to recommend a medication for sedating an agitated patient or addressing the need to paralyze a patient receiving mechanical ventilation.

---

18. Inhaled medications

a. Recommend bronchodilators (ELE code: IIIG4a) [Difficulty: ELE: R, Ap, An]

b. Recommend corticosteroids (ELE code: IIIG4b) [Difficulty: ELE: R, Ap, An]

c. Recommend mucolytics and proteolytics (ELE code: IIIG4c) [Difficulty: ELE: R, Ap, An]

Bronchodilators and corticosteroids usually are given to patients with COPD or asthma. The patient with a secretion problem usually will be given a mucolytic. Review the discussion in Chapter 9 that relates to the above types of inhaled medications.

d. Administer medications (Code: IIID5 a and b) [Difficulty: ELE: R, Ap; WRE: An]

An inhaled medication can be given through the ventilator by adding the dispenser into the inspiratory limb of the ventilator circuit. If a heat-moisture exchanger is used, it must be removed. A metered-dose inhaler (MDI) can be given by adding a modified actuator into the circuit. In some cases, a reservoir is included with the actuator. Press the canister into the actuator to dispense the medication into the circuit before the next breath is delivered. (See Chapter 8 for further discussion of MDIs.) A liquid medication must be given by adding small-volume nebulizer (SVN) into the circuit (see Figure 15-29). A length of small-bore oxygen tubing is connected between the nipple on the SVN and the outlet nipple on the ventilator. Turning on the ventilator's nebulizer control diverts some of the patient's tidal volume through the nebulizer. The medication is nebulized only during inspiration, and no change in delivered tidal volume or oxygen percentage is noted. Make sure that the nebulizer is turned off after the medication has been delivered. Typically the nebulizer then is removed, or bypassed, as is shown in Figure 15-29. A heat-moisture exchanger can be added back into the circuit after the treatment is completed.

MODULE G

Weaning the patient from the ventilator and extubation

1. Interpret the results of bedside spirometry and lung mechanics (Code: IB10e and n) [Difficulty: ELE: R, Ap; WRE: An]

Indications that the patient can tolerate weaning should include some, if not all, of the criteria listed in Box 15-5. The patient need not pass each and every criterion. However, the more the patient can attain, the more likely he or she is to wean successfully. Individual physicians and practitioners may favor some of these conditions over others and may include other factors not listed. Review the discussion on bedside spirometry earlier in this chapter and in Chapter 4, if needed.

Some patients do not wean successfully even though objective criteria indicate that they should. Conversely, some patients wean successfully even when objective criteria indicate otherwise. Keep in mind that each patient must be evaluated individually. Look at the objective criteria and how the patient actually performs during weaning.

2. Recommend procedures for weaning the patient (WRE code: IIIG1d) [Difficulty: An]

3. Independently initiate procedures for weaning (Code: IIIF2i12) [Difficulty: ELE: R, Ap; WRE: An]

4. Initiate and modify weaning procedures (Code: IIID7) [Difficulty: ELE: R, Ap; WRE: An]

Each of the five methods presented here has its advocates and a body of clinical evidence to show that it is a valid weaning technique. The practitioner must evaluate the patient before recommending any particular weaning method. The patient also must be evaluated during the weaning trial to determine whether the method chosen is meeting his or her needs. The practitioner must be prepared to discontinue weaning if the patient is failing and must be ready to try another weaning approach to help ensure success.

a. Ventilator discontinuance

Ventilator discontinuance is used widely with patients who have been ventilated for a short period and now are fully prepared to breathe on their own (Figure 15-31, A). When the patient is stable, awake, and alert and meets the criteria listed in Box 15-5, he or she can be prepared for weaning. The patient should be instructed about weaning, should be suctioned, and should be put in Fowler's or semi-Fowler's position if possible. The ventilator circuit is disconnected, and an aerosol and oxygen mix is breathed in through a T-piece (Briggs adapter) with reservoir (see

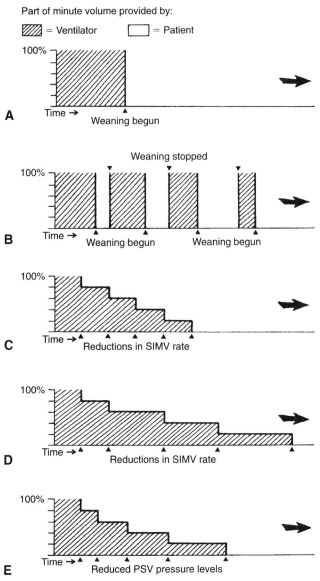

Figure 15-31 A through E, Options for weaning a patient from a mechanical ventilator. *PSV,* Pressure support ventilation; *SIMV,* synchronous intermittent mandatory ventilation.

Figure 6-36). The oxygen percentage should be the same as originally inspired or up to 10% higher, depending on the patient's PaO_2 level on the ventilator.

Ventilator discontinuance and weaning begin at the same moment. The patient goes from having the ventilator provide 100% of the minute volume needed to providing none of it. The patient should be watched continuously because he or she is now breathing totally independently. Vital signs and respiratory mechanics should be measured every 5 to 10 minutes throughout the procedure. If the patient's condition deteriorates, ventilator therapy is reestablished. After a rest period, intermittent ventilator discontinuance or another mode of weaning might be tried. If the patient is stable, an ABG sample should be taken after about 20 minutes. Alternatively, pulse oximetry and end-tidal carbon dioxide can be monitored. If the blood gas results are acceptable and the patient appears stable, the weaning is continued, or the patient can be extubated. Approximately 75% of patients who tolerate this procedure can be extubated.

b. Intermittent ventilator discontinuance

This method is used after the previously mentioned method proves less than successful. The patient is started on the ventilator on a schedule of intermittent weaning periods and rest periods (Figure 15-31, B). The method shown has a cycle of lengthening weaning periods and shortening rest periods. This goes on until the patient is weaning for an extended period, as was discussed earlier. Another method involves a cycle of set rest periods (commonly 0.5 to 1 hour) and lengthening weaning periods as the patient becomes stronger. Again, blood gas values should be monitored after about 20 minutes of weaning. The weaning period can be extended as long as the patient is stable or until extubated.

c. Regular steps in SIMV weaning

As was discussed earlier, SIMV was developed originally as a ventilating mode and has become a widely used weaning mode. It allows the patient a more gradual transition toward totally providing all of the WOB. SIMV seems to work especially well in weaning patients who have been ventilator dependent for an extended period. By gradually taking over more of the WOB, the patient reconditions respiratory muscles that may have atrophied through lack of use. The patient also is gaining self-confidence that complete weaning will occur. An additional benefit is that all ventilator alarm systems are functional, and the patient does not need to be watched directly as closely as in the two previously mentioned weaning methods.

This particular SIMV weaning pattern can be applied to a patient who is stable and is making rapid progress (Figure 15-31, C). The weaning pattern might involve reducing the SIMV rate in increments of about 2 per minute on a set time schedule. About 20 minutes after the SIMV rate is reduced, blood gas values should be monitored. The patient's respiratory mechanics are monitored closely. It is important to calculate the patient's spontaneous minute volume (rate × tidal volume). It should be approximately the same volume as was subtracted from the ventilator-delivered minute volume. The process continues as long as the patient tolerates each decrease in the SIMV rate. The stable, strong patient can be weaned rather quickly down to an SIMV rate of 2 to 4 times/min. The decision often is made at this point to use a T-piece, as was discussed earlier, or to extubate the airway.

d. Irregular steps in SIMV weaning

This method is applied when the regular SIMV method is unsuccessful. Often the patient starts out on a cycle of regular reductions in SIMV rate. This goes on until a point is reached at which the patient has a setback and cannot tolerate any further reduction in the SIMV rate. The rate may be kept at that level for an extended period until the patient is ready for a further decrease (Figure 15-31, D). Additional decreases in the IMV rate proceed as the patient tolerates them. No attempt is made to set up a regular pattern of reducing the rate.

It may be necessary to increase the rate to higher previous levels if the patient has a serious setback. One possible cause that may prevent the SIMV rate from decreasing is resistance to breathing through the demand valve and breathing circuit. A trial on a T-piece (which offers no resistance) may prove to be the final step in weaning. If this fails for the patient, the reason is probably the resistance caused by the endotracheal tube. The pressure support weaning method then should be tried on the patient.

e. Weaning by pressure support ventilation

The PSV mode is available on most modern electrically powered and microprocessor ventilators. It can be used as the newest weaning method (Figure 15-31, E). When it is used as a weaning method, the pressure support level is reduced gradually. Decreasing pressure support steps of 2 to 5 cm water are made commonly. The patient has to increase the WOB gradually to inspire a tidal volume. Blood gas values and respiratory mechanics should be evaluated after each decrease in the pressure support level. A modest pressure support level of 2 to 5 cm water is maintained to overcome any resistance of the endotracheal tube. If the patient does well during an extended trial of minimum pressure support, extubation is performed unless the endotracheal tube is needed for other reasons.

The criteria listed in Box 15-5 can be used in evaluating any patient who is being weaned by any of these methods. General signs that the patient is not tolerating weaning include anxiety, agitation, a large increase or decrease in respiratory rate, angina, tachycardia, an increase in premature ventricular contractions or other serious dysrhythmias, bradycardia, hypertension, hypotension, cyanosis, hypoxemia, and hypercarbia with acidemia. The patient probably will not exhibit all of these signs. Some tend to be seen together because they relate to the patient's WOB. Others appear to give conflicting signals of success or failure. It is the practitioner's responsibility to evaluate the patient's condition to determine whether weaning should be continued or ventilatory support resumed.

5. Recommend extubation (Code: IIIG1h) [Difficulty: ELE: R, Ap; WRE: An]

Extubation usually can be safely accomplished when the patient meets the following criteria:

- Has the desired bedside spirometry and vital signs listed in Box 15-5

- Has demonstrated the ability to breathe effectively for a clinically significant period as measured by the listed criteria
- Has acceptable blood gas results
- Is alert enough to protect his or her airway
- Can effectively cough out any secretions

It may be found that some patients need the endotracheal tube even though they no longer need ventilatory support. The tube provides a suctioning route if the patient is unable to cough out large amounts of secretions. The tube also protects the airway from the risk of aspiration in a comatose patient who may vomit.

6. Perform extubation (Code: IIIB9) [Difficulty: ELE: R, Ap; WRE: An]

The respiratory therapist must be competent to safely extubate a patient and care for the patient's needs after extubation. Review the full discussion in Chapter 12, if needed.

> **Exam Hint 15-20 (ELE, WRE)**
>
> Expect to see several questions that relate to evaluating a patient's ability to wean. These will include such information as initial bedside spirometry, arterial blood gas results, and vital signs. If a patient is able to wean, expect to make recommendations on which method(s) to use. Finally, expect to see questions related to evaluating a patient who is weaning. You will need to evaluate current bedside spirometry, arterial blood gas results, and vital signs. Make a decision to continue weaning, to change the weaning procedure, or to put the patient back on the ventilator. Review the content of Box 15-5.

> **Exam Hint 15-21 (ELE, WRE)**
>
> Be prepared to recommend extubation if a patient has weaned successfully and meets all extubation criteria. More information on this subject is provided in Chapter 12.

MODULE H
Respiratory care plan

1. Analyze the available information to determine the patient's pathophysiologic state (Code: IIIH1) [Difficulty: ELE: R, Ap; WRE: An]

2. Determine the appropriateness of the prescribed respiratory care plan and recommend modifications when indicated

a. Determine the appropriateness of the prescribed therapy and goals for the patient's pathophysiologic state (Code: IIIH3) [Difficulty: ELE: R, Ap; WRE: An]

b. Review the planned therapy to establish the therapeutic plan (Code: IIIH2a) [Difficulty: ELE: R, Ap; WRE: An]

c. Recommend changes in the therapeutic plan when indicated (Code: IIIH4) [Difficulty: ELE: R, Ap; WRE: An]

Be prepared to make recommendations on changing ventilator parameters based on the patient's pathologic condition, blood gas values, chest radiograph findings, breath sounds, and vital signs. Common recommendations follow.

> **Exam Hint 15-22 (WRE)**
>
> Past Written Registry Examinations have had questions about the management of patients with specific conditions such as increased ICP, COPD, CHF, ARDS, and pneumothorax. In addition, the Clinical Simulation Examination has at least one adult scenario on each of the following: a patient with COPD, a patient with trauma, a patient with cardiovascular disease, and a patient with neuromuscular or neurologic disease. The management of these patients is briefly discussed next.

---

1. Increased intracranial pressure (ICP)

ICP, the pressure within the cranium (skull), normally is less than 10 mm Hg. It is measured by placement of a catheter into the subarachnoid space, subdural space, or ventricular space. The most common cause of increased ICP is an acute head injury in which the brain is shaken. This is caused commonly by a closed head injury. Other causes of increased ICP include craniotomy for brain tumor resection and stroke (cerebral vascular accident [CVA]). Any significant increase in pressure within the skull will further injure the brain. Clinical experience has shown that when the ICP exceeds 20 mm Hg, the patient's outcome significantly worsens.

The A/C mode usually is selected with constant volume ventilation so that the patient is assured of a set minute volume if apnea occurs. It has been demonstrated that hyperventilating the patient to a $PaCO_2$ between 25 and 30 torr reduces the increased ICP. This is the result of the lowered carbon dioxide pressure, which causes cerebral vasoconstriction. Because the cerebral blood flow is decreased by hyperventilation, it is important to maintain the patient's PaO_2 in the 90 to 110 torr range.

2. Chronic obstructive lung disease

Patients with COPD usually are well known because of previous hospitalizations for acute exacerbations related to problems such as lung infection or heart failure. When the patient must be ventilated, it is important to maintain baseline "normal" blood gas values. This usually means accepting moderate hypoxemia and hypercarbia with a compensated respiratory acidosis. Ventilating the patient to provide textbook normal ABGs must be avoided. This is because the patient with COPD cannot maintain this level of breathing efficiency when ready to come off of the ventilator.

The A/C or SIMV mode may be used with a constant volume set or PC used to set the tidal volume. A patient with COPD must have the ventilator adjusted, including the addition of mechanical dead space, to maintain the patient's normally elevated $PaCO_2$ level. A PaO_2 of 60 to 70 torr usually is adequate. Keep the plateau pressure (alveolar pressure) less than 30 cm water to avoid overdistention of the patient's compliant lungs and resultant volutrauma.

If the patient has air trapping and auto-PEEP, a small amount of therapeutic PEEP may be added to help the patient exhale and to trigger the ventilator. Increase the therapeutic PEEP in 1-cm water steps until the patient is synchronized with the ventilator. Many patients with COPD need 5 cm water of PEEP or more. When the condition that caused the sudden deterioration is corrected, the patient should be weaned off of the ventilator as soon as possible to prevent atrophy of the ventilatory muscles.

3. Congestive heart failure

Patients with congestive heart failure (CHF) usually also have a pulmonary edema problem. This results in hypoxemia and low lung compliance. Mechanical ventilation with the A/C or SIMV mode with constant volume ventilation is needed to reduce the patient's WOB, deliver supplemental oxygen, and add therapeutic PEEP. Usually a pulmonary artery catheter is placed to measure pulmonary artery pressure (PAP), pulmonary capillary wedge pressure (PCWP), and cardiac output (CO). If the PEEP level is increased and the patient's cardiac output is decreased, the PEEP should be reduced to its previous level. The patient must be given a diuretic such as furosemide (Lasix) to increase urine output. The patient's heart function is improved by giving digitalis (Lanoxin). Closely follow the patient's cardiovascular values to monitor improvement after administration of a diuretic and digitalis. Reduce the PEEP and inspired oxygen as the pulmonary edema problem is corrected. See Chapter 9 for a discussion of medications and Chapter 5 for a discussion on hemodynamic monitoring, as needed.

3. Apply the ARDS-Net protocol (Code: IIID10) [Difficulty: ELE: R, Ap; WRE: An]

Acute respiratory distress syndrome (ARDS) is caused by a variety of pulmonary and circulatory conditions that result in nonhomogeneous damage to alveolar capillary membranes throughout the lungs. This results in noncardiac pulmonary edema with decreased pulmonary compliance and hypoxemia. Similar to the patient with CHF, the patient with ARDS needs mechanical ventilation to reduce the increased work of breathing, provide supplemental oxygen, and provide therapeutic PEEP. A pulmonary artery catheter is needed to follow the patient's cardiovascular status.

Unlike the patient with CHF, the patient with ARDS does not respond as favorably to diuretic and digitalis medications. The continued problem of low compliance and resulting high ventilating pressures have been linked to barotrauma/volutrauma. Recent research has led to the development of ARDS-Net lung protective strategies to prevent ventilator-associated lung injury. Following is a summary of the key recommendations; review the full document, as needed.

a. Small tidal volume ventilation

Initially, most patients with ARDS are started on the A/C or SIMV mode with constant volume ventilation. Unfortunately, many patients with severe ARDS cannot be managed in this manner. The stiff lungs result in a very high plateau pressure and risk of pulmonary barotrauma/volutrauma (also called shear stress). Recent studies have shown that the plateau pressure found in the alveoli (P_{plat}) must be kept at <30 cm water to avoid this serious complication. To lower a dangerously high alveolar pressure, the tidal volume must be reduced. Many clinicians recommend that the patient be switched from constant volume ventilation to pressure control ventilation (PCV) to do this. Recent evidence has shown a higher survival rate in patients with ARDS when the tidal volume was lowered from 12 mL/kg to 6 mL/kg of ideal body weight.

If the initial set of blood gases on PC with a small tidal volume does not show adequate oxygenation, the inspiratory time must be increased. Some patients with ARDS need an increased inspiratory time such that the I:E ratio is inverse. This results in pressure control inverse ratio ventilation (PCIRV). The advantages of PCIRV over conventional volume ventilation include the lowered peak airway pressure and the longer inspiratory time. The lowered peak pressure is thought to reduce the risk of volutrauma. The longer inspiratory time allows alveoli with long time constants of ventilation to fill and areas of atelectasis to reopen.

b. Permissive hypercapnia

The small tidal volumes used with PCIRV can result in failure to blow off carbon dioxide to a normal level. At times, this must be clinically accepted. Permissive hypercapnia involves allowing a $PaCO_2$ of 50 torr up to 100 to 150 torr. It is very important to prevent the carbon dioxide level from increasing too rapidly because it causes cerebral vasodilation and increases the patient's ICP. To minimize this risk, the $PaCO_2$ should not be allowed to increase faster than 10 torr/hr to a maximum of 80 torr. If the $PaCO_2$ must be allowed to increase to more than 80 torr, the rate of increase must be slower than 10 torr/hr. The high $PaCO_2$ also results in a respiratory acidosis. Keep the patient's arterial pH at ≥ 7.25 to avoid problems related to the acidosis. It may be necessary to administer intravenous bicarbonate to correct the respiratory acidosis. When the patient recovers, the $PaCO_2$ can be lowered gradually. If permissive hypercapnia was used for less than 24 hours, the $PaCO_2$ probably can be lowered by 10 to 20 torr/hr. If permissive hypercapnia was used for longer than 24 hours, or if bicarbonate was given to buffer the pH, the $PaCO_2$ must be lowered more slowly. It is important to monitor the patient's arterial pH throughout this process to prevent too rapid an increase.

c. Lung recruitment maneuver and inflection points

The purpose of a recruitment maneuver is to find the ideal amount of PEEP needed to keep the lungs open and to maintain the FRC (see Figure 4-14). When the FRC is maintained, the tidal volume can be delivered with the least amount of pressure. A secondary benefit of setting the ideal level of PEEP is that the patient can be oxygenated at the lowest inspired oxygen percentage. A lung recruitment maneuver has similarities to a Best PEEP/Optimum PEEP study to find the PEEP level needed to correct the low lung compliance, the severe hypoxemia, and the large shunt percentage that these patients have (see Figure 15-19).

Steps in the lung recruitment maneuver include the following:

1. Inflate the lungs as much as possible by applying a series of steps of increased baseline pressure. Lung volume and pressure should be plotted with the ventilator's graphics package, if possible. Maximally, 35 to 45 cm water pressure is applied against the lungs for 40 to 60 seconds. This baseline pressure increase is intended to open up any areas of atelectasis. As the pressure is increased, the opening pressure of the lungs is found. This corresponds to point **A** of Figure 15-16 when areas of atelectasis open up. As the pressure is maximized, the lungs become fully inflated. More pressure does little, if anything, to add more volume. This corresponds to point **B** of Figure 15-16.
2. The lungs are allowed to deflate through reduction of baseline pressure in a series of steps. The lung volumes and pressures should be graphed as

this is done. The purpose of this procedure is to find the pressure when most of the lung units begin to collapse. This corresponds to point C of Figure 15-16.

3. Finally, the lung recruitment maneuver is repeated to reopen any recently closed lung units.

When the recruitment maneuver is done on a modern microprocessor ventilator with graphics software and a monitor, set the unit to display a pressure/volume loop. A loop similar to the one shown in Figure 15-16 will be seen. Point A shows the inspiratory low inflection point and is found near the FRC. This identifies the pressure needed to open up alveoli and establish the patient's FRC. Point B shows the inspiratory high inflection point and is found near the total lung capacity. This identifies the highest lung volume and highest lung pressure that should be allowed. Note the "beaking" that occurs to the right of point B. Further pressure does not greatly increase tidal volume and can result in volutrauma to any overstretched alveoli. Many clinicians use the high inflection point as the maximum pressure allowed with PCV to deliver a tidal volume. The expiratory upper inflection point, C, represents the pressure below which atelectasis may occur.

There is controversy over how to best use the above information. Some feel that the minimum level of PEEP should be applied to minimize the risk of lung injury. This would correspond with a pressure at or above point A in Figure 15-16. Some feel that a higher PEEP level should be used to minimize shunting, but less than is shown in point B in Figure 15-16. The ARDS-Net group recommends that PEEP should be set above the expiratory high inflection point. This would be greater than point C of Figure 15-16 and would prevent alveolar collapse on exhalation.

d. Auto-PEEP recognition

If PCIRV is used, the inspiratory time must be reduced toward normal as lung compliance improves. Monitor the patient for air trapping and auto-PEEP if the expiratory time is too short (see Figure 15-3). Full exhalation of the tidal volume must be assured.

Exam Hint 15-23 (ELE, WRE)

Be prepared to make recommendations on changing ventilator parameters based on the patient's condition, blood gas values, chest radiograph films, breath sounds, and vital signs. This information can be found in this chapter and throughout this text.

4. Recommend the treatment of a tension pneumothorax (Code: IIIG1b) [Difficulty: ELE: R, Ap; WRE: An]

Recognize the signs of a pneumothorax on a mechanically ventilated patient (suddenly increasing peak and plateau pressures, hypoxemia, mediastinal shift to the side opposite the pneumothorax, hyperresonant percussion noted over the pneumothorax, and asymmetric chest movement on inspiration). Chest radiograph and physical examination of the patient will reveal whether air (or fluid) is found abnormally around the lung(s) or the heart.

Common causes of the pneumothorax include lung puncture during insertion of a central venous pressure (CVP) line via the subclavian vein, overinflated lungs from too large a tidal volume on the ventilator, punctured lung from a sharp broken rib, and thoracentesis.

If a patient has a tension pneumothorax, a pleural chest tube must be inserted on the affected side to remove the air and relieve the pressure within the chest. In an emergency, a large-gauge needle may be placed between the second and third ribs (second intercostal space) in the midclavicular line. These and related subjects are discussed in detail in Chapter 18. A nontension pneumothorax of greater than 10% often is treated by insertion of a pleural chest tube. In addition, a pleural chest tube is placed to remove blood or other fluid from the pleural space.

A pneumomediastinum, pneumopericardium, or pneumoperitoneum that puts the patient at risk also must be treated. A chest tube then is inserted into the area where the abnormal air is found. The same chest tube also would remove any abnormal collection of fluid. A pericardial chest tube usually is placed behind the heart to remove any blood that may leak out after open heart surgery is performed.

If the patient is being ventilated on a constant volume ventilator, the amount of air that is lost through the pleural chest tube can be calculated. This is done by subtracting the measured exhaled volume from the measured inhaled volume (the set tidal volume). The following equation demonstrates:

Inspired tidal volume = 500 mL
Exhaled tidal volume = −400 mL
100 mL of tidal volume is lost through the pleural chest tube.

It is not always possible to measure a consistent tidal volume when PCV or a similar mode is used. In a case like this, it is possible to make only a qualitative judgment on pleural air leak. In other words, if air is seen to bubble out through the pleural drainage system, an air leak is present. When the air stops bubbling, the pleural tear has healed.

See Chapter 18 for a complete discussion on pleural drainage systems.

Remember to get an ABG after every ventilator change that could result in a different PaO_2 (pulse oximetry or transcutaneous oxygen may be substituted) or $PaCO_2$ (end-tidal CO_2 or transcutaneous carbon dioxide may be substituted). Mixed venous blood gas values should also be obtained when possible.

Exam Hint 15-24 (WRE)

Usually one question deals with recognizing that a patient is losing tidal volume through a pleural chest tube or that a pneumothorax has developed. Know the signs and symptoms of a pneumothorax.

---

a. **Terminate the treatment or procedure based on the patient's response to therapy (Code: IIIF1) [Difficulty: ELE: R, Ap; WRE: An]**

b. **Recommend discontinuing the treatment or procedure based on the patient's response to therapy (Code: IIIG1i) [Difficulty: ELE: R, Ap; WRE: An]**

Physical responses to mechanical ventilation, as measured by the vital signs, can vary considerably. A patient who is anxious or angry or in pain will have an increase in vital signs. A patient who is relaxed has reduced WOB, and a patient whose blood gas values are now normal will have a return to normal vital signs. Watch carefully for the patient whose decrease in blood pressure coincides with a tachycardia. This patient may be having decreased venous return to the heart from increased intrathoracic pressure. Be prepared to stop a treatment or procedure related to mechanical ventilation if the patient has an adverse reaction to it.

5. Respiratory care protocols

a. **Develop any ventilator management protocol (Code: IIIH6b) [Difficulty: ELE: R; WRE: Ap, An]**

b. **Apply any ventilator management protocol (Code: IIIH8) [Difficulty: ELE: R, Ap; WRE: An]**

c. **Explain planned therapy and goals to the patient in understandable (nonmedical) terms to achieve the best results from the treatment (Code: IIIA6) [Difficulty: ELE: R, Ap; WRE: An]**

Because an intubated patient cannot speak, it is necessary to communicate by asking simple questions that can be answered by a *yes* nod or *no* shake of the head. Other methods of communication include a pad of paper and pencil and picture boards. It is not possible to predict how a patient will react to the initiation of mechanical ventilation or its prolonged need. Some patients react with relief and relax when the WOB is reduced. Others may become angry at the limitations imposed on them or become depressed.

   d. Monitor the outcome of the ventilator management protocol (Code: IIIH7b) [Difficulty: ELE: R, Ap; WRE: An]

   e. Communicate the outcome of therapy and change the treatment or procedure based on the protocol (Code: IIIA5) [Difficulty: ELE: R, Ap; WRE: An]

6. **Record and evaluate the patient's response to the treatment(s) or procedure(s), including the following**

   a. Record and interpret the following: heart rate and rhythm, respiratory rate, blood pressure, body temperature, and pain level (Code: IIIA1b4) [Difficulty: ELE: R, Ap; WRE: An]

   b. Record and interpret the patient's breath sounds (Code: IIIAb3) [Difficulty: ELE: R, Ap; WRE: An]

   c. Record and interpret the type of cough the patient has and the nature of the sputum (Code: IIIAb3) [Difficulty: ELE: R, Ap; WRE: An]

   d. Recheck any math work and make note of incorrect data (Code: IIIA1b2) [Difficulty: ELE: R, Ap; WRE: An]

7. **Communicate information relevant to coordinating patient care and discharge planning [e.g., scheduling, avoiding conflicts, sequencing therapies] (Code: IIIA2b) [Difficulty: ELE: R, Ap; WRE: An]**

BIBLIOGRAPHY

Aboussouan LS: Respiratory failure and the need for ventilatory support. In: Wilkins RL, Stoller JK, Kacmarek RM, editors: *Egan's fundamentals of respiratory care*, ed 9, St Louis, 2009, Mosby.

Aloan CA, Hill TV, editors: *Respiratory care of the newborn and child*, ed 2, Philadelphia, 1997, Lippincott Williams & Wilkins.

American Association for Respiratory Care: Clinical Practice Guideline: application of continuous positive airway pressure in neonates via nasal prongs or nasopharyngeal tube, *Respir Care* 39(8):817, 1994.

American Association for Respiratory Care: Clinical Practice Guideline: capnography/capnometry during mechanical ventilation, *Respir Care* 40(12):1321, 1995.

American Association for Respiratory Care: Clinical Practice Guideline: capnography/capnometry during mechanical ventilation: 2003 revision and update, *Respir Care* 48(3): 534, 2003.

American Association for Respiratory Care: Clinical Practice Guideline: endotracheal suctioning of mechanically ventilated adults and children with artificial airways, *Respir Care* 38(5):500, 1993.

American Association for Respiratory Care: Clinical Practice Guideline: evidence-based guidelines for weaning and discontinuing ventilatory support, *Respir Care* 47(1):69, 2002.

American Association for Respiratory Care: Clinical Practice Guideline: humidification during mechanical ventilation, *Respir Care* 37(8):887, 1992.

American Association for Respiratory Care: Clinical Practice Guideline: in-hospital transport of the mechanically ventilated patient: 2002 revision and update, *Respir Care* 47(6):721, 2002.

American Association for Respiratory Care: Clinical Practice Guideline: long-term invasive mechanical ventilation in the home—2007 revision & update, *Respir Care* 52(1):1056, 2007.

American Association for Respiratory Care: Clinical Practice Guideline: neonatal time-triggered, pressure-limited, time-cycled mechanical ventilation, *Respir Care* 39(8):808, 1994.

American Association for Respiratory Care: Clinical Practice Guideline: patient-ventilator system checks, *Respir Care* 37(8):882, 1992.

American Association for Respiratory Care: Clinical Practice Guideline: removal of the endotracheal tube—2007 revision & update, *Respir Care* 52(1):81, 2007.

American Association for Respiratory Care: Clinical Practice Guideline: selection of device, administration of bronchodilator, and evaluation of responses to therapy in mechanically ventilated patients, *Respir Care* 44(1):105, 1999.

American Association for Respiratory Care: Clinical Practice Guideline: ventilator circuit changes, *Respir Care* 39(8):797, 1994.

American Association for Respiratory Care: Consensus statement on the essentials of mechanical ventilation, *Respir Care* 37(9):1000, 1992.

American Association for Respiratory Care: Evidence-Based Clinical Practice Guidelines: care of the ventilator circuit and its relation to ventilator-associated pneumonia, *Respir Care* 48(9):869, 2003.

ARDS Network: Ventilation with lower tidal volumes as compared with traditional tidal volumes for acute lung injury and the acute respiratory distress syndrome patients, *N Engl J Med* 342(18):1301, 2000.

Banner MJ, Lampotang S: Clinical use of inspiratory and expiratory waveforms. In: Kacmarek RM, Stoller JK, editors: *Current respiratory care*, Philadelphia, 1988, BC Decker.

Barnes TA, editor: *Core textbook of respiratory care practice*, ed 2, St Louis, 1994, Mosby.

Bone RC: Pressure-volume measurements in detection of bronchospasm and mucous plugging in acute respiratory failure, *Respir Care* 21(7):620, 1976.

Boysen PG, McGough E: Pressure-control and pressure-support ventilation: flow patterns, inspiratory time, and gas distribution, *Respir Care* 33(2):620, 1988.

Branson RD, Campbell RS, Davis K Jr, et al: Altering flowrate during maximum pressure support ventilation (PSV_max): effects on cardiorespiratory function, *Respir Care* 35(11):1056, 1990.

Branson RD, Chatburn RL: Technical description and classification of modes of ventilator operation, *Respir Care* 37(9):1026, 1992.

Branson RD, Hess DR, Chatburn RL, editors: *Respiratory care equipment*, ed 2, Philadelphia, 1999, Lippincott Williams & Wilkins.

Branson RD, Hurst JM: Laboratory evaluation of moisture output of seven airway heat and moisture exchangers, *Respir Care* 32(9):741, 1987.

Burton GC, Hodgkin JE, Ward JJ, editors: *Respiratory care: a guide to clinical practice*, ed 4, Philadelphia, 1997, Lippincott Williams & Wilkins.

Cairo JM, Pilbeam SP: *Mosby's respiratory care equipment*, ed 8, St Louis, 2010, Mosby.

Campbell RS, Davis BR: Pressure-controlled versus volume-controlled ventilation: does it matter? *Respir Care* 47(4):416, 2002.

Chang DW: *Clinical application of mechanical ventilation*, ed 3, Albany, NY, 2006, Delmar.

Chatburn RL: A new system for understanding mechanical ventilation, *Respir Care* 36(10):1123, 1991.

Chatburn RL: Classification of mechanical ventilators, *Respir Care* 37(9):1009, 1992.

Dantzker DR, MacIntyre NR, Bakow ED, editors: *Comprehensive respiratory care*, Philadelphia, 1995, WB Saunders.

Dhand R: Ventilator graphics and respiratory mechanics in the patient with obstructive lung disease, *Respir Care* 50(2):246, 2005.

Drinker PA, McKhann CF III: Landmark perspective: the iron lung: first practical means of respiratory support, *JAMA* 256(11):1476, 1986.

Epstein SK: Extubation, *Respir Care* 47(4):483, 2002.

Epstein SK: Weaning from mechanical ventilation, *Respir Care* 47(4):454, 2002.

Evidence-based guidelines for weaning and discontinuing ventilator support, *Respir Care* 47(1):69, 2002.

Felix WR Jr, MacDonnell KF, Jacobs L: Resuscitation from drowning in cold water, *N Engl J Med* 304(14):843, 1981.

Fink JB, Hunt GE, editors: *Clinical practice in respiratory care*, Philadelphia, 1999, Lippincott Williams & Wilkins.

Fink JB, Tobin MJ, Dhand R: Bronchodilator therapy in mechanically ventilated patients, *Respir Care* 44(1):53, 1999.

Greer K: Hypothermia: a quiet killer, *Adv Respir Ther* Jan 15, 1990.

Gregg BL: Invasive mechanical ventilation. In: Wyka KA, Mathews PJ, Clark WF, editors: *Foundations of respiratory care*, Albany, NY, 2002, Delmar.

Gurevitch MJ: Selection of the inspiratory:expiratory ratio. In: Kacmarek RM, Stoller JK, editors: *Current respiratory care*, Philadelphia, 1988, BC Decker.

Hamel DS, Cheifetz IM: Capnography to optimize and minimize mechanical ventilation. In: Gravenstein JS, Jaffe MB, Paulus DA, editors: *Capnography: clinical aspects*, Cambridge, United Kingdom, 2004, Cambridge University Press.

Hess DR: Mechanical ventilation of the adult patient: initiation, management, and weaning. In: Burton GG, Hodgkin JE, Ward JJ, editors: *Respiratory care: a guide to clinical practice*, ed 4, Philadelphia, 1997, Lippincott Williams & Wilkins.

Hess DR, Branson RD: Mechanical ventilation. In: Hess DR, MacIntyre NR, Mishoe SC, et al, editors: *Respiratory care principles and practice*, Philadelphia, 2002, Saunders.

Hess DR, Kacmarek RM: *Essentials of mechanical ventilation*, ed 2, New York, 2002, McGraw-Hill.

Hess DR, McCurdy S, Simmons M: Compression volume in adult ventilator circuits: a comparison of five disposable circuits and a nondisposable circuit, *Respir Care* 36(10):1113, 1991.

Hill NS: Clinical application of body ventilators, *Chest* 90(6):897, 1986.

Hill NS, Eveloff SE, Carlisle CC, et al: Efficacy of nocturnal nasal ventilation in patients with restrictive thoracic disease, *Am Rev Respir Dis* 145(2):365, 1992.

Hirsch C, Kacmarek RM, Stanek K: Work of breathing during CPAP and PSV imposed by the new generation mechanical ventilators: a lung model study, *Respir Care* 36(8):815, 1991.

International Consensus Conferences in Intensive Care Medicine: Ventilator-associated lung injury in ARDS, *Am J Respir Crit Care Med* 160(6):2118, 1999.

Kacmarek RM: Noninvasive positive pressure ventilation. In: Wilkins RL, Stoller JK, Kacmarek RM, editors: *Egan's fundamentals of respiratory care*, ed 9, St Louis, 2009, Mosby.

Kacmarek RM: The role of pressure support ventilation in reducing work of breathing, *Respir Care* 33(2):99, 1988.

Kacmarek RM, Foley K, Cheever P: Determination of ventilatory reserve in mechanically ventilated patients: a comparison of techniques, *Respir Care* 36(10):1085, 1991.

Kacmarek RM, Hess D: Pressure-controlled inverse-ratio ventilation: panacea or auto-PEEP? *Respir Care* 35(10):945, 1990.

Kallet RH, Diaz JV: The physiologic effects of noninvasive ventilation. *Respir Care* 54(1):102, 2009.

Kirby RR: Modes of mechanical ventilation. In: Kacmarek RM, Stoller JK, editors: *Current respiratory care*, Philadelphia, 1988, BC Decker.

Kuhlen R, Rossaint R: The role of spontaneous breathing during mechanical ventilation, *Respir Care* 47(3):296, 2002.

MacIntyre NR: Setting the frequency-tidal volume pattern, *Respir Care* 47(3):266, 2002.

MacIntyre NR: Pressure support: inspiratory assist. In: Kacmarek RM, Stoller JK, editors: *Current respiratory care*, Philadelphia, 1988, BC Decker.

MacIntyre NR: Weaning from mechanical ventilatory support: volume-assisting intermittent breaths versus pressure-supporting every breath, *Respir Care* 33(2):121, 1988.

MacIntyre NR, Branson RD: *Mechanical ventilation*, ed 2, Philadelphia, 2009, Saunders.

Martz KV, Joiner JW, Rodger MS: *Management of the patient-ventilator system: a team approach*, ed 2, St Louis, 1984, Mosby.

Medhof BD: Invasive and noninvasive ventilation in patients with asthma, *Respir Care* 53(6):740, 2008.

Mehta S, Al-Hashim AH, Keenan SP: Noninvasive ventilation in patients with acute cardiopulmonary edema, *Respir Care* 54(2):186, 2009.

Nava S, Navalesi P, Gregoretti C: Interfaces and humidification for noninvasive mechanical ventilation, *Respir Care* 54(1):71, 2009.

Nilsestuen JO, Hargett KD: Using ventilator graphics to identify patient-ventilator asynchrony, *Respir Care* 50(2):202, 2005.

Pennock BE, Kaplan PD, Carlin BW, et al: Pressure support ventilation with a simplified ventilatory support system administered with a nasal mask in patients with respiratory failure, *Chest* 100(5):1371, 1991.

Pierson DJ: Indications for mechanical ventilation in adults with acute respiratory failure, *Respir Care* 47(3):249, 2002.

Pilbeam SP Cairo SP: *Mechanical ventilation: physiological and clinical applications,* ed 4, St Louis, 2006, Mosby.

Quan SF, Parides GC, Knoper SR: Mandatory minute volume (MVV) ventilation: an overview, *Respir Care* 35(9):898, 1990.

Radford EP Jr: Ventilation standards for use in artificial respiration, *J Appl Phys* 7:451, 1955.

Respironics: Guidelines for invasive applications with BiPAP systems, Carlsbad, CA, Philips Healthcare.

Respironics: Product literature on the suggested protocol for initiation of the BiPAP S/T or BiPAP S/T-D ventilatory support system, Carlsbad, CA, Philips Healthcare.

Saura P, Blanch L: How to set positive end-expiratory pressure. *Respir Care* 47(3):279, 2002.

Scanlan CL, Wilkins RL, Stoller JK, editors: *Egan's fundamentals of respiratory care,* ed 8, St Louis, 2003, Mosby.

Shapiro BA, Kacmarek RM, Cane RD, et al, editors: *Clinical application of respiratory care,* ed 4, St Louis, 1991, Mosby.

Shelledy DC: Discontinuing ventilatory support. In: Wilkins RL, Stoller JK, Kacmarek RM (eds): *Egan's fundamentals of respiratory care,* ed 9, St Louis, 2009, Mosby.

Shelledy DC: Initiating and adjusting ventilatory support. In: Wilkins RL, Stoller JK, Kacmarek RM (eds): *Egan's fundamentals of respiratory care,* ed 9, St Louis, 2009, Mosby.

Shelledy DC, Mikles SP: Newer modes of mechanical ventilation, I: pressure support, *Respir Manage* July/Aug 14, 1988.

Shelledy DC, Mikles SP: Newer modes of mechanical ventilation, II: mandatory minute volume ventilation, *Respir Manage* July/Aug 21, 1988.

Stoller JK: Establishing clinical unweanability, *Respir Care* 36(3):186, 1991.

Strumpf DA, Carlisle CC, Millman RP, et al: An evaluation of the Respironics BiPAP Bi-Level CPAP device for delivery of assisted ventilation, *Respir Care* 35(5):415, 1990.

The Acute Respiratory Distress Syndrome Network: Ventilation with lower tidal volumes as compared with traditional tidal volumes for acute lung injury and the acute respiratory distress syndrome, May 2000: http://www.nejm.org/ content/ browser/1.asp

Tobin MJ: Monitoring of pressure, flow, and volume during mechanical ventilation, *Respir Care* 37(9):1081, 1992.

Tobin MJ, Lodato RF: PEEP, auto-PEEP, and waterfalls, *Chest* 96(3):449, 1989.

Waldhorn RE: Nocturnal nasal intermittent positive pressure ventilation with bi-level positive airway pressure (BiPAP) in respiratory failure, Chest 101(2):516, 1992.

Waugh JB, Deshpande VM, Harwood RJ, Brown M: *Rapid interpretation of ventilator waveforms,* ed 2, Upper Saddle River, NJ, 2007, Pearson Prentice-Hall.

Whitaker K: *Comprehensive perinatal and pediatric respiratory care,* ed 2, Albany, NY, 1997, Delmar.

White GC: *Equipment theory for respiratory care,* ed 3, Albany, NY, 1999, Delmar.

Wright J, Gong H: "Auto-PEEP": incidence, magnitude, and contributing factors, *Heart Lung* 19(4):352, 1990.

SELF-STUDY QUESTIONS FOR THE ENTRY LEVEL EXAM

See page 598 for answers

1. A 40-year-old patient is brought to the emergency room after being in an automobile accident. She has broken ribs on her right side and a right-sided pneumothorax. Which of the following ventilators would you recommend for her?
   A. PR-2
   B. Bird Mark 7
   C. Servo-*i*
   D. Bird Mark 14

2. Your patient needs to be placed on a ventilator. His body weight is 86 kg (190 lb). The most appropriate uncorrected ventilator V_T would be:
   A. 800 mL
   B. 860 mL
   C. 1350 mL
   D. 500 mL

3. Two patients are brought into the emergency room simultaneously. One has taken an accidental overdose of sleeping pills and has respiratory center depression. The other has pneumonia and bronchitis and is coughing up large amounts of thick, yellow secretions. The airways of both are intubated, and they will undergo mechanical ventilation. You have available only a Bird Mark 7 and a Dräger E-4. Which would you recommend for the patient who has taken the overdose of sleeping pills?
   A. Bird Mark 7
   B. Dräger E-4
   C. Either is acceptable for either patient.
   D. Neither is acceptable.

4. An adult male patient is on the A/C mode with a ventilator V_T of 800 mL and a backup rate of 12 times/min. The physician would like to evaluate the patient's readiness to wean from the ventilator. Which of the following parameters indicate that weaning should be successful?
   1. Spontaneous V_T of 7 mL/kg of ideal body weight

2. V_D/V_T ratio of 0.4
3. Intrapulmonary shunt of 10%
4. VC of 9 mL/kg of ideal body weight
5. MIP of −15 cm H_2O
   A. 1, 2
   B. 3, 4, 5
   C. 1, 2, 3
   D. 2, 3, 4

5. The physician asks your opinion on which weaning method would be most successful in the patient with the weaning parameters listed in Question 4. His spontaneous V_T is 400 mL. You would recommend which of the following methods?
   A. T-piece and extubation in 30 minutes
   B. Intermittent ventilator discontinuance
   C. SIMV weaning
   D. PCV

6. An alert 25-year-old patient is receiving mechanical ventilation. She has a spontaneous V_T of 200 mL and the desire to breathe spontaneously. After oral surgery, she has an endotracheal tube that is smaller than the ideal size. Her PaO_2 level is 73 torr on 40% O_2. What ventilator mode would you recommend for her?
   A. PSV with PEEP
   B. CPAP
   C. SIMV with PSV and PEEP
   D. SIMV with PSV

7. Your patient is recovering from ARDS and is receiving 10 cm H_2O CPAP and 40% O_2. In evaluating the patient after 1 hour, you notice the following: His SpO_2 has dropped from 95% to 90%, his respiratory rate has increased from 14 to 23 breaths/min, and he is complaining of tiredness. You would recommend which of the following?
   A. Continue for another hour and reevaluate.
   B. Raise the CPAP level to 13 cm H_2O because the SpO_2 value has decreased.
   C. Decrease the CPAP level to 7 cm H_2O because the patient is becoming tired at the present level.
   D. Initiate SIMV with 10 cm PEEP.

8. Your patient has an HME in place for humidification purposes. You notice that the peak pressure has increased by 10 cm H_2O in the past hour. The nurse reported to you that the patient's secretions were difficult to suction the last time because they were rather thick. You would recommend which of the following?
   A. Switch the HME to a cool passover-type humidifier.
   B. Switch to a heated cascade-type humidifier.
   C. Have the nurse instill a few milliliters of normal saline solution before suctioning.
   D. Turn up the temperature on the HME.

9. Your ventilated patient with ARDS has the following blood gas values on 40% O_2: PaO_2 75 torr, $PaCO_2$

35 torr, and pH 7.43. She is on the A/C mode with a backup rate of 10 breaths/min and is assisting at a rate of 18 breaths/min. Her peak airway pressure is 65 cm H_2O, and her plateau pressure is 45 cm H_2O. She has developed a pneumothorax caused by the ventilating pressures. What would you suggest?
   A. Switch her to the PCV mode.
   B. Switch her to the SIMV mode.
   C. Switch her to the CPAP mode.
   D. Sedate her so that she does not assist.

10. The sensitivity control should be set at what level when the patient is being ventilated on the A/C mode?
    A. 0 cm H_2O
    B. −1 to −2 cm H_2O
    C. −5 cm H_2O
    D. 1 to 2 cm H_2O

11. In preparing for a mode change from A/C to SIMV, the following must be done:
    1. Turn the sensitivity control off.
    2. Inform the patient of the change in ventilator function.
    3. Turn off the ventilator's sigh control.
    4. Add 5 cm H_2O of therapeutic PEEP to reduce the WOB.
    5. Remove any mechanical dead space from the patient's breathing circuit.
    A. 1, 3, 4
    B. 3, 4
    C. 2, 4, 5
    D. 2, 3, 5

12. Which of the following indicates that the patient is not tolerating PEEP?
    1. Increased Cst
    2. Decreased Cst
    3. Increased intrapulmonary shunt
    4. Stable heart rate
    5. Decreasing blood pressure
    A. 1, 3, 5
    B. 2, 3
    C. 3, 4
    D. 2, 3, 5

Use the following information for questions 13 and 14: Your ventilated patient has an exhaled V_T of 800 mL. Because of refractory hypoxemia, 8 cm of PEEP therapy is started. The peak pressure is 40 cm H_2O, and the static or plateau pressure is 30 cm H_2O. The compliance factor has been determined to be 3 mL/cm H_2O.

13. Calculate the Cst for this patient.
    A. 22 mL/cm H_2O
    B. 32 mL/cm H_2O
    C. 27 mL/cm H_2O
    D. 17 mL/cm H_2O

14. Calculate the Cdyn for this patient.
    A. 32 mL/cm H_2O
    B. 20 mL/cm H_2O

C. 25 mL/cm H_2O

D. 21 mL/cm H_2O

15. Your patient is being ventilated by a volume-cycled ventilator that has a circuit with an external exhalation valve. The nurse calls you to evaluate the patient because the alarm is going off. When you arrive, you notice that the patient's chest is barely moving during a control breath, the peak pressure does not rise above 3 cm H_2O, and the exhaled V_T spirometer shows the set V_T when the control breath is delivered. The most likely cause of these findings is:

    A. The machine is self-cycling

    B. The inspiratory and expiratory limbs of the circuit are reversed at the cascade humidifier

    C. The tubing to the exhalation valve is disconnected

    D. The spirometer is out of calibration

16. Expiratory retard would be indicated in a patient with:

    A. Pulmonary edema

    B. Air trapping on exhalation

    C. Pleural effusion

    D. Pneumothorax

17. All of the following parameters indicate the need for intubation and mechanical ventilation EXCEPT:

    A. V_C of less than 10 mL/kg of ideal body weight

    B. MIP of less than −20 cm H_2O

    C. $P(A − a)O_2$ on 100% O_2 of 40 torr

    D. V_D/V_T of 0.7

18. Your patient with post-polio syndrome is being ventilated with a BiPAP system and has an IPAP level of 15 cm water and an EPAP level of 5 cm water. She complains of being short of breath. You check her V_T and find that it has dropped. How should the tidal volume be restored?

    A. Lower the IPAP level.

    B. Lower the EPAP level.

    C. Raise the IPAP level.

    D. Raise the EPAP level.

19. You are working with a patient with obstructive sleep apnea who is receiving bilevel NPPV through a nasal mask. During a sleep period, you notice that he is snoring. You would recommend the following ventilator adjustment:

    A. Increase the respiratory rate.

    B. Increase the upper pressure level.

    C. Increase the lower pressure level.

    D. Loosen the nasal mask so that it is not as tight on the patient's face.

20. You are working with an 80-kg (176-lb) patient who is apneic after suffering a stroke. He is being ventilated with the A/C mode and has the following settings:

$\dot{V}_E$	8 L
Rate	10/min
I : E ratio	1 : 3
Inspired O_2	40%
Mechanical dead space	200 mL

The ABG results show the following:

PaO_2	70 torr
$PaCO_2$	50 torr
pH	7.33
HCO_3^-	24 mEq/L

Which of the following would you recommend?

    A. Decrease the mechanical dead space.

    B. Decrease the patient's $\dot{V}_E$.

    C. Change the I : E ratio to 1 : 2.

    D. Add 5 cm H_2O PEEP.

21. It is noticed that a patient's peak pressure has increased from 20 cm water to 40 cm water without a change in static pressure. Possible causes of this include which of the following?

    1. **Retained secretions**

    2. **Pleural effusion**

    3. **Bronchospasm**

    4. **Pulmonary edema**

    A. 2, 4

    B. 1, 2

    C. 1, 3

    D. 3, 4

22. Which of the following will have the greatest impact on increasing the mean airway pressure?

    A. Increasing the inspiratory flow

    B. Adding 5 cm H_2O PEEP

    C. Removing 0.5 second of inflation hold

    D. Increasing the expiratory time by 0.25 second

23. If your ventilator-dependent patient has a large amount of thick tracheal secretions, it is best to:

    A. Use a cascade-type humidifier warmed to body temperature

    B. Use an HME for his or her humidity needs

    C. Use no humidification system so that the secretions will dry out to some extent

    D. Either B or C is acceptable.

24. All of the following are needed to assemble a free-standing CPAP system EXCEPT:

    A. An exhaled volume spirometer

    B. A low-pressure or disconnect alarm

    C. Water traps in the inspiratory and expiratory tubing

    D. A device to create the CPAP pressure

25. A pediatric patient is receiving volume-controlled ventilation with a tidal volume of 250 mL. The patient's breath sounds are clear, but the expiratory flow is seen on the monitor to not return to baseline before the next breath. How could this be interpreted?

    A. Presence of auto-PEEP

    B. Too small a tidal volume

    C. Decreasing lung compliance

    D. Normal airway resistance

26. The following values are found on an adult patient receiving volume-cycled ventilation with the A/C mode:

Tidal volume	500 mL
Peak flow	45 L/min (0.75 L/sec)
Peak pressure	40 cm H_2O
Plateau pressure	20 cm H_2O
PEEP	5 cm H_2O

    Calculate the patient's airway resistance (cm H_2O/L/sec).
    A. 27
    B. 800
    C. 15
    D. 0.4

27. A 16-year-old patient with severe asthma has been receiving nebulized albuterol (Proventil) treatments through the ventilator over the last 12 hours. What can the respiratory therapist recommend to best evaluate his response?
    A. Breath sounds
    B. Chest radiograph
    C. Check airway resistance changes
    D. Check lung compliance changes

28. A 75-year-old male with congestive heart failure has been receiving noninvasive bilevel ventilation over the past 24 hours. The diuretic drug furosemide (Lasix) has been given several times. What is the best way to evaluate how the patient's lung function is responding?
    A. Compare the patient's admission weight vs. current weight.
    B. Compare lung compliance measurements at the start of therapy and now.
    C. Compare airway resistance measurements at the start of therapy and now.
    D. Evaluate breath sound changes over the past 24 hours.

29. Following open heart surgery, a patient is receiving mechanical ventilation. She needs to have a pacemaker inserted in the cardiac procedures lab. It is expected that she will be back in the intensive care unit within an hour or two. How should ventilatory support be provided during this time?
    A. Microprocessor-type ventilator
    B. Manual ventilation with a resuscitation bag
    C. Negative-pressure ventilator
    D. Pressure-cycled transport ventilator

30. A patient with emphysema is receiving mechanical ventilation with the following settings:

Mode	A/C
Set tidal volume	600 mL
Set rate	12
Total rate	12
F_1O_2	0.30
I:E ratio	1:2

    During a ventilator check, you measure the patient's exhaled tidal volume at 500 mL. What can be done to help the patient exhale more completely?
    A. Change to the pressure control mode.
    B. Change to a larger endotracheal tube.
    C. Increase the expiratory time.
    D. Decrease inspiratory flow.

31. Following abdominal surgery, a patient is awakening gradually from anesthesia. Her ventilator settings are as follows:

Mode	SIMV
Set tidal volume	550 mL
Spontaneous tidal volume	400 mL when awake
Set rate	12
Total rate	16 when awake
F_1O_2	0.30
Inspiratory flow	40 L/min

    When awake, she uses accessory muscles and her breathing is not synchronized with the ventilator. What can be done to improve this with a goal of weaning her?
    A. Increase the inspiratory flow to 50 L/min.
    B. Decrease the set tidal volume.
    C. Give her more pain medication.
    D. Give her more oxygen.

32. An adult patient with myasthenia gravis is receiving mechanical ventilation with these settings:

Mode	A/C
Set tidal volume	550 mL
Set rate	10
Total rate	15
F_1O_2	0.40
Inspiratory flow	60 L/min

    His blood gas values are all within the normal range. While performing patient-ventilator rounds, you notice that the patient is making 24 breathing efforts/min and is using inspiratory accessory muscles. What should be done?
    A. Increase the oxygen percent.
    B. Increase the inspiratory flow.
    C. Increase the set rate to 15.
    D. Increase the sensitivity.

33. An unconscious adult patient has been received in the Emergency Department after suffering a stroke. The physician asks for your recommendation for the ventilator tidal volume to use with the patient who weights 73 kg (160 lb). What should be recommended?
    A. 1000 mL
    B. 700 mL
    C. 500 mL
    D. 320 mL

34. A 6-year-old near-drowning patient will be started on mechanical ventilation. What should be the initial respiratory rate?

A. 14/min
B. 20/min
C. 50/min
D. 80/min

35. A 50-year-old, 75-kg (165-lb), male patient has just returned from open heart surgery and has been placed on the mechanical ventilator with the following settings:

Mode	Assist/control
Set tidal volume	700 mL
Set rate	12
Total rate	12
F_IO_2	0.50
I:E ratio	1:3

After 45 minutes, he has the following arterial blood gas values:

pH	7.50
$PaCO_2$	30 torr
PaO_2	115 torr
HCO_3^-	28 mEq/L
BE	+1 mEq/L

What should be done in this situation?
A. Decrease the tidal volume to 500 mL.
B. Decrease the oxygen to 40%.
C. Decrease the respiratory rate to 10/min.
D. Increase the respiratory rate to 14/min.

36. A patient with bilateral pneumonia is receiving mechanical ventilation with the following settings:

Mode	PC
Set tidal volume	650 mL
Set rate	14
F_IO_2	0.50
I:E ratio	1:2
PEEP	10 cm H_2O

The nurse is concerned that his SpO_2 value drops from 94% to 85% when suctioned. How can this be prevented?
A. Give him 100% oxygen before suctioning.
B. Perform suction only once an hour.
C. Use the largest suction catheter available.
D. Increase the PEEP level to 15 cm H_2O before suctioning.

37. A 40-year-old, 60-kg (132-lb) patient is recovering from ARDS. Her current ventilator settings are as follows:

Mode	Pressure control
Set tidal volume	400 mL
Set rate	12
Total rate	18
F_IO_2	0.40
I:E ratio	1:3

She has the following arterial blood gas values:

pH	7.42
$PaCO_2$	37 torr
PaO_2	85 torr

HCO_3^-	25 mEq/L
BE	+1 mEq/L

She has no complications and is conscious and cooperative. Her spontaneous tidal volume is 300 mL and vital capacity is 800 mL. What should be recommended at this time?
A. Maintain the current situation.
B. Increase the set rate.
C. Decrease the tidal volume.
D. Change to the SIMV mode.

38. An adult male is recovering from a flail chest injury and the physician wants to wean him from the ventilator. The patient is intubated with a 7.0-mm ID endotracheal tube and is breathing with support of the SIMV mode. When the set rate was decreased from 8 to 6/min, the patient became tired. How can the patient's work of breathing be decreased?
A. Increase the flow through the ventilator during SIMV breaths.
B. Nebulize a bronchodilator medication.
C. Add pressure support ventilation.
D. Maintain the set respiratory rate at 8.

39. A 75-year-old, 75-kg (175-lb), male patient who suffered a heart attack is receiving mechanical ventilation with the following settings:

Mode	PC plus pressure support
Set tidal volume	800 mL
Set rate	12
Total rate	18
F_IO_2	0.80

The physician is concerned that the patient may be developing pulmonary edema. These arterial blood gas values were recorded while the patient was on the ventilator:

pH	7.45
$PaCO_2$	32 torr
PaO_2	50 torr
HCO_3^-	22 mEq/L
BE	−3 mEq/L

What should be done to help manage the patient?
A. Increase the oxygen to 100%.
B. Add mechanical dead space.
C. Increase the set rate to 18/min.
D. Add 5 cm water PEEP therapy.

40. A 42-year-old patient was accidentally given an overdose of morphine for pain after surgery. Because the drug caused hypoventilation, she was intubated and started on mechanical ventilation in the assist/control mode. The morphine now has been reversed and the patient is awake. She has the following bedside spirometry values:

Respiratory rate	16/min
Vital capacity	2300 mL
Tidal volume	400 mL
Maximum inspiratory pressure	−55 cm H_2O

What should be done at this time?

A. Reassess the patient in 4 hours.

B. Change to the SIMV mode.

C. Remove the endotracheal tube.

D. Place the patient on a T-piece for weaning.

SELF-STUDY QUESTIONS FOR THE WRITTEN REGISTRY EXAM   *See page 623 for answers*

1. PCIRV is indicated in which of the following conditions?
   A. Asthma
   B. Chronic bronchitis
   C. Pulmonary contusion
   D. ARDS

2. Mean airway pressure is defined as:
   A. P_{peak} minus the plateau pressure
   B. P_{peak} divided by inspiratory time
   C. The average pressure throughout the breathing cycle
   D. Tidal volume divided by peak pressure

3. Clinical conditions that cause decreased lung compliance include:
   1. Pulmonary edema
   2. Pulmonary fibrosis
   3. Emphysema
   4. ARDS
   A. 1, 2
   B. 2, 3
   C. 1, 2, 4
   D. All of the above

4. MMV ventilation is:
   1. Similar to A/C ventilation
   2. Indicated when a patient with an unstable respiratory drive is weaned
   3. Designed to make sure that at least a minimum minute volume is delivered
   4. A substitute for CPAP
   A. 2, 3
   B. 1
   C. 3
   D. 1, 4

5. The U.S. Food and Drug Administration has approved high-frequency ventilation for management of all of the following situations EXCEPT:
   A. Laryngoscopy
   B. Near-drowning
   C. Bronchopleural fistula
   D. Bronchoscopy

6. Weaning should be terminated when:
   1. The patient's rapid, shallow breathing index is 120
   2. Cardiac dysrhythmias occur
   3. The patient's $PaCO_2$ is 60 torr
   4. The patient's PaO_2 is 70 torr on 40% oxygen
   A. 1, 3
   B. 2, 4

   C. 2, 3, 4
   D. 1, 2, 3

7. If a patient has just returned from surgery for a left pneumonectomy, the ventilator-delivered tidal volume should be:
   A. Less than normal based on ideal body weight
   B. The same as normal based on ideal body weight
   C. Larger than normal based on ideal body weight
   D. The same volume as delivered before surgery

8. A negative-pressure ventilator is indicated for all the following types of patients EXCEPT:
   A. ARDS
   B. Neuromuscular defects
   C. Kyphoscoliosis
   D. COPD in acute failure

9. The parameters found with an ideal optimal PEEP study are:
   1. Pulmonary compliance improves
   2. PaO_2 increases
   3. Percentage shunt decreases
   4. Pulmonary vascular resistance increases
   5. Pulmonary vascular resistance decreases
   6. Blood pressure decreases and heart rate increases
   A. 2, 4, 6
   B. 1, 2, 3, 5
   C. 2, 3, 5, 6
   D. 1, 2, 3, 4

10. What would be a patient's static compliance (Cst) if the corrected tidal volume is 600 mL, the ventilator's peak pressure is 65 cm water, the plateau pressure is 48 cm water, and there is 12 cm water of PEEP?
    A. 9 mL/cm water
    B. 11 mL/cm water
    C. 13 mL/cm water
    D. 17 mL/cm water

Use the following information for questions 11 and 12: Your ventilated patient has an exhaled tidal volume of 700 mL. Because of refractory hypoxemia, 6 cm of PEEP therapy is started. The peak pressure is 35 cm water, and the static or plateau pressure is 25 cm water. The compliance factor has been determined to be 4 mL/cm water.

11. Calculate the static compliance (Cst) for this patient.
    A. 19 mL/cm water
    B. 24 mL/cm water
    C. 28 mL/cm water
    D. 32 mL/cm water

12. Calculate the dynamic compliance (Cdyn) for this patient.
    A. 16 mL/cm water
    B. 19 mL/cm water
    C. 24 mL/cm water
    D. 32 mL/cm water

13. When preparing to ventilate a patient with HFJV, it is necessary to have all of the following EXCEPT:
    A. Spirometer to measure tidal volume
    B. Jet injector line
    C. High-pressure oxygen source
    D. Humidifier

14. Over the course of an 8-hour shift, the respiratory therapist notices that a patient receiving constant volume ventilation has had an increase in peak pressure from 25 to 40 cm water. What could have caused this change?
    1. Airway resistance decreased
    2. Lung compliance increased
    3. Airway resistance increased
    4. Lung compliance decreased
    A. 3
    B. 4
    C. 3, 4
    D. 1, 2

15. A 45-year-old patient has developed ARDS. The physician asks the respiratory therapist for the best ventilator adjustment to reduce the patient's intrapulmonary shunting. The therapist should recommend:
    A. Increasing the inspiratory time
    B. Increasing the sigh volume
    C. Decreasing the respiratory rate
    D. Increasing the PEEP

16. A trauma patient has a pleural chest tube to the left lung. A volume-cycled ventilator is delivering an inspiratory tidal volume of 800 mL. The expiratory tidal volume is shown to be 600 mL. What could best explain the volume difference?
    A. Air leak through the chest tube
    B. Deflated endotracheal tube cuff
    C. Miscalibrated spirometer
    D. Bronchospasm and auto-PEEP

17. In a patient with ARDS, the indication to switch from volume-cycled ventilation to pressure-cycled ventilation is:
    A. Peak pressure of 30 cm water or greater
    B. Lung compliance less than 30 mL/cm water
    C. Plateau pressure of 30 cm water or greater
    D. Peak pressure and plateau pressure total 30 cm water

18. A 70-kg (154-lb) patient with a stroke and increased intracranial pressure is being mechanically ventilated in the A/C mode with the following settings:

Minute ventilation	8.4 L
I:E ratio:	1:2
F_IO_2	0.35
Rate	12
Mechanical dead space	150 mL

    His ABG results are as follows:

pH	7.30
$PaCO_2$	51 torr
HCO_3^-	24 mEq/L
PaO_2	107 torr

    On the basis of this information, it would be most appropriate to recommend:
    A. Decreasing the F_IO_2
    B. Decreasing the minute ventilation
    C. Increasing the respiratory rate
    D. Removing the mechanical dead space

19. The chest radiograph of a patient receiving mechanical ventilation reveals atelectasis in both bases. In addition, the patient's breath sounds are diminished bilaterally, and she has a low-grade fever. Which of the following ventilator adjustments should the respiratory therapist recommend?
    A. Increasing the flow rate
    B. Lengthening the expiratory time
    C. Increasing the ventilator frequency
    D. Increasing the ventilator sigh volume

20. When permissive hypercapnia is being used to help manage a patient with ARDS, the following should be remembered:
    1. Bicarbonate may be given to increase the pH if needed.
    2. The carbon dioxide level is allowed to increase in a controlled manner.
    3. The pH should be kept between 7.45 and 7.35.
    4. The pH should be kept greater than 7.25.
    5. The $PaCO_2$ should be kept between 40 and 50 torr.
    A. 1, 2, 4
    B. 3, 5
    C. 2, 4
    D. 2, 5

21. Your adult patient has the desire to breathe spontaneously and has a tidal volume that is 4 mL/kg of ideal body weight. Because of facial trauma from an automobile accident, she has a 6.5-mm ID endotracheal tube. She also had lung contusions in the crash. Her PaO_2 is 63 torr on 55% oxygen. What ventilator mode(s) would you recommend for her?
    A. A/C with flow-by for triggering the ventilator
    B. Low-level pressure support ventilation with PEEP
    C. SIMV with low-level pressure support and PEEP
    D. SIMV with high-level pressure support (PSV_{max})

22. An apneic 60-kg (132-lb) patient is being ventilated with the PC mode. Her ventilator settings are:

Tidal volume	700 mL
Rate	10/min
Oxygen	60%
Mechanical dead space	100 mL

Her ABG shows:

PaO_2	66 torr
$PaCO_2$	55 torr
pH	7.32
Base excess	0

Considering this information, all of the following individual ventilator adjustments would improve her ABG values EXCEPT:

A. Increase the respiratory rate to 14/min
B. Increase the tidal volume to 800 mL
C. Change to an SIMV mode with a rate of 10/min
D. Remove the mechanical dead space

23. Indications that the patient is tolerating SIMV include all of the following EXCEPT:

A. The respiratory rate is increased
B. The heart rate is stable
C. The blood gas results are stable
D. Accessory muscles of ventilation are not being used

24. Your 55-kg (120-lb) female patient is being ventilated with an SIMV rate of 10, tidal volume of 600 mL, 10 cm water of therapeutic PEEP, and 35% inspired oxygen. She has an 8.0-mm inner diameter tracheostomy tube. Her spontaneous tidal volume is 350 mL, and the rate is 10/min. The most recent ABG shows PaO_2 95, $PaCO_2$ 42, and pH 7.40. What would you recommend?

A. Reduce the SIMV rate to 3.
B. Reduce the PEEP to 7 cm water.
C. Increase the SIMV rate to 12.
D. Add 10 cm of pressure support.

25. Five adult patients are being weaned from mechanical ventilation. Their bedside spirometry values are shown below.

	f	$\dot{V}_E$ (L)	V_T (mL)	FEV_1 (mL/kg)	MIP (cm Water)
Patient 1	7	2.45	350	5	−35
Patient 2	12	5.44	501	10	−30
Patient 3	15	8.25	550	15	−20
Patient 4	37	11.1	300	13	−15
Patient 5	40	17.0	425	7	−15

Which of the following patients may be ready for extubation?

A. Patients 1 and 2
B. Patients 1 and 4
C. Patients 2 and 3
D. Patients 3 and 5

26. The measurements below are obtained on a patient while he is being mechanically ventilated:

	6 PM	8 PM
Total respiratory rate	14	14
PEEP, cm water	8	8
P plateau, cm water	15	15
P peak, cm water	30	45
Compliance, mL/cm water	40	40

In this situation, the most appropriate action would be to:

A. Increase therapeutic PEEP
B. Administer a bronchodilating agent
C. Administer a diuretic agent
D. Administer a paralyzing agent

27. When working with a patient who recently had a bowel resection and is receiving a paralyzing medication to prevent fighting against the ventilator, it is important to:

A. Give the patient caffeine as a central nervous system stimulant
B. Give the patient a sedative medication for pain
C. Give the patient a narcotic medication for pain
D. Talk quietly because the patient is probably sleeping

28. A patient with a closed head injury and increased ICP is being ventilated mechanically in the A/C mode with an FIO_2 of 0.3, a rate of 12, and a tidal volume of 700 mL. Her ABG results are shown:

pH	7.44
$PaCO_2$	35 torr
PaO_2	295 torr

The physician orders a $PaCO_2$ of 25 torr for the patient. What should the respiratory therapist change on the ventilator to accomplish this?

A. Add 100 mL of mechanical dead space.
B. Increase the tidal volume by 100 mL.
C. Change to the PC mode.
D. Decrease the ventilator rate to 10/min.

29. An 80-kg (176-lb) man with bilateral pneumonia is being ventilated in the PC mode. The following data are available:

	8 AM	12 PM
Set respiratory rate	12/min	12/min
Total respiratory rate	16/min	26/min
Exhaled tidal volume	800 mL	600 mL
Inspiratory pressure	28 cm water	28 cm water

What is the most appropriate thing to do at this time?
A. Sedate the patient.
B. Increase the set respiratory rate.
C. Add 5 cm PEEP.
D. Increase the inspiratory pressure.

30. A 17-year-old girl has been admitted with status asthmaticus and placed on a Dräger Evita 4 ventilator. The physician wants to know if she has any auto-PEEP. Which ventilator waveform would be best for determining whether the patient has any auto-PEEP?
A. Maximum voluntary ventilation tracing
B. Flow/volume loop
C. Flow/time
D. Pressure/time

31. An adult patient will be receiving noninvasive ventilation (NIV) at night in her home. The nasal mask has been applied and these NIV parameters set: IPAP of 15 cm H_2O, EPAP of 4 cm H_2O, rate of 14/min, 30% oxygen. After trying the NIV system for 10 minutes, the patient states that she is not getting enough air. What is the first thing to do to eliminate the patient's shortness of breath?
A. Increase the rate to 16 per minute.
B. Increase the oxygen to 40%.
C. Increase the IPAP to 20 cm H_2O.
D. Increase the EPAP to 8 cm H_2O.

32. After suffering multiple trauma from an automobile accident, a 43-year-old male patient is recovering. Mechanical ventilation has been needed for 5 days, and weaning is being tried for the first time. After breathing on a T-piece for 40 minutes, the patient has the following arterial blood gas values while breathing 40% oxygen:

pH	7.30
$PaCO_2$	54 torr
PaO_2	65 torr
HCO_3^-	26 mEq/L
BE	+2 mEq/L
SpO_2	91%

Bedside spirometry values are as follows:

	Start of Wean	After 40 Minutes
Vital capacity	1100 mL	700 mL
Tidal volume	400 mL	300 mL
Respiratory rate	14/min	28/min
Maximum inspiratory pressure	−26 cm H_2O	−15 cm H_2O

Based on this information, what should be recommended?
A. Return the patient to mechanical ventilation.
B. Extubate and give the patient 50% oxygen.
C. Extubate and begin PEEP therapy treatments every 4 hours.
D. Continue to monitor the patient's weaning trial.

33. An adult patient with ARDS has developed a pneumothorax during volume-oriented mechanical ventilation. The physician has decided to change the patient to high-frequency oscillation. The following HFO parameters have been set:

Frequency	4 Hz
Amplitude	20 cm water
I:E ratio	1:2
Oxygen	60%
PEEP	8 cm water

After 50 minutes of HFO, the patient has the following blood gas values:

pH	7.31
$PaCO_2$	52 torr
PaO_2	66 torr
HCO_3^-	27 mEq/L
BE	+2 mEq/L
SpO_2	92%

What should the respiratory therapist recommend be done?
A. Increase the PEEP to 15 cm water.
B. Increase the amplitude to 25 cm water.
C. Change the I:E ratio to 1:1.
D. Continue to monitor the patient.

16 Mechanical Ventilation of the Neonate

Note 1: This book is written to cover every item listed as testable on all *Entry Level Examination (ELE)*, *Written Registry Examination (WRE)*, and *Clinical Simulation Examination (CSE)*.

The listed code for each item is taken from the National Board for Respiratory Care's (NBRC) **Summary Content Outline for CRT (Certified Respiratory Therapist) and Written RRT (Registered Respiratory Therapist) Examinations** (http://evolve.elsevier.com/Sills/resptherapist/). For example, if an item is testable on both the ELE and WRE, it will simply be shown as (Code: . . .). If an item is only testable on the ELE, it will be shown as (ELE code: . . .). If an item is only testable on the WRE, it will be shown as (WRE code: . . .).

Following each item's code will be the difficulty level of the questions on that item on the ELE and WRE. (See the Introduction for a full explanation of the three question difficulty levels.) **Recall [R]** level questions typically expect the exam taker to recall factual information. **Application [Ap]** level questions are harder because the exam taker may have to apply factual information to a clinical situation. **Analysis [An]** level questions are the most challenging because the exam taker may have to use critical thinking to evaluate patient data to make a clinical decision.

Note 2: A review of the most recent Entry Level Examinations (ELE) has shown an average of one question (out of 140), or <1% of the exam, will cover continuous positive airway pressure (CPAP) or mechanical ventilation of the neonate. A review of the most recent Written Registry Examinations (WRE) has shown an average of two questions (out of 100), or 1% of the exam, will cover continuous positive airway pressure (CPAP) or mechanical ventilation of the neonate. Of the 10 tested scenarios of the Clinical Simulation Examination, expect one neonatal patient and one pediatric patient. CPAP or mechanical ventilation may be involved in both situations. Be sure to review neonatal and pediatric assessment items in Chapter 1.

MODULE A

Perform continuous positive airway pressure to support ventilation or recommend modifications in ventilatory support based on the patient's response

1. Initiate and adjust an elevated baseline pressure: continuous positive airway pressure (CPAP) breathing (Code: IIID2d) [Difficulty: ELE: R, Ap; WRE: An]

a. Physiologic effects

Continuous positive airway pressure (CPAP) and positive end-expiratory pressure (PEEP) increase the patient's functional residual capacity (FRC). In neonates, the most common cause of a decreased FRC is infant respiratory distress syndrome (RDS). This condition is caused by the lack of surfactant in the lungs of the premature neonate. The neonate with RDS has relatively airless lungs that are prone to atelectasis. This results in hypoxemia. In addition, each tidal volume breath requires a greater than normal inspiratory effort (Figure 16-1). The restoration of FRC in the neonate increases its PaO_2, decreases the percentage of shunt, narrows the alveolar to arterial difference in oxygen, and reduces its work of tidal volume breathing. CPAP must be used with caution in neonates with persistent pulmonary hypertension (PPHN) of the newborn. An excessive amount of pressure in the alveoli compresses the capillary bed. This decreases pulmonary blood flow, which in turn increases blood flow through the patent ductus arteriosus and worsens the problem.

b. Indications, contraindications, and hazards

CPAP is indicated for any condition that results in an unacceptably low PaO_2 secondary to a decreased FRC. Some neonates respond so well to CPAP that mechanical ventilation is not needed. In addition, CPAP has been used to keep open the airways of infants with tracheal malacia or other conditions in which the airways collapse abnor-

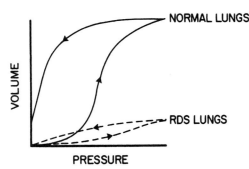

Figure 16-1 Pressure-volume curves for normal neonate and for one with infant respiratory distress syndrome (RDS). Normal neonate's lungs inhale a relatively large tidal volume at low pressure. Note how when the same pressure is placed against the lungs of an infant with RDS, the tidal volume is much smaller. To get a normal tidal volume, the RDS infant must generate a much greater negative pressure. *(From Carlo WA, Martin RJ:* Pediatr Clin North Am *33:221, 1986.)*

mally. In general, contraindications include any CPAP-related condition that results in a worsening of the patient's original status. Some neonates cannot tolerate CPAP and progressively hypoventilate as the pressure level is increased. Clinical judgment is needed to decide how high the PaCO₂ should be allowed to rise before discontinuing the CPAP and beginning mechanical ventilation. In general, the PaCO₂ should not be greater than 50 torr as long as the pH is at least 7.25. An absolute contraindication is apnea resulting in hypoxemia and hypotension. These infants should be mechanically ventilated. Box 16-1 gives a complete listing of indications, contraindications, and hazards.

Exam Hint 16-1 (ELE, WRE)

There is typically a question about the indications to start CPAP, the initial CPAP setting, or making a CPAP adjustment.

---

c. Initiation

Before starting CPAP, a set of baseline arterial blood gases should be taken. Transcutaneous oxygen monitoring or pulse oximetry may be substituted in some clinical situations if oxygenation is the only parameter that must be measured. The neonate's vital signs should also be recorded. Assemble the CPAP circuit and pressure device. The decision must be made whether to apply the CPAP above the epiglottis (Figures 16-2 and 16-3) or to intubate the infant and apply the CPAP within the trachea. Nasal CPAP (NCPAP) or nasopharyngeal tube CPAP (NP-CPAP) are both widely used to apply pressure from above the

---

BOX 16-1 Indications, Contraindications, and Hazards of CPAP Therapy

INDICATIONS
Infant respiratory distress syndrome (RDS)
Atelectasis
Pulmonary edema
Apnea of prematurity
Tracheal malacia
Recent extubation
Transient tachypnea of the newborn
Physical examination shows some, if not all, of the following:
    Respiratory rate 30%-40% greater than normal
    Substernal and suprasternal retractions
    Nasal flaring
    Expiratory grunting
    Cyanosis
    Chest radiograph shows atelectasis or pulmonary edema
Arterial blood gases showing:
    PaO₂ less than 50 torr on 60% or more oxygen
    Adequate ventilation with a PaCO₂ less than 50 torr and pH greater than 7.25
Weaning from mechanical ventilation when the intermittent mandatory ventilation (IMV) rate is about 4-12/min, the pulmonary condition is improved, blood gases show acceptable PaCO₂, and there is acceptable PaO₂ on PEEP. The CPAP level is set to match the level of PEEP used on the ventilator.

CONTRAINDICATIONS
Prolonged apnea leading to hypoxemia and hypotension (begin mechanical ventilation)
Untreated pneumothorax or other evidence of a pulmonary gas leak
Unstable cardiovascular status such as bradycardia and hypotension
Inadequate ventilation with a PaCO₂ greater than 50 torr and pH less than 7.25
Unilateral pulmonary problem: untreated congenital diaphragmatic hernia
Nasal CPAP should not be used on a patient with cleft palate, choanal atresia, or tracheoesophageal fistula

HAZARDS
Persistent pulmonary hypertension of the newborn (PPHN)
Increased intracranial pressure that can cause intraventricular hemorrhage
Decreased cardiac output
CPAP may be ineffective if the neonate weighs less than 1000-1200 grams

---

epiglottis. The neonate or infant must have an endotracheal tube placed to apply CPAP within the trachea. Among the factors to be considered are the neonate's gestational age and weight, the amount of secretions that need to be suctioned, the pulmonary problem, and the likelihood of mechanical ventilation eventually becoming necessary. More mature and larger infants with few

Figure 16-2   A, Nasal CPAP is delivered through a set of prongs and placement system. Shown is a Kendall Health Argyle CPAP prong and headgear set. **B,** Nasopharyngeal CPAP is delivered through a shortened endotracheal tube. Shown are 2.5, 3.0, and 3.5 mm ID endotracheal tubes that have been cut off at the proximal end and attached to the ventilator adapter. Always select the prongs or tube that are the proper size to fit the neonate's airway. *(From Cario J, Pilbeam S:* Mosby's Respiratory Therapy Equipment, *ed 8, St Louis, 2010, Mosby.)*

Figure 16-3   An assembly for supporting nasal CPAP prongs in an infant. *(Modified from advertisement of Stayflex tubing system from Ackrad.) (From Sills JR:* Respiratory care registry guide, *ed 1, St Louis, 1994, Mosby.)*

secretions and relatively stable pulmonary conditions will most likely have CPAP applied above the epiglottis by nasal prongs or nasopharyngeal tube. In contrast, less mature and smaller infants (less than 1000 to 1200 g) who need suctioning and have relatively unstable pulmonary conditions will probably be intubated. Mechanical ventilation can then be easily started if needed.

CPAP is usually started at about 4 to 5 cm water pressure whether the pressure is applied above or below the epiglottis. The inspired oxygen percentage is usually kept at the previously set level. It is important to make only one change at a time so that each adjustment in care can be evaluated for its own effect. For example, if you simultaneously increased the oxygen percentage by 10% and started 5 cm water of CPAP, it would not be known whether the increase in PaO_2 was from the additional oxygen, the CPAP, or both. Usually the long-term inspired oxygen is limited to 40% to 50% because of concern of the possibility of pulmonary oxygen toxicity.

d. Monitor and adjust alarm settings (ELE Code: IIIG3g) [Difficulty: ELE: R, Ap, An]

Depending on the clinical situation, CPAP can be administered through a freestanding, improvised system or through a mechanical ventilator set on the CPAP mode. A variety of alarms and monitoring systems should be used to ensure the patient's safety. Patient monitors should have visual and audible alarms and include the following:

- Pulse oximeter or transcutaneous oxygen monitor. Either should alarm if the patient's oxygen falls below the set, safe level.
- Electrocardiogram monitor. It should have alarm limits set for high and low heart rate.

Equipment should have visual and audible alarms and include the following features:

- A low pressure alarm in case >2 cm water pressure is lost due to a leak or disconnection. For example, CPAP is set at 6 cm water and a leak drops the pressure to 3 cm water.
- A high pressure limiting valve that prevents an accidental dangerous high pressure in the system from being applied to the patient's airways. If this pressure limit is reached the alarm will be activated.
- An oxygen analyzer set to alarm if the patient's ordered inspired oxygen percentage is set below the ordered percentage.

e. CPAP adjustment

Blood gases and vital signs must be evaluated at the starting CPAP level. The heart rate, blood pressure, and respiratory rate should be stable or improved. Wait at least 10 minutes after a change in CPAP before getting an arterial blood gases sample. See Table 16-1 for the recommended blood gas limits. In general, the PaO_2 should be kept between 60 and 70 torr, $PaCO_2$ less than 50 to 55 torr, and pH at least 7.25. If the PaO_2 is too low and the patient's vital signs are acceptable, the CPAP may be increased in a step of 1 to 2 cm water. The vital signs and blood gases should then be reevaluated. In addition, the neonate's work of breathing can be indirectly assessed. Improved lung function will be demonstrated by seeing decreased respiratory rate, retractions, expiratory grunting, and nasal flaring. If necessary, the process of adding CPAP and reassessing the patient can be continued. The maximum CPAP level in a neonate is generally held to be 10 cm water; the maximum CPAP level in an infant is generally held to be 15 cm water.

Mechanical ventilation is usually indicated if more than these maximum CPAP pressures are needed to correct hypoxemia. Depending on the patient, even levels less than these maximum CPAP pressures may not be well tolerated. The infant may become exhausted from exhaling against the back pressure of the CPAP system. That is seen clinically as decreased chest movement from the smaller tidal volume. The $PaCO_2$ will probably increase. It may be neces-

TABLE 16-1   Commonly Recommended Blood Gas Goals for CPAP and Mechanical Ventilator Therapy

	Age of Neonate	
	Less Than 72 Hours	Greater Than 72 Hours
PaO_2 (torr)	60-70	50-70
$PtcO_2$ (torr)	Greater than 50,* less than 90*	Greater than 40,* less than 90*
SpO_2	92%-96%	92-96%
$PaCO_2$ (torr)	35-45†	45-55
$PtcCO_2$ (torr)	May be used after correlation with $PaCO_2$ as discussed in Chapter 3.	
pH	7.25-7.45	7.25-7.45

*$PtcO_2$ values may be used after they have been shown to correlate within 15% of the PaO_2 from an arterial blood gas.
†With CPAP, this value may be increased to 50 to 55 torr as long as the pH is at least 7.25.
NOTE: Keep the PaO_2 no greater than 80 torr in the premature neonate to reduce the risk of retinopathy of prematurity.

sary to place the infant on mechanical ventilation to decrease the work of breathing and then add PEEP to maintain the FRC. When nasal prongs or a nasopharyngeal tube are used, CPAP pressures of greater than 8 cm water may cause the infant's mouth to open. This results in the loss of CPAP. A crying infant also opens its mouth and loses the CPAP. In either case, the CPAP pressure gauge drops to zero or fluctuates below the set pressure.

f. Independently initiate weaning from CPAP (Code: IIIF2i12) [Difficulty: ELE: R, Ap; WRE: An]

As the patient improves, it is necessary to reduce the CPAP level so as not to cause pulmonary barotrauma. The pressure level can be reduced in steps of about 2 cm water. The vital signs and blood gases should be reassessed after each step. The apparatus is usually removed when the CPAP level is down to 2 to 4 cm water. The infant is then placed into an oxyhood at the same oxygen percentage as before or 5% to 15% higher. If the infant has an endotracheal tube that is needed for suctioning or a secure airway, the pressure is usually left at 2 to 4 cm water. After extubation, the infant is placed into an oxyhood as before. Alternatively, the neonate may be weaned to a high flow nasal cannula and then to a traditional, low-flow nasal cannula. See Chapter 6 for more discussion on the high-flow nasal cannula.

If the infant was breathing more than 50% oxygen while on the CPAP, it may be more important to lower the oxygen before decreasing the CPAP level. The following guidelines may prove helpful when deciding whether to first lower the oxygen percentage or the CPAP level:

- If the patient has been breathing more than 50% oxygen for more than 48 hours and has stable vital signs without any pulmonary barotrauma, decrease the oxygen first. Lower the inspired oxygen in 5% to 15% steps, and check the oxygenation level after each reduction. Attempt to get the oxygen down to 40%, if possible. Then decrease the CPAP level.

- If the patient is breathing 50% oxygen or less and has unstable vital signs or pulmonary barotrauma, decrease the CPAP first. After the CPAP is reduced (or removed entirely) and the patient is stable, reduce the inspired oxygen percentage.

Exam Hint 16-2 (ELE, WRE)

Know the indications to switch from CPAP to mechanical ventilation.

MODULE B

Perform mechanical ventilation to achieve adequate artificial ventilation or recommend modifications in ventilatory support based on the patient's response

1. Select a mechanical ventilation

a. Recommend changing the type of ventilator to be used on the patient (Code: IIIG3i) [Difficulty: ELE: R, Ap; WRE: An]

b. Independently change the type of ventilator to be used on the patient (Code: IIIF2i9) [Difficulty: ELE: R, Ap; WRE: An]

Historically, most neonatal patients requiring life support receive time-triggered, pressure-limited, time-cycled mechanical ventilation (TPTV). These ventilators are pneumatically powered with electrical controls and alarm systems. They are used in the IMV mode and feature a continuous flow of gas from which the neonate can breathe spontaneously. TPTV units are pressure limited to prevent an excessive peak airway pressure and can have therapeutic PEEP added. Furthermore, they are capable of reaching the Food and Drug Administration (FDA) limited rate of 150 breaths/min. The majority of neonatal and small pediatric patients can be effectively ventilated on these types of units.

High-frequency ventilation (HFV) with a small tidal volume has been approved by the FDA for use in the rescue of neonates with RDS and a bronchopulmonary fistula or pulmonary interstitial emphysema (PIE) who fail under conventional TPTV ventilation. HFV has also been used in the short-term support of neonates with a congenital diaphragmatic hernia until corrective surgery can be performed.

Volume-cycled ventilators are commonly used on infants who weigh more than 10 kg (22 lb). The most recent generation of conventional volume-cycled ventila-tors can be used to deliver a tidal volume as small as 2 to 3 mL. They often have chest wall sensor systems that note movement and match that breathing effort with a machine delivered breath. Volume-oriented ventilation can also be performed with a neonatal TPTV-type ventilator if the patient is apneic. This technique is discussed later.

When selecting a ventilator, it is important to choose one that offers the features needed to ventilate the patient. For example, if real-time graphics are needed to evaluate the patient's response to a ventilator adjustment, the proper unit will be needed. Any selected ventilator must be able to meet the typical tidal volume goal for a neonatal of 4 to 6 mL/Kg or small pediatric patient of 6 to 8 mL/Kg. A patient receiving HFV for an FDA-approved pulmonary problem has a smaller tidal volume goal.

2. Adjust the ventilator settings.

a. Initiate and adjust continuous mechanical ventilator settings (Code: IIID2b) [Difficulty: ELE: R, Ap; WRE: An]

b. Recommend changes in mechanical ventilation to modify ventilator techniques (Code: IIIG3e) [Difficulty: ELE: R, Ap; WRE: An]

c. Independently modify ventilator techniques (Code: IIIF2i5) [Difficulty: ELE: R, Ap; WRE: An]

With traditional neonatal TPTV, a set tidal volume is not ordered and cannot be measured. With volume-cycled ventilation of a pediatric patient, the tidal volume is ordered just as it is with an adult patient. Typically the therapist is expected to set the following ventilator controls based on a protocol or the patient's condition and response to the ventilator: sensitivity, flow, I:E ratio, alarms, and humidified gas temperature. Specific examples of ventilator settings, based on pathological problem, will be presented next.

d. Sensitivity

1. Observe the patient for signs of ventilator-patient dyssynchrony (Code: IIIE5b) [Difficulty: ELE: R, Ap; WRE: An]

2. Independently adjust the ventilator to improve patient synchrony (Code: IIIF2i1) [Difficulty: ELE: R, Ap; WRE: An]

There is no sensitivity control on traditional continuous flow TPTV-type neonatal ventilators. The IMV mode is used with these units. Newer ventilators have the ability to sense a neonate's respiratory effort and trigger a machine delivered breath. Some units sense a change in flow through the ventilator circuit when the neonate inspires. Other ventilators make use of electrocardiogram-type leads on the neonate's chest to sense a change in electrical impedance (skin resistance) when the neonate makes an inspiratory effort. A child on a volume-cycled ventilator should have the sensitivity set at about −1 to −2 cm water pressure. No matter which method the ventilator uses to sense the patient's respiratory effort, the neonate or child should not have to work hard to trigger a machine tidal volume.

e. Flow

Flow is adjusted to set the inspiratory time, the I:E ratio, or to meet the patient's needs to better synchronize breathing efforts with the ventilator. The flow should be increased if the patient appears to be attempting to inhale faster than the ventilator is delivering the tidal volume.

f. I:E ratio

1. Independently adjust the I:E ratio settings (Code: IIIF2i4) [Difficulty: ELE: R, Ap; WRE: An]

2. Recommend changes in mechanical ventilation to reduce auto-PEEP (Code: IIIG3l) [Difficulty: ELE: R, Ap, An]

The I:E ratio is adjusted to ensure that the patient can inhale in as physiologically appropriate a manner as possible and can completely exhale the inspired tidal volume. A ventilator with real-time graphics can reveal the presence of auto-PEEP (incomplete exhalation). In most situations, auto-PEEP can be reduced or eliminated by increasing expiratory time or reducing the tidal volume. In addition, suctioning out secretions and the administration of an aerosolized bronchodilator in a patient with bronchospasm can reduce air trapping and auto-PEEP.

g. Alarms

Alarm systems are different for each type of ventilator. Generally speaking, they are set with a safety margin of ±10% from the patient's normal ventilator settings. A variation of greater than 10% results in an audible or visual alarm condition.

h. Humidified gas temperature

The goal for most patients is to minimize their humidity deficit by giving gas that is humidified and warmed to near body temperature. It is common to have the gas warmed to 90° to 95° F (about 35° C). It should be measured in the inspiratory limb of the circuit as close to the patient as possible.

A review of the literature dealing with neonatal critical care shows that there are few universally accepted strategies for the use and modification of CPAP/PEEP and mechanical ventilation. The discussion presented here is an attempt to describe what are widely accepted approaches to neonatal TPTV and related therapy. The approach used in this discussion focuses on adjusting the ventilator and treating a neonate based on its pathologic problem.

3. Indications for mechanical ventilation

All authors agree that apnea is an absolute indication for mechanical ventilation. A general indication is any condition that causes respiratory failure. This is usually documented by unacceptable arterial blood gases. Box 16-2 lists indications for mechanical ventilation.

Math Review

TIME CONSTANTS OF VENTILATION

Note: This concept has not been directly tested by the NBRC. It is hoped that understanding the concept of time constants as used here and in the later text will help the reader understand lung pathology and why certain ventilator adjustments are made.

It is important in any patient requiring mechanical ventilation to consider both the patient's lung-thoracic compliance and airway resistance when setting inspiratory and expiratory times. This is especially important in neonates because, in comparison with adults, they are less compliant and have greater resistance. In addition, neonates are usually ventilated at faster rates. As a review, the respective lung-thoracic compliances (C_{LT}) and airway resistances (R_{AW}) of normal adults and infants are shown here:

Adult lung-thoracic compliance: 100 mL/cm water pressure (0.1 L/cm water pressure)

Neonatal lung-thoracic compliance: 5 mL/cm water pressure (.005 L/cm water pressure; about 20 times stiffer than in an adult)

Adult airway resistance: 2 cm water/L/sec

Neonatal airway resistance: 20 to 40 cm water/L/sec (about 10 to 20 times more resistance to airflow than in an adult)

The placement of an endotracheal tube to facilitate mechanical ventilation results in a total pulmonary resistance ranging from 50 to 150 cm water/L/sec. The time constant of ventilation (Tc or time constant of the respiratory system T_{RS}) is calculated as the product of compliance and resistance:

Time constant in seconds = compliance (L/cm water)
$$\times \text{resistance (cm water/L/sec)}$$

For example, using these values for a spontaneously breathing normal neonate, its time constant is calculated as

$$Tc = \text{compliance} (.005 \text{ L/cm water})$$
$$\times \text{resistance} (30 \text{ cm water/L/sec})$$
$$= .005 \times 30 \text{ seconds}$$
$$= .15 \text{ seconds}$$

BOX 16-2 Common Indications for the Initiation
of Mechanical Ventilation

RESPIRATORY FAILURE
PaO₂ less than 50-60 torr despite maximal CPAP therapy (about
10 cm water) and 60% or more inspired oxygen
PaCO₂ greater than 60 torr and pH less than 7.25

NEUROLOGIC
Complete apnea
Apneic periods leading to hypoxemia and bradycardia
Intracranial hemorrhage
Drug depression
Muscular dystrophies

PULMONARY CONDITIONS
Infant respiratory distress syndrome (RDS)
Diffuse pneumonia
Pulmonary edema
Meconium aspiration
Diaphragmatic hernia
Prophylactic use
Cyanotic congenital cardiac defect
Persistent pulmonary hypertension of the newborn (PPHN)
Near drowning
Postoperatively after major thoracic or abdominal surgery

Figure 16-4 Graphic presentation of the percentage of
inspiratory and expiratory volume and pressure in comparison
with time constants of ventilation. *(From Chatburn RL:* Respir
Care *36:569, 1991.)*

Although technically impractical to measure the time
constant of ventilation at the bedside, the concept is
important because it relates to two important clinical considerations during mechanical ventilation. First, it relates
to the pressure that develops at the alveolar level as the
tidal volume is delivered. For each time constant, progressively more of the peak inspiratory pressure (PIP) is
applied within the alveoli (Figure 16-4). As can be seen,
at three time constants, 95% of the PIP is applied to the
alveoli. At five time constants, virtually the entire PIP is
applied at the alveolar level. Second, the time constant
relates to how rapidly the lung recoils to baseline (FRC)
during an exhalation. As shown in Figure 16-4, it takes
three time constants to exhale 95% and five time constants
to completely exhale.

The clinical significance of this relates directly to
the pulmonary condition of the patient. Infants with stiff
lungs and normal resistance, as found in RDS, have a
short time constant. Alveolar pressure quickly increases to
match the peak inspiratory pressure. The lungs then
rapidly recoil during exhalation so that there is little
chance of air trapping. Infants with normal compliance
and increased resistance, as found in meconium aspiration, have a long time constant. It takes a relatively long
time for the alveolar pressure to reach the PIP. Also, a relatively long time is needed for the exhalation to be complete. For this reason, these infants are at risk for air
trapping and auto-PEEP.

4. Initiation and adjustments based on the patient's condition

a. Patients with normal cardiopulmonary function

Patients with normal cardiopulmonary function may
need mechanical ventilation because of apnea from anesthesia, paralysis, or a neurologic condition. The initial
TPTV ventilator parameters for this type of patient are
listed in Box 16-3. Once mechanical ventilation is established, it is important to evaluate the patient's blood
gases, vital signs, breath sounds, and any other pertinent
clinical information before changing any ventilator
parameters.

BOX 16-3 Common Mechanical Ventilator
Parameters for Neonates with
Normal Lungs

Delivered tidal volume: 6-8 mL/kg (this may be estimated by
calculation if the neonate is apneic and the pressure limit is
not reached until the end of the inspiratory time)
Pressure limit (peak inspiratory pressure or PIP): 10-20 cm water
Frequency: 10-20/min
I:E ratio: 1:2 to 1:10
Inspiratory time (T₁): at least 0.4 seconds
Expiratory time (T_E): at least 0.5 seconds
PEEP: none unless 2-4 cm water is added to replace "epiglottal
PEEP"
Inspiratory flow: sufficient to see the chest move and hear bilat-
eral breath sounds during the inspiration; 5-8 L/min com-
monly used; or start with at least twice the infant's estimated
minute volume (respiratory rate x estimated tidal volume of
7 mL/kg); check the blood gases for the PaCO₂.
Oxygen percentage: 40%

As the patient recovers and begins to breathe spontaneously, it will probably be necessary to reduce the ventilator-delivered minute volume. This encourages the child to breathe more because the final goal is to completely wean and extubate the patient. The most accepted way to reduce the ventilator-delivered minute volume is to reduce the ventilator rate. A reduction of about 10% is a good starting place but must be tailored to meet the patient's needs. The tidal volume is maintained as originally set. Obtain a set of blood gases in 10 to 20 minutes (or follow the transcutaneous or pulse oximetry values), and check the patient's vital signs to see how well the adjustment is tolerated.

If the blood gases show an elevated $PaCO_2$, the ventilator-delivered minute volume must be raised. Do this by increasing either the alveolar ventilation or respiratory rate. Alveolar ventilation can be increased by increasing either the inspiratory flow or the pressure limit (if it has been reached) to increase the tidal volume. The ventilator rate may be increased if the flow and pressure limit cannot be increased. An increase of about 10% is a good starting place but must be tailored to meet the patient's needs. As before, blood gases and vital signs should be monitored after every change to see if the increase is well tolerated and accomplishing what was intended.

If the blood gases show that the $PaCO_2$ is lower than desired, the ventilator-delivered minute volume must be decreased. The first parameter to adjust is usually the rate. Try decreasing the rate by about 10% and check another set of blood gas values. If other parameters need to be reduced, try decreasing the peak inspiratory pressure, inspiratory flow, or inspiratory time about 10% to decrease the tidal volume. Again, check the blood gas values after every adjustment.

If the blood gases show that the PaO_2 is higher or lower than necessary, the oxygen percentage must be adjusted. An increase or decrease of about 5% is a good starting place but must be adjusted as needed. If the patient does not respond to the increased oxygen as expected, the patient should be reevaluated. It may be necessary to reclassify him or her into one of the following categories.

Math Review

CALCULATION OF ESTIMATED TIDAL VOLUME DURING TPTV MECHANICAL VENTILATION

The NBRC examination content outline does not specifically list estimated tidal volume calculations. However, the information may be useful in understanding concepts presented later in the text.

If the neonatal patient receiving TPTV is apneic and neither assisting nor fighting against the ventilator-delivered breath, it is possible to calculate an approximate tidal volume. This is referred to as volume-oriented ventilation. The following formula is used:

$$\text{Calculated tidal volume} = (T_I \times \dot{V}) - Vc$$

In which

T_I = inspiratory time

(It is important that either the pressure limit is not reached or the pressure limit is reached at the same time inspiratory time is completed. If the pressure limit is reached before the inspiratory time limit is reached, part of the inspiratory time is spent as an inflation hold, and no additional tidal volume is delivered.)

$\dot{V}$ = inspiratory flow rate on the ventilator in mL/sec

Vc = volume compressed in the circuit and ventilator

(This is found by multiplying the peak inspiratory pressure by the manufacturer's stated compliance factors for the circuit and ventilator.)

For example, estimate the delivered tidal volume for an apneic 5 kg infant. The ventilator parameters are inspiratory flow of 5.5 l/min, frequency of 20/min, I:E ratio of 1:3, inspiratory time of 0.75 seconds, and expiratory time of 2.25 seconds. Peak inspiratory pressure (PIP) is 15 cm water. The internal compliance of the ventilator is 0.4 mL/cm water, and the circuit compliance factor is 1.6 mL/cm water.

$$\text{Calculated tidal volume} = (T_I \times \dot{V}) - Vc$$

In which:

T_I = .75 seconds

$\dot{V}$ = 5.5 L/min. This is converted to mL/sec by dividing the flow in L/min by 60 seconds. So 5.5 L/min = .092 L/sec or 92 mL/sec:

Vc = 0.4 + 1.6 mL/cm water = 2 mL/cm water = 2 mL/cm water × 15 cm water PIP = 30 mL

Therefore,

$$
\begin{aligned}
\text{Calculated tidal volume} &= (0.75 \text{ sec.} \times 92 \text{ mL/sec}) - 30 \text{ mL} \\
&= (69 \text{ mL}) - 30 \text{ mL} \\
&= 39 \text{ mL. (This is within the ideal} \\
&\quad \text{tidal volume range of 30 to} \\
&\quad \text{40 mL[based on 5 kg} \\
&\quad \text{weight} \times 6 \text{ to 8 mL/kg])}
\end{aligned}
$$

It must be emphasized that this is only a calculated tidal volume. Leaks in the system, a decrease in the patient's compliance, or an increase in the patient's resistance decreases the true tidal volume. Conversely, an increase in the patient's compliance or a decrease in the patient's resistance increases the true tidal volume. Also, if the pressure limit is reached before the inspiratory time is completed, less volume than expected will be delivered. This is because part of the inspiratory time is spent as an inflation hold and no additional tidal volume is delivered (Figure 16-5). Finally, the infant must be completely passive during the delivery of the breath.

b. Patients with decreased lung compliance and normal airway resistance such as infant respiratory distress syndrome (RDS)

Although RDS in infants weighing less than 1000 g is the most common cause of decreased lung compliance with

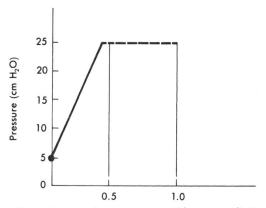

Figure 16-5 Pressure-time curve seen with pressure limit set at 25 cm water and inspiratory time being increased from 0.5 to 1 second. Pressure limit is reached when inspiratory time is about 0.5 second. As inspiratory time is increased to 1 second (or greater), the pressure limit is held at 25 cm water resulting in a "square wave" pressure curve. *(From Betis P, Thompson JF, Benjamin PK: Mechanical ventilation. In: Koff PB, Eitzman DV, Neu J: Neonatal and pediatric respiratory care, ed 2, St Louis, 1993, Mosby.)*

normal airway resistance, stiff lungs are also found in patients with other lung conditions such as pneumonia and pulmonary edema (Figure 16-6). The greatest challenge presented in the care of these infants is to oxygenate them without causing oxygen toxicity or pulmonary barotrauma. Common recommendations for the initial ventilator settings are listed in Box 16-4. As discussed earlier, blood gases, vital signs, and so forth must be monitored after the infant is placed on the ventilator. Any further adjustments can then be determined and evaluated by another set of blood gases and vital signs.

The issue of time constants of ventilation helps to better explain the various options available for adjusting the ventilator. As presented earlier, the time constant of ventilation (T_c or time constant of the respiratory system

---

BOX 16-4 Common Mechanical Ventilator Parameters for Neonates with Low Compliance and Normal Resistance

Delivered tidal volume: 6-8 mL/kg

Pressure limit: 20-25 cm water (this may need to be increased up to 35-40 cm water)

Frequency: 30-60/min (this may need to be raised up to 150/min)

I:E ratio: 1:2 (this may eventually need to be altered to an inverse I:E ratio)

Inspiratory time (T_I): between 0.4 and 0.7 seconds (this may need to be increased)

Expiratory time (T_E): at least 0.5 seconds (this may need to be decreased)

PEEP: 2-4 cm water initially (this may need to be increased up to 8-10 cm water)

Inspiratory flow: sufficient to see the chest move and hear bilateral breath sounds during the inspiration; 5-8 L/min commonly used; as a general rule, the faster the rate is, the higher the flow must be to deliver an adequate tidal volume; check the blood gases for the $PaCO_2$

Oxygen percentage: 40% (this may need to be increased to keep the SpO_2 greater than 92%)

CHILD	INFANT	SICK INFANT	
300	16	14	TIDAL VOLUME ml
75	5	8.5	DEAD SPACE ml
21	36	70	RESPIRATORY RATE /min.
68	4.4	1.0	COMPLIANCE (ml/cm H₂O)
5.8	29	26	RESISTANCE (cm H₂O/liter/sec.)
9	6	5	DIAMETER of TRACHEA (mm)

Figure 16-6 Comparison of the lung volumes and capacities of a 6-year-old child, normal infant, and an infant with IRDS. Note relatively high compliance and low resistance of a normal child compared with an infant, and infant with RDS compared with normal infant. *(From Chatburn RL, Lough MD. Mechanical ventilation. In: Lough MD, Doershuk CF, Stern RC, editors: Pediatric respiratory therapy, ed 3, St Louis, 1985, Mosby.)*

T_{RS}) is calculated as the product of compliance and resistance. For example, using the following values for a mechanically ventilated neonate with RDS, its time constant is calculated as

T_c = compliance (.001 L/cm water because the lungs are less compliant) × resistance (100 cm water/L/sec because the infant is intubated). Simplify as follows:
= .001 × 100 second
= .1 seconds (Compare this with a Tc of .15 for a normal, spontaneously breathing neonate.)

Neonates with RDS have a relatively short time constant; therefore the tidal volume and ventilating pressure are delivered rather quickly to the lungs. However, because the lungs are so stiff, there is usually no problem with the tidal volume being fully exhaled as long as five time constants are allowed. An expiratory time of at least 0.5 seconds is usually set initially. The various options available for increasing oxygenation are discussed on the following pages.

1. Administer oxygen

a. Recommend changes in mechanical ventilation to enhance oxygenation (Code: IIIG3b) [Difficulty: ELE: R, Ap; WRE: An]

b. Administer oxygen (ELE Code: IIID6) [IIID6] [Difficulty: ELE: R, Ap, An]

c. Independently modify mechanical ventilation to enhance oxygenation (Code: IIIF2i2) [Difficulty: ELE: R, Ap; WRE: An]. Up to 100% oxygen can be given to the neonate in the short term. Hypoxemia cannot be tolerated and supplemental oxygen is usually the best way to correct it. See Chapter 15 for equations that can be used to predict the oxygen percentage change needed to correct the patient's hypoxemia. Although hypoxemia cannot be tolerated, there are several limiting factors. First, it is commonly held that giving more than 50% oxygen for more than 48 to 72 hours increases the risk of pulmonary oxygen toxicity. Second, if more than 80% oxygen is given, some poorly ventilated alveoli will have all of the oxygen absorbed from them, leading to denitrogenation absorption atelectasis. Third, keep the neonate's PaO_2 below 80 torr to minimize the risk of retinopathy of prematurity (ROM). Fourth, if the hypoxemia is caused by a decreased FRC because of the lack of surfactant and small lung volumes, increasing the oxygen will not markedly increase the PaO_2. Other solutions, such as adding PEEP, altering the I:E ratio to lengthen the inspiratory time, and giving surfactant must be used. These will be discussed later.

2. Increased inspiratory flow

a. Recommend changes in mechanical ventilation to improve alveolar ventilation (Code: IIIG3c) [Difficulty: ELE: R, Ap; WRE: An]

b. Independently modify mechanical ventilation to improve alveolar ventilation (Code: IIIF2i3) [Difficulty: ELE: R, Ap; WRE: An]. With TPTV-type ventilators, increasing the flow increases the tidal volume until the pressure limit is reached.

Increasing the tidal volume should result in an increased PaO_2 and is likely to reduce the $PaCO_2$. If the pressure limit is reached, the delivered tidal volume is held in the lungs for the duration of the inspiratory time. This acts as an inflation hold and should also increase the PaO_2. The mean airway pressure is raised by holding the tidal volume in the lungs. (See Figure 16-7 for the pressure waveforms seen during low-flow and high-flow conditions.) Under high-flow conditions, the pressure waveform takes on a characteristic square shape (square wave) because the pressure limit is reached. This pattern of ventilation is currently widely used with these types of patients.

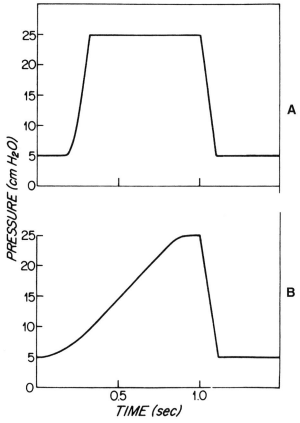

Figure 16-7 Comparison of pressure-time curves showing influence of inspiratory flow when the pressure limit is set at 25 cm water pressure. **A,** Curve at high flow rate. Pressure limit is reached very early in the inspiratory time with resulting "square wave" flow pattern. **B,** Curve at low flow rate. Pressure limit is not reached until inspiratory time is almost 1 second. *(From Chatburn RL, Lough MD. Mechanical ventilation. In: Lough MD, Doershuk CF, Stern RC, editors: Pediatric respiratory therapy, ed 3, St Louis, 1985, Mosby.)*

3. Increased inspiratory time leading to inverse ratio ventilation

As with increasing the flow, increasing the inspiratory time increases the tidal volume until the pressure limit is reached. If the pressure limit is reached, any increased inspiratory time acts as inflation hold. This also raises the mean airway pressure and should result in an increased PaO_2. (See Figure 16-5 for the pressure waveform change as the inspiratory time is increased.)

Some authors have advocated an increased inspiratory time as an important way to improve oxygenation. This has led to the use of inverse I:E ratios of up to 3:1 (.33) or 4:1 (.25) to produce an adequate PaO_2. The inspiratory time should be increased in small time increments and followed in 10 to 20 minutes with a blood gas to determine if the desired improvement in oxygenation was achieved. Inspiratory time is increased only as long as necessary to result in a satisfactory PaO_2. Great care must be taken to adjust expiratory time, respiratory rate, or both when a prolonged inspiratory time is used. Obviously, expiratory time must be reduced to keep the same rate as the inspiratory time is increased, or the rate must be reduced as the inspiratory time is increased if the expiratory time cannot be reduced. Care must be taken to ensure that the tidal volume is fully exhaled to avoid auto-PEEP.

As the neonate's lung compliance improves, the inspiratory time must be decreased for two reasons. First, the alveolar pressure is more readily transmitted throughout the lungs and may decrease venous return to the heart. That results in a decreased cardiac output. Second, the more normal lungs are more prone to barotrauma or volutrauma. The inspiratory time should be decreased in small time increments and followed with a set of blood gases to be sure that the neonate is not hypoxemic.

4. Initiate and adjust an elevated baseline pressure: positive end-expiratory pressure (PEEP) (Code: IIID2d) [Difficulty: ELE: R, Ap; WRE: An]

Positive end-expiratory pressure (PEEP) increases the patient's functional residual capacity (FRC) by preventing a complete exhalation to the baseline (atmospheric) pressure. Because PEEP increases the FRC, it is more effective at increasing the PaO_2 than increasing the tidal volume, inflation hold, or an inverse I:E ratio. See Table 16-1 for the recommended guidelines for arterial blood gas values in neonates. If the patient needs more than 50% oxygen to keep the desired PaO_2, PEEP should be started; unless there is a contraindication to its use. Often, the proper level of therapeutic PEEP can result in an acceptable PaO_2 with no more than 50% oxygen being inhaled.

As discussed in regard to CPAP therapy, PEEP is usually started out at 4 to 5 cm water. A blood gas is then checked and, if necessary, more PEEP is added in 1 to 2 cm water increments. It is rare for more than 7 cm of PEEP to be needed. Another blood gas should be checked for PaO_2 after every addition of pressure. PEEP has the greatest impact on raising the mean airway pressure of all the options presented here. For that reason, excessive PEEP may cause a decreased venous return to the heart and decreased cardiac output. It also may cause barotrauma resulting in pulmonary interstitial emphysema (PIE), pneumothorax, or pneumomediastinum. Care must be taken to carefully evaluate the patient after each increase in PEEP. Watch for a sudden deterioration in the patient's condition as a sign of a pulmonary air leak. As the patient's PaO_2 improves, the PEEP level should be reduced in steps of about 1 to 2 cm water. As always, recheck the blood gases with each adjustment.

Exam Hint 16-3 (ELE, WRE)

Initiate or increase CPAP or PEEP if more than 50% oxygen is needed to maintain a PaO_2 of greater than 50 torr.

---

5. Increased pressure limit

To deliver a larger tidal volume, it may become necessary to increase the pressure limit when it is reached by the peak inspiratory pressure (PIP). It may also be necessary to raise the pressure limit to restore the original tidal volume after the addition of PEEP. This is because the original tidal volume is reduced when PEEP is added and the PIP reaches the pressure limit. This is shown in Figure 16-8. To restore the original tidal volume, the pressure limit (and PIP) must be increased by the same amount as the added PEEP. It is important to remember that as PEEP is reduced, the pressure limit must also be reduced by the same amount. This maintains the original tidal volume.

6. Increased respiratory rate

Increasing the ventilator respiratory rate increases the minute volume and probably raises the PaO_2 and lowers the $PaCO_2$. Patients with stiff lungs and short time constants of ventilation often respond well to an increased respiratory rate. To that end, some authors advocate using a rate of up to 150/min on a conventional time-triggered, pressure-limited, time-cycled mechanical ventilator, if necessary. (It should be noted that the Food and Drug Administration [FDA] has set the upper rate limit of 150/min on these units.) A rate of greater than 150/min is termed *high-frequency ventilation* (HFV) and requires a special ventilator.

Figure 16-8 Pressure-time curve showing effect of addition of PEEP on tidal volume. Initially, tidal volume is delivered by pressure difference of 30 cm water (difference between 0 and 30 cm water pressure). With addition of 5 cm water PEEP, pressure difference is reduced to 25 cm water (difference between 5 and 30 cm water pressure). This results in less tidal volume being delivered. *(From Burgess WR, Chernik V: Respiratory therapy in newborn infants and children, ed 2, New York, 1986, Thieme.)*

7. Initiate and select appropriate settings for high-frequency ventilation (HFV) (Code: IIID4) [Difficulty: ELE: R, Ap; WRE: An]

High-frequency ventilation (HFV) involves the use of a ventilator respiratory rate that is much greater than commonly needed. The FDA defines HFV as a rate of more than 150/min. Because of this FDA definition of HFV, conventional neonatal TPTV ventilators are not considered high-frequency ventilators. Several manufacturers have developed ventilators capable of rates significantly greater than 150/min. One of these must be used when HFV is indicated. The FDA has also set some guidelines for the appropriate use of HFV. See Box 16-5 for the clinical indications for HFV. The most commonly encountered problem is with a premature neonate with infant respiratory distress syndrome (RDS), a homogenous lung

---

BOX 16-5   Common Clinical Indications for the Use of High-Frequency Ventilation in Infants and Children

Severe hypoxemia and hypercarbia unresponsive to conventional ventilation techniques
    Infant respiratory distress syndrome (RDS)
    Acute respiratory distress syndrome (ARDS)
    Pneumonia
    Aspiration syndromes
    Pulmonary hemorrhage
Conventional ventilation with a persistent pulmonary air leak
    Pneumothorax
    Bronchopleural fistula
    Pulmonary interstitial emphysema (PIE)
    Pneumomediastinum
    Pneumoperitoneum
Persistent pulmonary hypertension of the newborn (PPHN)
Pulmonary hypoplasia
Bronchoscopy, laryngoscopy, or tracheal surgery

---

disease causing low compliance. If the RDS patient is failing despite optimal conventional mechanical ventilation and has a mean airway pressure of greater than 15 cm water, high-frequency ventilation is indicated.

Despite the FDA guidelines, many respiratory therapists consider a rate of greater than 40/min on a neonatal patient to be HFV. When a conventional TPTV ventilator is used to deliver a respiratory rate of up to 150/min, the term high-*frequency positive pressure ventilation* (HFPPV) is used. Experience has shown that many RDS infants can be successfully managed with conventional TPTV ventilator set to deliver a small tidal volume at a rate between 40 and 150/min. However, when these methods fail, true HFV is needed.

Ventilator manufacturers have developed two different technologies for delivering FDA-defined HFV. The first is called *high-frequency jet ventilation* (HFJV). With HFJV, small jets of gas are directed down the patient's endotracheal tube. These gas jets entrain additional gas into the tube. The two combined volumes of gas make up the patient's tidal volume. The patient exhales passively because of normal lung recoil. The second method is called *high-frequency oscillation* (HFO) or *high-frequency oscillatory ventilation* (HFOV). With HFO, a pumping device (piston, diaphragm, or sound speaker) actively pushes a small tidal volume into the patient from a continuous flow of gas (called bias flow) passing through the circuit and by the endotracheal tube. HFO technology can deliver very high rates because the patient actively exhales the delivered tidal volume. This active exhalation is created by the back stroke of the pumping device that pulls the tidal volume out of the patient's airways and lungs. See Table 16-2 for a comparison of HFV methods and characteristics.

Initial HFV settings depend on the patient's diagnosis, clinical situation, current conventional ventilator settings, and the type of high-frequency ventilator to be used. Generally speaking, the initial HFV settings include a tidal volume large enough to see chest movement and a continuation of the patient's original mean airway pressure, PEEP level, and oxygen percentage. The I:E ratio should be set at 1:2 and the high-frequency rate should be between 10 and 15 Hertz (Hz) depending on the infant's body weight. (A Hz is defined as 1 respiratory cycle/sec; 60 respiratory cycles/min. For example, a rate of 600/min is 10/sec or 10 Hz.) After the patient is stabilized on HFV, arterial blood gases should be drawn and analyzed, vital signs assessed, and a chest radiograph obtained. In a patient without a pulmonary air leak, a chest radiograph finding of lung expansion to T8 to T9 on the right hemidiaphragm, without intercostal bulging, is believed to show the best lung volume. Once established, the HFV rate is seldom changed. Adjustments in tidal volume are made by increasing or decreasing what is referred to as either drive pressure (with HFJV) or amplitude (with HFO). Increasing drive pressure/amplitude increases the tidal volume and decreases the carbon dioxide level. The

TABLE 16-2	High-Frequency Ventilation Features and Characteristics		
	HFPPV	**HFJV**	**HFO**
Rate (1-2.5 Hz) (4-10 Hz) (5-50 Hz)	60-150/min	240-660/min	300-3000/min
V_T (>dead space) (approx. dead space) (<dead space)	3.5 mL/kg	2.5 mL/kg	1.3 mL/kg
I/E ratio	1:3-1:2	1:3-1:2	1:3-1:2
Technical application	Conventional ventilator	Special ventilator	Special ventilator
F_IO_2	0.21-1.0	0.21-1.0	0.21-1.0
PEEP	0-20	0-20	0-20
Expiration	Passive	Passive	Active
Gas movement	Bulk flow	Bulk flow	*See below

HFJV, High-frequency jet ventilation; *HFO*, high-frequency oscillation; *HFPPV*, high-frequency positive pressure ventilation. Hz (Hertz) = 1 respiratory cycle/second.
*There are several theories on how gas movement occurs with HFO. See a dedicated mechanical ventilation textbook for a discussion on them.

patient's oxygenation should also improve as the mean airway pressure is increased. Decreasing drive pressure/amplitude decreases the tidal volume and increases the carbon dioxide level. If the patient's oxygenation should decrease too much, additional therapeutic PEEP may be needed. See Table 15-1 for high-frequency ventilation guidelines with infant and adult patients. See Figure 16-9 for a protocol on initiation and adjustment of HFO. Figure 16-10 shows a protocol for weaning from HFO.

Exam Hint 16-4 (WRE)

If a patient with RDS is failing with conventional mechanical ventilation, high-frequency ventilation is indicated.

---

8. Recommend the instillation of exogenous surfactant (Code: IIIG4j) [Difficulty: ELE: R, Ap; WRE: An]

The primary problem with a premature neonate with RDS is the lack of surfactant, a phospholipid, to reduce the surface tension in the alveoli. In 1991 the FDA approved the use of exogenous surfactant that can be directly instilled into the lungs of RDS neonates. Exosurf Neonatal (a synthetic product), Survanta and Infasurf (both bovine lung extract), and Curosurf (a pig lung extract) have been successfully used clinically. These drugs have proven very beneficial to premature neonates with inadequate natural surfactant. After the drug is administered, the patient's lung compliance improves dramatically. When this improvement occurs, be prepared to rapidly reduce the ventilator-delivered oxygen percentage, rate, pressure limit, and PEEP. The PIP will need to be reduced to keep the same tidal volume. Failure to reduce PIP and PEEP could result in too large a tidal volume and functional residual capacity that could cause pulmonary barotrauma.

Exam Hint 16-5 (WRE)

Recent Written Registry Exams have included a question about the application or modification of HFV. Know that increasing the amplitude results in a larger tidal volume and a reduction in the patient's $PaCO_2$. Reducing the amplitude would have the opposite effect.

Exam Hint 16-6 (WRE)

Recent Written Registry Exams have included a question about the exogenous surfactant being indicated in a neonate with RDS.

Each of the options discussed in this section has its advocates; however, it seems logical that the best possible care would come from the proper application of each option when it is best suited to the patient's condition. To that end, Chatburn, Waldemar, and Lough (1983) have developed a rather comprehensive approach to the adjustment of the various ventilator parameters to optimize the care of the RDS infant. They use the initial and subsequent blood gas results to direct the various ventilator changes that have been discussed. Because of the complexity of the logic in the algorithm, it is recommended that their articles, listed in the references, be read to fully appreciate its use.

c. Patients with increased airway resistance and normal lung compliance such as meconium aspiration syndrome (MAS)

Although meconium aspiration is a commonly seen cause of increased airway resistance, it is also seen in infants with excessive airway secretions or bronchospasm. These neonates usually have normal lung compliance and their clinical problem is getting enough air into and out of the lungs. The meconium or other obstruction causes uneven airflow and results in hypoxemia, air trapping, auto-PEEP,

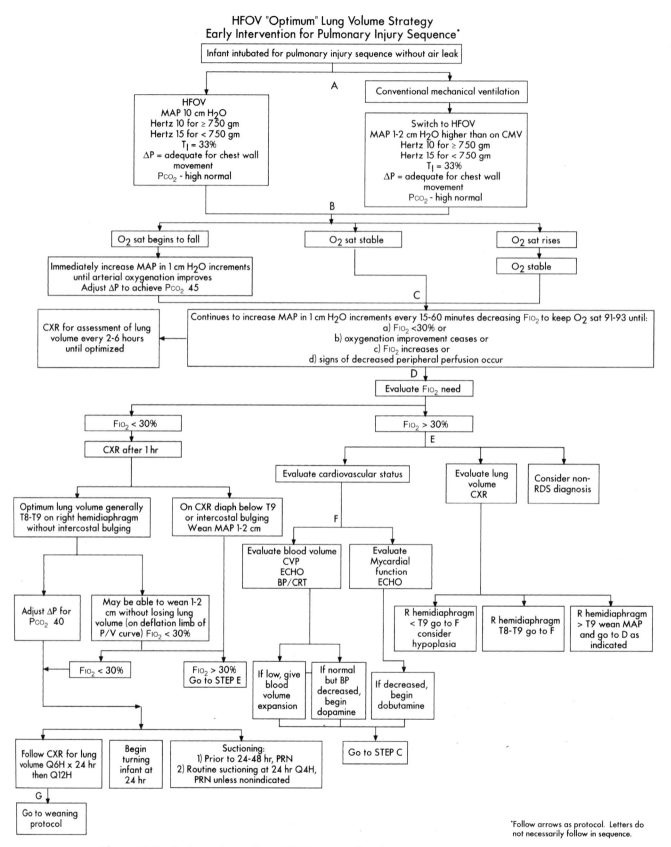

Figure 16-9 Optimum lung volume HFOV strategy flowchart. *(From Minton S, Gerstmann D, Stoddard R: Cardiopul Rev, Yorba Linda, Calif, 1995, Sensormedics Corp. PN 770118-001.)*

HFOV "Optimum" Lung Volume Strategy
Pulmonary Injury Sequence Without Air Leak
Weaning Strategy

Figure 16-10 HFOV flowchart for weaning from optimum lung volume strategy. *(From Minton S, Gerstmann D, Stoddard R:* Cardiopul Rev, *Yorba Linda, Calif, 1995, Sensormedics Corp. PN 770118-001.)*

and an increased risk of barotrauma or volutrauma. Because of these issues, there are two key clinical goals. The first is to minimize turbulence during inspiration by reducing the inspiratory flow rate as much as possible. The second is to give a long enough expiratory time to prevent air trapping. Common recommendations for the ventilator settings are listed in Box 16-6. As discussed earlier, blood gases, vital signs, and so forth must be monitored after the infant is placed on the ventilator. Listen to the breath sounds to detect the end of exhalation and a pause before the start of the next inspiration. This is to ensure that the exhalation has been complete and there is no air trapping that would lead to auto-PEEP. Any further adjustments can then be determined and evaluated by another set of blood gases and vital signs.

Look again at the issue of time constants of ventilation to better understand the various options for adjusting the ventilator. Using the following values for a mechanically ventilated neonate with meconium aspiration, its time constant is calculated as follows:

BOX 16-6 Common Mechanical Ventilator Parameters for Neonates with Increased Airway Resistance and Normal Lung Compliance

Delivered tidal volume: 6-8 mL/kg

Pressure limit: less than 20 cm water

Frequency: 20-40/min

I:E ratio: 1:3 to 1:10

Inspiratory time (T_I): between 0.4 and 0.7 seconds (this may need to be increased)

Expiratory time (T_E): at least 0.5 seconds (this may need to be increased)

PEEP: 2-4 cm water if needed

Inspiratory flow: sufficient to see the chest move and hear bilateral breath sounds during the inspiration. 5-8 L/min commonly used

Oxygen percentage: 40% (this may need to be increased to keep the SpO_2 greater than 92%)

Tc = compliance (.005 L/cm water) × resistance
(150 cm water/L/second because the infant is intubated and has an obstructive problem).

Simplify as follows:

$$Tc = .005 \times 150 \text{ second}$$

$$= .75 \text{ second}$$

(Compare this with a Tc of 0.15 for a normal, spontaneously breathing neonate and a Tc of 0.1 for a ventilated infant with RDS.)

This relatively long time constant means that the tidal volume and peak inspiratory pressure are rather slowly delivered to the alveoli. There is little chance of causing barotrauma or volutrauma from high ventilating pressures; however, it takes a fairly long inspiratory time to deliver an adequate tidal volume. Care must be taken to provide enough expiratory time for the tidal volume to be exhaled completely. Briefly then, the challenge is to deliver an adequate tidal volume to maintain acceptable blood gases at a rate slow enough to prevent air trapping on exhalation.

In general, the inspiratory flow and rate are kept low, inspiratory and expiratory times are kept relatively long, and the I:E ratio should favor a long time for complete exhalation. Furthermore, it is important to frequently suction the airway to remove meconium or secretions. Postural drainage and percussion are also provided to mobilize the secretions so that they can be suctioned out. Usually these procedures and the natural breakdown of meconium result in reduced airway resistance within a few days. Ventilatory support can then be lessened.

d. Patients with persistent pulmonary hypertension of the newborn

Persistent pulmonary hypertension of the newborn (PPHN) is also referred to as persistent pulmonary hypertension (PPH), persistent fetal circulation (PFC), or persistence of the fetal circulation. Infants with PPHN present clinically with an elevated pulmonary artery pressure and a right-to-left shunt through a patent ductus arteriosus (PDA) or the foramen ovale. Therefore, their oxygenation fluctuates greatly. The problem may be seen right after birth or up to 24 hours later. PPHN seems to result from fetal hypoxemia and acidosis. These, in turn, are caused by or associated with maternal drug addiction, infection, preeclampsia, abruptio placenta, postterm gestation, oligohydramnios, and meconium staining or aspiration. The following four tests are done to help confirm the diagnosis:

1. Hyperoxia test

This is the first test and is done after an arterial blood gas has shown a low PaO_2. The test involves having the patient inspire 100% oxygen for about 10 minutes and obtaining a second arterial blood gas. If the PaO_2 does not improve to more than 50 torr, a fixed right-to-left shunt is proven. The shunt may be from PPHN or a cyanotic heart defect. If the PaO_2 does go over 100 torr, the neonate probably has parenchymal lung disease and should be treated accordingly.

2. Preductal and postductal arterial blood sampling

Simultaneously draw and then analyze (1) a blood gas sample from the right radial or brachial artery to check the preductal PaO_2, and (2) a blood gas sample from the left brachial, left radial, either femoral artery, or the umbilical artery catheter to check the postductal PaO_2. Compare the results. A drop in saturation from preductal to postductal blood of greater than 10% or a drop in PaO_2 of greater than 15 to 20 torr indicates shunting. For example, a preductal PaO_2 of 70 torr and a postductal PaO_2 of 45 torr indicates significant shunting. This same test may be performed noninvasively with either transcutaneous oxygen monitoring or pulse oximetry monitoring. The $PtcO_2$ monitors should be placed over the right upper chest for preductal blood and left upper chest, abdomen, or either thigh for postductal blood. Pulse oximetry monitors should be placed on the right hand for preductal blood and left hand or either foot for postductal blood. Again, a greater than 15 to 20 torr drop in preductal to postductal $PtcO_2$ or a greater than 10% drop in saturation in preductal to postductal SpO_2 confirms a significant shunt.

It is important to note that if the neonate has a shunt through the foramen ovale instead of the ductus arteriosus, this test will be negative. The preductal and postductal oxygen levels will be the same. Shunting through the foramen ovale is seen in as many as 50% of PPHN babies.

3. Hyperoxia-hyperventilation test

The infant is manually ventilated with 100% oxygen at a rate and pressure adequate to significantly reduce the carbon dioxide level. When this "critical $PaCO_2$" (usually between 20 and 30 torr) is reached, the pulmonary artery pressure drops, the lungs are better perfused, and the PaO_2 improves. Although the patient's color will likely change from cyanotic to pink and the $PtcO_2$ and SpO_2 values will improve, the test is confirmed by a postductal PaO_2 of greater than 80 torr. The critical $PaCO_2$ value, ventilation rate, and manometer pressure on the manual ventilator should be recorded. These values can be used later to set the mechanical ventilator parameters.

4. Doppler echocardiography

This procedure can be used to identify an intracardiac shunt through the foramen ovale, shunt through a patent ductus arteriosus, or evidence of increased right ventricular pressure as a sign of pulmonary hypertension.

Any infant who shows signs of PPHN, such as positive results to any of these tests or the need for more than 70%

oxygen to prevent hypoxemia, should be considered for hyperventilation therapy. The goal is to reduce pulmonary artery hypertension and thus reduce shunting and improve the PaO_2. This is accomplished by hyperventilating the patient to his or her critical $PaCO_2$. Box 16-7 lists common ventilator parameters used to treat persistent pulmonary hypertension. Once the proper ventilator settings are found and the blood gas goals are met, the patient is maintained at this level for 1 or more days. It is often necessary to pharmacologically paralyze the infant with pancuronium bromide (Pavulon) or a similar drug to ensure that the patient's breathing is synchronized with the ventilator. This is especially important when high ventilator rates are needed. After about 24 hours, the ventilator is adjusted to increase the $PaCO_2$ by 1 to 2 torr. If the peak inspiratory pressure is greater than 45 cm water it should be reduced first. A blood gas is drawn to see if the PaO_2 is stable and if the $PaCO_2$ increased the desired small amount. If this first reduction in support is tolerated, it may be slowly followed by further reductions. Each step back from hyperventilation should be small so that the $PaCO_2$ increases only by 1 to 2 mm Hg each time.

As this happens, the patient should be supported in every other way. The medication tolazoline (Priscoline) is a pulmonary vasodilator that has proven to be successful in about one of six neonates with PPHN. Watch for signs of pulmonary barotrauma or bronchopulmonary dyspla-sia from the high peak pressures and oxygen percentages required with these patients.

5. Inhaled nitric oxide

a. **Independently change the mode of administer of nitric oxide (Code: IIIF2e1) [Difficulty: ELE: R, Ap; WRE: An]**

b. **Perform exhaled nitric oxide measurement (WRE Code: IB9k) [Difficulty: WRE: R, Ap]**

c. **Interpret the results of exhaled nitric oxide measurement (WRE Code: IB10k) [Difficulty: WRE: R, Ap, An]**

d. **Independently adjust the flow or concentration of nitric oxide (Code: IIIF2e2) [Difficulty: ELE: R, Ap; WRE: An].** Inhaled nitric oxide (iNO) gas has been approved for use as a pulmonary artery vasodilator in neonates with persistent pulmonary hypertension of the neonate (PPHN) and increased pulmonary vascular resistance. Clinical improvement is often seen when a neonate with PPHN or RDS inhales a small amount of nitric oxide. It is important to keep the concentration of iNO as low as possible to achieve this clinical improvement. The upper limit of a therapeutic dose of iNO is less than 20 parts per million (ppm). This is because nitric oxide combines with oxygen to form nitrogen dioxide (NO_2). A level of nitrogen dioxide greater than 10 ppm can cause cell damage, hemorrhage, and pulmonary edema leading to death. As the NO_2 increases, it causes an increase in the patient's methemoglobin level. Therefore, the serum level of this nonfunctional form of hemoglobin must also be monitored. Patients who receive iNO are usually also receiving mechanical ventilation. In addition, special iNO measurement and delivery systems are needed and levels of inspired oxygen, nitric oxide, and nitrogen dioxide must be measured. As the patient's PPHN improves, the level of iNO can be reduced. This is commonly done by reducing the iNO concentration in steps of 50%. For example, if 20 ppm was the original dose on nitric oxide, it would be reduced in steps of 10 ppm, then 5 ppm, and so on until there is 1 ppm or less. The neonate is assessed at each decreasing step to be sure that the pulmonary hypertension does not increase.

BOX 16-7   Common Mechanical Ventilator Parameters to Treat a Neonate with Persistent Pulmonary Hypertension

Delivered tidal volume: 6-8 mL/kg initially. 8-10 mL/kg may be needed to hyperventilate the neonate

Pressure limit: 20-25 cm water; use as little pressure as possible but be prepared to raise up to 35 cm water to deliver an adequate tidal volume

Frequency: 60-100/min may be needed to decrease the $PaCO_2$ to the critical level of probably between 20 and 30 mm Hg; a rate of up to 150/min has been used

I:E ratio: 1:2 (this depends on the respiratory rate needed to decrease the carbon dioxide level)

Inspiratory time (T_I): Between 0.4 and 0.7 seconds (this must be decreased at higher respiratory rates)

Expiratory time (T_E): at least 0.5 seconds (this must be decreased at higher respiratory rates)

PEEP: none if possible to lower the mean airway pressure and prevent crushing of the pulmonary capillary bed; 2-4 cm water may be used if needed

Inspiratory flow: sufficient to see the chest move and hear bilateral breath sounds during the inspiration; 5-8 L/min commonly used initially; flow must be increased at higher respiratory rates

Oxygen percentage: up to 70%-100% to keep the postductal PaO_2 greater than 55 torr and ideally between 115 and 120 torr

---

Exam Hint 16-7 (ELE, WRE)

Know that inhaled nitric oxide is indicated in a patient with PPHN and how to interpret the patient's response to iNO.

---

e. **Patients with bronchopulmonary dysplasia.** The neonate who develops bronchopulmonary dysplasia (BPD) is usually born prematurely with a low birth weight. He or she is a survivor of RDS but has suffered serious lung damage in the process. It is controversial whether high peak pressures, high mean airway pressures, high inspired oxygen percentages, or a combination of these factors is the main cause of BPD. It is important to try to minimize all of them so that new lung tissues can grow to replace lung tissue that has been damaged. It is important to try to wean these infants as quickly as possible to avoid further ventilator-induced damage. If acceptable blood gases can be maintained with a ventilator rate of less than 15/min, the infant may be extubated. Nasal CPAP may be used to help maintain the PaO_2. See Box 16-8 for the commonly recommended ventilator settings for a BPD patient.

A number of medications are used to help optimize the patient's pulmonary function. Methylxanthines such as aminophylline or caffeine are beneficial as respiratory stimulants. There is further evidence that they help to strengthen the diaphragm and decrease muscle fatigue. The diuretic furosemide (Lasix) has been widely reported to improve lung compliance and airway resistance by decreasing any pulmonary edema fluid. Remember that patients receiving furosemide must be given a potassium-chloride supplement to replace what is lost through the kidneys. Some authors have reported the use of cortico-steroids to be helpful in weaning because of increased pulmonary compliance. This possible advantage must be balanced against the known problems associated with the prolonged use of the medication. Finally, a dietary supplement of vitamin E may increase lung healing. It is hoped that the use of surfactant replacement therapy early in the treatment of the RDS neonate will reduce the incidence of BPD.

BOX 16-8   Common Mechanical Ventilator Parameters for Neonates with Bronchopulmonary Dysplasia

Delivered tidal volume: 6-8 mL/kg

Pressure limit: as low as possible and not to exceed 25 cm water

Frequency: as low as possible to maintain the $PaCO_2$ between 35 and 45 torr; some authors report accepting a $PaCO_2$ as high as 55 to 65 torr to minimize the need to increase peak and mean pressures

I:E ratio: 1:2 to 1:10

Inspiratory time (T_I): between 0.3 and 0.7 seconds

Expiratory time (T_E): at least 0.5 seconds to allow for a complete exhalation

PEEP: no more than 2-4 cm water

Inspiratory flow: sufficient to see the chest move and hear bilateral breath sounds during the inspiration; 5-8 L/min commonly used initially

Oxygen percentage: as low as possible to keep the PaO_2 between 55 and 65 torr; some authors report accepting a PaO_2 as low as 35 torr to minimize the need to increase peak and mean pressures; it must be noted that a PaO_2 below 55 torr increases the risk of pulmonary hypertension

---

5. Monitor the mean airway pressure to evaluate the patient's response to respiratory care (ELE Code: IIIE9) [Difficulty: ELE: R, Ap, An]

Mean airway pressure (Paw) is the average pressure over an entire breathing cycle. A number of current neonatal and adult ventilators are able to calculate the value. Paw is influenced by both the patient's lung thoracic compliance (C_{LT}) and airway resistance (R_{AW}). If the ventilator settings are unchanged, a decrease in compliance or an increase in resistance will result in an increase in the mean airway pressure. This is because in a neonatal ventilator, the pressure limit is reached earlier and held for the duration of the inspiratory time. Conversely, if the patient's compliance increases or the resistance decreases, the Paw will decrease. It is important to further evaluate the patient when a change in Paw is noticed. This is because the new pressure by itself does not show you whether there has been a change in compliance, resistance, or both. Any treatments that improve lung compliance and reduce airway resistance are shown by a reduced mean airway pressure.

In general, an increase in mean airway pressure increases the patient's oxygenation. This is because the alveoli are kept open longer, allowing more time for diffusion and preventing alveolar collapse. If alveolar ventilation is improved, the $PaCO_2$ will also be reduced. There is clinical evidence that a mean airway pressure of 12 or more cm water pressure is associated with an increased risk of pulmonary barotrauma and decreased cardiac output. This is especially true if PEEP is increased to raise the Paw. Watch the patient closely whenever a ventilator change is made that increases the Paw. A sudden deterioration in cardiopulmonary function may be caused by a pneumothorax. A reduction in urine output, an increased heart rate, and decreased blood pressure are often seen when the cardiac output is reduced. The mean airway pressure should be reduced if either of these situations is seen. To prevent these complications, it is necessary to reduce the mean airway pressure whenever the patient's compliance improves.

Usually the mean airway pressure is the result of the patient's lung compliance, airway resistance, and the various ventilator settings. The initial mean airway pressure should be considered along with the ventilator settings when interpreting the first set of arterial blood gases. Based on the blood gas results, ventilator adjustments may be needed. Note the Paw at each adjustment.

A number of ventilator control adjustments influence the patient's mean airway pressure. (See Figure 16-11 for several examples of airway pressure tracings based on ventilator control changes.) If the patient's compliance and resistance are stable, the Paw will be *increased* by the following: (1) an increased inspiratory flow, (2) an increased pressure limit (assuming the pressure limit has been previ-

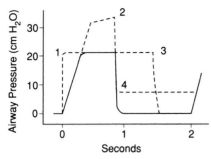

Figure 16-11   Pressure-time tracings showing four different ventilator settings that can be used to increase mean airway pressure. *1*, Inspiratory flow is increased. *2*, Pressure limit is increased. *3*, Inspiratory time is increased. This also changes the I : E ratio by reducing expiratory time if rate is kept the same. *4*, PEEP is added. *(In: Harris TR: Physiologic Principles. Goldsmith JP, Karotkin EH, editors: Assisted ventilation of the neonate, Philadelphia, 1981, WB Saunders.)*

ously reached), (3) an increase in PEEP, (4) an increased inspiratory time (assuming no change in ventilator rate and a decreased expiratory time), and (5) a decreased expiratory time (assuming an increased ventilator rate). These ventilator adjustments should result in an increased PaO_2 and possibly a decreased $PaCO_2$. Measure blood gases to be sure of the patient's response.

If the patient's compliance and resistance are stable, the Paw will be *decreased* by the following:
- A decreased inspiratory flow
- A decreased pressure limit (assuming the pressure limit has been previously reached)
- A decrease in PEEP
- A decreased inspiratory time (assuming no change in ventilator rate and an increased expiratory time)
- An increased expiratory time (assuming a decreased ventilator rate)

These ventilator adjustments may result in a decreased PaO_2 and possibly an increased $PaCO_2$. Measure blood gases to be sure of the patient's response.

It should be noted that of all the various controls that have an influence on the mean airway pressure, PEEP has the greatest impact. There is usually a one-for-one relationship between the addition or removal of PEEP and the resulting $P\overline{aw}$. For example, the $P\overline{aw}$ is 10 cm water when 5 cm water of PEEP is added. The resulting $P\overline{aw}$ is seen to become 15 cm water. If 2 cm of PEEP is removed the $P\overline{aw}$ will drop to 13 cm water.

6. Ventilator alarm systems

a. Check and adjust alarm systems (ELE Code: IIIE9) [Difficulty: ELE: R, Ap, An]

b. Monitor and adjust alarm systems (ELE Code: IIIG3g) [Difficulty: ELE: R, Ap, An]

All alarm systems must function properly, so test all audible and visual alarms. The respiratory therapist should be familiar with the most widely used neonatal ventilators and those that can be used with pediatric as well as adult patients. It is common practice to set most ventilator alarms at ± 10% from the set value.

If the patient is on a CPAP system, the low-pressure or disconnection alarm should be set to alarm if the pressure drops about 2 cm water below the set level. For example, if the patient is on 8 cm water CPAP, the alarm setting should be set at 6 cm water.

Many types of alarm systems have a timer that can be set to delay when the alarm sounds. For example, if the neonatal patient has a ventilator rate of 30/min, the cycling time between mandatory breaths is 2 seconds. The delay should be set so that the alarm sounds in 1 to 2 seconds after a mandatory breath fails to be delivered. If the patient is on a CPAP system, the timer may be set for no delay or a short delay after the CPAP pressure drops below the set value. Always adjust all alarm systems to fit the clinical situation and the patient's condition.

7. Ventilator flow, volume, and pressure graphic waveforms

a. Select ventilator graphics e.g., waveforms, scales (Code: IIID3) [Difficulty: ELE: R, Ap; WRE: An]

A patient who has been intubated and placed on a modern mechanical ventilator with a microprocessor and graphics software can have ventilator flow, volume, and pressure waveforms visualized on the monitor. Usually these parameters can be individually selected and paired up for comparison (such as pressure versus volume) or compared versus time (such as volume versus time). Select the parameters that best provide the data to help explain the patient's situation. Some units allow the information to be stored in memory or printed out. Compare current information with any past data.

b. Perform the procedure to measure ventilator graphics (e.g., pressure or volume) (WRE Code: IB9o) [Difficulty: WRE: R, Ap, An]

Because not every ventilator can provide waveform information, the correct unit must be selected for the patient. For example, the Drager Babylog 8000 has the monitor and graphics software built into the unit. Follow the ventilator manufacturer's guidelines to direct the unit to create the desired flow, volume, or pressure waveforms.

c. Interpret ventilator graphics e.g., pressure/volume (WRE Code: IB10o) [Difficulty: WRE: R, Ap, An]

Ventilator flow, volume, and pressure waveforms offer much clinically useful information. For example, expiratory flow can be monitored to look for air trapping and auto-PEEP. As discussed earlier, this is a concern if the neonate has obstructive airway disease or if a high respiratory rate is being used. Volume can be monitored as an indicator of improving or worsening lung compliance. Pressure can also be monitored as it relates to improving or worsening lung compliance. Less pressure is needed to deliver the desired tidal volume if the patient's lung compliance is improving. Conversely, more pressure is needed to deliver the desired tidal volume if the patient's lung compliance is worsening. Chapter 15 and this chapter include examples of waveform tracings.

d. Recommend changes in mechanical ventilation based on ventilator graphics (Code: IIIG3h) [Difficulty: ELE: R, Ap; WRE: An]

e. Independently adjust mechanical ventilation based on ventilator graphics (Code: IIIF2i8) [Difficulty: ELE: R, Ap; WRE: An]

As discussed earlier, be prepared to make adjustments in the ventilator as indicated by graphics. For example, if air trapping and auto-PEEP are observed, be prepared to increase the expiratory time, decrease the inspiratory time, or decrease the tidal volume to ensure that there is a complete exhalation.

8. Prevent procedure-associated hypoxemia by oxygenating the patient before and after suctioning and equipment changes (ELE Code: IIID9) [Difficulty: ELE: R, Ap, An]

Chapter 13 discusses the suctioning procedure and steps that should be taken to prevent hypoxemia during suctioning. Older children can be given 100% oxygen during suctioning or equipment changes. Children younger than 6 months of age should have their oxygen percentage increased by 10% to 20% for the procedure.

MODULE C
Mechanical ventilation and CPAP equipment

1. Ventilators

As discussed in Chapter 15, the literature produced by the manufacturers and the descriptions used in many standard texts break the various ventilators into more categories than used by the NBRC. To avoid confusion, this text uses the NBRC's more simplified terminology. A pneumatically powered ventilator is defined here as powered by compressed gas. It may be electrically controlled with electrical alarm systems. Fluidic ventilators are defined here as being pneumatically powered and partially or completely controlled by fluidic methods. Fluidic controls make use of compressed gas for cycling and other ventilator functions. Both of these types of neonatal ventilators use compressed air and oxygen that go to an air-oxygen mixer (blender) to determine the inspired oxygen. The gas then goes to a flow meter where the continuous flow per minute through the ventilator circuit is set. Depending on the ventilator, either compressed air or oxygen are used to drive the other control functions in fluidic ventilators.

An electrically powered ventilator is defined here as being electrically powered and controlled. Compressed air and oxygen go to a blender where the inspired oxygen is set. A microprocessor ventilator is defined here as being controlled by a microprocessor; it may be pneumatically or electrically powered. All of these types of ventilators are limited to the 150 breaths/min maximum rate set by the FDA. A high-frequency ventilator is capable of delivering a respiratory rate of more than 150/min. CPAP can be delivered through the types of ventilators described previously, manufactured CPAP-only units, or through a freestanding, assembled component system.

a. Manipulate pneumatic ventilators by order or protocol (Code: IIA6a) [Difficulty: ELE: R, Ap; WRE: An]

1. Get the necessary equipment for the procedure

It is beyond the scope of this text to discuss in detail the functions of pneumatic ventilators and the following types of ventilators. Refer to the manufacturer's literature for specific information. Examples of neonatal pneumatic ventilators include the Babybird, Babybird 2, Bio-Med MPV-10, BEAR Cub BP2001, and Healthdyne 105. They are used to deliver conventional TPTV mechanical ventilation to the majority of neonatal and pediatric patients. The Bio-Med device MVP-10 is an example of a pediatric transport ventilator.

2. Put the equipment together and make sure that it works properly

3. Troubleshoot any problems with the equipment

Make sure that the air and oxygen high-pressure hoses are screwed tightly into the air-oxygen blender. A gas leak is heard as a whistling or hissing sound. If either gas source is cut off to the blender, its alarm will sound.

b. Manipulate fluidic ventilators by order or protocol (Code: IIA6a) [Difficulty: ELE: R, Ap; WRE: An]

1. Get the necessary equipment for the procedure

The Sechrist IV-100B and IV-200 ventilators are pneumatically powered and electrically and fluidically controlled.

2. Put the equipment together and make sure that it works properly

3. Troubleshoot any problems with the equipment

Fluidic ventilators are prone to the same kind of problems with leaking high-pressure air and oxygen hoses as pneumatic ventilators. In addition, they are very sensitive to obstructions. Make sure that all inlet filters are intact and free of debris.

c. Manipulate electric ventilators by order or protocol (Code: IIA6a) [Difficulty: ELE: R, Ap; WRE: An]

1. Get the necessary equipment for the procedure

The following are examples of electrically powered (and microprocessor controlled) ventilators that can deliver a tidal volume small enough for a neonatal patient: Newport Breeze, Maquet Servo *i*, and Drager Evita XL.

2. Put the equipment together and make sure that it works properly

3. Troubleshoot any problems with the equipment

Make sure that the electrical power source is secure. Do not use a unit that does not power up or operate properly.

d. Manipulate a microprocessor ventilator by order or protocol (Code: IIA6a) [Difficulty: ELE: R, Ap; WRE: An]

1. Get the equipment necessary for the procedure

The Drager Babylog 8000 Plus, Puritan Bennett 840, VIP Bird, and VIP Bird Gold are electrically and pneumatically powered and controlled by a microprocessor. The LifeCare PLV-102 and Nelcor Puritan Bennett Companion 2801 are microprocessor controlled and electrically powered. They are home care ventilators that can deliver tidal volumes small enough for pediatric patients (50 mL).

2. Put the equipment together and make sure that it works properly

All ventilators must have a stable electrical supply. Both the LifeCare PLV-102 and the Nelcor Puritan Bennett Companion 2801 must have a home oxygen source if more than room air is required by the patient. An oxygen analyzer should also be added into the patient circuit because the oxygen percentage varies with a changing respiratory rate or tidal volume.

3. Troubleshoot any problems with the equipment

Microprocessor ventilators typically come with self-diagnostic software. If a problem is detected, the unit will display it on the monitor. There is little to repair with these units at the bedside. Occasionally a computer chip must be replaced.

e. Manipulate high-frequency ventilators by order or protocol (WRE code: IIA6c) [Difficulty: WRE: R, Ap]

1. Get the necessary equipment for the procedure

The Bunnell Life Pulse High-Frequency Ventilator provides high-frequency jet ventilation (HFJV). The Sensor-Medics 3100A High-Frequency Oscillatory Ventilator and Infrasonics Infant Star 950 Ventilator are examples of high-frequency oscillator (HFO) ventilators.

2. Put the equipment together and make sure that it works properly

The following are needed for proper assembly of a HFJV: (1) a pressurized oxygen source, (2) a pressurized air source, (3) an air-oxygen proportioner (blender), (4) a pressure regulator for controlling the patient's peak pressure, (5) an injector line to add the jet volume to the endotracheal tube (Figure 15-20), and (6) an intravenous infusion pump to supply a steady drip of water to the jet ventilator injector line for nebulization.

An HFO ventilator needs the following basic accessories for assembly: (1) a pressurized oxygen source, (2) a pressurized air source, (3) an air-oxygen proportioner (blender), and (4) a passover or cascade-type humidifier, and (5) a low-compliance patient circuit designed specifically for the ventilator.

3. Troubleshoot any problems with the equipment

Make sure that gas sources are stable, all tubing connections are tight, and humidification systems are functioning properly. Because the patient's tidal volume is very small, it cannot be accurately measured. Any leaks will result in an undetectable loss of delivered tidal volume.

2. Manipulate ventilator breathing circuits by order or protocol (ELE code: IIA11c) [Difficulty: ELE: R, Ap, An]

a. Get the necessary equipment for the procedure

Conventional neonatal ventilators use a circuit that has all of the standard features of an adult circuit as discussed in Chapter 15. Commonly, disposable single-patient-use corrugated plastic circuits are used. They are inexpensive and meet the needs of most patients. Condensation is drained out into water traps that are placed at low points in the natural draping of the inspiratory and expiratory limbs of the circuit. If excessive moisture is a problem or if the gas temperature must be maintained within a narrow range, a heated-wire circuit may be used. These types of circuits are built with a heated wire either loosely threaded through the lumen or coiled within the tubing itself. They are integrated with the humidification system and a servo unit for automatic temperature regulation. Because of the added wiring, these disposable circuits are considerably more expensive than the simple circuits used with most patients. A heat-moisture exchanger (HME) is usually only used with children because the tidal volume must be greater than the dead space of the HME. If a HME is used for passive humidification, it is added between the patient's endotracheal tube and the Y of the ventilator circuit.'

Be aware that corrugated circuits have a relatively high internal resistance and compressible volume. The corrugations lead to gas turbulence that increases as the flow is raised. When the tubing is warmed, it becomes more stretchable. This stretch results in more tidal volume lost to the circuit instead of being delivered to the patient.

When high flow rates and ventilating pressures are needed, as in HFV, a smooth bore and low compressible volume circuit is used instead of the standard disposable type. A special circuit made of noncompliant tubing is needed with the SensorMedics 3100A ventilator. In addition, to complete an HFJV circuit, a Hi-Lo Jet endotracheal tube or special endotracheal tube adapter is needed to deliver the jetted gas and add the entrained gas for the tidal volume. These are shown in Chapter 15.

b. Put the equipment together and make sure that it works properly

c. Troubleshoot any problems with the equipment

Conventional neonatal ventilator circuits are basically the same as adult circuits with an inspiratory limb and an expiratory limb. Water traps are usually added. An obvious difference is the smaller diameter so that there is less compressible volume. Some are smooth bore to minimize gas turbulence, and some have a heated wire running through them to keep a constant temperature and eliminate condensation. It is important that a heated-wire circuit be used only with the servo-controlled humidifier for which it is designed. Mixing circuits and humidifiers can lead to either overheating or underheating problems. Furthermore, do not cover a heated-wire circuit with a blanket. The circuit should not be allowed to touch the patient to avoid burns. If the patient is inside an incubator with a radiant warmer, the circuit's temperature probe must be kept outside.

An added feature is a third small-bore tubing for measuring the proximal airway pressure. The tube runs from the patient Y to the proximal airway pressure nipple on the ventilator. Make sure that all the connections are tight to prevent gas leaks.

d. Recommend a change in the patient breathing circuit (ELE code: IIIG3j) [Difficulty: ELE: R, Ap, An]

As discussed previously, there are situations when a special circuit should be used rather than a standard corrugated plastic circuit. A heated-wire circuit should be used if the patient needs to have the gas temperature and humidity level kept within a narrow range. If the patient is changed to a high-frequency ventilator, a special circuit designed for the ventilator must be used.

Ventilator circuits should not be changed routinely for infection control purposes. Current guidelines recommend that they be changed only when visibly soiled. A heat-moisture exchanger may be used for at least 48 hours. Change it whenever it is visibly soiled or contains sputum or blood.

Exam Hint 16-8 (ELE)

Current guidelines on the prevention of ventilator associated pneumonia (VAP) state that a ventilator or CPAP circuit should not be routinely changed. The circuit should be changed when visibly soiled (i.e., secretions or blood).

---

3. Manipulate continuous positive airway pressure (CPAP) devices (Code: IIA2) [Difficulty: ELE: R, Ap; WRE: An]

a. Get the necessary equipment for the procedure

Nasal CPAP devices are widely used with neonates who are born prematurely and have RDS. Their immature lungs lack sufficient surfactant and need the CPAP pressure to keep the alveoli open. Often, nasal CPAP meets the patient's needs so that endotracheal intubation and mechanical ventilation can be avoided. Nasal CPAP works with neonates because they are obligate nose breathers.

Nasal CPAP is associated with the hazards of gastric distension and reflux aspiration. These occur when the airway pressure forces air into the stomach. A gastric tube is usually inserted to vent the air out. There are two different devices for administering nasal CPAP. A nasopharyngeal tube is actually an endotracheal tube that has been cut shorter (see Figure 16-2, B). Select a tube that is the largest that can be easily inserted into the patient. Nasal prongs come in short and long versions (see Figure 16-2, *A*); both types involve prongs that fit into both nostrils. The prongs come in different diameters so that the proper size can be found to fit the internal diameter of the infant's nares.

b. Put the equipment together and make sure that it works properly

Follow the manufacturer's instructions for assembly of the CPAP device and CPAP circuit. See Figures 16-2 and 16-3 as well as the illustration of the CPAP circuit in Chapter 15 for general assembly guidance.

c. Troubleshoot any problems with the equipment (WRE Code: IIA2) [Difficulty: Ap]

A sudden drop in the CPAP level to zero indicates a disconnection at the patient or somewhere in the breathing circuit. Check all connections and reassemble the break. The patient may need to be manually ventilated while the problem is corrected.

If the CPAP level drops more than 2 cm of water pressure during an inspiration, the flow is inadequate and should be increased. Flow is also inadequate if the patient shows an increased use of accessory muscles of respiration or appears to have an increased work of breathing. Too high a flow is seen by an inadvertently high level of CPAP or the appearance that the patient is having a difficult time exhaling. A common problem with small diameter tubes like these is mucous plugging. A plugged tube may result in a backup of gas and can increase CPAP; however, depending on the CPAP system, there may be no change in pressure. Careful patient monitoring is important. Watch for a decrease in a drop in oxygenation, an increase in the respiratory rate, or retractions as signs of airway obstruction. Suction to clear out the mucous plug or remove the tube and place a new one.

4. Manipulate a continuous positive airway pressure (CPAP) circuit by order or protocol (ELE code: IIA2) [Difficulty: Ap]

a. Get the necessary equipment for the procedure

The general discussion and an illustration related to CPAP systems was presented in Chapter 15. Freestanding neonatal systems are similar to those used with adults. All currently available neonatal ventilators offer a CPAP mode. This allows the practitioner to easily switch the intubated neonate from IMV to CPAP without the need to set up new equipment. Humidification options are similar to those for mechanical ventilation. A heated Cascade-type or wick-type humidifier can be used to provide moisture to the inhaled gas.

b. Put the equipment together and make sure that it works properly

c. Troubleshoot any problems with the equipment (WRE Code: IIA2) [Difficulty: Ap]

The previous discussion about putting together and fixing problems with the CPAP device applies to the CPAP circuit.

d. Recommend a change in the patient breathing circuit (ELE code: IIIG3j) [Difficulty: ELE: R, Ap, An]

CPAP circuits should not be changed routinely for infection control purposes. Current guidelines recommend that they be changed only when visibly soiled (sputum or blood).

Exam Hint 16-9 (ELE)

A variable CPAP level indicates insufficient flow or a leak. A sudden drop in CPAP level to zero indicates a disconnection within the circuit or at the patient connection.

5. Manipulate humidification equipment by order or protocol (ELE code: IIA3) [Difficulty: ELE: R, Ap, An]

a. Get the necessary equipment for the procedure

The general discussion of humidification equipment was presented in Chapters 8 and 15. See the figures there and the general discussion for set-ups in ventilator and CPAP breathing circuits. Both heated humidifiers and heat-moisture exchangers are used with pediatric patients. Heated passover-type humidifiers systems are preferred with neonates.

b. Put the equipment together and make sure that it works properly

c. Troubleshoot any problems with the equipment

Again, see Chapters 8 and 15 for assembly and troubleshooting of humidification systems. With a Cascade-type of passover-type humidifier, the gas temperature is usually maintained close to the neonate's body temperature to maintain a neutral thermal environment. Make sure that the water level is kept in the recommended range to properly humidify the gas.

6. Perform quality control procedures for mechanical ventilators (Code: IIC5) [Difficulty: ELE: R, Ap; WRE: An]

Follow the manufacturer's guidelines for quality control procedures on mechanical ventilators. The microprocessor ventilators usually have a software package that performs self-diagnostic tests on the unit. If a problem is found it is displayed on the monitor. Obviously the ventilator should deliver the volume, flow, and pressure that is set on the control. Do not use a ventilator that fails a quality control check.

MODULE D
Respiratory care plan

1. Analyze the available information to determine the patient's pathophysiologic state (Code: IIIH1) [Difficulty: ELE: R, Ap; WRE: An]

Refer to Chapter 1 or earlier in this chapter for a detailed discussion on neonatal assessment. A brief discussion of the most common neonatal pulmonary conditions requiring mechanical ventilation was presented earlier in this chapter.

2. Determine the appropriateness of the prescribed therapy and goals for the patient's pathophysiologic state (Code: IIIH3) [Difficulty: ELE: R, Ap; WRE: An]

Specific recommendations for ventilatory support for the various pulmonary conditions were given earlier in the chapter.

a. Recommend changes in the therapeutic plan when indicated (Code: IIIH4) [Difficulty: ELE: R, Ap; WRE: An]

In many cases, time-triggered, pressure-limited, time-cycled (TPTV) mechanical ventilation with the IMV mode is utilized. An infant who is attempting to exhale when the IMV breath is being delivered is said to be "bucking" or "fighting" the ventilator. This problem is almost unavoidable because the IMV breaths are difficult to synchronize on the majority of neonatal ventilators. If the asynchrony between the infant's efforts and the ventilator is too great, there is an increased risk of hypoxemia and barotrauma or volutrauma. Carefully evaluate the patient to determine if the patient is breathing rapidly because of pain or improper adjustment of the ventilator. Make sure that the flow, rate, pressure limit, and so forth are correctly set for the patient's condition.

As discussed earlier, the ventilator must be adjusted to maintain desired arterial blood gas goals. It may be necessary to change from CPAP, to conventional ventilation modes, to high-frequency ventilation as the patient's condition changes.

b. Recommend sedation and/or use of muscle relaxant(s) (Code: IIIG1c) [Difficulty: ELE: R, Ap; WRE: An]

Sedation or paralysis should be considered only after all other causes of asynchrony have been ruled out. In many cases, when the ventilator is appropriately adjusted, the patient breathes in synchrony with it. If this cannot be achieved, sedation or paralysis must be considered.

Antianxiety agents are not typically used with neonates. Morphine sulfate or other opiates are typically used for pain but other less powerful medications may also be tried. If the patient must be paralyzed, pancuronium (Pavulon), atracurium (Tracrium), and vecuronium (Norcuron) are commonly used. Remember that these paralyzing agents have no effect on the patient's ability to feel pain or to be afraid of what is happening. Pain medications must be given as necessary.

c. Recommend discontinuing treatment or procedure based on the patient's response (Code: IIIG1i) [Difficulty: ELE: R, Ap; WRE: An]

d. Terminate the treatment or procedure if the patient has an adverse reaction to it (Code: IIIF1) [Difficulty: ELE: R, Ap; WRE: An]

Be prepared to stop a particular treatment or change in ventilator parameter if the patient has an adverse reaction to it. Physical assessment is vitally important because a neonate or small child cannot communicate how he or she feels about the care being provided.

3. Recommend the treatment of a pneumothorax (Code: IIIG1b) [Difficulty: ELE: R, Ap; WRE: An]

A chest radiograph and physical examination of the neonate will reveal if abnormal air or fluid is found around the lung(s) or heart. When transillumination of the chest is performed, any free air around the lung will be identified through the chest wall as a halo of light with a nonuniform shape. A nontension pneumothorax of greater than 10% is often also treated by inserting a pleural chest tube. If a patient has a tension pneumothorax, a pleural chest tube *must* be inserted to remove the air and relieve the pressure within the chest. A pleural chest tube is also placed to remove blood or other fluid from the pleural space. Chapter 18 has specific information that relates to treating a pneumothorax.

A pneumomediastinum, pneumopericardium, or pneumoperitoneum that puts the patient at risk must also be treated. A chest tube is then inserted into the area where the abnormal air is found. The same chest tube also removes any abnormal collection of fluid. A chest tube is usually placed behind the heart to remove any blood that should leak out after open-heart surgery.

If a neonate is being ventilated on a constant volume ventilator, the amount of air that is lost through the pleural chest tube can be calculated. This is done by subtracting the measured exhaled volume from the measured inhaled volume. For example:

Inspired tidal volume =   40 mL
Exhaled tidal volume = −30 mL
100 mL of tidal volume is lost through the pleural chest tube

It is not possible to measure tidal volume when the neonate is ventilated by any other means. In a case like this, it is only possible to make a qualitative judgment on pleural air leak. In other words, if air is seen to bubble out through the pleural drainage system, an air leak is present. When the air stops bubbling, the pleural tear has healed. See Chapter 18 for a complete discussion on pleural drainage systems.

4. Weaning from the ventilator

a. Recommend weaning from mechanical ventilation (Code: IIIG1g) [Difficulty: ELE: R, Ap; WRE: An]

As the neonate's condition improves, weaning must be considered. Indications of improvement include acceptable blood gas results, improved chest radiograph, and stable vital signs.

b. Initiate and modify weaning procedures (Code: IIID7 and IIIF2i12) [Difficulty: ELE: R, Ap; WRE: An]

Specific steps in increasing ventilator support were discussed earlier with each of the types of common pathologic conditions and the various modes of ventilation. In general, ventilator support should be reduced in the opposite manner that it was increased. Remember to evaluate the patient's arterial blood gas values and vital signs before and after making a change in the ventilator parameters. If the patient's condition deteriorates, the ventilator setting(s) should be placed as before. General steps in weaning ventilator support in a patient receiving traditional time-triggered, pressure-limited, time-cycled mechanical ventilation (TPTV) include the following:

1. Reduce the oxygen percentage in 2% to 5% steps down to 40% or less, while meeting the oxygenation goal (see Table 16-1).
2. Once the patient is receiving 40% or less oxygen, the PEEP level can be decreased in 1 to 2 cm water increments. The goal is a PEEP level of 3 to 4 cm water while meeting the oxygenation goal.
3. Next, peak inspiratory pressure (PIP) can be reduced in 1 to 2 cm water increments. The goal is a PIP of 15 to 18 cm water. The patient's arterial blood gas goals must be met (see Table 16-1).
4. The ventilator rate can now be reduced in steps of 1 to 5 breaths per minute. The patient's spontaneous breathing rate should increase as the ventilator rate is reduced.

The goal is a ventilator rate of less than 10/minute. Arterial blood gas goals must continue to be met.
5. Depending on the patient's tolerance of the above steps, the patient may be maintained on CPAP or given a spontaneous breathing trial.

5. Extubation

a. Recommend extubation (Code: IIIG1h) [Difficulty: ELE: R, Ap; WRE: An]

If the patient is stable with low pressure CPAP or a spontaneous breathing trial of 30 to 120 minutes, and the endotracheal tube is not needed for a suctioning route, the endotracheal tube can be removed.

b. Perform extubation (Code: IIIB9) [Difficulty: ELE: R, Ap; WRE: An]

The following additional steps are generally taken to ensure an appropriate, safe extubation:
1. Feedings should be withheld for several hours to reduce the risk of aspiration.
2. Perform an endotracheal tube "leak test" by delivering a mandatory breath and auscultating a leak at the neonate's larynx. An audible leak indicates the absence of laryngeal edema. If a leak cannot be heard, the neonate should be given a treatment of aerosolized racemic epinephrine to reduce the edema. Do not extubate a patient with laryngeal edema because it is likely that the endotracheal tube will need to be put back in.
3. Hyperoxygenate the neonate.
4. Suction the trachea and the oral pharynx.
5. Deliver a large tidal volume breath and remove the endotracheal tube when the lungs are full.
6. Suction the mouth as needed.
7. Provide supplemental oxygen by face mask or nasal cannula.
8. Follow-up arterial blood gases and frequent monitoring of vital signs and breath sounds should be done after extubation.
9. Be prepared to reintubate if the patient's condition deteriorates or a suctioning route is needed.

BIBLIOGRAPHY

AARC Clinical Practice Guideline: application of continuous positive airway pressure to neonates via nasal prongs or nasopharyngeal tube, *Respir Care* 39:817, 1994.

AARC Clinical Practice Guideline: application of continuous positive airway pressure to neonates via nasal prongs, nasopharyngeal tube, or nasal mask—2004 revision and update, *Respir Care* 49(9):1100, 2004.

AARC Clinical Practice Guideline: care of the circuit and its relation to ventilator-associated pneumonia. *Respir Care* 48:869, 2003.

AARC Clinical Practice Guideline: evidence-based guidelines for weaning and discontinuing ventilatory support. *Respir Care* 47:69, 2002.

AARC Clinical Practice Guideline: humidification during mechanical ventilation, *Respir Care* 37:887, 1992.

AARC Clinical Practice Guideline: neonatal time-triggered, pressure-limited, time-cycled, mechanical ventilation, *Respir Care* 39:808, 1994.

AARC Clinical Practice Guideline: patient-ventilator system checks, *Respir Care* 37:882, 1992.

AARC Clinical Practice Guideline: removal of the endotracheal tube—2007 revision & update. *Respir Care* 52:81, 2007.

AARC Clinical Practice Guideline: surfactant replacement therapy, *Respir Care* 39:824, 1994.

AARC Clinical Practice Guideline: ventilator circuit changes, *Respir Care* 39:797, 1994.

Aloan CA, Hill TV: *Respiratory care of the newborn and child*, ed 2, Philadelphia, 1997, JB Lippincott-Raven.

Avery ME, Tooley WH, Keller JB et al: Is chronic lung disease in low birth weight infants preventable? A survey of eight centers, *Pediatr* 79:26, 1987.

Barnhart SL, Czervinske MP: *Perinatal and pediatric respiratory care*, Philadelphia, 1995, WB Saunders.

Betit P, Thompson J: Neonatal and pediatric respiratory care. In: Wilkins RL, Stoller JK, Kacmarek RM, editors: *Egan's fundamentals of respiratory care*, ed 9, St Louis, 2009, Mosby.

Boros SJ, Matalon SV, Ewald R et al: The effect of independent variations in inspiratory-expiratory ratio and end expiratory pressure during mechanical ventilation in hyaline membrane disease: the significance of mean airway pressure, *J Pediatr* 91:794, 1977.

Branson RD, Hess DR, Chatburn RL: *Respiratory care equipment*, ed 2, Philadelphia, 1999, Lippincott Williams & Wilkins.

Burgess WR, Chernick V: *Respiratory therapy in newborn infants and children*, ed 2, New York, 1986, Thieme.

Cairo JM, Pilbeam SP: *Mosby's respiratory care equipment*, ed 8, St Louis, 2009, Mosby.

Carlo WA, Martin RJ: Principles of neonatal assisted ventilation, *Pediatr Clin North Am* 33:221, 1986.

Cavanagh K: High frequency ventilation of infants: an analysis of the literature, *Respir Care* 35:815, 1990.

Chang DW: *Clinical application of mechanical ventilation*, ed 2, Albany, NY, 2001, Delmar.

Chatburn RL: High frequency ventilation: a report on a state of the art symposium, *Respir Care* 29:839, 1984.

Chatburn RL: Principles and practice of neonatal and pediatric mechanical ventilation, *Respir Care* 36:569, 1991.

Chatburn RL, Lough MD: Mechanical ventilation. In: Lough MD, Doershuk CF, Stern RC, editors: *Pediatric respiratory therapy*, ed 3, St Louis, 1985, Mosby.

Chatburn RL, Waldemar AC, Lough MD: Clinical algorithm for pressure-limited ventilation of neonates with respiratory distress syndrome, *Respir Care* 28:1579, 1983.

Coghill CH et al: Neonatal and pediatric high-frequency ventilation: principles and practice, *Respir Care* 36:596, 1991.

Gagnon C, Simoes J: The management of the mechanically ventilated infant receiving pancuronium bromide (Pavulon), *Neonatal Network*, pp 20-24, Dec 1985.

Goldberg RN, Bancalari E: Bronchopulmonary dysplasia: clinical presentation and the role of mechanical ventilation, *Respir Care* 31:591, 1986.

Goldberg RN, Bancalari E: Therapeutic approaches to the infant with bronchopulmonary dysplasia, *Respir Care* 36:613, 1991.

Goldsmith JP, Karotkin EH: *Assisted ventilation of the neonate*, ed 2, Philadelphia, 1996, WB Saunders.

Hess DR, Kacmarek RM: *Essentials of mechanical ventilation*, New York, 1996, McGraw-Hill.

HIFI Study Group: High-frequency oscillatory ventilation compared with conventional mechanical ventilation in the treatment of respiratory failure in preterm infants, *N Engl J Med* 320:88, 1989.

Jobe A: Surfactant treatment for respiratory distress syndrome, *Respir Care* 31:467, 1986.

Koff PB, Eitzman DV, Neu J: *Neonatal and pediatric respiratory care*, ed 2, St Louis, 1993, Mosby.

MacIntyre NR, Branson RD: *Mechanical ventilation*, ed 2. Philadelphia, 2009, WB Saunders.

Milner AD, Hoskyns EW: High frequency positive pressure ventilation in neonates, *Arch Dis Child* 64:1, 1989.

Miyagawa CI: Sedation of the mechanically ventilated patient in the intensive care unit, *Respir Care* 32:792, 1987.

Nicks JJ, Becker MA: High-frequency ventilation of the newborn: past, present, and future, *Respir Ther* 4(4), 1991.

Pilbeam SP, Cairo JM: *Mechanical ventilation: physiological and clinical applications*, ed 4, St Louis, 2006, Mosby.

Schmidt JM: Nitric oxide therapy in neonates: adding to the arsenal, *Respir Ther* 7:37, 1994.

Smith I: The impact of surfactant on neonatal intensive care unit management, *Respir Ther* 4(4):22-26, 1991.

Spear ML, Spitzer AR, Fox WW: Hyperventilation therapy for persistent pulmonary hypertension of the newborn, *Neonatal Intensive Care: Perinatology/Neonatology* 9:27, 1985.

Tobin MJ: What should the clinician do when a patient "fights the ventilator"? *Respir Care* 36:395, 1991.

Whitaker K: *Comprehensive perinatal and pediatric respiratory care*, ed 3, Albany, NY, 2001, Delmar.

White GC: *Equipment theory for respiratory care*, ed 4, Albany, NY, 2005, Delmar.

SELF-STUDY QUESTIONS FOR THE ENTRY LEVEL EXAM   *See page 601 for answers*

1. The neonate less than 72 hours old with pulmonary problems should have its PaO_2 kept in the ____ range on the lowest possible inspired oxygen level.
   A. 40-45 torr
   B. 45-50 torr
   C. 60-70 torr
   D. 80-90 torr

2. If you observe that your patient has apnea spells leading to bradycardia, you should:
   A. Start CPAP.
   B. Start mechanical ventilation.
   C. Start an aerosolized bronchodilator.
   D. Give endotracheal surfactant.

3. An actively moving neonate is receiving 7 cm water CPAP by nasal prongs with 40% oxygen at a flow of 4 liters/minute. It is noticed that the CPAP pressure is variable between 4 and 7 cm water. What is the most likely cause of this?
   A. The patient is taking more shallow breaths.
   B. The patient's breathing rate has decreased.
   C. There is a leak when the neonate turns its head.
   D. Someone has accidentally changed the oxygen percentage.

4. You are taking care of a newborn who has aspirated meconium. You would recommend which of the following ventilator settings:
   A. I:E of 1:2
   B. I:E of 2:1
   C. I:E of 1:4
   D. I:E of 1:1

5. A premature neonate with a low Apgar score is demonstrating hypoxemia, intercostals retractions, and expiratory grunting noises. What is the best way to correct these problems?
   A. Nebulize albuterol.
   B. Suction the neonate.
   C. Instill surfactant into the airway.
   D. Give supplemental oxygen.

6. Your patient with pneumonia needs regular suctioning. You notice that her ventilator circuit has blood-streaked sputum in it. What should be done?
   A. Put in a heat-moisture exchanger.
   B. Change the circuit.
   C. Flush out the sputum with normal saline.
   D. Put in a closed airway suctioning system.

7. A 28-week gestational age neonate has the following arterial blood gas values while breathing 60% oxygen in an oxyhood: PaO_2 48 torr, $PaCO_2$ 45 torr, and pH 7.35. What should be done in this situation?
   A. Increase the oxygen to 70%.
   B. Begin mechanical ventilation.
   C. Intubate and begin CPAP at 4 cm water.
   D. Begin nasal CPAP at 4 cm water.

8. A hypoxic newborn has been diagnosed with PPHN and is receiving 80% oxygen. What should be recommended to improve its condition?
   A. Inhaled nitric oxide.
   B. Instill surfactant.
   C. Decrease the oxygen percentage to 70%.
   D. Inhaled 80/20 mix of heliox.

STUDY QUESTIONS FOR THE WRITTEN REGISTRY EXAM

See page 626 for answers

1. If CPAP is administered through an endotracheal tube, the child should be extubated when the CPAP pressure is:
   A. 0-2 cm water
   B. 2-4 cm water
   C. 4-6 cm water
   D. 6-8 cm water

2. The time to switch a patient from CPAP to mechanical ventilation is indicated by:
   1. CPAP of 8 to 10 cm water with a resulting PaO_2 of less than 50 torr
   2. F_IO_2 of 0.8 or more resulting in a PaO_2 of less than 50 torr
   3. $PaCO_2$ of greater than 60 torr
   A. 1
   B. 2
   C. 1, 2
   D. 1, 2, 3

3. Identify the rationale for the use of pressure limiting or "square wave ventilation" in a patient with RDS.
   1. It increases the $PaCO_2$.
   2. It limits the peak pressure.
   3. It decreases the PaO_2.
   4. It increases the patient's oxygenation.
   5. The tidal volume is held for a period of time.

   A. 1, 2, 3
   B. 1, 3
   C. 1, 2, 4
   D. 2, 4, 5

4. Hyperventilation is recommended in which of the following types of patients?
   A. Meconium aspiration
   B. PPHN
   C. RDS
   D. Infant with normal lung compliance

5. A neonate has meconium aspiration syndrome. Increasing the pressure limit on the ventilator increases the patient's risk of:
   A. ROP
   B. Oxygen toxicity
   C. Pneumothorax
   D. Tracheoesophageal fistula

6. Given the following choices, which would you select to increase the PaO_2 in a neonate with pneumonia who is supported on a standard pressure-limited type ventilator?
   1. Increase inspiratory time.
   2. Increase the pressure limit if it is reached.
   3. Decrease flow.
   4. Increase PEEP.
   5. Decrease the IMV rate.

A. 1, 5

B. 2, 3

C. 3, 4

D. 1, 2, 4

7. If you increase PEEP without increasing the pressure limit by the same amount, the patient's:

A. Minute volume will increase.

B. Tidal volume will decrease.

C. $PaCO_2$ will decrease.

D. Tidal volume will increase.

8. All of the following are indications for HFV EXCEPT:

A. Cleft palate before surgical correction

B. PPHN

C. RDS unresponsive to conventional ventilation

D. Mechanical ventilation patient with unresolved pneumothorax

9. High-frequency oscillatory ventilation is being used with a neonate with RDS. The following settings are in use: 50% oxygen, rate 700/minute, amplitude 10 cm water, and 4 cm water PEEP. The patient's $PaCO_2$ is 52 torr. What should be recommended to correct the carbon dioxide level?

A. Increase the amplitude.

B. Decrease the amplitude.

C. Increase the PEEP level.

D. Increase the inspiratory time.

10. A premature newborn is becoming progressively more hypoxic and tachypneic despite being in an oxyhood with 50% oxygen. The decision is made to begin CPAP. What initial pressure should the respiratory therapist recommend?

A. 0-2 cm water

B. 2-3 cm water

C. 4-5 cm water

D. 6-8 cm water

11. A neonate with PPHN is being mechanically ventilated and has responded favorably to 10 ppm of iNO and surgical correction of a patent ductus arteriosus. What should be done now?

A. Wean from the ventilator.

B. Initiate CPAP.

C. Decrease the inhaled nitric oxide to 5 ppm.

D. Discontinue the inhaled nitric oxide.

12. A patient with RDS has been receiving CPAP at 8 cm water and 60% oxygen. The following arterial blood gases are found: PaO_2 48 torr, $PaCO_2$ 58 torr, and pH 7.23. What should be done now?

A. Initiate volume cycled ventilation.

B. Increase CPAP to 10 cm water.

C. Increase the inspired oxygen to 70%.

D. Begin high-frequency ventilation.

17

Home Care and Pulmonary Rehabilitation

Note 1: This book is written to cover every item listed as testable on the *Entry Level Examination (ELE), Written Registry Examination (WRE),* and *Clinical Simulation Examination (CSE).*

The listed code for each item is taken from the National Board for Respiratory Care's (NBRC) **Summary Content Outline for CRT (Certified Respiratory Therapist) and Written RRT (Registered Respiratory Therapist) Examinations** (http://evolve.elsevier.com/Sills/resptherapist/). For example, if an item is testable on both the ELE and the WRE, it will simply be shown as: (Code: . . .). If an item is only testable on the ELE, it will be shown as: (ELE code: . . .). If an item is only testable on the WRE, it will be shown as: (WRE code: . . .).

Following each item's code will be the difficulty level of the questions on that item on the ELE and WRE. (See the Introduction for a full explanation of the three question difficulty levels.) **Recall [R]** level questions typically expect the exam taker to recall factual information. **Application [Ap]** level questions are harder because the exam taker may have to apply factual information to a clinical situation. **Analysis [An]** level questions are the most challenging because the exam taker may have to use critical thinking to evaluate patient data to make a clinical decision.

Note 2: A review of the most recent Entry Level Examinations (ELE) has shown an average of 3 questions (out of 140), or 2% of the exam, will cover Home Care and Pulmonary Rehabilitation. A review of the most recent Written Registry Examinations (WRE) has shown an average of 5 questions (out of 100), or 5% of the exam, will cover Home Care and Pulmonary Rehabilitation. The Clinical Simulation Examination is comprehensive and may include everything that should be known by an advanced level respiratory therapist.

MODULE A

Patient and family teaching

1. Assess a patient's learning needs (Code: 1B6) [Difficulty: ELE: R, Ap; WRE: An]

It is very important to determine what the patient understands about his or her cardiopulmonary condition and its treatment. If the patient is found to need additional teaching in some area, it should be incorporated into the respiratory care plan. See Chapter 1 for more discussion on teaching methods.

2. Explain the planned therapy and goals to a patient in understandable terms to achieve optimal therapeutic outcomes (Code: IIIA6) [Difficulty: ELE: R, Ap; WRE: An]

Determining the patient's ideal therapeutic goals is best done with a team approach. The patient's physician, nurse, and respiratory therapist should work together. The first consideration should be the patient's diagnosis. Next, determine whether the patient's condition is permanent, improving, or worsening. Objective information such as arterial blood gas results, pulmonary function testing results, chest radiographs, sputum production, and vital signs must be evaluated. The patient's physical capabilities must also be considered when establishing therapeutic goals. It is also important to evaluate the patient's mental state. Is the patient emotionally ready to be discharged home and learn about self-care or start a rehabilitation program? Each patient's therapeutic goals must be individualized. If the patient is not physically or emotionally ready to take care of himself or herself, the family or a paid care provider is needed.

The patient and family must understand the therapeutic goals and how they are to be achieved. Effective teaching methods include the following steps:

1. Speak at the patient's and family's level of understanding. Medical language usually reserved for peer discussions is not understandable to people without a medical background, yet using overly simple explanations can be insulting to someone who is intelligent or well educated, or both. In either case, the important information will not be perceived as intended. Give the patient written instructions as needed.
2. Frequently ask the patient and family whether they have any questions, and then answer them.
3. Have the patient and family explain back to you in their own words how they understand what you just described.
4. Have the patient and family demonstrate back to you all procedures and techniques.
5. Reteach anything that is misunderstood.

6. Retest the patient and family as needed.
7. Document in the patient's chart what has been instructed.

3. Counsel a patient and family concerning smoking cessation (Code: IIIK6) [Difficulty: ELE: R, Ap; WRE: An]

Absolute proof exists that smoking causes emphysema, chronic bronchitis, lung cancer, and heart disease. These conditions occur in the smoker who directly inhales the smoke as well as in the nonsmoking spouse and children who inhale secondhand smoke. Asthmatic patients often find that their bronchospasm is worsened when they inhale tobacco smoke. Obviously it is important that any patient with a smoking-related cardiopulmonary disease cease smoking. The patient's family must also stop smoking. Continued exposure to tobacco smoke harms the patient.

Because the nicotine found in tobacco is highly addictive, many patients find that they cannot stop smoking without having withdrawal symptoms such as agitation and craving for a cigarette. To aid in smoking cessation, it is often helpful to meet with a group of people who also are trying to stop. This group support helps the patient feel less alone in his or her efforts to stop smoking. The patient's physician also must be involved in this process.

If the patient has been unable to stop smoking because of withdrawal symptoms, it is likely that he or she is addicted to nicotine. A nicotine replacement system that allows gradual withdrawal greatly aids in smoking cessation. Although no smoking cessation plan works in every case, the highest percentage of patients are able to stop smoking if they have a combination of psychological support and a gradual reduction in nicotine intake.

Several well-established nicotine replacement and reduction systems currently exist. All are available without prescription. The Commit lozenge is held in the mouth to release a controlled amount of nicotine. Nicotine polacrilex (Nicorette) is a gum that is chewed by the patient to release a dose of nicotine. The Nicotrol Inhaler allows the user to inhale nicotine through a device shaped like a cigarette. Nicotine transdermal patches are another nicotine reduction system. ProStep, Nicoderm, and Habitrol are three brands of patches that, when placed onto the skin, allow a set amount of nicotine to be absorbed. With these systems, the patient starts with a relatively high dose of the drug and, over a period of weeks, transitions through a series of patches with less and less nicotine. It is critical that the patient not smoke while using one of these systems. Patients who continue to smoke run the risk of a nicotine overdose, which increases the risk of myocardial infarction.

Another option involves the patient taking a medication to change how the brain reacts to nicotine. Zyban (bupropion HCl) alters the brain's chemistry so that nicotine craving is reduced. It was originally found helpful in the care of patients with depression. Chantix (varenicline) is incorporated into the nicotine receptors of the brain. As a result, nicotine withdrawal cravings are reduced and if the patient "cheats" by smoking, there is no nicotine stimulating effect. Both medications require a physician's prescription.

Some patients experience problems with nicotine replacement and reduction systems. The transdermal patch can cause skin irritation. If this happens, the patch should be moved to another site. Some patients report insomnia or strange dreams while wearing a nicotine patch at night. Patients with this problem should remove the patch before sleeping.

Exam Hint 17-1 (WRE)

Most past examinations have included a question related to recommending a nicotine replacement system to a patient wishing to stop smoking or the possible side effects of the nicotine system.

4. Counsel a patient and family in health management (Code: IIIK4) [Difficulty: ELE: R, Ap; WRE: An]

The respiratory therapist should have a solid understanding of the pathophysiology of the commonly found cardiopulmonary and cardiovascular conditions. This includes, but is not limited to asthma, emphysema, chronic bronchitis, pneumonia, pulmonary fibrosis, cystic fibrosis, right and left heart failure, stroke, and neuromuscular diseases. Be prepared to teach the patient and family about the patient's disease, its cause, and its medical management.

MODULE B
Home respiratory care services

1. Interview the patient to determine the presence of dyspnea, sputum production, and exercise tolerance (Code: IB5c) [Difficulty: ELE R, Ap; WRE: An]

The following subject areas and questions can help the therapist to further determine the patient's exercise tolerance and activities of daily living:

a. Personal grooming

- Do you get short of breath when dressing?
- What is the most difficult part of dressing?
- Are you able to wash your hair regularly?
- (For men) Are you able to shave regularly?
- Does using extra O_2 help you to do these things without getting as short of breath?

b. In-home activities

- Can you go up and down stairs without getting short of breath?
- Can you walk through your home without getting short of breath?
- Can you cook and prepare nutritious meals?
- Does using extra O_2 help you do these things without getting as short of breath?

c. Out-of-home activities

- Can you go shopping without getting short of breath?
- What clubs, church, or other organizations do you attend regularly?
- Can you do yard or garden work?
- Do you have a pet dog that you walk through the neighborhood?
- Does using extra O_2 help you do these things without getting as short of breath?

See Chapter 1 for the discussion on interviewing a patient about sputum production. The patient with chronic and severe cardiopulmonary disease may describe a very restricted and limited lifestyle. Extra O_2 may have only limited benefit. The patient with chronic, but moderate, cardiopulmonary disease can live a somewhat limited but full lifestyle. Extra O_2 may help greatly at times when the patient becomes short of breath. The otherwise healthy patient with an acute cardiopulmonary disease should describe a previously full and enjoyable lifestyle. Extra O_2 may be needed now, but it is hoped that it will not be needed upon recovery.

2. Interview a patient to determine his or her social history (e.g., smoking, substance abuse) (Code: IB5e) [Difficulty: ELE: R; WRE: Ap]

The patient's family and social life is an important consideration in discharge planning with the patient and family. Whether the patient is an adult or a child, it is important to know about his or her home life. Probably no one knows more about the patient or cares more about his or her well-being than the immediate family. Very close friends can assist the family or even replace a nonexistent one. The following questions can be asked of an adult patient and family:

- Have you ever smoked? If yes, for how long? How many packs of cigarettes a day?
- Have you used illegal drugs? What have you used? For how long?
- Is your spouse able to help you at home?
- Do you have other family members who can help you at home?
- Can neighbors or family friends help you at home?
- Do you belong to any clubs or church? Can you get to them?

- Do you garden, have a pet, or do any hobbies at your home?

The following questions can be asked of the family of a minor child:

- Do both parents live at home? If not, with whom does the child live? Do both parents care for the child?
- Can any siblings help care for the child?
- Do you have other family members who can help you care for the child at home?
- Can neighbors or family friends help you care for the child at home?
- Does the child belong to any clubs or church? Can you get the child to them? Can they help you care for the child at home?
- Can you get the child to and from school?

The answers to these types of questions may lead you to think of other questions about the patient's family and social life. Consider the patient's disease or condition and the answers that are given to determine a discharge plan that minimizes any disturbances in family life.

The home environment is an important consideration in discharge planning with the patient and family. Barriers to the patient's mobility and complete recovery must be identified so that they can be eliminated or minimized. Ideally, the patient's home environment is determined by visiting the patient's home; however, the following questions also can be asked in the hospital:

- How many floors does your home have?
- Do you have to go up a set of stairs to get into your home?
- Is your bedroom on the main floor?
- If your bedroom is upstairs, can it be relocated to a room on the main floor?
- If your bedroom were relocated to the main floor, would it be easy for you to get to a bathroom and the kitchen?
- Does anyone who lives with you smoke?
- Is there anything else in or around your home that puts smoke or dust into the air?

The answers to these types of questions may lead to other questions about the patient's home environment. Consider the patient's disease or condition and the answers that are given to determine a discharge plan that minimizes any inconveniences or barriers.

3. Interview the patient to determine his or her nutritional status (ELE code: IB5d) [ELE difficulty: R]

Patients who have been ill for more than a few days should be suspected of suffering from malnutrition and/or dehydration to some degree. The longer they have been ill and not eating and drinking, the worse their condition will be. Ask the following questions of the patient or family:

- How long have you been sick?
- Were you able to eat and drink normally before you became sick?
- How long has it been since you were able to drink normally? Do you feel thirsty now?
- How long has it been since you were able to eat normally? Do you feel hungry now?
- Is it more difficult to cough out your secretions now than before you became sick?

4. Instruct the patient and family to assure safety and infection control (Code: IIIK7) [Difficulty: ELE: R, Ap; WRE: An]

Evaluate the following aspects of the patient's home environment:

- Does the patient live alone or have a spouse or companion to help provide care? Make sure that telephone numbers to relatives, helpful neighbors, the patient's physician, ambulance service, local hospital, pharmacy, and any other support services are posted by each telephone.
- Ensure that all respiratory care equipment is cleaned (see Chapter 2 for suggestions on methods of disinfection) and functioning properly.
- Check that home oxygen systems are working properly. If the patient has an oxygen concentrator, confirm that the filters are cleaned and that the alarms are set and working. Ensure that an oxygen cylinder, regulator, and oxygen delivery system are working properly as a backup system if the oxygen concentrator fails.
- Have the patient centrally locate all necessary items for daily living. The patient should avoid unnecessary stair climbing. It might be recommended that the patient convert the living room, if it is located near the kitchen and bathroom, into a bedroom. Clothing can be modified with Velcro fasteners, snaps, or zippers if the patient cannot use buttons easily. Shoes can be put on more easily with a long-handled shoehorn. Avoid shoes with laces. A long-handled comb or brush makes grooming easier.
- The kitchen should be modified so that all commonly used equipment is on the counter. Everyday dishes, utensils, and foods should be placed so that they can be easily reached in cabinets and drawers within an arm's reach. The patient should not have to bend over, stoop down, or climb onto a footstool to get anything that is needed.
- The bathroom may need handholds added to the walls by the toilet and shower or tub for extra security when using these facilities. A shower chair can be added so that the patient can sit while bathing. A handheld shower head might make bathing easier.
- Check the home for airborne irritants. Smoking by the patient or anyone else in the home must be stopped. The patient should avoid contact with other forms of indoor pollution such as aerosol sprays, paints, varnishes, and dust. A high-efficiency particulate air (HEPA) filtration system is best for removing indoor airborne pollutants and irritants. Indoor kerosene-fueled space heaters should not be used because they release carbon monoxide.
- The patient should avoid contact with any known allergens, people who smoke, or substances that have resulted in a bad reaction.

5. Home sleep apnea management

a. Perform overnight pulse oximetry (Code: IB9q) [Difficulty: ELE: R; WRE: Ap, An]

b. Interpret the results of overnight pulse oximetry (Code: IB10q) [Difficulty: ELE: R, Ap; WRE: An]

While it less expensive to perform overnight pulse oximetry in the home than polysomnography in the hospital, most patients who are suspected of having sleep-disordered breathing will be evaluated in the hospital. See the discussion on sleep-disordered breathing and overnight pulse oximetry in Chapter 18.

c. Initiate treatment for sleep disorders (e.g., CPAP) (WRE code: IIIK9) [WRE difficulty: Ap, An]

See Chapter 18 for the discussion on treatment for sleep disorders. CPAP systems are presented in Chapters 15 and 18.

6. Apnea monitoring

a. Initiate and adjust sleep apnea monitors (WRE code: IIIK2) [WRE difficulty: Ap]

b. Perform apnea monitoring (Code: IB9p) [Difficulty: ELE: R, Ap; WRE: An]

Apnea monitoring is indicated in an infant who has documented periods of apnea of prematurity resulting from an immature central nervous system. This condition is most commonly seen in infants younger than 35 weeks' gestational age. The usual monitoring guidelines include apneic periods that last longer than 20 seconds and are associated with bradycardia with a heart rate of less than 100 beats/min. Hypoxemia is often demonstrated by cyanosis, pallor, or documented desaturation through pulse oximetry. In addition, the infant may show marked limpness, choking, or gagging. Other conditions such as intracranial hemorrhage, patent ductus arteriosus, upper airway obstruction, hypermagnesemia, infection, and maternal narcotic agents, for example, should be ruled out before apnea of prematurity is confirmed. If this is the infant's problem, it is usually outgrown by the time the infant is 40 weeks' postconceptional age. Home apnea monitoring is not indicated in normal infants, in preterm infants without symptoms of apnea, or to test for sudden infant death syndrome (SIDS). See Box 17-1 for guidelines on starting and stopping home apnea monitoring.

Apnea monitors currently in use sense respiratory efforts through the changing electrical impedance measured through the chest wall as the infant breathes. Impedance is resistance to the flow of electricity through the skin and other organs. The monitor transmits a small, constant electrical current that results in a voltage across the two electrodes on the infant's chest. As the infant breathes and the chest wall expands and contracts, a resulting change in voltage occurs. This fluctuation is measured and interpreted as inhalation and exhalation. Similarly, smaller voltage changes are measured with each

heartbeat. This is measured and interpreted as the heart rate.

The following are desirable features on a home apnea monitor: (1) ability to store and display events for later analysis, (2) identification of breathing patterns and apnea periods, (3) identification of heart rate patterns, (4) estimation of tidal volume, and (5) identification of hypoxemia by pulse oximetry. Assembling a home apnea monitor involves placing the electrodes properly on the infant's chest, turning on the monitor, and setting the proper high and low limits for the alarms.

Two electrodes are usually placed where the greatest amount of movement occurs during breathing. Most often, this is on the infant's upper chest between the nipples and armpits (Figure 17-1). With older infants, the electrodes might have to be placed on the sides over the lower ribs. Occasionally one electrode is placed on the chest and the other on the infant's abdomen. Some monitoring systems require that a Velcro belt be placed around the infant over the electrodes to secure their positions. (Obviously this works only if both electrodes are on the chest.) Other systems employ electrodes with an adhesive. In either case, for best results, the infant's chest should be washed with mild soap and water and dried before the electrodes are placed. This results in the best electrical conduction. Do not use baby oils, lotions, or powders over the electrode sites. Attach the lead wires to the electrodes. These connect to the patient cable that is then connected to the monitor. Occasionally static electricity causes some interference with the signal. A third chest electrode is then added to act as a ground wire.

The monitor should be plugged into a working electrical outlet and turned on. Set the unit to charge the internal battery so that it can be made portable for later use. Confirm that the infant's respiratory and heart rates are being sensed and displayed. If pulse oximetry is a feature

---

BOX 17-1   Guidelines for Starting and Stopping Home Apnea Monitoring

INDICATIONS TO START HOME APNEA MONITORING

Infant has experienced one or more apparent life-threatening apnea events.

Infant is preterm and symptomatic of apnea.

Infant is a sibling of two or more SIDS victims.

Infant has central nervous system–based hypoventilation.

INDICATIONS TO STOP HOME APNEA MONITORING

Two to three months have passed without a significant number of alarms.

Two to three months have passed without an apnea episode.

Infant can tolerate stress of illnesses (e.g., nasopharyngitis) or immunizations (e.g., diphtheria-pertussis-tetanus [DPT]) without apnea episodes.

SIDS, Sudden infant death syndrome.

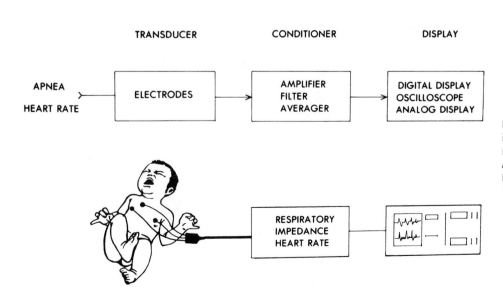

TRANSDUCER   CONDITIONER   DISPLAY

APNEA
HEART RATE → ELECTRODES → AMPLIFIER FILTER AVERAGER → DIGITAL DISPLAY OSCILLOSCOPE ANALOG DISPLAY

RESPIRATORY IMPEDANCE HEART RATE

Figure 17-1 Block diagram for impedance apnea and heart rate monitor. *(From Lough MD. In Lough MD, Williams TJ, Rawson JE, editors: Newborn respiratory care, St Louis, 1979, Mosby.)*

on the unit, the probe should be properly placed on the infant, and an SpO_2 value should be displayed. Set the high and low alarm values according to the physician's orders or established protocols. For example:

1. Set the apnea alarm to trigger after 20 seconds.
2. Set the low heart rate alarm to trigger if the heart rate is less than 100 beats/min.
3. If available, set the pulse oximeter alarm to trigger if the SpO_2 value decreases to less than 90%.
4. If available, set the high heart rate alarm to trigger if the heart rate is greater than 150 beats/min.

Multiple alarms provide for a greater margin of patient safety. They also indicate what physiologically deteriorates first in the infant. These backup alarm systems are important because the apnea monitor senses chest wall movement, not air movement. It is possible for the infant to have an upper airway obstruction and continue to make breathing attempts; therefore the apnea monitor will not alarm because the chest wall is moving. The bradycardia or desaturation alarms will signal that the infant is in trouble.

It is critically important that the parent(s) know(s) about the infant's medical condition. They need to understand how the monitor functions and what to do if the alarms sound. They should demonstrate their knowledge of the monitor's functions and be given written instructions about the monitor. The parents should not be more than 10 seconds away from the infant at any time, which means that the infant will not be apneic for more than 30 seconds (20-second alarm delay and 10 seconds for the parents to respond). The parents must know how to give tactile stimulation to the infant, use the manual resuscitator, call for emergency help, and perform infant cardiopulmonary resuscitation.

c. Interpret apnea monitoring results (Code: IB10p) [Difficulty: ELE: R, Ap; WRE: An]

Alarm situations fall into two basic categories: patient alarms and equipment alarms. Patient alarms mean that the infant either is apneic, has a heart rate below or above an acceptable level, or is desaturated. One, any two, or all three alarms may be triggered. Other than the audible alarm, a visual alarm flashes to show the problem(s), and the recording device keeps track of the events. The parents should be instructed first to care for the infant, and then, when the infant is back to normal, the alarms can be reset.

Three types of equipment alarms are found: electrode or lead problem, low battery, or monitor failure. The unit should have different visual and audible alarms for equipment failure so that the family does not mistakenly believe that the infant is in trouble. An electrode or lead problem alarm usually occurs because the electrode fell off of the infant or the lead became disconnected. The family should be taught how to fix these types of problems. A low battery

alarm indicates that time is limited for the monitor to function on battery power. The family should be instructed to plug the monitor into a functioning electrical outlet, and the unit should be set to recharge the battery. A monitor failure alarm indicates a serious internal problem with the monitor. It is not functioning properly and should not be used. The family should be instructed to observe the infant continuously and call the home care company for a replacement monitor.

Apnea monitors in current use record and store the alarm situations discussed previously. The information can usually be downloaded into a computer for a visual display of breathing and heart rate patterns, equipment problems, and the dates and times of their occurrences. The therapist or physician should review all these data to determine what kinds of problems the patient experienced.

7. Modify respiratory care procedures for use in the home (Code: IIIK8) [Difficulty: ELE: R, Ap; WRE: An]

8. Monitor and maintain all respiratory care equipment used in the home (ELE code: IIIK1) [ELE difficulty: R, Ap]

Home care equipment is essentially the same as that found in any hospital. The same types of equipment problems can occur in the patient's home as in the hospital. Those who wish to learn more about specific brands of home care equipment are referred to the several excellent books that discuss respiratory care equipment or the manufacturer's literature. Review, if necessary, the respiratory care procedures presented in this or other respiratory care books because they can be performed in the home care setting as well as in the hospital.

Exam Hint 17-2 (ELE)

Past examinations have included questions on the maintenance of O_2 concentrators for low-flow oxygen in the home and the use of backup sources of O_2 when an O_2 concentrator fails. In addition, questions have been asked about how to treat a home care patient whose nasal cannula has no flow. Telephone instructions include having the patient place the cannula under water to check for bubbling, tightening all tubing connections, confirming that gas is flowing from the O_2 concentrator, cleaning the concentrator's filters, replacing a defective cannula, and switching to an O_2 cylinder if the concentrator has malfunctioned.

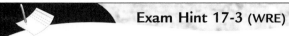

Exam Hint 17-3 (WRE)

Past examinations have included a question related to home respiratory care equipment. Examples include (1) recommendation of the use of an oxygen-conserving nasal cannula and oxygen concentrator for the economic delivery of low-flow oxygen; (2) recommendation of the maintenance of an oxygen concentrator (cleaning its filters) and the use of a backup source of oxygen (switching to an oxygen cylinder) when an oxygen concentrator fails; and (3) provision of telephone instructions to a home care patient whose nasal cannula has no flow. This includes having the patient place the cannula under water to check for bubbling, tightening all tubing connections, confirming that gas is flowing from the oxygen concentrator, or replacing a defective cannula.

MODULE C
Pulmonary rehabilitation

1. Interview the patient to determine the presence of dyspnea, sputum production, and exercise tolerance (Code: IB5c) [Difficulty: ELE: R, Ap; WRE: An]

The following subject areas and questions will help you to further determine the patient's exercise tolerance and activities of daily living (ADLs):

a. Personal grooming

- Do you get short of breath when dressing?
- What is the most difficult part of dressing?
- Are you able to wash your hair regularly?
- Are you (men) able to shave regularly?
- Does using extra oxygen help you to do these things without getting as short of breath?

b. In-home activities

- Can you go up and down stairs without getting short of breath?
- Can you walk through your home without getting short of breath?
- Can you cook or prepare nutritious meals?
- Does using extra oxygen help you to do these things without getting as short of breath?

c. Out-of-home activities

- Can you go shopping without getting short of breath?
- What clubs, church, and other organizations do you attend regularly?
- Can you do yard or garden work?
- Do you have a pet dog that you walk through the neighborhood?

- Does using extra oxygen help you to do these things without getting as short of breath?

If necessary, review the discussion on sputum production in Chapter 1. The patient with chronic and severe cardiopulmonary disease will describe a very restricted and limited lifestyle. Extra oxygen may have only a limited benefit. The patient with chronic, but moderate, cardiopulmonary disease is able to live a somewhat limited but full lifestyle. Extra oxygen may help greatly at times when the patient becomes short of breath. The otherwise healthy patient who has an acute cardiopulmonary disease should describe a previously full and enjoyable lifestyle. Extra oxygen may be needed now but not on recovery.

2. Timed walk test (e.g., 6-minute walk)

A timed walk test has become a widely used standard for measuring a patient's success in a pulmonary rehabilitation program. The usual timed walk test involves having the patient walk as far as possible in 6 minutes. An alternative is to have the patient walk as far as possible in 12 minutes. In either timed walk test, the distance covered is the key outcome measured.

a. Perform a 6-minute walk (Code: IB9h) [Difficulty: ELE: R; WRE: Ap, An]

A 6-minute walk procedure involves the therapist having a patient walk as far as possible in 6 minutes and noting the distance covered. (Or, the distance that can be covered in a 12-minute walk test.) A timed walk test is easy to perform, is generally well tolerated, and directly relates to pulmonary rehabilitation activities. See the discussion on stress testing in Chapter 18 for information on evaluating a patient before a walk test and contraindications to exercise testing that may apply to a patient performing a timed walk.

Ideally, repeated tests should be performed at the same time each day and at least 2 hours after a meal. Basic equipment for the walk test includes a straight hallway at least 100 feet long that is marked at intervals for distance, a stopwatch, and a pulse oximeter. Record the temperature in the hallway. Be aware of two outside factors that can alter a patient's performance. First, the so-called practice or learning effect can alter performance. The practice effect means that with repeated attempts, the patient will probably walk farther each time. Therefore the patient should perform at least two 6-minute timed walks that are measured and reported. The patient may rest for about 15 minutes between each walk test. Second, positive encouragement and feedback from the respiratory therapist can boost the patient's walking distance. Therefore when and how encouragement is given need to be standardized with all patients. See Box 17-2 for a recommended 6-minute walk protocol.

BOX 17-2 Suggested Protocol for a 6-Minute Timed Walk Test

1. *Pretest activities:* Have the patient take all normal preexercise medications, such as an inhaled bronchodilator. If the patient has been prescribed supplemental oxygen, such as a nasal cannula and portable oxygen system, it should be used during the test. Measure the patient's vital signs, pulse oximeter value, and peak flow value (if indicated). Have the patient rank his/her dyspnea (shortness of breath) on the 10-point Borg Scale.* Record this information.

2. Instruct the patient about the timed test, including: "The test involves you walking as far as you can, back and forth in this hallway, for 6 minutes. I'll be checking your oxygen level (with a pulse oximeter), asking you how you are doing, and encouraging you during your walk. If you need to rest you can; but, try to walk as far as possible. I'll periodically tell you how much time is left. When I tell you the test is finished, stand where you are. There will then be a 15 minute rest period. You will then repeat the test. If possible, after another 15-minute rest period, I would like you to repeat the test a third time." Ask the patient to repeat back to you the key points of the test so that you know he/she understands the procedure.

3. Place the patient at the starting point. Make sure that both you and the patient are ready to begin.

4. Tell the patient to start walking and start the stopwatch. During the first timed walk the respiratory therapist will keep pace with the patient to monitor the pulse oximeter value and evaluate the patient's overall appearance.

5. At 30-second intervals the therapist will offer the patient words of encouragement, such as the following: "You're doing fine." "Keep up the good work."

6. Tell the patient when 2 minutes and 4 minutes have lapsed. At 6 minutes, tell the patient to stop.

7. In general, stop the test at any time if the patient's pulse oximeter reading drops below 88% saturation or 4% below the starting value. (The physician may set specific criteria for stopping the test.) If ordered, supplemental oxygen may be started or increased to maintain the desired oxygen saturation.

8. Immediately after the test:
   a. Check the patient's vital signs and pulse oximeter value.
   b. Ask the patient to rate his/her dyspnea on the 10-point Borg Scale.
   c. Ask the patient what limited his/her walking distance, for example, shortness of breath, wheezing, leg or chest pain.

9. Document the test results. Make note of the above items. Record the walked distance. If the patient stopped to rest, note when it occurred and how long the patient needed to rest.

10. Tell the patient to rest for 15 minutes and the test will be repeated.

11. Repeat the above steps for the second 6-minute walk test. If possible, the test should be repeated a third time. NOTE: If the patient did not desaturate during the first timed walk, it may not be necessary for the respiratory therapist to accompany the patient and monitor pulse oximetry values during the second and third walks.

12. Forward all information to the physician for a formal interpretation.

---

*The 10-point Borg Scale allows the patient to assign a numeric value of 1 to 10 to his/her feeling of dyspnea. A large poster of the Borg Scale is placed so the patient can easily see it during the walk test. Before and after the test the patient is asked to rate his/her dyspnea. For example, a score of 1 indicates very slight dyspnea, 5 is severe dyspnea, and 10 is maximal dyspnea.

b. Interpret the results of a 6-minute walk (Code: IB10h) [Difficulty: ELE: R, Ap; WRE: An]

Research has shown that patients participating in a pulmonary rehabilitation program will usually show an increase in their timed walk distance. The following indicates that the patient is making progress:

- The patient has an increase in the 6-minute (or 12-minute) walk distance.
- The patient subjectively feels that he or she is doing as well as can be expected. The patient is motivated to try new things.
- Symptoms are reduced or at least under control.
- Cardiopulmonary function tests and blood gases show improvement. Even a slowing in the patient's former rapid rate of decline is a good sign.

The following indicate that the patient's health is deteriorating:

- The patient's 6-minute (or 12-minute) walk distance has decreased.
- He or she subjectively feels worse. The patient is afraid to try new things.
- Symptoms are worse. The patient feels dyspneic at less exertion than previously.
- The sputum has changed. It may be thick and harder to expectorate or have changed color to yellow or green. The patient may be expectorating more than before, or less if there is decreased movement of secretions.
- Cardiopulmonary function tests and blood gases are worse. The patient may need more supplemental oxygen, an increase in aerosolized bronchodilator medication, or other cardiopulmonary medications.

c. General considerations in a graded exercise program

NOTE: While the following information is not specifically listed as testable by the NBRC, past Written Registry Examinations have included questions pertaining to it.

The patient's physical condition must be evaluated before designing an exercise program. Besides chronic obstructive pulmonary disease (COPD), the patient may have other conditions that further limit his or her ability to safely participate in a rehabilitation program. See Box 17-3 for the suggested assessment parameters. If the patient is too ill or too limited in ability, he or she should not be placed into a rehabilitation program.

Although the patient's physical condition is the most important factor to evaluate from a safety point of view, other aspects of the patient's life also must be reviewed. These include a nutritional evaluation, a psychosocial evaluation, and a vocational evaluation. Because these areas are beyond the scope of practice of most respiratory therapists, the physician must refer the patient to other experts. In addition, any patient who is still smoking must be enrolled in a smoking cessation program.

Similar to preparing a patient for home care, all aspects of the patient's physical condition information must be evaluated. Each patient must have an individualized program and be physically and emotionally prepared to begin the rehabilitation program. As discussed next, the patient is placed into either an open- or a closed-end program format. The starting and ending points of the

---

BOX 17-3   Patient Evaluation before Starting a Pulmonary Rehabilitation Program

History
Complete physical examination
Chest radiograph
Resting diagnostic electrocardiogram
Complete blood count
Serum electrolytes
Urinalysis
Arterial blood gases
Theophylline level
Sputum analysis
Pulmonary function tests
  Spirometry
  Lung volume study
  Diffusion capacity
  Before and after bronchodilator study
Pulmonary stress test including
  Electrocardiogram
  Blood pressure
  Heart rate
  Respiratory rate
  Pulse oximetry
  Maximum ventilation
  Oxygen consumption
  Carbon dioxide production
  Respiratory quotient

See Chapter 4 for information on pulmonary function testing and Chapter 18 for information on cardiopulmonary stress testing.

---

program are determined based on the patient's physical condition, heart rate target, and stress test results.

A graded exercise program is an individually structured sequence of events that is designed to safely increase the patient's exercise tolerance. It is a critical component of any pulmonary rehabilitation program. In 1942 the Council of Rehabilitation defined rehabilitation as "the restoration of the individual to the fullest medical, mental, emotional, social, and vocational potential of which he/she is capable" (Hodgkin, 1993). In 1974 The American College of Chest Physicians' Committee on Pulmonary Rehabilitation adopted the following:

Pulmonary rehabilitation may be defined as an art of medical practice wherein an individually tailored, multidisciplinary program is formulated which through accurate diagnosis, therapy, emotional support, and education, stabilizes or reverses both the physio- and psychopathology of pulmonary diseases and attempts to return the patient to the highest possible functional capacity *[italics added] allowed by his pulmonary handicap and overall life situation (Petty, 1975).*

It further states: "In the broadest sense, pulmonary rehabilitation means providing good, comprehensive respiratory care for patients with pulmonary disease."

The patient with pulmonary disease who is inactive because of his or her condition experiences a slow deterioration in overall body function. It is well-known that physical activity is important for general health. Box 17-4 lists the effects of inactivity.

The remainder of this discussion focuses on how to start a patient in a graded exercise program and to monitor the patient's progress. (Note that the education of the patient about normal and abnormal lung function, respiratory care procedures, and medications, for example, is addressed in earlier sections of this book and in other textbooks dedicated solely to pulmonary rehabilitation.)

d. Benefits of an exercise program

The benefits of the exercise program must be stressed to the patient to gain his or her acceptance of it. If the patient does not believe that the program will make his or her life better, it will not be followed. In 1981 the American Thoracic Society Executive Committee adopted the following as principle objectives of pulmonary rehabilitation:

- To control and alleviate as much as possible the symptoms and pathologic complications of respiratory ailments
- To teach the patient how to achieve optimal capability for carrying out his or her ADLs

Most authors agree with the following general therapeutic goals:

- The primary goal is to increase the patient's functional ability as much as possible. This can best be accomplished by determining what the patient wants to be able to do with his or her life on a daily

---

BOX 17-4   Effects of Inactivity

METABOLISM

Decreased metabolic rate, decreased protein catabolism, negative nitrogen balance, decubitus ulcers, imbalance of cellular electrolyte levels, and gastrointestinal hypomotility

PSYCHOSOCIAL

Decreased learning ability, decreased motivation to learn, decreased retention of new material, decreased problem-solving ability, exaggerated or inappropriate emotional reactions, perceptual and motor changes, and increased somatic concerns

RESPIRATORY SYSTEM

Decreased movement of secretions, decreased use of respiratory muscles, and development of microatelectasis and infection

MUSCULAR SYSTEM

Loss of normal muscle tone, decreased muscle efficiency, increased local muscle oxygen consumption, rapid onset of fatigue, and contracture

CARDIOPULMONARY SYSTEM

Decreased cardiac output, venous stasis, thromboembolism, and pulmonary emboli

SKELETAL SYSTEM

Osteoporosis, reabsorption of calcium from the bone, and increased incidence of compression fractures

---

From May DF: *Rehabilitation and continuity of care in pulmonary disease,* St Louis, 1991, Mosby.

basis. From this list of ADLs, a series of short- and long-term goals can be developed. One of the primary short-term goals should be that the patient feels better. He or she should be able to control or reduce any symptoms. This alone improves the patient's quality of life. Make sure that the patient's goals are realistic and can be reached. The family must be involved with any major decision making. Often it is helpful to break a large goal down into several smaller tasks so that the patient and family receive frequent positive feedback.

- Improve the patient's self-image. This should occur after the first goal is reached. The patient should experience less anxiety and depression and also feel better about himself or herself.
- Increase the patient's ability to exercise. This may depend on the level of the patient's disability. In general, the worse the patient's lung disease, the less able the patient is to increase his or her exercise level.
- Decrease the frequency and length of any hospitalizations.
- Prolong the patient's life by the proper use of oxygen and other respiratory care modalities.

Note that the benefits did not list an improvement in the patient's cardiopulmonary condition. Numerous studies have documented that pathologic changes seen in COPD do not improve despite the patient being in a rehabilitation program. It is important that the therapist correct any misunderstanding of this.

Exam Hint 17-4 (WRE)

Past examinations have included one or two questions related to identifying the goals or benefits, or both, of a pulmonary rehabilitation program.

---

e. Individualized graded exercise program

The program format and features may vary considerably. Minimally, the patient's physician should specify four parts to the exercise prescription: mode, intensity, duration, and frequency. The following program formats and suggestions are typical of what might be ordered.

f. Program format

There are two basic types of formats. Each has its own advantages and disadvantages depending on the limitations and preferences of the patient. The open-end format allows the patient to enter and progress through the program at his or her own pace. Because each patient's goals are individualized, the time of their accomplishment is relatively unimportant as long as progress is being made. The program facilitator (often a respiratory therapist) acts as a coordinator. This may include ensuring that educational materials are available for the patient, exercise equipment is available, and the patient's questions are answered. The patient may stay in the program until the last goal is achieved. The advantages of this program are that it is self-directed and can be adjusted if the patient has a schedule conflict. The disadvantage of this program is that no group support or involvement with other people who have COPD is included.

The closed-end format involves the program facilitator setting up a formal schedule of educational topics and exercise sessions. These group events commonly last from 1 to 3 hours and may occur from one to three times per week. The whole program can vary in length from 8 to 16 weeks, depending on the content. These events are attended by a group of patients who share a common problem and have common goals to address. One major advantage of this program is that most patients do better when they have peers to ask for emotional support. The facilitator will probably find that it is easier to schedule speakers when a established time frame can be set. The disadvantages of this program relate to the loss of individual goals and attention. If a patient misses a session, he or she will have to wait for the topic to be repeated at the next program. If the group is too large, the facilitator may not have time to help a patient with an individual goal.

g. Strength training

Many patients are so weak from years of relative inactivity that they must regain muscle strength before pursuing increased endurance. The specific muscle groups that need strengthening can be determined by physical examination. In general, the large muscle groups of the legs and arms and inspiratory muscles must be strengthened.

Before beginning strength training, the patient must perform calisthenics for about 10 minutes as a "warm-up." It is important to stretch the muscles and joints and increase circulation before starting more vigorous activity. See Figure 17-2, groups 1 to 7, for a series of progressively more demanding calisthenic exercises. All patients should at least be able to perform the calisthenics shown in groups 1 and 2 for a warm-up. The patient must focus on breath control (pursed-lip breathing) during the warm-up period to avoid dyspnea.

Arm and leg strengthening can be done in a variety of ways for about 10 minutes. Typically, a 1- or 2-lb weight is used. Barbell weights can be held as the arms are moved to the back, front, sides, and overhead to strengthen the arms, shoulders, and chest and back muscles. Ankle weights can be worn. The legs are then moved to the back, front, and sides; the legs can be lifted with the knees bent; or the initial calisthenics can be repeated with added weight. The abdominal muscles can be strengthened by having the patient lie on his or her back and placing a 2-lb weight on the abdomen. The patient then concentrates on maintaining breath control against the added weight.

Inspiratory muscle strengthening is done in two ways. First, the patient is told to take in a deep sigh and hold it for a brief time. This both stretches the rib cage and increases the workload of the primary and secondary inspiratory muscles. The deep sigh should be repeated several times. Second, the patient uses a specific inspiratory muscle training device. The PFLEX device is popular because it is inexpensive and can be gradually adjusted to increase the workload as the patient improves. Review the discussion in Chapter 7 and see Figure 7-1.

Finally, the patient should spend about 10 minutes in "cool-down" activities. This may involve more light calisthenics or slow walking. The cool-down period allows the body to return to a slower metabolic rate while still maintaining good circulation to the arms and legs. This helps to eliminate any lactic acid that might have accumulated in the muscles during the more vigorous exercise. Increased lactic acid may cause some muscle aches after exercise. Inform the patient that some muscle soreness may be felt the next day. It can be relieved by taking an antiinflammatory medication such as aspirin if the physician approves.

BOX 17-5 Guidelines for Strength and Endurance Training

STRENGTH TRAINING

This involves a low number of repetitions of a high-intensity activity, such as lifting weights.

A warm-up period involving calisthenics should be carried out for about 10 min.

The following strengthening program should last about 10 min:

Three sets of 10 to 15 repetitions of an activity should be performed.

Each set is followed by a rest period of a few minutes.

The patient should work at 85% to 90% of the maximum capacity of the muscles being exercised.

Follow with a cool-down period involving calisthenics for about 10 min.

The patient should exercise every other day (for example, Monday, Wednesday, and Thursday).

This program may precede or be done simultaneously with an endurance program.

It takes 4 to 8 weeks for improved strength to be realized.

ENDURANCE TRAINING

This involves a high number of repetitions of a relatively low-intensity activity, such as walking.

A warm-up period involving calisthenics should be carried out for about 10 min.

The patient should do the following:

Exercise continuously for about 20 to 30 min.

Exercise at a level that results in the target heart rate being maintained.

Follow with a cool-down period involving calisthenics for about 10 min.

The patient should exercise every other day (for example, Tuesday, Thursday, and Saturday).

This program may follow or be done simultaneously with a strength program.

It takes 4 to 8 weeks for improved endurance to be realized.

Modified from May DF: *Rehabilitation and continuity of care in pulmonary disease*, St Louis, 1991, Mosby.

See Box 17-5 for specific guidelines for a strength training program.

It is helpful, but not necessary, for the patient to have access to professional body building equipment found in many gymnasiums. In addition, a physical therapist is helpful in designing a training program.

h. Endurance training

Endurance training is designed to improve the patient's stamina to perform essential ADLs. It accomplishes this by improving the functioning of the patient's cardiopulmonary and cardiovascular systems. When these systems perform better, they can meet the patient's need for

Group 1 Exercises

Figure 17-2   Modified calisthenic exercises. In all groups, the figure to the left is the starting point. The figures to the right show the sequence of steps in the exercise. The patient can adjust the pace of exercises to either increase or decrease the energy that is expended. In general, most patients choose 10 to 15 repetitions per minute. Exercises shown in groups 1 and 2 are useful during the warm-up period of either a strength or an endurance program. Exercises shown in groups 3 and 4 are more demanding and can be used for muscle reconditioning by many patients in an endurance program. The most demanding exercises are those shown in groups 5, 6, and 7. Patients with only moderate disability may be able to progress to this level for further muscle conditioning. *(From May DF:* Rehabilitation and continuity of care in pulmonary disease, *St Louis, 1991, Mosby.)*

increased oxygen delivery to and carbon dioxide removal from exercising muscles.

Endurance training must be preceded by the patient performing calisthenics for about 10 minutes as a warm-up. Just as in strength training, it is important to stretch the muscles and joints and increase circulation before starting more vigorous activity. See Figure 17-2, groups 1 through 7, for a series of progressively more demanding calisthenic exercises. All patients should be able to at least perform the calisthenics shown in groups 1 and 2 for a warm-up.

Patients who can perform the activities shown in groups 3 and 4 gain some endurance training as well. Some very debilitated patients may not be able to perform at this higher level. Some less debilitated patients will eventually be able to advance to the highest levels. The patient must focus on breath control (pursed-lip breathing) during the warm-up period to avoid dyspnea.

The actual endurance exercise that is selected must meet the patient's needs. He or she can walk, use a treadmill, ride a bicycle ergometer, swim, or do a combination of these. The method that is selected must be both practi-

Group 2 Exercises

Figure 17-2, cont'd

cal and fun for the patient. For this reason, walking is usually the main activity; however, the upper body should not be ignored. An arm ergometer, rowing machine, or barbell weights can be used for upper-body endurance.

A key concept of the endurance program is that the patient must exercise at a level great enough to increase the heart rate to a predetermined level. The increased heart rate (HR) reflects the increased metabolic rate and work being performed by the patient. The target heart rate must be maintained for 20 to 30 minutes to have any muscle training effect. Exercising at a lower heart (and metabolic) rate is not as beneficial. Exercising at a higher heart rate may be dangerous to the patient. Karvonen's formula is used to determine the target heart rate for endurance training:

Target heart rate (HR) = (% intensity [maximum HR − resting HR]) + resting HR

In which:

Target HR = the target HR for the exercise period
% intensity = 60% to 80%

Maximum HR = maximum HR determined by either of the following formulas:

   a. Maximum HR = 220 − age of the patient

   b. Maximum HR = 210 − (age of the patient × 0.65)

   Resting HR = the patient's resting HR

EXAMPLE

Determine the target HR for a 50-year-old patient (of either gender) who is enrolled in an endurance training program. The patient has a resting HR of 80 beats/min.

Group 3 Exercises

Figure 17-2, cont'd

The patient's maximum heart rate is 170 (220 − 50 for the patient's age = 170).

$$\text{Target HR} = (\% \text{ intensity}[\text{maximum HR} - \text{resting HR}]) + \text{resting HR}$$

$$
\begin{aligned}
\text{Lowest target HR} &= (0.60[170-80])+80 \\
&= (0.60[90])+80 \\
&= (54)+80 \\
&= 134 \text{ beats/min}
\end{aligned}
$$

$$
\begin{aligned}
\text{Highest target HR} &= (0.80[170-80])+80 \\
&= (0.80[90])+80 \\
&= (72)+80 \\
&= 152 \text{ beats/min}
\end{aligned}
$$

The range of target HRs for this patient is 134 to 152 beats/min. The patient must monitor his or her HR during the exercise period to make sure that it stays within this range. This is most easily accomplished by feeling the radial or carotid pulse and counting heartbeats for a 15-second period, and then multiplying by 4 to find the HR for 1 minute.

Finally, as in strength training, the patient should spend about 10 minutes in "cool-down" activities. This may involve light calisthenics or slow walking. As discussed earlier, the cool-down period allows the body to return to a slower metabolic rate while still maintaining good circulation to the arms and legs. This helps to eliminate any lactic acid that may have built up in the muscles during the endurance exercise. See Box 17-5 for specific guidelines for an endurance training program.

Group 4 Exercises

Figure 17-2, cont'd

MODULE D

Respiratory care plan

1. Analyze available information to determine the patient's pathophysiologic state (Code: IIIH1) [Difficulty: ELE: R, Ap; WRE: An]

The respiratory therapist should have a solid understanding of the pathophysiology of commonly found cardiopulmonary and cardiovascular conditions. These include, but are not limited to, asthma, emphysema, chronic bronchitis, pneumonia, pulmonary fibrosis, cystic fibrosis, right and left heart failure, stroke, and neuromuscular disease. The scope of this text prevents a full discussion of these conditions; the reader is referred to the many excellent pathology textbooks that are available.

In addition, review the information presented in Chapters 1, 3, 4, and 5. These chapters discuss bedside patient assessment, blood gas interpretation, pulmonary function

Group 5 Exercises

Figure 17-2, cont'd

testing, and hemodynamic monitoring that the NBRC has determined to be testable on the Entry Level Examination and Written Registry Examination. Be prepared to evaluate areas such as vital signs, breath sounds, blood gas values, pulmonary function results, and cardiac study results to determine the patient's condition.

a. Determine the appropriateness of the prescribed therapy and goals for the patient's pathophysiologic state (Code: IIIH3) [Difficulty: ELE: R, Ap; WRE: An]

The patient's physical condition must be evaluated before a home care or rehabilitation program is designed. Besides the patient's primary cardiopulmonary diagnosis, the patient may have other conditions that further limit his or her ability to safely participate. For example, diabetes and kidney failure are common maladies seen in patients with lung or heart disease. If the patient is too ill or too limited in ability, he or she should not be placed into a home care or rehabilitation program.

b. Review the planned therapy to establish the therapeutic plan (Code: IIIH2a) [Difficulty: ELE: R, Ap; WRE: An]

Determination of the patient's ideal therapeutic goals is best accomplished with a team approach. The patient's physician, nurse, and respiratory therapist should work together. The first consideration should be the patient's diagnosis. Then, it should be determined whether the patient's condition is permanent, improving, or worsening. Objective information such as arterial blood gas results, pulmonary function testing results, chest x-ray

Group 6 Exercises

Figure 17-2, cont'd

film findings, sputum production, and vital signs must be evaluated. The patient's physical capabilities should be considered when establishing therapeutic goals. The therapist must also evaluate the patient's mental state. Is the patient emotionally prepared to return home and be taught about self-care or start a rehabilitation program? The therapeutic goals for each patient must be individualized. If the patient is not physically or emotionally ready to take care of himself or herself, the family or a paid care provider is needed. Following are common therapeutic goals:

- The primary goal is to improve the patient's functional ability as much as possible. This can best be accomplished by determining the patient's life goals. From this, a list of attainable short- and long-term goals can be developed. One of the primary short-term goals should be that the patient feels better. He or she should be able to control or reduce any symptoms. Make sure that the patient's goals are realistic and can be reached. The family needs to be involved with any major decision making. Often, it is helpful to break a large goal down into several smaller tasks. In this way, the patient and family receive frequent positive feedback.
- Improve the patient's self-image. This should follow when the first goal is reached.
- Enhance the patient's ability to exercise. How this is approached may depend on the level of the patient's disability. In general, the worse the patient's lung disease, the less able the patient is to increase his or her exercise level.
- Decrease the frequency and length of any hospitalizations.

Group 7 Exercises

Figure 17-2, cont'd

- Prolong the patient's life through the proper use of O_2 and other respiratory care modalities.

c. Recommend changes in the therapeutic plan when indicated (Code: IIIH4) [Difficulty: ELE: R, Ap; WRE: An]

Be prepared to evaluate the patient's condition and make suggestions for changing goals and methods. The thera-pist must have a thorough understanding of the patient's condition and individual goals to evaluate the progress. Objectively consider the patient's physical, emotional, and social condition. The therapist must also listen to the patient's subjective opinion about his or her situation. Be prepared to make recommendations to the patient and attending physician for modifying the goals according to the patient's changing condition.

The following signs indicate that the patient is stable or making progress:

- The patient subjectively feels that he or she is doing as well as can be expected. The patient is motivated to try new things.
- Symptoms are reduced or at least under control.
- Cardiopulmonary function tests and blood gases show improvement. Even a slowing in the patient's formerly rapid rate of decline is a good sign.
- The patient reports an increase in the distance that can be walked at his or her own pace.
- The patient has an increase in the 6- or 12-min walking distance.

The following indicate that the patient's health is deteriorating:

- He or she subjectively feels worse. The patient is afraid to try new things.
- Symptoms are worse. The patient feels dyspnea at less exertion than before.
- The sputum has changed. It could be thick and harder to expectorate or could have changed color to yellow or green. The patient may be expectorating more than before, or less if there is decreased movement of secretions.
- Cardiopulmonary function tests and blood gases are worse. The patient may need increased O_2, more aerosolized bronchodilator, or other cardiopulmonary medications.
- The patient cannot walk or perform as much work as before without worsening of symptoms.

d. Educate the patient and family in health management (Code: IIIK4) [Difficulty: ELE: R, Ap; WRE: An]

Effective teaching methods include the following:

- Speak at the patient's and family's levels of understanding. Medical language usually reserved for peer discussions is not typically understood by people without a medical background. However, use of overly simple explanations can be insulting to someone who is intelligent or well educated. In either case, the important information is not received as intended. Give the patient written instructions as needed.
- Frequently ask the patient and family whether they have any questions; then answer them.
- Have the patient and family repeat in their own words what they were just told to ensure understanding.
- Have the patient and family demonstrate all procedures and techniques.
- Reteach anything that is misunderstood.
- Retest the patient and family as needed.
- Document in the patient's chart what has been taught.

The therapist should be able to implement a patient's health management program. For example, the patient may have a home care program to manage emphysema, asthma, cystic fibrosis, or congestive heart failure. In addition, the therapist should monitor the patient's compliance with the program. For example, is the patient faithfully following the smoking cessation program, or has he or she "cheated"? Is the patient following the asthma control program by monitoring his or her peak flow and adjusting inhaled medications according to the physician's order?

e. Terminate the treatment or procedure based on the patient's response to therapy (Code: IIIF1) [Difficulty: ELE: R, Ap; WRE: An]

The respiratory therapist should know the complications and hazards of any patient care activity that is performed. These were discussed in the previous chapters. Be prepared to stop the treatment or procedure if the patient has an adverse reaction to it. Additionally, be prepared to recommend to the physician that the treatment or procedure be discontinued if it is likely to result in additional adverse reactions.

f. Recommend discontinuing the treatment or procedure based on the patient's response to therapy (Code: IIIG1i) [Difficulty: ELE: R, Ap; WRE: An]

Be prepared to recommend that a treatment or procedure be discontinued. See the previous chapters for discussion on when respiratory care procedures should be discontinued.

2. Develop the home care and pulmonary rehabilitation protocols (Code: IIIH6b) [Difficulty: ELE: R; WRE: Ap, An]

3. Apply the home care and pulmonary rehabilitation protocols (Code: IIIH8) [Difficulty: ELE: R, Ap; WRE: Ap]

4. Monitor the outcomes of home care and pulmonary rehabilitation protocols (Code: IIIH7b) [Difficulty: ELE: R, Ap; WRE: An]

Respiratory care protocols may be used at home as well as in the hospital. An oxygen therapy protocol can be implemented that uses the patient's pulse oximetry values to adjust the oxygen percentage or flow up or down. For example, keep the patient's SpO_2 less than 95% but greater than 85%. A second protocol may be using inhaled sympathomimetic bronchodilators based on the patient's peak flow results.

The patient's physical condition must be evaluated before designing a home care or rehabilitation program. Besides the primary diagnosis, the patient may have other conditions that further limit his or her ability to participate safely. If the patient is too ill or too limited in ability, he or she should not be placed into a home care or rehabilitation program.

Although the patient's physical condition is the most important factor to evaluate from a safety point of view, other aspects of his or her life also must be reviewed. These include a nutritional evaluation, a psychosocial evaluation, and a vocational evaluation. Because these areas are beyond the scope of practice of most respiratory therapists, the physician must refer the patient to other experts.

Be prepared to evaluate the patient's condition and make suggestions for changing goals or methods, for example. The therapist must have a thorough understanding of the patient's condition and individual goals to evaluate his or her progress toward meeting them. Objectively consider the patient's physical, emotional, and social condition. The therapist also must listen to the patient's subjective opinion about his or her situation. Be prepared to make recommendations to the patient and attending physician for modifying the goals depending on the patient's changing condition.

5. Record and evaluate the patient's response to the treatment(s) or procedure(s), including the following:

a. **Record and interpret the following: heart rate and rhythm, respiratory rate, blood pressure, body temperature, and pain level (Code: IIIA1b4) [Difficulty: ELE: R, Ap; WRE: An]**

b. **Record and interpret the patient's breath sounds (Code: IIIAb3) [Difficulty: ELE: R, Ap; WRE: An]**

c. **Record and interpret the type of cough the patient has and the nature of the sputum (Code: IIIAb3) [Difficulty: ELE: R, Ap; WRE: An]**

d. **Recheck any math work and make note of incorrect data (Code: IIIA1b2) [Difficulty: ELE: R, Ap; WRE: An]**

Review the previous chapters for relevant information on assessment as needed.

6. Communicate information

a. **Communicate information regarding the patient's clinical status to appropriate members of the health care team (Code: IIIA2a) [Difficulty: ELE: R, Ap; WRE: An]**

b. **Communicate information relevant to coordinating patient care and discharge planning (Code: IIIA2a) [Difficulty: ELE: R, Ap; WRE: An]**

c. **Interact with a case manager (Code: IIIK5) [Difficulty: ELE: R, Ap; WRE: An]**

Before the patient is discharged, it is vital that there be effective coordination between the hospital and the home care company. Typically, the discharge plan would include the following:

- Patient evaluation that determines the patient is ready for discharge. The patient needs to have recovered sufficiently to leave the hospital.
- Determination of the best place for the patient to go for further recovery and the necessary patient care resources. It must be determined whether the patient can go home or should be transferred to an extended care facility. If the patient is to be discharged home, it must be determined whether the family can provide the necessary care. If not, home care respiratory therapists and nurses will have to be scheduled for home visits.
- Determination that the patient's financial resources are adequate. If not, social services will have to be contacted to work with the patient's insurance company or other financial support agencies.

d. **Communicate the results of therapy and alter the therapy by protocol(s) (Code: IIIA5) [Difficulty: ELE: R, Ap; WRE: An]**

The home care respiratory therapist must be able to alter care based on the patient's respiratory care protocols. Inform the patient's nurse or physician and the supervising therapist if any serious questions or problems occur with the patient. Routine communication should occur as needed between home care and hospital caregivers.

BIBLIOGRAPHY

American Association for Respiratory Care: Clinical Practice Guideline: Oxygen therapy in the home or alternate site health care facility—2007 revision & update, *Respir Care* 52:1063, 2007.

American Association for Respiratory Care: Clinical Practice Guideline: Discharge planning for the respiratory care patient, *Respir Care* 40:1308, 1995.

American Association for Respiratory Care: Clinical Practice Guideline: Long-term invasive ventilation in the home, *Respir Care* 40:1313, 1995.

American Association for Respiratory Care: Clinical Practice Guideline: Providing patient and caregiver training, *Respir Care* 41:658, 1996.

American Association for Respiratory Care: Clinical practice guideline: Pulmonary rehabilitation, *Respir Care* 47(5):617, 2002.

American Association for Respiratory Care: Clinical Practice Guideline: Suctioning the patient in the home, *Respir Care* 44:99, 1999.

American Association for Respiratory Care: Clinical Practice Guideline: Exercise testing for evaluation of hypoxemia and/or desaturation: 2001 revision & update, *Respir Care* 44:514, 2001.

Bell CW, Blodgett D, Goike C, et al: *Home care and rehabilitation in respiratory medicine,* Philadelphia, 1984, Lippincott.

Belman MJ, Wasserman K: Exercise training and testing in patients with chronic obstructive pulmonary disease, *Basics Respir Dis* 10(2):1-6, 1981.

Branson RD, Hess DR, Chatburn RL: *Respiratory care equipment,* ed 2, Philadelphia, 1999, Lippincott Williams & Wilkins.

Cairo JM, Pilbeam, SP: *Mosby's respiratory care equipment,* ed 8, St Louis, 2009, Mosby.

Christopher KL: At-home administration of oxygen. In Kacmarek RM, Stoller JK, editors: *Current respiratory care,* Toronto, 1988, BC Decker.

Connors G, Hilling L, editors: *American Association of Cardiovascular and Pulmonary Rehabilitation: guidelines for pulmonary rehabilitation programs,* Champaign, Ill, 1993, Human Kinetics.

Des Jardins T, Burton GG: Clinical manifestations and assessment of respiratory disease, ed 5, St Louis, 2006, Mosby.

Edge RS: Infection control. In Barnes TA, editor: *Respiratory care practice,* St Louis, 1988, Mosby.

Eubanks DH, Bone RC: *Comprehensive respiratory care,* ed 2, St Louis, 1990, Mosby.

Farzan S, Farzan D: *A concise handbook of respiratory disease,* ed 4, Stamford, Conn, 1997, Appleton & Lange.

Gardner DD and Wilkins RL: Patient education and health promotion. In Scanlan CL, Wilkins RL, Kacmarek Rm, editors: *Egan's fundamentals of respiratory care,* ed 9, St Louis, 2009, Mosby.

Gilmartin M: Transition from the intensive care unit to home: patient selection and discharge planning, *Respir Care* 39:456, 1994.

Gourley DA: Respiratory home care. In Wyka KA, Mathews PJ, Clark WF, editors: *Foundations of respiratory care,* Albany, NY, 2002, Delmar.

Heuer AJ and Scanlan CL: Respiratory care in alternative sites. In Scanlan CL, Wilkins RL, Kacmarek RM, editors: *Egan's fundamentals of respiratory care,* ed 9, St Louis, 2009, Mosby.

Hodgkin JE: Home care and pulmonary rehabilitation. In Kacmarek RM, Stoller JK, editors: *Current respiratory care,* Toronto, 1988, BC Decker.

Hodgkin JE, Celli BR, Connors GL: *Pulmonary rehabilitation: guides to success,* ed 3, Philadelphia, 2000, Lippincott Williams & Wilkins.

Hodgkin JE, Connors GA: Pulmonary rehabilitation. In Burton GG, Hodgkin JE, Ward JJ, editors: *Respiratory care: a guide to clinical practice,* ed 4, Philadelphia, 1997, Lippincott, Williams and Wilkins.

Holden DA, Stelmach KD, Curtis PS, et al: The impact of a rehabilitation program on functional status of patients with chronic lung disease, *Respir Care* 35:332, 1990.

Jones PW: Measurement of breathlessness. In Hughes JMB and Pride NB, editors: *Lung function tests: physiological principles and clinical applications,* London, 2000, W. B. Saunders.

Kwiatkowski CA, Tougher-Decker R, O'Sullivan-Maillet J: Nutritional aspects of health and disease. In Scanlan CL, Wilkins RL, Stoller JK, editors: *Egan's fundamentals of respiratory care,* ed 7, St Louis, 1999, Mosby.

Lewis ML, Hagarty EM, Lawlor B: Home respiratory care. In Fink JB, Hunt GE, editors: *Clinical practice in respiratory care,* Philadelphia, 1999, Lippincott Williams & Wilkins.

Lucas J, Golish JA, Sleeper G, et al: *Home respiratory care,* Norwalk, Conn, 1988, Appleton & Lange.

MacIntyre NR: Pulmonary rehabilitation. In Hess DR, MacIntyre NR, Mishoe SC, et al, editors: *Respiratory care principles and practices,* Philadelphia, 2002, WB Saunders.

May DF: *Rehabilitation and continuity of care in pulmonary disease,* St Louis, 1991, Mosby.

McInturff SL, O'Donohue WJ Jr: Respiratory care in the home and alternate sites. In Burton GG, Hodgkin JE, Ward JJ, editors: *Respiratory care: a guide to clinical practice,* ed 4, Philadelphia, 1997, JB Lippincott.

Mulligan SC, Masterson JG, Devane JG, et al: Clinical and pharmacokinetic properties of a transdermal nicotine patch, *Clin Pharmacol Ther* 47:331, 1990.

Nett LM: The physician's role in smoking cessation, *Chest Suppl* 97(2):28s, 1990.

Petty TL: Pulmonary rehabilitation, *Basics Respir Dis* 1975.

Petty TL: Pulmonary rehabilitation: better living with new technology, *Respir Care* 30:98, 1985.

Petty TL, Nett LM: *Enjoying life with emphysema,* Philadelphia, 1987, Lea & Febiger.

Pulmonary rehabilitation: official American Thoracic Society statement, *Am Rev Respir Dis* 124:663, 1981.

Rennard SI, Daughton D: Transdermal nicotine for smoking cessation, *Respir Care* 38:290, 1993.

Sobush D, Dunning M, McDonald K: Exercise prescription components for respiratory muscle training: past, present, and future, *Respir Care* 30:34, 1985.

Taylor C, Lillis C, LeMond P: *Fundamentals of nursing: the art and science of nursing care,* ed 2, Philadelphia, 1993, JB Lippincott.

White GC: *Equipment theory for respiratory care,* ed 4, Albany, NY, 2005, Delmar.

Wilkins RL, Dexter JR: *Respiratory disease: a case study approach to patient care,* ed 2, Philadelphia, 1998, FA Davis.

Wyka KA: Cardiopulmonary rehabilitation. In Wilkins RL, Stoller JK, Kacmarek RM, editors: *Egan's fundamentals of respiratory care,* ed 9, St Louis, 2009, Mosby.

Wyka KA: Pulmonary rehabilitation. In Wyka KA, Mathews PJ, Clark WF, editors: *Foundations of respiratory care,* Albany, NY, 2002, Delmar.

1. After instructing a home care patient on the use of her small volume nebulizer, you want to be sure that she understands how to fill and clean it. How could you confirm this?
    1. Have the patient demonstrate use of the nebulizer to you.
    2. Have the patient's boyfriend demonstrate use of the nebulizer to you.
    3. Have the patient answer your questions about the nebulizer.
    4. Have the patient tell you how the equipment is assembled and cleaned.
    A. 1, 3, 4
    B. 1, 2
    C. 3, 4
    D. 2, 3, 4

2. Your patient with chronic obstructive pulmonary disease (COPD) is starting a pulmonary rehabilitation program and taking her first 6-minute walk test. If she should desaturate, at what pulse oximeter reading would supplemental oxygen be indicated?
    A. <96%
    B. <90%
    C. <88%
    D. <84%

3. A home care patient tells you that she cannot feel any O_2 coming to her nasal cannula from the O_2 concentrator. You would do all of the following EXCEPT
    A. Refill the humidifier bottle with sterile water
    B. Place the cannula prongs under water to see if there is any bubbling of gas
    C. Tighten all the equipment connections
    D. Switch the patient to her tank of O_2

4. On surveying a patient's home, you notice that four steps lead to the front door. The patient's bedroom is upstairs, and his wife smokes about one pack of cigarettes a day. You would recommend all the following EXCEPT
    A. The patient's wife should stop smoking
    B. The patient should use a cane when climbing stairs
    C. The patient's bedroom should be moved downstairs
    D. A ramp should be added to facilitate entering through the front door

5. When first visiting a home care patient's house, the therapist should evaluate all of the following to attempt to eliminate risks associated with the patient's performance of daily activities:
    1. Bathroom facilities, including an assessment of ease of getting into and out of the shower or bathtub
    2. Television and remote control for operation
    3. Kitchen facilities, including all cooking and eating utensils placed within arm's reach
    4. Properly cleaned HEPA filtration system
    A. 1
    B. 1, 2, 3, 4
    C. 3, 4
    D. 1, 2

6. In attempts to determine the daily exercise tolerance of a male COPD patient, all of the following questions might be asked EXCEPT
    A. How far can you walk your pet dog around the yard?
    B. Are you able to shave every day?
    C. Is your wife or a relative able to drive you to the grocery store?
    D. How many flights of stairs can you climb before you have to stop?

7. The main goal of a pulmonary rehabilitation program should be to
    A. Reduce the amount of sputum coughed out every day
    B. Return the patient to his or her highest possible level of functioning
    C. Reduce the amount of supplemental O_2 needed
    D. Increase the patient's appetite to achieve weight gain

8. Your patient and her husband are both smokers. She is about to be discharged after treatment for bronchitis. Which of the following would you recommend?
    1. She should stop smoking.
    2. She should see her physician to get help to stop smoking.
    3. Her husband should stop smoking.
    4. She should switch to her husband's brand of cigarettes to reduce the conflict between them.
    A. 1, 2
    B. 3
    C. 1, 2, 3
    D. 1, 2, 3, 4

1. The therapeutic goals of a rehabilitation program include all the following *except*
   A. Decreased hospitalizations
   B. Reversal of lung disease
   C. Increase the patient's energy level
   D. Increase the patient's ability to perform ADLs

2. A home care patient calls to say that he cannot feel any oxygen coming out of the nasal cannula. The oxygen concentrator is making odd cycling noises. What should the respiratory therapist recommend?
   A. Reset the circuit breaker on the concentrator and call back in an hour.
   B. Switch the cannula to a liquid oxygen system at a higher flow rate than the concentrator.
   C. Switch the cannula to an oxygen cylinder at the same flow rate as the concentrator.
   D. Disassemble the concentrator, and clean out the air filter.

3. An open-end format exercise program should be recommended to a patient who has an unpredictable work and social schedule because of the following:
   1. Members of the exercise group can offer support to each other.
   2. It is self-directed by the patient.
   3. The facilitator can easily plan group activities.
   4. The patient can adjust the schedule of activities if necessary.
   A. 2, 4
   B. 1, 3
   C. 4
   D. 2, 3

4. All of the following are indications for monitoring infant apnea at home *except*
   A. Surgically repaired cleft palate
   B. Apnea periods lasting 25 seconds
   C. Two older siblings who died of SIDS
   D. Premature infant with apnea periods and bradycardia

5. The components of a strength training program include
   1. Cool-down period
   2. Strengthening exercises performed daily
   3. Warm-up period
   4. Strengthening exercises performed every other day
   5. Exercises performed for 20 to 30 minutes continuously
   A. 1, 2
   B. 3, 4, 5
   C. 2, 3, 5
   D. 1, 3, 4

6. You are supervising a patient who is participating in an endurance training rehabilitation program. Her target heart rate is between 130 and 150 beats/min. She is exercising on a bicycle ergometer, and her heart rate is 167 beats/min. What would you advise her to do?
   A. Exercise only until she begins to perspire.
   B. Continue exercising if she feels that she can handle the workload.
   C. Exercise a maximum of 10 minutes each day.
   D. Slow down on the ergometer until her heart rate decreases to the target level.

7. Home apnea monitoring can usually be discontinued when all the following conditions exist *except*
   A. Thirty days have passed without the infant having an apnea episode
   B. The infant received a diphtheria-pertussis-tetanus (DPT) immunization without any consequences
   C. Three months have passed without any alarms sounding
   D. Two months have passed without an apnea episode

8. A pulmonary rehabilitation patient is ordered to perform a 6-minute walk to improve her endurance. The patient should be instructed to
   A. Ride a bicycle ergometer for 6 minutes, and note the distance pedaled
   B. Walk as quickly as possible for 3 minutes, and double the distance covered
   C. Walk as far as possible in 6 minutes, and note the distance
   D. Walk as far as possible in 1 minute, and multiply the distance by 6

9. The respiratory therapist is working with a group of COPD patients who need to begin a pulmonary rehabilitation program. A closed-end program would be best for the group for all of the following reasons *except*
   A. Group members can offer emotional support to each other
   B. The program facilitator can direct group activities
   C. Learning activities can be optimally sequenced
   D. Each patient can easily adjust activities if a scheduling conflict arises

10. A COPD patient who is trying to quit smoking is using a nicotine patch. He complains of skin irritation on his arm where the patch is placed and difficulty sleeping. The respiratory therapist should recommend the following:
    1. Apply a topical cortisone cream to the irritated skin.

2. Move the patch to another area.
3. Take a sleeping pill.
4. Remove the patch before going to bed.
5. Drink a beer or a glass of wine before going to bed.
   A. 4, 5
   B. 2, 4
   C. 1, 3, 4
   D. 1, 2, 4, 5

11. A patient receiving public aid is being discharged. The physician has ordered 2 L/min of home oxygen as needed for shortness of breath. Which of the following should be set up in the home?
    A. A bank of H tanks and simple oxygen mask
    B. Liquid oxygen system with air entrainment mask
    C. Oxygen concentrator with oxygen-conserving cannula
    D. A portable, shoulder-bag oxygen tank and a regular nasal cannula

12. A 50-year-old patient with COPD is a participant in an exercise program. Which of the following are expected benefits of the program?
    1. Improved pulmonary function studies
    2. Fewer hospitalizations
    3. More exercise tolerance
    4. Reversal of lung disease
    A. 1, 2
    B. 2, 3
    C. 1, 2, 3
    D. 1, 2, 3, 4

18 Special Procedures

Note 1: This book is written to cover every item listed as testable on the *Entry Level Examination (ELE), Written Registry Examination (WRE),* and *Clinical Simulation Examination (CSE).*

The listed code for each item is taken from the National Board for Respiratory Care's (NBRC) **Summary Content Outline for CRT (Certified Respiratory Therapist) and Written RRT (Registered Respiratory Therapist) Examinations** (http://evolve.elsevier.com/Sills/resptherapist/). For example, if an item is testable on both the ELE and the WRE, it will simply be shown as: (Code: . . .). If an item is only testable on the ELE, it will be shown as: (ELE code: . . .). If an item is only testable on the WRE, it will be shown as: (WRE code: . . .).

Following each item's code will be the difficulty level of the questions on that item on the ELE and WRE. (See the Introduction for a full explanation of the three question difficulty levels.) **Recall [R]** level questions typically expect the exam taker to recall factual information. **Application [Ap]** level questions are harder because the exam taker may have to apply factual information to a clinical situation. **Analysis [An]** level questions are the most challenging because the exam taker may have to use critical thinking to evaluate patient data to make a clinical decision.

Note 2: A review of the most recent Entry Level Examinations (ELE) has shown an average of 3 questions (out of 140), or 2% of the exam, will cover special procedures. A review of the most recent Written Registry Examinations (WRE) has shown an average of 6 questions (out of 100), or 6% of the exam, will cover special procedures. The Clinical Simulation Examination is comprehensive and may include everything that should be known by an advanced level respiratory therapist.

MODULE A

Patient transportation

1. Participate in intrahospital patient transport (Code: III 13b) [Difficulty: ELE: R, Ap; WRE: An]

2. Participate in land or air patient transport outside of the hospital (Code: III 13a) [Difficulty: ELE: R; WRE: Ap, An]

Be prepared to perform, during patient transport, all the respiratory care practices and procedures that have been described in this and other texts. It is extremely important that all equipment and supplies be accounted for before leaving the patient's room for the next location. This is especially true if the patient is being moved to another hospital. Obviously, once interhospital transport is under way it is not possible to obtain an item that was forgotten. To help ensure that this does not happen, it is wise to have a checklist of everything that may be needed. In addition, all equipment must be checked for proper function. Calculate the duration of the oxygen cylinders at expected liter flows. Make sure that batteries and light bulbs work and have spare batteries and light bulbs.

If mechanical ventilation will be needed, select a unit that is lightweight and portable and has solid-state circuitry. For intrahospital transport, many respiratory care departments use pneumatically powered units. Typically, for interhospital transport, an electrically powered unit is selected. Make sure that it can be powered by both alternating current (AC) and direct current (DC) from batteries. If the ventilator will be used for a helicopter or unpressurized cabin fixed-wing aircraft, it must be able to deliver an intermittent mandatory ventilation (IMV)/synchronous intermittent mandatory ventilation (SIMV) mode through a demand valve rather than through a reservoir system. The ventilator controls and positive end-expiratory pressure (PEEP) should not be adversely affected by changes in atmospheric pressure during ascent and landing. Be prepared to provide ventilatory support with a bag-mask system if the mechanical ventilator should fail.

3. Participate in the medical emergency team (MET) (e.g., rapid response team) (Code: III 13d) [Difficulty: ELE:R, WRE: Ap, An]

Respiratory therapists need to be prepared to respond to individual emergency cases such as a cardiopulmonary resuscitation (CPR) or trauma victim. In addition, there are three mass casualty disaster scenarios that would require respiratory therapists to help care for a large number of casualties. These could be accidental or terrorism incidents.

The first is airborne chemical exposure to the lungs and skin. This could include lung-damaging agents (e.g., ammonia, chlorine, and phosgene gases); blistering agents of the skin, eyes, and mucous membranes (e.g., sulfur mustard [mustard gas] and phosgene); blood agents that block oxygen's metabolism (e.g., hydrogen cyanide and cyanogen chloride); and nerve agents that block the breakdown of acetylcholine (e.g., organophosphate pesticides). In all cases, the first action is to remove the victim from the toxic area. First responders must wear a hazardous materials suit to protect themselves before entering the toxic area to remove any victims. Once a victim is taken to a safe area, specific treatment is based upon the type of chemical exposure. Then the victim will receive other supportive measures such as supplemental oxygen, airway management, and mechanical ventilation.

Second is exposure to airborne infectious agents such as the viruses that cause avian flu and severe acute respiratory syndrome (SARS) or the spores that cause anthrax. In these cases the victim must be treated by caregivers who are wearing personal protective devices such as an N95 mask or a powered air protection respirator (PAPR). See Chapter 2 for the guidelines on airborne infection control precautions.

The third scenario would be trauma from explosion, gun fire, or train wreck, for example. The most severely injured victims would have trauma to the head, neck, chest, and/or abdomen. Many would require intubation and mechanical ventilation. Airway management and intubation are covered in Chapters 12 and 18; mechanical ventilation is covered in Chapters 15 and 16.

4. Participate in disaster management (Code: III I3c) [Difficulty: ELE:R, WRE: Ap, An]

Respiratory therapists are an important group of health care professionals who respond to local emergencies and take part in mass casualty/disaster planning. They should be part of a hospital's disaster management team. The local hospital is linked to a regional disaster management team that further connects to the state system and finally the national system. Currently, in anticipation of a catastrophe that could overwhelm a local or regional medical system, the federal government has established the Strategic National Stockpile (SNS). If there should be a locally overwhelming need for supplies or equipment, the state government would submit a request to the appropriate division of the Centers for Disease Control and Prevention. The following items can be dispatched by the SNS and received within 1 day:

- Uni-Vent Eagle 754 ventilators or LP10 ventilators and ancillary supplies for pediatric or adult patients (NOTE: The LP10 has not been manufactured since 2006.)
- Intubation supplies
- Oxygen masks and nasal cannulas
- Suction machines and suction catheters
- Medications used to help manage ventilated patients: sedatives, analgesics, and neuromuscular blockers

Other respiratory care related supplies and oxygen supply systems must be provided locally. Be prepared to perform any and all respiratory care practices and procedures listed in this book or in other respiratory care textbooks.

Exam Hint 18-1 (WRE)

Usually one question on the examination deals with the effects of increased altitude when flying in an unpressurized helicopter or airplane. Remember that as altitude increases, barometric pressure (P_B) decreases. Decreased barometric pressure directly leads to a decrease in the alveolar pressure of oxygen (PAO_2), which results in a decrease in the patient's arterial pressure of oxygen (PaO_2). In addition, as barometric pressure decreases at increased altitude, gases within the patient (stomach and intestine, pneumothorax, and lung) expand. The air within the endotracheal tube cuff expands, and the delivered tidal volume increases. This requires adjustments in the ventilator settings. Later, when the aircraft descends to land, the increased barometric pressure results in a decrease in the cuff volume, the tidal volume, and the patient's internal gas volumes. Be prepared to adjust the ventilator again.

MODULE B

Assist the physician with patient care and related procedures

1. Assist with moderate (conscious) sedation (Code: IIIJ7) [Difficulty: ELE: R, Ap; WRE: An]

The phrase moderate (or conscious) sedation refers to the administration of a sedative agent that calms a patient during a medical procedure (for example, cardioversion or bronchoscopy) but does not cause the patient to lose consciousness. The sedated patient can be stimulated to cooperate and follow commands during the procedure. Typically the patient has no memory of the procedure after it is completed.

Medications in the benzodiazepine group are preferred for conscious sedation and given intravenously. Currently midazolam (Versed) is preferred but diazepam (Valium) is also commonly used. When the patient's procedure is completed, these medications can be reversed by intravenous flumazenil (Romazicon). Another option is to intravenously administer the narcotic agent fentanyl (Duragesic, Sublimaze) for rapid sedation. After the procedure is completed, naloxone (Narcan) is given intravenously to reverse the effects of fentanyl. There is more discussion of these and other sedative agents in Chapter 9, Pharmacology.

The respiratory therapist must be prepared for the possibility of the patient being overdosed with a sedative agent. This could result in a decreased respiratory rate and tidal volume or apnea. Safety guidelines require either a nurse or a respiratory therapist to monitor the patient's breathing, pulse oximetry values, heart rate, blood pressure, and electrocardiogram. The therapist must be prepared to administer supplemental oxygen or begin bag-mask ventilation if needed.

2. Assist with the insertion of venous or arterial catheters (WRE code: IIIJ6) [Difficulty: WRE: An]

Chapter 5, Advanced Cardiopulmonary Monitoring, contains discussions on preparation, care, and maintenance of central venous, arterial, and pulmonary artery lines. Review the chapter if needed.

Each hospital or physician may have a prescribed way that the catheter insertion procedure is performed. The general steps are listed here:

1. Inform the patient of the procedure and have the patient sign the medical release form if time permits.
2. Have a sedative or pain-relieving agent administered if needed.
3. If necessary, shave body hair from the insertion site.
4. Don a sterile mask, cap, gown, and gloves according to protocol.
5. Disinfect the insertion site with a Betadine (iodine) soaked sterile 4 × 4 inch gauze pad. Place the pad at the center of the insertion site, and move it in a widening spiral away from the center. This step should be repeated with a second gauze pad. Let the Betadine dry.
6. Protect the area around the insertion site with a sterile fenestrated surgical drape.
7. Prepare the sterile field where the catheter, scalpel, supplies, and so forth will be placed. Have a local anesthetic such as Xylocaine (lidocaine) available in a syringe with needle. The physician will inject this into the insertion site.
8. Assist the physician into his or her sterile mask, cap, gown, and gloves.
9. Obtain the properly sized catheter for the procedure or patient.
10. Assist the physician with the procedure as needed. This may include connecting the catheter to the tubing system, flushing the catheter and tubing system, and inflating the balloon on a pulmonary artery catheter.
11. Make any adjustments in the patient's respiratory care equipment as needed.
12. Dispose of any used supplies and so forth after the procedure is completed.
13. Tend to the patient's comfort.

3. Assist with ultrasound (ELE code: IIIJ9) [Difficulty: ELE: R]

The ultrasound (also called a sonogram or ultrasonography) procedure uses a transducer to send soundwaves through the soft tissues of the body. A lubricating gel is placed on the skin so that there is good sound transmission from the transducer into the patient. Depending on the density of the tissues and fluids, the soundwaves bounce off and are received back to the transducer. The sound energy is converted to electrical energy to produce a two-dimensional image of the various organs. Ultrasound can be very useful in the following areas of interest to respiratory therapists:

- Helps locate arteries and veins, visualize blood flow through the vessels, and determine blood pressure.
- Obstetric ultrasound will help to establish the number of fetuses and their size, the amount of amniotic fluid present, and the location of the placenta(s).
- Helps determine if a neonate has suffered a cerebral hemorrhage.
- Heart sonograms will provide information on cardiac structure and blood flow through the chambers and valves.
- Locates pleural fluid to help guide needle placement for a thoracentesis.
- Identifies the movement of the hemidiaphragms.
- A very small transducer can be placed via bronchoscopy into a bronchus. This procedure has been used to identify a bronchial wall tumor and affected local lymph nodes to help guide a biopsy procedure.

Note that the lungs themselves cannot be properly imaged with ultrasound because they are air-filled. The ultrasound procedure is noninvasive and safe with no patient side effects.

4. Assist with cardioversion (Code: IIIJ8) [Difficulty: ELE: R, Ap; WRE: An]

Cardioversion (or countershock) refers to deliberately sending a direct current (DC) electrical shock through the patient's heart. Its purpose is to suppress an abnormal heartbeat so that the normal pacemaker at the sinoatrial (SA) node assumes control. This is accomplished if a great enough electrical current is sent through the chest wall to cause the depolarization of a critical mass of myocardial cells. After this, the SA node should take over as the pacemaker, provided that the heart muscle is oxygenated and not too acidotic. Two different types of cardioversion exist: defibrillation (also called unsynchronized cardioversion) and synchronized cardioversion. Both were introduced in Chapter 11 for the treatment of specific arrhythmias.

Defibrillation is performed in an emergency situation (see Figure 11-41). Patients who need to be defibrillated include those who have ventricular tachycardia or ventricular flutter (see Figures 11-38 and 11-39) when they are pulseless, unresponsive, or hypotensive or patients who have pulmonary edema and ventricular fibrillation (see Figure 11-40). Because the fastest possible action is needed, no attempt is made to synchronize the defibrillation shock with the heart's rhythm. While cardiopulmonary resuscitation (CPR) is being performed, the defibrillator unit is prepared. The defibrillating paddles (large positive and negative electrodes) are placed on the patient's right anterior and left lateral chest wall. The physician or other qualified person (respiratory therapist, registered nurse, or paramedic) performing the defibrillation should call out, "Stand clear." All other medical personnel should stand back from the patient and the bed and not touch anything that is electrically grounded. When the buttons on the paddles are pushed, the shock is administered. If it is successful, the patient's heartbeat returns to normal sinus rhythm. If the initial shock is unsuccessful, CPR is continued. The defibrillator is then recharged for another attempt as quickly as possible. Box 18-1 shows the sequence of increasingly more powerful countershocks that can be given.

Synchronized cardioversion is similar in some ways to defibrillation. An electrical shock is sent by two paddles through the heart to suppress paroxysmal atrial tachycardia, atrial flutter, atrial fibrillation, or hemodynamically stable ventricular tachycardia (see Figures 11-25, 11-26, and 11-27) so that the SA node assumes control. Its major difference from defibrillation is that the electrical shock is administered automatically by the defibrillator after an R wave is recognized by the electrocardiogram (ECG) monitor (see Figure 11-5). The ECG electrodes must be in place and the best lead (often lead II) selected to show a clear, strong, upright R wave. The defibrillator unit is programmed for synchronized cardioversion. The physician holds the paddles on the patient's right anterior and left lateral chest wall. When the discharge buttons are pushed on the paddles, the shock is sent after the next R wave is identified by the ECG monitor.

Cardioversion is not considered an emergency; however, it is performed as quickly as possible so that the patient does not stay in the abnormal rhythm any longer than necessary. Synchronized cardioversion is performed only if medical treatment with antiarrhythmia drugs or carotid artery massage has no effect. Because these patients are usually conscious, they should be sedated with diazepam (Valium), midazolam (Versed), or a similar medication. Patients who are hypotensive or already unconscious should not be sedated.

The respiratory therapist's role in cardioversion may include the following:
- Making sure that the ECG electrodes are properly positioned for either monitoring or diagnosing the rhythm, as the physician requires

---

BOX 18-1   Wattage Used in Synchronous Cardioversion and Defibrillation

SYNCHRONIZED CARDIOVERSION OF AN INFANT
0.5-1.0 J (watt-seconds) per kg
Stepwise increases in energy should be used if the initial shock fails to convert the rhythm.

SYNCHRONIZED CARDIOVERSION OF AN ADULT
Atrial flutter and paroxysmal atrial tachycardia: 50-100 J
Stepwise increases in energy should be used if the initial shock fails to convert the rhythm: 200, 300, 360 J.

ATRIAL FIBRILLATION
Stepwise increases in energy should be used if the initial shock fails to convert the rhythm: 200, 300, 360 J.

VENTRICULAR TACHYCARDIA WITH A REGULAR FORM AND RATE WITH OR WITHOUT A PULSE
100 J
Stepwise increases in energy should be used if the initial shock fails to convert the rhythm: 200, 300, 360 J.

VENTRICULAR TACHYCARDIA WITH AN IRREGULAR FORM AND RATE
200 J
Stepwise increases in energy should be used if the initial shock fails to convert the rhythm: 300, 360 J.

DEFIBRILLATION
Infant
2 J/kg
4 J/kg for second and succeeding attempts

Adult
200 J on first attempt
200-300 J on second attempt
Up to 360 J on third and succeeding attempts

J, joules. 1 joule = 1 watt-second of power.

- Making sure that the ECG monitor and electrocardiograph are working properly
- Making sure that the ECG lead that results in a strong R wave is selected; usually the R wave is upright in lead II
- Charging the defibrillator to the power level ordered by the physician
- Adding the electrode cream to the electrode paddles to decrease the skin's resistance to electricity
- Being prepared to keep a patent airway, manually ventilate the patient's lungs, or begin chest compressions, if necessary

5. Bronchoscopy

Bronchoscopy is a procedure that involves looking directly into the patient's tracheobronchial airways. The physician can perform a number of diagnostic and therapeutic tasks under direct vision. (See Box 18-2 for uses, limitations, and risks of bronchoscopy.)

a. Recommend a diagnostic bronchoscopy procedure to evaluate hemoptysis or atelectasis (Code: IC3) [Difficulty: ELE: R, Ap; WRE: An]

Hemoptysis commonly is caused by blunt chest trauma or a bleeding bronchial tumor. Segmental or lobar atelectasis is commonly caused by an aspirated foreign body or a bronchial tumor. As listed in Box 18-2, bronchoscopy can be used to help diagnose and manage these problems.

b. Recommend a bronchoalveolar lavage (Code: IC5) [Difficulty: ELE: R, Ap; WRE: An]

A bronchoalveolar lavage (BAL) (also called bronchopulmonary lavage) is a diagnostic procedure most commonly performed if lung cancer or infection is suspected and expectorated sputum specimens are inconclusive. The BAL procedure involves introducing sterile saline through the open channel of a flexible fiberoptic bronchoscope into a specific segment or bronchus. The fluid and any loose alveolar cells or bacteria are then suctioned out through the bronchoscope. The removed materials are sent to the laboratory for cytologic and microbiologic studies.

BOX 18-2 Uses, Limitations, and Risks of Bronchoscopy

RIGID BRONCHOSCOPY

Diagnostic Use
Biopsy of tumors within the main airway

Therapeutic Uses
Treatment of massive hemoptysis by cold-saline lavage or placement of a Fogarty catheter to occlude the airway
Removal of foreign body in infants and small children
Aspiration of inspissated secretions and mucous plugs

Limitations
Cannot be used for observing or treating problems beyond the left or right mainstem bronchus
Cannot be used with patients with disease or trauma of the cervical spine who cannot hyperextend their necks
Cannot be used with patients with disease or trauma of the jaw who cannot open their mouths wide enough to pass the tube

FIBEROPTIC BRONCHOSCOPY

Diagnostic Uses
Search for the origin of a positive sputum cytologic result
Evaluate lung lesions and perform transbronchial biopsy of lung tissue (should be done only under fluoroscopic control)
Stage lung cancer preoperatively
Investigate unexplained hemoptysis, unexplained cough, localized wheeze, or stridor
Search for the cause of unexplained paralysis of a vocal cord or hemidiaphragm
Search for the cause of superior vena cava syndrome, chylothorax, or unexplained pleural effusion
Assess airway patency and investigate suspected bronchial tear or other injury after thoracic trauma

Investigate a suspected tracheoesophageal fistula
Investigate problems related to an endotracheal tube such as tracheal damage, airway obstruction, or tube placement
Obtain mucus for identification of pathogens
Investigate suspected injury secondary to inhaled superheated gas and smoke from an enclosed fire
Investigate suspected injury secondary to the aspiration of gastric contents
Perform bronchoalveolar lavage

Therapeutic Uses
Remove secretions or mucous plugs that cannot be cleared by other methods
Remove small foreign bodies
Remove abnormal endobronchial tissue or foreign material by forceps or laser techniques

INCREASED RISKS RELATED TO RIGID OR FIBEROPTIC BRONCHOSCOPY
Recent myocardial infarction or unstable angina
Unstable cardiac arrhythmia
Partial tracheal obstruction
Unstable bronchial asthma
Severe hypoxemia
Hypercarbia
Pulmonary hypertension (risk of hemorrhage after biopsy)
Bleeding disorder (risk of hemorrhage after biopsy)
Lung abscess (airway may be flooded with purulent material)
Pulmonary infection from contaminated equipment
Pneumothorax from transbronchial biopsy
Respiratory failure requiring mechanical ventilation of the patient

c. Assist with the bronchoscopy procedure (Code: IIIJ2) [Difficulty: ELE: R, Ap; WRE: An]

Typical duties of the respiratory therapist during bronchoscopy may include the following:

1. Inform the patient of the procedure. Have the patient sign the medical release form if not already done. Ask the patient if he/she has eaten within the last 6 hours. (If the patient has recently eaten, the procedure will have to be rescheduled.)
2. Have a sedative such as midazolam (Versed) or diazepam (Valium) administered for conscious sedation, if needed.
3. Nebulize a topical anesthetic, such as 4% lidocaine (Xylocaine), to the airway.
4. Check the fiberoptic unit for proper function: working light source, working thumb control to flexible tip, working adjustable eyepiece focus, and patency of the suction and biopsy channel.
5. Check the functioning of the biopsy brush and forceps.
6. Set up and monitor the patient's ECG.
7. Monitor the patient's vital signs.
8. Place the pulse oximeter on the patient and monitor.
9. Administer oxygen via a nasal catheter or the suction and biopsy channel on the unit.
10. Collect all suctioned material or other specimens for culture and sensitivity.
11. Perform biopsies and brushings for cytology.
12. Operate any photographic equipment.
13. If the patient is being mechanically ventilated during fiberoptic bronchoscopy, perform the following:
    - Place a bronchoscopy adapter between the endotracheal tube and Y of the circuit. This keeps a seal around the bronchoscopy tube to minimize any decrease in tidal volume.
    - Place a bite block into the patient's mouth so that the endotracheal tube and fiberoptic catheter cannot be bitten.
    - Watch for an increase in the peak pressure from the increased resistance to airflow caused by the bronchoscopy tube.
    - Be prepared to make adjustments in inspired oxygen, respiratory rate, flow, and set tidal volume if there is a leak.
    - Be prepared to switch from conventional volume ventilation to high-frequency jet ventilation if needed.
14. Assess the patient after the procedure:
    - Check vital signs and auscultate breath sounds every 15 minutes for 1 hour, then every 2 hours for 4 hours, then as ordered.
    - Monitor cough for hemoptysis, especially after a biopsy procedure.
    - Suction secretions if needed.
    - Provide for pain relief if needed.
15. Use a glutaraldehyde disinfecting solution (Cidex) on the equipment between patient procedures.

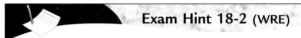

Exam Hint 18-2 (WRE)

Usually one question on the examination asks about indications for bronchoscopy or hazards related to the procedure.

d. Manipulate a bronchoscope by order or protocol (Code: IIA27) [Difficulty: ELE: R; WRE: Ap, An]

1. Get a bronchoscope for the planned procedure

The rigid bronchoscope is a straight, hollow, stainless-steel tube (Figure 18-1). It has a distal light source so that the airway can be seen and a side port for providing oxygen or mechanical ventilation to the patient. The right and left mainstem bronchi can be observed by passing a mirror through the main channel. A hook or net can be passed through the main channel into the trachea or either bronchus to remove a foreign body. The rigid bronchoscope is preferred for the treatment of massive hemoptysis or to remove a foreign body.

Flexible fiberoptic bronchoscopy (FFB) uses a smaller diameter flexible tube with two sets of fiberoptic bundles that shine light into the airway and allow viewing of the airway. It has gained wide popularity because it is better tolerated by the patient and allows for better visualization

Figure 18-1 A rigid tube bronchoscope being inserted into a patient's trachea. Note how the head and neck must be hyperextended. *(From Simmons KF: Airway care. In Scanlan CL, Spearman CB, Sheldon RL, editors:* Egan's fundamentals of respiratory care, *ed 5, St Louis, 1990, Mosby.)*

and collection of specimens from smaller bronchi (Figures 18-2 and 18-3). The adult bronchoscopy tube is about 5- to 6-mm outer diameter (OD), and the pediatric tube is about 3-mm OD. The small diameter and ability to guide the catheter allow the operator to look into the bronchus to each lung segment (segmental bronchi). The fiberoptic bronchoscope is preferred over the rigid one when the patient is being mechanically ventilated or has disease or trauma to the skull, jaw, or cervical spine. As shown in Figure 18-2, a photo connection allows the assistant either to take still photographs of pulmonary anatomy or to videotape the entire procedure.

A limitation of the pediatric unit is that there is no channel outlet for suctioning purposes. This is because of its small size. If a patient has an obstructing bronchial tumor, a special laser fiberoptic bronchoscope is used to burn part of the tumor. This enables the patient to breathe more easily, but this procedure is not a cure for the cancer.

2. Put the equipment together and make sure that it works properly

The fiberoptic bronchoscope is preassembled (see Figure 18-2 for its primary features). If photographing or videotaping is planned, the camera must be attached

Figure 18-2 A flexible fiberoptic bronchoscope with its components and special features. *(From Wilkins RL, Stoller JK, Kacmarek RM: Egan's fundamentals of respiratory care, ed 9, St Louis, 2009, Mosby.)*

Figure 18-3 A flexible fiberoptic bronchoscopy procedure being performed on a patient. *(From Williams SF, Thompson JM: Respiratory disorders, St Louis, 1990, Mosby.)*

at the photo connection. Have a central or portable suctioning system set up with suction tubing. In addition, the following steps must be used to check for proper functioning:

1. Make sure the light source shines through to the distal end of the bronchoscope.
2. Look through the eyepiece. Point the distal end of the bronchoscope at a close object, and adjust the lens to bring it into focus.
3. Adjust the thumb control to bend the distal tip.
4. Pass biopsy forceps or brush through the channel port to the outlet.
5. Make sure the suction tubing connects to the channel port.

3. Troubleshoot any problems with the equipment

If the light source does not work, you must check the manufacturer's equipment manual to help determine if the problem could be something simple such as a burned-out light bulb or a more serious problem. Similarly, problems with the camera equipment can be resolved by checking the manufacturer's equipment manual.

Failure to pass a biopsy forceps or brush through the channel port probably means that an obstruction such as dried blood or tissue is present. Try applying suction through the channel port to clear out the debris. It also may be helpful to squirt sterile distilled water from a syringe through the channel. Try suctioning again or pushing the biopsy forceps through the channel. If alternating suction, instilling water, and pushing the forceps through the channel does not dislodge the debris, the unit cannot be used. Try soaking the bronchoscope in water to soften the debris before repeating these processes. If the channel cannot be cleared, the unit must be sent back to the manufacturer for repairs.

6. Thoracentesis

a. Recommend a thoracentesis to treat a pleural effusion (WRE code: IC14) [Difficulty: WRE: R, Ap, An]

Thoracentesis (also called thoracocentesis) is the surgical puncture of the chest wall and pleural space with a needle to aspirate pleural fluid for therapeutic or diagnostic purposes. Thoracentesis is performed as a therapeutic procedure to remove air or fluid that has accumulated in the pleural space and is causing the patient pain, dyspnea, hypoxemia, or a combination of these symptoms. Thoracentesis also is performed as a diagnostic procedure to obtain a fluid sample for analysis to diagnose the cause of a pleural effusion. Pleural fluid may be a transudate that results from congestive heart failure, cirrhosis, nephrotic syndrome, or hypoproteinemia. Pleural fluid may also be an exudate that results most often from inflammatory,

infectious, or neoplastic diseases of the pleura or lung. Other causes of an exudate include pulmonary infarction, chest trauma, drug hypersensitivity, and collagen vascular disease.

b. Assist with a thoracentesis procedure (Code: IIIJ3) [Difficulty: ELE: R, Ap; WRE: An]

The respiratory therapist may be responsible for preparing the patient, disinfecting the puncture site, setting up the sterile field, and preparing the equipment and supplies. Each hospital or physician may have a prescribed way of doing this. If the patient had a previous thoracentesis procedure, review the patient's chart for information on the nature of the removed fluid. Be prepared to compare the previously removed fluid with the fluid being removed at this time. The general steps listed here apply to a thoracentesis procedure and a percutaneous needle biopsy of the pleura and lung (described below):

1. Inform the patient of the procedure. Have him or her sign the medical release form if not already done.
2. Have a sedative or pain-relieving agent administered if needed.
3. Position the patient sitting on the side of the bed and leaning on the overbed table as shown in Figure 18-4. Alternatively, the patient may straddle a chair and rest his or her arms and head on the

Figure 18-4 Technique for thoracentesis. The patient sits up and leans on the overbed table. The pleural fluid is withdrawn through the needle by the syringe and then directed into the collection jar.

back of the chair. The patient who cannot sit up is positioned on his or her side with the unaffected lung down on the bed.

4. If necessary, shave the insertion site clear of body hair.

5. Put on a sterile mask, cap, gown, and gloves according to protocol.

6. Disinfect the insertion site with a Betadine (iodine) soaked sterile 4 × 4 inch gauze pad. Place the pad at the center of the insertion site, and move it in a widening spiral away from the center. This step should be repeated with a second gauze pad. Let the Betadine dry.

7. Protect around the insertion site with a sterile fenestrated surgical drape.

8. Prepare the sterile field with needed supplies such as 1% Xylocaine and a variety of needles and syringes. NOTE: A Curity Thoracentesis Tray or other prepackaged tray will contain the supplies that will most commonly be used.

9. Assist the physician into his or her sterile mask, cap, gown, and gloves.

10. Assist the physician with the procedure as described in the following steps.

11. Make any adjustments in the patient's respiratory care equipment as needed.

12. Dispose of any used supplies and so forth after the procedure is completed.

13. Tend to the patient's comfort.

General steps in the removal of pleural fluid:

1. Check the patient's chest x-ray for the location of the pleural fluid (or targeted tissue for a needle biopsy) and its relationship to the ribs and other tissues.

2. Inform the patient not to move or cough during the procedure so that accidental needle damage to the pleura or lung can be avoided.

3. The physician will anesthetize the thoracentesis site as shown in Figure 18-5, *A* and *B*.

4. The physician will insert a large-gauge needle (often 16 gauge) with attached 50-mL syringe into the pleural fluid (see Figure 18-5, *C*). (A cutting needle is used during a needle aspiration of pleural or lung tissue.)

5. The sample is then aspirated. If there is more than 50 mL of pleural fluid, the two-way valve or three-way stopcock, rubber hose, and collection tube are assembled to remove the fluid (see Figure 18-4).

6. The needle is removed and a bandage is placed over the puncture site.

7. Place the patient with the unaffected side down on the bed for 1 hour.

8. Observe the patient for dizziness and cyanosis. Frequently check the patient's pulse oximeter valve. Assess the patient's vital signs according to hospi-

---

BOX 18-3   Common Complications of Thoracentesis

Infection
Hemothorax
Subcutaneous emphysema
Air embolism
Pneumothorax
Sudden mediastinal shift from removal of a large amount of pleural fluid (usually greater than 1500 mL in an adult)
Unstable vital signs from the sudden mediastinal shift
Pulmonary edema from the sudden reexpansion of the lung and mediastinal shift

---

tal policy. Auscultate frequently for diminished breath sounds over the affected lung as a sign of pneumothorax. The physician should order a chest x-ray to check for pneumothorax. (See Box 18-3 for the commonly seen complications of a thoracentesis or needle biopsy.)

9. Evaluate the gross appearance of the fluid that has been removed. A *transudate* is found when the fluid is clear, serous, or light yellow. It contains few cells of any kind. This is most commonly found in patients with congestive heart failure and pulmonary edema. A *chylothorax* is found when the fluid is opalescent or pearly white in color. Chyle is lymphatic fluid that drains into the pleural cavity when the thoracic duct is blocked. This could be caused by injury to the neck or a tumor that invades the thoracic duct. A *hemothorax* is found when the pleural fluid is bloody (sanguineous or serosanguineous). Chest wall injury or puncture is the usual cause. An *empyema* is found when the fluid is thick and puslike with a foul odor. The patient usually has a bacterial infection of the lung and/or pleura, and infected fluid has entered the pleural space. In all cases, the collected pleural fluid sample should be sent to the laboratory for detailed analysis.

10. Send the collected sample to the laboratory for analysis.

c. Assist with percutaneous needle aspiration biopsies of the lung

Percutaneous aspiration of pleural tissue or lung tissue involves a cutting needle being inserted through the chest wall into the target tissue(s) and the tissue sample being removed. The general procedure for a needle aspiration is described in the preceding section with the thoracentesis procedure.

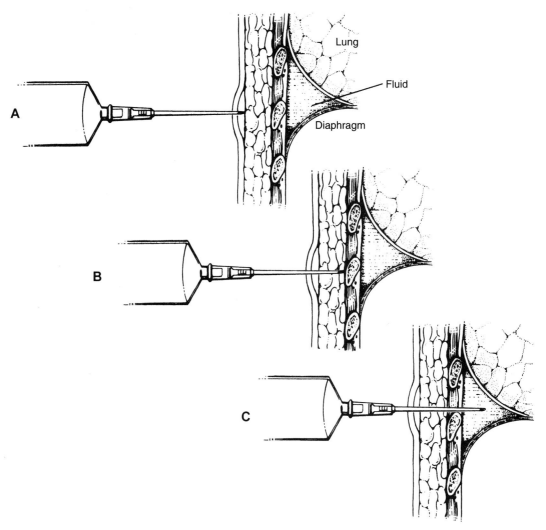

Figure 18-5   Anesthetizing the needle insertion site and performing a thoracentesis. **A,** A 25-gauge needle is used to inject Xylocaine into the thoracentesis puncture site until the skin is raised. **B,** A 22-gauge needle is used to inject Xylocaine into the periosteum of the rib and surrounding tissues. The properly anesthetized patient should feel no pain during the thoracentesis. **C,** A 22- or larger-gauge aspirating needle is pushed through the numbed tissues, over the top edge of the rib, and into the pleural space. The fluid sample can now be aspirated. *(From Martin L:* Pulmonary physiology in clinical practice: the essentials for patient care and evaluation, *St Louis, 1987, Mosby.)*

A pleural biopsy is indicated when exudative fluid is found during a thoracentesis procedure. The cause could be from an infection, including tuberculosis, or a lung tumor. Additionally, a pleural biopsy is indicated when a chest x-ray shows a pleural tumor or unexplained pleural thickening. A cutting needle is inserted into the parietal pleura to withdraw a specimen for analysis.

A lung biopsy is indicated when a chest x-ray or a computed tomography (CT) scan indicates pulmonary parenchymal disease. A tissue sample is needed to determine if the cause is lung cancer, granuloma, infection, or sarcoidosis. A cutting needle is inserted through the parietal and visceral pleura to withdraw a specimen of suspicious lung tissue for analysis.

7. Management of a pneumothorax

a. Treat a tension pneumothorax (Code: III I2) [Difficulty: ELE: R, Ap; WRE: An]

In an emergency when the patient has a tension pneumothorax and rapidly worsening vital signs, the trapped pleural air must be rapidly removed from the chest. This is done by inserting a large-bore needle (16 gauge or larger) through the second or third intercostal space in the midclavicular line of the affected lung. Place the needle over the top of the rib to avoid injury to the blood vessels and nerves below the ribs. The intrapleural air leaves the chest, allowing the lung to expand. A pleural chest tube is then inserted for a long-term solution to the problem. If necessary, review the discussion in Chapters 1 and 15 on the signs and symptoms of a pneumothorax.

b. Assist with chest tube insertion (Code: III J5) [Difficulty: ELE: R, Ap; WRE: An]

A chest tube (also called tube thoracostomy) may be inserted into either one or both pleural spaces around the lungs, the mediastinal space, or the pericardial space around the heart. This procedure is indicated when air or fluid, or both, in any of these spaces interferes with normal lung or heart function. Box 18-4 lists the indications for the insertion of a chest tube.

In addition to chest tube insertion, the patient is often given 100% oxygen by a nonrebreather mask for two reasons. The first is to treat the patient for hypoxemia. Second, if pure oxygen enters the pleural space through a tear in lung tissue, it will be quickly absorbed into the blood. This allows the lung to expand faster than if the patient was breathing a lower percentage of oxygen.

General steps in inserting a pleural chest tube follow:

1. Check the patient's chest radiograph for the location of the air or fluid in the pleural space and its relation to the ribs and other tissues.
2. Prepare the patient as described in the thoracentesis procedure. The patient is usually positioned to lie on his or her back or with the lung of the unaffected side down on the bed.
3. The physician anesthetizes the tube insertion site as shown in Figure 18-5, *A* and *B*.
4. The physician creates an opening into the patient's chest wall to place the chest tube (Figure 18-6). A

BOX 18-4   Indications for the Insertion of a Chest Tube

PLEURAL SPACE (SEE FIGURE 18-6, D)
Tension pneumothorax
Greater than a 10% to 20% simple pneumothorax
Hemothorax
Empyema
Pleural effusion
Chylothorax

MEDIASTINAL SPACE
Free air
Free blood or other fluid

PERICARDIAL SPACE (SEE FIGURE 18-7)
Cardiac tamponade
Pneumopericardium

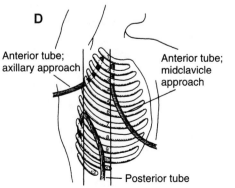

Figure 18-6   Technique for inserting a pleural chest tube. **A,** Anatomic landmarks. **B,** Dissecting through the tissues with a hemostat. **C,** Using a finger to widen the opening and ensure that the lung has not been punctured. **D,** Proper tube placement. Air is removed by a tube that is placed toward the apex of the lung. Fluid is removed by a tube placed toward the posterior base of the lung.

tube to remove air is placed into one of two places and then advanced toward the apex of the lung. With a midclavicular approach, the tube is placed over the top edge of a rib into the second to fourth intercostal space. With a midaxillary approach (preferred site), the tube is placed over the top edge of a rib into the fourth to sixth intercostal space. A tube to remove *fluid* is placed over the top edge of the rib into the sixth to eighth intercostal space. It is inserted at the midaxillary line and advanced toward the posterior base of the lung. Mediastinal or pericardial tubes are placed via an opening below the xiphoid process and positioned posterior to the heart (Figure 18-7). This is most commonly done during open heart surgery.

5. The tube is secured by sutures and covered with a sterile 4 × 4 inch gauze pad and tape.
6. The other end of the tube is connected to the drainage system (discussed later).
7. Place the patient with his or her back against the bed or with the unaffected side down on the bed. The physician may want the head of the bed elevated or flat.
8. Observe the patient for dizziness, cyanosis, and changes in heart rate and respiratory rate. (See Box 18-4 for the most commonly seen complications.)

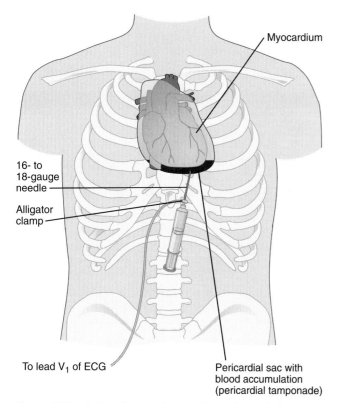

Figure 18-7 Pericardiocentesis procedure. *(From Black JM, Hawks JH: Medical-surgical nursing, clinical management for positive outcomes, ed 8, St Louis, 2009, Saunders.)*

Labels in figure:
Myocardium
16- to 18-gauge needle
Alligator clamp
To lead V_1 of ECG
Pericardial sac with blood accumulation (pericardial tamponade)

Exam Hint 18-3 (ELE, WRE)

Every past examination has included at least one question that relates to identifying a patient having a tension pneumothorax, requiring the insertion of a large-bore needle or a pleural chest tube. Know the indications of a tension pneumothorax, including sudden deterioration of vital signs and hypoxemia, decreased breath sounds over the affected lung, decreased chest wall movement over the affected lung, hyperresonant percussion noted over the affected lung, and shift of the mediastinal structures away from the affected lung. See Figure 1-2 for a chest radiograph showing a pneumothorax.

---

c. Manipulate a pleural drainage system by order or protocol (ELE code: IIA21) [ELE difficulty: R, Ap, An]

1. Select a pleural drainage system

Modern drainage systems consist of either three or four chambers or sections designed to regulate the vacuum level, hold any drained fluids, prevent any outside air from entering the patient's thorax, and act as a pressure-relief valve in case the vacuum regulator should fail. Argyle and Pleur-evac are two well-known manufacturers. The systems for draining the pleural space are discussed here, but the principles are the same for draining the mediastinal and pericardial spaces.

2. Assemble a pleural drainage system, ensure that it works properly, and identify any problems with it

Refer to Figure 18-8 for the assembly and operation of the three-chamber drainage system. The four-chamber drainage system is shown in Figure 18-9 and is discussed concurrently.

   a. Vacuum level. The operation of the wall or central vacuum systems was discussed in Chapter 13. It is common practice to set a partial vacuum of −15 to −20 cm H_2O pressure to the pleural space.

   b. Suction control. The suction control chamber is dry when the unit is unpacked. Follow the manufacturer's instructions for adding the correct amount of water. The proper water level is generally 15 to 20 cm high and results in that level of vacuum being applied to the patient's pleural space.

   It is normal to have room air drawn into the opening on top and bubbling through the water column. This corresponds to bottle or chamber C in Figure 18-9. The constant air bubbling causes the water level to gradually decrease from evaporation. Water must be added occasionally.

Figure 18-8   Three-chamber pleural drainage systems.
A, Homemade three-chamber drainage system. The depth that the suction column tube is placed under water determines the level of vacuum that will be applied against the patient's pleural space. **B,** Schematic drawing of a modern manufactured three-chamber drainage system. *(From Shapiro BA, Kacmarek RM, Cane RD et al: Clinical application of respiratory care, ed 4, St Louis, 1991, Mosby-Year Book. Used by permission.)*

Figure 18-9   Four-chamber pleural drainage systems. *Top,* Homemade four-chamber drainage system. The depth that the suction column tube in chamber C is placed under water determines the level of vacuum that will be applied against the patient's pleural space. *Bottom,* Schematic drawing of a modern manufactured four-chamber drainage system. The fourth chamber acts to vent high-pressure air if the vacuum should be turned off or malfunction. *(Modified from Pilbeam SP, Deshpande VM: Chest tubes and pleural drainage,* Curr Rev Respir Ther *5:151, 1983. Used by permission.)*

c. Water seal. The water-seal chamber, which corresponds to chamber B in Figure 18-9, is a safety feature. It is dry when unpacked. Follow the manufacturer's directions regarding the amount of water to add. Typically, the water-seal tube should be filled with about 2 cm of water through which any patient air can bubble. As indicated by the arrows, it is designed to permit air to leave the patient's chest cavity. (Air also will be seen bubbling when fluid enters the drainage collection chamber and displaces some of its air.) However, room air cannot be drawn "backward" through the water to enter the chest if the vacuum fails or is disconnected.

The water-seal chamber must be checked regularly to see if any air is bubbling through from the patient's chest. If so, the patient has an active air leak. If the chest tube has been placed into the pleural space, it shows that the patient has an unhealed pneumothorax or bronchopleural fistula. If the chest tube has been placed into the mediastinum or pericardium, it indicates that air is leaking through a tear in the lung structures to these areas. When the air leak stops, it indicates that the tissues have healed over the tear.

d. Drainage collection. The drainage collection chamber, which corresponds to bottle or chamber A in

Figure 18-9, is designed to hold any fluid that is removed from the pleural space. It is divided into several sections that are demarcated for volume measurement. The volume that has accumulated in the chamber should be recorded each hour. A sudden, significant increase in the amount of drainage should be called to the physician's attention. This is especially important if the patient is losing blood. Note the color of the drainage. Blood is obviously red, chyle is white, pus from an empyema is yellow or green, and pleural effusion fluid is a straw-yellow color. The whole drainage system must be replaced when the drainage collection chamber becomes filled.

e. Pressure-relief valve on the four-chamber system. This additional chamber is a safety feature and is seen on four-chamber systems such as those shown in Figure 18-9, chamber D. Its purpose is to act as an escape route for any gas leaking from the patient if the vacuum system is accidentally turned off or disconnected. Without the relief valve, air pressure from a pneumothorax might increase to a dangerous level. Instead, the air and pressure are released. In three-chamber systems, the pressure has to build up to the point that water in the suction control chamber "geysers" out before the pressure is relieved.

3. Troubleshoot any problems with the pleural drainage system

A number of problems can occur with chest drainage systems. The practitioner must understand how the systems are designed to work and how to recognize and correct any problems. See Table 18-1 for examples of problems and their correction. Figure 18-10 lists important considerations when assessing the patient who is connected to a chest drainage system.

Exam Hint 18-4 (ELE)

Remember that a pleural drainage system is operating properly when air leaking from a pneumothorax is seen bubbling through the water seal. Most examinations have a question concerning this or some other aspect of managing a patient with a pleural drainage system.

---

8. Assist with an intubation (Code: IIIJ1) [Difficulty: ELE: R, Ap; WRE: An]

The procedure for a therapist (or physician) performing oral endotracheal intubation was discussed in Chapter 12. The following discussions are limited to assisting an anesthesiologist or other trained physician in performing a nasal endotracheal intubation. Most commonly, the respiratory therapist is the assistant. This procedure is usually only carried out on spontaneously breathing patients. See Box 18-5 for indications and contraindications and Box 18-6 for complications of nasal

TABLE 18-1	Troubleshooting Problems with Chest Drainage Systems
Problem	**Corrective Action**
Drainage system is cracked open or drainage tubing is permanently disconnected from the drainage system	If the patient has a leaking pneumothorax: Leave the tube open to room air so the pleural air can be vented out. As quickly as possible, place the distal end of the tubing into a glass of water to create a water seal. If the patient does not have a leaking pneumothorax, clamp the distal end of the tube to prevent room air from being drawn into the pleural space. In either case, attach the tube to a new drainage system as soon as possible.
No bubbling through the suction control chamber	Increase the vacuum pressure. Correct any leak in the system.
Water is spouting out of the suction control chamber (three-bottle system)	Turn on the vacuum. Remove obstruction inside tubing between vacuum and drainage system.
Air leak through the water-seal chamber	Check the patient for a pneumothorax; report a new air leak to the physician. Check for a hole in the drainage tube, a loose connection between the tube and the drainage system, or if a fenestration in the tubing has pulled out of the chest wall.
Fluid has filled a dependent loop in the tubing	Drape the tubing so that are no loops or kinks
No change in drainage	Check for loops or kinks in tube. Carefully milk the tube to remove any clots. Do not rapidly strip the chest tube.
Drainage collection chamber is full	Prepare another unit, clamp the tube while making the exchange, and unclamp the tube after the new unit is functioning.

ASSESSING THE PATIENT ON CHEST DRAINAGE

PATIENT

Subjective
Ease of breathing?
Anxiety?
Chest discomfort?
Level of understanding?

Breathing
Rate?
Regularity?
Depth?
Ease?
Breath sounds?

ENTRY SITE

Dressing intact?
Drainage?
Subcutaneous
  emphysema?

TUBING

Tight, taped connections?
Kinks, compression?
Dependent loops?

DRAINAGE UNIT CHAMBERS

Suction source
If no control chamber:
Set at ordered level?

If control chamber:
Set so gentle, con-
  tinuous bubbling
  occurs?

Suction control
Filled to appropriate level?
Gentle, continuous
  bubbling?
Open to atmosphere?

If suction off:
Tubing detached from
  air vent

Water seal
Filled to appropriate level?
Bubbling?
Fluctuations?

If not on suction:
Air vent open?

Drainage collection
Volume?
Type?
Rate?
Chamber below chest
  level?

BOB JACKSON

Figure 18-10 Assessing the patient's chest drainage. *(From Erickson RA: Chest drainage, II, Nursing89 19[6]:47-49, 1989. Used by permission.)*

BOX 18-5 Indications and Contraindications for Nasal Endotracheal Intubation

GENERAL INDICATIONS FOR ENDOTRACHEAL INTUBATION
• Provide a secure, patent airway
• Provide a route for mechanical ventilation
• Prevent aspiration of stomach or mouth contents
• Provide a route for suctioning the lungs
• General anesthesia

INDICATIONS FOR NASAL INTUBATION
• Patient has a cervical spine abnormality or injury
• Use of muscle relaxants may cause a complete loss of the airway
• Limited movement of the cervical spine or mandible
• Lower facial injury or surgery

CONTRAINDICATIONS FOR NASAL INTUBATION
• Basilar skull fracture
• Nasal tumors
• Deviated nasal septum
• Severe coagulation disorder

---

endotracheal intubation. Two different procedures are used for passing an endotracheal tube by the nasal route: blind nasotracheal intubation and direct vision nasotracheal intubation.

a. Blind nasotracheal intubation

Be prepared to assist in blind nasotracheal intubation by positioning the patient properly in a sitting or supine position, providing supplemental oxygen or manual ventilation to the patient, selecting the proper endotracheal tube, making sure the cuff properly inflates and deflates, and securing the tube. Often, the physician orders spraying 1% phenylephrine or 0.25% racemic epinephrine into the patient's nares. These medications constrict the blood vessels. This dilates the nasal passages, makes intubation easier, and also reduces the risk of bleeding. Often, 2% to 4% lidocaine (Xylocaine) is sprayed into the nares for its local anesthetic effect. The distal end of the endotracheal tube is usually also covered with a sterile, water-soluble lubricant for easier insertion (K-Y Brand Jelly), or lido-

---

BOX 18-6   Complications of Nasal Endotracheal Intubation

GENERAL COMPLICATIONS
- Reflex laryngospasm
- Perforation of the esophagus or pharynx
- Esophageal intubation
- Bronchial intubation
- Reflex bradycardia
- Tachycardia or other arrhythmias from hypoxemia
- Hypotension
- Bronchospasm
- Aspiration of tooth, blood, gastric contents, laryngoscope bulb
- Laceration of pharynx or larynx
- Nosocomial infection
- Vocal cord injury
- Laryngeal or tracheal injury from the tube or the excessive cuff pressure
- Mucosal bleeding
- Trauma to the larynx during an attempted blind intubation
- Sinusitis

COMPLICATIONS AFTER EXTUBATION
- Reflex laryngospasm
- Aspiration of stomach contents or oral secretions
- Sore throat
- Hoarseness
- Laryngeal edema (postintubation croup)

---

caine ointment can be used to lubricate the tube and numb the nasal passage.

This procedure is done without the aid of a laryngoscope and blade to visualize the patient's anatomy and expose the trachea. However, other supplies will be needed. See Box 12-4 for a general list of equipment needed for intubation. The general steps in the procedure are listed here:

1. Place the patient in the sniffer's position. Apply supplemental oxygen by mask and monitor the patient's vital signs and pulse oximeter value.
2. Select the nasal passage that is the most open by feeling which one has the most airflow.
3. Select the proper endotracheal tube by size and style and check its cuff. See Table 12-1 for the proper tube size based on the age of the patient. It may be necessary to place a smaller than ideal size tube because the nasal passage is smaller than the oral passage. The tube should be very flexible and have a bevel that opens to the nasal septum of the selected naris. This is to minimize trauma as the tube is inserted.
4. Estimate the depth the tube will be advanced from the external naris to enter the larynx. In an adult male, this will be to about the 28-cm line on the tube. In adult females, this will be to about the 26-cm line on the tube. In other cases, this will be from the external naris to the earlobe.
5. As described previously, prepare the nasal passage and tube for the insertion.
6. Remove the supplemental oxygen and monitor the patient.
7. Gently advance the tube through the medial turbinate. The angle of approach may be adjusted but the tube should not be forced.
8. Advance the tube to less than the predetermined depth in step 4. With one ear positioned at the end of the tube, listen and feel for air movement on exhalation. On inspiration, carefully advance the tube through the oropharynx and into the larynx.
9. A cough with expiratory airflow through the tube usually confirms its placement into the trachea. The cuff needs to be past the vocal cords (see Figure 18-11). If there is no cough or airflow, the tube has likely entered the esophagus. Withdraw the tube until airflow can be heard and felt. Reposition the patient's head and neck and advance the tube on inspiration again. Confirm the tube is properly placed into the trachea.

Figure 18-11 An intubation guide stylet. The flexible tip can be guided by pulling or pushing on a ring attached to a wire running to the distal end. Once the end of the guide is directed into the trachea the endotracheal tube is slipped over it. After the intubation the guide is withdrawn. *(Modified from Heffner JE: Managing difficult intubations in critically ill patients, Respir Management 19[3], 1989.)*

10. Inflate the cuff to a safe pressure. Apply supplemental oxygen to the endotracheal tube.

11. Auscultate for equal, bilateral breath sounds to confirm the tube is within the trachea. Secure the endotracheal tube. Check vital signs and the pulse oximeter reading.

12. Order a chest radiograph to confirm the position of the endotracheal tube.

Because blind nasotracheal intubation can be challenging, several different devices can aid in this intubation procedure. The physician may choose to place a so-called trigger tube (see Figure 12-25) into the patient. This special endotracheal tube has a wire placed into it along the inside curve to the tip. The wire is pulled when the tube is near the larynx to bend the tip more anteriorly and aim it into the trachea. A flexible lighted stylet can be passed through the tube so that the light source is at the distal tip. The light shines through the skin over the larynx. When this is seen, the tube is advanced and the stylet is removed. A fiberoptic bronchoscope (Figure 12-31) can be placed through the tube and guided into the patient's trachea. The tube is then advanced and the bronchoscope removed. Another choice is the intubation guide. This is a stylet with a flexible tip that can be bent through a proximal handle (performed by the physician) (Figure 18-11). The intubation guide is passed through and beyond the distal end of the endotracheal tube. When the guide is in the oropharynx, the tip can be bent in an anterior direction and directed into the trachea. The tube is then advanced over the guide and into the trachea. The guide is then removed.

b. Direct vision nasotracheal intubation

The respiratory therapist assists in direct vision nasotracheal intubation by positioning the patient properly, providing supplemental oxygen or manual ventilation to the patient, obtaining the endotracheal tube, ensuring that the cuff properly inflates and deflates, and securing the tube. Often 1% phenylephrine or 0.25% racemic epinephrine is sprayed into the nares. These medications constrict the blood vessels. This dilates the nasal passages, makes intubation easier, and also reduces the risk of bleeding. Often 2% to 4% lidocaine (Xylocaine) is sprayed into the nares for its local anesthetic effect. A sterile, water-soluble lubricant (K-Y Brand Jelly) is added to the distal end of the tube for easier insertion. Alternatively, lidocaine ointment can be used to lubricate the tube and numb the nasal passage.

This procedure is different from blind nasotracheal intubation in that intubation equipment is used to visualize the patient's anatomy and see the glottis. See Box 12-4 for a general list of equipment needed for intubation. A Magill forceps is needed but a hard stylet is not. Prepare a laryngoscope handle and the physician's choice of either a straight or a curved blade (see Figures 12-29 and 12-30). The general steps in the procedure are listed here:

1. Place the patient in the sniffer's position. Apply supplemental oxygen by mask and monitor the patient's vital signs and pulse oximeter value.

2. Select the nasal passage that is the most open by feeling which one has the most airflow. Select the proper endotracheal tube by size and style and check its cuff. See Table 12-1 for the proper tube size based on the age of the patient. It may be necessary to place a smaller than ideal size tube because the nasal passage is smaller than the oral passage. The tube should be very flexible and have a bevel that opens to the nasal septum of the selected naris. This is to minimize trauma as the tube is inserted.

3. Estimate the depth the tube will be advanced from the external naris to enter the larynx. In an adult male this will be approximately to the 28-cm line on the tube. In adult females this will be to about the 26-cm line on the tube. In other cases this will be from the external naris to the earlobe.

4. As described previously, prepare the nasal passage and tube for the insertion.

5. Remove the supplemental oxygen and monitor the patient.

6. Gently advance the tube through the medial turbinate. The angle of approach may be adjusted but the tube should not be forced.

7. Advance the tube to less than the predetermined depth in step 4. Look into the patient's mouth for the tip of the tube in the oropharynx. If necessary, advance the tube so that the cuff is completely visible.

8. Grasp the laryngoscope handle with the left hand and carefully advance the laryngoscope blade along the right side of the patient's mouth. Move the tongue to the left side (see Figure 12-34).

9. Advance the blade under the epiglottis and lift at a 45-degree angle toward the patient's chest. To avoid injury to the patient's front teeth, DO NOT pull back on the handle and blade.

10. Observe the patient's open larynx (see Figure 12-36). Hold the Magill forceps with the right hand. Grasp the endotracheal tube proximal to the cuff to avoid damaging it (see Figure 18-12).

11. When the patient inhales, use the Magill forceps to pull the tip of the endotracheal tube between the vocal cords and into the larynx. The respiratory therapist may need to push on the end of the endotracheal tube to help advance it. The cuff needs to be inserted past the vocal cords (see Figure 18-13).

12. Carefully remove the laryngoscope blade and Magill forceps.

Figure 18-12 Direct vision nasotracheal intubation. Note that the Magill forceps and laryngoscope and blade are both used. The Magill forceps is used to grasp the tip of the endotracheal tube and pull it anterior into the trachea. *(From Shapiro BA, Harrison RA, Cane RD: Clinical application of respiratory care, ed 4, St Louis, 1991, Mosby.)*

Figure 18-13 Properly placed nasotracheal tube. *(From Shapiro BA, Harrison RA, Cane RD: Clinical application of respiratory care, ed 4, St Louis, 1991, Mosby.)*

13. Inflate the cuff to a safe pressure. Apply supplemental oxygen to the endotracheal tube.
14. Auscultate for equal, bilateral breath sounds to confirm the tube is within the trachea. Secure the endotracheal tube. Check vital signs and pulse oximeter reading.

15. Order a chest radiograph to confirm the position of the endotracheal tube. See the complete discussion in Chapter 12 about confirming the location of the tube.

Be aware that nasal intubation can be difficult in some patients. It may be necessary to perform oral intubation (discussed in Chapter 12) or perform a tracheostomy to ensure a safe airway.

9. Assist with a tracheostomy procedure (Code: IIIJ4) [Difficulty: ELE: R, Ap; WRE: An]

A tracheostomy is a surgical opening in the anterior tracheal wall. The opening is usually placed below the cricoid cartilage and through the second, third, or fourth ring of tracheal cartilage (Figure 18-14, *A*). The term tracheotomy is used to describe the surgical procedure itself (the two terms are often used interchangeably).

Historically, most tracheostomy procedures were performed in the operating room under sterile conditions. When the respiratory therapist is called to assist at the bedside, it is usually because of a patient emergency. The emergency situation commonly involves an upper airway obstruction, such as that caused by facial trauma, or a surgical patient in which an endotracheal tube cannot be placed by either the oral or the nasal route. Because of time constraints, the full sterile technique may be bypassed in favor of a clean technique. The physician's preference and the situation itself dictate how the procedure is performed. The respiratory therapist also may be called to assist in the procedure when the patient is already intubated. Usually this involves an unstable patient who requires long-term mechanical ventilation. Because of the patient's critical condition, the physician makes the decision to perform the tracheostomy at the bedside rather than in the operating room. The respiratory therapist may be responsible for positioning the patient properly, providing supplemental oxygen or ventilation to the patient, monitoring the patient, obtaining the tracheostomy tube, ensuring that the cuff properly inflates and deflates, and securing the tube. In addition, the respiratory therapist or nurse will be responsible for preparing the patient, disinfecting the tracheostomy site, and setting up the sterile field around the site as well as the equipment and supplies needed for the procedure. Each hospital or physician may have a prescribed way that this is done. The general steps in the surgical tracheostomy procedure and the percutaneous dilational tracheostomy procedures are listed here:

1. Inform the patient of the procedure, and have him or her sign the medical release form.
2. Have a sedative or pain-relieving agent administered if needed.
3. If necessary, trim or shave the insertion site clear of body hair.

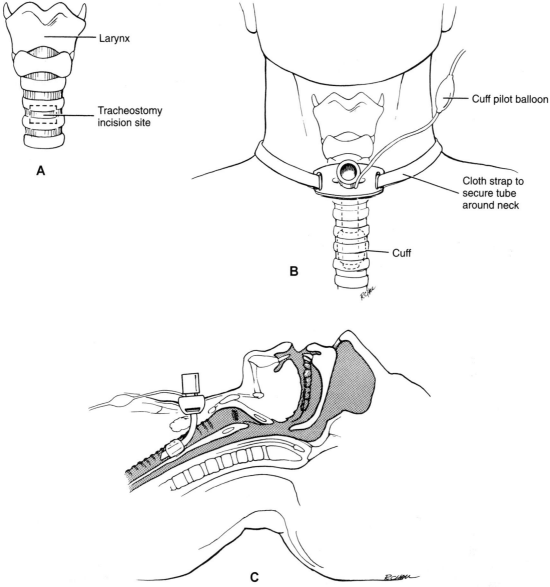

Figure 18-14   Anatomy of the larynx and insertion of a tracheostomy tube. **A,** Close-up of the larynx and the tracheostomy incision site. **B,** Anterior cut-away view of the tracheostomy tube after its insertion. **C,** Lateral cut-away view of the tracheostomy tube after its insertion. *(From Eubanks DH, Bone RC: Comprehensive respiratory care: a learning system, ed 2, St Louis, 1990, Mosby.)*

4. Put on a sterile mask, cap, gown, and gloves according to protocol.

5. Disinfect the insertion site with an iodine (Betadine) soaked sterile 4 × 4 inch gauze pad. Place the pad at the center of the insertion site, and move it in a widening spiral away from the center. This step should be repeated with a second sterile gauze pad. Let the iodine dry.

6. Protect the area around the insertion site with a sterile fenestrated surgical drape.

7. Prepare the sterile field with the tracheostomy tube, scalpel, supplies, and so forth. Have a local anesthetic such as lidocaine (Xylocaine) available in a syringe with needle. The physician injects this into the insertion site.

8. Assist the physician into his or her sterile mask, cap, gown, and gloves.

9. Get the proper size tracheostomy tube (see Table 12-1). Make sure the cuff inflates and deflates properly.

10. Assist the physician with the procedure as needed.
   - **Surgical procedure:** If the patient is already intubated, withdraw the endotracheal tube after the tracheostomy opening has been created and the physician is ready to place the tracheostomy tube into the opening.

- **Percutaneous dilational tracheostomy:** If the patient is already intubated, withdraw the endotracheal tube but keep the tip within the larynx. Temporarily adjust the ventilator settings if there is a significant leak. The physician will insert a large-gauge needle between the first and second tracheal rings to create an opening into the trachea. The physician can then select from two methods to enlarge the initial opening. In the first, a guidewire is inserted through the needle into the trachea. The needle is removed and a series of rapidly increasing diameter dilators are passed over the guidewire. In the second method, a single dilator of gradually increasing diameter is slid over the guidewire into the trachea. (Examples of the single, tapered dilators are Ciaglia Blue Rhino, Balloon Ciaglia Blue Rhino, PercuTwist, and T-Dagger.) With either method, a stoma large enough to accept the tracheostomy tube has to be created.

11. Insert the tracheostomy tube into the tracheal opening. Inflate the cuff to a safe pressure. Make any adjustments in the patient's respiratory care equipment as needed, such as modifying the oxygen percentage, changing the oxygen delivery apparatus, or adjusting the mechanical ventilator settings.

12. Auscultate for equal, bilateral breath sounds to confirm the tube is within the trachea. Secure the tracheostomy tube. Check vital signs and pulse oximeter reading.

13. Order a chest radiograph to confirm the position of the endotracheal tube.

14. Dispose of any used supplies and so forth after the procedure is completed.

15. Tend to the patient's comfort. A pain-relieving medication may be needed.

See Chapter 12 for further discussion on the indications for the various airway routes and when to routinely change a tracheostomy tube. Table 18-2 lists the common complications of a tracheostomy.

TABLE 18-2 | Common Complications of a Tracheostomy

Complication	Approximate Time of Onset
Bleeding	During and after surgery for up to 24 hr; if possible, do not replace the first tube for 2 to 3 days
Pneumothorax	During the procedure
Infection of the stoma or lungs	Usually seen after second day
Subcutaneous or mediastinal emphysema	May be seen during the procedure or at any later time

MODULE C

Exercise testing

1. Stress testing

a. Perform stress testing (e.g., ECG, pulse oximetry) (Code: IB9t) [Difficulty: ELE: R, Ap; WRE: An]

Stress testing is performed to determine a patient's limits to exercise. The limiting factor(s) to exercise provide(s) much information about a patient's medical condition. Box 18-7 lists the indications for stress testing. Before starting a stress test the patient's chart should be reviewed for information on any previous stress testing. It is important to know the type of testing that was performed, how the patient tolerated it, and what caused the patient to stop the test. Review the physician's evaluation of the test results and the patient's diagnosis.

Stress testing is the intentional exercising of the patient to the point of exhaustion or physiologic deterioration, when the test must be stopped because the patient cannot continue. Because of this, the procedure is inherently risky to the patient. It is imperative that the patient be carefully evaluated before, during, and after the procedure. An informed consent statement must be signed by the patient before beginning the test. A physician should be present during the test along with the therapist and possibly a nurse.

Despite the risks involved in the procedure, a stress test is an important diagnostic or clinical evaluation tool for many patients (Table 18-3). Box 18-8 lists the steps in

---

BOX 18-7 | **Indications for Exercise Testing**

Evaluation of nonspecific dyspnea on exertion

Evaluation of the patient's ventilatory response to increased work

Evaluation of the patient's need for supplemental oxygen

Serial testing of the patient to help in evaluating the response to therapy, medication, smoking cessation, or a rehabilitation program

To determine the presence and/or nature of ventilatory limits to exercise, such as decreased flows, increased or decreased lung volumes, and/or decreased diffusing capacity

To determine the presence and/or nature of cardiovascular limits to exercise, such as heart rate, cardiac output, arrhythmias, blood pressure, and/or angina pectoris

To determine the presence and/or nature of muscular limits to exercise such as general deconditioning or decreased local perfusion

Preoperative assessment for a lung resection or transplantation

Assessment for the degree of impairment for disability evaluation

Assessment of an apparently healthy adult more than 40 years old before starting a vigorous exercise program

TABLE 18-3 Exercise Intolerance: Differentiating between Heart Disease, Lung Disease, and Deconditioned Muscles

Parameter	Heart Disease	Lung Disease	Deconditioned Muscles
VO_{2max}	D*	D	D
Heart rate reserve	D	I	I
Breathing reserve	N	D	N
Exercise PaO_2 or SpO_2	N	D	N
VO_2 at anaerobic threshold	D	N	D
VO_2/heart rate	D	N	N
Exercise $P(A-a)O_2$	N	I	N
Exercise V_D/V_T	N	I	N
Exercise electrocardiogram	Abnormal	Normal	Normal
Common chief complaint	Chest pain	Dyspnea Bronchospasm	Leg fatigue or cramps

Based on a table in Sue D: Exercise testing and the patient with cardiopulmonary disease. In Goldman AL, editor: *Problems in pulmonary disease*, 2(1), 1986.

*Abbreviations: *D*, decreased; *I*, increased; *N*, normal.

BOX 18-8 Patient Evaluation Before Exercise Testing

History of acute or chronic illness leading to the need for stress testing

General physical exam

Resting 12-lead electrocardiogram to exclude unexpected cardiac disease

Chest x-ray

Laboratory studies for complete blood count and levels of serum electrolytes

Spirometry with measurement of flows, all lung volumes and capacities, and maximum voluntary ventilation

Carbon monoxide diffusing capacity

Pulse oximetry or arterial blood gases for PaO_2 measurement

Before and after bronchodilator spirometry studies if the patient is using an inhaled beta$_2$-adrenergic medication or has a history of exercise-induced asthma

---

BOX 18-9 Contraindications to Exercise Testing

ARTERIAL BLOOD GASES

PaO_2 less than 50 mm Hg when breathing room air

SpO_2 less than 85% when breathing room air

PULMONARY

Severe pulmonary hypertension

Recent pulmonary embolism

Untreated or unstable asthma

$FEV_{1.0}$ less than 30% of predicted

CARDIOVASCULAR

Myocardial infarction within the last 4 weeks

Dissecting thoracic or abdominal aortic aneurysm

Dissecting ventricular aneurysm

Thrombophlebitis

Systemic embolism

Uncontrolled hypertension

Unstable angina pectoris

Second-degree or third-degree heart block

Atrial arrhythmias with a rapid ventricular response

Frequent premature ventricular contractions or other life-threatening ventricular arrhythmias

Congestive heart failure with pulmonary edema

Severe aortic stenosis

Acute pericarditis

Resting diastolic blood pressure greater than 110 mm Hg or resting systolic blood pressure greater than 200 mm Hg

Neuromuscular disorders that prevent or limit the testing Orthopedic disorders that prevent or limit the testing

---

the patient work-up before testing can be safely performed. Box 18-9 lists the contraindications to exercise testing. Patients with any of these problems are too ill to be jeopardized by the procedure.

1. Commonly measured patient parameters specific to exercise testing metabolic equivalent of basal metabolic rate

A person who is sleeping or totally relaxed is consuming the minimum number of calories and the least amount of oxygen to stay alive. The minimum amount of carbon dioxide is being produced as a waste product of metabolism. He or she is said to be at basal metabolic rate (BMR). At BMR a person consumes about 3.5 mL of oxygen/kilogram of body weight/minute. Multiplying this value by the person's body weight produces the metabolic equivalent of basal metabolic rate for oxygen, or MET, as it is abbreviated. The average adult at BMR consumes about 250 mL of oxygen/minute and produces about 200 mL of carbon dioxide/minute. Obviously, the more active a person is the more calories and oxygen are consumed and the more carbon dioxide is produced. Often a person's exercise limit is quantified in terms of how many METs he or she can perform. For example, light household cleaning might be 2 METs of exercise while competitive swimming might be 8 to 10 METs of exercise.

2. Respiratory quotient and respiratory exchange ratio

Respiratory quotient (RQ) is the ratio, at the cellular level, of the amount of carbon dioxide produced in 1 minute to the amount of oxygen consumed in 1 minute. It must be readily apparent that it is impossible to directly measure the RQ because it studies cellular metabolism; however, the same gases can be easily measured in the lungs.

A metabolic study is performed to evaluate a patient's oxygen consumption in 1 minute ($\dot{V}O_2$) and carbon dioxide production in one minute ($\dot{V}CO_2$) for the assessment of a patient's metabolism at rest or during exercise, or as part of a general nutritional assessment. The bedside testing procedure is called *indirect calorimetry* and involves collecting the patient's exhaled gases to send them through a rapid O_2 analyzer and CO_2 analyzer. In a normal, healthy person the cellular metabolic processes, lung function, and cardiovascular function are working properly. As can be seen in Figure 18-15, this results in a cellular respiratory quotient (RQ) of 0.80 and a resulting respiratory exchange ratio (R) measured at the lung of 0.80. This indicates normal oxygen consumption and carbon dioxide production. The calculation is shown in the following equation.

Sick patients will often have an R value of greater than 0.80. This can be the result of the patient's diet. However, in many sick patients, the high R value is because of the inability of the lungs to remove carbon dioxide (many COPD patients) or insufficient oxygen delivery to the

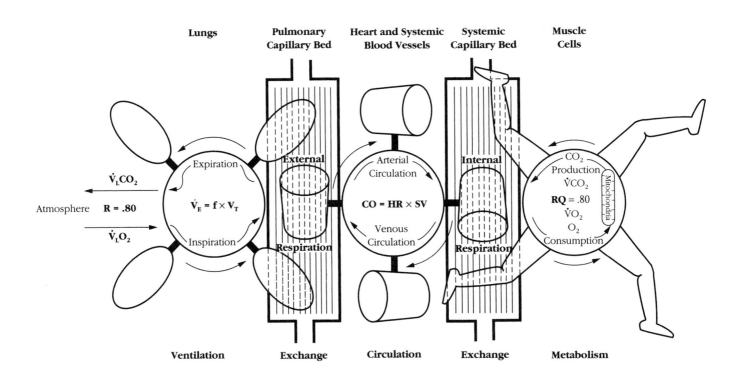

| Lungs | Pulmonary Capillary Bed | Heart and Systemic Blood Vessels | Systemic Capillary Bed | Muscle Cells |

R = Respiratory Exchange Ratio $\dot{V}_E$ = Minute Ventilation of Breathing   CO = Cardiac Output
RQ = Respiratory Quotient   f = Frequency of Breathing (Respiratory Rate)   HR = Heart Rate
                                   V_T = Tidal Volume of Breathing   SV = Stroke Volume

Figure 18-15   Representation of the interconnected relationships between the pulmonary system, the cardiovascular system, and the tissues of the body to show the processes of oxygen delivery and consumption and carbon dioxide production and exhalation. Note how the relationship of oxygen consumption and carbon dioxide production in the mitochondria of the cells results in a respiratory quotient (RQ) of 0.80 and the intake of oxygen and exhalation of carbon dioxide by the lungs result in a matching respiratory exchange ratio (R) of 0.80. This allows indirect calorimetry to be used to evaluate a patient's metabolism at rest and during exercise to assess the pulmonary system, cardiovascular system, and muscle function. *(From Madama VC: Pulmonary function testing and cardiopulmonary stress testing, ed 2, Albany, Delmar Publishers, 1998.)*

tissues. Tissue hypoxia results in anaerobic metabolism with resulting lactic acid production. This lactic acid, in turn, converts to excessive carbon dioxide. Even a healthy person can have an increased R value during heavy exercise with a stress test.

The respiratory exchange ratio (R or RER) is the ratio, at the alveolar level, of the amount of carbon dioxide produced in 1 minute to the amount of oxygen consumed in 1 minute. The volume of these two gases is determined through indirect calorimetry, as discussed previously. Using the oxygen consumption and carbon dioxide volumes discussed earlier, the R (or RQ) of a resting adult would be calculated as:

$$R = \frac{V_{CO_2}}{V_{O_2}} = \frac{200 \text{ mL } CO_2}{250 \text{ mL } O_2} = 0.80$$

The R value (and RQ) of 0.80 remains quite steady during light to moderate exercise (see Figure 18-15). A normal, healthy person can quite easily increase the amount of oxygen consumed and eliminate the extra carbon dioxide produced during exercise. This is what is seen during aerobic metabolism when all body systems are functioning smoothly. It is only during heavy exercise that the body has difficulty coping and must eventually stop.

3. Maximum oxygen consumption and maximum carbon dioxide production

The maximum oxygen consumption (V_{O_2max}) is the highest oxygen consumption attainable by a person. Men have a greater capacity for oxygen consumption than women, and both genders have a natural decline with age. The oxygen consumption at less than a maximum level is recorded as the volume in milliliters of oxygen used in 1 minute and abbreviated as V_{O_2}. The maximum carbon dioxide production (V_{CO_2max}) is the highest carbon dioxide production attainable by a person. The carbon dioxide production at less than a maximum level is recorded as the volume in milliliters of CO_2 produced in 1 minute and abbreviated as V_{CO_2}. Healthy, athletic people can increase their V_{O_2} and V_{CO_2} values by 8 to 10 times their basal metabolic rate.

4. Anaerobic threshold

Anaerobic threshold (AT) is the highest oxygen consumption during exercise, above which a sustained lactic acidosis occurs. When an exercising patient hits the anaerobic threshold, he or she will demonstrate a sudden increase in respiratory rate and tidal volume (minute volume). This is an attempt by the patient to exhale the sudden excess of carbon dioxide produced as a result of anaerobic metabolism—the inability to get enough oxygen to the exercising muscles.

If the patient's oxygen consumption and carbon dioxide production values are graphed during heavy exercise when AT is reached, it will be seen that the patient

has a respiratory exchange ratio of 1.0. This indicates equal values for both gases. An R value of 1.0 is reached in most people during heavy exercise at about 50% to 60% of the V_{O_2max}. At this exercise level insufficient oxygen reaches the muscles, resulting in the formation of lactic acid. This then converts to additional carbon dioxide until the level of CO_2 production equals (or exceeds) the level of oxygen consumption. Most healthy people can continue to exercise vigorously for a short time with an R value of 1.1 to 1.2 until they must stop. Elderly persons or patients with cardiopulmonary disease are rarely intentionally stressed to the anaerobic threshold.

5. Maximum heart rate

The maximum heart rate (HR_{max}) is the highest heart rate that a person should be able to achieve. Either of the following prediction equations for maximum heart rate in beats per minute can be used (the standard deviation for these formulas is ±10 to 15 beats/minute):

$$HR_{max} \text{ for males and females} = 210 - (0.65 \times \text{age in years})$$

or

$$HR_{max} \text{ for males and females} = 220 - (\text{age in years})$$

Because it is obviously hazardous to exercise anyone to their maximum heart rate for a prolonged time, a lower target heart rate is usually calculated. Initially, a target heart rate of 60% to 70% of maximum is often used. Later, as the patient becomes better conditioned, the target heart rate may be raised.

There are many other concepts and formulas that may be studied by the student who wishes to learn more and become more skilled in performing and interpreting stress tests.

6. Exercise equipment

Whether the patient is exercising on a treadmill or a bicycle, it is very informative to perform indirect calorimetry by analyzing the patient's exhaled gases for oxygen and carbon dioxide. There are two different types of systems for this. One utilizes a mixing chamber from which the patient's gases are periodically analyzed. The other is a breath-by-breath system that samples and analyzes each exhaled breath (see Figure 18-16). The measured patient parameters in both systems usually include the following: (a) fraction of exhaled oxygen (F_EO_2), (b) fraction of exhaled carbon dioxide (F_ECO_2), (c) respiratory rate, (d) exhaled gas temperature, (e) exhaled volume, and (f) time from the start of the test.

a. Treadmill. The treadmill is a motorized continuously looped belt combined with a ramp. The belt's speed may be adjusted from the stopped position to 1.5 to 10 miles per hour (great enough to exhaust a trained runner). The ramp may be adjusted from flat (0% grade) to sloped (30% grade) (great enough to require the patient to run to

Figure 18-16 Schematic drawing of a breath-by-breath system for gas analysis during exercise testing. Gas is taken continuously from the sampling port. The gas sample in combination with the pneumotachometer information is integrated by the computer to yield data on average mixes of sealed oxygen (F_EO_2) and carbon dioxide (F_ECO_2), respiratory rate, tidal volume, minute volume, VO_2, VCO_2, and respiratory quotient. The insert shows a single breath. During inspiration, the oxygen percentage increases and carbon dioxide percentage decreases. During expiration, the oxygen percentage decreases and carbon dioxide percentage increases. There is an unavoidable delay as the gas flows to the analyzer to determine the gas concentrations and send the data to the computer for display. The information that is displayed will still be on a breath-by-breath basis but not synchronized with the patient's real-time breathing efforts. *(From Ruppel G: Manual of pulmonary function testing, ed 9, St Louis, 2009, Mosby.)*

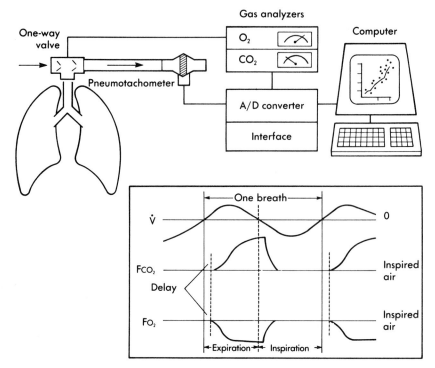

keep from falling off the back of the treadmill). There is a railing for the patient to hold if necessary. Commonly there is also an emergency button that the patient can hit to stop the unit. Adjunct equipment is nearby for monitoring the electrocardiogram, exhaled gases, and so forth (see Figure 18-17). The treadmill has an advantage over the bicycle ergometer in that it trains the patient's muscles that are needed for walking. This is an important practical consideration for most patients. However, it is more difficult to quantitate the exercise test results from a treadmill compared to a bicycle because the patient's stride and mechanics of walking vary as the speed increases.

b. Bicycle ergometer. The bicycle ergometer is a stationary bicycle with seat, handle bars, and electronics for calculating distance, effort, and so forth. The electromechanical units as shown in Figure 18-18 have electronic brakes to increase the patient's workload. Although less practical in training muscles for everyday tasks such as walking, the ergometer allows for easier workload adjustments and calculation of the exercise test results. Other exercise methods such as an arm ergometer or a rowing machine are rarely performed on patients.

7. Exercise protocols

There are a number of exercise protocols that may be followed. Basically they fall into one of the two following test categories and may be performed on either a treadmill or a bicycle ergometer.

a. Progressive multistage test. This test is designed to examine the effects of rapidly increasing workloads on the cardiopulmonary system. A steady state may or may not be reached because the goals are to trend the measured exercise parameters and find the maximum workload. The following parameters are measured: maximum oxygen consumption, maximum carbon dioxide production, maximum minute ventilation, and maximum heart rate. This is a less exhausting test than the steady state and may be repeated if necessary. This test may be used for its own purposes or to establish maximum workloads before having the patient perform the steady-state test.

Patients with known or suspected cardiac disease use a version of the progressive multistage test called the Modified Bruce Protocol. Its goal is to rapidly increase the patient's workload until a target heart rate of 85% of predicted is reached. To accomplish this, the speed and angle of the treadmill are increased every 3 minutes until the target heart rate is reached or the patient feels the need to stop.

b. Steady-state test. This test is designed to measure cardiopulmonary parameters under steady metabolic conditions. Commonly these levels are 50% and 75% of the predicted maximum oxygen consumption. The following parameters are measured: oxygen consumption, carbon dioxide production, minute ventilation, and heart rate. This is a more exhausting test than the progressive multistage test because it takes longer. It usually is not repeated the same day.

8. General steps in the procedure

1. Explain the procedure to the patient. Answer any questions. Show the patient how to stop the test in case of

Figure 18-18 An electromechanical bicycle ergometer with controls for electronic braking, pedaling resistance, test timer, meters for pedaling frequency in revolutions per minute (RPM), and external workload in watts. *(Courtesy Medical Graphics Inc., St Paul, Minn. In Ruppel G:* Manual of pulmonary function testing, *ed 5, St Louis, 1991, Mosby.)*

Figure 18-17 Exercise equipment usually consists of a treadmill *(left)* and indirect calorimeter (also called a metabolic cart *[right]*) for analysis of exhaled oxygen and carbon dioxide. The operator can control the treadmill's speed and angle of incline to vary the amount of work the patient performs. During the exercise test, the indirect calorimeter measures the patient's respiratory rate, tidal volume, and exhaled gas concentrations. *(Courtesy Medical Graphics, Inc., St Paul, Minnesota. In: Ruppel G:* Manual of pulmonary function testing, *ed 5, St Louis, 1991, Mosby.)*

an emergency. Develop a hand signal system so that the patient can approve an increase in workload (thumb up) or warn you of the need to stop the test (thumb down).

2. Set up the following monitoring equipment on the patient:
   - Electrocardiogram with chest leads placed as usual and limb leads moved to the shoulder areas and lower abdominal areas
   - Pulse oximetry monitor for SpO_2 or (rarely) arterial line for monitoring PaO_2, other blood gas values, and continuous blood pressure
   - Arm cuff and sphygmomanometer for automatic or manual blood pressure monitoring if an arterial line is not inserted
   - Mouthpiece with one-way valves or head hood to gather exhaled gases for analysis
3. Have the patient breathe normally through the system and take a set of baseline parameters. Tell the patient to warm up on the equipment by exercising at a low level (approximately 25% of VO_{2max}). Take a set of parameters. NOTE: Steps 4, 5, and 6 are for the steady-state test. With the progressive multistage test, the patient will exercise at a given level for only a few minutes before moving to a higher work level.
4. Begin the test by having the patient exercise at a predetermined moderate level (approximately 50% of VO_{2max}) for 5 to 8 minutes. Take a set of parameters in the last 1 to 2 minutes.
5. Increase the workload (approximately 75% of VO_{2max}) and have the patient exercise at this level for 5 to 8 minutes. Take a set of parameters in the last 1 to 2 minutes. Alternatively, the patient may be given a short rest period or low exercise period between the steps of increased workload.
6. Repeat step 5, if necessary, at a higher workload until the patient is exhausted or cannot continue because of one of the conditions listed in Box 18-10.
7. Have the patient exercise at a low level for several minutes during a cool down/recovery period. It is important to monitor the patient during the recovery period because a sudden drop in blood pressure and

---

BOX 18-10   Indications for Stopping an Exercise Test

ARTERIAL BLOOD GASES

PaO_2 decreasing to less than 55 mm Hg

Acidosis with or without a rise in the $PaCO_2$ level

SpO_2 less than 83% or <4% less than the baseline value

PULMONARY

Exercise-induced bronchospasm

Severe dyspnea

CARDIOVASCULAR

20 mm Hg fall in systolic blood pressure below the baseline value

Systolic blood pressure greater than 250 mm Hg

Diastolic blood pressure greater than 120 mm Hg

Onset of angina pectoris

Frequent premature ventricular contractions (PVCs)

Ventricular tachycardia

ST-segment depression or elevation of more than 1 mm

Onset of second-degree or third-degree heart block

Onset of left or right bundle branch block

EQUIPMENT

Monitoring equipment failure

Unavailability of CPR equipment and defibrillator

MISCELLANEOUS

Request by patient, light-headedness, mental confusion, or headache

Muscle cramping

Nausea or vomiting

Sweating and pallor

Cyanosis

Exercise electrocardiogram

Heart disease

Bronchospasm

Deconditioned muscles

---

fainting are known to occur if exercise should stop too quickly. Note how long it takes for the patient to return to baseline conditions.

b. Interpret the results of stress testing (e.g., ECG, pulse oximetry) (Code: IB10t) [Difficulty: ELE: R, Ap; WRE: An]

1. In a healthy person the following physiologic changes can be expected

a. Tidal volume, respiratory rate, and minute volume. All patients will find the combination of tidal volume and respiratory rate that allows the most efficient ventilation. Patients with normal, healthy lungs will increase their tidal volume to about 60% of their vital capacity. They will then increase the respiratory rate to produce the maximum ventilation possible. Patients with obstructive airways disease are flow-limited and cannot increase their respiratory rate adequately. They attempt to raise their tidal volume to increase their minute volume but must stop exercising earlier than predicted. Patients with restrictive lung disease cannot increase their tidal volume as expected. Instead, they increase their respiratory rate to raise their minute volume. They too must stop exercising earlier than predicted.

b. Heart rate, stroke volume, and cardiac output. At low and moderate workloads the stroke volume increases from about 80 mL to 110 mL in healthy adults. Increases in heart rate account for the rest of the increase in cardiac output from low to heavy exercise. The heart rate increases are almost parallel with the increases in VO_2 values (see Figure 18-19). A patient with a diseased left ventricle or heart block would be unable to increase cardiac output sufficiently when exercising and must stop earlier than predicted.

c. Oxygen consumption, carbon dioxide production, and respiratory quotient. Both oxygen consumption and carbon dioxide production will increase linearly with low and moderate exercise. The respiratory quotient will remain at approximately 0.80 or increase slightly. As the subject exercises at levels closer and closer to the VO_{2max}, the muscles are progressively starved for oxygen. This results in local anaerobic metabolism with lactic acid production. Lactic acid in turn converts to carbon dioxide. Because of this added CO_2, the respiratory center is stimulated to increase ventilation even more than expected. Eventually this fails to keep up with the increased production and the CO_2 level increases. The anaerobic threshold is identified when oxygen consumption equals carbon dioxide production and the respiratory quotient reaches 1.0.

d. Blood gases and pH. PaO_2, $PaCO_2$, and pH will remain stable in the normal ranges during low and moderate exercise. The cardiopulmonary system is able to deliver adequate oxygen to the tissues and remove sufficient carbon dioxide to keep the body functioning properly. However, at high levels of work, a lactic acid buildup occurs and a progressive metabolic acidosis is seen. This forces the patient to decrease the exercise level. Some may need to stop. Patients with cardiopulmonary disease will not be able to exercise heavily because they can provide only very limited increases of oxygen to the muscles or eliminate the extra carbon dioxide produced during even moderate exercise. Figure 18-19 shows the parameter changes seen as a healthy individual exercises from a low to a maximal level.

c. Limitations caused by abnormal physiology

Patients who are forced to stop exercising at a lower than predicted workload will probably fall into one of the fol-

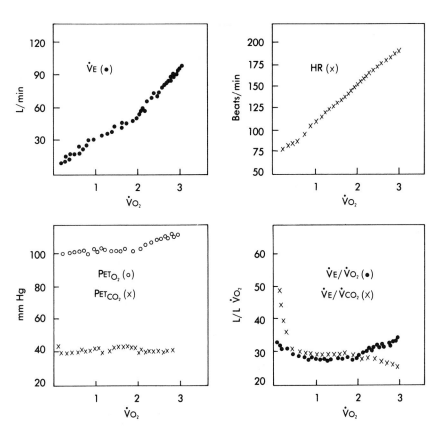

Figure 18-19   Exercise data showing 30-second averages from a normal, healthy adult subject. Heart rate increases linearly as workload is increased and is not the limiting factor in this exercise test. The other three graphic displays show that the anaerobic threshold (AT) occurs at 2 L/min of $\dot{V}O_2$. The following key points should be noted: (a) minute volume (V_E) increases sharply at AT; (b) end-tidal carbon dioxide ($P_{ET}CO_2$) and the ventilatory equivalent for carbon dioxide (V_E/VCO_2) both decrease at the AT, which shows a disproportionate increase in CO_2 production secondary to lactic acid formation; and (c) end-tidal oxygen ($P_{ET}O_2$) and the ventilatory equivalent for oxygen (V_E/VO_2) both increase at the AT. *(From Ruppel G:* Manual of pulmonary function testing, *ed 9, St Louis, 2009, Mosby.)*

lowing three broad categories. Box 18-10 lists conditions that would require that the stress test be stopped. Table 18-3 lists parameters that will help in differentiating between deconditioned muscles, pulmonary limitations, or cardiac limitations as the reason that exercise had to be stopped.

1. Deconditioned muscles

Normal, healthy people are quite commonly seen in this category. They are deconditioned from lack of exercise. These people are able to do quite well in a training program if there are no underlying cardiopulmonary limitations.

2. Pulmonary limitations

As discussed earlier, patients with obstructive airways disease or restrictive lung disease have limited ventilatory reserve. This limits their exercise tolerance even if they have a normal cardiovascular system. If the limitation is due to bronchospasm, this may be treated by inhaling a bronchodilator before exercising. These patients may also be able to increase their exercise tolerance if given supplemental oxygen to prevent desaturation.

3. Cardiovascular limitations

Patients with a damaged or diseased left ventricle, heart block, exercise-induced angina because of coronary artery disease, hypertension, and so forth are unable to exercise to expected levels. Medical or surgical intervention may enable them to increase their work level.

2. Oxygen titration

a. Perform oxygen titration with exercise (Code: IB9i) [Difficulty: ELE: R, Ap; WRE: An]

Oxygen titration with exercise involves determining the amount of supplemental oxygen needed by a patient with cardiopulmonary disease to keep the SpO_2 value at no less than 93% during an exercise period. Many of the principle considerations for this procedure are the same as those discussed during the 6-minute walk exercise discussed in Chapter 17 and earlier in this module. See Box 18-7 for the patient indications for this procedure. Patient evaluation before testing is presented in Box 18-8 and contraindications to testing are listed in Box 18-9.

The patient's history will indicate that he or she is hypoxemic at rest or becomes so during exercise. Therefore, the patient's oxygen level must be monitored, along with the vital signs and electrocardiogram, during the oxygen titration with exercise procedure. Minimally, continuous pulse oximetry must be done. However, it is preferred to have arterial blood gas samples taken at rest and during peak exercise. While single samples can be taken, it is preferable to place an arterial catheter into the radial artery. The respiratory therapist's duties will probably include monitoring the patient, changing the oxygen flow (likely by nasal cannula), and adjusting the exercise equipment.

The physician will determine the patient's exercise workload at a given oxygen flow or percentage. It is preferable to measure the workload and heart rate (as a percentage of predicted) at each supplemental oxygen level. At each workload level, make note of the patient's inspired oxygen flow or percentage, vital signs, and pulse oximeter reading. Ideally, obtain an arterial blood gas sample at the peak workload level. The overall goal of the procedure is to keep the patient's SpO_2 <93% at an increased exercise level.

b. Interpret the results of oxygen titration with exercise (Code: IB10i) [Difficulty: ELE: R, Ap; WRE: An]

When the physician or patient decides to stop the procedure there must be a record of the workload level, inspired oxygen flow or percentage, vital signs, and pulse oximeter reading. An arterial blood gas sample should be taken to send to the laboratory for analysis. Note the reason that the test was stopped. See Box 18-10 for indications to stop an exercise test.

Based on the physician's interpretation of the data, a plan will be developed so that the patient can safely exercise with a prescribed amount of supplemental oxygen. The patient will need to be instructed about the meaning of the test results, the exercise plan, and how to assess his or her response during exercise. This may be done as part of a pulmonary rehabilitation program.

MODULE D
Sleep-disordered breathing

1. Recommend sleep studies (Code: IC13) [Difficulty: ELE: R, Ap; WRE: An]

A sleep apnea study (cardiopulmonary sleep study or polysomnography) is performed to determine whether the patient has sleep-disordered breathing. Furthermore, it can help to determine the type of disorder and monitor the patient's response to treatment. Box 18-11 lists the indications for a polysomnography sleep study.

2. Review data on sleep study results (e.g., diagnosis, treatment) (WRE code: IA10) [Difficulty: WRE: R, Ap]

The following procedures are usually performed before the sleep study:

1. History of the problem from the viewpoint of both the patient and the patient's bed partner

---

> **BOX 18-11 Indications for a Cardiopulmonary Sleep Study**
>
> Patient with COPD whose awake PaO_2 is <55 torr but who has pulmonary hypertension, right heart failure (cor pulmonale), or polycythemia
>
> Patient whose awake PaO_2 is <55 torr without continuous supplemental oxygen and who must have the proper oxygen flow rate set for sleeping at night; overnight sleep ear oximetry should be performed
>
> Patient with restrictive ventilatory impairment secondary to chest wall or neuromuscular disturbances who also has chronic hypoventilation, polycythemia, pulmonary hypertension, disturbed sleep, morning headaches, or daytime somnolence and fatigue
>
> Patient with awake $PaCO_2$ <45 torr who also has polycythemia, pulmonary hypertension, disturbed sleep, morning headaches, or daytime somnolence and fatigue
>
> Patient with snoring, obesity, and other symptoms indicating disturbed sleep pattern
>
> Patient with excessive daytime sleepiness or sleep-maintenance insomnia
>
> Patient with nocturnal cyclic bradytachyarrhythmias, atrioventricular conduction abnormalities while asleep, or increased abnormal ventricular beats compared with those when awake

2. Physical examination, including neck, upper airway, blood pressure, heart rate, and respiratory rate and pattern
3. Arterial blood gas (ABG) results or pulse oximetry results
4. Hemoglobin level
5. Thyroid function
6. Chest and upper airway radiograph examinations; may include a computed axial tomographic scan of the upper airway if obstructive sleep apnea is suspected
7. ECG

The following physiologic parameters are usually measured during a polysomnography sleep study:
- Pulse oximetry for O_2 saturation. An ear or bridge-of-nose oximetry probe is recommended. Finger oximetry is not recommended because the unit may fall off during patient movement.
- Sleep stages through an electroencephalographic (EEG) recording of brain wave activity and an electro-oculographic (EOG) recording of eye movements.
- Inspiratory and expiratory airflow by nasal thermistor, pneumotachograph, or end-tidal CO_2 analyzer.
- Inspiratory and expiratory effort by respiratory inductive plethysmography. (Some may prefer to have the patient swallow a transducer to measure

esophageal pressure changes.) This is to look for paradoxical thoracoabdominal movements during obstructive apnea episodes.

- Body position related to normal and abnormal breathing patterns.
- Periodic arm and leg movements.
- ECG for monitoring heart rate and arrhythmias.

3. Initiate treatment for sleep disorders (e.g., CPAP) (WRE code: IIIK9) [Difficulty: WRE: Ap, An]

Apnea is the cessation of breathing for 10 seconds or longer. Sleep apnea is diagnosed when a patient experiences at least 30 apneic periods during 6 hours of sleep. In addition, the patient will likely have episodes of hypopnea. These harmful, and potentially fatal, problems that lead to repeated episodes of hypoxemia must be treated, as discussed in the following sections.

4. CPAP/BiPAP titration

a. Perform CPAP/BiPAP titration during sleep (Code: IB9v) [Difficulty: ELE: R, Ap; WRE: An]

b. Interpret the results of CPAP/BiPAP titration during sleep (Code: IB10v) [Difficulty: ELE: R, Ap; WRE: An]

During polysomnography, the EEG tracing should confirm that the apneic periods occur during both of the major sleep stages. The first stage is called *non–rapid eye movement* (non-REM) sleep and starts soon after the person loses consciousness. The second stage is called *rapid eye movement* (REM) sleep and follows the non-REM stage. Normally people cycle through both stages about every 1 to 1.5 hours during the night. This normal cycle of sleep is important for both mental and physical health. People with disturbed sleep do not dream as they should and are not physically rested when they awaken. Whether the patient was evaluated by overnight pulse oximetry (OPO) or polysomnography, the results lead to one of the following classifications for sleep apnea.

1. Obstructive sleep apnea

Obstructive sleep apnea (OSA) results when the patient's upper airway is obstructed despite continued breathing efforts (Figures 18-20 and 18-21). Patients with this problem often exhibit the following symptoms: loud snoring (reported by the bed partner), morning headache, excessive daytime sleepiness, depression or other personality changes, decreased intellectual ability, sexual dysfunction, bed-wetting (nocturnal enuresis), or abnormal limb movements during sleep.

Obstructive sleep apnea is associated with the following: middle-age men, obesity, short neck, hypothyroidism, testosterone administration, myotonic dystrophy, temporomandibular joint disease, narrowed upper airway from excessive pharyngeal tissue, enlarged tongue (macroglossia), enlarged tonsils or adenoids, deviated nasal

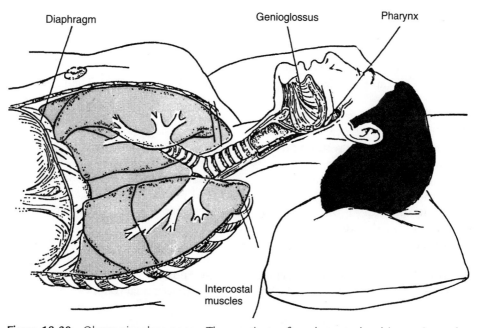

Figure 18-20 Obstructive sleep apnea. These patients often obstruct when lying supine and the genioglossus muscle of the tongue fails to oppose the negative force on the airway during an inspiration. *(From Des Jardins TL, Burton GG: Clinical manifestations of respiratory disease, ed 2, St Louis, 1990, Mosby.)*

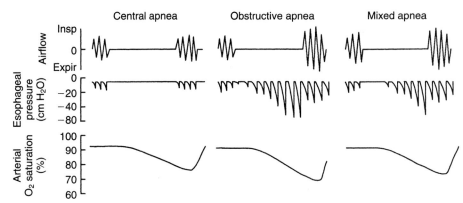

Figure 18-21 Typical patterns of airflow, esophageal pressure (or respiratory inductive plethysmography) showing respiratory effort, and arterial oxygen saturation produced by central, obstructive, and mixed sleep apnea. Central apnea shows a lack of respiratory effort resulting in no airflow. Obstructive apnea shows a continued respiratory effort but no airflow because of the airway obstruction. Mixed apnea begins with an initial lack of respiratory effort (central apnea). Later, breathing efforts are made but there is no airflow because of the airway obstruction (obstructive apnea). Arterial desaturation results from all three types of apnea. When the desaturation becomes great enough and the carbon dioxide level high enough, the patient (hopefully) awakens enough to breathe again. *(From Des Jardins TL, Burton GG: Clinical manifestations and assessment of respiratory disease, ed 5, St Louis, 2006, Mosby.)*

septum, recessed jaw (micrognathia), goiter, laryngeal stenosis or web, or pharyngeal neoplasm. Management of patients with obstructive sleep apnea may include any of the following:

- Losing weight
- Sleeping on either side or the abdomen; do not sleep in the supine position
- Wearing a continuous positive airway pressure (CPAP) mask or bilevel positive airway pressure (BiPAP) mask
- Performing surgery to open the airway: mandibular advancement, palatopharyngoplasty, or tracheostomy
- Taking protriptyline (Triptil, Vivactil) to decrease REM sleep (when most obstructive episodes occur)
- Having the patient wear a tongue-retaining device to prevent it from obstructing the pharynx
- Having the patient wear a neck collar to keep the head and neck aligned with the body

a. CPAP and BiPAP titration. CPAP and BiPAP have become essential components of the treatment plan for obstructive sleep apnea. The positive upper airway pressure generated by CPAP or BiPAP will act as a "splint" to keep the soft tissues of the upper airway from blocking the oropharynx (see Figure 18-20). Part of the CPAP or BiPAP titration process involves finding a mask or other appliance that fits the patient properly. The appliance should fit the patient's face tight enough to prevent air leaks but without causing skin irritation. See Figure 15-23 and the related discussion on CPAP and BiPAP masks.

The goal of CPAP titration is to find the proper pressure to eliminate obstructive sleep apnea episodes.

Remember that CPAP only supports the soft tissues of the oropharynx. It does not support tidal volume breathing. Before starting the CPAP titration process, the patient must be assessed, have the CPAP system put on, and fall asleep. When the respiratory therapist recognizes an apnea episode, the CPAP system is activated. The CPAP pressure is gradually increased from zero until the apnea episodes are eliminated over the sleep period. Most adults will need between 7.5 and 12.5 cm H_2O pressure of CPAP to eliminate obstructive apnea. The patient is assessed throughout the polysomnography sleep study.

BiPAP is also called bilevel ventilation because it involves using a lower pressure and a higher pressure to support the patient's breathing. The goal of BiPAP is to find the proper pressure to eliminate obstructive sleep apnea episodes and to support tidal volume breathing. As stated previously, the patient is assessed, has the BiPAP system put on, and falls asleep. During BiPAP titration, the lower pressure (known as expiratory positive pressure airway pressure [EPAP]) acts like CPAP to open the soft tissues of the airway. The higher pressure (known as inspiratory positive pressure airway pressure [IPAP]) is set to help deliver a tidal volume. When the respiratory therapist recognizes an apnea episode, the BiPAP system is activated. Both EPAP and IPAP pressures are gradually increased from zero until the apnea episodes are eliminated over the sleep period. Most adults will need between 7.5 and 12.5 cm H_2O pressure of EPAP to eliminate obstructive apnea. The IPAP pressure is then gradually increased until the tidal volume goal is reached. The patient is assessed throughout the polysomnography sleep study.

b. Interpretation of the results of CPAP or BiPAP. When the proper level of CPAP or BiPAP is determined, the following benefits should be found:

- There should be no apneic episodes.
- There should be fewer hypopneic episodes.
- There should be no paradoxical thoracoabdominal movements.
- There should be no snoring.
- The patient's sleeping pattern should return to normal.

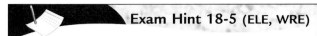

Exam Hint 18-5 (ELE, WRE)

There is often a question about the use of CPAP to treat obstructive sleep apnea.

2. Central sleep apnea

Central sleep apnea is diagnosed when the respiratory center of the medulla fails to signal the respiratory muscles for breathing to occur. The patient makes no respiratory effort, and no air movement occurs (see Figure 18-21). Patients with this problem often exhibit normal weight, mild snoring, insomnia, and lesser levels of daytime sleepiness, depression, or sexual dysfunction than found in the obstructive sleep apnea patient.

Central sleep apnea is associated with primary alveolar (idiopathic) hypoventilation (Ondine's curse), muscular dystrophy, bilateral cervical cordotomy, bulbar poliomyelitis, encephalitis, brainstem infarction or neoplasm, spinal surgery, or hypothyroidism. Management of patients with central sleep apnea may include the following:

- Negative pressure ventilation for sleeping
- Intubation or tracheostomy and positive pressure ventilation if the patient has acute ventilatory failure
- Phrenic nerve pacemaker

3. Mixed sleep apnea

Mixed sleep apnea is diagnosed when the patient shows evidence of both central and obstructive apnea. The patient usually first stops all breathing efforts (central apnea). After some time, the patient makes attempts to breathe but cannot because the upper airway is blocked (obstructive apnea) (see Figure 18-21). Patients with mixed sleep apnea may show a variety of symptoms and traits from those listed earlier. Clinical management may

include any of the treatments mentioned that prove to be effective. This includes the patient using a CPAP or BiPAP system to correct the obstructive sleep apnea.

Whatever the cause of the sleep apnea, it must be treated. If the apnea is left to continue its pathologic course, a number of problems may develop, such as pulmonary hypertension, cor pulmonale, polycythemia, cardiac arrhythmias, and even unexplained nocturnal death. At the very least, the patient's personal, family, and social life will suffer.

5. Overnight pulse oximetry

a. Perform overnight pulse oximetry (Code: IB9q) [Difficulty: ELE: R; WRE: Ap, An]

Because of the cost involved in a polysomnography study, overnight pulse oximetry (OPO) has been studied as a less expensive way to determine desaturation from sleep apnea. OPO can be performed in the patient's home or in the hospital setting. The respiratory therapist may be responsible for preparing the patient and setting up the equipment and supplies. Each hospital or physician may have a prescribed procedure. The general steps are listed here:

1. Inform the patient of the procedure, and have him or her sign the medical release form.
2. Attach the pulse oximeter, ECG leads, and other monitoring equipment to the patient.
3. Calibrate the equipment, and make sure it is working properly.
4. Record the patient's parameters during the course of a 6-hour or longer sleep period. The patient also may be recorded by videotape and audiotape during the sleep period.
5. Make any adjustments in the patient's respiratory care equipment as needed.
6. Dispose of any used supplies after the procedure is completed.
7. Tend to the patient's comfort.

b. Interpret the results of overnight pulse oximetry (Code: IB10q) [Difficulty: ELE: R; WRE: Ap, An]

Apnea is the cessation of breathing for 10 seconds or longer. Sleep apnea is diagnosed when a patient experiences at least 30 apneic periods during 6 hours of sleep. Numerous studies have shown that OPO can be used to screen patients with moderate to severe sleep apnea. These patients will have experienced at least 10 apnea episodes per hour in which their SpO_2 levels decreased at least 4% from baseline to less than 90%. In cases where the OPO results are difficult to interpret, polysomnography is needed. If the patient is found to have obstructive sleep apnea, a CPAP or BiPAP system will be needed to help correct the problem.

Exam Hint 18-6 (ELE, WRE)

Know how to differentiate between the clinical signs of obstructive and central sleep apnea. Usually a question is asked about identifying that a patient has obstructive sleep apnea. The key is to recognize that the patient will not be moving any air despite making breathing efforts. Nasal CPAP should be used to treat the patient's condition.

MODULE E
Respiratory care plan

1. Analyze the available information to determine the patient's pathophysiologic state (Code: IIIH1) [Difficulty: ELE: R, Ap; WRE: An]

See the previous topics for discussion of the patient's disease state.

2. Determine the appropriateness of the prescribed therapy and goals for the patient's pathophysiologic state (Code: IIIH3) [Difficulty: ELE: R, Ap; WRE: An]

a. Terminate the treatment or procedure based on the patient's response to therapy (Code: IIIF1) [Difficulty: ELE: R, Ap; WRE: An]

Patient safety should always be an important consideration during the treatment or procedure. Specific concerns were discussed with each of the topics in this chapter. Be prepared to stop the treatment or procedure if the patient has an adverse reaction to it. In addition, be prepared to recommend to the physician that the treatment or procedure be discontinued if it is likely to result in additional adverse reactions.

b. Recommend discontinuing the treatment or procedure based on the patient's response to therapy (Code: IIIG1i) [Difficulty: ELE: R, Ap; WRE: An]

There are typically three reasons for a patient's treatment to be discontinued. First, the patient has recovered and no longer needs the treatment or procedure. It is expensive and wasteful to perform unnecessary treatments. Second, the patient has had an adverse reaction and is likely to have an adverse reaction every time the treatment or procedure is repeated. Third, the patient's condition is terminal, and the patient or responsible family member wants all treatment to be stopped.

MODULE F
Quality assurance and quality control

1. Develop a quality improvement program (Code: IIIH6a) [Difficulty: ELE: R; WRE: Ap, An]

The broad concept of quality assurance (QA) can be viewed as a personal and departmental philosophy that ensures constant improvement in production and service. A number of ways exist to approach the subject. A key to QA is understanding what the respiratory care department should do for the patients, the physicians, the nurses, and other allied health professionals, as well as for the hospital. Once these objectives are determined, the QA program can be instituted. Minimally, the following can be done:

- Make sure that all respiratory care equipment is working properly or, if malfunctioning, is repaired.
- Audit the patient's medical records to determine if all ordered services were performed. If not, find out why.
- Communicate with patients during their hospitalization and after discharge to determine their impressions of the care they received.
- Communicate with the physicians, nurses, and so forth to assess if their needs for optimizing patient care are being met.
- Work with the hospital administration to find ways to contain unnecessary costs, expand into new areas as opportunities arise, and so forth.

2. Perform respiratory care quality assurance (Code: IIIH5) [Difficulty: ELE: R, Ap; WRE: An]

Any of the procedures or activities discussed in this chapter should be evaluated to help ensure that the best practices are being followed.

3. Record and monitor quality assurance data by using accepted statistical methods (Code: IIC8) [Difficulty: ELE: R, Ap; WRE: An]

Be able to calculate mean (average), median (middle value in a series of numbers), and mode (most common value). Consult a math book to review these calculations, if necessary.

4. Monitor the outcomes of quality improvement programs (Code: IIIH7a) [Difficulty: ELE: R; WRE: Ap, An]

Quality improvement (QI) refers to the processes used to identify areas for improvement in patient care services. QA refers to any evaluation of services provided and the results achieved as compared with accepted standards. These standards are developed through a process called benchmarking in which agreement is reached on fair and reasonable patient care criteria and outcomes. Previous chapters contain information on quality control procedures in the NBRC areas listed earlier.

5. Recheck any math work and make note of incorrect data (Code: IIIA1b2) [Difficulty: ELE: R, Ap; WRE: An]

Exam Hint 18-7 (WRE)

Usually one question deals with the general concept of quality assurance (QA). The question could relate to gathering the appropriate information to determine whether a respiratory care procedure is making a difference in patient care. For example, is a change in the aerosolized bronchodilator protocol improving patient compliance or resulting in fewer patient days in the hospital?

BIBLIOGRAPHY

AARC Clinical Practice Guideline: Fiberoptic bronchoscopy assisting, *Respir Care* 38:1173, 1993.

AARC Clinical Practice Guideline: Management of airway emergencies, *Respir Care* 40:749, 1995.

AARC Clinical Practice Guideline: Polysomnography, *Respir Care* 40:1236, 1995.

AARC Clinical Practice Guideline: Exercise testing for evaluation of hypoxemia and/or desaturation: 2001 revision & update, *Respir Care* 46: 514, 2001.

AARC: Clinical Practice Guideline: In-hospital transport of the mechanically ventilated patient: 2002 revision and update, *Respir Care* 47(6):721, 2002.

Anderson HL, Bartlett RH: Respiratory care of the surgical patient. In Burton GG, Hodgkin JE, Ward JJ, editors: *Respiratory care: a guide to clinical practice*, ed 3, Philadelphia, 1991, JB Lippincott.

Arand DL and Bonnet, Sleep-disordered breathing, in Burton GC, Hodgkin JE, and Ward JJ (eds): *Respiratory Care: A Guide to Clinical Practice*, ed 4. Philadelphia, Lippincott-Raven Publishers, 1997.

Barnes TA, editor: Core textbook of respiratory care practice, ed 2, St Louis, 1994, Mosby.

Branson RD, Hess DR, Chatburn RL, editors: *Respiratory care equipment*, ed 2, Philadelphia, 1999, Lippincott Williams & Wilkins.

Brutinel WM, Cortese DA: Fiberoptic bronchoscopy. In Burton GC, Hodgkin JE, Ward JJ, editors: *Respiratory care: a guide to clinical practice*, ed 4, Philadelphia, 1997, Lippincott-Raven.

Byhahn C, Wilke JH, Halbig S, et al: Percutaneous tracheostomy: Ciaglia Blue Rhino versus basic Ciaglia technique of percutaneous dilational tracheostomy. *Anesthesia & Analgesia*: 2000: 91: 882-886.

Cairo JM: Sleep diagnostics. In Cairo JM, Pilbeam SP, editors: *Mosby's respiratory care equipment*, ed 8, St Louis, 2009, Mosby.

Chadha TS, Schneider AW, Tobin MJ et al: Noninvasive monitoring of breathing patterns during wakefulness and sleep, *Respir Ther* 27-40, May/June 1985.

Chavis AD, Grum CM: Fiberoptic bronchoscopy with mechanical ventilation, *Choices Respir Manage* 21:4, 1991.

Chavis AD, Grum CM: Pulmonary procedures during mechanical ventilation, *Choices Respir Manage* 21:29, 1991.

Coppolo DP, Brienza LT, Pratt DS, May JJ: A role for the respiratory therapist in flexible fiberoptic bronchoscopy, *Respir Care* 30:323, 1985.

Curity thoracentesis tray package insert, Kendall Hospital Products, Boston, Mass.

Decker MJ, Smith BL, Strohl KP: Center-based vs. patient-based diagnosis and therapy of sleep- related respiratory disorders and role of the respiratory care practitioner, *Respir Care* 39(4):390-400, 1994.

Deshpande VM, Pilbeam SP, Dixon RJ: *A comprehensive review in respiratory care*, East Norwalk, Conn, 1988, Appleton & Lange.

Des Jardins TL: *Clinical manifestations and assessment of respiratory disease*, ed 5, St Louis, 2006, Mosby.

Downey III R, and Dexter JR, Assessment of sleep and breathing, in Wilkins RL, Krider SJ, and Sheldon, editors: *Clinical assessment in respiratory care*, ed 3, St. Louis, 1995, Mosby.

Epstein LJ, Dorlac GR: Cost-effectiveness analysis of nocturnal oximetry as a method of screening for sleep apnea-hypoventilation syndrome, *Chest* 113:97, 1998.

Erickson RS: Mastering the ins and outs of chest drainage: I, *Nursing* 19:37, 1989.

Erickson RS: Mastering the ins and outs of chest drainage: II, *Nursing* 19:47, 1989.

Eubanks DH, Bone RC: *Comprehensive respiratory care: a learning system*, ed 2, St Louis, 1990, Mosby.

Fischback F: *A manual of laboratory & diagnostic tests*, ed 6, Philadelphia, 2000, Lippincott Williams & Wilkins.

Garay SM: Therapeutic options for obstructive sleep apnea, *Respir Management* 17(4):11-17, 1987.

Guidelines for fiberoptic bronchoscopy, *ATS News* 12:14, 1986.

Howard TP: Foreign body extraction by means of combined rigid and flexible bronchoscopy: a case report, *Respir Care* 33:786, 1988.

Indications and standards for cardiopulmonary sleep studies, *Am Rev Respir Dis* 139:559-568, 1989.

Johnson MD: Noninvasive monitoring. In Aloan CA, Hill TV, editors: *Respiratory care of the newborn and child*, ed 2, Philadelphia, 1997, Lippincott-Raven.

Kendall Hospital Products, Curity Thoracentesis Tray (package insert), Boston, Mass.

Khoury JB, Radtke RA: Sleep assessment. In Hess DR, MacIntyre NR, Mishoe SC, et al, editors: *Respiratory care principles and practices*, Philadelphia, 2002, WB Saunders.

Kilkenny LA, Fernandes KS, Strollo PJ Jr: Disorders of sleep. In Wilkins RL, Stroller JK, Kacmarek RM, editors: *Egan's fundamentals of respiratory care*, ed 9, St Louis, 2009, Mosby.

Lewis CA, Eaton TE, Fergusson W, et al: Home overnight pulse oximetry in patients with COPD: more than one recording may be needed, *Chest* 123:1127, 2003.

Lewis RM: Airway care. In Fink JB and Hunt GE: *Clinical practice in respiratory care*, Philadelphia, 1999, Lippincott Williams & Wilkins.

Lough MD: Newborn respiratory care procedures. In Lough MD, Williams TJ, Rawson JE, editors: *Newborn respiratory care*, St Louis, 1979, Mosby.

Madama VC: *Pulmonary function testing and cardiopulmonary stress testing*, ed 2, Albany, Delmar Publishers, 1998.

Malitino EM: Strategic national stockpile: overview and ventilator assets, *Respir Care* 53:91, 2008.

Mathewson HS: Drug therapy for obstructive sleep apnea, *Respir Care* 31(8):717-719, 1986.

Mims BC: You can manage chest tubes confidently, *RN* 48:39, 1985.

Mishoe SC: The diagnosis and treatment of sleep apnea syndrome, *Respir Care* 32(3):183-201, 1987.

Muskat PC: Mass casualty chemical exposure and implications for respiratory failure, *Respir Care* 53:58, 2008.

Netzer N, Eliasson AH, Netzer C, Kristo DA: Overnight pulse oximetry for sleep-disordered breathing in adults, *Chest* 120:625-633, 2001.

Peters RM: Chest trauma. In Moser KM, Spragg RG, editors: *Respiratory emergencies*, ed 2, St Louis, 1982, Mosby.

Phillipson EA: Breathing disorders during sleep, *Basics Respir Dis* 7(3):1-6, 1979.

Plevak DJ, Ward JJ: Airway management. In Burton GC, Hodgkin JE, Ward JJ, editors: *Respiratory care: a guide to clinical practice*, ed 4, Philadelphia, 1997, Lippincott-Raven.

Podnos SD, Chappell TR: *Hemoptysis: a clinical update*, Respir Care 30(11):977-985, 1985.

Rapaport DM: Techniques for administering nasal CPAP, *Respir Management* 17(4):17-21, 1987.

Ruppel G: *Manual of Pulmonary Function Testing*, ed. 9. St. Louis, Mosby-Year Book, Inc., 2009.

Sachs S: Fiberoptic bronchoscopy. In Hess DR, MacIntyre NR, Mishoe SC, et al, editors: *Respiratory care principles and practices*, Philadelphia, 2002, WB Saunders.

Shapiro BA, Kacmarek RM, Cane RD, et al: *Clinical application of respiratory care*, ed 4, St Louis, 1991, Mosby.

Smalling T, Valente J: Examining laser surgery, *J Respir Care Pract* 11:93, 1998.

Whitaker K: *Comprehensive perinatal and pediatric respiratory care*, ed 2, Albany, NY, 1997, Delmar.

Williams SF, Thompson JM: *Respiratory disorders*, St Louis, 1990, Mosby.

SELF-STUDY QUESTIONS FOR THE ENTRY LEVEL EXAM

See page 602 for answers

1. Which of the following should the respiratory therapist evaluate to determine whether a patient's chest tube is functioning properly and removing pleural air?
   A. Fluid is present in the collection chamber.
   B. The vacuum level is set at −15 cm H_2O.
   C. Air is bubbling in the water-seal chamber.
   D. Air is bubbling in the suction control chamber.

2. Your patient is being mechanically ventilated when the nurse calls you to evaluate the patient's condition. You discover that her breath sounds are absent over the left lung field, the left-sided percussion note is hyperresonant, and peak airway pressures have increased from 40 to 65 cm H_2O. What would you recommend?
   A. Place a pleural chest tube into the right side.
   B. Increase the V_T to better inflate the atelectatic left lung.
   C. Change the mode to synchronous intermittent mechanical ventilation from assist/control.
   D. Place a pleural chest tube into the left side.

3. You notice that air is bubbling through the water seal of the patient's pleural drainage system when she coughs. This tells you that
   A. The vacuum has to be increased
   B. Air is still leaking through a tear in the lung
   C. The proper level of vacuum has been set
   D. There is a leak in the system

4. After a sleep study has been performed, your patient is given a diagnosis of obstructive sleep apnea. His physician asks for your advice on the best method of management. You would recommend that
   A. The patient should use nasal CPAP when sleeping
   B. The patient should sleep with an oropharyngeal airway to keep the tongue forward in the mouth
   C. The patient should always sleep on his back
   D. A tracheostomy should be performed, and the patient should be placed on a volume-cycled ventilator to sleep

5. An adult patient with obstructive sleep apnea and frequent pulse oximetry desaturations is fitted with a nasal CPAP system. A pressure of 7 cm H_2O is set. After the CPAP system is set up, the patient's SpO_2 value stays above 90%. How should the results be interpreted?
   A. The CPAP system has corrected the patient's problem.
   B. Greater CPAP pressure is needed.
   C. Improved gas flow is needed through the CPAP system.
   D. The delivered oxygen percentage should be increased.

6. Your mechanically ventilated patient is going to have a flexible fiberoptic bronchoscopy performed. Of what kinds of considerations must you be aware?

1. The V_T must be monitored for a leak.
2. The inspiratory flow resistance will increase.
3. The inspiratory pressure will decrease.
4. The inspiratory pressure will increase.
   A. 1, 2
   B. 3
   C. 2, 3
   D. 1, 2, 4

7. During the transport of your patient with a pneumothorax, the chest tube drainage system is pulled off of the drainage tubing and cracked open. Your best response is to
   A. Clamp the tube near the patient's chest at once
   B. Hold the distal end of the tubing a few centimeters below the surface of a bottle of sterile water or saline
   C. Leave the tube open to the atmosphere
   D. Have the patient perform the Valsalva maneuver until a new system can be set up

8. When preparing to assist the physician with the cardioversion of a patient, you must check the following:
   1. A strong R wave should be seen on the ECG monitor.
   2. The charge level should be set as ordered.
   3. The electric paddles should be kept clean for the best possible conduction.
   4. Ensure that the ECG electrodes are attached properly.
   A. 1, 3
   B. 1, 2, 4
   C. 3, 4
   D. All of the above

9. A 6-year-old patient has aspirated a tooth that was dislodged during a sporting event. The chest x-ray film shows the tooth to be lodged in the right mainstem bronchus; the neck x-ray film is normal. What would you recommend as the best way to quickly remove the tooth?
   A. Flexible fiberoptic bronchoscopy (FFB)
   B. Positive expiratory pressure breathing (PEP)
   C. Rigid tube bronchoscopy
   D. Postural drainage therapy (PDT)

10. A patient is referred for a sleep study. The attending physician wants to know which parameters are measured during the study. You would measure all of the following EXCEPT
    A. SpO₂
    B. ECG
    C. Inspiratory and expiratory breathing efforts
    D. ABG values

11. Your patient is performing an exercise test and has the following signs and symptoms: systolic blood pressure of 260 mm Hg, cyanosis, headache, and dizziness. Which of the following would you recommend?
    A. Continue the test until the patient's respiratory exchange ratio reaches 1.1.
    B. Stop the test.
    C. Continue the test until the patient complains of shortness of breath.
    D. Continue the test at a lower work level.

12. A patient is performing a stress test. Which of the following respiratory exchange ratio values would confirm that the patient has reached the anaerobic threshold?
    A. 0.8
    B. 0.9
    C. 1.0
    D. 1.1

13. You are assisting a physician with a surgical tracheostomy procedure on a patient with an oral endotracheal tube. When should you withdraw the endotracheal tube?
    A. After the tracheostomy tube has been inserted
    B. After the cuff of the tracheostomy tube has been inflated
    C. As the tip of the tracheostomy tube is placed into the stoma
    D. Before the stoma is made

14. A medical student is assigned to care for a patient with a smoking history and who is suspected of having emphysema. She asks for recommendations on what tests might be used to help determine the diagnosis. You would recommend all of the following EXCEPT
    A. Pulmonary function testing
    B. Chest radiograph
    C. Chest ultrasound
    D. Arterial blood gases

SELF-STUDY QUESTIONS FOR THE WRITTEN REGISTRY EXAM   *See page 628 for answers*

1. All the following should be done when preparing to helicopter transport an adult patient requiring mechanical ventilation EXCEPT
   A. Select a heated cascade-type humidification system
   B. Calculate the duration of the oxygen cylinder that will be used
   C. Select a ventilator that uses a demand valve IMV system rather than one with an external reservoir IMV system
   D. Select a lightweight and portable ventilator

2. A 60-year-old patient with a smoking history and recurrent bouts of left lung pneumonia has a persistent chest radiograph shadow in the left lower lobe area. Despite 2 days of postural drainage with percussion and incentive spirometry, the haziness has not cleared. What should be recommended next?
   A. Nebulize a bronchodilator medication.
   B. Perform rigid tube bronchoscopy.
   C. Perform flexible fiberoptic bronchoscopy.
   D. Nebulize hypertonic saline to induce a cough.

3. Which of the following conditions is first treated by placing a large-bore needle at the midclavicular line through the second or third intercostal space?
   A. 5% pneumothorax
   B. Pleural effusion
   C. Hemothorax
   D. Tension pneumothorax

4. A patient was found to have a $\dot{V}O_2$ value of 2000 mL and a $\dot{V}CO_2$ value of 1700 mL during an exercise test. Calculate her respiratory exchange ratio (R).
   A. 0.85
   B. 1.18
   C. 2000
   D. 3700

5. An intubated patient receiving mechanical ventilation will be transported from Chicago to Denver by an airplane with an unpressurized cabin. A pressure-cycled transport ventilator will be used. What should be monitored during the flight?
   1. Increased cuff volume
   2. Decreased tidal volume
   3. Hypoxemia
   4. Increased tidal volume
   5. Fluid retention
   A. 1, 3, 4
   B. 2, 3, 5
   C. 2, 3
   D. 1, 4

6. A mechanically ventilated patient is having a central venous line inserted by the subclavian vein route. He coughs vigorously. Within 1 minute the peak pressure on the ventilator increases significantly, and the SpO_2 value is progressively decreasing. Chest percussion demonstrates a hyperresonant sound over the right side of the chest, and breath sounds are diminished on the right side. What is the most important thing to do at this time?
   A. Complete the insertion of the central venous pressure (CVP) line.
   B. Insert a pleural chest tube on the right side.
   C. Get a chest radiograph.
   D. Compare the peak and plateau pressures on the ventilator.

7. A conscious adult patient with atrial fibrillation is being prepared for synchronous cardioversion. Which of the following should be recommended?
   1. **Administer midazolam (Versed) before starting.**
   2. **Administer flumazenil (Romazicon) before starting.**
   3. **Charge the defibrillator to 100 J.**
   4. **Charge the defibrillator to 360 J.**
   5. **Set the ECG machine to lead II.**
   6. **Have a manual resuscitator on standby.**
   A. 2, 3
   B. 1, 2, 4
   C. 1, 3, 5
   D. 1, 3, 5, 6

8. All of the following may be done by a respiratory therapist during a tracheostomy procedure EXCEPT
   A. Insert the tracheostomy tube into the new stoma
   B. Disinfect the surgical site
   C. Check for proper functioning of the tracheostomy tube
   D. Withdraw the endotracheal tube when the stoma is ready for the tracheostomy tube

9. A respiratory therapist is assisting an anesthesiologist in a direct vision nasotracheal intubation of a patient. All of the following equipment will be needed EXCEPT
   A. Magill forceps
   B. Laryngoscope handle with blade
   C. Sterile, water-soluble lubricant
   D. Lubricated hard stylet

10. Calculate the maximum heart rate for a 55-year-old woman who is about to undergo a stress test.
    A. 55 beats/minute
    B. 174 beats/minute
    C. 265 beats/minute
    D. 275 beats/minute

11. What would be expected of a patient's ventilation efforts during light exercise that progresses to moderate exercise?

A. It decreases as $\dot{V}O_2$ increases.

B. It decreases as carbon dioxide production increases.

C. It increases as workload levels increase.

D. It remains constant in normal subjects as workload levels increase.

12. While performing a sleep study the respiratory therapist noticed the following information: the respiratory inductive plethysmography reading indicates chest and abdominal movement, the nasal thermistor shows no air movement, and the patient's pulse oximeter value drops to 85%. After 35 seconds the patient snores loudly, rolls on his side, and resumes normal breathing. What best describes the patient's problem?

A. Central sleep apnea

B. Airway obstruction

C. Cheyne-Stokes respiration

D. Hyperventilation

13. You are assisting in performing a thoracentesis of a mechanically ventilated patient. She cannot sit up on the edge of the bed because of weakness. You would recommend the following position for the procedure:

A. Lying with the abnormal side down on the bed

B. Lying face down on the bed

C. Supine on the bed with the head down 30 degrees

D. Lying with the normal side down on the bed

14. After assisting with a thoracentesis where 1400 mL of straw-colored yellow fluid was removed, the patient complains of shortness of breath and has increased heart and respiratory rates. What would you recommend to further evaluate the patient's reaction to the procedure?

1. **Measuring pulse oximetry value**

2. **Obtaining a chest x-ray**

3. **Sending the fluid to the laboratory for analysis**

4. **Removing additional fluid**

A. 1

B. 1, 2

C. 3

D. 3, 4

15. You are about to assist in the bronchoscopy of a patient with COPD and suspected lung cancer. She is quite nervous before the procedure and conscious sedation will be done. All of the following drugs could be used to help in managing her sedation EXCEPT

A. Diazepam (Valium)

B. Fluticasone (Flovent)

C. Flumazenil (Romazicon)

D. Midazolam (Versed)

Answer Key for the Entry Level Exam Self-study Questions

For specific page cross-references for each answer, refer to the Evolve site.

Chapter One: ANSWER KEY FOR THE ENTRY LEVEL EXAM SELF-STUDY QUESTIONS

1. **C.** From a legal point of view, a charting error should never be obliterated. Simply correct and initial the correct information. Only the person making the error should correct it.
2. **C.** Bronchial breath sounds are not normal in the right lower lobe and indicate consolidation of the alveoli. Neither pneumothorax nor pleural effusion can be identified by bronchial breath sounds.
3. **B.** Never give an overdose of a medication. Personally contact the physician to clarify the error. (Rarely, a larger than usual dose of medication is given under special circumstances. The physician must make it clear that he or she is aware of the large dose and wants it delivered.)
4. **D.** The patient's history of injury and crepitus indicates air under the skin. The air under her skin would have to come from a lung tear.
5. **A.** All of the patient's symptoms point to a bacterial pneumonia problem. The other options may have some but not all of the noted symptoms.
6. **C.** The patient is reacting with anger to his diagnosis of cancer. He should be evaluated for emotional state. The other problems should not cause anger.
7. **A.** The correct two questions relate to the patient's level of consciousness and understanding. The first question relates to the patient's understanding of *time*. The third question relates to the patient's understanding of *place*. The fifth question relates to the patient's understanding of *person*.
8. **C.** Orthopnea relates to the patient's inability to lie down and breathe comfortably. Extra pillows are needed to raise the head and body. The other questions relate to other areas of assessment.
9. **A.** An infant's chest is basically round in dimension.
10. **B.** Diminished breath sounds mean that less air than normal is entering an area. A tracheal shift to the side of the diminished breath sound indicates less air in the lung. Both of these point to atelectasis.
11. **B.** Left-sided pneumonia and pneumothorax both result in decreased movement on that side. Emphysema and congestive heart failure would not cause a one-sided change in movement. Right-sided pneumonia would result in less movement on the right side.
12. **C.** Inspiratory stridor is the only listed breath sound that can be heard with the unaided ear. It is a respiratory emergency.
13. **D.** Only Cheyne-Stokes respiration fits the description.
14. **B.** The high air pressure found with a tension pneumothorax causes the mediastinal contents to be shifted to the opposite side and the diaphragm on the affected side to be depressed. These drastic changes can cause the patient's vital signs to deteriorate rapidly.
15. **A.** A pleural friction rub is identified as a localized area of abnormal grating breath sound; it is often localized to an area of pain on breathing.
16. **B.** Fluid overload causes the jugular veins to be distended. Dehydration may result in the jugular veins being flat. Emphysema and hypertension should not have any effect on the jugular veins.
17. **C.** Tactile fremitus would be reduced in pneumothorax and COPD because the lung is overinflated. A pleural effusion would block and decrease the sounds coming from the lung.
18. **C.** It is appropriate to ask about advance directives, such as a DNR order, for a patient with a fatal illness. Eating and bowel habits are not essential to know at this time. He will be given new orders for medications during his stay in the hospital, so it does not matter if he brought his medications with him.
19. **A.** It is important to assess the patient's level of pain from the broken ankle. Severe pain should be managed with increased medication. The other issues are less important to assess unless there is an apparent problem.
20. **B.** All listed conditions except bilateral lower lobe pneumonia would shift the mediastinum. Because bilateral lower lobe pneumonia affects both lungs, the mediastinum would stay centered properly.
21. **A.** It is most likely that a patient with respiratory distress would show an *increased* respiratory rate.

Chapter Two: ANSWER KEY FOR THE ENTRY LEVEL EXAM SELF-STUDY QUESTIONS

1. **B.** A glutaraldehyde solution soak for 10 hours is the only way listed to sterilize plastic equipment without damaging it. Putting plastic equipment into a steam autoclave causes it to melt and be destroyed. Pasteurization or soaking the equipment in an alcohol solution disinfects but does not sterilize the equipment as needed.

2. **A.** A hot water wash with detergent will remove secretions and other debris from the equipment. Soaking the equipment in white vinegar (acetic acid) will kill many of the microorganisms commonly found on home care equipment. The heat generated in an oven under the broiler will melt plastic used in a small-volume nebulizer and other respiratory care equipment. Rinsing the equipment in salt water will not make a significant difference in killing microorganisms. In addition, the dried salt crystals may plug up the capillary tube of a nebulizer.

3. **D.** Steam autoclaving is the only method listed that is acceptable for sterilizing the bacteria filter of a ventilator. Glutaraldehyde solutions will damage the filter medium and will make the filter useless.

4. **C.** The equipment must be resterilized because living spores of *Bacillus subtilis* indicate that the sterilization process was not successful. Other microbes also may have survived. Because of this concern, the equipment should not be used. Aeration of the equipment will not sterilize it, and 70% alcohol will not remove the spores from the equipment or sterilize it.

5. **A.** Acetic acid is found in white vinegar. It is inexpensive and available in any grocery store. Realize that acetic acid is not a powerful disinfectant and does not kill most pulmonary pathogens. Acid glutaraldehyde and ethylene oxide systems are too expensive to use in a home. Warm, soapy water can be used to clean secretions from equipment but does not disinfect it.

6. **C.** Pasteurization is the least expensive way to disinfect large amounts of the plastic equipment used in respiratory care departments. Steam autoclave and dry heat are used to sterilize, not disinfect, equipment. In addition, the high temperatures used with these methods melt the plastic tubing and oxygen masks. Seventy percent ethyl alcohol is used only to wipe off the surfaces of large equipment items for disinfection.

7. **B.** Ethylene oxide gas should be used on an IPPB machine because it sterilizes the unit without causing any damage. Pasteurization and glutaraldehyde involve solutions that damage the internal structures of any IPPB machine. The heat of steam autoclaving melts any plastic or rubber components of the unit and seriously damages the machine.

8. **D.** It is recommended that patients with cardiopulmonary conditions, like COPD, get an influenza vaccination each fall. In patients with preexisting conditions, the flu can be a very serious illness. Routine vaccination is also recommended for those older than 50 years of age. The flu is a seasonal problem through the fall and winter months. So, the vaccination should be given in September or October. There is no indication that the patient has been exposed to tuberculosis or has a throat infection.

Chapter Three: ANSWER KEY FOR THE ENTRY LEVEL EXAM SELF-STUDY QUESTIONS

1. **B.** A modified Allen's test is used to determine whether adequate perfusion exists through the ulnar artery in case the radial artery should become occluded. This would ensure that the hand is still well perfused. The Allen's test is used to determine adequate perfusion through the radial artery. Adequate arm blood pressure does not ensure adequate perfusion of the hand, should the radial artery become blocked. The $P(A-a)O_2$ test does not measure local perfusion.

2. **A.** Blood gas analysis through a CO-oximeter gives the most accurate results in that the unit can detect COHb. The other three choices cannot measure COHb level. Additionally, pulse oximetry and $PtcO_2$ monitoring do not give CO_2 or pH values.

3. **C.** The described test and its results are of a positive modified Allen's test. This positive result means that the patient has adequate ulnar circulation.

4. **C.** When a blood sample is not quickly cooled in ice-water, the living tissue will continue to consume O_2 and produce CO_2. The increased CO_2 level will decrease the pH value.

5. **D.** All of the listed conditions would warrant a blood gas analysis because they all deal with significant oxygenation and/or CO_2 removal issues.

6. **A.** Standard Precautions necessitate that gloves be worn on both hands when blood may be contacted by either hand. Additionally, the eyes should be protected from possible blood splashes.

7. **B.** Review Table 3-3 on page 87 for the categories of hypoxemia.

8. **B.** Shapiro and associates (1994) have stated that an acute rise in CO_2 of 20 mm Hg results in a drop in pH of 0.10 unit. So, an acute rise in CO_2 of 10 mm Hg would result in a drop in pH of 0.05 unit.

9. **D.** A PaO_2 value of less than 80 torr is uncorrected hypoxemia. A compensated respiratory acidosis is indicated by the increased $PaCO_2$ value coupled with an increased bicarbonate level and increased base excess found with a normal pH. (Review Table 3-2 on page 87 and Table 3-8 on page 90.)

10. **B.** A PaO_2 value greater than 80 torr with supplemental O_2 is corrected hypoxemia. An uncompensated metabolic acidosis is indicated by the normal $PaCO_2$ value coupled with decreased bicarbonate concentration and decreased base excess found with an acidotic pH. (Review Table 3-2 on page 87 and Table 3-8 on page 90.)

11. **C.** Normal oxygenation is indicated because the patient's PaO_2 level is elevated as a result of hyperventilation ($PaCO_2$ value of 20 torr). An uncompensated respiratory alkalosis is indicated by the low $PaCO_2$ value coupled with normal bicarbonate concentration and normal base excess found with an alkalotic pH. (Review Table 3-2 on page 87 and Table 3-8 on page 90.)

12. **A.** A PaO_2 level of less than 80 torr is uncorrected hypoxemia. A combined metabolic and respiratory acidosis is indicated by the increased $PaCO_2$ value coupled with decreased bicarbonate level and decreased base excess found with an acidotic pH. (Review Table 3-2 on page 87 and Table 3-8 on page 90.)

13. **C.** A PaO_2 value of less than 80 torr is uncorrected hypoxemia. A compensated respiratory alkalosis is indicated by the decreased $PaCO_2$ value coupled with decreased bicarbonate concentration and decreased base excess found with a normal pH. (Review Table 3-2 on page 87 and Table 3-8 on page 90.)

14. **C.** An $S\bar{v}O_2$ value of 75% is normal and correlates with normal tissue oxygenation. A $P\bar{v}O_2$ value of 30 torr indicates tissue hypoxia. Normal ABG values do not necessarily correspond to normal tissue oxygenation values. (See Table 3-11 on page 91.)

15. **B.** Two SDs are considered "in control" with a blood gas analyzer. (See Figure 3-8 on page 90.)

16. **C.** The patient's $PaCO_2$ value best correlates with her ventilatory status and level of fatigue. The other tests are of value but give less direct evidence of her ability to breathe effectively.

17. **B.** The results of an ABG measurement inform you of the patient's oxygenation status and $PaCO_2$ level. Pulse oximetry gives information only on oxygenation status. Pulmonary function tests do not give any information on the patient's PaO_2 and $PaCO_2$ levels. Additionally, a full set of pulmonary function tests can be very tiring for the patient.

18. **B.** Some pulse oximeters obtain inaccurate readings through the skin of darkly pigmented patients. Blocking outside light with an opaque wrap or moving the probe to a lightly pigmented area such as a fingertip (without nail polish) often results in accurate readings. (See Table 3-12 on page 94.)

19. **C.** The patient's approximate $PaCO_2$ value of 54 torr is found by dividing the $PtcCO_2$ value of 63 torr by the correlation factor of 1.4. (See page 100 for an example calculation.)

20. **B.** The patient's PAO_2 value (pressure of alveolar oxygen) can be calculated as follows:

$$PAO_2 = ([P_B - P_{H_2O}]F_IO_2) - \frac{PaCO_2}{0.8}$$
$$= ([750 - 54]0.5) - \frac{36}{0.8}$$
$$= ([696]0.5) - 45$$
$$= (348) - 45$$
$$= 303 \text{ torr}$$

21. **B.** The patient's $P(A-a)O_2$ value (difference between alveolar pressure and arterial pressure of oxygen) can be calculated as follows:

$$\text{The patient's } PAO_2 = 303 \text{ torr}$$

$$\text{The patient's } PaO_2 = -\frac{-60 \text{ torr}}{243 \text{ torr}}$$

22. **D.** The normal $P(A-a)O_2$ difference should be no more than 25 torr for a healthy person of this age. The patient's difference of 243 torr is far greater than normal. No indication is found that the blood gas analyzer needs recalibration. If a normal person was breathing 50% oxygen, the PaO_2 value would be much higher (about 275 torr) than this patient's PaO_2 value. The difference is much larger than normal for a patient of this age. (See Figure 3-17 on page 101.)

Chapter Four: ANSWER KEY FOR THE ENTRY LEVEL EXAM SELF-STUDY QUESTIONS

1. **D.** The MEP test is a measure of expiratory muscle strength. A value of +40 cm H_2O usually indicates enough strength for spontaneous breathing and the ability to cough effectively. The pressure should be sustained for a short time to ensure that the measurement is accurate.

2. **C.** African Americans have been shown to have an FVC that is 10% to 15% less than age- and height-matched Caucasians. Review the FVC discussion.

3. **D.** Review Figure 4-14 for volumes and capacities.

4. **A.** Flow at the midpoint of expiration normally is less than flow at the midpoint of inspiration, because the small airways are beginning to close at the halfway point of an expiratory effort. A flow-volume loop test cannot measure lung diffusion or RV to calculate the FRC.

5. **D.** A progressively declining VC and MIP indicate that the patient is getting weaker and her condition is getting worse. If her condition were improving, these tests would show increasing values. It is up to the respiratory therapist to ensure that the patient is performing the tests properly. If done properly, the test results will be valid. The MIP test is not used to help in the diagnosis of asthma, because it measures strength, not flow.

6. **C.** A differential-pressure pneumotachometer is portable enough to be taken to a patient's bedside. It can be used to determine a patient's tidal volume, FVC, and peak flow. A Stead-Wells water-seal spirometer is not typically moved, because it is large, and the water will be splashed about while it is moving. The device can be used for all three listed tests when done in the pulmonary function laboratory. A maximum inspiratory pressure manometer is used for the maximum inspiratory pressure (MIP) test. It may be reconfigured for a maximum expiratory pressure (MEP) test but cannot measure any gas flows. A body plethysmograph is far too large to move to a patient's bedside. However, it can be used for all three listed tests when they are done in the pulmonary function laboratory.

7. **C.** CO_2 buildup is not a problem with the FVC test, because the patient does not rebreathe his or her own gas for very long. A gas analyzer and kymograph are not used with an FVC test.

8. **A.** A bronchoprovocation study would be the best test for a patient with an unclear history or signs and symptoms of asthma. If the patient has any airway hypersensitivity, this test will cause a measurable decrease in expiratory flow. The other three tests can be used in the diagnosis of asthma but are not as specific to asthma as a bronchoprovocation study.

9. **C.** Emphysema is the only condition listed in which the CL would be increased. Normal compliance is 0.1 L (100 mL)/cm H_2O.

10. **A.** Review the calculation on page 112.

11. **C.** It has been determined that blowing out from TLC results in the greatest expiratory force. This is the recommended procedure.

12. **C.** V_T is estimated as 3 to 4 mL/lb (or 7 to 9 mL/kg) of ideal body weight, which results in a range of about 300 to 400 mL.

13. **B.** Alveolar ventilation is estimated by subtracting the patient's ideal body weight in pounds (170) from the V_T (580 mL).

14. **D.** The patient exhaled a normal percentage of his or her VC in 1 second. The other conditions would all result in a low value. Review the normal values discussed earlier in the chapter.

15. **B.** The FVC is the largest capacity that can be measured by spirometry.

16. **A.** The V_T would be seen as the repeated smallest volumes.

17. **D.** The VC is made up of these three volumes.

18. **B.** PF is directly related to height and indirectly related to age. When done properly, the PF will be seen at the start of an FVC effort, because that is when air is emptied from the upper airway.

19. **D.** Inconsistent high and low pressures are most likely the result of inconsistent effort. A leak would result in a consistently low value. A patient should have a consistent value starting from either the RV or the FRC.

20. **A.** Review the calculation on page 121.

Chapter Five: ANSWER KEY FOR THE ENTRY LEVEL EXAM SELF-STUDY QUESTIONS

1. **A.** The pulmonary artery catheter first enters the right atrium (RA) of the heart. It then follows the flow of blood through the heart by entering the right ventricle (RV). Next the catheter enters the pulmonary artery and the pulmonary artery pressure (PAP) is recorded. When the balloon at the tip of the catheter advances as far into the pulmonary artery as it can, it "wedges" in place. The resulting pressure is the called the pulmonary capillary wedge pressure (PCWP).

2. **C.** Stroke volume is the blood volume pumped by each ventricle with each heartbeat and has a range of 50 to 120 mL in the adult. Cardiac index (CI) is an indicator of the adequacy of perfusion of the body's tissues. Cardiac output (CO) is the output of blood for 1 minute. Afterload is the resistance to flow. It is caused by the level of tone in the blood vessels and the viscosity of the blood. (See Box 5-2 on page 160.)

3. **C.** This problem requires the calculation of the decimal fraction or percentage of dead space. To do so, place both the patient's arterial and end-tidal carbon dioxide values into this formula:

$$V_D/V_T = \frac{(Pa_{CO_2} - P_{\bar{E}CO_2})}{Pa_{CO_2}}$$

In which:

V_D/V_T or V_D = The patient's physiologic dead space

Pa_{CO_2} = The patient's arterial carbon dioxide pressure

$P_{\bar{E}CO_2}$ = The patient's average exhaled carbon
dioxide pressure

Calculate the V_D/V_T as follows:

$$V_D/V_T = \frac{(53-20)}{53}$$
$$= \frac{33}{53} = 0.62$$

The patient's V_D/V_T or V_D fraction can be recorded as 0.62 or 62%. (Note that this equation must be used when the patient's tidal volume is not known.)

4. **B.** This problem requires the calculation of the patient's dead space volume. To do so, place both the patient's arterial and end-tidal carbon dioxide values into this formula:

$$V_D = \frac{(Pa_{CO_2} - P_{\bar{E}CO_2})}{Pa_{CO_2}} \times \dot{V}_E$$

In which:

V_D = The patient's physiologic dead space

$\dot{V}_E$ = Average exhaled tidal volume

Pa_{CO_2} = The patient's arterial carbon dioxide pressure

$P_{\bar{E}CO_2}$ = The patient's average exhaled carbon
dioxide pressure

Calculate the V_D as follows:

$$V_D = \frac{(43-22)}{43}$$
$$= \frac{21}{43} \times 650 = .49 \times 650 \text{ mL} = 319 \text{ mL}$$

The patient's physiologic V_D volume equals 319 mL. (Note that this equation must be used when the patient's tidal volume is known.)

5. **A.** A normal adult's systemic vascular resistance (SVR) has a range of 900 to 1400 dynes/sec/cm^{-5}. This patient's SVR value of 600 dynes/sec/cm^{-5} is well below normal. This may result from vasodilation or hypovolemia. All of the other values are within normal range. (See Box 5-2 on page 160.)

6. **B.** If excessive fluid is given to a patient with congestive heart failure, the fluid is likely to accumulate in the pulmonary vessels because the left ventricle cannot pump effectively. This backup of fluid into the lungs will increase the pulmonary capillary wedge pressure. The patient should be monitored for pulmonary edema. If the patient develops pulmonary edema, a chest radiograph will show increased, rather than decreased, lung markings and fluid in the lungs. The patient's Pa_{O_2} level can be expected to decrease rather than increase if pulmonary edema develops. If fluid builds up from the left ventricle into the pulmonary vessels, the pulmonary artery pressure will increase along with the pulmonary capillary wedge pressure.

7. **D.** The patient's history and current situation suggest that a pulmonary embolism has developed. The V_D/V_T test should be performed to determine whether the patient's dead space has increased. If it has, this will match the clinical suspicion of a pulmonary embolism. It is doubtful that the patient's lung compliance will change if a pulmonary embolism occurred. There is no specific change in the electrocardiogram that corresponds with a pulmonary embolism or other sudden cause of shortness of breath. Chest radiograph changes are unlikely soon after a pulmonary embolism has occurred.

8. **A.** A capnograph is zero calibrated on room air because it contains only a trace of carbon dioxide. A capnograph cannot measure oxygen percentage or anesthetic gases. Either 5% or 10% carbon dioxide is often used for the second point (high point) in two-point calibration of the capnograph.

9. **A.** A PCWP level of 2 mm Hg is very low. (See Box 5-2 on page 160.)

10. **B.** The normal PAP level is about 25/10 mm Hg. The normal PCWP value is about 8 mm Hg. A PAP value of 30/15 mm Hg would be elevated. Normal arterial blood pressure is about 120/80 mm Hg. (Review the values in Box 5-2 on page 160.)

11. **C.** Infrared absorption is the main operating principle for bedside capnography units.

12. **D.** The difference between the PAP diastolic pressure of 12 mm Hg and the PCWP pressure of 8 mm Hg is 4 mm Hg.

13. **D.** The patient's estimated $PaCO_2$ value is 34 torr. It is found by adding the $PetCO_2$ value of 30 torr and the $P(a-et)CO_2$ gradient value of 4 torr. Review the math examples in the chapter, if necessary.

14. **B.** Patients with COPD have significant ventilation-to-perfusion mismatches. This results in increased dead space ventilation and shuntlike effects. The COPD patient would not be expected to have normal or decreased dead space.

15. **C.** An $S\bar{v}O_2$ level of 75% would be normal and indicate normal tissue oxygenation. Values of less than 75% saturation would indicate tissue hypoxia. A saturation of 90% is far higher than that needed in venous blood.

16. **B.** When ventilation and perfusion match well, as in a normal person, the gradient between the arterial carbon dioxide level and the exhaled carbon dioxide level is 2 to 3 torr with a range between 1 and 5 torr. A carbon dioxide level of less than this would indicate either no alveolar ventilation or no production of CO_2. Gradients of greater than 5 torr have been found in patients with significant ventilation/perfusion mismatching.

17. **A.** The patient's blood pressure of 115/78 mm Hg is within normal limits for an adult. Blood pressure cannot be used as an indicator of an intracranial bleed. (See Box 5-2 (Page 160) and review Chapter 1, if necessary.)

Chapter Six: ANSWER KEY FOR THE ENTRY LEVEL EXAM SELF-STUDY QUESTIONS

1. **A.** See the sample H-tank duration calculation given earlier in the chapter. Common errors include using the E-tank factor and failing to convert from minutes to hours by dividing by 60.

2. **B.** A patient with COPD who is hypercarbic and is breathing on hypoxic drive should be given supplemental O_2 with great care. Too much O_2 will result in too high an arterial O_2 level and will blunt the hypoxic drive. Hypoventilation will result in a rising CO_2 level. Pulmonary edema from O_2 toxicity would necessitate a high percentage of O_2 for an extended period. ROP is seen only in premature infants. Hyperventilation is not caused by breathing of supplemental O_2.

3. **A.** An oxygen tent will provide 35% oxygen to an alert 2-year-old patient without restricting normal movement. It is doubtful that an alert, active 2-year-old will keep either a nasal cannula or a simple mask in place as needed. In addition, the actual oxygen percentage cannot be measured through these devices. This child is too large for an incubator.

4. **D.** The reservoir tubing holds O_2 from which the patient can inspire. Losing the reservoir results in inhalation of room air and a decrease in the overall O_2 percentage. When set up properly, any exhaled CO_2 is blown clear from the reservoir tubing before the next inspiration.

5. **C.** No known condition of O_2-induced hyperventilation exists. Do not confuse this with O_2-induced hypoventilation, which needs to be monitored in some patients with COPD. See the rationale for Question 2.

6. **D.** Because the face tent is open on top and O_2 is heavier than room air, the O_2 in the face tent tends to "pour" out if the patient lies supine. When all is set up properly, CO_2 should not build up in a face tent, no matter the patient's position. A face tent should not influence a patient's V_T. Lying supine may result in decreased V_T.

7. **B.** The three listed items are all important for minimizing hypoxemia during a treatment or procedure. Increasing the O_2 by 20% will help to minimize hypoxemia, but it is appropriate to raise the percentage much higher.

8. **A.** Running two flowmeters at flush would put too much O_2 into the tent and probably would raise the percentage to a far greater extent than ordered. In addition, the noise level would be high, which could be harmful to the child's hearing. Closing any source of leaks would help keep the O_2 level stable. The analyzer may be malfunctioning and may be reporting a low value.

9. **D.** When properly operating, a partial-rebreathing mask's reservoir bag should not collapse during inspiration. Raise the O_2 flow so that the bag stays at least two-thirds full during inspiration. Hypoxic patients usually breathe in at whatever pattern and rate is most

efficient for them. It may be counterproductive to try to have the patient breathe differently. A nasal cannula cannot deliver as high an O_2 percentage as can be delivered by the partial-rebreathing mask.

10. **B.** The reservoir membrane is defective, so the cannula should be replaced. The O_2 flow should not be increased because this would give the patient more O_2 than is intended. Decreasing (or increasing) the O_2 flow will not unstick a defective reservoir membrane. Changing to an air entrainment mask would be a possible remedy if a replacement cannula did not exist.

11. **B.** An air entrainment mask (high-flow delivery system) is designed to provide enough flow of the prescribed O_2 percentage (fixed concentration) at any patient rate, V_T, and so forth. The other three devices do not provide enough flow to deliver a consistent, known O_2 percentage.

12. **A.** A properly fitting nonrebreathing mask with enough flow to keep the reservoir bag inflated will deliver the highest O_2 percentage of all available devices.

13. **C.** A Bourdon flowmeter is the only unit that will accurately indicate the flow when it is laid horizontally. The others read accurately only in a vertical position.

14. **D.** Review the information on pinholes in Table 6-3 on page 201.

15. **B.** Review the sample E-tank duration calculation in this chapter. Common errors include using the H-tank factor and failure to convert from minutes to hours by dividing by 60.

16. **C.** Covering the air entrainment ports on an air entrainment mask will result in the patient's receiving a higher O_2 percentage than is desired. In addition, the total flow will be decreased.

17. **D.** Because a major obstruction exists in the transtracheal oxygen catheter, it should be replaced, but first the patient must switch her oxygen delivery system to a nasal cannula. Attempts to force out the obstruction by doubling the oxygen flow or forcing the saline or cleaning rod through the catheter can result in injury to the trachea.

18. **D.** The patient's current blood gases show unacceptable hypoxemia with a PaO_2 of 47 torr and an SaO_2 of 80%. Increasing the patient from 2 to 3 L/min through the transtracheal oxygen catheter should help to correct the situation. The patient should be monitored for a possible increasing carbon dioxide level as well as an improving oxygen level. Changing the patient to 24% oxygen by an air entrainment mask probably will not change his actual inspired oxygen percentage. In addition, no indication that the transtracheal oxygen catheter has failed is reported. The patient's ventilation is stable, with no indication that bilevel mask ventilation is needed. Changing the patient to a nonrebreathing mask with 10 L/min of oxygen is potentially dangerous. This much oxygen may blunt his hypoxic drive to breathe.

19. **A.** Adding 100 mL of aerosol tubing as a reservoir will help to maintain the patient's inspired O_2 percentage. No clear reason exists for changing the patient's O_2 percentage by protocol, and no physician order exists to do so. Changing the flow probably will not stabilize the patient's O_2 percentage without the added reservoir tubing. A comatose patient will not follow instructions to "not breathe so deeply."

20. **D.** A high-flow nasal cannula should be able to provide enough oxygen to the patient to correct her hypoxemia. In addition, she should keep it on because it will not make her feel claustrophobic. A traditional nasal cannula is not run at over 6 L/min of oxygen. It could be dangerous to sedate a hypoxic patient. It is likely that the CPAP mask also will make her feel claustrophobic.

21. **C.** A nonrebreather mask with reservoir bag is the best way to deliver heliox because it will provide for all of the patient's inspiratory flow needs. A partial-rebreather mask with reservoir bag is not a sealed system. Room air will be entrained, which will reduce the patient's helium and oxygen percentages. A high-flow nasal cannula is designed to provide oxygen, not heliox mixes. There is no indication at this time that mechanical ventilation is needed. In addition, several technical challenges are associated with providing heliox through most mechanical ventilators.

Chapter Seven: ANSWER KEY FOR THE ENTRY LEVEL EXAM SELF-STUDY QUESTIONS

1. **C.** Switching the patient from a flow displacement to a volume displacement incentive spirometer lets her see the results of her breathing efforts. This should help to motivate her to keep trying.

2. **D.** IS is the most reasonable treatment for atelectasis at this time. The other three options are more equipment and labor intensive and therefore are more expensive.

3. **D.** An initial IS goal of twice the V_T is widely accepted as a starting volume. A bedside IC may be less than that measured under laboratory conditions.

4. **B.** It is widely accepted that an IS breath should be performed 10 times/hr while the patient is awake. Less often would be beneficial but not ideal; more often is probably not of any added benefit.

5. **D.** Tingling fingers and dizziness are signs of acute hyperventilation. Relaxing and breathing normally will restore the CO_2 level.

6. **A.** A pinched breathing tube is the simplest reason for the obstruction. No special flow resistance features exist on these units.

7. **C.** Multiply the volume in 1 second by the number of seconds that the ball is elevated to calculate the inhaled volume. (900 cc/sec × 1.5 sec = 1350 cc)

8. **D.** Because the patient is comfortable breathing at the current resistance level, it is reasonable to have him work a little harder by breathing through the next smallest hole.

9. **C.** Pursed-lip breathing should help the patient regain control over his breathing and be able to calm down. The patient should not be encouraged or allowed to change his own oxygen flow. This is potentially dangerous. The PFLEX unit is indicated only to help strengthen inspiratory muscles. It will not help to reduce dyspnea. The variable backpressure created by blowing through the Flutter valve unit will only help to mobilize secretions. It will not help to reduce dyspnea.

10. **A.** The PFLEX unit (and other similar units from other manufacturers) is designed specifically to help strengthen the inspiratory muscles. Maximal inspiratory pressure (MIP) and maximal expiratory pressure (MEP) are bedside spirometry tests to identify a patient's respiratory accessory muscle strength at that time. Neither is intended to exercise the patient's muscles to increase his or her strength over time. Trendelenburg positioning is used in some surgical procedures and in some postural drainage positions. Although the patient may have to work harder to breathe with his or her head down, this position is not used to increase respiratory muscle strength.

Chapter Eight: ANSWER KEY FOR THE ENTRY LEVEL EXAM SELF-STUDY QUESTIONS

1. **C.** The patient's signs and symptoms indicate hyperventilation. The easiest way to correct this situation is to have the patient breathe more slowly (and/or less deeply). If the patient continues to breathe in the same pattern, the hyperventilation will continue. Although albuterol may cause tachycardia, it is unlikely to cause dizziness and tingling fingers in the patient. If the patient is advised to breathe deeper and faster, the hyperventilation will get worse.

2. **A.** Adding 100 mL of aerosol tubing as a reservoir will help to increase the amount of inhaled medication and maintain the patient's inspired O_2 percentage. Increasing the flow of oxygen will make the nebulizer dispense the medication more quickly and waste more of it. Decreasing the oxygen flow may result in the nebulizer not working properly and could decrease the patient's O_2 percentage. If the patient were told not to breathe deeply, less medication would be inhaled into the lungs.

3. **D.** An MDI with holding chamber is the only practical way, from among those presented, to deliver this type of medication to a small child. A DPI necessitates an inspiratory flow that is too high for a small child. Holding chambers are not used with a DPI.

4. **D.** Increasing the gas flow on the nebulizer will increase the total amount of water that is nebulized and delivered to the mist tent. Mist tents are supposed to have a hole at the top of the tent canopy to allow the excess gas and aerosol to exit. Only oxygen tents, not mist tents, have the hole closed on the top of the tent canopy. This ensures that the oxygen tent has the highest possible oxygen percentage. Remember, a mist tent does not deliver supplemental oxygen. Lowering the temperature on the refrigeration unit will further cool the infant but will not affect the amount of aerosol delivered into the mist tent.

5. **B.** Upper (larger) airway deposition is enhanced by V_T breathing at a normal speed and in a normal pattern. A slowly inhaled IC (inspiratory capacity) would increase the change of deposition of medication in smaller airways, not larger airways.

6. **C.** An ultrasonic nebulizer generates the greatest quantity of aerosol particles from among the listed choices. An aerosol mask is appropriate for an adult. A hand-held nebulizer used every 4 hours does not deliver enough aerosol fast enough to help the patient, as the ultrasonic nebulizer would. A mist tent is not appropriate for an adult. A cascade-type humidifier does not deliver an aerosol that meets the patient's needs.

7. **D.** The cascade-type humidifier that is heated to near body temperature will provide almost 100% of the patient's body humidity needs. All the other devices are much cooler than body temperature and provide a lower humidity level.

8. **C.** The small, uniform droplet size produced by the ultrasonic unit is a reason for its use. It should not be used to nebulize all medications because vibrations of the ultrasonic unit may break down the drug.

9. **C.** An unheated bubble-type humidifier delivers humidity at room temperature or cooler. All of the

other units deliver humidity or aerosol at a warmer temperature.

10. **D.** The absolute humidity of 44 mg/L is found in the airways of a person at normal body temperature.

11. **A.** Condensation will occur because the saturated air is heated to above room temperature and will cool down as it goes through the tubing. The air will stay saturated with water vapor despite the cooling.

12. **C.** Backpressure on the humidifier will make the pop-off valve whistle. Pinched tubing could cause this. The delivered O_2 flow does not affect the pop-off valve. If a leak occurs between the reservoir jar and the top of the humidifier, the gas will not leak out of the pop-off valve.

13. **B.** An infant with laryngotracheobronchitis (LTB, or croup) usually is best managed with a *cool*, bland aerosol. This helps to reduce swelling in the large airways. Body temperature aerosol is delivered to a patient with a tracheostomy or thick (viscous) secretions to minimize the patient's humidity deficit. A hypothermic patient is given body temperature or warmer aerosol to speed up warming.

14. **D.** A nebulizer will fail because of too little water in the reservoir, a clogged jet, or a clogged capillary line to the reservoir. Air entrainment nebulizers do not have one-way valves. O_2 flows down a capillary tube in a bubble-type humidifier.

15. **D.** Particles in the 1- to 3-μm range will penetrate to the alveoli. All other sizes will affect the airways.

16. **C.** Low water level in the couplant chamber will cause the light to flash. No other indicators help with troubleshooting.

17. **C.** Wastewater should be emptied out of the tubing to prevent contamination. The water level in the reservoir jar has nothing to do with water in the tubing.

18. **D.** The three listed criteria all indicate that the patient's inhaled air is saturated completely with water vapor at body temperature.

19. **B.** The best way for the patient to deposit an aerosol in small airways and alveoli is to slowly inhale an IC with a breath-hold when the lungs are full. A rapidly inhaled V_T tends to deposit aerosol in the larger airways.

20. **A.** Any of the following will result in delivery of less or no aerosol: (1) If the nebulizer is not tightly screwed into the DISS connector on the flowmeter, the gas will leak and will not go through the nebulizer; (2) if the nebulizer jet is obstructed, no aerosol will be created; (3) if the water level is below the refill line on the nebulizer's reservoir jar, no water will be drawn up the capillary tube to the jet and baffle; therefore no aerosol will be created; or (4) if the capillary tube is obstructed, the water in the reservoir jar will not be drawn up to the jet and baffle. However, if the water level is *above* the refill line on the nebulizer's reservoir jar water, water will be drawn up the capillary tube to the jet and baffle. Aerosol will be generated if everything else is functioning normally.

Chapter Nine: ANSWER KEY FOR THE ENTRY LEVEL EXAM SELF-STUDY QUESTIONS

1. **A.** Lasix is a diuretic and is known to cause patients to urinate large amounts of potassium. The loss of potassium can result in cardiac arrhythmia. Giving more Lasix could worsen the loss of potassium. No indication is given that the patient has a life-threatening arrhythmia that needs to be defibrillated. No indication exists to give epinephrine.

2. **C.** Caffeine citrate (Cafcit) is known to be a respiratory center stimulant in infants and will stimulate breathing. This should help to prevent the apnea spells. Xylocaine is a local anesthetic agent. It is used to numb an injury or to stop cardiac arrhythmias, such as premature ventricular contractions (PVCs). Prostigmin is used to reverse the paralyzing effects of nondepolarizing neuromuscular blocking agents such as Pavulon. Isoetharine HCl is a short-acting sympathomimetic bronchodilator. It does not simulate breathing.

3. **A.** Morphine is indicated to relieve severe, acute pain. In addition to controlling the pain, morphine will sedate the patient. Advil is not effective against severe pain. Anectine is a paralyzing medication. Atrovent is a parasympatholytic (anticholinergic) medication.

4. **C.** QVAR is an inhaled corticosteroid that is widely used to treat asthma. Narcan is a reversing agent for morphine and related opium-based drugs. Prostigmin is a reversing agent for nondepolarizing neuromuscular blocking agents. Solu-Medrol is a steroid taken by pill or intravenously for systemic effects.

5. **B.** Combivent combines a sympathomimetic (albuterol) agent and a parasympatholytic (ipratropium) agent for effective bronchodilation. Vanceril is an inhaled corticosteroid medication and Singulair is a leukotriene blocker. Atrovent is a parasympatholytic agent and Intal is a mast cell stabilizer. Serevent is a

long-duration sympathomimetic agent and Advair is a corticosteroid.

6. **A.** MicroNefrin will stimulate the α-receptors in the mucous membrane of the patient's airway to cause vasoconstriction and reduce edema. Mucomyst is a mucolytic. Xopenex and Isoetharine HCl are sympathomimetic agents with no α-receptor effect.

7. **B.** Mucomyst is an effective mucolytic for most patients. Dopamine is a vasoconstrictor used to raise blood pressure. Intal is used to prevent an asthma attack. Hypotonic saline is not known as an effective mucolytic.

8. **C.** The physician should be contacted because 5 mL is too large a dose of Proventil. A respiratory therapist should know not to give this large a dose even if the order is written. A respiratory therapist should not alter a written order from a physician or presume to know what a physician might want to do.

9. **C.** Pulmozyme is indicated in patients with cystic fibrosis who have pulmonary infection and thick secretions. A normal saline solution is not the most effective option for liquefying secretions. Mucomyst has no effect against purulent secretions with bacterial DNA. In addition, Mucomyst is not currently recommended by aerosol or tracheal instillation in this patient with cystic fibrosis.

10. **D.** Review the first two drug dosage calculations shown in Module C to see how to set up this problem.

11. **C.** It is commonly accepted that an aerosolized bronchodilator treatment should be stopped if the patient's pulse rate increases by 20% or more (from 85 to ≥102 beats/min).

12. **C.** Tremor, headache, nervousness and irritability, and tachycardia are all known possible adverse effects.

13. **A.** Brovana is a long-duration medication indicated in stable patients with bronchospasm. The other medications are all sympathomimetic bronchodilators with a shorter duration of action.

14. **B.** Hypertonic (10%) saline is commonly used to induce a sputum sample in patients with tuberculosis. The other saline solutions will not be as effective. Pulmozyme is indicated in patients with cystic fibrosis who have purulent secretions.

15. **A.** Xopenex is a fast-acting sympathomimetic bronchodilator that should help to prevent a bronchospasm reaction from Mucomyst. Sterile water and normal saline are not bronchodilators and can cause bronchospasm in some asthmatic patients. Nembutal is a barbiturate.

16. **D.** Aminophylline is recognized as a medication that may be beneficial to a patient with status asthmaticus after inhaled bronchodilators and corticosteroids have been given. If a fast-onset sympathomimetic bronchodilator such as albuterol (in Combivent) has not been effective, it is doubtful if Proventil (more albuterol) or Brethaire would be effective. In addition, the patient is already tachycardic. Foradil is a long-acting sympathomimetic bronchodilator that is not given for a fast effect.

17. **B.** Pirbuterol (Maxair) is a fast-onset sympathomimetic bronchodilator. It may be used as a "rescue" inhaler during an asthma attack but is not used to prevent an asthma attack. Intal, Accolate, and Zyflo are all used as prophylactic agents to prevent an asthma attack. Intal stabilizes mast cells to prevent the release of leukotriene agents. Accolate and Zyflo block the effect of released leukotriene agents.

18. **C.** Treatment should be stopped because the patient's heart rate has increased by more than 20%. Monitor the patient's heart rate to find out if it returns to normal; chart the results. Only the physician can order a change in type of medication or medication amount. Only the physician can terminate treatment. Adding more saline to the medication will dilute the mixture but not reduce the amount of medication the patient receives. The same adverse reaction will probably happen again.

19. **D.** Decreasing the dose of Proventil is reasonable because it may be causing the patient's heart rate to increase. Adding saline will not reduce the total amount of medication that the patient will receive. There is no need to stop the treatment at this point based on the 15% increase in her heart rate.

20. **D.** Romazicon reverses a barbiturate medication, and Narcan reverses a narcotic medication in the patient. Intropin is used to raise blood pressure. Anectine is a depolarizing neuromuscular blocking agent. Valium is a barbiturate.

21. **D.** Review the third and fourth drug dosage calculations shown earlier in the chapter to see how to set up this problem. (Module C)

22. **A.** The patient's treatment can be continued because his heart rate has not increased by at least 20% from the baseline. The therapist cannot change a medication or decrease a medication amount without the physician's approval.

23. **B.** Ampicillin is used against gram-positive bacteria. Virazole is used against RSV. Garamycin and TOBI are used against gram-negative bacterial pneumonia.

24. **A.** Virazole has been approved by the Food and Drug Administration for the treatment of RSV. NebuPent is nebulized and Bactrim is given systemically against *P. carinii*. Garamycin is used against gram-positive bacteria.

Chapter Ten: ANSWER KEY FOR THE ENTRY LEVEL EXAM SELF-STUDY QUESTIONS

1. **C.** PEP therapy has been shown to help in mobilizing secretions. In addition, some PEP units can be coupled with an SVN to more efficiently deliver the medication. Incentive spirometry does not help with secretion mobilization or medication delivery. IPPB *may* help with medication delivery if the patient cannot properly perform the SVN treatment. However, no indication of this problem exists. The benefits of improperly positioning a patient for PDT are questionable. (See Box 10-5 on page 296.)

2. **D.** Manual percussion should be performed with a cupped hand and relaxed wrist and elbow joints.

3. **C.** Vibration should be performed only on expiration. Most people cannot vibrate at a faster rate than about 3 cycles/second.

4. **C.** There is no reason that a bedridden patient with a small vital capacity cannot have CPT. Head-down positions place a patient with a recent stroke or known increased intracranial pressure at risk for further brain damage. A patient who has just eaten should not be placed in a head-down position because of the risk of vomiting. (See Box 10-7 on page 297.)

5. **A.** Regular turning is an easy and inexpensive way for the patient to alter his breathing pattern and to move the VT into different lung segments. This helps to prevent atelectasis. PEP and IPPB may be needed, but only after regular turning has been shown to be ineffective. CPAP is not indicated for the treatment of simple atelectasis from inactivity.

6. **D.** The lateral basal, superior, and posterior basal segments are all located in the right lower lobe where the infiltrates are located. The apical segment is located in the upper lobe, and the medial segment is located in the middle lobe. (Review Figure 10-1 on page 289.)

7. **C.** A bedside spirometer is not needed because the patient's exhaled volume does not need to be measured. In addition, a spirometer cannot be connected to the unit for volume measurement. All of the other listed items are needed. The variable orifice resistor is needed to set the level of expiratory resistance. A pressure manometer is needed to determine that the expiratory pressure is kept in the 10- to 20-cm water range. A small volume nebulizer with reservoir is needed to deliver the albuterol. (See Figure 10-17 on page 299.)

8. **B.** Many references indicate that percussion and vibration are beneficial in mobilizing large quantities of secretions. Review Box 10-2 on page 287 for contraindications for percussion and vibration.

9. **A.** Review Figure 10-4 on page 290 for the recommended position to drain the anterior basal segment of the right lower lobe.

10. **A.** When the patient exhales through a larger hole, the pressure should decrease and the expiratory time should shorten. Review Box 10-8 on page 297 for the steps to be followed in the PEP therapy procedure. Having the patient exhale faster or exhale through a smaller hole increases the pressure and expiratory time. A bronchodilator medication has not been ordered for the patient.

11. **C.** Because an empyema is a collection of pus in the pleural cavity, it cannot be drained through postural drainage. The other options are all indications for postural drainage. See Box 10-1 on page 286 for the indications.

12. **C.** Neither manual nor mechanical percussion or vibration should be performed over female breast tissue. (See Box 10-2 on page 287.)

13. **B.** It is likely that the patient coughed secretions into the unit. Check for an obstruction. If one is present, it must be removed. A cotton swab or warm running water should remove any secretions. The patient blows out (does not breathe in) through the Flutter valve. It is not an incentive spirometer device. Removing the steel ball from the device will prevent it from working as intended. If the patient blows out hard, the obstruction may be blown deeper into the unit.

14. **A.** Hypoxemia is the only possibility for the problem from among those listed. A full stomach does not cause vagal stimulation that results in PVCs. The patient's symptoms of SOB and PVCs do not correspond with increased intracranial pressure or increased venous return to the heart.

15. **A.** Switching to an electrically powered percussor is the only workable option from among those provided. A pneumatically powered percussor does not have batteries or an electrical cord. The way that the percussor gradually lost function indicates that the tank did not have any compressed O_2 with which to run the unit.

16. **D.** Try another type of pad on the percussor to determine whether it is more comfortable for the patient. A flat one is probably best for the lower back. The patient is not having a reaction to the head-down position and does not need to sit up. No indication exists that the patient is hypoxic. Increasing the speed on the percussor is likely to increase the skin irritation.

17. **B.** It is unnecessarily risky to set the HFCWO controls at maximal speed and pressure to start a patient's treatment. It could be uncomfortable and the patient could be injured. Start the treatment at the lowest rate and pressure and let the patient increase the rate and pressure as needed. The patient should sit upright for the treatment to be most effective. The pumping unit and vest must be connected with the air hoses.

Chapter Eleven: ANSWER KEY FOR THE ENTRY LEVEL EXAM SELF-STUDY QUESTIONS

1. **B.** See Figure 11-36 on page 331 for a tracing and explanation of a PVC.
2. **B.** Current CPR guidelines state that effective ventilation can be achieved by an endotracheal tube, mouth-to-valve resuscitator, or manual resuscitator. A pneumatic (demand-valve) resuscitator is not recommended for use because it is difficult to control the delivered tidal volume and air tends to be forced into the patient's stomach.
3. **A.** ECG monitoring is justified because the patient's signs and symptoms could indicate a cardiac problem. An exercise program is not indicated in this situation and could be dangerous for the patient. A peak flow test is not indicated now and would not help with the diagnosis of exercise-induced asthma. It is best to wait at least 10 minutes after putting O_2 on a patient before drawing an ABG sample to check on the patient's O_2 level.
4. **B.** Defibrillation is indicated if the patient has VT and is without pulse or blood pressure. The patient should then be evaluated for full CPR efforts. The other options would delay effective treatment.
5. **C.** See Figure 11-36 on page 331 for a tracing of a PVC and explanation. *Unifocal* means that all of the PVCs originate from a single area. *Multifocal* means that PVCs originate from more than one area.
6. **C.** A portable defibrillator must be with the patient in case it is needed. The other items are useful for monitoring but offer no way to treat a life-threatening arrhythmia.
7. **A.** Direct instillation into the patient's airways and lungs offers the fastest way to administer the medications when an IV line is not available.
8. **D.** Defibrillation should be performed as quickly as possible when a patient is in VF. Figure 11-40 shows another example. All of the other options delay effective treatment.
9. **C.** Reversing the arm electrodes results in the heart's electrical signal being received by the ECG machine in the opposite direction of normal. This results in reversal of the ECG signal. A loose electrode or shivering would cause different types of artifacts. Miscalibration would not cause inversion of the QRS complex.
10. **B.** The first step in a suspected CPR situation is to assess the patient. CPR should be performed only when needed.
11. **C.** The jaw-thrust maneuver should be a safe way to open the airway of a patient with a known or suspected cervical spine injury. The patient's head should not be tilted back because of the possibility of spine injury. Nasal intubation and tracheostomy should be performed, if needed, only after the jaw-thrust maneuver has been tried.
12. **C.** "Look, listen, and feel" for air movement to determine breathlessness. Feeling with a hand for chest movement is helpful. However, both hands should be used to hyperextend and support the patient's neck and head.
13. **A.** A 5- to 10-second check of the brachial pulse should be done to determine pulselessness because an infant's pulse is more difficult to check at the carotid or femoral sites.
14. **B.** A mouth-to-valve device allows for quick ventilations without risk to the rescuer from the patient. Mouth-to-mouth ventilation should be avoided if possible in this situation. The other options would unnecessarily delay ventilations.
15. **D.** The current BCLS guidelines indicate a compression:ventilation of 30:2 for one rescuer. The other three options do not follow current guidelines with an adult. With an unintubated infant or child, two rescuers would use a compression:ventilation ratio of 15:2.
16. **A.** All are correct except that the air/O_2 intake valve should not open when the resuscitation bag is squeezed. This allows the gas to escape rather than be directed to the patient.
17. **D.** The femoral site is recommended because it is a large artery that should be relatively easy to hit and is away from the patient's chest during compressions.
18. **C.** It is easy and quick to check the valve for proper position. Fix the valve if necessary, and attempt to ventilate the patient again. Because the patient's pulse has not yet been checked, there is no indication that chest compressions are needed. Getting a lateral neck radiograph will greatly delay (probably fatally) ventilating the patient. There is not yet an indication that the patient needs abdominal thrusts to clear an airway obstruction. If the patient cannot be ventilated by the fixed mouth-to-valve resuscitation device, check for an obvious obstruction in the mouth or throat. Reposition the head, and attempt to ventilate again. If the patient still cannot be ventilated, then perform abdominal thrusts.
19. **D.** Current BCLS guidelines indicate that two rescuers should use 100 compressions: 8 to 10 ventilations per minute with an intubated patient. A 3:1 ratio is used on a neonatal patient. The other two options do not follow current guidelines for two rescuers with any patient.

Chapter Twelve: ANSWER KEY FOR THE ENTRY LEVEL EXAM SELF-STUDY QUESTIONS

1. **C.** Common problems with intubation equipment include a loose or burned-out light bulb in the laryngoscope blade or depleted batteries in the handle. Replacing the blade with one that is larger or smaller than appropriate would make the intubation procedure more difficult and dangerous. A plastic handle cannot be used with a stainless-steel blade.

2. **D.** An oropharyngeal airway is indicated to open the airway of an unconscious patient, protect the airway of a patient with seizures, and prevent an oral endotracheal tube from being bitten. A patient with a tracheostomy does not need an oral airway because he or she is not breathing through the mouth. An oropharyngeal airway probably should not be inserted into the mouth of a patient with a traumatic jaw injury because of the risk that further injury could occur.

3. **C.** A cuff pressure of up to 35 cm H_2O should be safe for a patient with a normal blood pressure. A cuff pressure of greater than 35 cm H_2O (>25 mm Hg) is likely to place the patient at risk for damage to the mucous membrane of the trachea.

4. **D.** All of these may be used, along with listening for bilateral breath sounds, to confirm the location of the endotracheal tube. An end-tidal carbon dioxide monitoring system (capnograph) or disposable carbon dioxide detector such as the Easy Cap may be used to detect exhaled carbon dioxide. If the tube is placed within the esophagus, no carbon dioxide will be found. An EDD can be attached to the endotracheal tube. After the bulb has been squeezed, it inflates with air from the patient's lungs if the tube is within a major airway. Laryngeal palpation during tube insertion allows the tube to be felt as it passes through the larynx. Remember that these three methods differentiate only between airway and esophageal intubation. They do not detect a tube that has been inserted too deeply and has entered a mainstem bronchus (usually the right). A neck and chest radiograph shows the tube entering the larynx and its tip within the trachea (or a bronchus). Observation of bilateral chest movement is valuable because equal movement correlates with tracheal intubation and ventilation of both lungs.

5. **A.** If the tip of the tracheostomy tube has been placed into the subcutaneous tissues the patient will not be able to ventilate at all. The tube must be immediately withdrawn. Because the tracheotomy site is below the larynx, it does not matter if the patient has closed her epiglottis over the trachea. She still can breathe through the tracheostomy tube. It is unlikely that the new cuff requires any more air than the previous one.

Even if this were the case, the patient should still be able to breathe through the tube. It should not be possible to place a tracheostomy tube into a patient's esophagus.

6. **D.** A 9.0-mm-ID oral endotracheal tube is appropriate for a large adult male. Also, the oral tube is more appropriate than a nasal tube in an emergency situation. (See Table 12-1 on page 354 for tube sizes.)

7. **A.** A cuff pressure of 17 mm Hg should be safe. No need exists to increase the pressure or replace the tube.

8. **B.** A tracheostomy tube is indicated in a patient with trauma to the nose and mouth and an upper airway obstruction. All of the other airway devices would pass through the upper airway.

9. **B.** A 2.5-mm-ID tube would be most appropriate. (See Table 12-1 on page 354 for tube sizes.)

10. **C.** An adult woman normally has a 7.5 (or 8.0) mm ID endotracheal tube. Review Table 12-1 for the recommended sizes of endotracheal and tracheostomy tubes for patients of all sizes.

11. **C.** A disposable exhaled-CO_2 detector would be easy to use and would give an immediate indication if the tube were removed from the trachea. A capnography device is expensive and is not designed for easy use in a transport situation. Pulse oximetry will give information on O_2 saturation, not on CO_2 removal from the lungs. An ECG will not give immediate feedback on the patient's condition related to the tube. If the patient was accidentally extubated, both the pulse oximeter and the ECG devices would eventually give information indicating that the patient is in trouble. However, this information is not specific to the patient who has been extubated.

12. **B.** Bowel sounds should not be affected by the placement of a tracheostomy tube. It is highly unlikely that the tracheostomy tube would be accidentally placed into the esophagus, which can happen during the placement of an endotracheal tube. All other items should be monitored.

13. **A.** Placement of the endotracheal tube into the right mainstem bronchus would result in the absence of breath sounds over the left lung. Placement of the tube into the left mainstem bronchus would result in the absence of breath sounds over the right lung. Placement of the tube into the esophagus would result in the absence of breath sounds over both lungs. A right pneumothorax could result in absent breath sounds over the right lung, not over the left lung.

14. **C.** Everything listed except the Magill forceps would be needed. These forceps are only used during a

nasal intubation procedure. (Review Box 12-4 on page 367.)

15. **A.** A patient should be extubated when the lungs are full so that a full coughing effort can follow and clear any secretions in the airways. All of the other options would result in less volume in the patient's lungs.

16. **B.** The tracheostomy tube should be removed quickly if there is evidence that the tube is blocked. In addition, the tracheotomy tube should be replaced with a new one so that a secure airway is maintained.

17. **B.** Right bronchial intubation is indicated by the presence of the patient's breath sounds on the right side but diminished on the left side. There is no direct evidence of a left-sided pneumothorax. The exhaled CO_2 monitor is functioning properly because it is supposed to change color (from dark purple to yellow when exposed to exhaled carbon dioxide) during the breathing cycle. Even a small tidal volume should deliver equal air to both lungs and result in equal breath sounds over both lungs.

18. **A.** A double-lumen tube is indicated because she can receive independent lung ventilation through it. This mode of ventilation would allow her lung with atelectasis to be ventilated differently than her normal lung. None of the other tubes offer this option.

19. **C.** A wire-reinforced (armored) tube would prevent her from biting and collapsing the tube during a seizure. None of the other tubes offer this security.

20. **D.** Substituting a fenestrated tracheostomy tube for the standard tube allows her to breathe spontaneously through the upper airway when the inner cannula is removed. This allows her to talk, which can have a very positive emotional impact on the patient. It is probably going too far to remove the tracheostomy tube when she is off of the ventilator. This necessitates removing the tube, covering the stoma, and reinserting the tube later in the day. This can lead to damage to the tracheal tissue. In addition, if the patient's condition suddenly deteriorates while the tracheostomy tube is removed, no secure airway is available. Although a speaking-type tracheostomy tube allows her to speak while on the ventilator, it does not enable her to breathe through her upper airway when she is off of the ventilator as a fenestrated tube allows. Replacing the current 7.5-mm-ID tracheostomy tube with one that is 6.0-mm ID greatly increases the patient's work of breathing. This can fatigue the patient and delay her recovery.

21. **B.** A nasopharyngeal airway can be inserted to protect the nasal passage from damage by the suction catheter. An oropharyngeal airway should only be used in unconscious patients and does not protect the nasal passage. There was no mention of the patient having a tracheostomy.

22. **D.** It is best to remove the speaking valve to determine if that is the cause of the dyspnea. If the patient can now breathe comfortably, attach a new speaking valve to the button. If the patient still cannot breathe comfortably, remove the tracheostomy button and reassess the patient.

23. **B.** A laryngeal mask airway is commonly used in the operating room to provide a secure airway without an endotracheal tube. The Combitube is an emergency airway and is not employed in the operating room. Oropharyngeal and nasopharyngeal airways do not provide a secure airway. There is no indication for two nasopharyngeal airways to be used at once.

24. **A.** A newborn with macroglossia has a very enlarged tongue and is at risk of upper airway obstruction. The immediate situation may require a respiratory therapist to hold the jaw forward or insert an oropharyngeal or nasopharyngeal airway to maintain a patent airway. Surfactant, mechanical ventilation, and supplemental oxygen are not needed because newborns with macroglossia have normal lung function.

25. **B.** Absent breath sounds over the left lung and a tube depth mark of 29 cm both indicate that the endotracheal tube is inserted too deep. It has entered the right mainstem bronchus. The cuff should be deflated, the tube pulled back to the 24-cm mark at the front teeth, and the cuff reinflated. Check again for bilateral breath sounds to confirm that the tip of the tube is within the trachea. It is not necessary to check the chest radiograph to know that the tube is in the right mainstem bronchus. Pushing the tube deeper will only make it go further into the right mainstem bronchus. It is generally recommended that listening over the epigastric area be done after listening over the lung areas for breath sounds. While there is nothing wrong with listening over the stomach area, there is enough clinical evidence given to confirm the tip of the tube is in the right mainstem bronchus.

26. **A.** It could be challenging to place an oral endotracheal tube because the patient has a neck brace. Because of the neck injury, her head cannot be hyperextended. An anesthesiologist would need to be called to perform the intubation. A nasopharyngeal airway, oropharyngeal airway, or LMA can be easily inserted into the patient without the need to hyperextend her neck.

Chapter Thirteen: ANSWER KEY FOR THE ENTRY LEVEL EXAM SELF-STUDY QUESTIONS

1. **D.** Lukens traps are used only to get a sputum sample from a patient who cannot cough productively.

2. **D.** A closed-system suction catheter allows the patient to be ventilated and keep the PEEP level while suctioning is performed. This should help to prevent hypoxemia. Changing to a smaller or larger diameter open-airway suction catheter will not significantly improve the patient's situation. When the patient is taken off of the ventilator and suctioned, she will become hypoxemic. Additional PEEP will not prevent hypoxemia when the patient is taken off the ventilator.

3. **B.** It is commonly accepted that a suction catheter's diameter should not be greater than one-half the ID of the endotracheal tube. This ensures that the patient has room to breathe around the catheter.

4. **C.** Increasing the vacuum pressure from −60 to −80 mm Hg will result in the secretions being removed more quickly. The whole suctioning procedure usually is limited to 15 seconds. Suctioning for 20 seconds will remove more secretions but is also likely to cause hypoxemia. Suctioning more frequently will not prove effective if the suctioning level is too low at −60 mm Hg. A hospital's central vacuum system is more powerful than a portable one and will suction more effectively.

5. **A.** All patients should be preoxygenated before suctioning and given added O_2 after suctioning to quickly restore the presuctioning O_2 level. O_2 at 100% should be given unless a reason exists to give less.

6. **D.** Hyperextending the patient's head and neck (sniff position) helps open the airway so that the catheter can be inserted more easily into the trachea. Placing the patient in the semi-Fowler position helps the individual to take a deeper breath as needed.

7. **A.** The full (maximum) vacuum level is too great to be safely applied to a patient's airway.

8. **B.** A suction catheter with a Coudé tip may help guide the catheter either to the left or to the right mainstem bronchus. In adults, a straight catheter has a tendency to go down the right mainstem bronchus because it comes off of the trachea at the carina at a more acute angle than the does the left mainstem bronchus. (In newborns, no significant difference exists in the angles of the mainstem bronchi from the trachea.) As stated in answer 3, the diameter of the catheter should be no more than one-half the ID of the endotracheal tube. Any adult-size suction catheter is long enough to suction adequately. Increasing the time of suctioning puts the patient at risk for hypoxemia.

9. **D.** The best course always is to replace a broken or defective piece of equipment.

10. **B.** If the equipment is properly assembled and does not have an air leak, the vacuum should reach the end of the catheter. The other three examples would result in failure of the vacuum to reach the end of the catheter.

11. **A.** More frequent suctioning is needed if the patient has more secretions. Suctioning for longer periods puts the patient at risk for hypoxemia. No indication exists (e.g., hypoxemia or therapeutic PEEP) that a closed-airway suction catheter is needed or would be more effective than a standard catheter. Nebulized atropine in a large enough dose reduces secretion production. However, a dose large enough to do this also is likely to cause tachycardia. Atropine is rarely given to control secretions other than in the operating room. A physician's order is needed to give this medication.

12. **D.** A larger suction catheter would not make any difference in restoring vacuum pressure. If the suctioning system is working properly, vacuum should be felt at the end of a catheter of *any* size. Problems with the other listed options could result in loss of vacuum.

13. **A.** The most reasonable course is to reduce the vacuum level slightly and assess how easily the secretions can be removed. Suctioning frequency should not be reduced unless fewer secretions are produced. The vacuum level need not be increased.

14. **B.** Because the patient is having an adverse reaction to the suctioning procedure, the suctioning time should be shortened. Changing to a catheter with a larger diameter increases the risk of trauma to the mucous membrane of the nasal passage. Inserting an oropharyngeal airway before suctioning may stimulate the gag reflex in a conscious patient. In addition, the airway may block the suction catheter, preventing it from passing through the patient's oropharynx to the larynx and trachea. Squirting 5 mL of saline down the suction catheter into the patient's trachea will probably trigger coughing. This could worsen the patient's distress with the whole procedure.

15. **D.** To seal the system and determine the set vacuum pressure, check the manometer while pinching off the connecting tubing. The system is not sealed off if the therapist just occludes the catheter tip; the thumb control valve is still open. Setting the vacuum control to maximum without sealing off the system allows air to leak, and the pressure cannot be measured. The system is not sealed off if the therapist just closes the thumb control valve on the catheter; the catheter tip opening is still open.

16. **A.** The only way to obtain an uncontaminated sputum sample is to place a Lukens trap between the suction catheter and the vacuum tubing. This way, the patient's secretions are collected in the Lukens trap after they have passed through the sterile suction catheter. Suctioning the patient's oropharynx with a sterile Yankauer suction catheter provides an oral sample, not a tracheal sample. The patient's mouth probably contains microorganisms besides those causing the pneumonia. Placing a Lukens trap between the vacuum tubing and the collection bottle would provide a contaminated sample, because unlike a suction catheter, the vacuum tubing is not sterile. The Lukens trap is designed to hold secretions and prevent them from becoming contaminated. It is not designed to hold a suction catheter.

Chapter Fourteen: ANSWER KEY FOR THE ENTRY LEVEL EXAM SELF-STUDY QUESTIONS

1. **C.** The sensitivity control on all IPPB units determines how much effort (negative pressure) the patient has to generate to trigger a breath. Pressure, flow, and terminal flow will adjust the functioning of the IPPB unit after the breath is started.

2. **C.** Terminal flow on a Bennett PR-2 unit is adjusted to attain additional flow at the end of an inspiratory effort. This added flow compensates for a small leak and cycles the unit to exhalation. Pressure, flow, and expiratory retard will adjust the functioning of the IPPB unit after the breath is started.

3. **D.** Pure O_2 is most clearly indicated in a patient with pulmonary edema and signs of hypoxemia. Room air (21% O_2) would not be very helpful. Intermediate levels of supplemental O_2 (40% or 80%) would be helpful but not as effective as pure O_2.

4. **D.** A cooperative patient with atelectasis should first be treated with a less expensive method such as IS. IPPB would be indicated in the other types of patients.

5. **B.** A face mask would allow a treatment to be given without injury to the lip ulcers. A mouthpiece cannot be held by a comatose patient. A Bennett seal would injure the lip ulcers. Intubation is unnecessarily invasive and risky.

6. **B.** A small negative pressure of −1 cm H_2O would not make the patient work harder than necessary to turn on the unit. A pressure of 0 cm H_2O would result in the self-cycling of the unit when ambient (room) barometric pressure is reached.

7. **A.** The needle on the pressure manometer bounces when the patient's inspiratory flow is greater than what is leaving the machine. Turn up the inspiratory flow from the unit for a smoother inspiratory effort by the patient. Decreasing flow would make the patient's situation worse. Increasing peak pressure will increase tidal volume only. Decreasing expiratory retard would alter the expiratory flow.

8. **A.** When the air-mix knob on a Bird unit is pushed in, only pure source gas (100% O_2) is given to the patient. Because no room air is entrained with the source gas, the overall total gas flow is decreased.

9. **B.** Adding expiratory retard adds some back-pressure to the patient's airways and allows for a more complete exhalation. Increasing inspiratory flow increases turbulence, and increasing system pressure increases tidal volume. Neither of these will help the patient's problem of air trapping. There is no indication that the patient is hypoxic and needs 100% oxygen.

10. **B.** A loose nebulizer medication jar would result in a hissing sound from the leaking air and a prolonged inspiratory time. If any of the hoses are misconnected, the IPPB machine will fail to function properly but the described problems will not be found. A missing bacteria filter does not cause any hissing sound or prolong the inspiratory time.

11. **D.** Decreasing the inspiratory flow would result in a longer inspiratory time. This is recommended to better distribute any inhaled medication. Decreasing peak pressure results in a smaller tidal volume and a shorter inspiratory time. Sensitivity has no effect on inspiratory time. If room air is entrained, the total flow will increase and inspiratory time will be shorter.

12. **C.** The 1993 *Clinical Practice Guideline* on IPPB recommends that an IPPB volume be at least 25% greater than a patient's spontaneous volume.

13. **C.** The patient's signs and symptoms indicate a pneumothorax. Treatment should be stopped, the patient evaluated, and the physician notified.

Chapter Fifteen: ANSWER KEY AND RATIONALE FOR THE ENTRY LEVEL SELF-STUDY QUESTIONS

1. **C.** The Servo-*i* is the only volume-cycled ventilator among those listed. It delivers a set V_T despite changes in the patient's pulmonary condition. The other ventilators are pressure cycled and cannot ensure a consistent V_T.

2. **B.** The minimal set V_T for a ventilated patient is 10 mL/kg. This would result in a set V_T of 860 mL (10 mL × 86 kg).

3. **A.** The patient with the drug overdose should be easily ventilated on a pressure-cycled ventilator such as the Bird Mark 7. The Dräger E-4 is a volume-cycled ventilator and should be reserved for the patient with serious pulmonary problems.

4. **C.** The first three listed patient parameters are close to normal. The other two items are not normal and do not indicate successful weaning.

5. **C.** SIMV would be the safest weaning method for this patient with an acceptable V_T but inadequate V_C or MIP. The ventilator will still provide intermittent deep breaths and alarms for safety. T-piece weaning offers no alarms, and the patient is not ready for extubation. PCV is not a weaning method.

6. **D.** SIMV offers intermittent deep breaths while allowing the patient to breathe spontaneously. PSV helps to overcome the Raw caused by the small endotracheal tube. PEEP is not needed to maintain her FRC and oxygenation. CPAP should not be used because it does not provide any support for the patient's breathing.

7. **D.** The information given indicates that the patient is tiring. SIMV decreases the patient's work of breathing by providing a set number of large V_T breaths. The patient can breathe between machine breaths as he wishes. Keep the same PEEP/CPAP level to maintain his FRC and oxygenation. Decreasing the CPAP causes a lower FRC and less oxygenation. Raising the CPAP level may increase FRC and oxygenation but does not help the patient's fatigue and work of breathing.

8. **B.** A heated cascade-type humidifier will do the best job of providing 100% relative humidity to the patient. Neither instilling a few milliliters of saline nor switching to a cool passover-type humidifier would do a good a job of adding moisture to the patient's secretions. HME devices can be heated only by the patient's warm exhaled gas.

9. **A.** The PCV mode will allow the therapist and the physician to lower her peak pressure. She should be able to ventilate without further injury to her lung(s). SIMV still will deliver the set V_Ts with high pressures. CPAP will not ventilate the patient at all. Sedation will not lower the high delivered ventilator pressures.

10. **B.** The sensitivity control should be set so that the patient has to begin an inhalation and generate a slightly negative pressure. A pressure of 0 cm H_2O or in the positive range will result in self-cycling of the ventilator to inspiration.

11. **D.** The patient should be told of any significant change in the ventilator unless a clinically based reason exists not to do so. (Page 382.) Sigh breaths are not used with SIMV because the mandatory breaths should be large enough to serve as a sigh. (Page 381.) Mechanical dead space should be removed because it could result in CO_2 retention during the patient's spontaneous breaths.

12. **D.** Too much PEEP will overstretch the lungs and result in decreased compliance. The overstretched lung areas compress their pulmonary capillaries, which causes blood to be diverted to other lung areas. This is likely to increase shunting. If the level of PEEP is too great, the lungs will compress the heart. This will reduce venous return to the heart. As a result, the cardiac output will drop, as will the blood pressure. (See Box 15-4 on page 450.)

13. **B.** Cst is calculated as follows:

$$C_{st} = \frac{\text{exhaled } V_T - \text{compressed volume}}{\text{plateau pressure} - \text{PEEP}}$$

Compressed volume = compliance factor × plateau pressure

$$(3 \text{ mL/cm } H_2O \times 30 \text{ cm } H_2O)$$

$$= \frac{800 \text{ mL} - 90 \text{mL}}{30 - 8}$$

$$= \frac{710 \text{ mL}}{22}$$

$$C_{st} = 32 \text{ mL/cm } H_2O$$

14. **D.** Cdyn is calculated as follows:

$$C_{dyn} = \frac{\text{exhaled } V_T - \text{compressed volume}}{\text{peak pressure} - \text{PEEP}}$$

Compressed volume = compliance factor × peak pressure

$$(3 \text{ mL/cm } H_2O \times 40 \text{ cm } H_2O)$$

$$= \frac{800 \text{ mL} - 120 \text{mL}}{40 - 8}$$

$$= \frac{680 \text{ mL}}{32}$$

$$C_{dyn} = 21 \text{ mL/cm } H_2O$$

15. **C.** Disconnecting the tubing to the external exhalation valve will cause it to fail, which causes the machine V_T to bypass the patient. A self-cycling ventilator would deliver the V_T to the patient. If the inspiratory and expiratory limbs of the circuit were reversed, no

volume would be delivered and the peak pressure alarm would sound. Even if the spirometer were out of calibration, the V_T would be delivered to the patient, and pressure would build in the system. (See Figure 15-20.)

16. **B.** Expiratory retard is indicated in a condition with air trapping on exhalation, such as asthma. The other three conditions do not interfere with exhalation.

17. **C.** The patient's oxygenation is normal. The other three parameters are not normal. (Review Box 15-1 on page 433.)

18. **C.** Increasing the IPAP (inspiratory positive airway pressure) level will lead to an increased tidal volume. If the IPAP level is decreased, the tidal volume will also decrease. The EPAP (expiratory positive airway pressure) level is similar to CPAP or PEEP in its effect on the patient's functional residual capacity (FRC). Therefore, EPAP is adjusted only to change FRC to affect the patient's oxygenation.

19. **C.** Increasing the lower pressure level will increase the CPAP pressure to open the patient's throat soft tissues and stop the snoring. A rate change will not affect the ventilator pressures. Increasing the upper pressure level will increase the V_T; it will not affect the lower pressure to stop the snoring. A face mask would be indicated if the patient did not tolerate the nasal mask or had a significant leak out of his mouth. He does not have these problems.

20. **A.** Decreasing the mechanical dead space will decrease the patient's CO_2 level. Decreasing the V_E will increase the CO_2 level. Neither changing the I:E ratio nor adding PEEP has any effect on CO_2 elimination.

21. **C.** Retained secretions and bronchospasm are Raw problems and cause only the peak pressure to increase. The other two conditions decrease C_{LT} and make the plateau pressure increase. The peak pressure increases as a result. (See Figure 15-9 on page 432.)

22. **B.** PEEP elevates the patient's baseline pressure and raises the Paw by the same amount. The other three options would decrease the Paw by increasing expiratory time.

23. **A.** An AARC Clinical Practice Guideline recommends the use of a cascade-type humidifier warmed to body temperature to help liquefy thick secretions. An HME should be used only if the patient has few secretions. The secretions should not be allowed to dry out. If they did, it would be very difficult to remove them by suctioning.

24. **A.** A spirometer is not needed because the patient's tidal volumes cannot be measured accurately while on the CPAP system. If a spirometer were incorporated into the CPAP system, it would register continuous flow rather than patient volumes. An alarm system is needed for patient safety, and water traps are used to keep the tubing clear. A pressure-generating device

must be added to set and maintain the CPAP level. (See Figure 15-28.)

25. **A.** Auto-PEEP (expiratory air trapping) is identified when the expiratory flow does not return to zero before the next ventilator tidal volume is delivered. The tidal volume size should not matter. The expiratory time should always be long enough for the patient to fully exhale a tidal volume of any size. Lung compliance cannot be determined by looking at the patient's expiratory flow pattern. The amount of airway resistance should not matter. The expiratory time should always be long enough for the patient to fully exhale the tidal volume regardless of airway resistance. (See Figure 15-7.)

26. **A.**

$$\text{Airway resistance (Raw)} = $$
$$= \frac{\text{Peak airway pressure} - \text{Plateau pressure}}{\text{Flow in L/sec}}$$
$$= \frac{40 \text{ cm H}_2\text{O} - 20 \text{ cm H}_2\text{O}}{0.75 \text{ L/sec}}$$
$$= \frac{20 \text{ cm H}_2\text{O}}{0.75 \text{ L/sec}}$$
$$= 27 \text{ cm H}_2\text{O L/sec}$$

27. **C.** If the bronchodilator therapy is effectively reversing the patient's bronchospasm, his airway resistance will be decreasing. Bronchodilator therapy will not have any effect on lung compliance. Although breath sounds should reveal less wheezing, each caregiver could interpret breath sounds differently. It is better to objectively evaluate a patient's airway resistance to determine whether the bronchodilator therapy is effective. Although a chest radiograph will show changes in a patient's lungs, it will not help to assess airway resistance.

28. **B.** If the diuretic medication is benefiting the patient, his lungs will dry out. This will result in improvement in lung compliance over time. Although a diuretic medication should improve his urine output and cause weight loss, this is not the best way to evaluate his pulmonary status. Pulmonary edema is a lung compliance problem, not an airway resistance problem. If the diuretic medication has improved his urine output and his lungs have dried out, breath sounds should improve. However, this is not the best way to quantitatively evaluate a patient's response to care.

29. **D.** A pressure-cycled transport-type ventilator will be able to provide effective ventilation through the transportation and the cardiac procedure. Manual ventilation is not recommended because, if the therapist should tire, the respiratory rate and tidal volume will decrease. A microprocessor-type ventilator is the most sophisticated and expensive unit available. It probably is not needed for the anticipated short period of time.

A negative-pressure ventilator is indicated only in stable patients with a neuromuscular disease. In addition, this type of ventilator does not allow for easy access to the patient's body.

30. **C.** Air trapping and auto-PEEP are corrected by increasing the expiratory time for a complete exhalation of the tidal volume. If the pressure control mode is used to deliver the same tidal volume and the other settings are kept the same, the patient still will have air trapping and auto-PEEP. Decreasing the inspiratory flow while keeping the same tidal volume and rate will result in an even shorter expiratory time. This will result in even more air trapping. It is unlikely that a larger endotracheal tube will help a patient with COPD to exhale more completely.

31. **A.** The use of accessory muscles and ventilator dyssynchrony indicate that the patient needs a faster breath. Increasing the inspiratory flow should help this. There is no indication that her tidal volume is too large. Too much pain medicine will sedate the patient and could make weaning difficult. Without a set of arterial blood gas values, there is no way to assess her oxygenation. The real issue here is the patient's desire for a faster tidal volume.

32. **D.** The difference between the patient's respiratory efforts (24) and total breaths (15) indicates that the ventilator is not sensing all of his efforts. Adjust the sensitivity control on the ventilator so that all of the patient's efforts result in ventilator breaths. The ABG values indicate that the patient is not hypoxemic. So, this cannot be the reason why his efforts are not triggering ventilator breaths. Although increasing the flow will deliver a faster tidal volume, it will not correct the difference between the patient's breathing efforts and the ventilator sensing those efforts. Increasing the set rate to 15 will only match the current total rate. The patient is making 24 respiratory efforts/min. The real problem is that the ventilator is not sensing all of his breathing efforts.

33. **B.** An initial tidal volume of 700 mL is appropriate because most patients require a ventilator-delivered tidal volume of about 10 mL/kg of ideal body weight. A tidal volume of 1000 mL is probably too large at almost 14 mL/kg of ideal body weight. A tidal volume of 500 mL is probably too small at less than 7 mL/kg of ideal body weight. A tidal volume of 320 mL is certainly too small at less than 5 mL/kg of ideal body weight.

34. **B.** Because children normally breathe faster than adults, a rate of 20/min is appropriate. A rate of 14 would be appropriate for an adult but is too slow for a child. A rate of 50 would be appropriate for a newborn infant and far too fast for a child. An initial rate of 80 is too fast for any patient. (See Table 1-2 on page 3.)

35. **C.** Decreasing the respiratory rate will allow the patient's carbon dioxide level to rise. This should correct the respiratory alkalosis. Although the patient's PaO$_2$ is higher than normal, it is not necessary to make a change in the oxygen percentage at this time. In addition, if the patient's carbon dioxide were to increase to the normal level, the PaO$_2$ would decrease. Increasing the respiratory rate will further decrease the carbon dioxide level. This could produce a dangerous respiratory alkalosis. Although decreasing the tidal volume will result in a higher PaCO$_2$ level, it is better to decrease the respiratory rate. The patient's tidal volume of 700 mL is appropriate at about 10 mL/kg of ideal body weight.

36. **A.** The patient should be given 100% oxygen before each suctioning procedure and afterward until he is stable again. Because cardiopulmonary risks are associated with PEEP, it should not be increased and decreased frequently for each suctioning episode. Suctioning should be done as often as necessary. If suctioning is performed less often than needed, secretions will accumulate in the patient's airways. The suction catheter should not be larger than one-half of the inner diameter of the patient's endotracheal tube. A larger catheter will block too much of the endotracheal tube, so that the patient cannot breathe around it.

37. **D.** As the patient recovers, it is appropriate to let her do some spontaneous breathing with the SIMV mode. Although there is no harm in keeping the current settings, switching her to the SIMV mode will let her begin to breathe spontaneously. She appears ready to do so. There is no need to increase the set rate. The patient is able to trigger additional breaths as she desires and has normal blood gas values. The tidal volume does not need to be decreased; it is set at about 7 mL/kg.

38. **C.** Pressure support usually is initiated to overcome a patient's increased work of breathing. In this case, a 7.0-mm ID endotracheal tube would increase the patient's workload because the tube is too small for an adult. Keeping the ventilator rate at 8/min is just enough to not exhaust the patient. However, it does not really solve the problem of increased work of breathing through a small endotracheal tube. Increased flow during machine breaths will not decrease the patient's spontaneous work of breathing. No evidence suggests that the patient has asthma or any condition that would cause bronchospasm.

39. **D.** The patient is exhibiting refractory hypoxemia. The best way to correct this problem is with PEEP therapy to reestablish the patient's functional residual capacity. If the patient is hypoxic while getting 80% oxygen, it is doubtful that giving 100% oxygen will make much difference. Increasing the set rate to 18 will only ensure that the patient is hyperventilated.

Mechanical dead space will correct the hyperventilation but will not correct the hypoxemia.

40. **D.** Because the patient has normal bedside spirometry values and is awake, she can have weaning procedures started. A T-piece would be appropriate because

she can fully support her own breathing. It is overly cautious to wait 4 more hours to reevaluate the patient or change to the SIMV mode. However, it is overly aggressive to extubate the patient without a weaning trial. (See Box 15-5 on page 466.)

Chapter Sixteen: ANSWER KEY FOR THE ENTRY LEVEL EXAM SELF-STUDY QUESTIONS

1. **C.** A PaO_2 in the range of 60 to 70 torr is adequate for a newborn infant. Less would result in unnecessary hypoxemia. A higher value is not needed and may increase the risk for retinopathy of prematurity (ROP). See Table 16-1 for all blood gas recommendations. (Table 16-1.)

2. **B.** Mechanical ventilation is indicated to support the patient's breathing when prolonged apnea spells lead to bradycardia. CPAP improves oxygenation but does not provide ventilation to support a patient with apnea spells. An aerosolized bronchodilator does not affect a patient in a way that corrects apnea. While endotracheal surfactant can help a neonate with respiratory distress syndrome (RDS), there is no indication of why the patient is having apnea spells.

3. **C.** A variable CPAP pressure indicates a leak in the system. In this case, most likely with the fit of the CPAP prongs into the neonate's nostrils. Smaller tidal volume or decreased respiratory rate should not have any effect on the CPAP level. The flow through the system should be the same without regard to the oxygen percentage set on the blender.

4. **C.** When meconium is aspirated, it causes a serious airway obstruction problem. For this reason, additional time is needed for the patient's tidal volume to be exhaled. Therefore, select the longest expiratory time possible. (Box 16-6.)

5. **C.** The neonate is premature with signs of respiratory distress syndrome (RDS). The best way to improve the patient's lung compliance and function is to administer exogenous surfactant. Albuterol has no effect on lung compliance. There are no signs of secretions that need to be suctioned out. Although supplemental oxygen may help to correct the hypoxemia, it does

nothing to correct the fundamental problem caused by RDS.

6. **B.** A ventilator circuit that is visibly soiled should be changed. This is because the blood or sputum in the circuit can act as a medium for bacterial growth. A heat-moisture exchanger provides passive humidification and is not intended as a place to collect sputum. Saline can be used to help with the suctioning procedure but is not recommended for flushing out sputum from a circuit. A closed airway suctioning system helps to prevent hypoxemia during suctioning but does not remove sputum from the circuit.

7. **D.** Nasal CPAP at 4 cm water is appropriate. There is no clear indication that the neonate needs to be intubated to provide the end-expiratory pressure. Most premature neonatal patients with moderate hypoxemia respond well to about 4 cm water pressure. Mechanical ventilation would only be needed if the neonate's hypoxemia did not respond to CPAP or if the carbon dioxide value increased significantly. Because the neonate is hypoxic on 60% oxygen, it is doubtful that 70% oxygen would result in a clinically significant improvement.

8. **A.** Inhaled nitric oxide (iNO) is a pulmonary artery vasodilator in neonatal patients with primary pulmonary hypertension of the newborn (PPHN). Its use should help to increase blood flow through the lungs and improve oxygenation. Although surfactant is indicated in a neonate the respiratory distress syndrome (RDS), this patient does not have that problem. Decreasing the oxygen percentage could make the patient more hypoxic and does not help PPHN. Heliox may help reduce the asthmatic patient's work of breathing but does not help PPHN.

Chapter Seventeen: ANSWER KEY FOR THE ENTRY LEVEL EXAM SELF-STUDY QUESTIONS

1. **A.** The best way to be sure that the patient understands the purpose of the equipment is to ask her questions about it and have her describe its function. Any misunderstandings then can be clarified. In addition, the patient should show that she has the necessary dexterity to operate the equipment.

2. **C.** Current guidelines recommend that supplemental oxygen be used during exercise when a patient's SpO_2 value drops <88%. Values between 96% and 90% are within the normal range. A value of <84% shows serious hypoxemia. The patient should not be allowed to become this hypoxemic if possible.

3. **A.** The level of water in the humidifier does not affect the ability of O_2 to flow through the O_2 delivery system. Tightening of all connections and placement of the cannula prongs under water reveal whether gas is flowing through the prongs. If no gas is flowing out from the O_2 concentrator, the nasal cannula should be switched over to the O_2 tank. (See the Entry Level Exam Hint on page 527.)

4. **B.** A cane should not be used without a documented need. The patient's life situation can improve if his spouse stops smoking, he minimizes climbing of stairs, and a front door ramp is added.

5. **D.** Many injuries occur in the bathroom and kitchen when weak patients fall while climbing into showers or tubs or onto chairs to reach high objects.

6. **C.** A patient's exercise tolerance is not evaluated by determining if a relative can drive the patient somewhere. Exercise tolerance can be assessed by determining the patient's ease or difficulty in performing specific tasks.

7. **B.** Restoring the patient to his or her highest possible functional capacity is the main goal of a rehabilitation program. All other goals are secondary to this.

8. **C.** The patient and her husband must both stop smoking. If she is the only one to quit, she will continue to inhale secondhand smoke from her husband. Her physician should be involved in her care to offer medical support and recommend group support.

Chapter Eighteen: ANSWER KEY FOR THE ENTRY LEVEL EXAM SELF-STUDY QUESTIONS

1. **C.** If air is seen to bubble in the water-seal chamber, it is known that vacuum is applied to the drainage system and the patient has pleural air (pneumothorax) that is being removed. The presence of fluid in the collection chamber confirms that the patient has pleural fluid that is being removed. It does not confirm that pleural air is being removed. A vacuum level of −15 cm H_2O is normal and should result in air bubbling in the suction control chamber. However, it does not confirm that pleural air is being removed.

2. **D.** The physical signs indicate that the patient has a left-sided pneumothorax; a pleural chest tube is indicated. Do not place a tube into the right pleural space. Increasing the V_T or changing the mode would not correct the problem.

3. **B.** An air leak through the water seal when the patient coughs indicates that the air is coming from the patient's lung. If a leak exists in the system, air will bubble through the water seal at all times. The vacuum level has no impact on the air leak from the patient.

4. **A.** Nasal CPAP would be indicated for the management of a patient with obstructive sleep apnea. An oropharyngeal airway would be indicated only in an obtunded patient with an obstructed upper airway. For many patients, sleeping on the back worsens the

obstruction. A tracheostomy and mechanical ventilation may be indicated in a patient with central sleep apnea if all other efforts have failed.

5. **A.** A normal SpO_2 value indicates that the CPAP system at 7 cm H_2O pressure has corrected the patient's problem. There is no need to raise the CPAP level because the patient's pulse oximetry value is normal. There is no indication of inadequate flow through the CPAP system. There is no need to raise the delivered oxygen percentage because the saturation is within the normal range.

6. **D.** Performing a bronchoscopy on a ventilated patient necessitates the use of a special bronchoscopy adapter between the endotracheal tube and the circuit. The bronchoscope is placed through the adapter, which may result in a V_T leak. In addition, the bronchoscope partially obstructs the endotracheal tube, which increases resistance and causes inspiratory pressure to increase.

7. **B.** The easiest way to seal the chest tube but allow air leaking from the patient to escape is to place the distal end of the tube under water. Clamping the tube does not allow any pleural air to escape. Leaving the tube open allows pleural air to escape but also allows room air to enter the pleural space. The Valsalva maneuver would require breath-holding by the patient for an

extended time and is not practical. (See Table 18-2 on page 564.)

8. **B.** Cardioversion requires a strong R wave on the ECG monitor, a proper electrical charge level, and proper placement of the ECG leads. The electrode paddles should be well covered with a conducting jelly to maximize the flow of current into the patient without a burn.

9. **C.** Rigid tube bronchoscopy is preferred in the removal of a large foreign body from a large airway. FFB may be used with a small foreign body or one that is in a smaller airway. PEP and PDT are not likely to dislodge a large foreign body such as a tooth. PDT with percussion may dislodge a foreign body. (See Box 18-2 on page 549.)

10. **D.** ABGs are not monitored during a sleep study because it is an invasive procedure and the patient would awaken as the blood sample is drawn. The other items are routinely monitored during a sleep study.

11. **B.** The test should be stopped because the patient's signs and symptoms indicate that he is not tolerating the procedure. A healthy person who does not have dangerous signs and symptoms may tolerate a respiratory exchange ratio of 1.1 for a short time; this patient should not be pushed to this point. This patient has several signs and symptoms showing intolerance and does not need to be pushed to complain of shortness of breath. While the patient may tolerate the stress test at a lower work level, it is safer to stop the test and evaluate the patient.

12. **C.** When indirect calorimetry is used to evaluate a patient's oxygen consumption and carbon dioxide production during a stress test, the anaerobic threshold is confirmed by a respiratory exchange ratio (R) of 1.0. See the calculation for question 4 of the Written Registry Exam Self-Study Questions. Before the R value reaches 1.0 the patient will dramatically increase his/her tidal volume and respiratory rate when the tissues are hypoxic and anaerobic metabolism occurs.

13. **C.** The endotracheal tube should be removed from the patient as the tracheostomy tube is to be placed into the stoma. This ensures that the patient has a secure airway throughout the procedure.

14. **C.** An ultrasound of the chest would not be helpful since sound waves do not reflect off of air-filled spaces such as the lungs. Pulmonary function tests would provide laboratory evidence of the patient's lung volumes and expiratory flow. A chest radiograph would illustrate if the lungs are hyperinflated. Arterial blood gases would show if the patient is hypoxemic and retaining carbon dioxide.

For specific page cross-references for each answer, refer to the Evolve site.

Chapter One: ANSWER KEY FOR THE WRITTEN REGISTRY EXAM SELF-STUDY QUESTIONS

1. **B.** Patients with emphysema usually have chest radiograph findings of increased AP diameter, depressed hemidiaphragms, and widened intercostal spaces that result from enlarged lungs, caused by air trapping. If the patient had pulmonary fibrosis, the lungs would be small rather than enlarged. If the patient had had an AP chest radiograph (rather than a PA), the lung finding would not be significantly changed. However, the heart size would be enlarged. The reported radiographic findings relate to lung problems, not heart problems. No report is made of the heart being enlarged or out of position.

2. **C.** Severe vomiting and diarrhea can result in significant loss of fluids and electrolytes. Her cardiac problems are likely the result of this. If an electrolyte abnormality is found, it must be promptly corrected by intravenous replacement. A urinalysis will be helpful for the evaluation of the patient's kidneys but is not needed at this time. An arterial blood gas analysis will be helpful to determine whether the patient's acid-base balance is altered. However, it is not needed at this time, because it will not guide the patient's clinical management. A complete blood count will not reveal any information that will guide the patient's care related to her cardiac arrhythmia.

3. **B.** The patient's history plus recent illness and worsening symptoms indicate a pulmonary infection. It is important to get a sputum sample for a culture-and-sensitivity study to determine the infectious organism and the antibiotic to fight it. Although the patient's illness may make him hypoxic, no information suggests that he has a home oxygen concentrator. A 6-minute walk test would cause unnecessary stress on the patient at this time. It will surely make him feel more short of breath. Although it may be interesting to know the position of the patient's hemidiaphragms, this will not help him with the current

problem; this procedure can be done later if indicated.

4. **D.** A normal term newborn should have a respiratory rate of 30 to 60 beats/min. All of the other listed vital signs are normal for a term newborn.

5. **D.** An Apgar score of 8 (of a maximum of 10) indicates that the newborn is in good condition and can be given to its mother. Review Table 1-17 for the scoring of the five Apgar signs. Because the newborn is in good condition, there is no need to give it or the mother oxygen or to begin bag-mask rescue breathing.

6. **A.** Laryngotracheobronchitis (croup) is a swelling of the mucous membrane below the vocal cords (subglottic area). This is often identified by a narrowing of the dark air column below the vocal cords. This pointed narrowing is sometimes referred to as the steeple sign or pencil sign. If the patient had aspirated a coin, a solid shape would be seen. In addition, the patient with an aspiration problem has a history of a sudden problem, not one of being sick for 2 days. Epiglottitis is a swelling of the airway above the vocal cords (supraglottic area). The upper airway radiograph shows haziness in the throat area with a normal tracheal air column. Bilateral upper lobe pneumonia appears on a chest radiograph as white shadows over both upper lung fields. The airway should show a normal, dark air column.

7. **A.** The young, healthy heart usually responds to a fluid overload situation by increasing its rate (tachycardia). The excessive intravenous fluid tends to leak out of the capillaries into the tissues in the dependent parts of the body, such as the feet and lower legs. The kidneys quickly put out the extra fluids, and a low urine specific gravity is found. It is highly unlikely that the heart will slow (bradycardia) in a fluid overload situation. Rather than a high urine specific

gravity indicating low urine output, the kidneys put out extra fluid, resulting in a low urine specific gravity.

8. **D.** A right-sided hemothorax pushes the mediastinum to the opposite side. A left-sided tension pneumothorax pushes the mediastinum to the opposite side. Right lower lobe atelectasis pulls the mediastinum to the affected side. Fibrosis of the left lung pulls the mediastinum to the affected side. Review Figure 1-5 if needed. If a patient has bilateral lower lobe pneumonia, both lungs are affected, therefore no shifting of the lungs or the mediastinum would be seen.

9. **C.** An enlarged left side of the heart in a 65-year-old patient is abnormal. The patient should be evaluated for left ventricular failure. An athletic heart is not significantly enlarged compared with a normal-sized heart. What makes it athletic is that it can pump more effectively with a higher than normal stroke volume. A left pleural effusion is identified by an obscured left costophrenic angle; a pleural air/fluid level may be seen. A left middle lobe infiltrate will have a distinctive shadow over the affected lung area, not the heart.

10. **A.** It is highly unlikely that a patient with ARDS, which results in small, stiff lungs and significant hypoxemia, would be breathing with a normal respiratory rate. A patient with these serious problems will likely show nasal flaring (to reduce airway resistance), intercostal retractions (because of the stiff lungs), and use of accessory muscles of inspiration (to assist the diaphragm in breathing).

11. **B.** The posteroanterior (PA) position has the radiographs penetrating from the back to the front of the patient. Because the heart is located behind the sternum, less distortion of its actual size appears on the radiograph. With the anteroposterior (AP) position, the radiographs penetrate from the front to the back of the patient. This results in the heart's shadow being abnormally enlarged on the film. The lateral and oblique chest radiograph views are indicated to help find the location of a tumor or other lung lesion. These views are not that useful in evaluating a patient with COPD and left ventricular failure.

12. **D.** It is best to obtain a chest radiograph, because the film will show whether the endotracheal tube is within the trachea (or esophagus or a mainstem bronchus) and where the tip of the tube is located within the trachea. Hearing stomach sounds during ventilation confirms only that the endotracheal tube is in the esophagus. Breath sounds also must be auscultated to confirm whether the tube is located within the trachea or a mainstem bronchus. Palpation of the larynx can be used during the initial intubation to confirm that the endotracheal tube has entered the trachea. It cannot be used to determine tube tip location within the trachea. Percussion of the patient's chest will not

help determine endotracheal tube location. Abnormal sounds can be from a variety of problems.

13. **A.** Both the blunting of the left costophrenic angle and the air/fluid level with a meniscus are consistent with a left pleural effusion (fluid in the intrapleural space). The patient's history also confirms this problem. Pulmonary edema or pneumonia of the left lung is seen on the radiograph film as a distinctive shadow within the lung field, not around it. Occasionally a pulmonary embolism results in a fluid leak within the lung and a localized shadow within the lung field, not around it.

14. **C.** Transillumination is an easy test for a pneumothorax in a newborn, because the chest wall is relatively thin. If a pneumothorax is present, a "halo" of light shines through the chest wall where the lung is collapsed. Abnormal arterial blood gas results will not be specific to a pneumothorax in this patient. An Apgar score is performed only shortly after a baby has been born to determine how it tolerated the birthing process. A thoracentesis would be performed to remove fluid from around the lung, which has not been shown.

15. **A.** A properly placed pulmonary artery (Swan-Ganz) catheter should have its tip located in either the right or left pulmonary artery (see Figure 1-6 and Chapter 5 for illustrations of this). A central venous pressure catheter (CVP) would be properly located in the superior vena cava. When a patient is going to have the perfusion of the coronary arteries checked, an arterial catheter passes through the aortic arch to reach them. The pulmonary artery catheter passes through the right ventricle to reach the pulmonary arteries.

16. **C.** Because the patient is competent and able to perform the procedure, it would be appropriate to begin a patient-driven protocol. The parent(s) should be involved in the care of a minor child. In this case, no need exists for a therapist or nurse to deliver the patient's inhaled medications. Although the parent could be taught to deliver the medication, it is not necessary because the child can do it.

17. **B.** See Table 1-17 for the five Apgar signs and how they are scored. In this example, all five signs would be rated at 1 point each, for a total score of 5 points.

18. **A.** Potassium is the most important electrolyte to monitor for several reasons. First, it affects the functioning of the heart's conduction system. Second, the serum level is relatively low compared with those of the other electrolytes. Third, potassium, in addition to sodium chloride, tends to be lost through the kidneys when a diuretic medication is given. In general, when a patient is given a diuretic medication, all of the serum electrolyte values should be closely watched. Be prepared to recommend replacement of electrolytes as needed.

19. **B.** The patient's signs and symptoms best fit those of a right-sided pneumothorax. Although it is possible for a patient to break a bone while lifting weights, this would not produce shortness of breath, a hyperresonant percussion note on the right side, and a tracheal shift to the left. An acute myocardial infarction could cause a sudden chest pain and shortness of breath but would not cause a hyperresonant percussion note on the right side or a tracheal shift to the left.

Chapter Two: ANSWER KEY FOR THE WRITTEN REGISTRY EXAM SELF-STUDY QUESTIONS

1. **A.** Poor hand-washing technique is the most common cause of *E coli*, *Staphylococcus aureus*, and *Streptococcus* bacterial infections. The fact that all infected patients have *E coli* infection points to a single person as the cause. In this case, it most likely would be the home respiratory therapist. It is very unlikely that the infections would result from poor manufacturing processes. These equipment and supply items are produced and sterilized under very demanding standards. If the patients' family members were the cause of the infections, it is likely that a variety of bacterial infections would be present—not just one.

2. **A.** Patients who are coughing should be sitting at least 3 feet away from anyone else to help prevent the spread of infection by droplets. In addition, coughing people should wear a surgical-type mask and should use facial tissues to cough into and to blow their nose. Used tissues should be disposed of safely.

3. **C.** An N-95 or higher face mask is worn by all caregivers who work with the patient to protect them from infected droplets. Airborne and Contact Precautions are used to minimize contact with infected droplets and surfaces in the patient's room. The patient needs to wear an N-95 mask only when transported outside of his/her room. The patient's room must have negative airflow compared with the hallway to prevent contaminated droplets from leaving.

4. **B.** The pneumovax vaccination is recommended for anyone older than 50 years of age and for anyone with a chronic cardiopulmonary disease. No current vaccination against SARS is available. A patient who needs continuous oxygen therapy should not be removing her nasal cannula for an hour at a time. In addition, glutaraldehyde is not typically used in the home care setting. This patient should not need a booster pneumovax vaccination until she is 65 years old.

5. **B.** A patient who is only suspected of having SARS is placed under Standard and Droplet Precautions until the disease is confirmed or ruled out. If SARS is confirmed, Airborne and Contact Precautions are added.

6. **D.** Infants need to be 6 months of age or older to receive the influenza vaccination. All health care workers should be vaccinated because of their high risk of contact with infected patients. Children and adults with chronic cardiopulmonary diseases should be vaccinated to prevent an exacerbation of their condition. Routine vaccination is recommended for everyone 50 years of age and older.

Chapter Three: ANSWER KEY FOR THE WRITTEN REGISTRY EXAM SELF-STUDY QUESTIONS

1. **C.** The $P(A-a)O_2$ value should be 15 torr or less in a normal person because of good matching of ventilation and perfusion. Therefore this patient's alveolar-arterial difference is increased. Review the example calculations in this chapter.

2. **C.** The point-of-care (POC) blood gas analyzer with expanded capabilities enables the patient to have arterial blood gases and serum electrolytes analyzed during transportation, if needed. A second-generation pulse will only provide data on oxygenation. There is no portable CO-oximeter currently available. While both of these systems would be valuable and provide information on the patient's oxygenation status if she had carbon monoxide poisoning, she does not have this problem. If a pressure transducer was added to her arterial catheter system her blood pressure could be monitored continuously and arterial blood samples could be taken for analysis. However, her blood pressure can be taken manually. In addition, arterial blood samples can be taken manually for analysis on the POC unit.

3. **A.** The sudden increase in the $PtcO_2$ value can be explained by the electrode being pulled loose from the skin, allowing room air to contact it. If the patient's oxygen percentage was decreased (less than 21% in room air), there would be a decrease in the $PtcO_2$ value. If the patient's pulmonary condition suddenly improved, her $PtcCO_2$ value would probably also have changed. If the patient was hyperventilating to raise her oxygen value, her carbon dioxide value would have decreased.

4. **D.** The results of the modified Allen's test performed on the patient's right wrist are abnormal. It took 25 seconds for the return of adequate circulation through the ulnar artery. No arterial blood sample should be taken from the right radial artery because of poor collateral circulation through the ulnar artery (see Figure 3-2). Check the circulation on the patient's left wrist by doing a modified Allen's test on it. Draw from the left radial artery if the test result is normal (less than 15 seconds for the return of circulation). The Allen's test is a test of circulation through the radial artery, whereas the modified Allen's test is a test of circulation through the ulnar artery.

5. **A.** A first-generation pulse oximeter value is of no use in evaluating a patient with carbon monoxide poisoning. This pulse oximeter technology is unable to distinguish carboxyhemoglobin from oxyhemoglobin; therefore the pulse oximeter value will show a higher oxygen saturation than is actually present in the patient. A 12-lead electrocardiogram is needed to help determine the cause of the patient's irregular pulse rate. The patient may have had a heart attack as the result of profound hypoxemia. To evaluate the patient's oxygenation accurately, an arterial blood sample should be drawn and analyzed with a CO-oximeter. A CO-oximeter can distinguish between carboxyhemoglobin and oxyhemoglobin, so that the patient's actual SaO_2 level can be determined. A Glasgow Coma Scale analysis should be done to evaluate the patient's neurologic status. The patient may have had a stroke as the result of profound hypoxemia.

6. **B.** A patient with septic shock who is receiving vasopressor therapy needs an arterial line to monitor blood pressure continuously. This is because the disease condition and the drugs result in considerable variation in blood pressure. A patient with ARDS who requires mechanical ventilation with PEEP needs frequent arterial blood sampling for gas analysis. Rather than puncture the patient's arteries for each sample, it is more humane and efficient to place an arterial line. In addition, the patient's blood pressure can be continuously monitored for the effects of PEEP. A patient with suspected (or actual) carbon monoxide poisoning does not usually need more than one or two arterial blood samples taken for the diagnosis and the evaluation of treatment effectiveness. An arterial line is not justified. A patient with anxiety-induced hyperventilation is not hypoxic and does not need an ABG sample analyzed.

7. **D.** The best way to assess the oxygenation status of a patient with carbon monoxide poisoning is to run an ABG sample through the CO-oximeter. The CO-oximeter is the only device that can accurately differentiate between carboxyhemoglobin and oxyhemoglobin (as well as other types of hemoglobin) and measure the amounts of each. Therefore it gives an accurate SaO_2 value. The first-generation pulse oximeter device is unable to distinguish between carboxyhemoglobin and oxyhemoglobin. This provides a false high value for SaO_2. The transcutaneous oxygen probe can be used to give an approximate tissue oxygen value. However, it is not the clinically accepted way to evaluate a patient with CO poisoning. Running an ABG sample through a standard blood gas analyzer results in measurements of oxygen and carbon dioxide concentrations and of pH. However, the SaO_2 value is calculated from the PaO_2 value. This can result in a falsely high value for the calculated SaO_2 level if the patient is receiving supplemental oxygen and has an elevated PaO_2 value (measured from the blood plasma).

8. **C.** Because the correlation factor between $PaCO_2$ and $PtcCO_2$ is 1.5, the solution to the problem requires that the patient's current $PtcCO_2$ value of 76 torr be divided by 1.5, as follows:

$$\text{Approximate } PaCO_2 = PtcCO_2 \text{ of 53 torr/1.5}$$
$$= 35 \text{ torr}$$

9. **D.** A PaO_2 level of less than 80 torr is uncorrected hypoxemia. A compensated respiratory acidosis is indicated by the increased $PaCO_2$ value coupled with an increased bicarbonate level and increased base excess found with a normal pH. (Review Table 3-2 on page 87 and Table 3-9 on page 90.)

10. **B.** A PaO_2 value of greater than 80 torr with supplemental oxygen is corrected hypoxemia. An uncompensated metabolic acidosis is indicated by the normal $PaCO_2$ value coupled with a decreased bicarbonate level and decreased base excess found with an acidotic pH. (Review Table 3-2 on page 87 and Table 3-9 on page 90.)

11. **C.** Normal oxygenation is indicated because the patient's PaO_2 level is elevated secondary to hyperventilation ($PaCO_2$ value of 25 torr). An uncompensated respiratory alkalosis is indicated by the low $PaCO_2$ value coupled with a normal bicarbonate concentration and normal base excess found with an alkalotic pH. (Review Table 3-2 on page 87 and Table 3-9 on page 90.)

12. **A.** A PaO_2 value of less than 80 mm Hg is uncorrected hypoxemia. A combined metabolic and respiratory acidosis is indicated by the increased $PaCO_2$ value coupled with a decreased bicarbonate level and decreased base excess found with an acidotic pH. (Review Table 3-2 on page 87 and Table 3-9 on page 90.)

13. **C.** A PaO_2 value of less than 80 mm Hg is uncorrected hypoxemia. A compensated respiratory alkalosis is indicated by the decreased $PaCO_2$ value coupled with a decreased bicarbonate level and decreased base excess found with a normal pH. (Review Table 3-2 on page 87 and Table 3-9 on page 90.)

14. **B.** A $P\bar{v}O_2$ value of 25 torr is quite low. A $P\bar{v}O_2$ value of 40 torr is normal, and a value below 30 torr usually indicates tissue hypoxemia. An $S\bar{v}O_2$ value of 80% is above the normal value of 75% and indicates above-normal tissue oxygenation. Review Table 3-11 if needed. Although a PaO_2 value of 55 torr and an SaO_2 value of 88% are below normal, they do not necessarily indicate tissue hypoxemia. Many patients with chronic lung disease live acceptable lives with values in this range. (Review Table 3-11 on page 91.)

15. **B.** Because the PO_2 level of room air is 150 torr, the only possible explanation for the dramatic increase in the patient's transcutaneous oxygen value has to be a leak of room air under the electrode. When the electrode is sealed to the patient's skin, the $PtcO_2$ value should decrease to the actual value. If the patient had a patent ductus arteriosus, a decrease in the $PtcO_2$ value would be found over the patient's left chest area and body. Usually a decrease in the $PtcO_2$ value over the right chest is not seen because this area receives preductal blood. An increased temperature inside the incubator would have no effect on the $PtcO_2$ value. However, a decrease in temperature inside the incubator could result in vasoconstriction and a resulting decrease in $PtcO_2$ value. Even if the patient's cardiac output and lung condition have improved, the $PtcO_2$ value is too high for a neonate breathing room air. (It is important also to realize that if a leak of room air occurs under the transcutaneous carbon dioxide electrode, a decrease in the $PtcCO_2$ value will be noted because room air contains virtually no carbon dioxide.)

16. **C.** Recheck the blood gas analyzer for a problem with the PO_2 electrode. A calculation of the patient's PAO_2 level shows that the maximum PaO_2 value the patient can have is 127 torr. Until an accurate PaO_2 value can be determined, no change should be seen in the patient's inspired oxygen percentage. Although no reason exists to doubt the pH and $PaCO_2$ values, no decision to maintain the patient on his or her present ventilator settings can be made until a correct PaO_2 value is obtained. No indication exists to hyperventilate this drug-overdose patient. Do not confuse this case with hyperventilation of a patient with a head injury and increased intracranial pressure.

Chapter Four: ANSWER KEY FOR THE WRITTEN REGISTRY LEVEL EXAM SELF-STUDY QUESTIONS

1. **D.** All of the data in the table indicate severe obstructive lung disease. The TLC and RV are both greater than 120% of predicted, indicating significant air trapping. All three flow measurements are far lower than predicted. If the patient had restrictive lung disease, the TLC and RV values would be smaller than predicted.

2. **C.** Patients with severe air trapping, as found with emphysema, take much longer than normal to "wash" the nitrogen out of their lungs. Often the test must be prolonged for several minutes past the usual 7-minute duration to eliminate enough nitrogen to complete the test. The nitrogen washout test requires the patient to breathe in 100% oxygen to displace the resident nitrogen found in the lungs. The respiratory exchange ratio has to do with oxygen consumption and carbon dioxide production; it has nothing to do with nitrogen elimination. Nitrogen is not active in metabolism. The normal amount of nitrogen found in the body is not significantly affected by the nitrogen washout test.

3. **B.** The unit should be calibrated before use. The lung diffusion test would be most affected in that the CO in the cigarette smoke would bind to the hemoglobin of the patient's blood. This results in a lower than true test result. The other tests are not affected by CO.

4. **D.** The inspiratory reserve volume (IRV) is found from the end of a tidal volume inspiration to the TLC. It represents the additional volume that can be inhaled after a normal tidal volume. Review Figure 4-14 if needed. Do not be confused by vital capacity efforts that look "upside down" compared with others. Review the various volume-time curve tracings in the chapter for extra practice determining volumes. Volume number 2 is the ERV. Volume number 3 is the vital capacity. Volume number 4 is the ERV and tidal volume combined. Volume number 1 is the tidal volume.

5. **B.** The expiratory reserve volume (ERV) represents the volume of air that can be exhaled after a normal tidal volume is exhaled. Review Figure 4-14 if needed. Do not be confused by vital capacity efforts that look "upside down" compared with others. Review the various volume-time curve tracings in the chapter for extra practice determining volumes. Volume number 1 is the tidal volume. Volume number 3 is the vital capacity. Volume number 4 is the ERV and tidal volume combined.

6. **B.** All patient flows, volumes, and capacities must be mathematically converted from atmospheric temperature, pressure, saturated (ATPS) to body temperature, pressure, saturated (BTPS) conditions. This results in the exhaled flows or volumes measured at room temperature being adjusted for the expansion of gas found at the patient's body temperature. Standard temperature, pressure, dry (STPD) conditions are used only with diffusing capacity tests. Atmospheric temperature, pressure, dry (ATPD) is not used for reporting any pulmonary function results.

7. **C.** It is necessary to place a carbon dioxide absorber in the PFT system when the patient has to breathe on a closed system for an extended period. Without one, the patient will rebreathe his or her own exhaled carbon dioxide. If too much water is around the spirometer bell, some splashing may occur. However, too much water will not cause the patient to feel short of breath. If nose clips were left off the patient, he or she may breathe through the nose instead of the mouth. This will not cause a feeling of shortness of breath.

8. **D.** A body plethysmography test for total lung capacity (TLC) will be the most accurate for a patient with severe emphysema, because it can measure the volume of *all* gas within the chest. This includes gas in damaged parts of the lungs that do not ultimately connect to larger airways and the outside atmosphere. The 7-minute nitrogen washout test and helium dilution test measure only the gas in areas of the lungs that connect to the larger airways and outside atmosphere. This may result in an undermeasurement of the patient's true lung volumes. The single-breath nitrogen washout test is not used to measure the TLC. It is used to assess the evenness of inspiratory and expiratory gas flow.

9. **B.** Patients with uncontrolled asthma will have increased airway inflammation. This causes an increase in exhaled nitric oxide (eNO). The exhaled nitric oxide analyzer can measure this level so that the physician is more aware of the patient's condition. To a lesser extent, patients with an exacerbation of their COPD will also have an increase in eNO. This technology has not been shown to be beneficial in patients with ARDS or asbestos exposure.

10. **B.** Because the FVC test lasts for only a few seconds, the patient will not rebreathe significant amounts of carbon dioxide; therefore a carbon dioxide absorber is not needed. In addition, in some pulmonary function systems, a carbon dioxide absorber slows the flow of exhaled gas and results in lower reported FVC values than are actually present. The PFT circuit must be airtight to prevent any leakage and resulting lower volumes and flows. Volume calibration is done by pumping a known volume (3 L) into and out of the spirometer. Any leak will result in a lower than expected volume being found. The kymograph should have its speed settings checked to make sure that the timing of the test is accurate.

11. **D.** All listed items must be avoided to ensure an accurate FVC test. Coughing causes variable flows and cuts off the full FVC volume. A leak results in a loss of volume. A weak patient effort results in a slower expiratory flow than the patient can optimally provide. When tests are done properly, they show consistent results. Excessive variability shows inconsistent patient effort.

12. **C.** A diffusion study measures carbon monoxide diffusion to evaluate oxygen diffusion across the alveolar-capillary membrane. It is not helpful in the diagnosis of asthma. The other three listed tests can be very useful in diagnosing asthma. With a before and after bronchodilator study, a patient with asthma who is responsive to inhaled bronchodilator medications shows improved flows after inhaling the medication. A patient with an asthma problem often reveals a distinctive flow-volume loop tracing (see Figure 4-10). A bronchoprovocation test usually produces a decreased expiratory flow in a patient with asthma.

13. **C.** Spirometry before and after inhalation of a bronchodilator is the best test to differentiate between asthma and emphysema. Most patients with asthma have some reversibility of the bronchospasm. Their spirometry should show improved expiratory flows after inhalation of a bronchodilating medication. Patients with emphysema have very little, if any, improvement in expiratory flows after inhalation of a bronchodilating medication. This is because the alveoli, and not the airways, are damaged. The other three listed tests may not show significant differences between patients with asthma and those with emphysema.

14. **D.** Tracing *D* shows a severe "scoop" during the expiratory part of the patient effort after the peak flow. This dramatic decrease in expiratory flow is characteristic of severe small airway obstruction. Tracing *A* shows a less severe decrease in expiratory flow after the peak flow. Tracing *B* shows a severely reduced peak flow that is characteristic of a fixed extrathoracic obstruction. Tracing *C* shows a normal flow-volume

loop. Review Figure 4-10 if needed for a comparison of different flow-volume loops.

15. **B.** Tracing *B* shows a severely reduced peak flow that is characteristic of a fixed extrathoracic obstruction. This might be caused by a laryngeal tumor, paralyzed vocal cord, or other upper airway problem. Tracing *D* shows a severe "scoop" during the expiratory part of the patient effort after the peak flow. This dramatic decrease in expiratory flow is characteristic of severe small airway obstruction. Tracing *A* shows a less severe decrease in expiratory flow after the peak flow. Tracing *C* shows a normal flow-volume loop. Review Figure 4-10 if needed for a comparison of different flow-volume loops.

16. **A.** Tracing *C* shows an increased peak flow compared with tracing *A* and correction of the expiratory "scoop"

seen in tracing *A*. In addition, the inspiratory flow on tracing *C* is greater than that on tracing *A*. All of these changes show significant improvement, indicating that the patient's condition is treatable. The patient's effort or lack of effort cannot be determined by looking at the two tracings. Tracing *C* is normal and does not justify another bronchodilator treatment.

17. **C.** The patient's value is increased, because the upper end of normal is 25 parts per billion (ppb). This would indicate increased airway inflammation, possibly from asthma. The analyzer should be calibrated before use, but there is no indication that this was not done or that the equipment is not functioning properly. The eNO test should always be performed first in a sequence. If other tests are performed first, the patient's eNO will be artificially increased.

Chapter Five: ANSWER KEY FOR THE WRITTEN REGISTRY EXAM SELF-STUDY QUESTIONS

1. **D.** The patient should be kept on 28% oxygen because the pulmonary vascular resistance decreased from 9 to 5 mm Hg/L/min and the PaO_2 increased from 57 to 63 torr when the patient was increased from 24% oxygen. The patient is not hypoxemic; there is no indication to begin mechanical ventilation. A bronchodilating agent such as albuterol may help the patient's breathing somewhat, but it is not effective at reducing pulmonary vascular resistance.

2. **C.** The patient's pulmonary vascular resistance can be determined by calculating the pulmonary artery diastolic pressure minus the pulmonary capillary wedge pressure (PAd-PCWP) as follows:

$$
\begin{array}{ll}
\text{PAd} & 20 \text{ mm Hg} \\
\text{PCWP} & \underline{-9 \text{ mm Hg}} \\
& 11 \text{ mm Hg}
\end{array}
$$

Because a normal PAd-PCWP gradient is no more than 5 mm Hg, this patient's value of 11 mm Hg indicates increased pulmonary vascular resistance. Even though the patient's PAP is elevated at 35/20 mm Hg, that pressure alone does not provide enough information to determine that the patient has right ventricular failure/cor pulmonale. An increased right ventricular pressure in a patient with COPD indicates right ventricular failure/cor pulmonale. Because the patient has a normal PCWP of 9 mm Hg she does not have left ventricular failure. This problem is identified by an

increased PCWP. This same normal PCWP of 9 mm Hg indicates normal blood volume. Hypovolemia is identified by a PCWP that is less than 4 mm Hg.

3. **A.** If a clot is at the tip of the catheter it will prevent the patient's blood pressure from being transmitted back to the transducer for measurement. By withdrawing the clot, the lumen of the catheter will be open and the blood pressure can be measured. If an air bubble is in the arterial line, the measured blood pressure will be less than actual. This is because the patient's blood pressure will partially collapse the gas bubble (Boyle's law) and transmit a lower pressure to the transducer. Withdrawing the air bubble allows the patient's blood pressure to be accurately transmitted to the transducer. If the ventilator's peak pressure is too high, the patient's cardiac output will be reduced. This will result in a drop in blood pressure that will be measured equally on both arms. There is no evidence that the patient has a ventricular septal defect. Even if a septal defect were present, the blood pressure would be the same in both arms.

4. **B.** There are two significant changes in the patient's parameters that indicate that the patient has a pulmonary embolism. First, the patient's pulmonary vascular resistance has almost tripled in 2 hours. Second, the patient's pulmonary artery diastolic pressure minus the pulmonary capillary wedge pressure (PAd-PCWP) difference has increased significantly.

	9:00 am	11:00 am
PAd	10 mm Hg	21 mm Hg
PCWP	−8 mm Hg	−10 mm Hg
	2 mm Hg	11 mm Hg
	(Normal)	(Increased)

The fact that both of these parameters have quickly increased significantly, combined with the sudden drop in the patient's oxygen level, indicates that a pulmonary embolism has developed. Because the patient's pulmonary capillary wedge pressure (PCWP) remains normal at 8 mm Hg and 10 mm Hg, pulmonary edema is not supported as a diagnosis. Pulmonary edema results in an increased PCWP. Pneumonia will result in hypoxemia. However, the other parameters do not match this diagnosis. Cardiac tamponade will decrease the patient's cardiac output but will not increase pulmonary vascular resistance or PCWP.

5. **A.** The increase in the patient's $P_{ET}CO_2$ level from 33 to 41 torr indicates that alveolar ventilation has decreased. There are no data that correlate with pulmonary edema (such as an increased pulmonary capillary wedge pressure). If the patient were hyperventilating, the $P_{ET}CO_2$ level would have decreased instead of increased. Also, the $PaCO_2$ value would have decreased. There are no data that correlate with an increased cardiac output (such as a decreased difference between the oxygen content of arterial blood and the oxygen content of venous blood).

6. **D.** It is necessary to "zero" the transducer by exposing it to local barometric pressure. Adjust the transducer so that it reads zero when exposed to room barometric pressure. The patient must lie flat in bed with the transducer at midchest level to give accurate blood pressure readings. If the patient sits up, the blood pressure will read low. If the patient's head is lower than his or her body, the blood pressure will read too high. Saline must fill the pressure tubing, transducer dome, and arterial catheter so that the patient's blood pressure is measured accurately. If air fills the transducer dome, it will be variably compressed based on the patient's systolic and diastolic blood pressure changes. This is the result of Boyle's law and results in a lower-than-actual blood pressure being measured.

7. **A.** The patient's history of vomiting and diarrhea would lead to a loss of body fluids. Hypovolemia correlates with tachycardia and all of the patient's low blood pressure values. High ventilating pressures can result in a drop in the cardiac output. This can cause the systemic blood pressure to drop, but is unlikely to result in all of the hemodynamic values being low. In addition, there is no information given that relates to the patient's ventilating pressures. There is no mention of the patient's breath sounds showing bronchospasm. Even if bronchospasm was present, it would not cause all of the low hemodynamic values. If the balloon on the catheter ruptured, there would be a small volume of gas released into the pulmonary circulation. This would act as a small gas embolism. Although not good for the patient, this small gas embolism is unlikely to cause a drop in all of the hemodynamic pressures.

8. **C.** A pressure transducer for blood pressure monitoring should be "zero" calibrated at the patient's midchest level. This will result in accurate blood pressure measurements. If the patient is below the level of the transducer, the measured blood pressure will be less than actual. Conversely, if the patient is above the level of the transducer, the measured blood pressure will be greater than actual. If an air bubble or clot was in the arterial catheter, the problem would not be resolved when the patient's position was changed. Although postural drainage positions can cause a decrease in blood pressure, this does not always occur or fit the circumstances in this situation.

9. **C.** The low PCWP value of 3 torr indicates hypovolemia. The best treatment would be to administer intravenous fluids. Other clues to hypovolemia include the high electrolyte values from dehydration. Review these values in Chapter 1, if necessary. Giving a diuretic would make the situation worse. More O_2 is not needed since the patient is not hypoxemic. It is doubtful that giving atropine to increase the heart rate would be very helpful to increase the low PCWP.

10. **A.** After treatment, the patient's $P\bar{v}O_2$ value has increased from 35 to 41 torr. This improvement is now within the normal range and would indicate that the patient has normal tissue oxygenation. If the patient had worsening heart failure or decreased tissue perfusion, the $P\bar{v}O_2$ value would have decreased to less than the original value of 35 torr.

11. **D.** If the patient has a ventricular septal defect, the oxygen level gradient from the right atrium to the right ventricle will be increased. This is because high-oxygen blood from the left ventricle will leak through the defect into the right ventricle. Capnography and dead space values will not specifically indicate a hole in the ventricular septum. It is insufficient to only check the $P\bar{v}O_2$ value from the pulmonary artery. This value will not provide a comparison with the oxygen value before the right ventricle.

12. **D.** A triple-lumen $ScvO_2$ CVP catheter is the only catheter that will provide the needed information. The CVP pressure will indicate fluid balance. The $ScvO_2$ level will indicate the patient's central venous oxygen saturation, which correlates with the patient's oxygen consumption.

13. **B.** Mrs. Decker should have an arterial line placed because of her diagnosis of sepsis and her unstable blood pressure. Mr. Boone's blood pressure is stable with the normal range. Mrs. Dylan's blood pressure is returning to normal as her dehydration is corrected. While Mr. Zawinal's blood pressure is slightly elevated, it is stable and he does not have a condition prone to hemodynamic instability.

14. **A.** While not as accurate a measurement as mixed venous oxygen saturation (SvO_2 %) at evaluating tissue oxygenation, an $ScvO_2$ value of 60% very likely indicates tissue hypoxia. The usual clinical goal is to keep the patient's $ScvO_2$ level ≥70%. The decreasing $ScvO_2$ value could indicate decreased cardiac output, not increased. There is no correlation between $ScvO_2$ level and pulmonary vascular resistance.

Chapter Six: ANSWER KEY FOR THE WRITTEN REGISTRY EXAM SELF-STUDY QUESTIONS

1. **A.** At a flow of 1 L/min, a molecular sieve oxygen concentrator delivers at least 90% oxygen to the patient. A portable LOX system is not needed if the patient is not actively and frequently mobile. A semipermeable membrane oxygen concentrator delivers only about 40% oxygen to the patient. A piston compressor is useful for delivering pressurized air to power a small-volume nebulizer. It does not deliver more than 21% oxygen (room air) to the patient.

2. **D.** A polarographic oxygen analyzer does not have a gas sampling capillary tube; the paramagnetic type does. The other four listed problems can cause a polarographic analyzer to fail. The probe has a membrane through which oxygen diffuses. It must not be torn and must not have water, blood, or mucus covering it. An adequate amount of electrolyte solution must be present within the probe for the oxygen-related chemical reaction to take place. A functional battery is needed to drive the chemical reaction within the electrolyte solution.

3. **D.** A properly applied and used nonrebreathing mask should deliver at least 60% O_2. Continuous positive-airway pressure is not indicated in a patient with CO poisoning; more than 40% O_2 should be delivered. A simple mask or face tent does not deliver as much O_2 as is provided by a nonrebreathing mask.

4. **B.** Carbogen will help to keep an open patent ductus arteriosus to maintain system circulation. Nitric oxide is indicated for pulmonary hypertension, not for HLHS. It would be dangerous to close the patent ductus arteriosus in this patient. Heliox is indicated for airway obstruction, not for HLHS.

5. **D.** A Thorpe-type flowmeter will read accurately if backpressure is placed upon the exit of gas. Thus, the flowmeter will read less than zero, as the outlet is partially and then completely blocked.

6. **C.** The patient's arterial blood gas results show her PaO_2 to be 84 torr. This is too high for many patients with COPD. It is likely that her hypoxic drive to breathe has become blunted. This has resulted in her hypoventilating, with an increasing carbon dioxide level and secondary drowsiness. Although it is not possible to know the patient's inspired oxygen percentage with a 6 L/min nasal cannula, this flow has resulted in a PaO_2 that is too high. It is best to switch her to an air entrainment mask so that a known low oxygen percentage (24%) can be administered. Then, she should be monitored closely for returning alertness, and another arterial blood gas sample should be obtained. This should be evaluated for a lower, but safe, PaO_2 and a lower $PaCO_2$. The patient should not be left on her present oxygen flow through the nasal cannula because of her unnecessarily high oxygen level, hypoventilation, increasing carbon dioxide level, and secondary drowsiness. Changing her from a cannula to a simple face mask at the same oxygen flow will not correct these problems. She needs to be awakened because her drowsiness is not the result of simple fatigue.

7. **A.** It is likely that the biopsy site has developed some edema, which is causing the shortness of breath and "tight" throat feeling. Giving the patient 20% oxygen and 80% helium should help to ease the patient's shortness of breath because helium is less dense than nitrogen. Commonly, a patient's head is put down 30 degrees when the patient's blood pressure is low; this is unlikely to ease a feeling of shortness of breathing. Carbogen (carbon dioxide and oxygen mix) stimulates the breathing center of the brain but will not relieve the patient's shortness of breath caused by laryngeal edema. The 7-minute helium dilution test is performed in the pulmonary function laboratory to measure the patient's residual volume. It is not intended to relieve the patient's feeling of shortness of breath from laryngeal edema.

8. **B.** The significant discrepancy between the pulse oximeter reading and the CO oximeter can be explained only by the patient's having carbon monoxide poisoning. In this situation, only the CO oximeter reading will be accurate. A CO oximeter reading of 73% indicates severe hypoxemia. Therefore the patient should be changed to a nonrebreather mask with enough flow to keep the reservoir bag inflated. This maximizes the inspired oxygen percentage to the

patient. Maintaining the simple oxygen mask at the present flow or decreasing the oxygen flow to the simple oxygen mask to 4 L/min will worsen rather than improve the patient's condition. Nothing indicates that the CO oximeter is malfunctioning and should be recalibrated.

9. **C.** Because the reservoir bag has collapsed, the flow of helium and oxygen must be increased. Ideally, the reservoir bag should not collapse by more than one-third on inspiration. Decreasing the flow of gas to the patient will worsen the problem of shortness of breath, not improve it. When flow of gas to the mask is inadequate, it does not matter if the patient is given 24% oxygen or is changed to a 30% oxygen and 70% helium mix. In addition, no indication that the patient is hypoxemic is noted.

10. **B.** Setting 4.4 L/min on the oxygen flowmeter will deliver 7 L/min of a 70/30 heliox mix. (See page 211 for the heliox factors and for examples of how to make this calculation.)

11. **B.** Inhaled nitric oxide (INOmax) is indicated to dilate the pulmonary vascular bed of a newborn with persistent PPHN. When the pulmonary vascular bed dilates, more blood flows through the lungs, and oxygenation should improve. Instillation of intratracheal surfactant is indicated only in a newborn with infant RDS. Surfactant therapy is not indicated in PPHN. Although PEEP increases the functional residual capacity of an infant with RDS and improves oxygenation, PEEP must be used with great care, if at all, in a newborn with PPHN. Ten centimeter water PEEP may overexpand the alveoli of a newborn with PPHN and prevent blood from flowing through the capillary bed. Oxygenation will worsen rather than improve. Carbogen (carbon dioxide and oxygen mix) may be harmful to a newborn with PPHN, because an increased carbon dioxide level further constricts the newborn's pulmonary vascular bed. Carbogen is indicated in a newborn with hypoplastic left-heart syndrome.

12. **A.** Heliox therapy should be helpful in reducing the patient's work of breathing. This should allow more time for the corticosteroid and aminophylline medications to begin working. Nitric oxide is a pulmonary vasodilator and is not indicated for status asthmaticus. Review Box 6-1 if needed. It is not ecessary at this time to go against a patient's wishes and begin mechanical ventilation without first trying heliox therapy. Absolutely no reason justifies allowing this patient to die of status asthmaticus! It should not be fatal if managed appropriately and aggressively.

13. **B.** Because the patient's PVR is now in the normal range, the concentration of nitric oxide can be reduced. The patient's PVR then should be reassessed. It is more prudent to wean off the nitric oxide level rather than discontinue the gas in one step. No need exists to increase the NO to 30 ppm because the patient's PVR is in the normal range. It also is possible that this level of NO could be toxic. Carbogen is not indicated for pulmonary hypertension.

14. **C.** The heliox factor for a 70% helium/30% oxygen mix is 1.6. To calculate the total flow of this heliox mix through an oxygen flowmeter, the following calculation is made: 8 L/min of gas observed on the oxygen flowmeter × 1.6 = 12.8 (13) L/min actual heliox gas flow.

15. **A.** A portable liquid oxygen system should have a long enough duration to provide her with oxygen for the trip. An "E" tank of oxygen could be awkward to take on the trip. It would be challenging to pre-stage oxygen tanks at various stores. The patient should not decrease her oxygen flow just to increase the duration of the "E" tank.

Chapter Seven: ANSWER KEY FOR THE WRITTEN REGISTRY EXAM SELF-STUDY QUESTIONS

1. **B.** The patient's symptoms indicate that she is hyperventilating. Having her inhale at a slower rate will cause her to retain more carbon dioxide while still taking in the desired deep breath. It is not necessary at this time to stop the treatment. However, it may be necessary to stop treatment if the hyperventilation symptoms return while the patient is breathing more slowly. Reducing her IS volume goal will not expand her lungs as deeply. The patient is more likely to hyperventilate if she breathes in a deeper volume at the original rate.

2. **D.** It is best to use common language when describing the basic purpose of a treatment. The phrase *bilateral basilar microatelectasis* is too technical for the average patient to understand. Limit technical discussions to other health care professionals. No evidence suggests that incentive spirometry will make a surgical wound heal faster. The topic of pneumonia should not be brought up at this time because the patient does not have it yet. There is no need to cause concern about a potential problem at this time in the teaching process.

3. **A.** Incentive spirometry is the simplest and least expensive way to correct a limited case of atelectasis. PEP therapy is indicated when a patient has difficulty mobilizing secretions. Nasotracheal suctioning is

limited to unconscious, uncooperative patients who cannot cough out their secretions. IPPB would be needed only if the patient could not adequately perform incentive spirometry. It is not needed yet.

4. **C.** No evidence suggests that incentive spirometry will increase cardiac output. Outcome measures indicating that incentive spirometry is improving lung function include normal lung fields on chest x-ray, increased arterial oxygen level, and improved breath sounds. All would indicate the opening of atelectatic alveoli.

5. **A.** According to Table 7-1, incentive spirometry is indicated in this patient at this time. In addition, a sustained maximal inspiration effort should be helpful. IPPB should be tried only if incentive spirometry is found to be ineffective. No evidence indicates that positive expiratory pressure therapy or postural drainage with percussion and vibration is needed at this time to help in mobilizing secretions.

6. **B.** If the patient inhales at a slower rate, she should be able to hold the inspiratory capacity longer. If her inspiratory capacity target is appropriate, she will not be able to inhale an additional 500 mL. There is no advantage to having her exhale faster. There is no

therapeutic reason to lower her target volume by 100 mL and raise her respiratory rate to 25 times per minute. Incentive spirometry is most effective at treating atelectasis when the inspiratory capacity is inhaled slowly and sustained for several seconds.

7. **C.** It is best to increase her goal by 500 mL because she can easily reach her current volume goal. Doubling her volume goal is too large of a step. It is best to increase volume goals gradually as the patient improves, so that progress can be seen. Switching to a flow displacement device with the same volume goal provides no benefit. The patient seems to be doing well with the self-directed protocol. So, there is no reason to change to IPPB at this time.

8. **C.** A patient with COPD should not attempt a normal cough because the high lung pressure generated may cause the airways to collapse. This could lead to air trapping.

9. **B.** Review Table 7-1 for the indications for IS.

10. **C.** Review the mathematical process presented earlier in this chapter and in Chapter 4 for the calculation of IC.

11. **C.** Normal vesicular breath sounds indicate normal lung expansion with no atelectasis.

Chapter Eight: ANSWER KEY FOR THE WRITTEN REGISTRY EXAM SELF-STUDY QUESTIONS

1. **A.** It is likely that a patient who has chronic bronchitis is always producing secretions. So, it is important to know if the volume has gone up or down recently. If the volume of secretions has gone down or the secretions are thicker, aerosol therapy may be helpful. Because the patient probably is taking pulmonary-related medications, it is important to know whether or not they are helping his breathing. If his medications are not effective, the physician should evaluate the patient and consider a change. Hours of sleep at night and exercise tolerance are important to know but do not related directly to secretions and the need for aerosol therapy.

2. **A.** A cascade-type humidifier can be used to deliver the desired 35% oxygen to the patient at the desired temperature to meet the neutral thermal environment requirements. An oxyhood will deliver the oxygen and humidity to the infant's head and will not be affected by the incubator portholes being opened for patient care. The incubator's low oxygen setting does not allow delivery of a precise oxygen percentage. It probably will provide about 40% oxygen, but the percentage will drop when the portholes are opened. There is no way to know the oxygen percentage that a 3-L/min nasal

cannula will deliver to an infant. The incubator's high oxygen setting does not allow a precise oxygen percentage to be delivered. It probably will provide about 80% oxygen, but the percentage will drop when the portholes are opened.

3. **C.** It is likely that this dehydrated patient also has dried secretions. When continuous aerosol therapy was started, her secretions absorbed the aerosol and swelled in size. The swollen secretions could block small airways, resulting in shortness of breath and crackles for breath sounds. Intravenous fluids should reduce her dehydration. Even if she were more dehydrated, this would not cause her new signs and symptoms. Although it is possible that her influenza may be getting worse, it is unlikely to result in these new signs and symptoms. Normal saline is a bland aerosol that should not cause any allergic reactions such as the ones the patient is demonstrating.

4. **B.** Incubators are not able to provide an exact and adjustable oxygen percentage to an infant. The two oxygen flow settings are not adjustable to control the delivered oxygen percentage. In addition, when the portholes are opened for patient care, the internal gas leaks out and the oxygen percentage drops. Incubators

are able to isolate an infant from the surrounding environment and to control the temperature and humidity around the infant.

5. **C.** Severe coughing and wheezing so quickly after the DPI medication is taken indicate an adverse reaction. Treatment should be stopped. The physician should be contacted about the possible need for an inhaled bronchodilator medication. Because it is possible that the rapidly inhaled breath triggered the cough and wheezing, the patient should not do it again. Slowly breathing through the DPI will not aerosolize the medication powder. No order states that more than the ordered dose of corticosteroid should be given. In addition, a corticosteroid is a controller-type medication and will not help a person with acute bronchospasm.

6. **C.** Placing the infant under a radiant warmer allows adequate contact with the patient for his or her many necessary medical procedures. The skin temperature probe allows the infant's temperature to be servo-controlled to prevent underheating or overheating. An oxygen hood will help to maintain the infant's head temperature but will not help with the rest of the body. Placing the infant inside an incubator will severely limit patient contact. It will be very difficult to maintain a steady temperature because the portholes are opened frequently. It will be difficult to try to maintain the incubator temperature based on occasional patient rectal temperature values. It would be acceptable to place the infant inside an incubator with a skin temperature probe if the unit could be kept closed. Unfortunately, this infant will need frequent contact for care and the portholes will have to be opened.

7. **A.** Humidity deficit will be *decreased* by aerosol therapy. Some patients with hypersensitive airways could have bronchospasm after inhaling a bland aerosol. Infants can become fluid overloaded with prolonged aerosol therapy. Dried secretions can absorb water and can swell up to block small airways.

8. **D.** A lung abscess is a serious infection. If the patient has this problem, the secretions would have a foul odor, would contain cellular debris, and would have a dark yellow or green color. If the secretions were collected and saved, they would settle out into three layers, as is shown in Figure 1-24. Review Table 1-13 and related discussion in Chapter 1, if needed. Specific gravity is performed on a urine specimen, not on secretions. Although some blood may be evident in secretions, a platelet count is not performed on a secretion sample.

Chapter Nine: ANSWER KEY FOR THE WRITTEN REGISTRY EXAM SELF-STUDY QUESTIONS

1. **A.** Flumazenil (Romazicon) is used to reverse the effects of the benzodiazepine-type sedative agents (Valium, Versed). There is no indication that the patient had been given a sedative. The other three drugs (Survanta, Infasurf, Curosurf) are used in surfactant replacement therapy in neonates with respiratory distress syndrome.

2. **B.** The patient's continued wheezing justifies more medication. The small increase in heart rate does not justify stopping the treatment. Vertolin will not be any more effective than Xopenex. Aminophylline is not indicated at this time. First, find out if more Xopenex causes bronchodilation.

3. **D.** A patient with status asthmaticus should be admitted to the intensive care unit. She will be monitored more closely in the ICU than on the pediatric floor, and she will be cared for by personnel who are accustomed to critically ill patients. Xopenex is a fast-onset bronchodilator that is indicated for continuous nebulization. Continuous ECG monitoring should be performed to observe tachycardia or arrhythmia. Continuous pulse oximetry should be performed to monitor oxygen level. Serevent is a slow-onset, long-duration bronchodilator that is indicated in stable patients with asthma.

4. **D.** A sedative agent will have a calming effect on a patient anxious about being unable to move or communicate while paralyzed on the ventilator. A sedative will not control pain or sustain a pharmacologic paralysis. Although a high enough dose of a sedative will put a patient to sleep and therefore prevent "fighting" the ventilator, that is not its primary purpose. In addition, if the patient is pharmacologically paralyzed, no need exists for any other medication to control the patient's breathing efforts.

5. **A.** Epinephrine has vasoconstricting properties (as well as properties causing bronchodilation and tachycardia) and should help to stop bleeding at the biopsy site. Intravenous heparin is contraindicated because it increases clotting time and will likely increase the bleeding. Albuterol (Proventil) is a very effective bronchodilator but has no effect on peripheral blood vessels. Lidocaine (Xylocaine) is used to stop cardiac arrhythmias but has no effect on peripheral blood vessels.

6. **D.** Hypertonic (1.8% to 20%) saline has been shown to be an effective mucolytic in patients with cystic fibrosis. Acetylcysteine (Mucomyst) is no longer recommended for cystic fibrosis patients because of possible complications from long-term use. Dornase alfa

(Pulmozyme) is not indicated in this patient because purulent (infected) secretions with DNA strands are not present. Normal (0.9%) saline will not be as effective a mucolytic as hypertonic saline.

7. **D.** Increasing the dose of albuterol should improve the patient's bronchodilation and result in an improved peak flow. Because the patient's peak flow is only 65% of personal best, the albuterol dose should not be maintained or decreased. Adding an intravenous corticosteroid to the patient's medications would require the home care patient to travel to the physician's office for injections. This is not a practical solution. In addition, no clear indication exists that intravenous corticosteroids are needed at this time.

8. **A.** Nebulized acetylcysteine (Mucomyst) has been found to decrease the viscosity (thickness) of mucoid secretions in patients with chronic bronchitis. Dornase alfa (Pulmozyme) has not been approved for use in patients with chronic bronchitis; it is only approved for patients with cystic fibrosis. Fluticasone (Flovent) is an inhaled corticosteroid; it has no effect on secretions. Flumazenil (Romazicon) is used to reverse the effects of benzodiazepine-type sedative drugs such as Valium or Versed. It has no effect on pulmonary secretions.

9. **A.** Flumazenil (Romazicon) is used to reverse the effects of benzodiazepine-type sedative agents (Versed, Valium). Rather than calming a patient, flumazenil is used to reverse the effects of oversedation. Pancuronium bromide (Pavulon) and succinylcholine (Anectine) are medications used to paralyze a patient. This will certainly result in the patient's breathing being controlled by the ventilator. Morphine sulfate (Duramorph) is given to control pain and will have a secondary benefit of sedating the patient if enough is given.

10. **A.** Adrenaline will cause vasoconstriction of the systemic blood vessels to raise the patient's blood pressure. In addition, the laryngeal blood vessels will constrict and reduce the airway swelling. Adrenaline is also a bronchodilator. Advil has some antiinflammatory properties but will not have any effect on the

patient's low blood pressure. Nebulized racemic epinephrine (microNefrin) is useful with upper airway edema but will not have enough systemic effect to raise the blood pressure significantly. Narcan is a reversing agent for the narcotic-type analgesics.

11. **D.** Tobramycin (TOBI) has been approved by the Food and Drug Administration (FDA) to prevent the development of *Pseudomonas aeruginosa* pneumonia in cystic fibrosis patients. Pentamidine (Pentam or NebuPent) has been approved by the FDA to prevent the development of *Pneumocystis carinii* pneumonia, not *Pseudomonas aeruginosa* pneumonia. Isoniazid (INH) is used to prevent or treat a *Mycobacterium tuberculosis* (TB) infection.

12. **B.** Ribavirin (Vibrazole) is given to stop the reproduction of respiratory syncytial virus (RSV). It is given by the SPAG II nebulizer. Racemic epinephrine (microNefrin) is a vasoconstricting drug and is given by small volume nebulizer to shrink edematous mucous membranes of the upper airway. Intratracheal beractant (Survanta) is given to a premature neonate with RDS. It would not be needed in this older patient who has recovered from the condition. Cromolyn sodium (Intal) is given by small volume nebulizer to prevent the onset of asthma. It is not effective against RSV.

13. **B.** NebuPent is given by small volume nebulizer (SVN) once every 4 weeks as a preventative agent for *Pneumocystis carinii* pneumonia. Bactrim is the preferred medication to treat an actual *Pneumocystis carinii* pneumonia infection. TOBI is given by SVN to treat a cystic fibrosis patient with *Pseudomonas aeruginosa* pneumonia. Relenza is given to treat influenza, a viral infection.

14. **A.** The potassium level of 3.4 mEq/L is lower than normal. Her PVCs could be caused by the hypokalemia. She should be given intravenous potassium to raise her K+ level into the normal range. Giving more diuretic medication and restricting her potassium could be dangerous. It would be best to continue 40% oxygen until her lung function has further improved. When her saturation is greater than 90%, the supplemental oxygen can be gradually reduced.

Chapter Ten: ANSWER KEY FOR THE WRITTEN REGISTRY EXAM SELF-STUDY QUESTIONS

1. **B.** By changing the expiratory resistance to a larger diameter orifice, the patient will be able to exhale more quickly. Telling the patient to blow out harder will increase the pressure within the system. This could increase the patient's discomfort. Changing the expiratory resistance to a smaller diameter orifice will further increase the expiratory time, not decrease it. Although

a PEP system can have oxygen added to it to power the nebulizer, no mention of one is made in the question. In addition, the use of supplemental oxygen to a nebulizer does not have any effect on the expiratory time of the patient. (See Figure 10-17 on page 299.)

2. **C.** Initially the patient should be taught to expectorate as hard as possible. If that is not possible because

of pain, a serial cough with low flows can be attempted. The patient should be given a pain medication so that a strong cough can be tolerated. It is important that the patient inhale deeply to have an effective cough. Pain will be lessened if the incision is supported with the patient's hands or a pillow. Inhaling and exhaling several times before coughing help the patient to build up to a large breath and prepare for the coughing effort.

3. **D.** The patient should sit up because tachycardia and dyspnea are definite indications of intolerance of the head-down position. It could be dangerous for the patient to continue in the head-down position for even 5 more minutes. The treatment should be stopped, and the patient should sit up rather than being turned to the other side. Give the patient supplemental oxygen only if it is determined that the patient is hypoxic after the patient sits up. (See Box 10-3 on page 288.)

4. **A.** It is reasonable to increase the PEP level from 5 to 10 cm water. Have the patient try this moderately increased pressure for several minutes, and evaluate the effectiveness of the patient's cough effort. The PEP level should not be increased to 15 cm water unless 10 cm water has been shown to be ineffective. Incentive spirometry is indicated for atelectasis or the prevention of atelectasis. It is not indicated for secretion clearance, as is PEP therapy. It is too early in the treatment to determine that PEP therapy should be discontinued.

5. **A.** To drain the lateral basal segment of the left lower lobe, the patient must be placed with the right side down on the bed and the head of the bed dropped 30 degrees. The other positions will not properly drain the left lower lobe. Review the postural drainage positions if needed. (See page 287 and Figure 10-3 on page 299.)

6. **A.** Review Figure 10-7 on page 291.

7. **D.** The Flutter is designed to cause rapid airway vibrations. These vibrations result in a rapid variation in airway pressure. This results in the airways rapidly dilating and then contracting to their resting diameter. These changes seem to loosen secretions so that they can expectorated more easily by the patient. Neither increased transpleural pressure nor increased intrapleural pressure has any effect on the mobilization of secretions.

8. **B.** PEP therapy will increase end-expiratory lung pressure. This should increase alveolar volume and prevent the development of atelectasis. Blow bottles are no longer in use because they have been shown to be ineffective in the management of atelectasis. A mechanical chest percussor can be used with CPT to help mobilize secretions. However, it does not have any benefit in preventing atelectasis. Inspiratory muscle training is beneficial in patients with chronic obstructive lung disease because they are usually deconditioned. This should be part of a general conditioning program. However, inspiratory muscle training has no direct effect on atelectasis and should not be confused with use of an incentive spirometer. (See Box 10-5 on page 296.)

9. **A.** The patient must sit up straight because the vest is ridged. To work best, it should have even contact with the patient's entire chest wall. This would not happen if the patient were lying on a side. It is best to have the patient start at the lowest rate and pressure to gain confidence in the unit and not risk injury. The HFCWO unit does not have a nebulizer.

10. **B.** The position described would be used to drain secretions from the patient's posterior segment of the right upper lobe. See Figure 1-8 on page 14 for the area of consolidation, Figure 10-1 for all lung segments, and Figure 10-3 on page 290 for the postural drainage position.

11. **C.** Hemoptysis indicates pulmonary trauma. The treatment should be stopped and the physician notified. No further treatment should be done until after the patient is assessed, and it is found safe to proceed with the treatment. (See Box 10-3 on page 288.)

12. **D.** According to the AARC *Clinical Practice Guideline* (1991), CPT (postural drainage, percussion, and vibration) should be discontinued when the patient is able to expectorate secretions without other assistance. Continuing the treatment and adding procedures are not necessary and may unnecessarily add to the patient's costs.

13. **D.** CPAP is indicated to increase a patient's functional residual capacity to improve oxygenation. It has no effect on secretions. OPEP therapy, the Flutter, the Acapella, and HFCWO have all been shown to be effective at mobilizing secretions. (Box 10-5 on page 296.)

14. **B.** The Acapella unit is inexpensive and easy for most patients to learn to use. HFCWO and IPV are expensive and complicated technologies. AD is not a form of high-frequency airway oscillation.

Chapter Eleven: ANSWER KEY FOR THE WRITTEN REGISTRY EXAM SELF-STUDY QUESTIONS

1. **D.** See page 323 for a listing of the identifying traits of normal sinus rhythm. See page 312 for Figure 11-5 showing a tracing of NSR and Table 11-1.

2. **D.** Sinus arrhythmia is shown in Figure 11-22 on page 323. Review the associated discussion if needed. In a patient receiving mechanical ventilation and PEEP, it is possible to put too much pressure on the heart, which reduces venous return. If the returning blood volume is decreased, the cardiac output also will decrease. The patient should be monitored and key people informed. It is too early to decide whether the PEEP level is too high and should be reduced. The physician should be consulted before making any change. Atropine will increase the patient's heart rate and is not indicated in this situation. No indication suggests that the patient has an arrhythmia that requires synchronized cardioversion.

3. **A.** ECG monitoring will not provide any useful information about peripheral perfusion. The patient could have a normal heart rhythm and have altered perfusion. Electrolyte disturbances, especially the potassium (K^+) level, can alter the heart's electrical conduction system. It is wise to monitor a patient with a known history of arrhythmias in case they return. Fast or excessive infusion of potassium can lead to serious arrhythmias that justify ECG monitoring.

4. **B.** The rhythm strip shows two identical premature ventricular contractions (unifocal PVCs). This, combined with the patient's history of sudden chest pain and shortness of breath, suggests a heart problem. A 12-lead ECG is indicted for the physician to be able to determine the patient's cardiac condition. Oxygen is indicated for the shortness of breath. In addition, the oxygen will help the heart if it is hypoxic. The patient's condition is not life threatening, and no need is seen for either synchronized cardioversion or defibrillation. A cardiac catheterization procedure is needed to identify any coronary artery blockages before angioplasty is indicated.

5. **C.** According to the current CPR guidelines, if an infant has a heart rate of less than 60/minute despite bag-mask ventilation with 100% oxygen, the rescuer should begin chest compressions. It is doubtful that adding PEEP or stimulation will increase the heart rate. In this situation, it is a waste of time and unnecessary to check the patient's pulse oximeter value.

6. **D.** Current ACLS guidelines state that atropine, epinephrine (both for bradycardia), and lidocaine (to suppress ventricular arrhythmias) can be given via the endotracheal tube during a CPR attempt if the patient

does not have a functioning IV line. Potassium chloride can be given only intravenously.

7. **A.** The rhythm strip shows ventricular fibrillation. The best way to treat this dangerous arrhythmia is to defibrillate the patient immediately. All of the other listed options are reasonable in a CPR attempt when appropriate. However, they are all secondary to treating the patient's ventricular fibrillation.

8. **C.** Interpretation of the patient's ABG results shows hyperventilation with a metabolic acidosis. Intravenous sodium bicarbonate should be given to correct the patient's acidosis. It is appropriate to keep the patient's PaO_2 at 210 torr during the CPR attempt to try to oxygenate the brain. Decreasing the respiratory rate or adding mechanical dead space to the manual resuscitator will increase the patient's carbon dioxide and further reduce the pH. If necessary, review arterial blood gas interpretation in Chapter 3.

9. **B.** Current ACLS guidelines state that atropine, epinephrine, and lidocaine can be given via the endotracheal tube during a CPR attempt if the patient does not have a functioning IV line. Intraosseous (within the bone) injection of CPR drugs is approved for neonatal resuscitation attempts. Intracardiac injection of CPR drugs is no longer performed. Currently CPR drugs are not given by nasal spray.

10. **A.** The patient's symptoms indicate a cardiac problem. It is wise to begin ECG monitoring quickly in case the patient has an arrhythmia. An ABG sample can be drawn after ECG monitoring has been started. A chest radiograph also can be done after ECG monitoring has been started. A capnometer value to check the patient's exhaled carbon dioxide value is not indicated at this time.

11. **C.** Pulseless ventricular tachycardia is a life-threatening arrhythmia. (See Figure 11-38 on page 331.) If the rate is so fast that a pulse cannot be felt, the cardiac output and blood pressure will be very low. The patient must be defibrillated as soon as possible to restore normal sinus rhythm. Second-degree heart block is treated with drugs or a pacemaker to speed the heart rate. Atrial flutter and sinus tachycardia are fast, but not life-threatening arrhythmias that are first treated with medications to slow the heart rate.

12. **C.** The newborn's vital signs and other clinical findings point to the need for manual ventilation with oxygen. Although directing oxygen to the neonate's face will be helpful, it does not go far enough to ensure adequate ventilation. It is too early to begin chest compressions. They will not be needed if the supplemental ventilation and oxygen cause the heart rate to increase. The neonate is in significant trouble,

and additional stimulation will not be enough to improve its breathing.

13. **B.** Intravenous naloxone (Narcan) can be given to reverse the sedating effect of the anesthetic drugs that passed from the mother to the infant. Epinephrine and atropine are cardiac stimulants, not breathing stimulants. Bag-mask ventilation may be needed but will not get the sedated infant to breathe by itself.

14. **D.** Giving intravenous epinephrine should increase the patient's heart rate and blood pressure. Lidocaine is given to suppress premature ventricular contractions (PVCs). Although the patient is bradycardic and hypotensive, chest compressions are not yet indicated. Because the patient is already being ventilated with supplemental oxygen, endotracheal intubation will not provide any significant improvement.

Chapter Twelve: ANSWER KEY FOR THE WRITTEN REGISTRY EXAM SELF-STUDY QUESTIONS

1. **C.** A tracheoesophageal fistula is a risk related to high cuff pressure; it would take several days to develop. The other complications would occur during placement of the tube. (See Box 12-6 on page 369.)

2. **D.** In an emergency situation it is fastest and easiest to place an oral endotracheal tube into most patients. A safe and secure airway can be assured within 20 to 30 seconds. An oropharyngeal airway only keeps the tongue from blocking the back of the throat. It does not provide a safe, secure airway. Hyperextending the patient's neck into the sniff position opens the airway but does not secure it from possible dangers such as vomiting and aspiration. Placing a nasal endotracheal tube requires an anesthesiologist and special equipment. This delay is unnecessary when oral endotracheal intubation can be done by a trained respiratory therapist.

3. **B.** A patient with a cervical spine injury should *not* have his or her neck hyperextended, as is needed during an oral intubation procedure. (See Box 12-5 on page 368.)

4. **A.** A mild case of stridor is first treated by nebulizing with the vasoconstrictor medication racemic epinephrine. This usually results in enough constriction of the throat's mucous membrane blood vessels to dilate the airway and correct the stridor. If this does not work, the patient may need to be intubated. A cricothyrotomy is only done to create an emergency airway opening if the patient's upper airway is obstructed by a foreign body or trauma. A tracheostomy is only performed if a long-term surgical airway opening is needed. This patient certainly does not need either of the latter two solutions to his or her problem.

5. **C.** Because the cuff pressure is so high on the small tracheostomy tube, it is best to replace the tube with one that is 8.5 mm ID. This is the correct size for an adult man. Increasing the tidal volume by 100 mL may deliver a larger tidal volume or it may just increase the leak around the tracheostomy tube. The actual problem is a tube that is too small for the patient's trachea. It is unsafe to increase the cuff pressure to seal the trachea and stop the tidal volume leak. Although the increased pressure overinflates the cuff to stop the leak, the circulation to the patient's tracheal mucosa is blocked and the mucosa can die. It is unsafe to deflate the cuff enough to reduce the cuff pressure to 15 mm Hg because the patient's tidal volume leak can worsen. (See able 12-1 on page 354.)

6. **B.** An adult patient usually has the proximal end of the tube at the 23- to 25-cm mark at the teeth for a midtracheal tube tip position. This, and the observation that the left side of the patient's chest is not moving as much as the right side, indicates that the tube has been pushed down into the right mainstem bronchus. The best thing to do is reposition the tube by suctioning the patient's airways and throat, deflating the cuff, withdrawing the tube about 4 cm, and reinflating the cuff. Of course, check for bilateral breath sounds, confirm a safe cuff pressure, and get a chest radiograph to complete the procedure. There is nothing to be gained by checking the abdominal radiograph because signs of vomiting and aspiration are not seen on it. Pneumonitis can be seen on a chest radiograph but not on an abdominal radiograph because an abdominal radiograph does not include the chest. Checking the patient's end-tidal carbon dioxide level demonstrates exhaled CO_2. However, this is not specific enough for this situation because the right lung can release carbon dioxide even if the left lung is not ventilated. Delivering a larger tidal volume breath does not inflate the left lung any better because the endotracheal tube has been pushed down the right mainstem bronchus.

7. **D.** All of the listed items can be used to confirm that the endotracheal tube is located within the trachea. Clinical experience has shown that the greater the

number of positive indicators, the more likely it is that the tube is properly located.

8. **C.** The patient should be reintubated because of the serious nature of the inspiratory stridor that is unresponsive to the inhaled vasoconstricting drug (racemic epinephrine), the low Spo_2 value, and the combative nature of the patient. An arterial blood gas value is not necessary because the Spo_2 value of 80% confirms hypoxemia. Getting the ABG sample and waiting for the results only delay the necessary intubation. Increasing the patient to 50% oxygen helps relieve the hypoxemia. However, once the patient is intubated and can breathe adequately, the Spo_2 value should increase to a safe level on the previous 40% oxygen. It could be very dangerous to administer a sedative medication to this patient. Sedating the patient further reduces the patient's ability to breathe through the narrowed airway.

9. **C.** A lateral neck x-ray film provides less useful information on proper placement of the endotracheal tube than is provided by a chest x-ray film. The presence of bilateral or at least right upper lobe breath sounds indicates proper tube placement.

10. **A.** A cuff pressure of 33 mm Hg is likely to obstruct blood and lymphatic flow to the tracheal soft tissues. This pressure does nothing to protect the vocal cords. In addition, the tracheostomy tube does not pass between the vocal cords.

11. **D.** When inserted into the esophagus, as is usually the case, the patient cannot vomit and the airway is maintained open. While the trachea is occasionally intubated with a Combitube, it is unintentional, and the patient can vomit. A Combitube is never placed through the nasal route. (See Box 12-2, Page 352.)

12. **B.** A nasopharyngeal airway can be easily inserted to push the tongue forward and open the airway. Prone positioning may cause the tongue to move forward and open the airway. More aggressive and invasive procedures, such as placing a tracheostomy button (or tube) or endotracheal intubation, should only be used if the first two options do not work.

13. **A.** A 7.0-mm nasotracheal tube would provide a secure airway and is the appropriate size for an adult female. Because of the nasal route, the tube should be smaller than that chosen for the oral intubation route. The Berman oropharyngeal airway device will support the tongue but does not provide a secure airway. The remaining two endotracheal tubes are too large for the patient whether an oral or nasal intubation is performed. (See Table 12-1 on page 354.)

14. **A.** With a fenestrated tracheostomy tube, when the inner cannula is removed and the cuff deflated, the patient can breathe through her natural upper airway and speak. At night, the inner cannula can be reinserted and the cuff inflated so that mechanical ventilation can be provided. It is impractical and possibly hazardous to switch a tracheostomy tube and tracheostomy button into and out of the patient twice a day. If the patient had an uncuffed tracheostomy tube, there would be a significant leak when she is put back onto the ventilator to sleep. It would be *fatal* to put the obturator into the tracheostomy tube without deflating the cuff. The patient's airway would be completely obstructed.

15. **A.** When the Combitube is placed into the esophagus, a gastric tube can be inserted into the stomach to empty it. The patient's lungs can be ventilated whether the tube is placed into the esophagus (as intended) or the trachea. Neither the Combitube nor the LMA can be placed by the nasal route. Unlike the LMA, the Combitube is not available in small pediatric sizes. (See Box 12-1 and Box 12-2.)

16. **A.** A cuff pressure of greater than 25 mm Hg (>35 cm H_2O) can obstruct blood flow to the mucous membrane of the trachea. The best solution is to replace the endotracheal tube with a larger one that can be sealed with a lower cuff pressure. Leaving the cuff pressure at 30 mm Hg or increasing the cuff pressure is likely to cause tracheal wall damage. Less cuff pressure would be safer but will result in a greater tidal volume leak. Increasing the respiratory rate only makes the leak occur more often.

17. **D.** A tracheoesophageal fistula could occur as a consequence of a high cuff pressure that blocks circulation to the tracheal mucosa. This problem is not caused by the intubation procedure itself. Tooth trauma, laceration of the pharynx, and esophageal intubation could occur during the intubation procedure. (See Box 12-6 on page 369.)

18. **D.** Reintubation is indicated by the patient's *severe* respiratory distress and inspiratory stridor. It would only be appropriate to administer a nebulized vasoconstricting drug (such as racemic epinephrine) if the patient had *mild* signs and symptoms. A bronchodilator medication has no vasoconstricting effects. While the patient may need supplemental oxygen, a cool aerosol will not correct the patient's dire situation.

Chapter Thirteen: ANSWER KEY FOR THE WRITTEN REGISTRY EXAM SELF-STUDY QUESTIONS

1. **C.** Suctioning an intubated patient does not simulate the gag reflex. The other listed items are important to know for patient safety and for legal reasons.

2. **D.** Suctioning removes secretions, as intended, as well as air (and its contained O_2) from the airways and lungs. This causes a transient drop in the patient's O_2 level. Vagal stimulation has no connection to hypoxic drive.

3. **D.** The commonly accepted practice is to limit the OD of a suction catheter to no more than one-half the ID of the endotracheal or tracheostomy tube. This allows the patient to breathe spontaneously around the catheter during the procedure. A smaller catheter may be used but will not remove as many secretions with each suctioning effort. This may result in the need to suction more frequently. Too frequent suctioning can result in a greater risk of trauma to the mucous membrane, hypoxemia, and vagal stimulation. A larger suction catheter prevents the patient from breathing around it. (Figure 13-3 and Table 13-1.)

4. **B.** Lubricating the tip of the catheter with sterile, water-soluble lubricating jelly helps the catheter to slide more easily through the patient's nasal passage. This should help to minimize the risk of trauma. Neither water nor saline is a good lubricant, because these drip off the catheter. A suction catheter should be flexible, not firm.

5. **D.** Suctioning is a *sterile* procedure. A clean-gloved hand is not sterile. The contaminated catheter should be replaced with a sterile one.

6. **A.** Suctioning of blood indicates that airway trauma has occurred. It is best to stop suctioning and monitor the patient. Only suction when there is a clear indication of retained secretions or blood. Tissue trauma can happen with a closed-airway suctioning system the same as with open-airway suctioning. There is no indication, such as thick secretions, for a saline lavage. There is no indication to change from an oral to a nasal route for the endotracheal tube. The tissue trauma is in the trachea or mainstem bronchi, not the upper airway.

7. **B.** If the Yankauer suctioning device hits the back of the patient's throat, gagging, retching, and vomiting can be induced. Bradycardia should not happen, because vagal stimulation does not occur with oropharyngeal suctioning. Hypoxemia should not occur, because oropharyngeal suctioning does not remove air (and oxygen) from the patient's lungs. Oropharyngeal stimulation should not produce any adrenergic stimulation or tachycardia.

8. **C.** Change to a 10 Fr catheter, because the 14 Fr catheter is too large for the endotracheal tube. (See Table 13-1 for the catheter and tube combinations that should be used.) A physician's order is needed to administer 10 cm H_2O PEEP. There is no indication that the patient is having any difficulties other than bradycardia during the suctioning procedure. Suctioning should be done as often as needed and not limited to twice per shift. The patient experiences bradycardia whenever she is suctioned because the catheter is too large. No indication is found that a catheter with a Coudé tip is needed to guide the catheter down the left (or right) mainstem bronchus. (See Table 13-1 for recommended catheter sizes.)

9. **C.** Because the patient experiences repeated serious hazards, suctioning should be discontinued. Switching to closed-airway suctioning may prevent hypoxemia and allow suctioning to be resumed. Because PEEP can have serious side effects, it should not be increased just for suctioning purposes. Because removing the patient from ventilatory support is the cause of the hypoxemia and related problems, shortening the duration of suctioning may lessen the hypoxemia. Increasing the frequency of suctioning exposes the patient to more frequent hypoxic episodes. It is safer to discontinue the suctioning procedure until a closed-airway suction system can be set up and used. Increasing the oxygen level from 80% to 100% is unlikely to prevent hypoxemia during suctioning. Again, it is safer to discontinue the suctioning procedure until a closed-airway suction system can be set up and used.

10. **D.** The greatest amount of negative pressure that can safely applied in any clinical situation is −150 mm Hg. Any greater negative pressure has been shown to cause airway tissue trauma, hypoxemia, and atelectasis. In general, use the least amount of suctioning pressure that effectively removes the patient's secretions.

Chapter Fourteen: ANSWER KEY FOR THE WRITTEN REGISTRY EXAM SELF-STUDY QUESTIONS

1. **D.** Pneumothorax, faintness and dizziness, and expectoration of blood indicate a serious patient problem. Treatment should be stopped, the patient evaluated, and help sought. It may be necessary to use a Bennett seal or face mask to get an airtight seal if the patient cannot seal his or her lips. The treatment can then be continued.

2. **B.** Adding expiratory retard is the only way to apply back-pressure to the patient's airways to attain more complete exhalations. This should help to reduce air trapping. Decreasing the flow will result in a longer inspiratory time but will not affect the expiratory flow of the tidal volume. Increasing the system pressure will deliver a larger tidal volume and could result in a worse air trapping problem. Adjusting the air-mix knob will change the oxygen percentage and inspiratory flow and will not improve the patient's air trapping.

3. **A.** The patient has a leak at the mouthpiece; correct it by switching to a face mask. Increasing the inspiratory flow will not correct the leak at the patient's mouth. Nose clips will not fix the patient's leak around the mouthpiece. There is no listed reason to switch the patient from IPPB to incentive spirometry.

4. **D.** Because the patient is calmer now, it is best to reduce the flow from the IPPB machine. This allows the delivered tidal volume and medication to be more equally delivered to all areas of the lungs. There is no need at this time to deliver a larger tidal volume. The goal is to deliver medication effectively to the lungs. Machine sensitivity is not a problem at this time.

5. **B.** The 1993 *AARC Clinical Practice Guideline* states that an IPPB-assisted breath should be at least 25% greater than the patient's spontaneous tidal volume. Considering the patient's condition, this would result in an initial IPPB breath goal of at least 450 mL (350 mL spontaneous tidal volume × 1.25 = 438 mL). The tidal volume can be increased later, as tolerated.

6. **A.** The 1991 *AARC Clinical Practice Guideline* on incentive spirometry states that IPPB should be used if the patient's IC is less than 33% of the preoperative value. It is doubtful if incentive spirometry would be effective since the patient's IC is so small. There is no indication of the need for nasotracheal suctioning, such as retained secretions. There is no indication of the need for a flutter treatment, such as retained secretions.

7. **C.** Expiratory retard cap setting 3 is best because the patient's tidal volume is adequate, wheezing is found only in the bases, and the patient is comfortable with the breath. The smaller settings (1 and 2) resulted in too long of an exhalation for patient comfort. With the largest setting (4) the patient's tidal volume decreased, wheezing was heard in all lobes, and the patient said that the lungs feel full.

8. **C.** Increasing the flow of gas to the patient will result in a more smooth delivery of tidal volume to the patient. This will be seen as a gradual, steady increase in the pressure. Increasing the target pressure will only deliver a larger tidal volume. It will not meet the patient's need for a faster breath. Increasing the sensitivity setting lets the patient start a breath easier but does not deliver a faster breath. If the patient inhales more quickly she will increase her work of breathing even more. If her breathing pattern is to be coached she should be told to inhale more slowly.

9. **A.** The best way to deliver a larger tidal volume is to deliver more pressure to the lungs. Decreasing the flow will only deliver the gas more slowly to the preset pressure. Less flow will not increase the tidal volume. Expiratory retard is only added if the patient has a problem with air trapping on exhalation. It will help with the exhalation of the delivered tidal volume but will not increase the size of the delivered tidal volume. If the patient inhales more forcefully, he or she will only increase the work of breathing because the flow will be inadequate.

10. **C.** The 2003 *AARC Clinical Practice Guideline* was used to determine this patient's minimum IPPB-delivered tidal volume. Steps in the calculation include:

    1. Convert the patient's body weight in pounds (lb) to kilograms (kg):

       $$\frac{180 \text{ lb}}{2.2 \text{ lb/kg}} = 81.82 \text{ kg (use 82 kg for this calculation)}$$

    2. Calculate the patient's predicted inspiratory capacity:

       Predicted IC = 50 mL × kg of ideal body weight

       Therefore, predicted IC = 50 mL × 82 kg = 4100 mL

    3. Calculate the patient's minimum IPPB-assisted tidal volume goal:

       Minimum IPPB goal = 0.33 × predicted IC
       = 0.33 × 4100 mL = 1353 mL

    Therefore a 1400-mL tidal volume is the best answer.

Chapter Fifteen: ANSWER KEY FOR THE ADVANCED SELF-STUDY QUESTIONS

1. **D.** ARDS results in stiff lungs that are at risk of volu-trauma if too large a tidal volume is forced into them. PCIRV is used with these patients because the peak pressure is limited to a safe level. The long inspiratory time used with PCIRV helps to oxygenate the patient. Asthma and chronic bronchitis are noted for high airway resistance, not stiffness of the lungs. These patients need a long expiratory time for complete exhalation. PCIRV would likely cause more air trapping because of the long inspiratory time and short expiratory time. A pulmonary contusion is a lung bruise from trauma. It is neither helped nor hindered by PCIRV.

2. **C.** Mean airway pressure is the average pressure throughout the breathing cycle. It is found by determining a series of inspiratory pressure and expiratory pressure points during short time intervals throughout a patient's breath cycle. See Figure 15-29 for an example. P_{peak} minus the plateau pressure gives a general indication of airway resistance. P_{peak} divided by inspiratory time is not used as a respiratory care calculation. Tidal volume divided by peak pressure is used to calculate dynamic compliance. See question 12 for an example.

3. **C.** Pulmonary edema, pulmonary fibrosis, and ARDS are all conditions in which the lungs become stiff. This results in decreased lung compliance and increased WOB. Emphysema is caused by loss of connective tissue within the lungs and results in increased lung compliance. As a result, the lungs are overinflated.

4. **A.** MMV ventilation is used to provide a secure minimum minute volume to unstable patients. Often, these patients have an unstable respiratory drive due to stroke or brain injury. MMV is a variation on SIMV; it does not allow the patient to trigger each breath as the A/C mode does. MMV is not like CPAP because MMV delivers mandatory tidal volume breaths.

5. **B.** Near-drowning patients are ventilated traditionally with the A/C or SIMV mode with a constant volume. HFV has been shown effective in ventilating patients with airway procedures such as laryngoscopy and bronchoscopy. HFO has been shown effective in patients with a bronchopleural fistula because the small tidal volumes and low driving pressures do not force gas out through the lung tear. This allows the tissues to heal.

6. **D.** Review the indications for ventilatory support in Box 15-1. These indications include a rapid, shallow breathing index of more than 105, a $PaCO_2$ of more than 55 torr, and cardiac dysrhythmias. The patient is not dangerously hypoxic with a PaO_2 of 70 torr.

7. **A.** Because the patient's left lung has been removed, he or she should have a delivered tidal volume that is about half of normal for two lungs. Giving a normal or larger than normal tidal volume for two lungs is likely to overdistend the patient's one remaining lung.

8. **A.** ARDS is characterized by very stiff lungs. A negative-pressure ventilator is unable to generate enough pressure to adequately ventilate any patient with low lung compliance. Also, an iron lung does not offer any modes other than control and cannot add PEEP. The other three conditions (neuromuscular defects, kyphoscoliosis, and COPD in acute failure) are not as challenging to ventilate. These patients are not intubated and require only assisted ventilation for a short period. Negative-pressure ventilation has been used successfully with these patients.

9. **B.** (See Box 15-3 on page 441 and Figure 15-19 on page 447 for information on the evaluation of an optimal PEEP study.) As PEEP establishes the patient's FRC, the pulmonary compliance should improve. Ventilation better matches perfusion, so that shunt will decrease and PaO_2 will increase. In addition, the patient's pulmonary vascular resistance (PVR) decreases as the lungs are properly ventilated and blood flow through them is normalized. If too much PEEP is applied, the lungs will be overstretched. This causes the PVR to increase and cardiac output to decrease as venous return to the lungs and heart is decreased. As a result, the patient's blood pressure decreases and heart rate increases.

10. **D.**

$$Cst = \frac{\text{Exhaled tidal volume} - \text{Compressed volume}}{\text{Plateau pressure} - \text{PEEP}}$$

In this situation, use the corrected tidal volume because the compressed volume has already been subtracted from the exhaled tidal volume. The following equation results:

$$Cst = \frac{600 \text{ mL}}{48-12}$$
$$= \frac{600 \text{ mL}}{36}$$

$$Cst = 17 \text{ mL/cm water}$$

11. **D.** Static compliance (Cst) is calculated as follows:

$$Cst = \frac{\text{Exhaled tidal volume} - \text{Compressed volume}}{\text{Plateau pressure} - \text{PEEP}}$$

Compressed volume = Compliance factor ×
Plateau pressure (4 mL/cm water × 25 cm water) = 100 mL

$$Cst = \frac{700\ mL - 100\ mL}{25 - 6}$$
$$= \frac{600\ mL}{19}$$

$$Cst = 32\ mL/cm\ water$$

12. **B.** Dynamic compliance (Cdyn) is calculated as follows:

$$Cdyn = \frac{Exhaled\ tidal\ volume - Compressed\ volume}{Peak\ pressure - PEEP}$$

Compressed volume = Compliance factor × Peak pressure
(4 mL/cm water × 35 cm water) = 140 mL

$$Cdyn = \frac{700\ mL - 140\ mL}{35 - 6}$$
$$= \frac{560\ mL}{29}$$

$$Cdyn = 19\ mL/cm\ water$$

13. **A.** HFJV involves the delivery of very small tidal volume breaths at a very high rate. It is impractical to try to measure these very small tidal volumes. The other three listed items plus a high pressure air source, suitable patient circuit, and the ventilator itself are needed for HFJV.

14. **C.** An increased airway resistance (caused by bronchospasm or airway secretions) causes the peak pressure to increase. A decrease in lung compliance (caused by pulmonary edema, pneumonia, or pleural effusion) causes the plateau pressure to increase. This, in turn, drives up the peak pressure. Without having both the peak and plateau pressures, there is no way to know more specifically what has caused the peak pressure to increase. If the lung compliance had increased or the airway resistance had decreased, the peak pressure would have decreased.

15. **D.** Therapeutic PEEP increases a patient's FRC. This increased lung volume enables better ventilation and perfusion matching. As a result, intrapulmonary shunting past underventilated alveoli is reduced. Increasing inspiratory time and sigh volume improves alveolar filling and may help to increase oxygenation. However, they do not increase FRC and therefore do not reduce shunting.

16. **A.** A 200-mL air leak through the pleural chest tube would explain the difference in delivered and returned tidal volumes. If the patient had a deflated endotracheal tube cuff, the delivered tidal volume would be decreased. The selected ventilator is microprocessor driven and has the ability to monitor itself. A warning of a system failure such as a miscalibrated spirometer would have occurred. No indication is noted that the patient has asthma or any condition causing bronchospasm. This ventilator has the ability to monitor auto-PEEP, and none is indicated.

17. **C.** Recent research has shown that alveolar overstretching and damage can occur when the plateau pressure is 30 cm water or greater. Therefore the patient should be switched from volume-cycled ventilation to pressure-cycled ventilation (pressure control) with a plateau pressure of no higher than 30 cm water. A high peak pressure may be caused by high airway resistance or lung stiffness. Lung compliance is calculated from tidal volume divided by plateau pressure. There is no direct connection between calculated lung compliance and alveolar overstretching. Both peak pressure and plateau pressure should be monitored. However, the combination has no direct connection to alveolar overstretching.

18. **D.** Interpretation of the patient's ABG results indicates hypercarbia and resulting respiratory acidosis. The best solution to the problem is to remove the 150 mL of mechanical dead space. There is no urgent need to decrease the patient's 35% oxygen because this is not a toxic amount. Decreasing the patient's minute volume further raises the carbon dioxide level and lowers the pH. Although increasing the respiratory rate would help to blow off some carbon dioxide, the best solution is to remove the dead space. After another set of ABGs is drawn and analyzed, the rate can be increased if still needed to blow off CO_2.

19. **D.** Atelectasis is best treated by giving the patient a larger sigh volume. This should help to open up alveoli that have collapsed or are prone to collapsing. Changing flow rate, expiratory time, and ventilator frequency have no impact on lung volume.

20. **A.** Permissive hypercapnia involves the gradual increasing of a patient's carbon dioxide level such that the pH does not become overly acidotic. It may be necessary to give the patient intravenous bicarbonate to keep the pH greater than 7.25. During permissive hypercapnia, the patient's $PaCO_2$ can increase to well above 50 torr, and the pH probably will decrease to below the normal range of 7.35.

21. **C.** SIMV allows the patient to breathe spontaneously when she wants to while still receiving support from the ventilator. A low level of pressure support should help to reduce her added WOB from the small endotracheal tube. Therapeutic PEEP is justified because of her PaO_2 measurement of only 63 torr on 55% oxygen. The A/C mode does not allow her to take any totally spontaneous tidal volume breaths. In addition, she would benefit from some therapeutic PEEP. A high level of pressure support (PSV_{max}) does not offer her the "safety net" of support offered by SIMV at this

stage of her recovery. Some therapeutic PEEP is needed.

22. **C.** Interpretation of the patient's ABG values shows an increased carbon dioxide level with resulting respiratory acidosis. An SIMV rate of 10/min does not increase the patient's baseline minute volume from the PC rate of 10. Because the patient is apneic, she will not be adding to the minute volume total. The patient's minute volume will be increased by both a higher respiratory rate and a larger tidal volume. Removing the mechanical dead space will prevent the patient from rebreathing her own carbon dioxide. All three of these options result in a lower $PaCO_2$ and correction of the low pH. Additionally, increasing the tidal volume probably will increase the PaO_2.

23. **A.** (Review Box 15-2 for indications of SIMV tolerance/intolerance if needed.) An increased respiratory rate (usually accompanied by a decreasing tidal volume) indicates that the patient is fatigued and needs more ventilator support. Review the rapid, shallow breathing index calculation shown in Box 15-1 if needed. Stable vital signs and blood gas values indicate good tolerance of the WOB. Lack of accessory muscle use indicates that the diaphragm is strong enough to ventilate the patient. (See Box 15-1 on page 433 and Box 15-2 on page 440.)

24. **B.** ABG results show adequate oxygenation; therefore the PEEP level can be reduced safely from 10 to 7 cm water. A decrease in SIMV rate from 10 to 3 is too large. A smaller rate of decrease from 10 to about 6 is more reasonable at this stage in the patient's recovery. ABG results show adequate ventilation. No need is seen to increase the SIMV rate at this time. No indication is present that the patient has an increased airway resistance problem that would justify the addition of pressure support. Her tracheostomy tube is of the appropriate size, and her spontaneous rate and tidal volume are adequate.

25. **C.** (See Review Box 15-5 on page 467 for indications of the ability to wean.) Only patients 2 and 3 have all parameters within the normal ranges listed. Patient 1 has a low respiratory rate, tidal volume, and forced expiratory volume in 1 second (FEV_1). Patient 4 has a fast respiratory rate, low tidal volume, and low MIP. Patient 5 has a fast respiratory rate, low FEV_1, and low MIP.

26. **B.** The only patient parameter that has changed significantly is the increase in P peak from 30 to 45 cm water. This can be caused only by an increase in airway resistance. Although several things can cause this (bronchospasm, secretions, biting or kinking of the endotracheal tube), the only option that fits is giving a bronchodilating agent. Increasing PEEP has no effect on airway resistance. A diuretic agent (such as

furosemide [Lasix]) would help to eliminate pulmonary edema and lower a patient's plateau pressure (P plateau). However, this value is unchanged, so no worsening is indicated. A paralyzing agent will not affect any of the recorded patient values. (See Figure 15-9 on page 432.)

27. **C.** Even though the patient is paralyzed and cannot request a medication for pain relief, the patient can feel the surgical pain. Paralyzing medications do not block touch (pain) or the other senses. A narcotic medication (morphine) is justified for pain relief. Caffeine does not have a role in the care of a patient who has been paralyzed pharmacologically. A sedative medication may be given to relieve any anxiety the patient may have, but it would not affect the patient's pain. Unfortunately, there is no easy way to tell when the paralyzed patient is awake or sleeping. Regardless, it is important to talk normally to the patient so that he or she knows what medical care is being given.

28. **B.** Increasing the tidal volume from 700 to 800 mL will decrease the patient's $PaCO_2$ toward the goal. Another ABG sample should be taken in 15 minutes to see if the ordered $PaCO_2$ of 25 torr has been achieved. Adding 100 mL of mechanical dead space will increase, rather than decrease, the patient's carbon dioxide level. Changing to the PC mode with the same settings will maintain the same minute volume and the same $PaCO_2$ as at present. Decreasing the ventilator rate from 12 to 10/min results in a higher rather than lower carbon dioxide level.

29. **D.** The decrease in patient tidal volume is significant. Probably the patient's lung compliance has worsened. The patient has increased his respiratory rate to make up for the lost minute volume. The best solution is to increase the pressure control inspiratory pressure to produce the previous tidal volume of 800 mL. Sedating the patient will result in a dramatic decrease in minute volume with resulting hypercarbia and hypoxia. Increasing the set respiratory rate will deliver a higher minute volume and will relieve the patient of some of the burden of triggering the ventilator. However, it will not correct the main problem—a decreased tidal volume. Without blood gas results to document hypoxia, no indication is found to add PEEP.

30. **C.** The flow/time tracing enables any auto-PEEP to be detected. (See Figure 15-7 on page 432 for the graphic.) The maximum voluntary ventilation tracing is done in the pulmonary function laboratory to evaluate a patient's overall breathing ability. It is not useful for detecting auto-PEEP. A flow/volume loop can be done on many microprocessor ventilators and is helpful in evaluating flow at the end of exhalation. However, the flow/time tracing is the best detector of

auto-PEEP. A pressure/time tracing (see Figure 15-4, top graphic, on page 426) is not helpful in detecting auto-PEEP.

31. **C.** Increasing the IPAP level from 15 to 20 cm H_2O will deliver a larger tidal volume to the patient. This should correct her feeling of not getting enough air. Increasing the EPAP level will increase the patient's functional residual capacity. However, this usually is done only when it is known that the patient has refractory hypoxemia. In addition, increasing the EPAP level, without increasing the IPAP level, will result in delivery of a smaller tidal volume. When the patient complained that she was not "getting enough air," she was referring to needing a large enough tidal volume. A faster respiratory rate will not give her what she wants. There is no indication that the patient is hypoxemic. The oxygen percentage should not be increased without knowledge of the patient's oxygenation.

32. **A.** The patient's blood gas results show hypoventilation and his spirometry results got worse after 40 minutes. Mechanical ventilation should be resumed for his safety. Extubation could be dangerous for the patient. He is not strong enough to breathe entirely on his own. PEP therapy will not support his breathing. The weaning trial should be stopped now because the patient is getting worse. He needs additional ventilatory support. (See Box 15-5 on page 467.)

33. **B.** The patient's carbon dioxide level is too high, causing a respiratory acidosis. The most effective way to increase alveolar ventilation to reduce the $PaCO_2$ is to increase amplitude. Increasing PEEP and changing the I:E ratio to 1:1 will improve oxygenation but will not blow off carbon dioxide.

Chapter Sixteen: ANSWER KEY FOR THE WRITTEN REGISTRY EXAM SELF-STUDY QUESTIONS

1. **B.** Extubation is performed with a CPAP level of 2 to 4 cm water because this small amount of pressure is typically the minimum used to maintain the neonate's normal functional residual capacity (FRC). A lower CPAP pressure while intubated would result in too little FRC and possibly hypoxemia. If a higher CPAP level is needed to treat a clinical problem, the patient should not be extubated.

2. **D.** All three listed items are indications to change from CPAP to mechanical ventilation. A neonatal patient who is receiving 8 to 10 cm water CPAP and 80% oxygen, and who is still hypoxemic, should have mechanical ventilation started.

3. **D.** Pressure limited "square wave ventilation" is widely accepted as the standard way to ventilate the majority of neonatal patients with RDS because it (1) limits the peak pressure to a predetermined safe level and (2) increases the patient's oxygenation by maintaining the peak pressure during a tidal volume breath for the duration of the inspiratory time.

4. **B.** It has been clinically shown that hyperventilation of the patient with PPHN causes pulmonary vasodilation. This improves the patient's condition by allowing more blood to pass through the pulmonary circulation to be oxygenated. Hyperventilation has not been shown to improve the other listed conditions.

5. **C.** Increasing the pressure limit on the ventilator increases the patient's tidal volume. This increased pressure and tidal volume can increase the risk of lung tissues being torn. This can result in a pneumothorax or other types of barotrauma or volutrauma. ROP is a complex condition related to prematurity and frequent swings in the patient's arterial blood oxygen and carbon dioxide levels. Oxygen toxicity is related to the patient inhaling a high percentage of oxygen for a prolonged period of time. A tracheoesophageal fistula can be the result of a developmental defect or caused by tissue damage from an endotracheal tube and nasogastric tube.

6. **D.** Increased inspiratory time keeps the alveoli open longer to improve oxygenation. If the pressure limit is increased, a larger tidal volume will be delivered and oxygenation will be improved. Additional PEEP increases the patient's FRC and improves oxygenation. If flow is decreased, the tidal volume will be decreased. This results in the oxygen level dropping. Decreasing the ventilator's IMV rate decreases the patient's minute volume. This results in the oxygen level dropping.

7. **B.** The patient's tidal volume is determined by the difference between the pressure limit and PEEP level. If the PEEP is increased without increasing the pressure limit, the difference between them decreases and the tidal volume decreases. Minute volume decreases, not increases, if the difference between the pressure limit and PEEP level is decreased. The patient's $PaCO_2$ increases, not decreases, if the tidal volume and minute volume decrease. Tidal volume decreases, not increases, when the difference between pressure limit and PEEP decreases.

8. **A.** An oral or nasal endotracheal tube is inserted into a patient's airway before a cleft palate is surgically repaired; a standard neonatal ventilator is used if needed. There is no special reason to use HFV. Patients

with all of the other clinical situations have been shown to benefit by HFV.

9. **A.** With HFO, the amplitude is directly related to the tidal volume. So increasing amplitude will increase the patient's tidal volume and reduce the $PaCO_2$. Decreasing the amplitude would have the opposite effect. Increasing PEEP would reduce the difference between the PEEP level and the amplitude (peak pressure). This would reduce the patient's tidal volume. The I : E ratio probably has little impact, in this situation, on the patient's carbon dioxide level.

10. **C.** It is common clinical practice to begin CPAP at 4 to 5 cm water pressure. Less than this is not likely to improve the patient's condition significantly. An initial CPAP of 6 to 8 cm water may not be needed to improve oxygenation and may result in cardiopulmonary complications. It is safer to start at 4 to 5 cm water, assess the patient, and determine if more CPAP is needed.

11. **C.** It is appropriate to wean the inhaled nitric oxide by decreasing the dose by 50%. Next, assess the patient to determine if the iNO can be further reduced. The patient should probably not be weaned from the ventilator or changed to CPAP until nitric oxide is no longer needed. Nitric oxide should be weaned down in steps of 50% rather than being abruptly discontinued.

12. **A.** The patient's arterial blood gas results show refractory hypoxemia and hypoventilation with respiratory acidosis. Conventional mechanical ventilation is indicated. This could be with either a volume-cycled ventilator or a pressure-cycled ventilator. Increasing CPAP may help to improve oxygenation but will not correct the hypoventilation. It is doubtful that increasing the oxygen percentage will correct the patient's refractory hypoxemia. High-frequency ventilation is not indicated until after conventional mechanical ventilation has been tried and shown to not be effective.

Chapter Seventeen: ANSWER KEY FOR THE WRITTEN REGISTRY EXAM SELF-STUDY QUESTIONS

1. **B.** Research has shown that lung disease cannot be reversed by a patient attending a rehabilitation program. However, a rehabilitation program can be expected to decrease a patient's number of hospitalizations, increase the patient's energy level, and increase the patient's ability to perform activities of daily living (ADLs). These are all worthy goals that will improve the quality of the patient's life.

2. **C.** The oxygen concentrator has failed. The patient should switch the cannula to an oxygen cylinder at the same flow rate as the concentrator. This delivers the needed oxygen supply to the patient until the therapist can repair the unit. It is not the patient's responsibility to perform equipment repairs, such as resetting the circuit breaker on the concentrator or disassembling the concentrator to clean the air filter. In addition, the patient should not have to risk discontinuation of ordered oxygen while waiting for an equipment update or for further assistance. The patient should not be told to increase the flow of oxygen through a liquid oxygen system above that ordered by the physician.

3. **A.** An open-end exercise program offers these two advantages: (1) it is self-directed by the patient, and (2) the patient can adjust the schedule of activities if necessary. A closed-end exercise program offers these two advantages: (1) members of the exercise group can offer support to each other, and (2) the facilitator can easily plan group activities.

4. **A.** A surgically repaired cleft palate has no connection with infant apnea. Apnea periods lasting 25 seconds, death of two or more older siblings from sudden infant death syndrome (SIDS), and a premature infant with apnea periods and bradycardia are all serious situations that indicate apnea monitoring. (See Box 17-1 on page 525.)

5. **D.** These three steps are needed in a strengthening program: (1) warm-up period, (2) strengthening exercises performed every other day, and (3) cool-down period after the strengthening exercises. Strengthening exercises should not be performed daily because the muscles that have been worked need a day to recover before exercising again. Endurance exercises should be performed for 20 to 30 minutes continuously, *not* strengthening exercises.

6. **D.** It would be safer to have the patient slow down on the ergometer until her heart rate decreases to the target level. The patient's target heart rate range is based on her age and physical conditioning. If the patient exercised only until she began to perspire, she would probably not gain any exercise benefit. As previously stated, the target heart rate range is based on the patient's age and physical conditioning. She should not continue exercising at this elevated heart rate even if she feels that she can handle the workload. The patient gains little benefit from exercising for a maximum of 10 minutes each day. Current guidelines dictate that a person should

exercise for 20 to 30 continuous minutes. (See Box 17-5 on page 531.)

7. **A.** Current guidelines dictate that an infant must have at least 2 to 3 months without an apnea episode, *not* 30 days without an apnea episode, to discontinue apnea monitoring. An infant can have apnea monitoring stopped if the other listed options are met. (See Box 17-1 on page 525.)

8. **C.** A 6-minute walk test requires that the patient walk as far as possible in 6 minutes and note the distance. It is hoped that as the patient's conditioning improves, her distance walked will increase. The patient must walk, rather than ride a bicycle ergometer, for 6 minutes.

9. **D.** It is only in an open-end format rehabilitation program that each patient can easily adjust activities if a scheduling conflict arises. In a closed-end format rehabilitation program, all group members do the same thing at the same time. This way they can offer emotional support to each other, and the program facilitator can direct group activities and optimally sequence learning activities.

10. **B.** Moving the patch to another area of skin allows the irritated area to heal. Removing the patch before going to bed removes the stimulating nicotine that has been preventing sleep. A physician, not a respiratory therapist, should make the recommendation to apply a topical cortisone cream to the irritated skin. Only a physician should make the recommendation that the patient take a sleeping pill. Although a patient may choose to drink a beer or a glass of wine before going to bed to help induce sleep, the respiratory therapist should not make this recommendation. If nicotine is preventing the patient from sleeping at night, it is best to remove the patch. Sleeping pills and alcohol can probably be avoided if the nicotine patch is removed at night.

11. **C.** An oxygen concentrator and oxygen-conserving cannula economically provide the necessary oxygen to the patient. A bank of H tanks is expensive to assemble and takes up more space than a concentrator. In addition, a nasal cannula is preferred over a simple oxygen mask to deliver 2 L/min of oxygen to a patient going home. A liquid oxygen system is more expensive to set up than a concentrator for a patient who will be using the system only during periods of shortness of breath. In addition, an air entrainment mask order must specify the patient's oxygen percentage (e.g., 24%, 28%). A portable oxygen tank does not provide a long enough duration of flow to the cannula if the patient has prolonged shortness of breath. An oxygen-conserving cannula is more economical than a regular cannula. (See the Written Registry Exam Hint on page 527. If necessary, review oxygen delivery systems in Chapter 6.)

12. **B.** Studies have shown that patients who complete a rehabilitation program can expect fewer hospitalizations and more exercise tolerance. Unfortunately, the patient cannot expect to experience clinically significant improvement in pulmonary function studies. This is because the lung damage sustained by COPD patients is not reversible.

Chapter Eighteen: ANSWER KEY FOR THE WRITTEN REGISTRY EXAM SELF-STUDY QUESTIONS

1. **A.** A heated cascade-type humidification system is inappropriate because the water will splash through the ventilator circuit and into the patient because of the constant motion during transport. A heat and moisture exchanger should be used instead. The oxygen cylinder duration should be calculated to be sure that sufficient oxygen is present for the trip. A demand valve IMV system should be chosen because it is not affected by altitude changes. A lightweight and portable ventilator is needed because the helicopter has a weight limit for equipment and passengers, and the chosen ventilator should be designed to tolerate the rough motion that can occur during a transport.

2. **C.** A flexible fiberoptic bronchoscopy is indicated for two reasons. First, the patient has a history of smoking and recurrent bouts of pneumonia of the left lung. Second, other treatment procedures have failed to produce improvement in the patient's chest radiograph. These facts should make one suspicious of a lung tumor. It is very doubtful that nebulizing a bronchodilator medication or hypertonic saline will make any difference in this patient's condition. No indication of bronchospasm or retained secretions is noted. A rigid tube bronchoscope cannot be used to visualize the left lower lobe bronchus because it is not flexible. It can be used only to view the trachea and right and left mainstem bronchi. (See Box 18-2 on page 549.)

3. **D.** A tension pneumothorax can be immediately treated by placing a large-bore (often 16 gauge) needle through the second or third intercostal space at the midclavicular line on the affected side. Later, a pleural chest tube should be inserted. Although a 5% pneumothorax is abnormal, it is probably not life-threatening. Sometimes the patient is given supplemental oxygen as needed and monitored. The pneumothorax gas may be reabsorbed into the tissues, and no other

treatment may be necessary. A pleural effusion or hemothorax requires a thoracentesis procedure to remove the fluid. This would probably be done through the lower area of the patient's back because the fluid is gravity dependent.

4. **A.** The respiratory exchange ratio (R) is calculated by placing the patient's $\dot{V}O_2$ and $\dot{V}CO_2$ values into the following equation:

$$R = \frac{\dot{V}CO_2}{\dot{V}O_2} = \frac{1700 \text{ mL}}{2000 \text{ mL}} = 0.85$$

5. **A.** According to Boyle's law, pressure and volume are inversely proportional. Therefore as barometric pressure decreases at increased altitude, the volume of gas in the patient's endotracheal tube cuff increases and the tidal volume increases. Despite the increased tidal volume, the patient is likely to become hypoxic because the alveolar pressure of oxygen (PAO_2) decreases and therefore the arterial pressure of oxygen (PaO_2) decreases as the barometric pressure decreases. The patient's tidal volume should be monitored and adjusted during the flight, and the pulse oximetry value should be monitored to assess for hypoxemia and the need to increase the inspired oxygen percentage. No link exists between fluid retention and change in barometric pressure. (See the Exam Hint on page 546.)

6. **B.** All of the stated signs indicate a tension pneumothorax. Because the patient's condition is rapidly deteriorating, it is most important to insert a pleural chest tube on the right side. Because it is very likely that the CVP needle pierced the lung and caused the pneumothorax, the procedure should be stopped at this time. Although a chest radiograph would be indicated if the patient's condition were stable, obtaining one now will unnecessarily delay inserting the needed chest tube. Nothing of clinical value is to be gained at this time by comparing the peak and plateau pressures on the ventilator. They will both increase because of the tension pneumothorax. This information only reinforces the previous signs, and performing this procedure now delays the needed chest tube. (See the Exam Hint on page 556.)

7. **D.** Before a conscious patient undergoes a cardioversion procedure, he or she should be given a sedative. The drug midazolam (Versed) is given intravenously for conscious sedation. The proper initial power setting for the first attempt at cardioversion of an adult patient with atrial fibrillation is 100 J (see Box 18-1). Set the ECG machine to lead II so that an upright R wave is detected by the unit. On occasion, the medication midazolam and shock from the cardioversion can cause a patient to stop breathing temporarily. For this reason, the respiratory therapist should have a manual resuscitator on standby and be ready to assist the patient's breathing. The drug flumazenil (Romazicon) is given intravenously after the procedure is finished to reverse the sedating effect of the midazolam. A defibrillator charge of 360 J is the maximum used to defibrillate a patient. It is far too high for a first attempt at cardioversion. (See Box 18-1 on page 548.)

8. **A.** The surgeon should insert the first tracheostomy tube into the stoma in case there is a problem. A respiratory therapist may replace a tracheostomy tube after the stoma is well established. The therapist may assist with the procedure by disinfecting the surgical site, checking the tube cuff, and withdrawing the endotracheal tube when the surgeon has created the stoma and is ready to insert the tracheostomy tube.

9. **D.** A stylet (lubricated or not) is not inserted into an endotracheal tube during a nasotracheal intubation procedure. This is because the tube should be kept flexible to follow the natural contours of the patient's airway anatomy. A stylet makes the endotracheal tube stiff and causes damage to the nasal passage. A Magill forceps is used to lift the tip of the tube for insertion into the trachea. A laryngoscope handle with blade is used as during an oral intubation procedure (see Figure 18-12). The tip of the endotracheal tube is lubricated so that it slides easily through the patient's nasal passage.

10. **B.** Maximum heart rate can be calculated by two different equations. Both are shown below for this 55-year-old patient. The first equation was used for this question.

$$\begin{aligned} HR_{max} \text{ for males and females} &= 210 - (0.65 \times \text{age in years}) \\ &= 210 - (0.65 \times 55) \\ &= 210 - (35.75) \\ &= 174.25 \end{aligned} \tag{1}$$

Round off to the nearest whole number for a maximum heart rate of 174 beats/minute.

$$\begin{aligned} HR_{max} \text{ for males and females} &= 220 - (\text{age in years}) \\ &= 220 - (55) \\ &= 165 \end{aligned} \tag{2}$$

By this alternate equation the patient's maximum heart rate would be 165 beats/minute.

11. **C.** Normally, as a person progressively exercises more vigorously, his or her ventilation efforts (larger tidal volume and faster respiratory rate) will increase proportionately. This is because the exercising muscles produce more carbon dioxide and require more oxygen. A decreasing or constant ventilation effort at increasing workload levels would be abnormal. The patient would soon have to stop exercising. Decreasing ventilation when carbon dioxide production

increases would result in respiratory acidosis. This would be markedly abnormal and cause the person to quickly stop exercising.

12. **B.** The lack of air movement, and related hypoxemia, while making respiratory efforts documents that the patient has an airway obstruction problem. If the patient had central sleep apnea he would have stopped making breathing efforts during the time when no air was moving. Cheyne-Stokes respiration is identified by cyclical increasing and decreasing of tidal volume breathes. There may or may not be short periods of apnea between the cycles. Hyperventilation can only be documented by a decreased arterial carbon dioxide level.

13. **D.** The normal lung should be down (i.e., in a dependent position) and the problem lung up during a thoracentesis. This will ensure that the good lung receives most of the air and blood for gas exchange.

14. **B.** Pulse oximetry will give you a fast analysis of the patient's oxygenation status. The chest x-ray will allow you to visualize how much the lung has expanded and if there is still fluid in the pleural space.

15. **B.** Fluticasone (Flovent) is an inhaled corticosteroid. It is not used as a sedating medication. Diazepam (Valium) and midazolam (Versed) are sedatives used in conscious sedation. Flumazenil (Romazicon) would be used as a reversing agent against Valium and Versed when the procedure is completed.

Index

631